Fundamental & Advanced
Nurs   kills

Fundamental & Advanced
Nursing Skills

Third Edition

GAYLENE BOUSKA ALTMAN

RN, PhD
Director, Nurse Education Specialist Training
Faculty, School of Nursing
University of Washington
Seattle, Washington

Contributing Editors

Patricia Kerestzes PhD, RN, CCRN
Assistant Professor of Nursing
Saint Mary's College
Notre Dame, Indiana

Mary A. Wcisel MSN, RN
Associate Professor, Nursing
Saint Mary's College
Notre Dame, Indiana

**DELMAR
CENGAGE Learning™**

Australia • Brazil • Japan • Korea • Mexico • Singapore • Spain • United Kingdom • United States

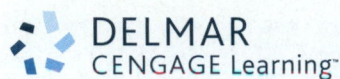

Fundamental and Advanced Nursing Skills
Third Edition
Author: Gaylene Bouska Altman

Director of Learning Solutions:
  Matthew Kane

Acquisitions Editor: Stephen Helba

Managing Editor: Marah Bellegarde

Senior Product Manager: Patricia Gaworecki

Editorial Assistant: Samantha Miller

Vice President, Career and Professional Marketing:
  Jennifer McAvey

Marketing Director: Wendy Mapstone

Senior Marketing Manager: Michele McTighe

Marketing Coordinator: Scott Chrysler

Production Director: Carolyn Miller

Production Manager: Andrew Crouth

Content Project Manager: Thomas Heffernan

Senior Art Director: Jack Pendleton

For product information and technology assistance, contact us at
Cengage Learning Customer & Sales Support, 1-800-354-9706

For permission to use material from this text or product,
submit all requests online at **www.cengage.com/permissions**
Further permissions questions can be e-mailed to
permissionrequest@cengage.com

Library of Congress Control Number: 2009922740

ISBN 13: 978-1-418-05233-1
ISBN 10: 1-4180-5233-7

Delmar
5 Maxwell Drive
Clifton Park, NY 12065-2919
USA

Cengage Learning is a leading provider of customized learning solutions with office locations around the globe, including Singapore, the United Kingdom, Australia, Mexico, Brazil, and Japan. Locate your local office at:
international.cengage.com/region

Cengage Learning products are represented in Canada by Nelson Education, Ltd.

For your lifelong learning solutions, visit **delmar.cengage.com**
Visit our corporate website at **cengage.com**.

Notice to the Reader

Publisher does not warrant or guarantee any of the products described herein or perform any independent analysis in connection with any of the product information contained herein. Publisher does not assume, and expressly disclaims, any obligation to obtain and include information other than that provided to it by the manufacturer. The reader is expressly warned to consider and adopt all safety precautions that might be indicated by the activities described herein and to avoid all potential hazards. By following the instructions contained herein, the reader willingly assumes all risks in connection with such instructions. The publisher makes no representations or warranties of any kind, including but not limited to, the warranties of fitness for particular purpose or merchantability, nor are any such representations implied with respect to the material set forth herein, and the publisher takes no responsibility with respect to such material. The publisher shall not be liable for any special, consequential, or exemplary damages resulting, in whole or part, from the readers' use of, or reliance upon, this material.

Printed in the United States of America
1 2 3 4 5 6 7 12 11 10 09 08

Dedication

Dr. Altman would like to dedicate this book and express a special thanks to her husband, Len, and her three children, Jonathan, Matthew, and Katherine, who exhibited patience and understanding during this project, and to all the staff and clients at the numerous health facilities who made this book possible. Furthermore, Dr. Altman dedicates this book to professional nurses, health care providers, clients, and families who will benefit from the application of knowledge presented in this publication.

Contents

CHAPTER 7 • OXYGENATION   865

CHAPTER 8 • CIRCULATORY   1001

CHAPTER 9 • SKIN INTEGRITY AND WOUND CARE   1181

Contributors

Patricia Abbott, RN, MSN, ARNP
University of Washington Medical Center
School of Nursing, University of Washington
Seattle, WA

Sharon Aronovitch, RN, PhD, CETN
Regents College
Albany, NY

Dale D. Barb, MHS, PT
Academic Coordinator of Clinical Education
Department of Physical Therapy
Wichita State University
Wichita, KS

Susan Weiss Behrend, RN, MSN
Fox Chase Cancer Center
Philadelphia, PA

Bethaney Campbell, RN, MN, OCN
University of Washington Medical Center
Seattle, WA

Curt Campbell
Integrated Health Services of Seattle
Seattle, WA

Nancy Chambers, RN, BSN
University of Washington Medical Center
Seattle, WA

Jung-Chen (Kristina) Chang, RN, MN, PhD
University of Washington
School of Nursing
Seattle, WA

Eileen M. Collins, MN, ARNP, AORN
School of Nursing
University of Washington
Seattle, WA

Cheryl L. Cooke, RN, MN
Student Services Coordinator
University of Washington
School of Nursing
Seattle, WA

Gayle C. Crawford, RN, BSN
Staff Nurse
University of Washington Medical Center
Seattle, WA

Mary Doyle, RN, MS
Maria College, Nursing Faculty
Niskayuna, NY

Eleonor U. de la Pena, BS
Northwest Asthma and Allergy Center
Seattle, WA

Jeanne Erickson, RN, MSN, AOCN
University of Virginia Cancer Center
Portsmouth, VA

Tom Ewing, RN, BSN
Hematology-Oncology
University of Washington Medical Center
Seattle, WA

Stacy Frish, RN, BSN
University of Washington Medical Center
Seattle, WA

Eva Gallagher, RN, BSN
Methodist Hospital
Minneapolis, MN

Susan Boyce Gilmore, RN, MN, CCRN
Lecturer, Biobehavior Nursing and Health Systems
University of Washington
School of Nursing
Seattle, WA

Hsiu-Ying Huang, RN, PhD
University of Washington
School of Nursing
Seattle, WA

Kimberly Hudson, RN, MN
University of Washington Medical Center
Seattle, WA

Karrin Johnson, RN
Health Care Project Manager
NRSPACE Software, Inc.
Bellevue, WA

Kimberly Sue Kahn, RN, MSN, FNP, AOCN
University of Virginia
Portsmouth, VA

Catherine H. Kelley, RN, MSN, OCN
Chimeric Therapies, Inc.
Palatine, IL

Carla A. Lee, PhD, ARNP, FAAN
Clarkston College
Omaha, NE

Kathryn Lilleby, RN
Clinical Research Nurse
Fred Hutchinson Cancer Research Center
Seattle, WA

Joan M. Mack, RN, MSN
Nebraska Medical Center
Omaha, NE

Patricia McDowell, RPPT
University of Washington Medical Center
Seattle, WA

Peter C. Meyer, RRT
University of Washington Medical Center
Seattle, WA

Marianne Frances Moore, RN, MSN
Clarkson Hospital
Omaha, NE

Agnes Morrison, RN, MSN
Department of Nursing
Thomas Jefferson University
Philadelphia, PA

Claretta D. Munger, MSN, ARNP
Newman Grove, NE

Susan Randolph, RN, MSN
Manager, Transplant Services
Coram Healthcare
Parkersburg, WV

Sally Ann Rinehart, RN, BSN
Nursing Lab Supervisor
Pacific Lutheran University
Tacoma, WA

Susan Rives, RN, BSN, OCN
CARE Center Coordinator
Martha Jefferson Hospital
Charlottesville, VA

Barbara Sigler, RN, MNEd, CORLN
Technical Publications Editor
Oncology Nursing Press, Inc.
Formerly: Clinical Nurse Specialist in
Otolaryngology—Head and Neck Surgery
University of Pittsburgh Medical Center
Pittsburgh, PA

Marilyn Stapleton, RNC, MS
Excelsior College
Albany, NY

Pam Talley, RN, PhD
University of Washington
School of Nursing
Seattle, WA

Hsin-Yi (Jean) Tang, RN, MS, PhD
School of Nursing
University of Washington
Seattle, WA

Samuel C. Taylor, RN
Assistant Nurse Manager, Orthopedics
Harborview Medical Center
Seattle, WA

Robi Thomas, MS, RN, AOCN
Clinical Nurse Specialist for Oncology
and the Pain Center
St. Mary's Mercy Medical Center
Grand Rapids, MI

Nancy Unger, RN, MN, MPH
University of Washington
Seattle, WA

Chandra VanPaepeghem, RN, BSN
University of Washington Medical Center
Seattle, WA

Debra A. Bovinett Wolf, RN, BSN, MPH
Roosevelt Pain Center
University of Washington Medical Center
Seattle, WA

Reviewers

Marie H. Ahrens, RN, MS: University of Tulsa, Tulsa, OK

Danette Birkhimer, RN, MS, OCN: College of Nursing, Ohio State University, Columbus, OH

Teri Boese, RN, MS: The University of Iowa, Iowa City, IA

Kathy Campbell: Maria College, Albany, NY

Brenda Cherry, RN, MSN, CCRN: DeKalb College, Decatur, GA

Pam Covault, RN, MS: Neosho County Community College, Ottawa, KS

Sandra E. Crowell, BSN, MSN: Wilcox College of Nursing, Middletown, CT

Linda Daley, RN, PhD: College of Nursing, Ohio State University, Columbus, OH

Laura Downes, RN, BSN, MSN,PhD: Springfield Technical Community College, Springfield, MA

Mary C. Doyle, BS, MS, CCRN: Maria College, Troy, NY

Carol Fowler Durham, RN, MSN: University of North Carolina—Chapel Hill, Chapel Hill, NC

Rebecca Gesler, RN, MSN: St. Catharine College, St. Catharine, KY

Deborah J. Gutshall, MSN, CRNP: Harrisburg Area Community College, Harrisburg, PA

Melinda Hamilton, RN, MSN: Pensacola Community College, Pensacola, FL

Cynthia Horvath, RN: Glens Falls Hospital, Glens Falls, NY

Valerie Howard, RN, MS: University of Pittsburg, School of Nursing, Venetia, PA

Bonnie Kirkpatrick, RN, MS, CNS: College of Nursing, Ohio State University, Columbus, OH

Clare Lamontagne, RN, MS: Springfield Technical Community College, Springfield, MA

Verlene Meyer, RN, MN: Walla Walla College, Portland, OR

Mary Moriarty Tarbell, RN, MSN: Springfield Technical Community College, Springfield, MA

Martha Nelson, RN, BSN, CETN, CCM: Florida Community College, University of North Florida, Jacksonville, FL

Joan C. Oliver, RN, EdD: Mt. Hood Community College, Gresham, OR

Marie Ostoyich, RN, MS, CDE: Hudson Valley Community College, Troy, NY

Diana Prouty, RN, MS: St. Luke's College, Kansas City, MO

Diane Sheets, RN, MS: College of Nursing, Ohio State University, Columbus, OH

Martha B. Spear, RN, MSN: Harrisburg Area Community College, Harrisburg, PA

Carol A. Vogt, RN, PhD: Cabarrus College of Health Sciences, Concord, NC

Barbara Voshall, RN, MS: Graceland University, Independence, MO

Health care is changing at an increasingly fast pace. The cumulative effects of sophisticated technology, an aging population of clients with chronic disease and long-term sequalae, an increasingly diverse population, and a growing nursing shortage challenge nurses today as never before. Often, nurses are placed in situations that demand an increased level of performance despite a decreased amount of support from the health care system.

Delmar's Fundamental & Advanced Nursing Skills Third Edition was revised with this nursing population in mind. This book was developed as a text and guideline to perform the skills used in daily nursing practice, and as a learning tool for new nurses. It was designed to be a usable volume, presenting concepts and actions clearly so that a nurse—whether a novice or experienced—may retain and master both the skill and the underlying rationale.

The third edition still serves this purpose. Nursing students, registered nurses, licensed practical/vocational nurses, physician assistants, nurse practitioners, certified aides, medical assistants, and any health care worker charged with performing common procedures will value the useful guidelines and principles discussed within this book.

This book contains over 200 nursing skills divided into 11 chapters that cover basic and advanced nursing procedures. The practitioner can follow the procedural- manual-type steps presented for each skill to improve competence and comfort levels in performing skills. Standards of nursing practice are maintained in each skill. Research-based knowledge has been incorporated into nursing interventions, especially where controversy may exist.

ORGANIZATION

Each skill is presented using the nursing process: assessment, diagnosis, planning, expected outcomes, implementation, and evaluation. The nursing process is a systematic method whereby nurses can make clinical decisions and delineate a course of action based on analysis of available data. The nursing process is continual and cyclic. Evaluation of the outcome incorporates a feedback loop leading to further assessment, decision making, and implementation of care.

North American Nursing Diagnosis Association (NANDA)

The diagnosis section of the text is based on NANDA's standardized list of nursing diagnoses. Using the input of practicing clinicians, NANDA has developed and refined a standardized list of diagnostic labels for use in the nursing process. Using the standardized list as a guideline, the practitioner interprets the assessment data and derives a diagnosis. The standardized diagnoses help guide client treatment by allowing the practitioner to identify rationales for client care and anticipate potential problems.

CLINICAL PRACTICE GUIDELINES FOR PERFORMING A PROCEDURE

In order to utilize this text to maximize learning, the authors have provided guidelines to follow before beginning the procedure and after the procedure is completed.

Before the Procedure

- **Practice the procedure with supervision in a clinical setting.**
- **Read the client's chart.**
- **Review the treatment plan or verify orders as necessary.**
- **Review the procedure.**
- **Assess the client and determine the appropriateness of the procedure.**
- **Take into consideration the client's/family's cultural and social background when deciding what to teach and when eliciting feedback.**
- **Employ the aid of a translator if there is a language barrier.**
- **Use visual aids such as flip charts, models, videos, if available, to explain procedure to client/family.**

- If family members are to be involved, **plan to instruct when they are present**, if possible.
- Client and/or family members should be provided with a written set of instructions to take home with them, if needed.
- Plan the procedure.

After the Procedure

- **Assess the client** and his/her response to the procedure.
- **Document the client's response.**
- **Change the treatment plan** as appropriate.

SPECIAL FEATURES AND LEARNING TOOLS

Step-by-Step Format. The implementation section is presented in a step-by-step format with rationales for each action included. The skill is broken down into simple, easy-to-follow steps with explanations for the underlying reasons for each action. This allows even the novice to perform the skill and understand why each step is necessary. The steps presented provide specific directions for performing each skill. However, institutional policies, client condition, environmental setting, and other variables may prompt modification of the interventions presented. When modifications are made, adherence to standards of practice and Standard Precautions must be maintained. Assess and evaluate the client throughout the procedure, modifying intervention as needed to maintain client safety and security. Rationales provide the scientific basis for each implementation. The rationale enables both the practitioner and client to understand the reason for each implementation, and thus the need to comply with protocols.

Real-life Photographs. The focus of this text is to present reality-based information with photographic examples from current clinical practice, rather than staged or rehearsed scenarios.

Real-World Anecdotes. Client situations drawn from experiences of the contributors or other practitioners add to the immediacy and practicality of the book.

Critical Thinking Skills. This feature offers performance-related scenarios to foster learning, decision making, and analytic thinking. These scenarios often help the reader anticipate possible negative outcomes involved in performing a skill and provide alternatives to avoid unwanted results.

Skill Variations. Variations for each skill are presented for geriatric and pediatric age groups, as well as home-care and long-term care settings, to allow for adaptation of the skills to various situations. For example,

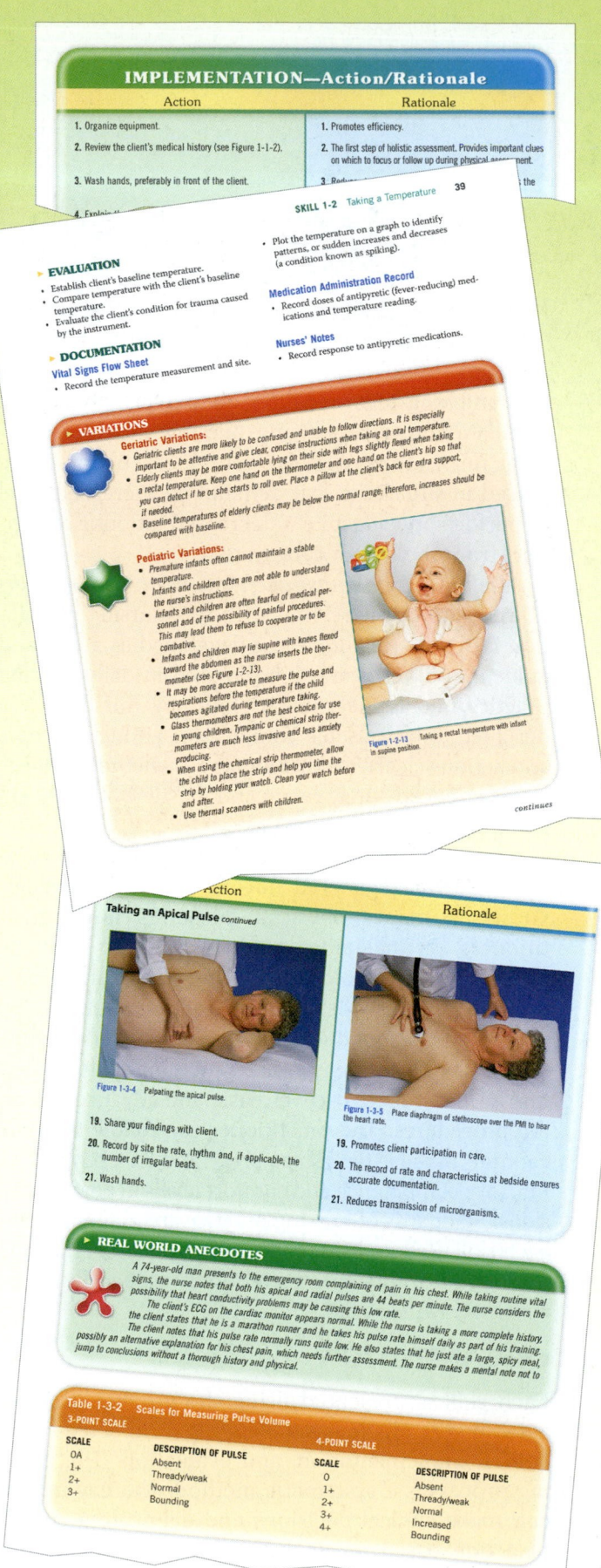

geriatric clients may require extra communication skills because of difficulty hearing or understanding. Pediatric clients may need psychosocial assessment of fear or anxiety, or require different sizes of equipment when performing the skill.

Common Errors and Nursing Tips. These are included to assist in improving client outcomes. These sections are presented by experienced nurses to aid and guide the novice practitioner through performing the skills, to help develop competency, and to prevent unwanted outcomes.

Equipment Needed. A list of common equipment needed is provided as an organizational tool to assist in preparation and setup. The equipment required may vary between institutions.

Estimated Time for Completion. The estimated time to complete a skill is identified to assist in planning and scheduling. The estimated time of completion should be used only as a general guide. Many factors, such as the skill of the practitioner, client cooperation, or degree of client illness, may affect the time required to accomplish a skill.

Client Education Needed. Client teaching should be routinely incorporated when performing skills. Client education is essential in promoting personal health responsibility and compliance. Education should be considered a routine part of most interventions. Informed clients are often less anxious, more cooperative, provide better histories, and are more proactive regarding their health care.

Delegation Tips, in a clear, direct manner, provide insights into what a nurse must know about the skill before it is delegated to ancillary personnel. Issues addressed include both technical concerns and legal/ethical aspects of care.

> **DELEGATION TIPS**
>
> The skill of temperature measurement often is delegated to ancillary personnel; however, the nurse retains responsibility for knowledge of the client's temperature and appropriate actions. The expectation is that ancillary personnel will have documented instruction and competency validation of their ability to:
> • Select the correct route for measurement of the temperature
> • Correctly position the client for measurement
> • Correctly perform the measurement according to established guidelines and record on the appropriate flow sheet (clinical record)
> • Recognize and report abnormal findings to the nurse

Special Considerations outline additional factors that may complicate issues or present a special hazard to either a client or nurse. These are issues that the nurse performing a procedure should be mindful of in caring for a client.

> **SPECIAL CONSIDERATIONS**
>
> • Never use your thumb to obtain a pulse because you may sense a beat from your own digital artery that can alter an accurate reading.
> • When using a Doppler to obtain a fetal heart beat, check the mother's pulse to ensure the beat you are hearing is indeed that of the fetus.
> • When preparing a client for surgery related to venous insufficiency of the lower extremities (i.e., femoral-popliteal bypass), it is essential to mark the pedal pulses with an "X." This facilitates locating the pulse during surgery to confirm circulation for the surgeon.

ALSO FROM DELMAR CENGAGE LEARNING

On-Line Skills and DVD-ROM

Nursing skills content comes in the format you want! Delivered on-line or in DVD-ROM format, got to *www.cengage.com/delmar* for complete information and a **FREE 30-Day Trial** visit. Look for the DVD-ROM icon at the beginning of each skill in the book.

Skills Checklist

(ISBN 10: 1-4180-5233-7)
(ISBN 13: 978-1-4180-5234-8)

Master your nursing skills! This clinical learning tool contains the step-by-step actions for every procedure found in *Fundamental and Advanced Nursing Skills,* Third Edition. These checklists were created to promote competence and confidence in performing basic and complex procedures used in every day nursing practice. Key features include:

• Easy to follow format
• Three categories to document performance: Able to perform, Able to perform with assistance, Unable to perform.
• Comment section is included with each step for constructive feedback and notes.
• Step-by-step approach allows the student to easily find the corresponding actions in core text

Acknowledgments

Dr. Altman would like to acknowledge the tireless efforts and contributions of the staff at Delmar, especially Stephen Helba, Patricia Gaworecki, and Thomas Heffernan.

Further appreciation is extended to the many nurses, contributing authors, and health care personnel who shared their knowledge and experience in writing the skills for this book.

Special recognition is given to the individuals in the photographs, and the clients, families, and health care personnel who so generously allowed staff to photograph them and record their giving and receiving care. During this very personal time photographers were allowed into their milieu.

GAYLENE BOUSKA ALTMAN, RN, PHD

Gaylene Bouska Altman, a faculty member at the University of Washington School of Nursing, is currently the codirector of the nursing education specialist training program. She has served as the director of the Learning Lab and the Center for Excellence in Nursing Education. Her role includes teaching and coordinating hands-on skills for the nursing courses. She holds a diploma in nursing from Marymount College, Salina, Kansas; a BSN from the University of Kansas, Lawrence; and both an MN and PhD from the University of Washington, Seattle. With more than 25 years of teaching experience, she has taught at both the undergraduate and graduate levels. Besides predominantly teaching at the University of Washington, Dr. Altman has also taught at Seattle University, Seattle Pacific University, and Catholic University (Washington, DC).

and has received numerous awards. Most recently Dr. Altman received the 2002 University of Washington School of Excellence in Undergraduate Teaching Award. With a background as an intensive care and coronary care nurse, she has taught courses ranging from fundamental to advanced practice. Her main emphasis has been to develop critical thinking strategies through case presentations. Dr. Altman was one of the pioneers in initiating coronary care units and a mobile coronary care system in the 1970s, in the state of Washington. Furthermore, she helped develop some of the early quality assurance programs implemented throughout the state. Dr. Altman's work has been published in numerous textbooks and journals. She has delivered presentations throughout the country and maintains membership in several professional organizations.

Physical Assessment

Physical Assessment

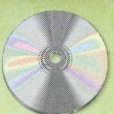

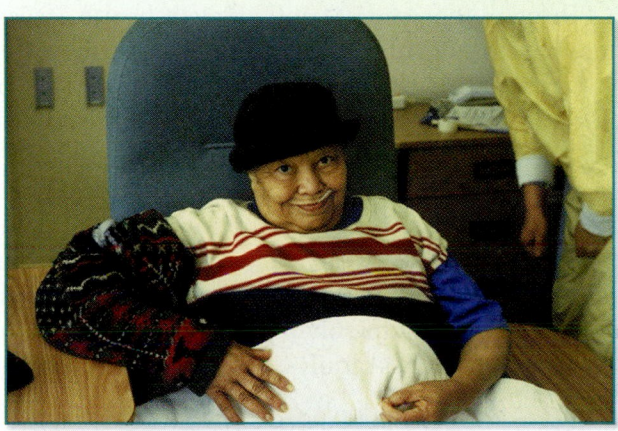

▶ OVERVIEW OF THE SKILL

A dynamic health assessment is the foundation of all nursing care, with physical assessment as part of every holistic health evaluation. Physical assessment builds on information obtained from the client's history. Assessment is the first step of the nursing process. It involves the orderly collection of objective information about the client's health status. Objective data are observable, measurable, and verifiable by more than one person. A fundamental systematic approach is used based on a combination of head-to-toe and body system assessments. These assessments are expanded as appropriate to the client's situation and setting. By using a systematic approach, one ensures that signs are not overlooked and that time is used efficiently. Through the process of data collection, meaningful information—including health status, actual and potential health problems, and areas of focus for priority health promotion—is identified. Physical assessment/examination is used in outpatient, inpatient, and home health services.

A complete and organized assessment is obtained by using a combination of head-to-toe and body system approaches in conjunction with the use of four basic techniques: inspection, palpation, percussion, auscultation (IPPA):

- Inspection: Observation (see, smell); starts during the health history and continues throughout the exam; always comes first (before you touch or listen); continues concurrently with PPA. First, note general observations and then specifics of each area proceeding from the outside to the inside.
- Palpation: Use touch to assess skin temperature, moisture, vibrations and organ or mass location, texture, shape, and size. Identify presence of pain, fluid, or crepitus. First use light touch (1 cm), then deep (4 to 5 cm), then rebound (deep with quick release). Compare symmetry for equality, such as the chest (e.g., respiratory vibrations—tactile fremitus).
- Percussion: Done to assess density or aeration. Audible sounds produced by tapping with the hyperextended middle finger on a surface with a quick, sharp wrist motion. Tap to produce vibration sounds from light to heavy. Compare areas and symmetry of the body, such as the chest. More solid areas will produce lower pitched sounds; more air-filled areas will produce higher pitched sounds. Sounds produced:

–Tympany: loud, high pitch, drum-like (example: gastric air bubble)

–Hyperresonance: very loud, low pitch, booming (example: emphysematous lungs)

–Resonance: loud, low pitch shallow (example: normal lungs)

–Dull: medium sound, mid-pitch (example: muscle, bone)

–Flatness: soft, short duration (example: muscle, bone)

- Auscultation: Listening direct (naked ear) and indirect (acoustic stethoscope or Doppler amplification). Analyzes intensity, pitch, duration, quality, and location. The bell analyzes low-pitched sounds, and the diaphragm analyzes high-pitched sounds.

A combined body system and body area approach focuses assessment by groupings:

- General Appearance: Examine appearance in the following groups: (1) skin, hair, and nails; (2) head, face, and lymphatic; (3) eye, ear, nose, mouth, and throat; (4) neck and upper extremities; (5) chest, breasts, and axillae; (6) thorax and lungs/respiratory system; (7) heart and cardiovascular system; (8) abdomen/gastrointestinal system; (9) genitalia/genitourinary system and anus.
- Lower Extremities: Musculoskeletal system (MBJB: muscles, bones, joints, and back assessment).
- Neurologic: Reflex, sensory, cranial, cerebral, cerebellar, neurodevelopmental, neuropsychiatric.

Internal genitalia, rectum, and prostate examinations are usually included in advanced assessment and will not be addressed here.

The IPPA organization can be combined by cephalocaudal (head-to-toe), general-to-specific, medial-to-lateral, and external-to-internal approaches within each category. The physical assessment is always correlated with the health history as well as with other assessments, such as laboratory or diagnostic data and/or developmental, psychosocial, family, and cultural assessment data. The nurse must also consider his or her own understanding of anatomy and physiology, basic nursing skills, and the nursing process. The educational preparation and clinical expertise of the nurse may, therefore, influence the extent to which the nurse participates in the physical assessment process.

► ASSESSMENT

1. Assess the environment, resources, and the client's medical condition **to determine a complete and systematic examination by reducing the possibility of overlooking important findings.**
2. Assess the client's history of previous physical assessments and the availability of previous data **to provide a baseline for comparisons.**
3. Assess the client's receptiveness to being examined **to help plan ways to reduce anxiety and improve compliance with the examination.**
4. Assess the client's understanding of the procedure **to help plan ways to reduce anxiety and improve compliance with the examination.**

► DIAGNOSIS

Disturbed Body Image

Risk for Situational Low Self-Esteem

Deficient Knowledge

Risk for Compromised Human Dignity

Risk for Delayed Development

Through the accurate and efficient health assessment process, normal, normal variant, and abnormal data are identified. The nurse can identify serious or life-threatening signs and critical assessment findings that require immediate attention. She or he can use the objective data obtained during the physical assessment process to contribute to problem-solving strategies that identify the client's current health status (acute, chronic, risk, and preventive). The nurse can institute problem-solving strategies to place the client and the client's family or community in optimal health status.

► PLANNING

Expected Outcomes:

1. Identify health parameters at multiple levels for total client management and to identify acute concerns and needs.
2. Identify serious, acute, or life-threatening abnormalities or critical assessment findings that require immediate attention.
3. Identify potential or chronic abnormalities that need planned intervention.
4. Monitor chronic stable problems to detect changes from baseline assessments.
5. Identify health risks, concerns, or needs. These include risks that are related to age, gender, environment, community, personal habits, or family history.
6. Respond to health maintenance needs, including monitoring the client's status and comparing findings with normal health parameters for age and gender. It also includes identifying normal variations of health that do not need intervention and providing routine or scheduled assessments, immunizations, preventive or palliative health care, and health education or anticipatory guidance.

Equipment Needed (see Figures 1-1-1A to 1-1-1H):

Equipment must be organized for easy accessibility. It is helpful to be able to reach each piece of equipment with one hand while the other is on the client. Warm hands with short fingernails are essential

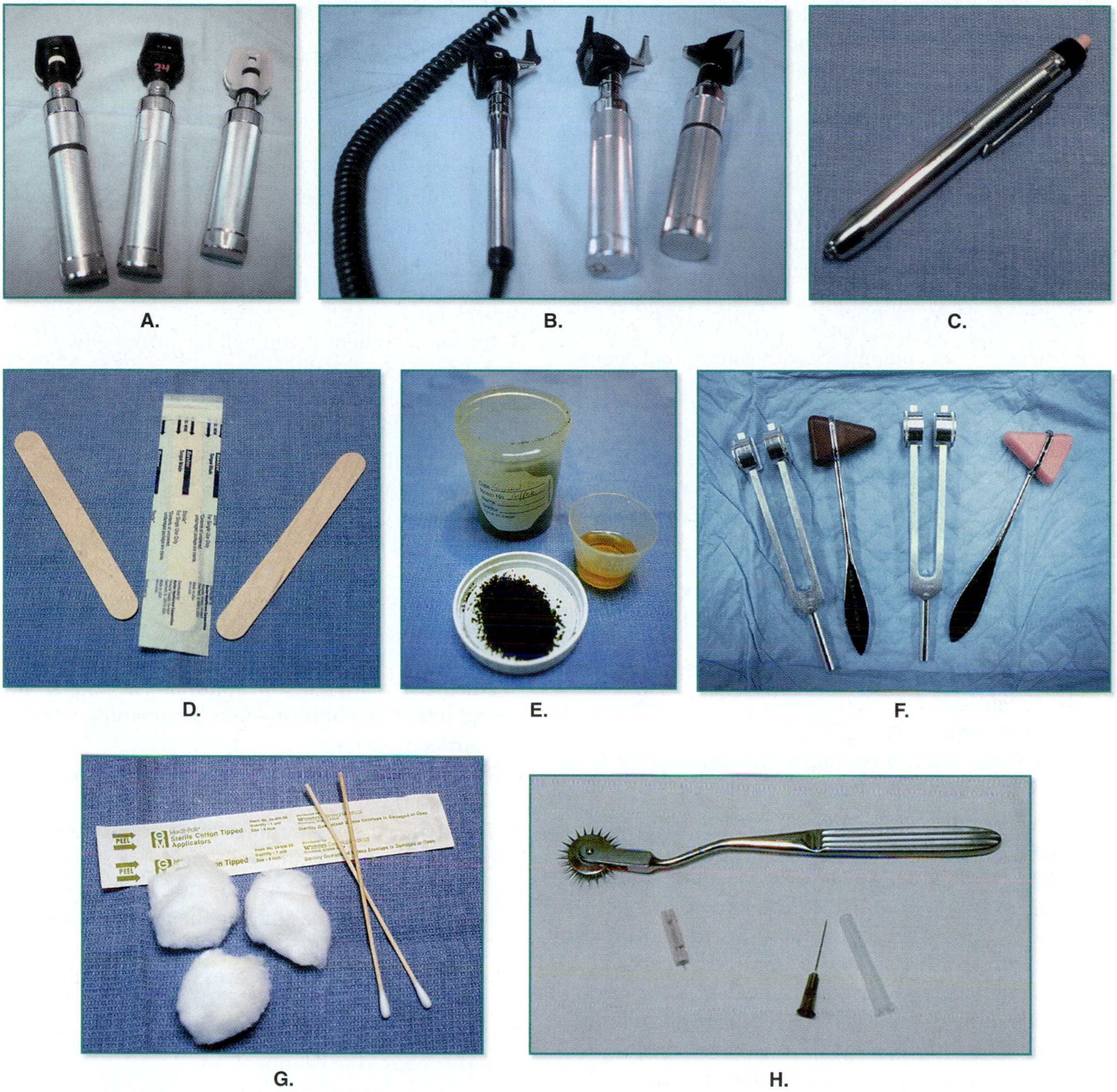

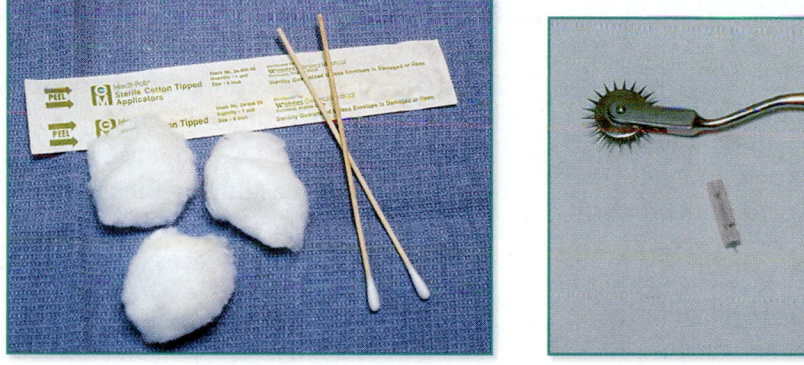
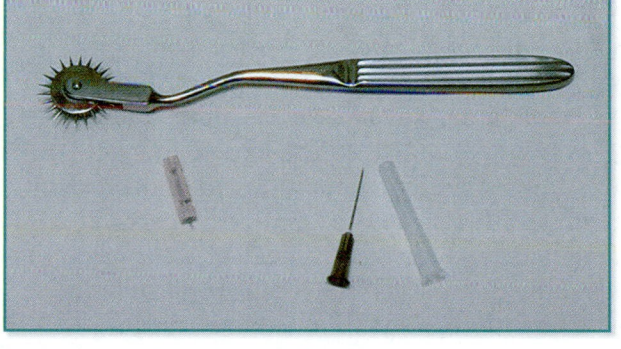

Figure 1-1-1 **A.** Ophthalmoscopes; **B.** Otoscopes; **C.** Penlight; **D.** Tongue depressors; **E.** Coffee grounds and orange extract; **F.** Tuning forks and reflex hammers; **G.** Cotton swabs and cotton balls; **H.** Sharp items used to assess sharp and dull sensations.

for performing a satisfactory physical examination. Equipment includes the following:

- Pen
- Assessment forms or paper to record notations as well as document findings
- Charts for recording height and weight (and head circumference for infants), age, gender, culture, and sometimes medical condition
- A well-lit, warm, private room or space

- Gown for client privacy and comfort (swimsuits work well with children and adolescents)
- Drape sheet or blanket for client privacy and comfort
- Thermometer: otic or oral/axillary digital is preferred
- Stethoscope: acoustic with bell and diaphragm; ideal tubing less than 35 cm long
- Watch with a second hand

- Sphygmomanometer and blood pressure cuff (bladder width to be 40% and length 80% to 100% of the upper arm circumference)
- Ophthalmoscope
- Vision charts: Illiterate (matching letters or objects), Snellen (far vision), Rosenbaum (near vision) pocket card, Ischara (color vision), or Titmus tester (includes all four), and pupil gauge (in mm)
- Otoscope with pneumatic tube
- Audio testing equipment: watch, tuning forks (minimum of one high-pitched, 512 Hz, and one low-pitched, 128 Hz), handheld audiometer, tympanometer, or full audiometry with soundproof room
- Nasal speculum with illumination. Optional headlamp with magnification
- Penlight
- Tongue depressors
- Nonsterile gloves (possibly sterile gloves as well)
- Glass of water
- Marking pen
- Measuring tape (with centimeters and inches), preferably cloth or plastic
- Water-soluble lubricant
- Guaiac card for occult blood
- Specimen cup
- Reflex hammer
- Neurologic "kit": temperature (test tubes of hot and cold), touch (cotton ball, hair pin, paper clip, safety pin, key, marble, coin, low-pitched tuning fork), taste (sweet—sugar, honey; sour—lemon, lime, vinegar; bitter—alum, quinine; salty—salt, saline), smell (coffee, lemon, orange extract, flowers, perfume, mouthwash). If making your own kit, be sure to use identical-appearing containers for each category and a cotton-tipped applicator or dropper for consistent application.
- Other (these items are helpful to have available although are not always used): slide, toothbrush (helpful to obtain skin scrapings), Wood's lamp, magnifying glass, small test tube, flashlight and transilluminator, head lamp, gooseneck lamp, Doppler (for amplification of body sounds), goniometer, Denver Developmental Screening Kit contents, Mini-mental status exam, fluid-resistant gowns, masks and eye covers

► CLIENT EDUCATION NEEDED:

1. Introduce yourself by name and title. In some cases you may need to describe your role as well.
2. Provide the client with an explanation of what is to follow ("I will be checking everything from your head to your toes") and an approximate time frame for the exam. It helps to tell children how they will know when you are done (e.g., "When I tell you to put your shoes back on").
3. Inform the client if you will be jotting down notations during the examination and how these notes will be used. This reassures confidentiality.
4. Before performing each step in the physical assessment process, inform the client of what to expect, where to expect it, and how you anticipate it will feel ("I don't think any of this will hurt, but be sure to tell me if it does").
5. Inform the client of what you are looking for and why as you perform your physical assessment. You can accomplish a great deal of education about the body, how it functions, and health prevention while performing your examination.
6. Teach skin self-examination as you evaluate the skin.
7. Teach breast self-examination as you examine breasts (male and female).
8. Teach testicular self-examination and self-checking for hernias during the genital exam.
9. Teach proper urinary hygiene and basics about sexually transmitted diseases (STDs) with the genital exam.
10. Reinforce good hygiene as you wash your hands and conduct the examination.

Estimated time to complete the skill: **Variable depending on the purpose and depth of the examination: average of 20–30 minutes**

Physical assessment skills are within the practice realm and licensure of the nurse. The nurse is responsible for instructing ancillary personnel to report any changes in the client's physical appearance or condition to the nurse for further assessment and evaluation. The nurse is responsible for instructing ancillary personnel to report any changes in the client's physical appearance or condition to the nurse for assessment.

IMPLEMENTATION—Action/Rationale

Action	Rationale
1. Organize equipment.	1. Promotes efficiency.
2. Review the client's medical history (see Figure 1-1-2).	2. The first step of holistic assessment. Provides important clues on which to focus or follow up during physical assessment.
3. Wash hands, preferably in front of the client.	3. Reduces transmission of microorganisms. Educates the client.
4. Explain the plan and procedure.	4. Educates the client. Reassures the client.
5. Assist the client to a sitting position, if possible.	5. Provides best access to begin examination.
6. Examine the client.	6. Collects information about health and disease.

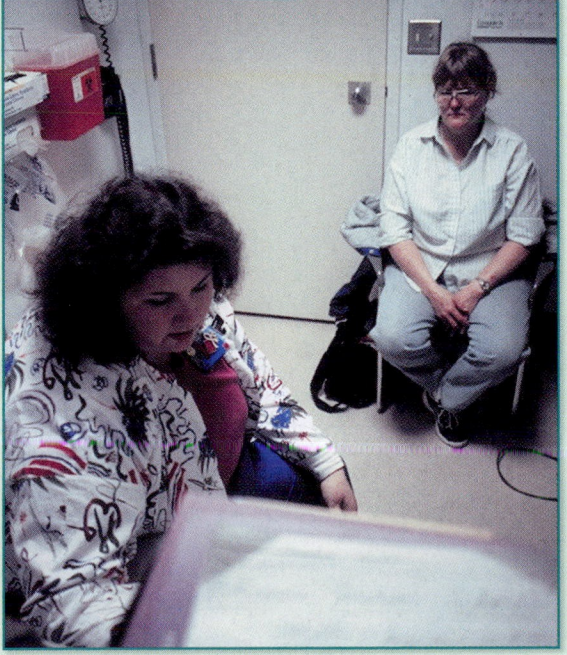

Figure 1-1-2 Review client history. Clients often are uncomfortable and anxious in the unfamiliar clinic setting. Establishing privacy and using words and body language to create a supportive environment help place the client at ease. Listen to the client's complaint, ask pertinent questions about symptoms and medical history, and write down key information.

continues

Action	Rationale
7. Present any appropriate findings. Ask for additional information. Answer the client's questions.	7. Provides closure for the examination and communicates information.
8. Schedule follow-up assessments, tests, or other appointments as needed.	8. Provides for follow-up care.
9. Clean, replace, and discard equipment appropriately.	9. Promotes efficiency, organization, and reduces microorganisms.
10. Wash hands.	10. Reduces the transmission of microorganisms.

Measurements and Overall Observations

Action	Rationale
11. Obtain baseline measurements and compare with normal data. Remember that normal values vary with age and normal temperatures do not rule out illness, especially with very young and elderly clients. Check height, weight, head circumference (check normal values based on age percentiles for infants to 24 months), and temperature (palpate skin temperature during examination as well).	11. Provides measurable objective data about health state or baseline data.
12. Measure the heart rate, rhythm, and volume; the respiratory rate and rhythm; and the blood pressure bilaterally.	12. Provides clues for additional observations or actions required later in the examination.
13. Check anthropometric measurements prn, body mass index (BMI), and so forth.	13. Body mass and height-weight proportion can be better indicators of illness than simple height and weight measurements.
14. Assess the overall appearance of the client in a "once over" evaluation before you begin the detailed examination. Look for clues to poor health, such as level of consciousness, personal hygiene, nutritional status, posture, gait, symmetry, appearance, and appropriateness of clothing. Listen to the quality and appropriateness of speech. Observe facial expressions, whether the client makes eye contact, and how comfortable the client is with interpersonal interaction. Assess whether age is congruent with appearance. Observe body fat, stature, motor movements, and body and breath odors. Assess dress, grooming, personal hygiene, speech, facial expressions, general mannerisms, mood, and affect. Look for signs of distress, as evident by breathing patterns, speech, facial expressions, perspiration, tension, guarding, bracing, and anxiety.	14. Provides objective clues about overall health state and clues to possible specific abnormalities to watch for later in the examination.

continues

Action	Rationale

Skin, Hair, and Nails Examination

15. Take a moment to assess initially and continue assessment as you perform the remainder of the exam.
    - Inspect: color, vascularity, lesions, ulcers, scars, hair distribution, nail shape and configuration, nail bed angles. Measure, describe, draw, and/or stage abnormalities.
    - Palpate: moisture, temperature, texture, turgor, capillary refill (normal capillary refill is less than 3 seconds), edema.

15. Detects normal variation and abnormalities. Establishes a baseline for future comparisons. Skin abnormalities, including crepitus, nodules, mobility, and hydration will provide clues to illness and are often indicators of systemic abnormalities.

Head, Face, and Lymphatics Examination

16. Inspect and palpate the head, face, and lymph nodes (see Figures 1-1-3 and 1-1-4). Proceed from front to back.

16. Confirms health and identifies signs and symptoms of illness or disease, infections, old or new trauma, or other abnormalities.

17. Head: Examine scalp, hair, and cranium (frontal-parietal-temporal-occipital). Examine fontanelles and sutures in newborns to 24 months. Head should be normocephalic and symmetric with no acromegaly, hydrocephalus, craniosynostosis, premature closure of sutures, masses, depressions, tenderness, or infestations.

17. Confirms health and identifies signs and symptoms of illness or disease, infections, old or new trauma, or other abnormalities.

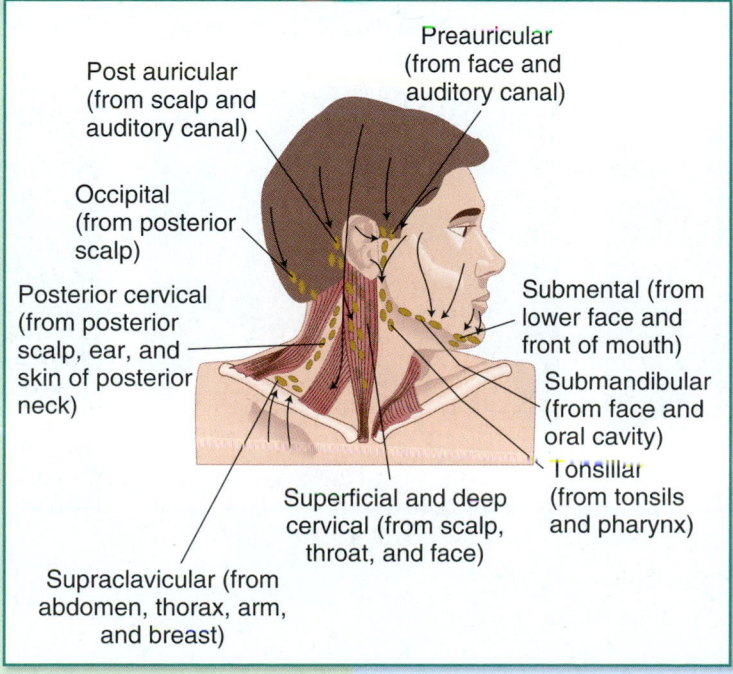

Figure 1-1-3   Lymph nodes of the head and neck. Arrows indicate drainage patterns.

continues

Action	Rationale

Head, Face, and Lymphatics Examination *continued*

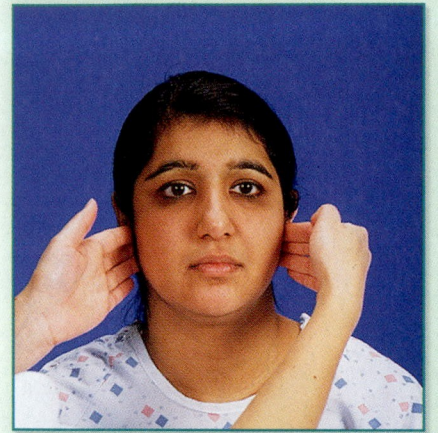

A. Preauricular

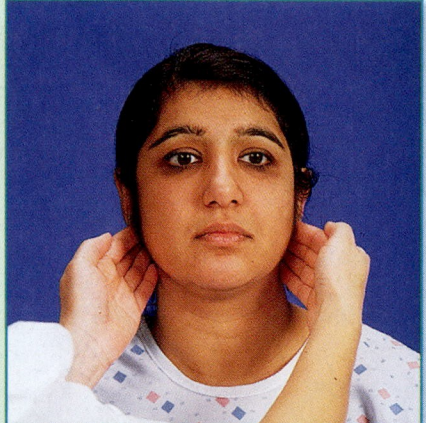

B. Postauricular

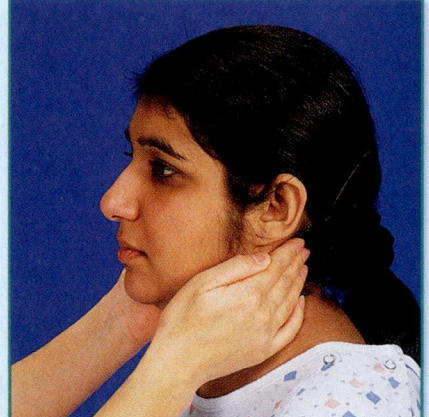

C. Occipital

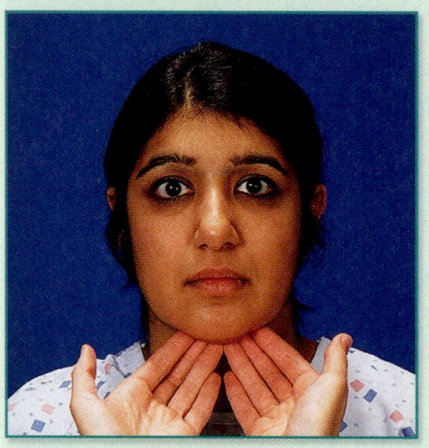

D. Submental

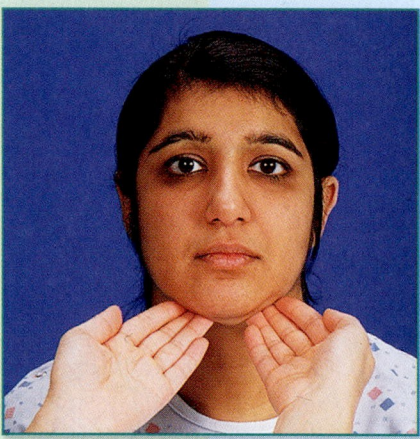

E. Submandibular

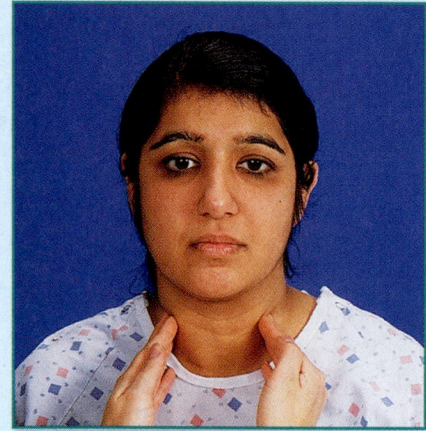

F. Anterior cervical chain

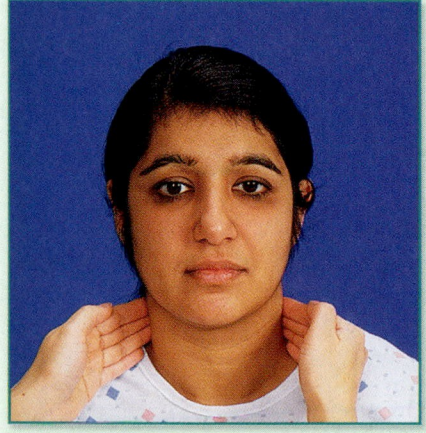

G. Posterior cervical chain

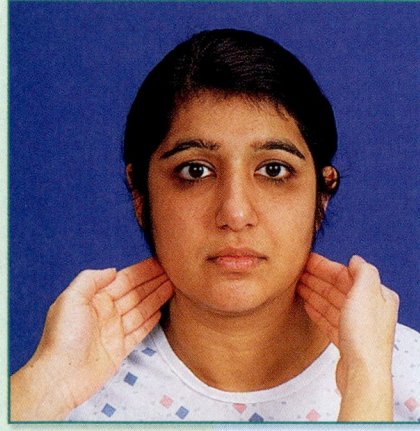

H. Tonsillar

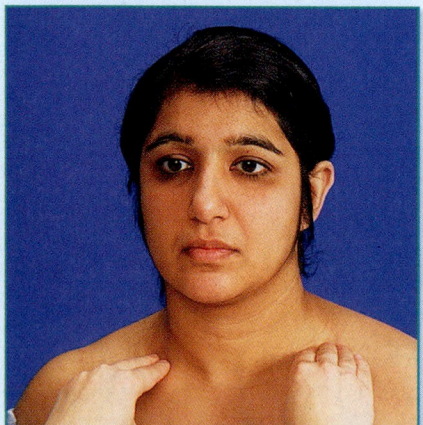

I. Supraclavicular

Figure 1-1-4   Palpation of lymph nodes.

continues

Action	Rationale
18. Lymph nodes: Examine preauricular, postauricular, occipital, submental, submandibular, anterior cervical chain, posterior cervical chain, tonsillar, supra-clavicular, and parotid. Lymph nodes should be less than 1 cm in size and nontender. Note that children may have multiple nodes less than 1 cm, especially postauricular, but these will be small, nontender, and movable.	**18.** Confirms health and identifies signs and symptoms of illness or disease, infections, old or new trauma, or other abnormalities.
19. Temporomandibular joint: Observe the motion of opening and closing the jaw. It should articulate smoothly without crepitus, clicking, or tenderness. There should be no sign of inflammation.	**19.** Confirms health and identifies signs and symptoms of illness or disease, infections, old or new trauma, or other abnormalities.
20. Face: Observe for shape, symmetry, and expression. Have the client smile, frown, raise eyebrows, wrinkle forehead, show teeth, purse lips, puff cheeks, press tongue into cheek, "cluck" tongue, and whistle. Inspect, percuss, and palpate frontal and maxillary sinuses. Use a wisp of cotton to assess tactile sensation over the trigeminal nerve sites and mandible bilaterally. Facial features should be symmetric with a naso-labial fold present bilaterally. Clients of Asian descent may have slanted eyes with inner epicanthal folds. Normal sounds should be resonant. No pain should be present on percussion or palpation. Abnormal findings include edema, disproportionate structures, or involuntary movements.	**20.** Confirms health and identifies signs and symptoms of illness or disease, infections, old or new trauma, or other abnormalities.

Eye, Ear, Nose, Mouth, and Throat Examination

Action	Rationale
21. Examine the client's eyes. Inspect and palpate external structures, including brows, lids, lacrimal gland, and puncta. Inspect eye position and palpebral fissures. Examine bulbar and palpebral conjunctivae, sclera, cornea, and iris. Assess for a corneal touch reflex.	**21.** Confirms health and identifies signs and symptoms of illness or disease. • Establishes the presence or absence of drooping, infection, or tumors. Confirms that the lid "meets" the iris, the lid margins are smooth, tears flow evenly instead of accumulating and "tearing up" the eye. • Establishes the presence or absence of inflammation of hair follicles, hemorrhages, discharge, discolorations, ectropion, swelling, edema, blepharitis, or dacryoadenitis. • Checks that the third cranial nerve (CN III) raises the lids symmetrically, and that the puncta are open and without inflammation.

continues

Action	Rationale

Eye, Ear, Nose, Mouth, and Throat Examination *continued*

22. Extraocular mobility: Check for Hirschberg's corneal light reflex by using the cover-uncover test. Check the six cardinal fields of gaze. Examine pupils, including size, shape, and response to light and accommodation, both direct and consensual. Examine the lens and retinal structures. First check for a red reflex with the ophthalmoscope set on "0." Move the diopter wheel to "1" to focus on anterior ocular structures and "2" to focus on posterior structures. Locate the retina, vessels, optic disk, and macula.

22. Checks that light reflects symmetrically from the center of corneas at 12 to 15 inches, and that the uncovered eye stays focused.
    - Checks the functions of CN III, IV, and VI.
    - Checks for the absence of tropia, phoria, or nystagmus.

23. Have the client identify an object, such as your finger, as it enters the visual fields from each of four directions. Normal movement is temporal 90 degrees, nasal 60 degrees, superior 50 degrees, and inferior 70 degrees (see Figure 1-1-5).

23. Checks the function of CN II.

24. Check for visual acuity, including near and far sight, primary colors, and Ishihara plates (see Figure 1-1-6).

24. Visual acuity tests are the last step in the eye examination so that physical abnormalities that might cause abnormal acuity will be detected first.

25. Examine the ears. Inspect and palpate the external ear, including alignment, pinna, tragus, lobule, and neck mastoid muscle. Observe the shape, color, and size of the ear.

25. Confirms health and identifies signs and symptoms of illness or diseases of the ear. Checks for normal alignment, that the top of the ear crosses an imaginary line from eye to occiput. Checks for abnormal findings of tags, excess wax, drainage, deformities, nodules, inflammation, pain, and a tender or "boggy" mastoid.

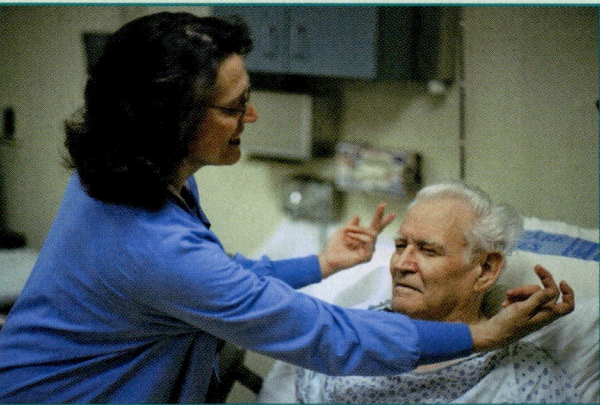

Figure 1-1-5   Have client identify the moment an object enters the visual field.

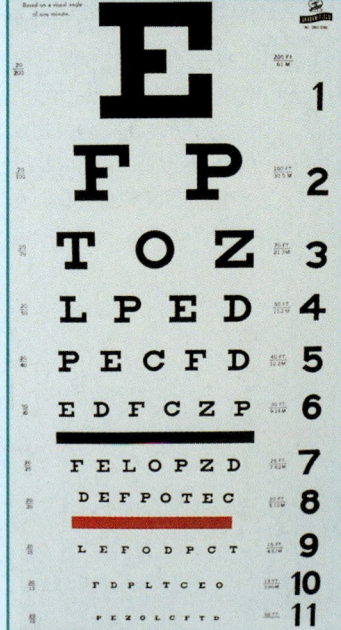

Figure 1-1-6   Snellen chart used to assess visual acuity.

continues

Action	Rationale
26. Proceed with an otoscopic assessment, starting with the ear canal. Identify landmarks, the tympanic membrane, and observe tympanic membrane movement. Use tympanometry if needed to confirm visual findings.	26. Establishes the quality of tympanic membrane (TM) movement, detects retractions, bulging, and abnormal or discolored middle ear fluid. Confirms if there are signs of infection, impaction, or other abnormalities.
27. Check the client's hearing acuity. Note responses to normal sounds. In an infant, observe for a startle reflex/bell response. In adults, conduct a voice/whisper or watch-tick test at 1 to 2 feet. Conduct Weber and Rhinne tests at 512 Hz.	27. Hearing acuity tests are the last step in the ear examination so that physical abnormalities that might cause abnormal acuity will be detected first.
28. Examine the nose. Inspect and palpate for nasal patency. Have the client inhale and exhale through each nostril. Observe the external surface, nasal mucosa, turbinates, and septum.	28. Confirms health and identifies signs and symptoms of illness or disease, including unusual or excessive discharge, damaged septum, polyps, tenderness, or nonclear drainage.
29. Have the client identify common odors.	29. Tests CN I (the olfactory nerve).
30. Examine the mouth, including the teeth, tongue, and throat (see Figure 1-1-7).	30. Confirms health and identifies signs and symptoms of illness or disease.
31. Inspect and count teeth.	31. Confirms the number and condition of teeth for age.
32. Inspect and palpate lips and frenula, gums, buccal mucosa, tongue protrusion and frenulum, salivary glands, hard and soft palates, tonsils, uvula position and movement, and arches. Inspect the naso-oropharynx.	32. Identifies lesions, color of membranes, abnormalities, cavities, odors, swelling, inflammation, swallowing difficulties, or hyperplasia.
33. Conduct gag reflex response, and taste tests for sweet, sour, bitter, and salt.	33. Tests cranial nerve functions.
34. Examine the neck. Inspect and palpate the trachea. Check that the trachea runs midline down the neck by examining the trachea at the suprasternal notch.	34. Confirms health and identifies signs and symptoms of illness or disease.

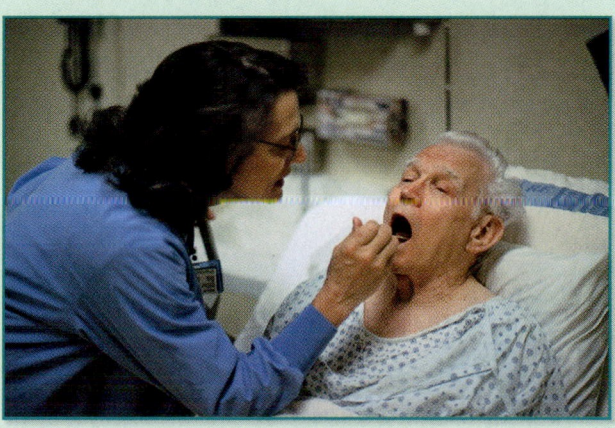

Figure 1-1-7 The mouth examination includes the teeth, tongue, throat, oral mucosa, and salivary glands.

continues

Action	Rationale
Eye, Ear, Nose, Mouth, and Throat Examination *continued*	
35. To examine the thyroid, observe the anterior neck slightly extended, then have the client flex the neck and swallow. Palpate the anterior neck, then palpate forward from the posterior. Identify tracheal rings, isthmus, thyroid cartilage, and gland lobes as the client is swallowing.	35. Checks for goiter, nodules, enlargement, or tenderness in the neck and thyroid.
36. Palpate the temporal and carotid pulses. Assess the quality, character, rhythm, and strength of the pulse.	36. Identifies signs and symptoms of cardiovascular illness or disease.
Upper Neuromuscular Examination	
37. Inspect and palpate muscles, bones, and joints. In general, evaluate from the periphery to the center of the body. Observe the configuration, symmetry, size, tone, and range of motion (ROM). Assess strength using resistive ROM.	37. Confirms health and identifies signs and symptoms of illness or disease.
38. Examine the cervical spine. Flex, extend, move lateral, and rotate the spine. Examine the spine for resistive strength by pushing your hand against the side of the client's face. Push left, right, back on the forehead, forward on the occiput, and down on the top of the head.	38. Checks the cervical spine, sternocleidomastoid, and trapezial baseline strength, integrity, and function.
39. Examine shoulders. Flex, hyperextend, abduct, adduct, turn in internal and external rotation, shrug, and push/pull against the shoulders.	39. Detects limitations of mobility, torticollis, pain, crepitus, nodules, lumps, or pulsations in the muscles, bones, and joints.
40. Examine elbows. Flex, extend, rotate, push, and pull each elbow.	40. Checks for tenderness and mobility.
41. Examine wrists. Flex, extend, and rotate each wrist.	41. Checks for tenderness and mobility. Detects the presence of carpal tunnel.
42. Examine hands by having the client grasp your hands with his/hers.	42. Checks for tenderness and mobility.
43. Examine fingers. Abduct and adduct the fingers. Perform finger-thumb opposition with counting and position sense.	43. Checks for tenderness and mobility.
44. Examine the epitrochlear lymph nodes, brachial and radial pulses, and bicep, tricep, and brachioradialis reflexes.	44. Confirms that lymph nodes are nonpalpable and nontender and that pulses are strong and regular. Checks neurologic reflexes.
Chest and Breast Examination	
(See Skill 1-8, Breast Examination)	
45. Inspect and palpate the breast, nipple, and areola. Palpate the axillary lymph nodes.	45. Confirms health and identifies signs and symptoms of illness or disease. Detects lumps, nodules, or discharge in tissue. Detects tenderness or lumps in axillary nodes, which drain the chest and breast.

continues

Action	Rationale
46. Calculate the Tanner stage of sexual maturity if appropriate.	**46.** The Tanner stage assesses appropriate breast development progression and status for age and provides an opportunity for teaching.
47. Repeat breast and axillae examination while the client is in the supine position.	**47.** Repeating the examination while the client is supine increases likelihood of early identification of abnormalities.

Back and Posterior Lung Examination

Action	Rationale
48. Inspect and palpate the skin.	**48.** Confirms health and identifies signs and symptoms of illness or disease.
49. Recheck the thyroid from the posterior position.	**49.** Gland lobules are easier to palpate from back.
50. Examine the cervical and thoracic spine (see Figure 1-1-8), the scapulae, and the rib cage. Observe the posterior thoracic expansion. Estimate the anteroposterior-to-transverse chest ratio. A normal ratio is 1:2.	**50.** Determines normal, normal variations, and abnormal findings in alignment, flexion, spinous processes, and paravertebral muscles. Checks that the scapulae are equal and that the rib cage is symmetric.
51. Feel for the presence of fremitus posteriorly and laterally. Compare sides.	**51.** Checks for fremitus either increased with consolidation, or decreased with hyperinflation of the lungs. Bilateral comparison enables the identification of differences.
52. Use indirect percussion at a minimum of four sites, preferably in regular intervals every 5 cm from top to bottom of lung fields. Move from superior to inferior and from lateral to spine.	**52.** Indirect percussion allows comparison of resonance bilaterally and checks for tenderness over the lungs and kidneys. The organized sequence of side-to-side and superior-to-inferior increases the possibility of detecting abnormalities.

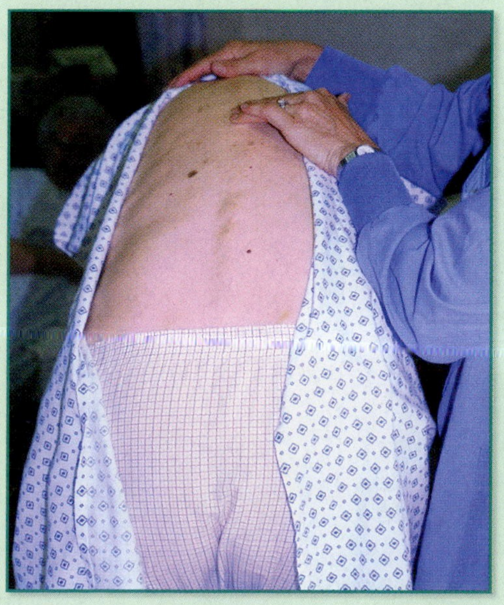

Figure 1-1-8 Examine the cervical and thoracic spine for alignment, flexion, and symmetry with the rib cage and scapulae.

continues

Action	Rationale
Back and Posterior Lung Examination *continued*	
53. Auscultate the lungs (see Figure 1-1-9) using a side-to-side sequence and moving down 2 to 5 cm at a time. Listen to inspiration and expiration at each site. Listen for vocal fremitus while the client makes "99" and sustained "ee" sounds.	53. Checks for bronchial noises over trachea, bronchovesicular sounds in the first and second intercostal spaces (ICSs), and vesicular sounds over the peripheral chest. Detects abnormal sounds of rales, rhonchi, or wheezes.
Thorax, Lungs, and Respiratory Examination	
54. Stand in front of the client.	54. Best position to examine anterior lungs.
55. Inspect and palpate the anterior chest. Observe position, chest movement, size, shape, and symmetry of the clavicles and ribs.	55. Confirms health and identifies signs and symptoms of illness or disease. Checks for barrel chest, pectus excavatum, pectus carinatum, or tripod "splinting" positions. Splinting positions indicate the client is compensating for decreased oxygenation.
56. Listen to the respiratory rate, including rhythm and depth of respirations. Compare rate with normal respiratory rates for the age of the client.	56. Checks for 2:1 timing of the exhale/inhale breathing cycle. Detects shortness of breath (SOB), and abnormal respiration patterns, including Cheyne-Stokes, tachypnea, hyperpnea, and hyspnea (see Figure 1-1-10).
57. Observe the diaphragmatic excursion, ICSs, respiratory muscles, respiratory effort, and expansion. Watch for pursed lips, cyanosis, or a cough. Note that abdominal breathing is normal from birth to 2 years of age.	57. Detects accessory muscle use or stridor.
58. Feel for tactile fremitus along the lung apexes and bases.	58. Detects fremitus, which is increased with consolidation or decreased with hyperinflation.
59. Use indirect percussion at intervals over ICSs, moving superior to inferior and lateral to spine. Percuss lung apexes and bases, and the cardiac border if appropriate. Note that percussion should be resonant over the lung, flat over bone, and dull over organs.	59. Side-to-side and superior-to-inferior organized approach increases the possibility of detecting abnormalities.

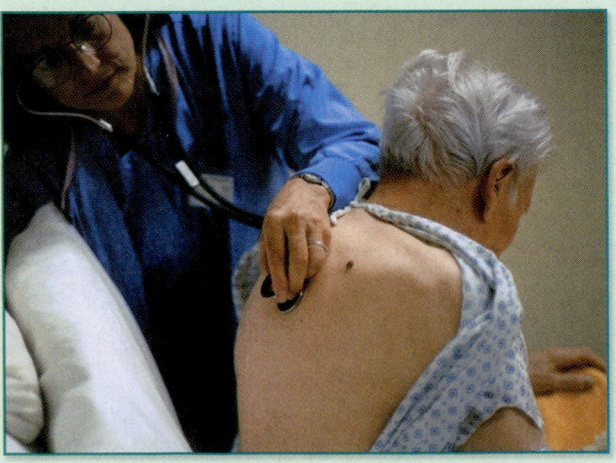

Figure 1-1-9 Auscultate the lungs, listening to inspiration and expiration at each site.

continues

Action	Rationale

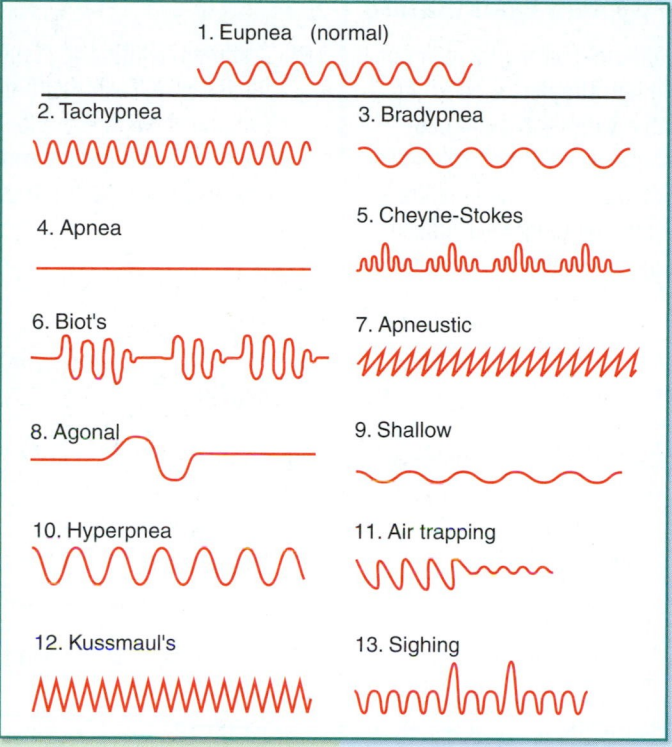

1. Eupnea (normal)

2. Tachypnea

3. Bradypnea

4. Apnea

5. Cheyne-Stokes

6. Biot's

7. Apneustic

8. Agonal

9. Shallow

10. Hyperpnea

11. Air trapping

12. Kussmaul's

13. Sighing

Figure 1-1-10　Normal and abnormal respiratory patterns.

60. Auscultate the anterior lung fields, using the same progression as the palpation procedure. Avoid listening over bone and breast tissue. Observe intensity, pitch, ratio, quality (see Figure 1-1-11).

Listen for vocal fremitus during "99" and sustained "ee" sounds (egophony or whispered pectoriloquy).

60. Checks for bronchial noises over trachea, bronchovesicular sounds to the left and right of the sternum in the first and second ICSs, and vesicular sounds over the peripheral chest. Detects abnormal sounds of rales, rhonchi, or wheezes.

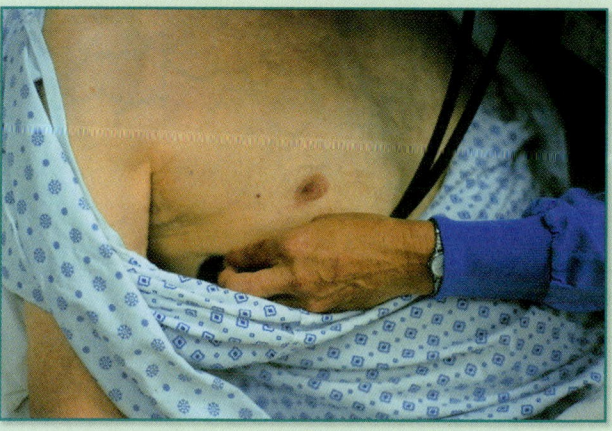

Figure 1-1-11　Auscultate the anterior lung fields. Listen for abnormal sounds, including rales, rhonchi, or wheezes.

continues

Action	Rationale
Heart and Cardiovascular System Examination	
61. Inspect and palpate the precordium. Identify the point of maximal intensity (PMI) at the mitral/apical area of the heart. This pulsation, associated with ventricular contraction, is located at the left fifth ICS. Confirm synchrony with the carotid pulse. The PMI may be visible in children and thin clients. Palpation of the PMI in large or muscular persons may require leaning the client forward or to the left side.	**61.** Confirms health and identifies signs and symptoms of illness or disease. Confirms the absence of cardiomegaly symptoms, visible thrills, heaves, and pulsations (except possibly 1 to 2 cm movements at mitral area during systole, especially in children, thin clients, or elderly clients).
62. Auscultate with the client sitting, then leaning forward. Listen with the diaphragm and then the bell.	**62.** The bell detects lower pitched sounds than the diaphragm.
63. Auscultate the apical heart rate and feel radial pulse at the same time. Identify rate, rhythm, regularity, amplitude, and difference between apical and radial pulses. Note carotid impulse with apical sound.	**63.** A difference in apical and radial pulse (pulse deficit) reflects difference in stroke volume with each beat. Irregular rates with pulse deficit may indicate atrial fibrillation, whereby disorganization exists between atrial and ventricular electrical activity.
64. Examine all valvular landmarks at least twice. First locate and identify the S_1, S_2, S_3, and S_4 heart sounds. Then listen for other sounds (murmurs, rubs, clicks, etc.). Auscultate in an orderly fashion from the apex to the base of the heart (or vice versa).	**64.** Systematic progression of the examination minimizes omissions. Detects normal physiology, as the S_1 closure of mitral and tricuspid valves signals the onset of systole. Detects any abnormal opening snap in early diastole, which could indicate mitral stenosis.
65. In the mitral area identify that S_1 is louder than S_2 with the diaphragm of the stethoscope, because the left heart pressure is greater than the right, and the mitral valve closes slightly before the tricuspid valve. Use the bell to listen for a possible S_3 sound (see Figure 1-1-12).	**65.** Detects S_3 sounds, which are early diastolic filling sounds from the ventricles, and could indicate diastolic gallop.
66. In the tricuspid area, identify that S_1 is louder than S_2 with diaphragm but that it is softer than at the mitral area. Listen for possible S_1 split that disappears when the client holds his or her breath. Listen for the S_3 sound with the bell.	**66.** Detects the normal aortic valve closure occurring slightly before the pulmonic valve closure during inspiration as more negative intrathoracic pressure causes an increase in venous return to the right side of the heart
67. In the pulmonic area identify that S_2 is louder than S_1, but softer than at aortic area. Note that physiologic splitting of S_2, which indicates closure of the semilunar valves at this site is normal. In the aortic area identify that S_2 is louder than S_1 with diaphragm.	**67.** Finds symptoms of abnormal splits, which are wide, fixed, or paradoxic.
68. Assess the epigastric, axillary, and Erb's point areas.	**68.** Assesses for signs of mitral valve prolapse, which are best heard at the epigastric location. Assesses for abnormal murmurs radiating to the axilla. Checks Erb's point, where both aortic and pulmonic murmurs may be heard.

continues

Action	Rationale

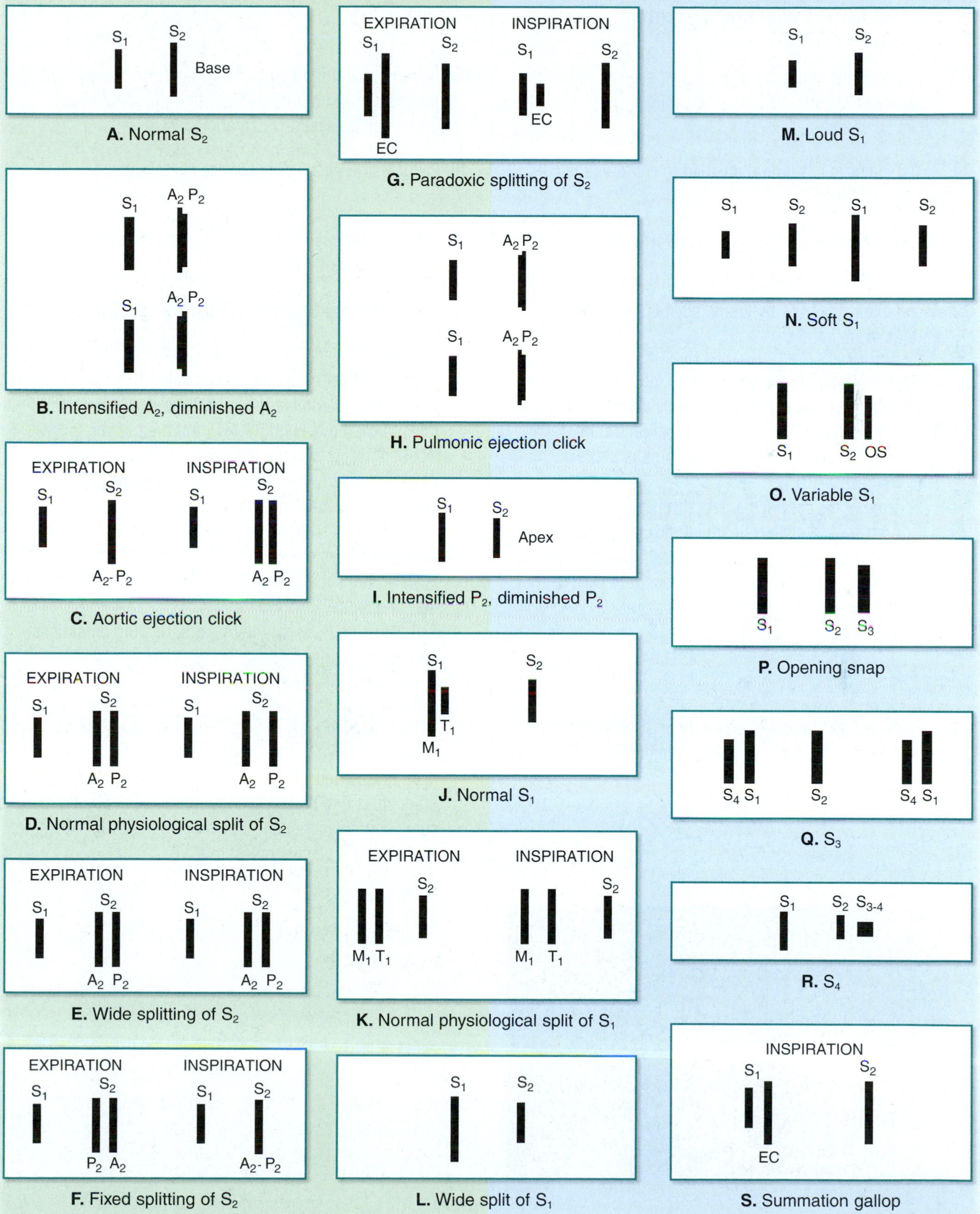
S_1 S_2 Base
A. Normal S_2
S_1 A_2 P_2
S_1 A_2 P_2
B. Intensified A_2, diminished A_2
EXPIRATION S_1 S_2 A_2-P_2 INSPIRATION S_1 S_2 A_2 P_2
C. Aortic ejection click
EXPIRATION S_1 S_2 A_2 P_2 INSPIRATION S_1 S_2 A_2 P_2
D. Normal physiological split of S_2
EXPIRATION S_1 S_2 A_2 P_2 INSPIRATION S_1 S_2 A_2 P_2
E. Wide splitting of S_2
EXPIRATION S_1 S_2 P_2 A_2 INSPIRATION S_1 S_2 A_2-P_2
F. Fixed splitting of S_2
EXPIRATION S_1 S_2 EC INSPIRATION S_1 EC S_2
G. Paradoxic splitting of S_2
S_1 A_2 P_2
S_1 A_2 P_2
H. Pulmonic ejection click
S_1 S_2 Apex
I. Intensified P_2, diminished P_2
S_1 T_1 M_1 S_2
J. Normal S_1
EXPIRATION S_2 M_1 T_1 INSPIRATION S_2 M_1 T_1
K. Normal physiological split of S_1
S_1 S_2
L. Wide split of S_1
S_1 S_2
M. Loud S_1
S_1 S_2 S_1 S_2
N. Soft S_1
S_1 S_2 OS
O. Variable S_1
S_1 S_2 S_3
P. Opening snap
S_4 S_1 S_2 S_4 S_1
Q. S_3
S_1 S_2 S_{3-4}
R. S_4
INSPIRATION S_1 S_2 EC
S. Summation gallop

Figure 1-1-12 Normal and abnormal heart sounds.

continues

Action	Rationale

Heart and Cardiovascular System Examination *continued*

69. Summarize the character of S_1 and S_2 sounds. Note the presence or absence of S_3 and S_4 (gallop), murmurs, rubs, clicks, or snaps.

69. S_3 can be normal in children, in the third trimester of pregnancy, and adults younger than 30 years of age. Other sounds need investigation.

70. Assist client to left lateral position to continue the cardiac examination.

70. Positions the heart closer to the chest wall.

71. Auscultate mitral and tricuspid sites with the bell.

71. Mitral and tricuspid abnormalities are heard best in the left lateral position.

72. Assist client to return to supine position and continue cardiac examination.

72. Facilitates next portion of cardiac examination.

73. Inspect and palpate the precordium. Identify the PMI at the mitral area and confirm synchrony with carotid pulse. Assess apical, carotid, temporal, brachial, radial, femoral, popliteal, posterior tibial, and dorsalis pedis pulses (see Figure 1-1-13).

Percuss the cardiac borders, if needed.

Auscultate the heart in supine position with bell, then with diaphragm. Check the mitral, tricuspid, pulmonic, aortic, and ectopic areas. Auscultate with bell for bruits at carotid and temporal pulse sites.

73. The PMI is best palpated in the supine position. Confirms the absence of visible thrills, heaves, and pulsations except possibly a small (1 to 2 cm) area at the mitral location during systole, especially in children, thin clients, and elderly clients. PMI may not be palpable in large and muscular clients.

The client's position determines which sounds are heard best. It is easier to hear some murmurs with the client in the supine position. The bell is best for detecting deeper sounds.

Notes unusual symmetry, rate, rhythm, pulsations, volume, or thrills of pulses.

Evaluates for cardiomegaly.

74. Raise the client's head to an angle of 30 to 45 degrees, and inspect the jugular vein distention (JVD).

74. Detects normal jugular vein distention, which is usually 1 to 2 cm above the sternal angle when the client's head is elevated 45 degrees and is usually absent at 90 degrees and distended when flat. Jugular vein pressure (JVP) measurement plus 5 cm will give an estimate of the central venous pressure (CVP).

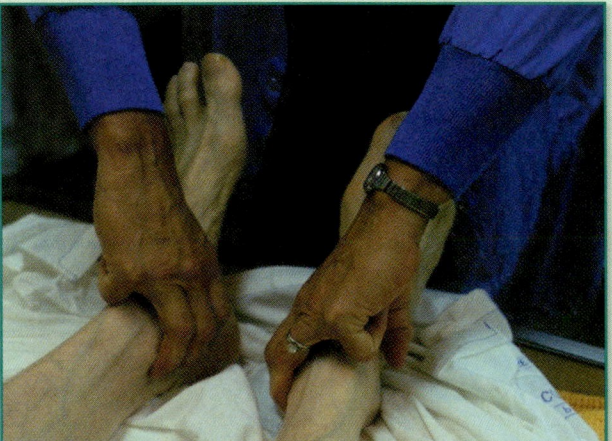

Figure 1-1-13   Assess for unusual symmetry, pulsations, volume, or thrills of pulses.

continues

Action	Rationale

Abdominal Examination

75. Inspect the size, contour, and symmetry of the abdomen. The normal abdomen is flat (except in young children), symmetric, without scars, striae, masses, nodules, peristalsis (except in very thin clients), or rectus ridge (except in young or thin clients). Note pigmentation, scars, striae, masses, nodules, the condition of the umbilicus, and any respiratory or peristaltic movement. Check the rectus abdominis muscle by having the client raise his or her head.

76. Auscultate with the diaphragm and then the bell. Listen for bowel sounds in each of the four quadrants: right lower quadrant (RLQ), right upper quadrant (RUQ), left upper quadrant (LUQ), and left lower quadrant (LLQ).

77. Percuss the RLQ, RUQ, gastric bubble, spleen, bladder, LLQ, LUQ, and liver span (see Figure 1-1-14).

Note that the spleen, located between the sixth and tenth rib, may go undetected. The gastric air bubble (LUQ) is lower pitched than tympany of the intestine. The tympany changes to dull at lower edge of liver, and lung resonance changes to dull at upper edge of liver. You may try to percuss the kidney posteriorly while the client is sitting, if needed.

78. Palpate all four quadrants superficially first then deep and rebound palpations to identify any discomfort, tenderness, or abnormalities. Check superficial abdominal reflexes in the LLQ, LUQ, spleen (use bimanual palpation), RLQ, RUQ, liver, aorta, kidney (use bimanual technique), and bladder (see Figure 1-1-14). Evaluate for guarding on expiration.

75. Confirms health and identifies signs and symptoms of illness or disease.

Aortic pulsations may be seen in epigastric area in thin clients. Newborn to 2 year olds breathe with their abdominal muscles, with no retractions of the intercostal muscles during inspiration, and a smooth rhythm. The umbilicus is normally depressed.

76. Auscultate before palpating, as sounds will change in response to touch.

Detects a normal frequency of sounds of 5 to 30 sounds per minute, or abnormal bruits, hums, or rubs.

77. Detects size and location of internal organs as tympany changes to dull over organs.

78. Checks for normal umbilical deviation toward the direction of palpation stroke.

Determines normal abdomen, which is smooth and soft with no masses, bulges, swelling, organomegaly, bladder distention, fluid retention, or pain. Locates normal findings of palpated liver edge, aortic pulsations, and lower pole of kidney.

Normal voluntary muscle guarding ceases on expiration.

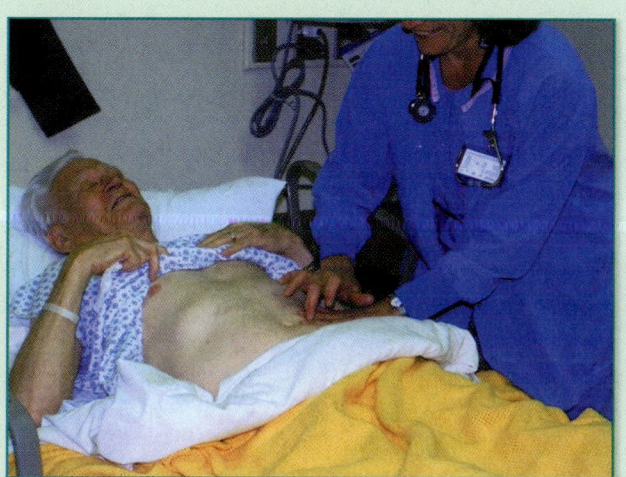

Figure 1-1-14 Percuss the abdomen to assess size and location of internal organs.

continues

Action	Rationale
Abdominal Examination *continued*	
79. Check femoral pulses and superficial and deep inguinal nodes.	79. Determines normal pulses, which are symmetric and even, with no bounding or thrills, and normal inguinal nodes, which are less than 1 cm, movable, and nontender.
External Genitalia Examination	
80. Assist client to modified or full lithotomy position.	80. Lithotomy position without stirrups is usually more comfortable for the client; however, both positions provide good visibility and access.
81. Inspect and palpate deep inguinal nodes.	81. Deep nodes are more easily palpated in this position.
82. Observe pubic hair distribution, color, and texture. Check the femoral and inguinal areas for hernias.	82. Confirms normal distribution of hair in an inverse triangle, and identifies abnormalities, including infestations, rashes, edema, condylomata, vesicles, varicose veins, discharge, odor, or bulges.
83. Calculate the Tanner stage of sexual maturity if appropriate.	83. The Tanner stage assesses appropriate genital development progression and status for age and provides an opportunity for teaching.
84. Check the skin and look for abnormalities. In women, examine the mons pubis, labia majora, labia minora, clitoris, urethral meatus, vaginal introitus, and perineum.	84. Checks for abnormal color, lesions, pain, trauma, abnormal size, imperforate introitus, odor, or discharge.
85. In men, check the cremasteric reflex (in infant), urethral meatus, penis (glans, foreskin, shaft), scrotum (transilluminate if hydrocele suspected), scrotal rugae, testicles, epididymis, spermatic cord, and external inguinal ring.	85. Confirms normal appearance, where the urethral meatus is located centrally, with dorsal vein prominence, a small amount of smegma, and the left scrotal sac lower than the right. Detects a nonretractable foreskin in an uncircumcised child. Checks for abnormal lesions, odor, swelling, inflammation, nodules, condyloma, vesicles, pustules, scaling, edema, phimosis, chordee (curvature), hernia, hydrocele, spermatocele, or varicocele.
86. Examine the anus. You may need to return the client to the left lateral position or have the client stand and lean elbows on the exam table to aide in visualization.	86. Confirms normal appearance of sacral dimpling, dark pink to brown color, puckered, and free of lesions, swelling, inflammation, tenderness, itching, fissures, rashes, masses, hemorrhoids, or skin tags.
Lower Extremity and Musculoskeletal Examination	
87. Assist the client down from the table to a standing position, if necessary.	87. To observe the client's ability to change position and assist for safety when needed.

continues

Action	Rationale

88. Have the client walk across the room while you observe his or her gait. Observe from the side profile, assessing cervical, thoracic, and lumbar curves. Look for differences in height of shoulders, iliac crests, and skin creases below the buttocks. Ask the client to bend forward as you observe the spine for any curvatures or deformities. Check the ROM of the spine. Have the client bend forward to touch toes (flexion), bend sideways (lateral bending), and then bend backward (extension). Stand beside the client for support if needed. Check rotation as the client twists from side to side.
 	
  Palpate the paravertebral muscles for tenderness and spasm.
	88. To observe whether gait is steady and assess whether the client is at risk for falls. The normal spine has concavities in the cervical and lumbar regions and a convexity in the thorax. If iliac crests are uneven, it is suggestive of unequal leg lengths. Scoliosis may be noted if there is deviation in the line from T1 to the gluteal cleft. Decreased spinal mobility may be noted in osteoarthritis as well as other conditions.
	
	  When a paravertebral muscle is in spasm it looks prominent, feels tight, and is tender to the touch.

89. Assist the client to the supine position.	89. Prepares for the next sequence in the examination.

90. Inspect and palpate the skin. Look at the skin color, check that capillary refill is less than 3 seconds, observe hair distribution, veins, temperature, and texture of skin.
 	
  Observe the size, shape, isometric muscle contraction, tone, and strength (using resistive ROM) of muscles.
	90. Detects skin atrophy, breakdown, edema, ulcerations, or varicose veins.
	
	  Determines that muscle shape is symmetric, with good tone. Detects atrophy, hypertrophy, flaccidity, spasticity, spasm, masses, or involuntary movements.

91. Inspect the joints. Palpate from periphery to center. Observe contour, periarticular tissue, neutral anatomic position, ROM (active and palpate passive), and strength (resistive motion). Also evaluate the hips. Have the client do a straight leg raise. Move the hips knee to chest, internal rotation, external rotation, abduction, and adduction. Listen carefully for a hip click in infants (Ortolani's sign).
 	
  Assess the knees. Check the tibiofemoral joints by flexing the knee 90 degrees and with thumbs palpate tibial margins and collateral ligament. Check knee flexion, extension, and strength.
 	
  For the ankles and feet, palpate the Achilles tendon, at rest, in dorsiflexion and plantar flexion, eversion and inversion. Check toe flexion, abduction, and adduction. Palpate metatarsophalangeal joints and interphalangeal joints.
 	
  Check popliteal, posterior tibial, and dorsalis pedis pulses.
	91. Confirms joints articulate in proper alignment and are free from swelling, nodules, pain, warmth, deformities, masses, crepitus, grating, or popping.
	
	  Evaluates for contractures, pain, or swelling.
	
	  Evaluates for clonus, varus, valgus, planus, deviations, and inflammation.

Neurologic Examination

92. Assist the client to a sitting position.	92. Prepares for the remainder of the neurologic examination.

93. Check for deep tendon reflexes, biceps, triceps, brachioradialis (if not done previously), patellar, and Achilles reflexes.
 	
  Check infantile reflexes, including rooting, suck, palmer grasp, tonic neck, stepping, plantar grasp, moro, Gallant, and Landau.
 	
  Check the Babinski reflex. A positive Babinski reflex is normal until a child is walking or reaches 18 months of age.
	93. Measures the degree and speed of response, from 0 (absent) to 41 (hyperactive), and the presence of clonus.
	
	  Observe fanning of toes with stroke of outer aspect of sole of foot from heel across ball.

continues

Action	Rationale
Neurologic Examination *continued*	
94. Examine the client's sensory abilities. Check for responses to skin sensations. Begin distally and move proximally. Touch fingers, hands, lower arms and toes, feet, legs, and abdomen as necessary. Be careful not to be "predictable." Alter the rate and rhythm of stimulation. Compare right-to-left and proximal-to-distal sensations. Check exteroceptive sensation, including light touch (use a cotton wisp), and sharp and dull (use a hair pin or paper clip). If the sharp/dull evaluation was abnormal, check temperature sensation as well. Check the proprioceptive sensations of vibration, motion, and position. Check the cortical sensations of stereognosis (coin, button, key, paper clip, etc.; different object in each hand), and graphesthesia. If needed, examine two-point discrimination and extinction. Normal distances vary with the body part tested. For example, fingers are approximately 5 mm, the hand or foot is 20 mm.	94. Confirms health and identifies signs and symptoms of illness or disease. Confirms normal sensory perceptions. Proximal nerve transmission must be functional for distal sensations to be present. Determines that client can feel stimuli, detect vibrations over bony prominences (which decreases after age 65), and identify changes in body position and motion. Clients should be able to identify objects with eyes closed.
95. Review and recheck the cranial nerves: CN I: Olfactory CN II: Optic CN III: Oculomotor CN IV: Trochlear CN V: Trigeminal motor and sensory CN VI: Abducens CN VII: Facial motor and sensory CN VIII: Acoustic cochlear and vestibular CN IX: Glossopharyngeal motor/sensory CN X: Vagus motor and sensory CN XI: Spinal accessory CN XII: Hypoglossal A helpful acronym for the cranial nerves is: **O**n **O**ld **O**lympic **T**owering **T**ops **A** **F**inn **A**nd **G**erman **V**iewed **S**ome **H**ops.	95. Identify normal versus abnormal functions: CN I: To verify the client is able to distinguish and identify odors with each nostril. CN II: To verify the client has normal visual acuity, visual fields, and a normal fundus or optic disk. CN III: Checks for normal pupil reactions, cardinal fields of gaze, and eyelid elevation. CN IV: Checks for normal extraocular movement. CN V: Checks for strength and function of temporalis and masseter muscles, trigeminal nerve sensation, including light pain, light touch, temperature, and corneal reflex. CN VI: Checks for normal extraocular movements, cardinal fields of gaze. CN VII: Checks facial movements (frown, raise eyebrows) symmetrical (no palsy), and tearing. CN VIII: Checks for normal hearing, Weber and Rinne tests. Checks vertigo, nystagmus, and good equilibrium. CN IX and CN X: Checks for uvula rise midline, speech clear, swallow, taste in posterior third of tongue. Gag present. CN XI: Checks for shoulders, trapezius, and sternocleidomastoid muscle movements. CN XII: Checks for clarity of speech and tongue movements.

continues

Action	Rationale
96. Evaluate the client's mental status. Check level of consciousness, orientation to person, time, place, general appearance, behavior, affect, speech, content, memory, logic, and abstract reasoning (describe proverb), judgment, spatial perception (copy figures, identify familiar sounds, identify right versus left body parts). Mentally summarize the mental status from earlier observations during the examination.	**96.** Identifies normal versus abnormal functions. Check that the client is awake, alert, and oriented to time and place, and exhibits appropriate behavior. Look for abnormal findings of drowsiness, lethargic, stuporous, comatose, or disoriented behaviors.
97. Examine cerebellar status: Conduct a finger-to-nose test (have the client use the index finger to touch your finger, held 18 inches away from the client, then have client touch nose). Have client repeat this movement, gradually increasing the speed. Observe the client's ability to cross the midline. Look for tremor, overshoot, and undershoot. Repeat with the other hand. Conduct a rapid alternating hand movements (RAHM) and note if the client exhibits smooth pronation-supination with increasingly rapid speed. Have the client touch fingers-to-thumb, and note whether he or she can touch thumb to each of the fingers of the same hand in rapid succession from index to fifth finger and back. Note that ability depends on age. Have the client touch heel-to-shin, foot taping RAHM, and foot "figure 8" movement tests. Determine whether the client can run heel down the shin of the opposite leg. Look for smooth rapid ankle extensions and rotation.	**97.** Confirms health and identifies signs and symptoms of illness or disease. Confirms cerebellar status by evaluating coordination, balance, and checking for smooth and harmonious movement.
98. Assist the client to a standing position.	**98.** Prepares the client for remainder of examination.
99. Inspect and/or palpate posture, weight-bearing and standing spine alignment, spinous processes, paravertebral muscles, and ROM (flexion, lateral bending, rotation, hyperextension). Perform a Romberg test. Have the client balance on one foot for 10 seconds. Repeat heel-to-shin test, and have client hop on each foot and do shallow knee bends.	**99.** Determines that shoulders and hips are level, scapulae and iliac crests are symmetric, toes and knees point forward, extremities are proportionate. Confirms that head spinous processes and gluteal cleft are in alignment. Checks for scoliosis, kyphosis, lordosis, or contractures.
100. Assess mobility by having the client perform a casual gait, toe and heel walk, tandem walk (forward and backward), step right, step left, walk briskly, and do jumping jacks (if client's condition permits).	**100.** Assesses cerebellar and developmental status as well as musculoskeletal structure and function. Checks that the posture and gait are erect, balanced, smooth, tandem for age with usually less than 1 to 2 inches between heel to toe steps. Estimates exercise tolerance for age and diagnosis.
101. Recheck heart and respiratory sounds after exercising. Compare with resting rates.	**101.** Checks for flow murmurs, cardiac rate, and recovery time.
102. Compare the client's status to age-appropriate standards for activities of daily living (ADLs), gross and fine motor function, speech and language, and personal-social interaction.	**102.** Confirms health and identifies signs and symptoms of illness or disease.

continues

Action	Rationale
Neurologic Examination *continued*	
103. Evaluate for psychiatric symptoms, including disturbed affect, aversive eye contact, symptoms of depression or anxiety, disrupted or confused thought processes, indications of delusional thoughts, and indications of suicidal thoughts.	103. Checks that verbal and nonverbal behavior is consistent and congruent, that there is no evidence of delusions, hallucinations, or suicidal ideations.

▶ REAL WORLD ANECDOTES

A nurse was performing a routine physical assessment on a client with chronic pulmonary disease, listening to lung sounds. She heard a rapid, irregular heartbeat as well. She reported her findings to the nurse practitioner, who ordered follow-up diagnostic tests. The client was later diagnosed with multifocal atrial tachycardia.

▶ EVALUATION

- Client relates history in logical, sequential manner. Questions are answered appropriately and without distraction. Client is able to easily and accurately recall history and facts.
- Explain findings to client within nurse's scope of practice and function.
- Formulate problem list reflecting findings.
- Generate intervention plan.

▶ DOCUMENTATION

Nurses' Notes

- All assessments and procedures must be completely documented according to institutional policy.
- Record under objective portion of assessment.
- Record in order of the category groupings used in the assessment.
- Record date and time of assessment.
- Identify information and historian.
- Indicate ability of client to assist with assessment.
- Record chief concern.
- List positive findings first, followed by significant negative findings, for each body system or body part examined.
- Record detailed description of assessment related to chief concern (need for visit).
- Record detailed description of abnormalities (positive findings).
- Record description of negative findings.

▶ CRITICAL THINKING SKILL

Introduction

The client knows his or her own body. Often, the client is the expert consultant.

Possible Scenario

A nurse was doing a routine physical exam. While the nurse was concentrating on the priorities in the exam, the client mentioned that he could feel a lump in his hamstring. He wondered if he had injured it jogging. Because the nurse was examining the client's lungs, he listened to the client's complaint, made a noncommittal comment, and continued with his assessment. The client did not bring up his concerns again.

Possible Outcome

One month later, this client was diagnosed with a rhabdomyosarcoma, a highly malignant soft tissue cancer most often seen in children. He underwent surgery, chemotherapy, and radiation, and continues to be evaluated for recurrence every 3 months.

Prevention

This man's survival was directly related to the stage of the disease at diagnosis. This cancer is often found when the client or a parent mentions feeling a lump. The nurse missed the abnormal finding, because he did not follow up on the client's comment. The nurse should have followed up on the complaint by asking for more specifics and history, examining the area carefully, and reporting the findings.

► **VARIATIONS**

Geriatric Variations:

- *Vital signs and measurements must be age-correlated to establish what "normal" is for an elderly client.*
- *Allow extra time for slower movement in an older client.*
- *An elderly client may need a warmer room to feel comfortable.*
- *You will find more "normal variations" in the geriatric population. This is especially true for skin conditions.*
- *History of ADLs needs to be assessed in view of visual, auditory, musculoskeletal, and neurologic findings.*
- *Any client with a change in neurologic function must be evaluated for dementia, depression, Alzheimer's disease, and Parkinson's disease.*
- *Make sure elderly clients can hear and understand what you want them to do when performing the neurologic part of the examination.*

Pediatric Variations:

- *Keep parents within view of the child.*
- *Infants and young children may be more comfortable being examined in a parent's lap. Sit facing the parent with your knees touching theirs to make a "table."*
- *Examine ear, nose, and throat last because the child may react to the invasiveness of the procedures.*
- *Allow the child some play time with your stethoscope or penlight. Clean these items before and after.*
- *Show the child the equipment before using it. Shine the otoscope light in the child's hand.*
- *Blow the air from the pneumatic tube. Sometimes demonstrating the procedure using a toy or doll helps make the child more comfortable.*
- *Give the child simple choices when possible. Do not bribe. Be honest.*
- *Allow children to cry or yell. Do not allow them to kick or bite.*
- *If there are two children to be examined, let them sit side by side and examine each body area on one and then on the other. You can enlist their cooperation by letting one child watch or help with the other child. Keep a careful recording of abnormal findings so you do not mix up who had what finding.*
- *Remember to thank the child for helping, cooperating, or just for coming in.*
- *Ask teens "private" questions by whispering or lowering your voice without drawing undue attention to the topic and without conveying the idea that certain topics should not be discussed with parents. You can act as a role model or help the child discuss "embarrassing" topics with the parents.*
- *Unclothe a child as you proceed with an examination rather than all at once. Shirt off, examine top half. Shirt on and pants off for bottom half. Leave underpants on, if possible.*
- *Examine the genitalia through a leg hole or by pulling the pants down halfway rather than taking off pants all the way. If you need to remove the underpants, let the child stand up on the table and hug a parent for balance while you perform the exam.*
- *Empower the child after the genital exam by asking the child to perform kicking motions of "exercise" while you check hips and knees. Sit the child up as soon as possible. Sit down to check reflexes, so that you are physically lower than the child, if possible.*

Home Care Variations:

- *The examination can be done in a bed, on a couch, on a kitchen table, or even on the floor. Ask the client for suggestions and decide the best location based on the age and flexibility of the client.*
- *Good lighting is more important than an optimum "table" or bed. Consider bringing extra lighting, such as a gooseneck lamp.*

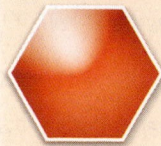

Long-Term Care Variations:

- *Examinations in the long-term care setting are usually performed with the client in bed. Be sure of good lighting and take your own equipment, if needed.*
- *Auditory and visual privacy is usually more of a problem in this setting. Anticipate schedules and be sure the staff and roommates know how much private time you need.*

► **COMMON ERRORS**

Possible Error:

Skipping seemingly insignificant areas and thereby missing significant information.

Prevention:

Allow enough time for the examination. Ask the client to communicate concerns. Have a systematic progression that covers all areas.

Possible Error:

Failing to follow the sequencing of techniques or omitting one of the techniques such as inspection or palpation.

Prevention:

Bring a checklist into the examination and follow it. Before moving on to the next part of the exam, review in your mind if you have covered all the techniques required to assess the current area.

► **NURSING TIPS**

- Vocalize "a" (like apple) versus "ah" (aw) to get higher uvula rise and better pharyngeal visualization.
- Measure chest circumference, divide by one-half, and subtract transverse diameter for anteroposterior (AP) measurement.
- If you detect rhonchi on auscultation, ask client to cough, then listen again. With infants and older children, check lung sounds after performing the gag reflex portion of the pharyngeal exam.
- The heart exam can be a good opportunity to teach the client about the heart. Ask the client to tell you about the heart, where it is located, its size, and its shape. Answer questions about "what a heart attack is" and teach about heart-healthy diet and exercise.
- Follow a specific order when conducting the heart examination: mitral, tricuspid, pulmonic, aortic, ectopic (epigastric and axillary), or vice versa. Remember the order with the mnemonic phrase "Mom Tries Pasta Again Every Evening." You may remember the four heart valves (in reverse order) using the phrase "A Poor Tired Monkey."
- Exercise may make flow murmurs easier to hear.
- Percuss up to lower edge of liver and down to upper edge. Start palpation 2 cm below lower percussed margin and "rock" up and under the rib to look for the edge.

► **SPECIAL CONSIDERATIONS**

- *Observe the client's affect. Provide an open attitude to facilitate receiving information that the client may want to share. A victim of domestic violence may wish to seek help so the examiner should be mindful of potential verbal and nonverbal cues. Clients who abuse alcohol or drugs usually will not readily admit this information; therefore, questions regarding alcohol and drug use can be incorporated into nutrition and medication history. Ask open-ended questions as a quick denial of alcohol or drug use may arrest further questioning. Clients may have health concerns that they wish to discuss. Always ask the reason for contacting a health care provider (routine checkup, s/s of concern) and if there are any further concerns before leaving the room.*
- *Note the client's stress level and realize that it may be a signal for further exam (i.e., cardiovascular).*
- *Breast exams may be performed in a variety of ways. You may use a "roll" method where the hand never leaves the breast. The finger pads roll back and forth across the breast from sternum to axilla and advance about an inch with each forward motion. Some practitioners believe this to be a more accurate approach because no area is missed, as when hands are raised to reposition in other methods. Most lumps are found behind the nipple and in the upper outer quadrant. Special attention should be paid to these areas during the exam.*

Taking a Temperature

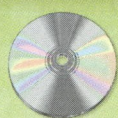

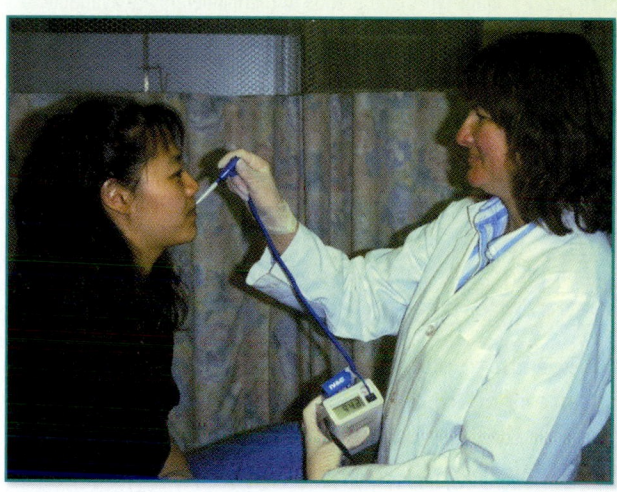

▶ OVERVIEW OF THE SKILL

Body temperature is a vital indicator of health status, and thus a critical parameter in nursing and medical evaluation of clients. Changes in body temperature can be an early indicator of diseases and the disease process. The efficacy of treatments can be evaluated by changes in temperature. Heat production increases with activity; however, considering the variation in internal heat production and the external environment, variations of the body's temperature maintain narrow limits. Temperature varies with age and the locations of assessment, that is, oral, rectal, or anxcillary (Table 1-2-1). When heat production exceeds heat loss, body temperature increases above the normal range, leading to pyrexia (fever). Pyrexia can be the result of an inflammatory response, a loss of body fluid, or prolonged exposure to high temperatures. Clients are stressed by their presenting conditions and further stressed by the hospital environment, thus more susceptible to nosocomial infections and elevated temperatures. Heat transfer occurs by radiation, conduction, convection, and evaporation. The body passively controls temperature as well as by neural feedback through sensors in the hypothalamus. When clients are exposed to temperatures lower than normal for a prolonged length of time, hypothermia occurs. This can be the result of immersion in cold water or exposure to the frigid weather. Injury to the hypothalamus can lead to the inability to regulate temperature. Accurate monitoring and recording of a client's temperature is essential for diagnosis, treatment, and continued monitoring of the client.

▶ ASSESSMENT

1. Assess body temperature for changes when exposed to pyrogens (endogenous or exogenous substances that cause fever) or to extreme hot or cold external environments **because such environments may indicate the cause of an infection**.
2. Assess the client for the most appropriate site to check temperature **to obtain an accurate reading**.
3. Confirm that the client has not consumed hot or cold food or beverage nor smoked for 15 to 30 minutes before the measurement **because these activities may alter the oral reading**. Confirm normal range of temperature for client.
4. Assess for mouth breathing and tachypnea **because both can cause an inaccurate oral reading**.
5. Assess for oral lesion, especially herpetic lesions **because herpes viruses are extremely contagious and require implementation of Standard Precautions of the Centers for Disease Control and Prevention. Clients with herpetic lesions should have their own glass thermometer or disposable thermometer to prevent transmission to others.**

▶ **DIAGNOSIS**

Ineffective thermoregulation. Temperature fluctuates between hypothermia and hyperthermia.

Ineffective Health Maintenance. The client may have increased risk of exposure to pyrogens (surgery, medical procedure, injury, or illness).

Risk for Infection. The client may have signs or symptoms of infection.

Hypothermia

Hyperthermia

Ineffective Thermoregulation

Deficient Fluid Volume

▶ **PLANNING**

Expected Outcomes:

1. An accurate temperature reading will be obtained.
2. The client will verbalize understanding of the reason for the procedure.

Equipment Needed (see Figure 1-2-1):

• Thermometer (one of the following)

—Electronic thermometer with disposable protective sheath

—Tympanic membrane thermometer with probe cover

—Disposable, single-use chemical strip thermometer

—Glass (mercury-free): oral or rectal at client's bedside usually color coded to avoid cross use.

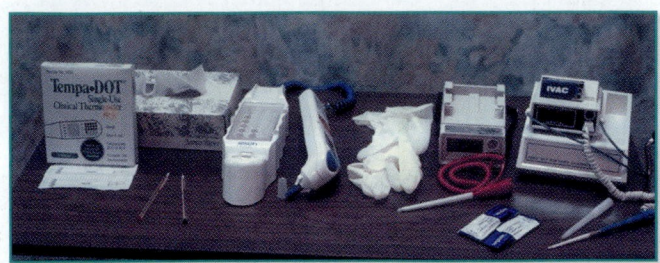

Figure 1-2-1 Many types and brands of thermometers are available to assess temperature.

• Lubricant for rectal and glass thermometer
• Two pairs of nonsterile gloves
• Tissues

▶ **CLIENT EDUCATION NEEDED:**

1. Explain to client why an accurate body temperature is needed.
2. Describe the equipment to the client and explain what to expect during the procedure.
3. Answer any questions and/or fears the client may have regarding the procedure.

Estimated time to complete the skill:
5–10 minutes

▶ **DELEGATION TIPS**

The skill of temperature measurement often is delegated to ancillary personnel; however, the nurse retains responsibility for knowledge of the client's temperature and appropriate actions. The expectation is that ancillary personnel will have documented instruction and competency validation of their ability to:

• Select the correct route for measurement of the temperature
• Correctly position the client for measurement
• Correctly perform the measurement according to established guidelines and record on the appropriate flow sheet (clinical record)
• Recognize and report abnormal findings to the nurse

IMPLEMENTATION—Action/Rationale

Action	Rationale
1. Review medical record for baseline data and factors that influence vital signs.	1. Establishes parameters for client's normal measurements, provides direction in device selection, and helps determine site to use for measurement. Vital signs are measured in the order of temperature, pulse, and respiration (TPR) and blood pressure (BP), usually without interruptions, to provide the nurse with an objective clinical database to direct decision making.
2. Explain to the client that vital signs will be assessed. Encourage the client to remain still and refrain from drinking, eating, and smoking, and to avoid mouth breathing, if possible.	2. Encourages participation, allays anxiety, and ensures accurate measurements. Cold or hot liquids and smoking alter circulation and body temperature. Mouth breathing can alter temperature.
3. Assess client's toileting needs and proceed as appropriate.	3. Prevents interruptions during measurements, communicates caring, and promotes client comfort.
4. Gather equipment.	4. Facilitates organized assessment and measurement.
5. Provide for privacy.	5. Decreases embarrassment.
6. Wash hands and apply gloves when appropriate.	6. Hands are washed before and after every contact with a client to reduce the transmission of microorganisms. Gloves are worn to avoid contact with bodily secretions and to reduce transmission of microorganisms.

Oral Temperature: Electronic Thermometer

Action	Rationale
7. Repeat Actions 1 to 6.	7. See Rationales 1 to 6.
8. Place disposable protective sheath over probe (see Figure 1-2-2).	8. Reduces transmission of microorganisms.
9. Grasp top of the probe's stem. Avoid placing pressure on the ejection button.	9. Pressure on the ejection button releases the sheath from the probe.
10. Place tip of thermometer under the client's tongue and along the gumline to the posterior sublingual pocket lateral to center of lower jaw (see Figure 1-2-3).	10. Sublingual pocket contains superficial blood vessels.
11. Instruct client to keep mouth closed around thermometer.	11. Maintains thermometer in proper place and decreases amount of time required for an accurate reading.
12. Thermometer will signal (beep) when a constant temperature registers (see Figure 1-2-4).	12. Signal indicates final temperature reading.

continues

Action	Rationale

Oral Temperature: Electronic Thermometer *continued*

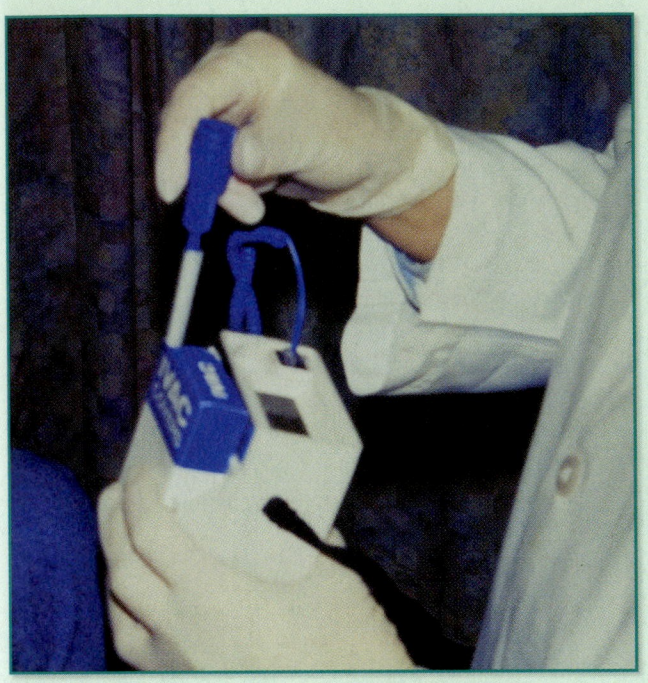

Figure 1-2-2 Place disposable sheath over probe.

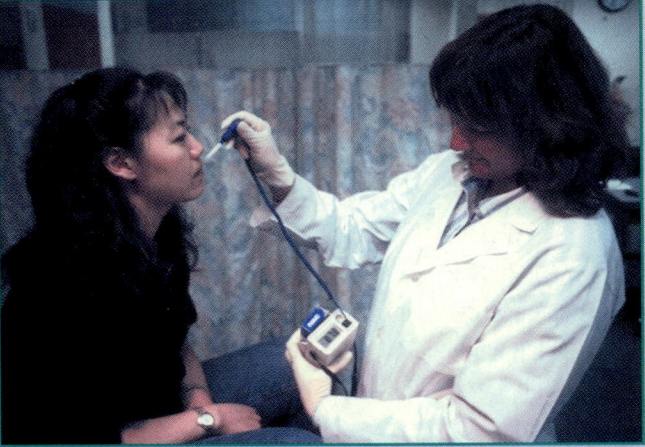

Figure 1-2-3 Place probe tip in the posterior sublingual pocket.

13. Read measurement on digital display of electronic thermometer. Push ejection button to discard disposable sheath into receptacle and return probe to storage well.

13. Reduces transmission of microorganisms. Ensures that the electronic system is ready for next use.

14. Inform client of temperature reading.

14. Promotes client's participation in care.

15. Remove gloves and wash hands.

15. Reduces transmission of microorganisms.

16. Record reading according to institution policies.

16. Accurate documentation by site allows for comparison of data.

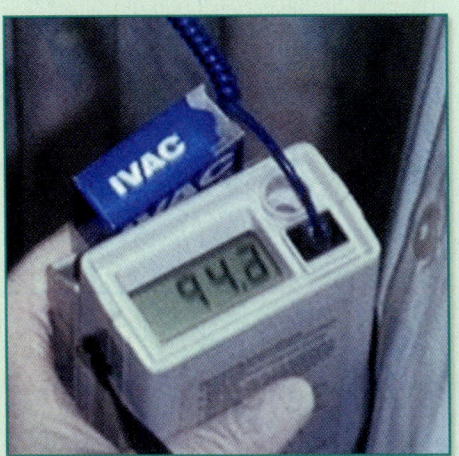

Figure 1-2-4 Listen for audible beep signal when temperature registers.

continues

Action	Rationale
17. Return electronic thermometer unit to charging base.	17. Ensures charging base is plugged into electrical outlet and ready for next use.
18. Wash hands.	18. Reduces transmission of microorganisms.

Tympanic Temperature: Infrared Thermometer

Action	Rationale
19. Repeat Actions 1 to 6.	19. See Rationales 1 to 6.
20. Position client in Sims' or sitting position.	20. Promotes access to client's ear.
21. Remove probe from container and attach probe cover to tympanic thermometer unit (see Figure 1-2-5).	21. Prevents contamination.
22. Turn client's head to one side. For an adult, pull pinna upward and back; for a child, pull down and back. Gently insert probe with firm pressure into ear canal (see Figure 1-2-6).	22. Provides access to ear canal. Gentle insertion prevents trauma to external canal. Firm pressure is needed to ensure probe will record an accurate temperature.
23. Remove probe after the reading is displayed on digital unit (usually 2 seconds).	23. Reading is displayed within seconds.
24. Remove probe cover and replace in storage container.	24. Protects damage to the reusable probe.
25. Return tympanic thermometer to storage unit.	25. Recharges batteries of unit for future use.
26. Record reading according to institution policy.	26. Promotes accurate documentation for data comparsion.
27. Wash hands.	27. Reduces transmission of microorganisms.

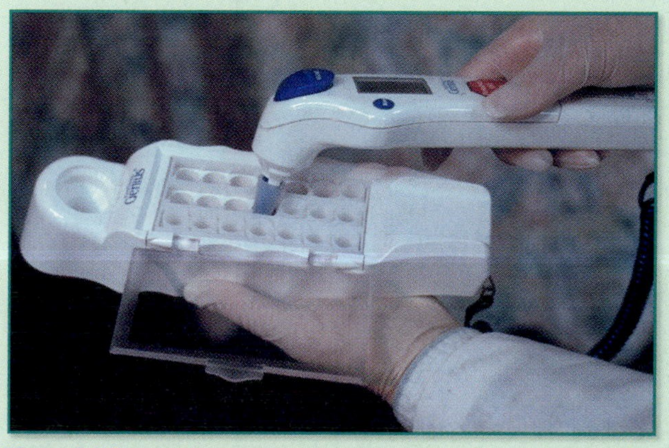

Figure 1-2-5 Attach disposable probe cover to unit.

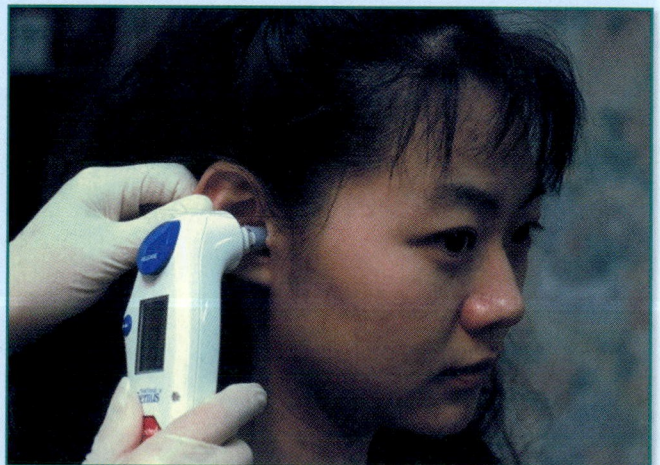

Figure 1-2-6 Insert temperature probe into ear canal.

continues

Action	Rationale
Using a "Tempa-Dot"	
28. Repeat Actions 1 to 6.	28. See Rationales 1 to 6.
29. Position the client in a sitting or lying position.	29. Promotes client's comfort, and promotes site access for all measurement.
30. Prepare Tempa-Dot according to directions (see Figure 1-2-7). • Oral measurement: Place Tempa-Dot under tongue as far back as possible. Have client press tongue down on thermometer and keep mouth closed for 60 seconds. Remove thermometer, read the last blue dot; ignore any skipped dot. • Axillary measurement: Place thermometer high in the armpit, vertical to the body, with dots against the torso. Lower client's arm to hold thermometer in place. Remove thermometer after 3 minutes.	30. Promotes accurate measurement and client safety.
31. Record temperature, indicate the method used, and discard the thermometer.	31. Nursing documentation, practice clean technique.
32. Wash hands.	32. Reduces transmission of microorganisms.
33. Repeat Actions 1 to 6.	33. See Rationales 1 to 6.
34. Position the client in a sitting or lying position with the head of the bed elevated from 45 degrees to 60 degrees for measurement of all vital signs except those designated otherwise.	34. Promotes comfort, and improves site access for all measurements. Activity and movement can elevate heart and respiratory rates.
Oral Temperature: Glass Thermometer (not commonly used)	
35. Repeat steps 1 to 6, then select correct color tip of thermometer from client's bedside container (see Figure 1-2-8).	35. Identifies correct device; a blue tip usually denotes an oral thermometer.

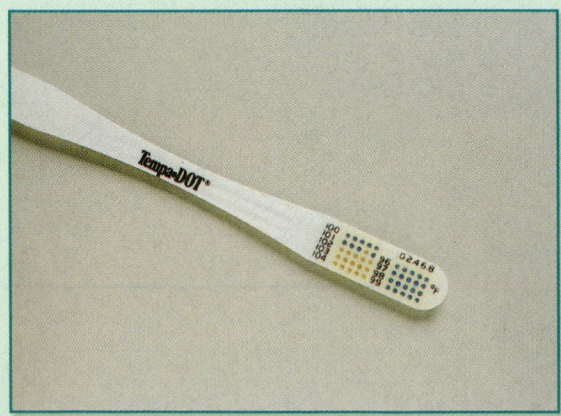

Figure 1-2-7   "Tempa-Dot" single-use disposable thermometer.

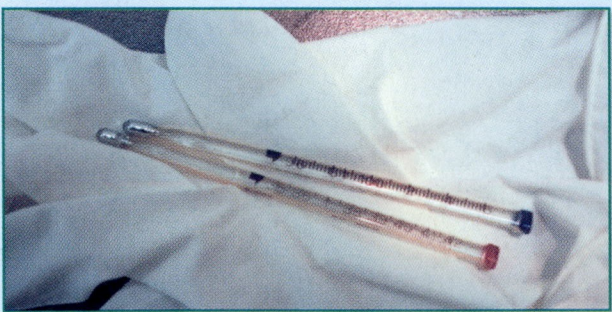

Figure 1-2-8   Oral (blue tip) and rectal (red tip) glass thermometers.

continues

Action	Rationale
36. Remove thermometer from storage container, hold at end away from bulb and cleanse under cool water.	**36.** Cleansing removes disinfectant, which can irritate oral mucosa. Cool water prevents expansion of the colored solution/mercury. Touching the bulb will heat the solution and cause an inaccurate reading.
37. Use a tissue to dry thermometer from bulb's end toward fingertips.	**37.** Wipe from area of least contamination to most contaminated area.
38. Read thermometer by locating colored solution or mercury level. It should read 35.5°C (96°F).	**38.** Thermometer must be below normal body temperature to ensure an accurate reading.
39. If thermometer is not below normal body temperature reading, grasp thermometer with thumb and forefinger and shake vigorously by snapping the wrist in a downward motion to move mercury to a level below normal.	**39.** Shaking briskly lowers level of mercury in column. Because glass thermometers break easily, make sure that nothing in the environment comes in contact with the thermometer when shaking it.
40. Place thermometer in client's mouth under the tongue and along the gumline to the posterior sublingual pocket. Instruct client to hold lips closed (see Figure 1-2-9).	**40.** Ensures contact with large blood vessels under the tongue. Prevents environmental air from coming in contact with the bulb.
41. Leave in place as specified by institution policy, usually 3 to 5 minutes.	**41.** Thermometer must stay in place long enough to ensure an accurate reading.
42. Remove thermometer and wipe with a tissue away from fingers toward the bulb's end (see Figure 1-2-10).	**42.** Mucus on thermometer may interfere with the effectiveness of the disinfectant solution. Wipe from area of least contamination to most contaminated area.
43. Read at eye level and rotate slowly until mercury level is visualized.	**43.** Ensures an accurate reading.
44. Shake thermometer down, cleanse glass thermometer with soapy water, rinse under cold water, and return to storage container.	**44.** Mechanical cleansing removes secretions that promote growth of microorganisms. Hot water may cause coagulation of secretions and cause expansion of mercury in the thermometer.

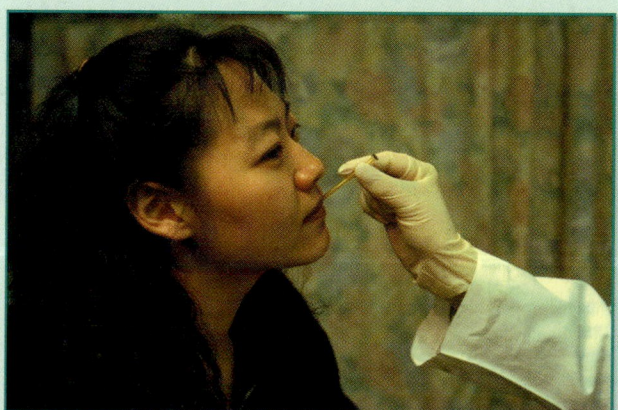

Figure 1-2-9 Place bulb of thermometer in the posterior sublingual pocket. Have client close his or her lips around thermometer.

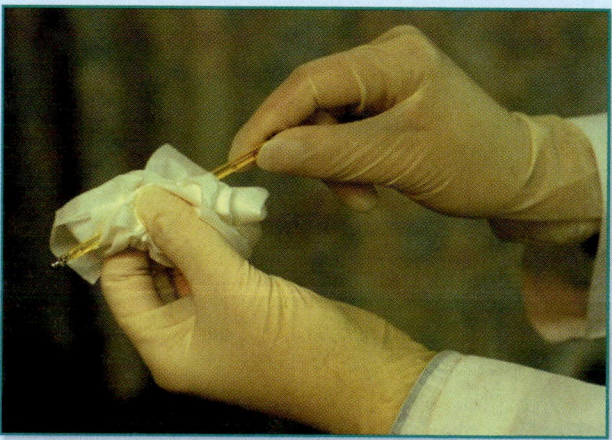

Figure 1-2-10 Wipe the thermometer with a tissue from fingertips to bulb end.

continues

Action	Rationale

Oral Temperature: Glass Thermometer
continued

45. Remove and dispose of gloves in receptacle. Wash hands.

46. Record reading according to institution policy.

47. Wash hands.

Rectal Temperature

48. Repeat Actions 1 to 6.

49. Place client in the Sims' position with upper knee flexed. Adjust sheet to expose only anal area.

50. Place tissues in easy reach. Apply gloves.

51. Prepare the thermometer.

52. Lubricate tip of rectal thermometer or probe (a rectal thermometer usually has a red tip or cap).

53. With dominant hand, grasp thermometer. With other hand, separate buttocks to expose anus (see Figure 1-2-11).

54. Instruct the client to take a deep breath. Insert the thermometer or probe gently into anus: infant, 1.2 cm (0.5 inches); adult, 3.5 cm (1.5 inches). If resistance is felt, do not force insertion.

55. Hold in place for 2 minutes.

56. Wipe off secretions on the glass thermometer with a tissue. Dispose of tissue in a receptacle.

57. Read measurement and inform the client of the temperature reading.

45. Reduces transmission of microorganisms.

46. Accurate documentation by site allows for comparison of data.

47. Reduces transmission of microorganisms.

48. See Rationales 1 to 6.

49. Proper positioning ensures visualization of anus. Flexing knee relaxes muscles for ease of insertion.

50. Tissue is needed to wipe anus after device is removed.

51. Ensures a smooth procedure and an accurate reading.

52. Promotes ease of insertion of thermometer or probe.

53. Aids in visualization of anus.

54. Relaxes anal sphincter. Gentle insertion decreases discomfort to client and prevents trauma to mucous membranes.

55. Prevents trauma to mucosa and breakage of glass thermometer.

56. Removes secretions and fecal material for visualization of mercury level. Prevents transmission of microorganisms.

57. Promotes client's participation in care.

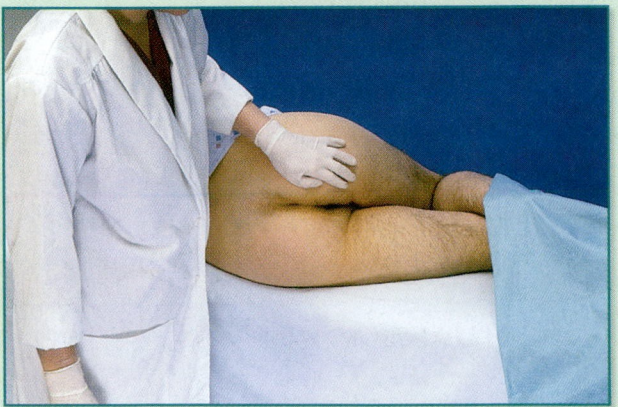

Figure 1-2-11   Preparation for the insertion of a rectal thermometer.

continues

Action	Rationale
58. While holding glass thermometer in one hand, use other hand to wipe anal area with tissue to remove lubricant or feces. Dispose of soiled tissue. Cover client.	58. Prevents contamination of clean objects with soiled thermometer, decreases skin irritation, and promotes client comfort. Prevents embarrassment.
59. Cleanse thermometer.	59. Reduces transmission of microorganisms.
60. Remove and dispose of gloves in receptacle. Wash hands.	60. Reduces transmission of microorganisms.
61. Record reading according to institution policy.	61. Accurate documentation by site allows for comparison of data.

Axillary Temperature

Action	Rationale
62. Repeat Actions 1 to 6.	62. See Rationales 1 to 6.
63. Remove client's arm and shoulder from one sleeve of gown. Avoid exposing chest.	63. Exposes axillary area.
64. Make sure axillary skin is dry; if necessary, pat dry.	64. Removes moisture and prevents a false low reading.
65. Prepare thermometer.	65. Ensures accurate use of thermometer.
66. Place thermometer or probe into center of axilla. Fold the client's upper arm straight down, and place arm across the client's chest.	66. Puts device in contact with axillary blood supply. Maintains the device in proper position.
67. Leave glass thermometer in place as specified by institution policy (usually 6 to 8 minutes). Leave an electronic thermometer in place until signal is heard.	67. Device must stay in place long enough to ensure an accurate reading. Signal indicates final temperature reading.
68. Remove and read thermometer.	68. Allows accurate reading of temperature.
69. Inform client of temperature reading.	69. Promotes client's participation in care.
70. Cleanse glass thermometer. Shake down thermometer, cleanse glass thermometer with soapy water, rinse under cold water, and return to storage container.	70. Prevents transmission of microorganisms and breakage of glass thermometer.
71. Assist the client with replacing the gown.	71. Promotes comfort.
72. Record reading according to institution policy.	72. Promotes accurate documentation for data comparison.
73. Wash hands.	73. Reduces transmission of microorganisms.

Disposable (Chemical Strip) Thermometer

Action	Rationale
74. Repeat Actions 1 to 6.	74. See Rationales 1 to 6.
75. Apply tape to appropriate skin area, usually forehead.	75. Tape must be in direct contact with the client's skin.
76. Observe tape for color changes.	76. Color indicates temperature reading (refer to the manufacturer's instructions).
77. Record reading and indicate method.	77. Promotes accurate documentation for data comparison.
78. Wash hands.	78. Reduces transmission of microorganisms.

continues

Action	Rationale

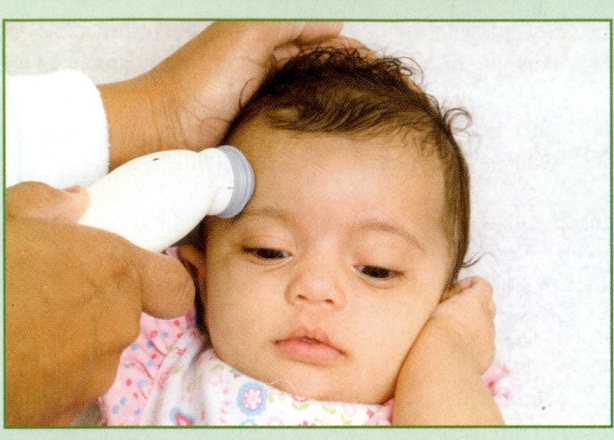

Figure 1-2-12   An arterial temporal scan thermometer.

Arterial Temporal Scan Thermometer (see Figure 1-2-12)

79. Repeat Actions 1 to 6.

79. See Rationales 1 to 6

80. Locate the client's exposed temporal artery. If the client has been lying on the side of the head, use the exposed artery.

80. Blood flow through the artery is the same temperature as blood flowing from the heart and, hence, is the best determinate of core body temperature. The temporal artery is only 2 mm beneath the skin. If the artery has been covered by a hat or the client has been lying on the side examined, heat will be retained in the skin.

81. Stroke the scanner head of the thermometer gently over the temporal artery.

81. Arterial temperature is fast and only requires a quick, gentle scan. A single scan takes 1,000 readings per second, thereby ensuring accuracy. Direct contact with the skin is needed for an accurate reading.

82. Record reading and indicate method.

82. Promotes accurate documentation.

83. Wash hands.

83. Reduces transmission of microorganisms.

▶ REAL WORLD ANECDOTES

The visiting nurse is making a routine visit to John, a diabetic client. John is a morbidly obese client with diabetic leg ulcers. The physician's orders are for routine wet-to-dry dressing changes and blood-glucose monitoring. While changing the dressing, the nurse notes that John says he is cold, yet his skin feels warm and looks flushed. His blood glucose is 310 mg/dL. There are no routine vital signs ordered, but the nurse feels that John may be seriously ill. John is chilling, and his teeth are chattering.

A glass thermometer is available, but the nurse feels John will not be able to hold it in his mouth firmly enough to get an accurate reading. Because he is obese, a rectal temperature would be difficult and time consuming. The nurse chooses to take an axillary temperature. The reading is 104°F. The nurse notifies John's doctor and John is admitted to the hospital with sepsis. In this case, "routine vital signs" became a critical assessment tool.

▶ EVALUATION

• Establish client's baseline temperature.
• Compare temperature with the client's baseline temperature.
• Evaluate the client's condition for trauma caused by the instrument.

▶ DOCUMENTATION

Vital Signs Flow Sheet

• Record the temperature measurement and site.

• Plot the temperature on a graph to identify patterns, or sudden increases and decreases (a condition known as spiking).

Medication Administration Record

• Record doses of antipyretic (fever-reducing) medications and temperature reading.

Nurses' Notes

• Record response to antipyretic medications.

▶ VARIATIONS

Geriatric Variations:

• *Geriatric clients are more likely to be confused and unable to follow directions. It is especially important to be attentive and give clear, concise instructions when taking an oral temperature.*
• *Elderly clients may be more comfortable lying on their side with legs slightly flexed when taking a rectal temperature. Keep one hand on the thermometer and one hand on the client's hip so that you can detect if he or she starts to roll over. Place a pillow at the client's back for extra support, if needed.*
• *Baseline temperatures of elderly clients may be below the normal range; therefore, increases should be compared with baseline.*

Pediatric Variations:

• *Premature infants often cannot maintain a stable temperature.*
• *Infants and children often are not able to understand the nurse's instructions.*
• *Infants and children are often fearful of medical personnel and of the possibility of painful procedures. This may lead them to refuse to cooperate or to be combative.*
• *Infants and children may lie supine with knees flexed toward the abdomen as the nurse inserts the thermometer (see Figure 1-2-13).*
• *It may be more accurate to measure the pulse and respirations before the temperature if the child becomes agitated during temperature taking.*
• *Glass thermometers are not the best choice for use in young children. Tympanic or chemical strip thermometers are much less invasive and less anxiety producing.*
• *When using the chemical strip thermometer, allow the child to place the strip and help you time the strip by holding your watch. Clean your watch before and after.*
• *Use thermal scanners with children.*

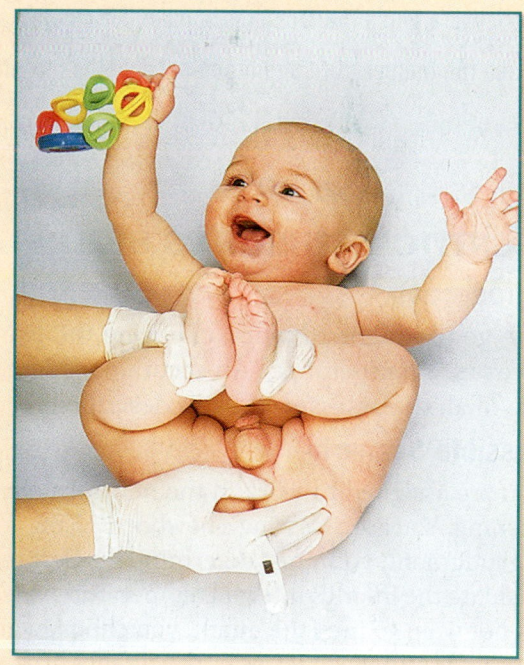

Figure 1-2-13   Taking a rectal temperature with infant in supine position.

continues

▶ **VARIATIONS** *(continued)*

Home Care Variations:
- *Working equipment may not be available in the home care setting. The nurse should come prepared with working equipment, including a thermometer appropriate to the client.*
- *The temperature and ventilation of the room may affect the client's temperature.*
- *Remember to bring the best type of thermometer for the client with you for your home health visit.*

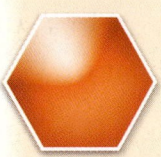

Long-Term Care Variation:
- *Long-term care clients more often have physical limitations that must be considered when choosing the route to use in measuring the internal temperature. When considering the route in a long-term care client, consider the possibility of a stoma where the rectum has been surgically closed or perhaps severe contractures that would make client positioning and cooperation difficult and painful.*

▶ **COMMON ERRORS**

Possible Error:

You are in a hurry and left the oral thermometer in the client's mouth for only 2 minutes.

Prevention:

Use the equipment and its signals such as the beep of the electronic thermometer. Know the recommended length of time to leave a glass thermometer in place for an oral, axillary, and rectal temperature.

Take the temperature again and observe the recommended time.

▶ **CRITICAL THINKING SKILL**

Introduction

Use good judgment when choosing the site used to measure a temperature. An accurate reading requires use of all the assessment skills described.

Possible Scenario

You are assigned to work in the newborn nursery this evening. You are assessing a newborn. Using your nursing judgment, you must determine the best method to evaluate the infant's internal temperature. Because you do not want to hurt the infant, you choose a glass thermometer and place it under the infant's arm.

Possible Outcome

Because this is the first temperature reading done on this client, it is an inaccurately low reading and fails to detect a problem. It also creates an incorrect baseline for future comparisons.

Prevention

You should realize that there are a number of factors that must enter into this decision. An oral temperature is contraindicated in newborns because they cannot follow instructions to keep their mouths closed and not bite the thermometer. An axillary temperature would be safe but would yield the least accurate reading. A tympanic reading would be less invasive than the rectal temperature and more comfortable for the infant, but it is less accurate in infants. The rectal temperature is the preferred method for assessing newborn temperatures. Not only is it the most accurate method available to nurses, but it also gives the nurse an opportunity to assess the structure and patency of the infant's anus, an important part of the newborn physical exam. Therefore, you should use the rectal thermometer to obtain an accurate reading.

► NURSING TIPS

- For the best comparison of the client's longitudinal temperature readings, the temperature should be taken at the same time every day using the same method.
- A temporal scan for body temperature captures the naturally emitted heat from the skin over the temporal artery and is a very accurate means of taking a noninvasive comfortable body temperature. Measure only the side of the head that is exposed, because any covering or pillows would cause a falsely high temperature.
- After giving antipyretic medication to a client, a temperature measurement should be taken 30 minutes after the intervention and then every 2 to 4 hours. Nursing intervention policy may vary across institutions.
- Oral, rectal, and tympanic temperature measurements are higher than axillary measurements because the measuring device is in contact with the mucous membrane.
- Rectal measurements are higher than oral measurements because of the seal created by the anal sphincter, which decreases contact with environmental influences.
- Avoid rinsing a glass thermometer in hot water. Hot water can cause the thermometer to expand and break.
- The client should not insert a rectal thermometer without assistance. Inappropriate application can cause tissue trauma.
- Continuous temperature monitoring can be done using a rectal probe, or a special urinary catheter.
- When checking the chart for trends in temperature, make sure the same measurement device was used. As noted in Table 1-2-1, the normal range varies according to the device used.

Table 1-2-1 Advantages and Disadvantages of Four Routes for Body Temperature Measurement

ROUTE	NORMAL RANGE	ADVANTAGES	DISADVANTAGES
ORAL			
Average 37.0° C or 98.6° F	36.0° to 38.0° C 96.8° to 100.4° F	Convenient; accessible	Safety: Glass thermometers with colored solution/mercury can be bitten and broken, causing client injury. Clients need to be alert and cooperative and cognitively capable of following instructions for safe use. Physical abilities: Clients need to be able to breathe through the nose and be without oral pathology or recent oral surgery; route not applicable for comatose or confused clients. Accuracy: Oxygen therapy by mask or ingestion of hot or cold drinks immediately before oral temperature measurement, affects accuracy of the reading.
RECTAL			
Average 0.7° C or 0.4° F higher than oral	36.7° to 38.7° C 100.4° to 100.8° F	Considered most accurate	Safety: Contraindicated following rectal surgery. Risk of rectal Valsalva's perforation in children less than 2 years of age. Risk of stimulating Valsalva's maneuver in cardiac clients. Physical aspects: Invasive and uncomfortable.

continues

Table 1-2-1 (continued)	Advantages and Disadvantages of Four Routes for Body Temperature Measurement		
ROUTE	NORMAL RANGE	ADVANTAGES	DISADVANTAGES
AXILLARY Average 0.6° C or 1° F lower than oral	35.4° to 37.4° C 95.8° to 99.4° F	Safe; noninvasive	Accuracy: Glass thermometer must be left in place for 5 minutes to obtain accurate measurement. Placement and position of thermometer tip affect reading.
TYMPANIC Calibrated to oral or rectal scales	See oral or rectal	Convenient; fast; safe; noninvasive. Does not require contact with any mucous membrane.	Accuracy: Research is inconclusive as to accuracy of readings and correlations with other body temperature measurements. Technique affects reading. Tympanic membrane is thought to reflect the core temperature.

▶ SPECIAL CONSIDERATIONS

- *Mercury thermometers should not be used because mercury is hepatotoxic. If your facility uses colored solution/ mercury thermometers, you must know the policy for management of broken thermometers as well as disposal of thermometers.*
- *If your client has a seizure disorder or is a mouth breather, you should avoid using a glass oral thermometer for temperature measurement.*
- *Taking a rectal temperature should be avoided when a client is receiving medication rectally or when diarrhea is present.*

Taking a Pulse

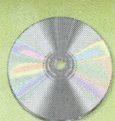

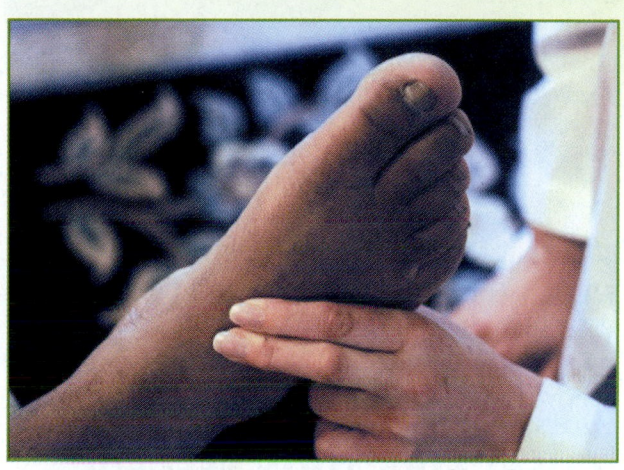

▶ OVERVIEW OF THE SKILL

Pulse assessment is the measurement of pressure pulsation created when the heart contracts and ejects blood into the aorta and, hence, the rest of the arterial vessels. The amplitude of the pulse reflects the stroke volume with each ejection. Assessment of pulse characteristics provides clinical data regarding the heart's pumping action and the adequacy of peripheral artery blood flow. The radial pulse is used most often for basic assessment; however, other site areas are used in total assessment and when specific areas of circulation are to be determined.

▶ PULSE-TAKING TECHNIQUES

Palpation

- Palpation of a pulse involves the index and middle fingers of one hand. Start with gentle pressure to locate the strongest pulsation, and then use firmer palpation for the counting. When counting, also assess the rhythm and quality of the pulse. Measure the pulse for 30 and 60 seconds, and then multiply the counts if need be to obtain the one-minute reading.

Auscultation

- Auscultation is usually used to assess the apical pulse. The apical pulse is the most accurate pulse, especially when the peripheral pulse is difficult to locate. Auscultation requires the stethoscope. The stethoscope should be equipped with a bell and a diaphragm. The diaphragm side is normally used for low-pitch sound, such as the normal heart sound, bowel sound, or breath sound; the bell side is used for high-pitch sound, such as murmur and abnormal heart sound.

Doppler

- An ultrasonic Doppler device is usually used when the pulse cannot be detected by palpation. The Doppler can detect the peripheral pulses in situations such as cardiopulmonary collapse in obese clients, infants with small arms, or clients with edema in which palpation of the pulse is difficult.
- A vendor-recommended conductive gel should be applied to the skin as a coupling medium for ultrasound transmission. The transmitting device (probe) is then placed over the artery to be assessed. The Doppler is usually equipped with both high- and low-frequency probes. A high-frequency (8- to 10-Hz) probe is usually used on the surface vessel sites. A low-frequency (2- to 3-Hz) probe is often used for deeper sites, such as obstetric assessment.
- The sounds can be amplified and heard through an earpiece or speaker attached to the device, assessing with low volume initially. Tilt the back

of the probe toward the hand at an angle of about 45 degrees. Search the area of the assessed artery and tilt the probe for best Doppler sounds. Adjust the sound volume control to a comfort level for counting.

▶ ASSESSMENT

1. Assess the need to monitor the client's pulse. **Certain diseases or conditions, such as history of heart disease or cardiac dysrhythmias, chest pain, invasive cardiovascular diagnostic tests, infusion of large volume of intravenous fluids, or hemorrhage, can cause an increased risk for alterations in pulse.**
2. Assess the pulse for rate, amplitude, contour, and regularity.
3. Assess for signs and symptoms of cardiovascular alterations, such as dyspnea, chest pain, orthopnea, syncope, palpitations, edema of extremities, cyanosis, or fatigue, **because these signs may indicate deficient cardiac or vascular function.**
4. Assess client for factors that may affect the character of the pulse, such as age, medications, exercise, change in position, or fever. **This enables the nurse to accurately assess for the significance of an alteration in pulse.**
5. Assess for the appropriate site for measuring pulse **so that the pulse will be accurate.**
6. Assess the baseline heart rate and rhythm in the client's chart **to compare it with the current measurement.**
7. Assess circulatory status by using appropriate site (Table 1-3-1) **because pulses may be affected by surgery, medical condition, arterial blood draws, or poor circulation.**

▶ DIAGNOSIS

Decreased Cardiac Output
Ineffective Cardiopulmonary Tissue Perfusion

▶ PLANNING

Expected Outcomes:

1. Pulse rate, quality, rhythm, and volume will be within normal range for the client's age group.
2. The client will be comfortable with the procedure and demonstrate an understanding regarding its importance.

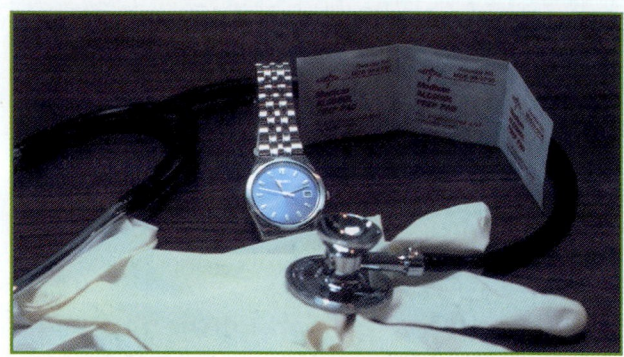

Figure 1-3-1   A watch with a second hand is used to count pulse. Use a stethoscope to assess apical pulse. Gloves and alcohol swabs reduce the transmission of microorganisms.

Equipment Needed (see Figure 1-3-1):

- Watch with a second hand
- Stethoscope
- Alcohol swab
- Gloves

▶ CLIENT EDUCATION NEEDED:

1. Ask the client to relax and sit or lie quietly while you assess the pulse rate.
2. Explain the normal pulse range when informing the client of their pulse rate. This eases the client's concerns regarding whether or not the rate is "normal."
3. If the client is taking any medications that affect pulse rate, this is a good time to review the name and purpose of this medication.
4. If taking a pulse at a site other than radial, explain to the client the reason for using an alternate site.
5. Have the client breathe normally through the nose, especially if taking an apical pulse. Breathing through the nose decreases breath sounds and makes the heart sounds easier to hear.

Estimated time to complete the skill:
5–10 minutes

Table 1-3-1   Pulse Point Assessment

PULSE POINT		ASSESSMENT CRITERIA

SITES OF THE PULSATION MEASUREMENT

SITE	LOCATION	
1. Temporal	Over the temporal bone, lateral to the eye, upper to the ear.	Accessible; used routinely for infants and when radial is inaccessible.
2. Carotid	Bilateral, under the lower jaw, beneath the sternomastoid muscles. Carotid pulse best represents the aortic pulse for its close location to the central circulation. Palpation of the carotid artery on the neck may cause stimulation of the carotid sinus and result in decrease of the pulse rate.	Accessible; used routinely for infants and during shock or cardiac arrest when other peripheral pulses are too weak to palpate; also used to assess cranial circulation.
3. Apical	Left ventricle, fourth to fifth intercostal space, on the midclavicular line.	Used to auscultate heart sounds and assess apical-radial deficit.
4. Brachial	Inner side between the groove of bicep and tricep muscles at the antecubital fossa.	Used in cardiac arrest for infants, to assess lower arm circulation, and to auscultate blood pressure.
5. Radial	On the thumb side, inner aspect of the wrist.	Accessible; used routinely in adults to assess character of peripheral pulse.
6. Ulnar	On the little finger side, outer aspect of the wrist.	Used to assess circulation to ulnar side of hand and to perform the Allen test.
7. Femoral	Below the inguinal ligament, in the anterior medial aspect of the thigh, midway to the anterior-superior iliac spine and symphysis pubis.	Used to assess circulation to legs and during cardiac arrest.
8. Popliteal	Behind the knee. Medial or lateral to the popliteal fossa.	Used to assess circulation to legs and to auscultate leg blood pressure.
9. Posterior Tibial	Inner side of the ankle, between the Achilles tendon and tibia.	Used to assess circulation to feet.
10. Pedal/Dorsal Pedal	Lateral to the extension tendon, from the great toe toward the ankle.	Used to assess circulation to feet.

► DELEGATION TIPS

The radial pulse assessment is often delegated to trained ancillary personnel; however, the nurse is responsible for knowing the results. Assessment of the apical pulse may be delegated to specially prepared staff. The assessment of peripheral circulation is delegated after proper training in the monitoring of peripheral sites for the presence of abnormal color, motion, or sensation in the extremity. The absence of pulses must be immediately reported for further assessment by the nurse, and the nurse is responsible for reviewing the data collected in a timely manner and revalidating the results, if indicated. The institution's policy should clearly indicate the training and validation requirements before the nurse delegates the monitoring of apical pulses and peripheral vascular assessments on stable clients. These tasks should not be delegated if the client is unstable.

IMPLEMENTATION—Action/Rationale

Action	Rationale

Taking a Radial (Wrist) Pulse

1. Wash hands.

2. Inform client of the site(s) at which you will measure pulse.

3. Flex client's elbow and place lower part of arm across chest.

4. Support client's wrist by grasping outer aspect with thumb.

5. Place your index and middle fingers on inner aspect of client's wrist over the radial artery and apply light but firm pressure until pulse is palpated (see Figure 1-3-2).

6. Identify pulse rhythm.

7. Determine pulse volume.

8. Count pulse rate by using second hand on watch (see Figure 1-3-3).
    For a regular rhythm, count number of beats for 30 seconds and multiply by 2.
    For an irregular rhythm, count number of beats for a full minute, noting number of irregular beats.

---

1. Reduces transmission of microorganisms.

2. Encourages participation and allays anxiety.

3. Maintains wrist in full extension and exposes artery for palpation. Placing client's hand over chest will facilitate later respiratory assessment without undue attention to your action. (It is difficult for any person to maintain a normal breathing pattern when someone is observing and measuring.)

4. Stabilizes wrist and allows for pressure to be exerted.

5. Fingertips are sensitive; as a result, they facilitate palpation of pulsating pulse. The nurse may feel his or her own pulse if palpating with the thumb. Applying light pressure prevents occlusion of blood flow and pulsation.

6. Palpate pulse until rhythm is determined. Describe as regular or irregular.

7. Quality of pulse strength is an indication of stroke volume. Describe as normal, weak, strong, or bounding.

8. An irregular rhythm requires a full minute of assessment to identify the number of inefficient cardiac contractions that fail to transmit a pulsation, referred to as a "skipped" or irregular beat.

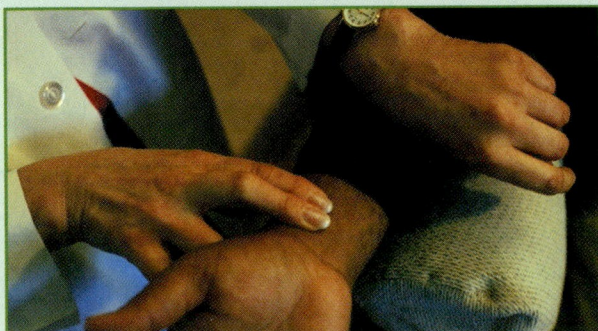

Figure 1-3-2   Place index and middle fingers over radial artery.

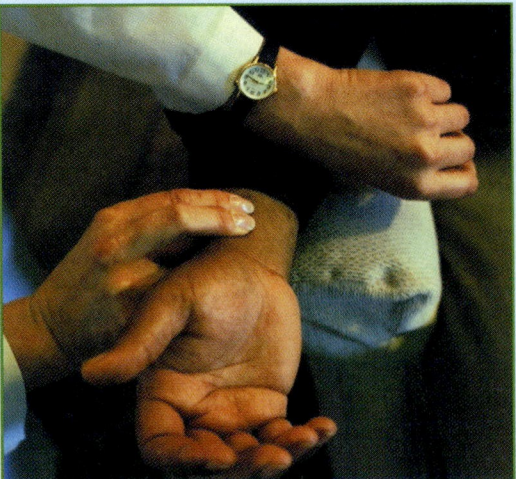

Figure 1-3-3   Count pulse rate for 30 seconds. Multiply by 2.

continues

Action	Rationale
Taking an Apical Pulse	
9. Wash hands.	**9.** Reduces transmission of microorganisms.
10. Raise client's gown to expose sternum and left side of chest.	**10.** Allows access to client's chest for proper placement of stethoscope.
11. Cleanse earpiece and diaphragm of stethoscope with an alcohol swab.	**11.** Decreases transmission of microorganisms from one health care practitioner to another (earpiece) and from one client to another (diaphragm).
12. Put stethoscope around your neck.	**12.** Ensures stethoscope is nearby for frequent use.
13. Locate apex of heart: • With client lying on left side, locate suprasternal notch. • Palpate second intercostal space to left of sternum. • Place index finger in intercostal space, counting downward until fifth intercostal space is located. • Move index finger along fourth intercostal space left of the sternal border and to the fifth intercostal space, left of the midclavicular line to palpate the point of maximal impulse (PMI) (see Figure 1-3-4). • Keep index finger of nondominant hand on the PMI.	**13.** Identification of landmarks facilitates correct placement of the stethoscope at the fifth intercostal space in order to hear point of maximal impulse. Ensures correct placement of stethoscope.
14. Inform client that you are going to listen to his or her heart. Instruct client to remain silent.	**14.** Elicits client support. Stethoscope amplifies noise.
15. With dominant hand, put earpiece of the stethoscope in your ears and grasp diaphragm of the stethoscope in palm of your hand for 5 to 10 seconds.	**15.** Dominant hand facilitates psychomotor dexterity for placement of earpiece with one hand. Heat warms metal or plastic diaphragm and prevents startling client.
16. Place diaphragm of stethoscope over the PMI and auscultate for sounds S_1 and S_2 to hear a "lub-dub" sound (see Figure 1-3-5).	**16.** Movement of blood through the heart valves creates S_1 and S_2 sounds. Listen for a regular rhythm (heartbeats are evenly spaced) before counting.
17. Note regularity of rhythm.	**17.** Establishment of a rhythmic pattern determines length of time to count the heartbeats to ensure accurate measurement.
18. Start to count while looking at second hand of watch. Count the "lub-dub" sound as one beat: • For a regular rhythm, count rate for 30 seconds and multiply by 2. • For an irregular rhythm, count rate for a full minute, noting number of irregular beats.	**18.** Ensures sufficient time to count irregular beats.

continues

Action	Rationale

Taking an Apical Pulse *continued*

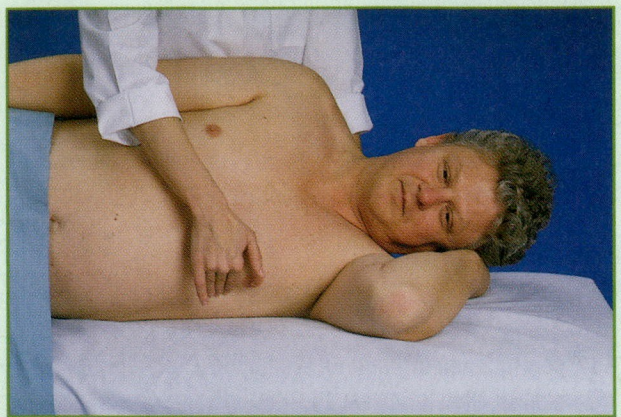

Figure 1-3-4   Palpating the apical pulse.

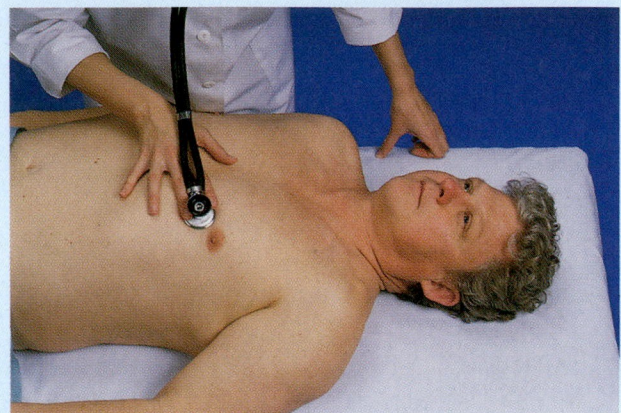

Figure 1-3-5   Place diaphragm of stethoscope over the PMI to hear the heart rate.

19. Share your findings with client.	19. Promotes client participation in care.
20. Record by site the rate, rhythm and, if applicable, the number of irregular beats.	20. The record of rate and characteristics at bedside ensures accurate documentation.
21. Wash hands.	21. Reduces transmission of microorganisms.

▶ REAL WORLD ANECDOTES

A 74-year-old man presents to the emergency room complaining of pain in his chest. While taking routine vital signs, the nurse notes that both his apical and radial pulses are 44 beats per minute. The nurse considers the possibility that heart conductivity problems may be causing this low rate.

The client's ECG on the cardiac monitor appears normal. While the nurse is taking a more complete history, the client states that he is a marathon runner and he takes his pulse rate himself daily as part of his training. The client notes that his pulse rate normally runs quite low. He also states that he just ate a large, spicy meal, possibly an alternative explanation for his chest pain, which needs further assessment. The nurse makes a mental note not to jump to conclusions without a thorough history and physical.

Table 1-3-2 Scales for Measuring Pulse Volume			
3-POINT SCALE		**4-POINT SCALE**	
SCALE	DESCRIPTION OF PULSE	SCALE	DESCRIPTION OF PULSE
0A	Absent	0	Absent
1+	Thready/weak	1+	Thready/weak
2+	Normal	2+	Normal
3+	Bounding	3+	Increased
		4+	Bounding

▶ **EVALUATION**

- Compare client's pulse with baseline rate, amplitude, and rhythm to detect any changes (see Table 1-3-2).
- If pulse is irregular or abnormal, ask another nurse to check the pulse and then report to health care provider.
- Evaluate pulse site (see Table 1-3-1) as required by client's condition and compare bilateral pulses. Example: For clients with poor peripheral circulation in the lower extremities, compare both pedal/dorsal or both posterior tibial pulses.

▶ **DOCUMENTATION**

Nurses' Notes and/or Flow Sheet

Record:

- Pulse rate
- Observations regarding regularity, volume, or rate
- New irregularities in pulse reported to the client's health care provider

▶ **CRITICAL THINKING SKILL**

Introduction

A pulse deficit is a condition in which the apical pulse is greater than the radial pulse rate. A pulse deficit exists when the heart is not ejecting enough blood volume to initiate a peripheral pulse wave. If left untreated, this can lead to serious complications. Check for a pulse deficit if the amplitude of pulsation is not the same with each beat. Check an apical pulse and assess any ECG changes. Because a client may not have a strong stroke volume with each beat, further cardiac assessment is needed.

Possible Scenario

You are taking a radial pulse on a client who was admitted to the coronary care unit. The client's pulse volume is weak and thready. The radial pulse is slow and irregular. You are concerned and take an apical pulse as well. His apical pulse is faster than his radial pulse and is regular. You check the nursing record, but see no mention of this finding.

Possible Outcome

You chart your findings and report them immediately to the client's physician. He confirms your finding of a pulse deficit and orders immediate intervention to increase this client's cardiac ejection volumes.

Prevention

Remember that the nature of the pulse volume, rate, and regularity is a valuable tool in assessing a client's overall health and in diagnosing disease states.

▶ **VARIATIONS**

Geriatric Variations:

- *Tremors in geriatric clients can interfere with evaluating the radial pulse accurately.*
- *An apical or carotid pulse might be the better option in older clients.*

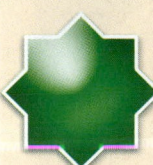

Pediatric Variations:

- *Radial pulses on infants are not reliable because of the small size of the client and the rapid heart rate normal in infants. A temporal or apical pulse is preferable.*
- *The PMI in an infant is usually located at the third to fourth intercostal space near the sternum.*
- *A child may be more comfortable sitting on a parent's lap while having his or her pulse assessed.*
- *A curious child may be more cooperative if able to listen to his or her own heart with a stethoscope.*

continues

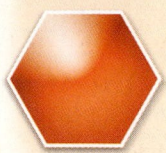

► **VARIATIONS** *(continued)*

Home Care Variations:

- *The home care environment can be distracting for the nurse and the client. The television and loud music can make it difficult to hear an apical pulse and can artificially elevate the client's pulse rate.*
- *Be sure that the client is sitting or lying quietly before taking the pulse.*
- *Clients can be taught to assess their own pulse, especially when taking cardiac medications.*

Long-Term Care Variation:

- *The relative immobility of most long-term-care clients puts them at risk of decreased peripheral circulation. Pedal pulses are an important part of the nursing examination in long-term-care clients.*

► **COMMON ERRORS**

Possible Error:

You count the pulse of a client with a cardiac arrhythmia for 15 seconds and then multiply the rate by 4 to obtain a 1-minute pulse rate.

Prevention:

Count the heart rate for at least 30 seconds to increase the probability of noting irregularities. Some irregularities do not occur in intervals of less than 15 seconds. Occasional premature beats or brief runs of supraventricular tachycardia can be missed.

Count the pulse for a full minute, noting the regularity or irregularity of the beats.

► **NURSING TIPS**

- Warm the bell of the stethoscope with your hands before placing it on the client's chest.
- Take a carotid pulse on only one side of the neck at a time to prevent cerebral blood flow impairment (see Figure 1-3-6).
- When taking pedal pulses, a firm touch is generally preferable to reduce any tickling sensations.
- A Doppler device may be necessary to detect a pulse on elderly or obese clients.

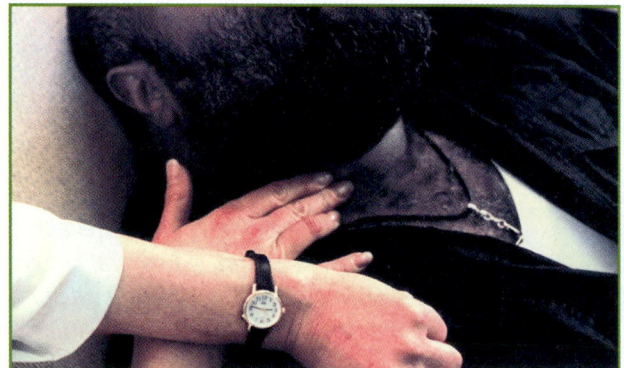

Figure 1-3-6   Take a carotid pulse on only one side of the neck at a time.

► **SPECIAL CONSIDERATIONS**

- *Never use your thumb to obtain a pulse because you may sense a beat from your own digital artery that can alter an accurate reading.*
- *When using a Doppler to obtain a fetal heart beat, check the mother's pulse to ensure the beat you are hearing is indeed that of the fetus.*
- *When preparing a client for surgery related to venous insufficiency of the lower extremities (i.e., femoral-popliteal bypass), it is essential to mark the pedal pulses with an "X." This facilitates locating the pulse during surgery to confirm circulation for the surgeon.*

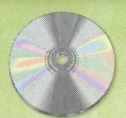

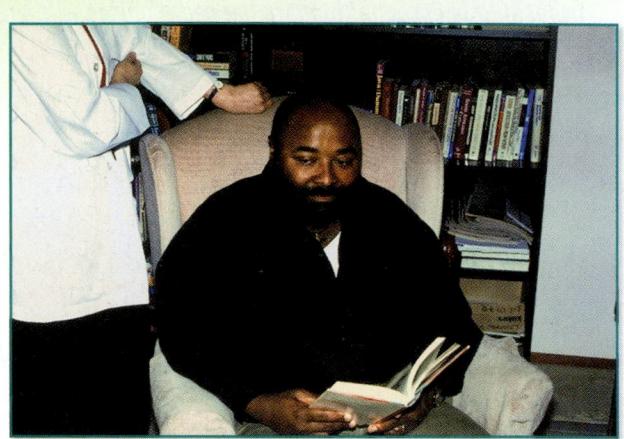

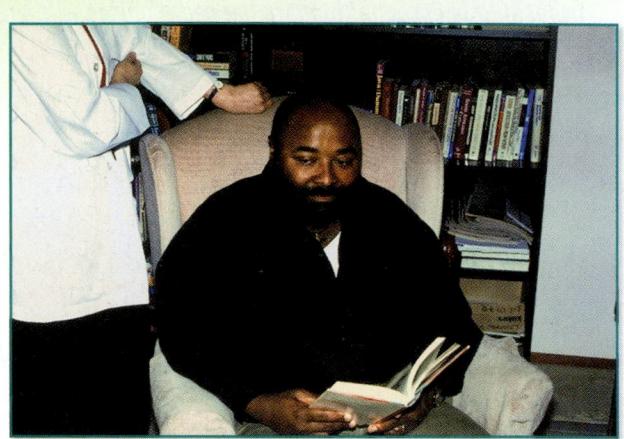

SKILL 1-4

Counting Respirations

▶ OVERVIEW OF THE SKILL

Respiratory assessment includes the measurement of the breathing pattern. Assessment of respirations provides clinical data regarding the critical respiratory status of clients and can reflect changes or be the result of changes in arterial blood gases.

Normal breathing is slightly observable, effortless, quiet, automatic, and regular. It can be assessed by observing chest wall expansion and bilateral symmetric movement of the thorax or by placing the back of the hand next to the client's nose and mouth to feel the expired air.

When assessing respiration, ascertain the rate, depth, and rhythm of ventilatory movement. Assess the rate by counting the number of breaths taken by the client per minute. Note the depth and rhythm of ventilatory movements by observing for the normal thoracic and abdominal movements and symmetry in chest wall movement. Normal respirations are characterized by a rate ranging from 12 to 20 breaths per minute and vary with age and conditioning.

One inspiration and expiration cycle is counted as one breath. You can observe the rise and fall of the chest wall and count the rate by placing the hand lightly on the chest to feel it rise and fall. Count the number of respirations for a 30-second interval and multiply by 2 if respirations are regular and even. If the client is experiencing any respiratory difficulty, count the rate for a full minute.

When the chest wall moves, so do the lungs, because the lungs are attached to the inner wall of the thoracic cavity by the outer layer of the pleura (lining of the chest cavity). The movement of the chest wall should be even and regular, without noise and effort. On inspiration, the chest changes shape and expands as the rib cage is raised and the diaphragm is lowered. Before inspiration, the pressure inside the chest cavity is negative (24.5 to 29.0 mm Hg below atmospheric pressure). Air flows along the concentration gradient from a higher atmospheric pressure to the lower intrathoracic pressure.

The opposite action occurs with expiration. The muscles relax, causing the rib cage to lower and the diaphragm to rise, compressing the chest. Intrathoracic pressure decreases to 23 to 26 mm Hg to allow the air to escape into the atmosphere.

Different respiratory wave patterns are characterized by their rate, rhythm, and depth. Eupnea refers to easy respirations with a normal rate of breaths per minute that are age specific. Bradypnea is a respiratory rate of 10 or fewer breaths per minute. Hypoventilation is characterized by shallow respirations. Tachypnea is a respiratory rate greater than 24 breaths per minute. Hyperventilation is characterized by deep, rapid respirations. Hyperpnea occurs with exercise when respirations are increased in depth and rate. Sighing is a protective physiologic mechanism for expanding small airways not used with normal breathing.

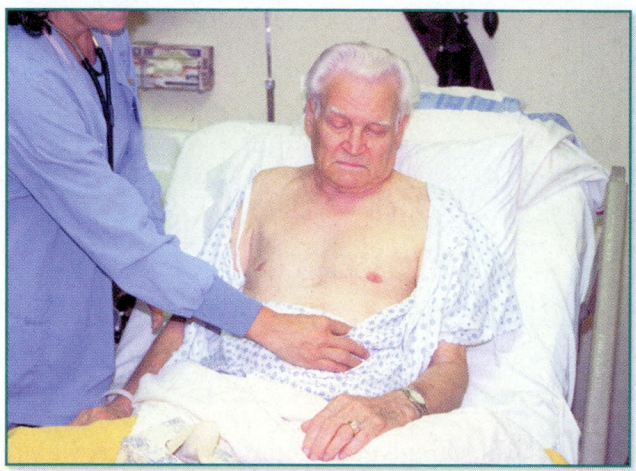

Figure 1-4-1 Observe the movement of the chest wall and assess the quality and depth of respiration. Place your hand below the diaphragm to feel if the client is using his diaphragm instead of expanding his chest wall to bring air into the lungs.

The nurse can also observe alterations in the movement of the chest wall: costal (thoracic) breathing occurs when the external intercostal muscles and the other accessory muscles are used to move the chest upward and outward; diaphragmatic (abdominal) breathing occurs when the diaphragm contracts and relaxes as observed by movement of the abdomen. Dyspnea refers to difficulty in breathing as observed by labored or forced respirations through the use of accessory muscles in the chest and neck to breathe. Dyspneic clients are acutely aware of their respirations and complain of shortness of breath (see Figure 1-4-1).

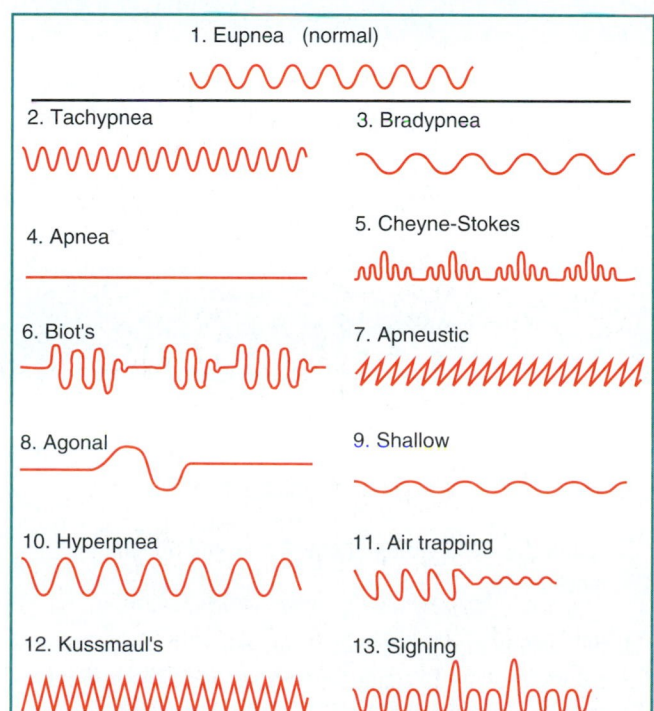

Figure 1-4-2 Normal and abnormal respiratory patterns.

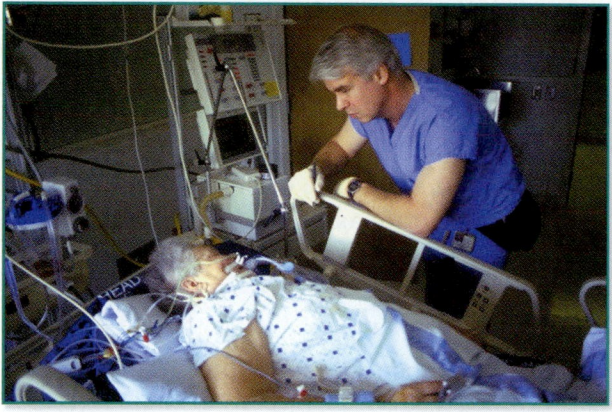

Figure 1-4-3 When assessing respirations, observe skin color and level of consciousness as well as respiratory rate and rhythm.

Respiratory alterations may cause changes in skin color as observed by a bluish appearance of the nailbeds, lips, and skin. The bluish color (cyanosis) results from reduced oxygen levels in the arterial blood. Changes in the level of consciousness (restlessness, anxiety, and dyspnea) may also occur with decreased oxygen levels. Clients with orthopnea may assume a forward-leaning position or may have to stand to increase the expansion capacity of the lungs.

Metabolic alterations, such as diabetic ketoacidosis, can cause Kussmaul's respirations, which are abnormally deep but regular.

Apnea is the cessation of breathing for several seconds. Persistent apnea is called respiratory arrest. Irregular rhythm with alternating periods of apnea and hyperventilation is called Cheyne-Stokes respirations (see Figure 1-4-2). The cycle begins with slow, shallow breaths that gradually increase to abnormally deep and rapid respirations, which then gradually slow and return to shallow breathing followed by apnea. This is common in dying clients (see Figure 1-4-3).

▶ **ASSESSMENT**

1. Assess the movement of client's chest wall **to see whether it is equal bilaterally, if the movement is labored, or if the client is using accessory muscles to breathe.**
2. Assess the rate of respirations to identify slow, rapid, or irregular respirations or even periods of apnea.
3. Assess the depth of the client's breaths **to monitor shallow, deep, or uneven respirations. Think whether there might be something influencing the client's respirations: Is the client in pain, frightened, talking, or smoking?**
4. Assess for risk factors such as fever, pain, anxiety, diseases, or trauma to the chest wall **that**

may alter the respirations because certain conditions may cause increased risk of alterations in respirations.

5. Assess for factors that normally influence respirations such as age, exercise, anxiety, pain, smoking, medications, or postural changes **so that an accurate assessment can be made.**

▶ DIAGNOSIS

Impaired Gas Exchange

Impaired Spontaneous Ventilation

Ineffective Airway Clearance

Ineffective Breathing Pattern

▶ PLANNING

Expected Outcomes:

1. An accurate evaluation of a client's respiratory rate and character will be obtained.
2. The respiratory rate and character will be normal.

Equipment Needed (see Figure 1-4-4):

• Watch with a second hand
• Stethoscope

▶ CLIENT EDUCATION NEEDED:

1. Instruct the client about the reason for assessing respirations.

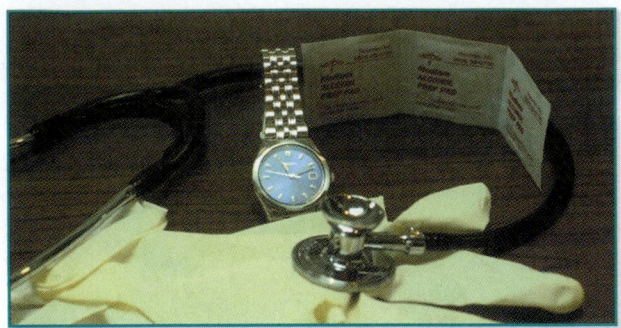

Figure 1-4-4   A watch with a second hand is used to assess respirations.

2. Teach the caregiver to count respirations while the client is not aware.
3. Instruct the caregiver to contact the nurse if there is an alteration in the client's respirations.
4. Teach clients to notify their caregiver or nurse when they feel a change in their respirations.
5. Clients who have decreased ventilation may benefit from being taught deep-breathing and coughing techniques.

Estimated time to complete the skill:
3 minutes

▶ DELEGATION TIPS

The skill of respiratory rate measurement is often delegated to properly trained ancillary personnel; however, the nurse is responsible for this information and appropriate action. Respiration counts greater than 30 (adult) or 60 (child) should immediately be reported to the nurse for further assessment.

IMPLEMENTATION—Action/Rationale

Action	Rationale
1. Wash hands.	1. Reduces transmission of microorganisms.
2. Be sure chest movement is visible. Client may need to remove heavy clothing.	2. Facilitates observation of chest wall and abdominal movements.
3. Observe one complete respiratory cycle. If it is easier, place the client's hand across the abdomen and your hand over the client's wrist.	3. Helps determine what constitutes a breath. Helps to determine what to count. Hand rises and falls with inspiration and expiration.

continues

Action	Rationale
4. Start counting with first inspiration while looking at the second hand of a watch (see Figure 1-4-5). • Infants and children: count for 1 minute. • Adults: count for 30 seconds and multiply by 2. If an irregular rate or rhythm is present, count for one full minute.	**4.** Respiratory rate is one complete cycle (inspiration and expiration). • Infants and children usually have an irregular rate.
5. Observe character of respirations: • Depth of respirations by degree of chest wall movement (shallow, normal, or deep) • Rhythm of cycle (regular or interrupted)	**5.** Reveals volume of air movement into and out of the lungs.
6. Replace client's gown if needed.	**6.** Prevents embarrassment and chilling.
7. Record rate and character of respirations.	**7.** Record rate and characteristics at bedside to ensure accurate documentation.
8. Wash hands.	**8.** Reduces transmission of microorganisms.

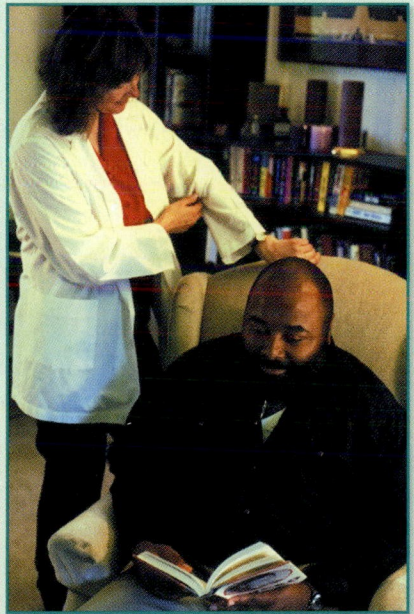

Figure 1-4-5   Count inspirations for a full 30 seconds.

▶ REAL WORLD ANECDOTES

It is 6:00 a.m. and morning medication administration is well underway. The nurse caring for Carl enters the room to take his vital signs before giving him a dose of digoxin. Carl is still sleeping, and the nurse completes the pulse assessment without waking him. While attempting to count respirations, she notes that Carl has stopped breathing. She feels for a pulse, which is still strong. After 45 seconds, Carl once again takes a breath. The nurse notes in Carl's chart that he appears to have sleep apnea. She leaves a note for Carl's physician regarding her observations and notes to herself the importance of counting respirations for at least 30 seconds.

▶ EVALUATION

- Evaluate client's respirations as a baseline value.
- Compare respirations with baseline to detect any alterations.

▶ DOCUMENTATION

Vital Signs Flow Sheet

- Record respiratory rate.

Nurses' Notes

- Record depth, rhythm, and character of respirations.
- Report a respiratory rate outside the normal age range, an irregular rhythm, inadequate depth, or any abnormal characteristics such as dyspnea.

▶ CRITICAL THINKING SKILL

Introduction

Assessing, but not correctly interpreting, abnormal respirations can lead to misdiagnosis or lack of treatment for a client.

Possible Scenario

While assessing clients at the beginning of the shift, the nursing student notes that Mr. Johnson, a diabetic, is lethargic. He responds to her greeting by asking where his baseball glove is. His respiration rate is 40 breaths per minute, and his respirations are deep. His breath has a fruity odor. At the shift report, the nurse reported that he was alert and oriented with normal vital signs.

Possible Outcome

The student is glad that Mr. Johnson seems interested in his hobbies again, and seems to be so calm. She is reassured by his deep breathing and is glad he was able to drink some apple juice. She leaves the room. Thirty minutes later, the respiratory therapist comes in and notes that Mr. Johnson is having Kussmaul's respirations and notifies Mr. Johnson's nurse. She instructs the student nurse to check Mr. Johnson's blood-glucose level while she urgently notifies his physician of the serious deterioration in his condition. Failure to catch this change in Mr. Johnson's condition could have led to his death.

Prevention

Any vital signs outside normal limits need assessment and interpretation. The rapid change in this client's condition should further alert the nurse to trouble. Any significant or rapid change in a client's condition should be noted and reported immediately to the client's physician. In this case, the client was exhibiting Kussmaul's respirations (a marked increase in rate and depth of respiration), which is associated with severe diabetic acidosis.

▶ VARIATIONS

Geriatric Variations:

- *Geriatric clients may be confused, restless, or eager to talk, so it may be difficult to get an opportunity to count quiet, at-rest respirations.*
- *Ask the client to sit quietly while you take his or her pulse or perhaps distract the client with television or other activities.*

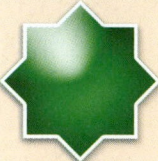

Pediatric Variations:

- *Counting respirations in small children should be done by observation.*
- *Give a small child a toy or something to distract the child while you count respirations.*
- *Infants or newborns at risk for respiratory arrest may need an apnea monitor at home.*

Home Care Variations:

- *Be sure the client is able to sit quietly while you take vital signs to ensure an accurate reading.*
- *Assess the home for factors that may influence breathing, such as ventilation or gas fumes.*

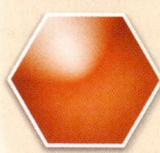

Long-Term Care Variation:

- *Clients with long-term respiratory disease are often very aware of any changes to the air space around them. Do not stand in front of clients because it may cause them to feel as if you are cutting off their air supply, which could increase their respiratory rate and anxiety.*

> **COMMON ERRORS**

Possible Error:

You take a resting respiration measurement of a client who is late for his appointment and who just walked up three flights of stairs instead of taking the elevator.

Prevention:

Be sure the client has at least 5 to 10 minutes to sit and rest to allow vital signs to return to a resting state.

> **NURSING TIPS**

- Try not to stand directly in front of the client while counting respirations. Some clients feel as though it is harder to breathe when someone stands directly in front of them.
- Fear, pain, and anger can easily raise the respiratory rate. If these emotions are present, consider assessing the rate again at a later time when the client appears calmed.
- If possible, clients should not be aware you are counting their respirations, because such awareness may alter the respiratory rate. Placing your hand on the client's wrist gives the appearance of taking a pulse and turns the client's attention away from your respiratory assessment.

> **SPECIAL CONSIDERATIONS**

- *Respirations are obtained in a variety of ways. The nurse might cross the client's hand across his or her chest as the pulse is obtained and then linger to count respirations. This is very helpful with shallow breathers or those whose respirations are not immediately visible.*
- *Be aware of the individual differences in breathing rate. Some clients, such as athletes, might be trained to breathe at a lower rate, for example, at 6 breaths per minute. In respiration assessment, use the individual baseline and the established individual record for respiration evaluation.*

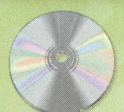

SKILL 1-5

Taking Blood Pressure

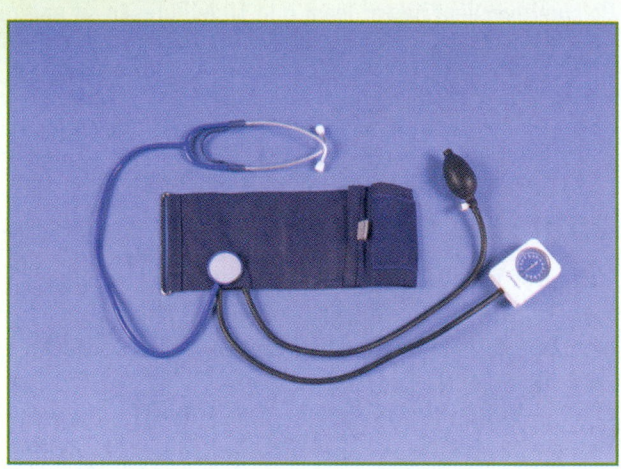

▶ OVERVIEW OF THE SKILL

Blood pressure refers to the pressure exerted on arterial vessels by circulating blood. Blood pressure measurement is one of the critical vital sign measurements and is performed as part of the physical examination, at initial assessment, and as part of routine vital signs assessment. Accurate measurement of blood pressure is essential to ascertain risk of disease and/or hemodynamic changes related to acute or chronic changes in health status. Depending on the client's condition, the blood pressure is measured by either a direct or indirect technique.

The indirect (non-invasive) method requires use of the sphygmomanometer and stethoscope for auscultation and palpation. The most common site for indirect blood pressure measurement is the client's arm over the brachial artery. When the client's condition prevents auscultation of the brachial artery, alternative sites can be auscultated. When pressure measurements in the upper extremities are not accessible, the popliteal artery, located behind the knee, is the site of choice. Blood pressure also can be assessed in other sites, such as the radial artery in the forearm and the posterior tibial or dorsalis pedis artery in the lower leg. Because it is difficult to auscultate sounds over the radial, tibial, and dorsalis pedis arteries, these sites are palpated to obtain a systolic reading.

The direct method requires an invasive procedure in which an intravenous catheter with an electronic sensor is inserted into an artery and the artery-transmitted pressure is displayed on an electronic monitor.

Hypotension is defined as a systolic blood pressure less than 90 mm Hg or 20 to 30 mm Hg below the adult client's normal systolic pressure. Orthostatic hypotension or postural hypotension refers to a sudden decrease of 25 mm Hg in systolic pressure and a decrease of 10 mm Hg in diastolic pressure when the client moves from a lying to a sitting position or from a sitting to a standing position.

High blood pressure is defined in an adult as a systolic pressure of 140 mm Hg or greater and/or a diastolic pressure of 90 mm Hg or greater. Refer to Table 1-5-1 for guidelines from the American Heart Association.

▶ ASSESSMENT

1. Assess the condition of the potential blood pressure site **so that a site with an injury or surgery proximal to the site can be avoided.**
2. Assess the artery for any compromise to it **so that compressing the artery briefly will not cause a decrease in circulation.**
3. Assess the distal pulse **to check whether it is intact and palpable.**
4. Assess the circumference of the extremity for the right size cuff to be used **so an accurate reading can be obtained**.
5. Assess for factors that affect blood pressure, such as age, anxiety, fear, medications, smoking,

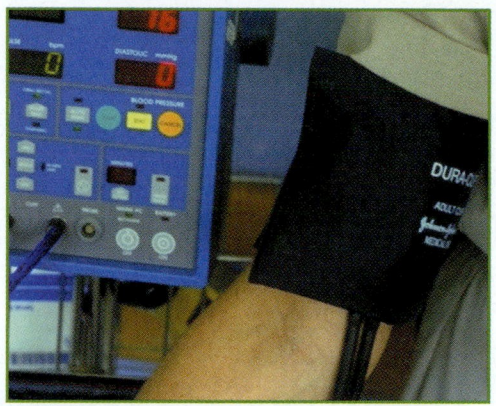

Figure 1-5-1   Be aware of blood pressure-related factors such as age, anxiety, and medications, before taking a blood pressure reading.

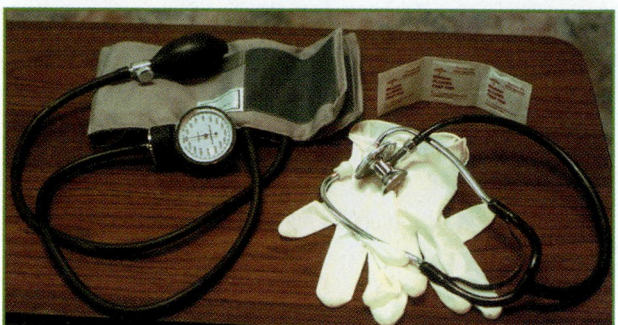

Figure 1-5-2   Sphygmomanometer, stethoscope, and gloves should be used.

eating, or exercising within 30 minutes before blood pressure assessment, and postural changes **so that an accurate reading can be obtained.**

6. Determine client's baseline blood pressure by reading the medical record **so that a comparison can be made with each blood pressure reading** (see Figure 1-5-1).

▶ DIAGNOSIS

Ineffective Cardiopulmonary Tissue Perfusion

Decreased Cardiac Output

Knowledge Deficient of Blood Pressure Control

▶ PLANNING

Expected Outcomes:

1. An accurate estimate of the arterial pressure at diastole and systole will be obtained.
2. Blood pressure is within normal range for the client.
3. Client will be able to understand why the blood pressure is taken and what it means.

Equipment Needed (see Figure 1-5-2):

- Stethoscope
- Sphygmomanometer/bladder with mercury column or aneroid dial
- Gloves
- Alcohol swabs

▶ CLIENT EDUCATION NEEDED:

1. Teach the client to refrain from eating, drinking, or smoking 30 minutes before the procedure.
2. Ask the client to sit or lie down in a warm, quiet room.
3. Ask the client to rest for 5 minutes before taking the measurement.
4. Calmly explain the procedure.
5. Advise the client regarding the correct size blood pressure cuff to use at home for his or her individual anatomy.
6. Advise the client to take his or her blood pressure at the same site using the same cuff for consistency.
7. Teach the client that the "top number" in a blood pressure reading is always higher than the "bottom number."

Estimated time to complete the skill:
5 minutes

Table 1-5-1	Blood Pressure Guidelines		
	NORMAL	**PREHYPERTENSION**	**HYPERTENSION**
SYSTOLIC	Less than 120 mm Hg	129–139 mm Hg	140 mm Hg or greater
DIASTOLIC	Les than 80 mm Hg	80–90 mm Hg	90 mm Hg or greater

IMPLEMENTATION—Action/Rationale

Action	Rationale

Auscultation Method Using Brachial Artery

1. Wash hands.

2. Determine which extremity is most appropriate for reading. Do not take a pressure reading on an injured or painful extremity or one in which an intravenous line is running.

3. Select a cuff size appropriate for the client. Estimate by inspection, or measure with a tape, the circumference of the bare upper arm at the midpoint between the shoulder (acromion) and the elbow (olecranon process) (see Figure 1-5-3).

4. Have the client's bared arm resting on a support so the midpoint of the upper arm is at the level of the heart. Extend the elbow with palm turned upward.

5. Make sure the bladder cuff is fully deflated and the pump valve moves freely. Place the manometer so the center of the mercury column or aneroid dial is at eye level and easily visible to the observer.

1. Reduces transmission of microorganisms.

2. Cuff inflation can temporarily interrupt blood flow and compromise circulation in an extremity already impaired artery or a vein receiving intravenous fluid.

3. The bladder inside the cuff should encircle 80% of the arm in adults and 100% of the arm of children less than 13 years of age. If in doubt, use a larger cuff to ensure equalization of pressure on the artery and accurate measurement.

4. Blood pressure increases when the arm is below the level of the heart and decreases when the arm is above the level of the heart.

5. Equipment must be visible and function properly to obtain an accurate reading.

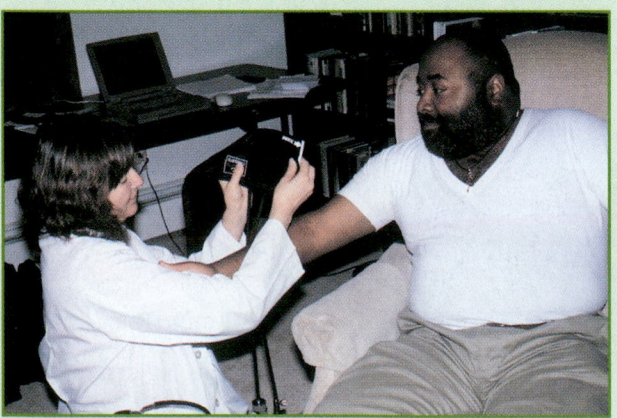

Figure 1-5-3 Select proper cuff size. An obese client may need a larger size cuff to obtain an accurate reading.

continues

Action	Rationale

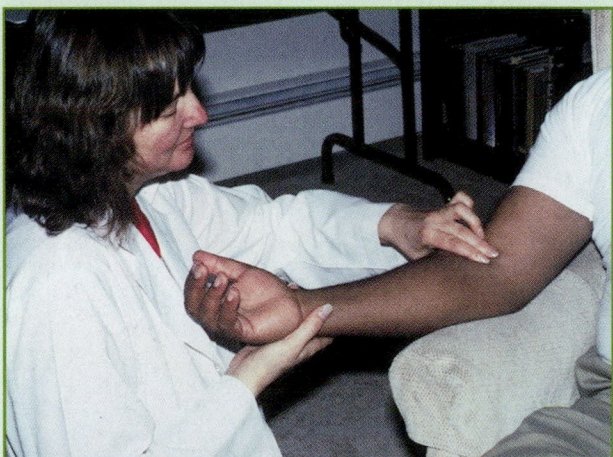

Figure 1-5-4   Palpate the brachial artery to determine placement of the stethoscope.

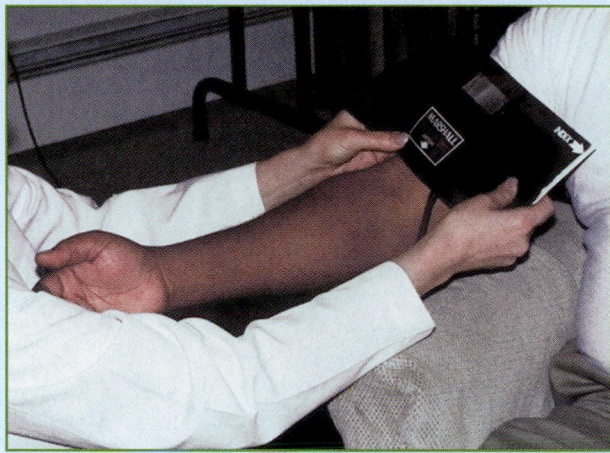

Figure 1-5-5   Center the blood pressure cuff over the brachial artery.

6. Palpate the brachial artery, in the antecubital space, and place the cuff so that the midline of the bladder is over the arterial pulsation. Next, wrap and secure the cuff snugly around the client's bare upper arm. The lower edge of the cuff should be 1 inch (2 cm) above the antecubital fossa (bend of the elbow), where the head of the stethoscope is to be placed (see Figures 1-5-4 and 1-5-5).

6. Ensures even pressure distribution over the brachial artery. Rolling up the sleeve may form a tourniquet around the upper arm. Always use a bare arm.

7. Inflate the cuff rapidly to 70 mm Hg and increase by 10-mm increments while palpating the radial pulse. Note the level of pressure at which the pulse disappears and subsequently reappears during deflation.

7. The palpatory method provides the necessary preliminary approximation of systolic blood pressure to ensure an accurate reading. When frequent measurements are required, such as every 15 minutes, the palpatory method is generally not incorporated with each pressure check.

8. Insert the earpieces of the stethoscope into the ear canals with a forward tilt to fit snugly.

8. The bell, the low-frequency position of the stethoscope, enhances sound transmission from chest piece to ears.

9. Relocate the brachial artery with your nondominant hand and place the bell of the stethoscope over the brachial artery pulsation. The bell should be held firmly in place, ensuring that the head is in direct contact with the skin and not touching the cuff (see Figure 1-5-6).

9. Sound is heard best directly over the artery. Wedging the head of the stethoscope under the edge of the cuff results in considerable extraneous noise and may cause an inaccurate reading.

10. With the dominant hand, turn the valve clockwise to close. Compress the pump to inflate the cuff rapidly and steadily until the manometer registers 20 to 30 mm Hg above the level previously determined by the palpation (see Figure 1-5-7).

10. Prevents air leaks during inflation. Ensures the cuff is inflated to a pressure greater than the client's systolic pressure.

continues

Action	Rationale

Auscultation Method Using Brachial Artery
continued

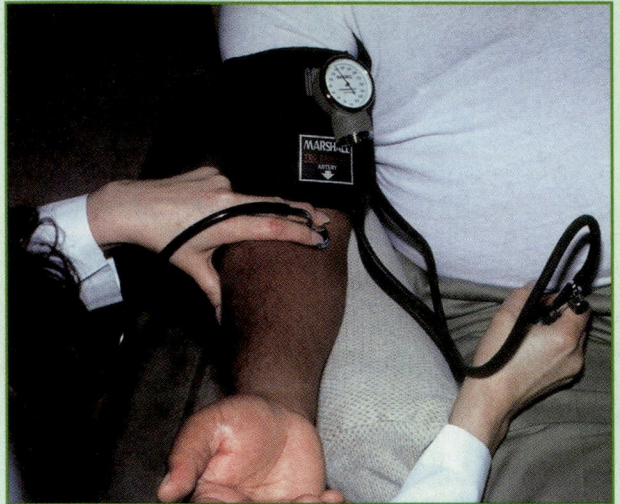

Figure 1-5-6 The stethoscope chest piece should not touch the blood pressure cuff.

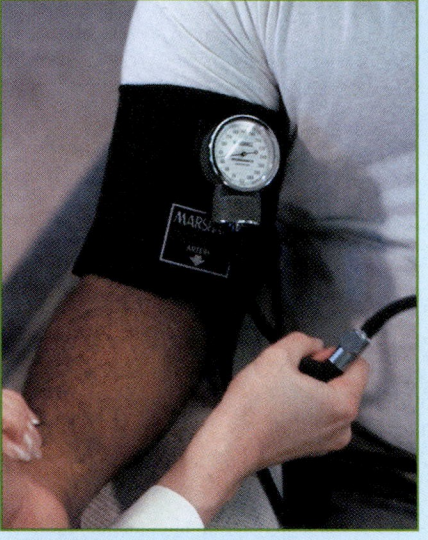

Figure 1-5-7 Compress the pump to inflate the blood pressure cuff.

11. Partially unscrew (open) the valve counterclockwise to deflate the bladder at 2 mm/sec while listening for the appearance of the five phases of the Korotkoff sounds. Note the manometer reading for these sounds.
    I   A faint, clear tapping sound that increases in intensity can be heard.
    II Swishing sound.
    III Intense sound.
    IV Abrupt, distinctive muffled sound.
    V   Sound disappears.
       (See Table 1-5-2 for more information about Korotkoff's sounds.)

11. Maintains constant release of pressure to ensure hearing first systolic sound. Identify manometer readings for each of the five phases.
    • Identify two consecutive tapping sounds to confirm systolic reading.
    • The American Heart Association (2002) recommends using Phase IV as the diastolic level in children younger than 13 years of age. Although five phases of Korotkoff sounds have been identified, most clients emit only two clearly distinct sounds (phase I and V), identified as the systolic and diastolic sounds.

12. After the last Korotkoff sound is heard, deflate the cuff slowly for at least another 10 mm Hg to ensure that no other sounds are audible; then, deflate rapidly and completely (see Figure 1-5-8).

12. Prevents arterial occlusion and client discomfort from numbness or tingling.

13. Allow the client to rest for at least 30 seconds and remove cuff. (A measurement should be repeated after 30 seconds and the two readings averaged. It may be done in the same or opposite arm) (American Heart Association, 2002).

13. Releases trapped blood in the vessels. Ensures accurate measurement.

14. Inform the client of the reading.

14. Promotes client's participation in health care.

continues

Action	Rationale

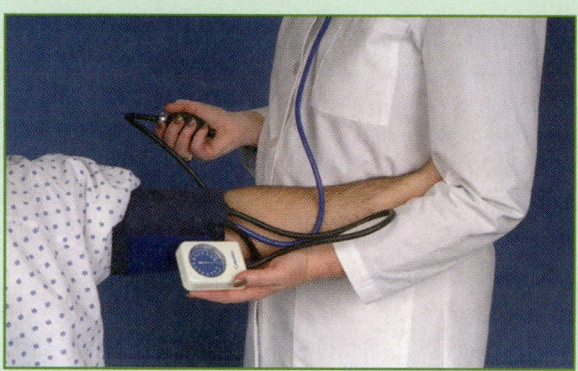

Figure 1-5-8 Deflate the cuff completely and wait at least 2 minutes before taking a second reading.

15. The systolic (Phase I) and diastolic (Phase V) pressure should be immediately recorded, rounded off (upward) to the nearest 2 mm Hg. (In children and when sounds are heard nearly to the level of 0 mm Hg, the Phase IV pressure should also be recorded.)

16. If appropriate, lower bed, raise side rails, and place call light in easy reach.

17. Put all equipment in proper place.

18. Wash hands.

15. Ensures accuracy.

16. Promotes the client's safety.

17. Fosters maintenance of equipment.

18. Reduces transmission of microorganisms.

Table 1-5-2   Korotkoff's Sounds Correlated to Pressure Dynamics

PHASE	PRESSURE DYNAMICS
I: Clear, soft tapping that increases to a thud or loud tap (systolic sound)	Ventilation—the inflow and outflow of air between the atmosphere and the lung alveoli
II: Tapping changes to a soft, swishing sound.	Circulation—the quantity of blood flowing through the lungs equals that flowing through systemic circulation
III: Clear tapping sound returns.	
IV: Muffled, blowing sound (diastolic sound in children or physically active adults)	Diffusion—the exchange of oxygen and carbon dioxide between the alveoli and the blood
V: Disappearance of muffled, blowing sound (second diastolic sound)	Transport—the carrying of oxygen and carbon dioxide in the blood and body fluids to and from the cells
	Regulation—the neurogenic system that adjusts the rate of alveolar ventilation to meet the demands of the body

▶ REAL WORLD ANECDOTES

Scenario 1

While Mrs. Price's blood pressure is being taken, she complains of pain in her arm. When Mrs. Price is questioned regarding the pain, she reports that about 5 years earlier she broke her shoulder and her arm has been sensitive ever since. When asked why she had not communicated this to the nurse before the blood pressure reading, Mrs. Price indicated that she assumed the nurse knew best. Be aware of individual client variations, especially when performing routine tasks.

Scenario 2

Mr. Johnson came to the occupational health nurse at his company to have his blood pressure checked as part of a company-wide campaign. His reading was very high. Upon further discussion, he told the nurse that he had just had a very frustrating argument over some purchase orders with a customer at lunch. He was stuck in traffic and had to run in from the parking lot to make this appointment. The nurse asked him to sit quietly for a few minutes, then took his blood pressure a second time. It was much lower and within normal limits. Clients who have recently eaten, ambulated, or experienced an emotional upset will have a falsely high blood pressure reading.

▶ EVALUATION

- Evaluate the blood pressure reading for accuracy by comparing with the medical record.
- Evaluate the client's blood pressure for being within the normal range.
- Identify variations in the client's blood pressure of more than 5 to 10 mm Hg from one arm to the other.
- Evaluate if the client's blood pressure changes significantly when he or she stands up.
- Report abnormal measurements to charge nurse or health care provider.

▶ DOCUMENTATION

Vital Signs Flow Sheet

Record:
- The blood pressure measurement
- The site where recording was done
- The method of obtaining the pressure (auscultation or palpation)

▶ CRITICAL THINKING SKILL

Introduction

The routine of taking a blood pressure reading may become a mindless task. It is an important physical assessment tool.

Possible Scenario

Paul is a morbidly obese middle-aged client. He has a history of Type II diabetes and hypertension. He is being admitted to the hospital for observation of his blood sugar and blood pressure. You are performing his admission evaluation, including the taking of vital signs. You use a blood pressure cuff that is in the room to take Paul's blood pressure, even though it barely covers his arm.

Possible Outcome

Your reading shows a drastically elevated blood pressure—the admitting orders call for transfer to intensive care and Nipride therapy for a blood pressure this high. The client reports that when he took his pressure earlier in the day it was much lower. You ask another nurse to check Paul's blood pressure, who notes that the cuff you used is too small for Paul's arm and brings the correct size cuff from the nurses' station. This reading is much lower. Subsequent readings with the correct-sized cuff show no immediate intervention is necessary.

Prevention

A blood pressure reading must be accurate to be an effective diagnostic tool. Taking a blood pressure reading on obese clients with an average-sized adult cuff can give a falsely elevated reading. In addition, a blood pressure cuff that is too small for the client's arm will often come unfastened as it is inflated. Be sure to use the correct-sized cuff for the client.

▶ VARIATIONS

Geriatric Variations:
- The systolic blood pressure may be overestimated by the indirect method of measurement because of sclerotic, calcified vessels. If the brachial artery is readily palpable, even when the cuff is inflated and the blood flow is interrupted (positive Osler's sign), then the measurement may not be accurate. Under these circumstances, an incorrect diagnosis of hypertension may be made. Direct measurement should be used for confirmation.
- Postural hypotension is often observed in elderly clients.
- Elderly clients may have lost muscle mass, and their upper arms may be quite thin. Be sure to adjust the cuff size to accommodate the client's arm.
- Many elderly clients have a history of hypertension and are taking antihypertensive medications.

Pediatric Variations:
- Determine the diastolic pressure as Phase IV in children younger than 13 years of age because the Korotkoff sounds are often heard through the entire period of deflation.
- The palpatory method is often used for approximating systolic pressure in small children and infants; however, the measurement may be 5 to 10 mm Hg lower than the level measured by auscultation.
- Small children may be uncooperative with the procedure and need the assistance of a parent or adult to hold still.
- A cuff that fits adequately may not be available to ensure that the bladder completely encircles the limb. It may be preferable to use the popliteal artery when taking a child's blood pressure.
- Blood pressure varies with size as the child reaches adolescence.
- Take a blood pressure reading first before anxiety- or pain-producing procedures.

Home Care Variations:
- Use the same blood pressure cuff the client normally uses for home readings.
- Compare the client's home readings to a reading obtained with a cuff that you know is properly calibrated.
- Assess the client's financial ability to buy his or her own sphygmomanometer.
- Consider use of an electric blood pressure cuff if the client has a hearing deficit.

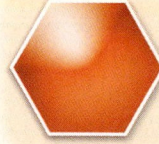

Long-Term Care Variation:
- Be aware of any injuries, disease processes, or medical devices (such as stents) that may contraindicate a blood pressure reading at the chosen site.

▶ COMMON ERRORS

Possible Error:

When taking a blood pressure reading, the cuff is low enough on the arm that the stethoscope bell must be slid underneath the bottom edge of the cuff to be properly placed over the artery.

Using the wrong cuff size for pediatric, bariatric, or very thin clients.

Prevention:

Make sure to use the correct-sized cuff and that it is positioned correctly on the client to prevent the stethoscope from contacting the cuff. If you find that it is incorrectly applied, remove the cuff, assess cuff size, and reapply the correct-sized cuff, fitting it firmly on the upper arm so that the antecubital space is visible. Repeat the blood pressure reading.

▶ **NURSING TIPS**

- Do not take a blood pressure over clothing or on an arm with an arteriovenous shunt, intravenous line, or if the client has a history of surgery or injury to the breast, axilla, or arm.
- The tubes extending from the blood pressure cuff bladder are not always centered on the bladder itself. It is not accurate to assume that the area between these tubes represents the center of the cuff bladder. Be sure to center the bladder by palpating the bladder itself.
- False high readings occur when the mercury column in the manometer is not positioned flat on a firm surface, when it is read above eye level, or when the extremity is below the heart's apex level.
- False low readings occur when the extremity is above the heart's apex level, when the cuff is too wide for the extremity, or when the mercury column in the manometer is read below eye level.
- If the nurse fails to recognize the auscultatory gap, the temporary disappearance of sounds at the end of Korotkoff's Phase I and beginning of Phase II, the systolic pressure is read at a false low.
- There are many different types and brands of blood pressure measurement devices. Become familiar with the ones with which you will be working.
- If an electronic blood pressure device is used, be sure to assess the accuracy of the machine. Use the same equipment when comparing a client's blood pressure.
- Avoid latex pressure cuff if client has history of latex allergy. Best practices are never to use latex pressure cuffs.

▶ **SPECIAL CONSIDERATIONS**

- *Pulsus paradoxus, also called paradoxic pulse, is an abnormal decrease (more than 10 mm Hg) in the systolic pressure and a decrease in pulse wave amplitude during inspiration. An excessive decrease may be a sign of tamponade, adhesive pericarditis, severe lung disease, heart failure, or other conditions.*
- *Ask the client what his or her normal blood pressure is, and use it not only as a gauge for cuff inflation but as an opportunity to teach the client about healthy blood pressure values.*
- *A child's blood pressure may vary with age. A very low diastolic pressure is not always indicative of underlying cardiac disease.*
- *An alternative method when taking a blood pressure reading in a very small infant, when Doppler or automated oscillometric equipment is unavailable, is the flush method. The American Heart Association (2002) defines this as follows: "placing a suitable cuff on the arm or leg, raising the limb, and wrapping the extremity distal to the cuff firmly with an elastic bandage until it is drained of blood and blanches. The limb is then lowered to heart level, the cuff is rapidly inflated, and the bandage is removed. As the pressure in the cuff is gradually reduced, flushing of the limb indicates the level at which the flow returns. This level corresponds to mean blood pressure but is inaccurate in infants with anemia, hypothermia, or edema."*
- *Blood pressure should be taken in the alternate arm in clients who have recently had a mastectomy with extensive axillary node dissection or other surgical procedure involving the arm or shoulder. In dialysis clients, the alternate arm should be used when the client has an arteriovenous fistula.*

Weighing a Client, Mobile and Immobile

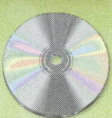

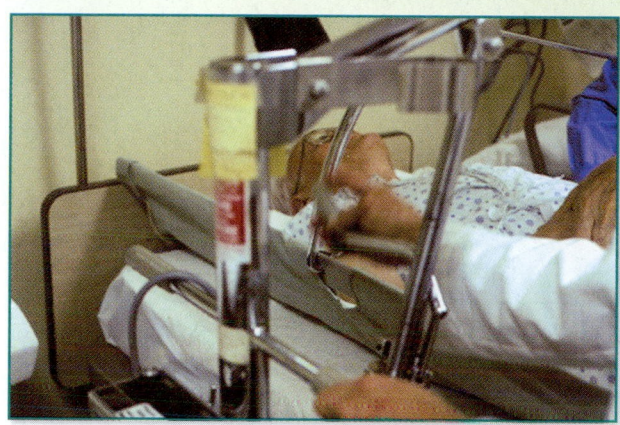

▶ **OVERVIEW OF THE SKILL**

A client's weight is an essential piece of data used in monitoring health status and in evaluation of the response to a variety of therapies. Changes in a client's weight could necessitate an alteration in the assessment and intervention plans. An accurate weight is important, therefore, to ensure appropriate care.

▶ **ASSESSMENT**

1. Assess the client's ability to stand independently and safely on a scale. **Consider factors requiring the use of a sling scale: the client is somnolent or comatose; paralyzed; too weak to stand; or unsteady when standing.**
2. Determine whether clothing is similar to that worn during previous weight measurement **to help determine accuracy of the new weight.**

▶ **DIAGNOSIS**

Imbalanced Nutrition: More than Body Requirements

Imbalanced Nutrition: Less than Body Requirements

Excess Fluid Volume

Deficient Fluid Volume

▶ **PLANNING**

Expected Outcomes:

1. Health care provider obtains accurate weight.
2. Client incurs no injuries.
3. Client maintains privacy.

Equipment Needed:

- Scale bed; standing electronic or balance scale (see Figure 1-6-1); or sling scale (see Figure 1-6-2)
- Recommended disinfectant
- 1 to 3 other staff members to assist when using sling scale
- Plastic cover for sling scale
- Gloves (when applicable)

▶ **CLIENT EDUCATION NEEDED:**

1. When using the standing electronic scale, instruct the client not to step onto the scale until the digital display reads zero.
2. When using the sling scale, incorporate clients as you go through the procedure. Provide instructions when asking clients to turn and be sure to inform clients before lifting.
3. Instruct clients in the correct way to monitor weight at home, that is, by weighing themselves without clothes first thing in the morning after voiding.
4. Remind clients that, when weighing themselves at home, they use the scales on the same, even hard surface (kitchen or bathroom tile, hardwood floor).

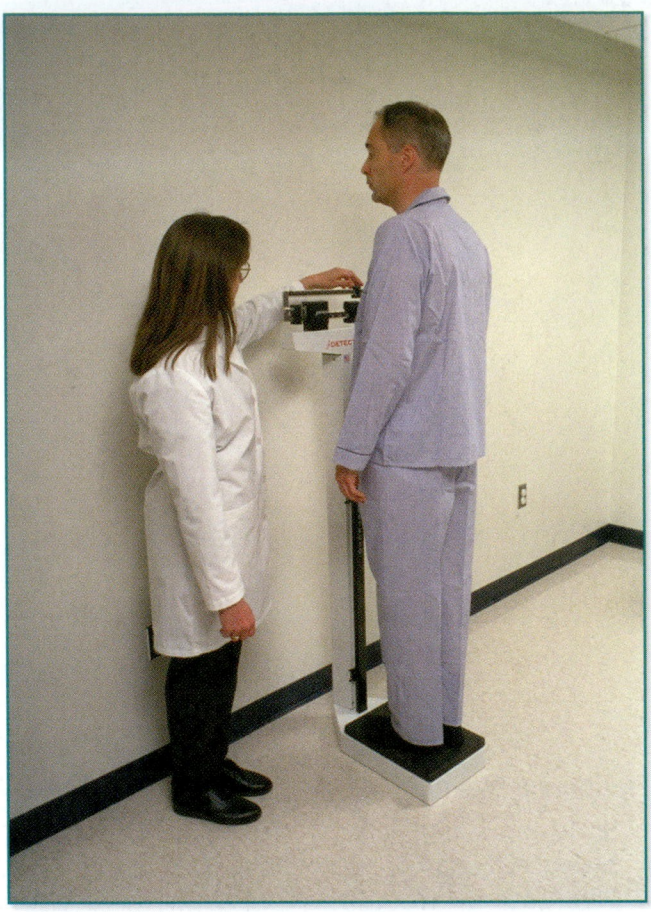

Figure 1-6-1   The standing balance scale is used to weigh ambulatory clients.

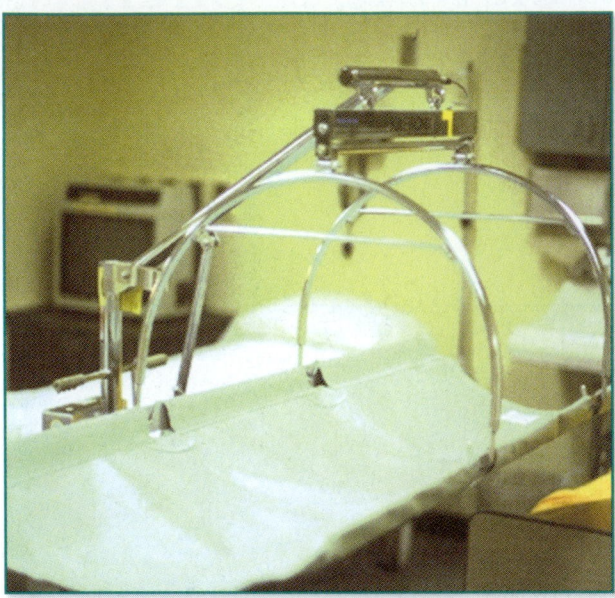

Figure 1-6-2   The sling scale is used to weigh clients in bed.

Estimated time to complete the skill:
3 minutes when using standing scale
10 minutes when using sling scale

▶ DELEGATION TIPS

The skill of weighing the mobile and immobile client is routinely delegated to trained ancillary personnel.
   The personnel should be instructed to do the following:
- Select the correct scale for measurement.
- Properly and safely position the client for measurement.
- Correctly and safely perform the measurement according to established guidelines and record on the appropriate flow sheet (clinical record).
- Recognize and report abnormal findings promptly to the nurse.

IMPLEMENTATION—Action/Rationale

Action	Rationale
Standing Scale	
1. Wash hands.	1. Reduces transmission of microorganisms.
2. Introduce yourself to the client and explain the action you are going to perform.	2. Builds rapport; involves the client in care.

continues

Action	Rationale
3. Place the scale near the client.	3. Reduces risk of fall or injury.
4. Turn on the scale and calibrate it to zero.	4. Ensures accurate reading.
5. Ask client to remove shoes if necessary step up on the scale, and stand still (see Figure 1-6-3). *Electronic scale:* Read weight after digital numbers have stopped fluctuating. *Balance scale:* Slide the larger weight into the notch most closely approximating the client's weight. Slide the smaller weight into the notch such that the balance rests in the middle. Add the two numbers to read the client's weight.	5. Obtains weight. Reading is not accurate when the numbers are still fluctuating. Weights on scale must be balanced to obtain accurate reading.
6. Ask the client to step down. Assist the client back to the bed or chair, if necessary.	6. Reduces risk of injury if client needs assistance.
7. Wipe the scale with appropriate disinfectant.	7. Reduces risk of spread of infection.
8. Wash hands.	8. Reduces transmission of microorganisms.

Sling Scale

Action	Rationale
9. Wash hands and put on gloves if appropriate.	9. Reduces risk of nosocomial infection.
10. Introduce yourself to the client and explain what you would like the client to do.	10. Builds rapport; involves the client in care.

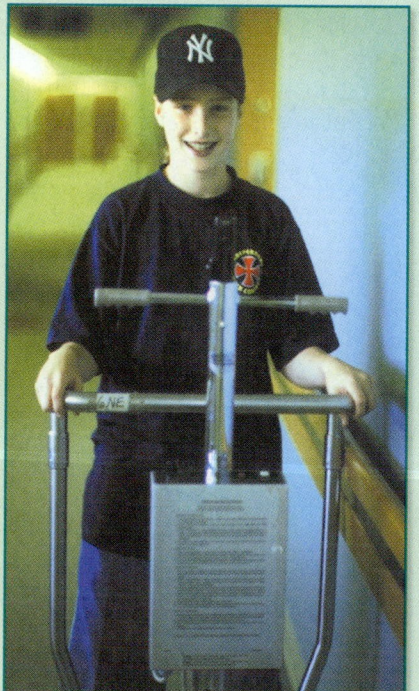

Figure 1-6-3 Have client stand straight and still while on the standing scale to obtain accurate measurements of weight and height.

continues

Action	Rationale
Sling Scale *continued*	
11. Place plastic covering on sling if available (can usually be ordered in bulk from the manufacturer).	11. Reduces risk of spreading infection between clients.
12. Remove pillows. Turn the client to one side and place half of sling on bed next to the client, with remaining half rolled up against the client's back (see Figure 1-6-4).	12. Most accurate weight will be obtained by leaving no other bedding between the client and sling.
13. Turn the client to the other side, and unroll the rest of the sling so it lays flat beneath the client.	13. Turning in this manner maximizes client comfort.
14. Roll the scale over the bed such that the legs of the scale are underneath the bed (see Figure 1-6-5). Open and lock the legs of the scale.	14. Ensures equipment is being used safely to reduce risk of injury.
15. Turn on scale and calibrate to zero.	15. Ensures accurate reading.
16. Lower arms of the scale and slip hooks through holes in sling (see Figure 1-6-6).	16. Attaches sling to scale to obtain weight.
17. Pump scale until sling rests completely off the bed (see Figure 1-6-7).	17. Ensures accurate weight.
18. Remind the client to remain still. Read weight after digital numbers have stopped fluctuating (see Figure 1-6-8).	18. Reading is not accurate when the numbers are still fluctuating.
19. Lower the client back to bed and remove arms of the scale from sling (see Figure 1-6-9).	19. Prepare for removal of sling.
20. Unlock legs, return to their original position, and remove scale from bed.	20. Allows for removal of equipment that obstructs proximity to the client, thereby facilitating removal of the sling.
21. Turn the client on one side, roll up sling, and then turn client to the other side.	21. Facilitates removal of the sling.

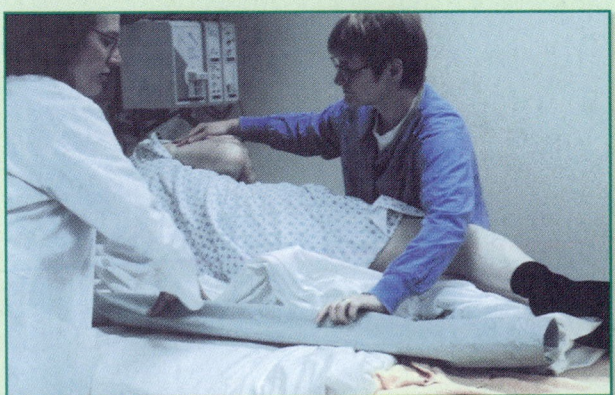

Figure 1-6-4   Turn client on one side and place sling on the bed.

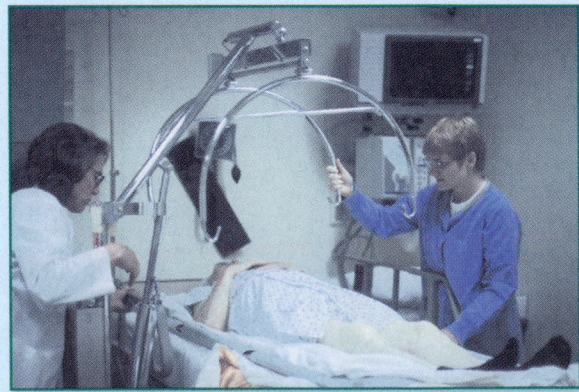

Figure 1-6-5   After unrolling the rest of the sling under the client, move the scale into position over the bed.

continues

Action	Rationale

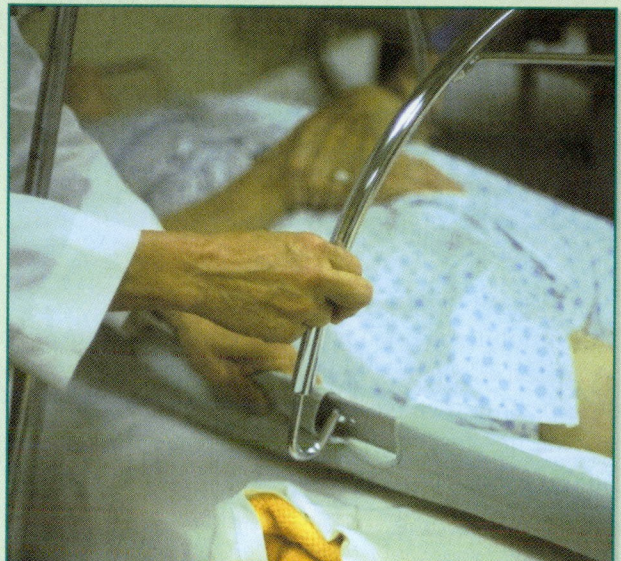

Figure 1-6-6   Attach the hooks through the holes in the sling.

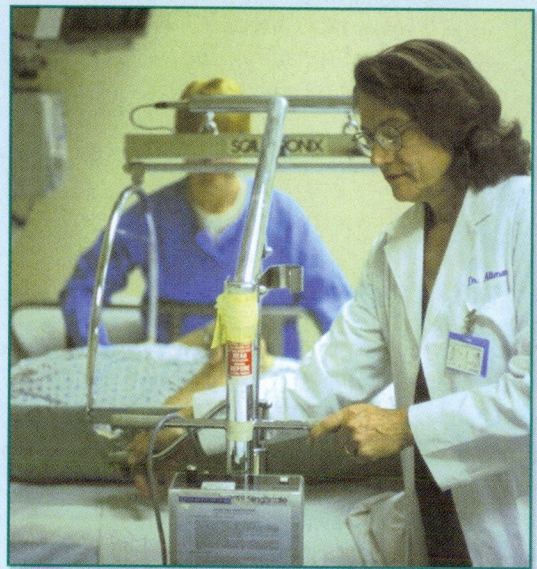

Figure 1-6-7   Pump the scale until the sling lifts completely off the bed.

22. Realign the client with pillows and covers.

23. Remove plastic covering from the sling and discard as per hospital policy.

24. Remove gloves.

25. Wash hands.

22. Ensures comfort and privacy.

23. Reduces risk of spread of infection.

24. Reduces risk of nosocomial infection.

25. Reduces transmission of microorganisms.

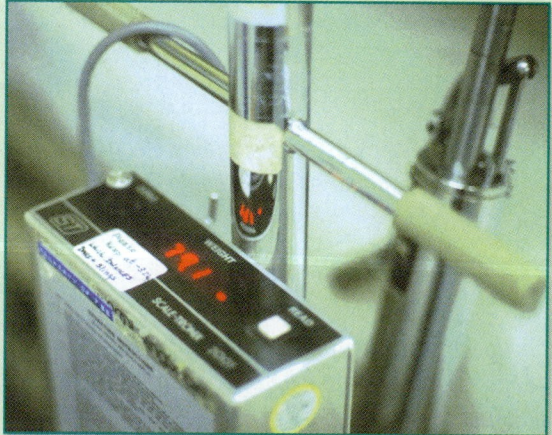

Figure 1-6-8   Read the weight after the numbers have stopped fluctuating.

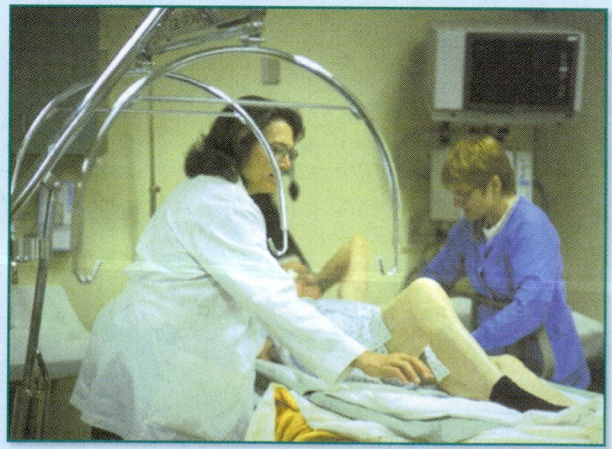

Figure 1-6-9   Lower the client back to the bed and remove the sling.

► **REAL WORLD ANECDOTES**

A client was called back to the exam room area. The nurse wanted to check the client's weight on the standing scale in the hallway. The client was very upset that the nurse wanted to weigh her with her shoes on, which would add pounds to her weight. The nurse needed to hear that this individual was concerned and embarrassed about being overweight.

► **EVALUATION**

- Compare weight obtained to previously recorded weight. Repeat weight if large discrepancy is noted.
- If large discrepancy still remains, notify appropriate health care team members.

► **DOCUMENTATION**

Vital Signs Flow Sheet

- Record the date, time of day, type of scale used, and the weight of the client on the appropriate flow sheet or electronic medical record (EMR).

► **CRITICAL THINKING SKILL**

Introduction

Dramatic weight fluctuation may be a reflection of improper technique.

Possible Scenario

An immobile client has just been weighed using an over-the-bed scale. The nurse is alarmed that the client seems to have lost 20 pounds in 2 days. She records her findings in the nurses' notes and alerts the nurse practitioner.

Possible Outcome

The nurse practitioner comes and repeats the weight. She finds the client has actually gained a pound. Upon reviewing her technique, the nurse realizes that she probably did not lift the scale sling high enough to clear the bed, thereby resulting in an inaccurate weight.

Prevention

Lift the sling high enough so that no part of the client touches the bed. Double-check any large change in weight with no apparent cause.

► **VARIATIONS**

Geriatric Variation:

- *Elderly clients may need more assistance when moving to the scale. Consider using a sling scale if the client is too unsteady to stand independently.*

Pediatric Variation:

- *Pediatric scales are necessary to weigh infants. Follow the same steps as for a standing electronic scale, except place the infant on the scale after ensuring calibration and elicit the caregiver's assistance in calming and distracting the child.*

Home Care Variations:

- *When using a client's own scale, assess its proper functioning and use it in a consistent manner to ensure accuracy. For example, weigh the client using the scale on the same hard, even surface for each reading (e.g., bathroom or kitchen tile, hardwood floor).*
- *If you bring your own scale to a home visit, compare the two scales before recording weights from the different scales on the same flow sheet.*
- *Home scales may need to be adjusted so they read "0" when there is no weight on the scale.*

continues

▶ VARIATIONS *(continued)*

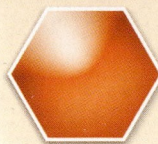

Long-Term Care Variations:
- *Establish an appropriate weigh schedule for the long-term care client. It is easy to forget to weigh a client. Keeping an accurate weight will help monitor long-term gains or losses.*
- *Keeping a current weight will establish a baseline to compare with future changes.*

▶ COMMON ERRORS

Possible Errors:

Weight obtained differs greatly from previously recorded weight.

Prevention:

Be sure the scale is appropriately calibrated before use. Recalibrate the scale and repeat the weight.

Possible Errors:

The sling scale begins to tip when the client is lifted off the bed.

Prevention:

Be sure to open the legs of the scale to broaden its support base. Lower the client, check scale legs, and open them if necessary.

▶ NURSING TIPS

- Weigh clients at the same time each day to enhance accuracy.
- Weigh clients in similar clothing each time to avoid unnecessary discrepancies.

- In an unfamiliar setting, check the bed. Some have a built-in scale.
- If a battery-operated electronic scale is used, plug it in between uses to keep the battery charged.

▶ SPECIAL CONSIDERATIONS

- *If the situation permits, use the same scale each time to ensure the measurement validity.*
- *When using the sling scale, it is important to assess the environment because the hooks that slide through the holes can easily catch on surrounding objects.*
- *Be aware of added lines, dressings, and bedding when trying to gauge an accurate weight.*
- *Many types of scales are on the market. Check directions for accurate use and calibration.*

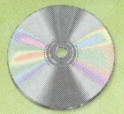

Measuring Intake and Output

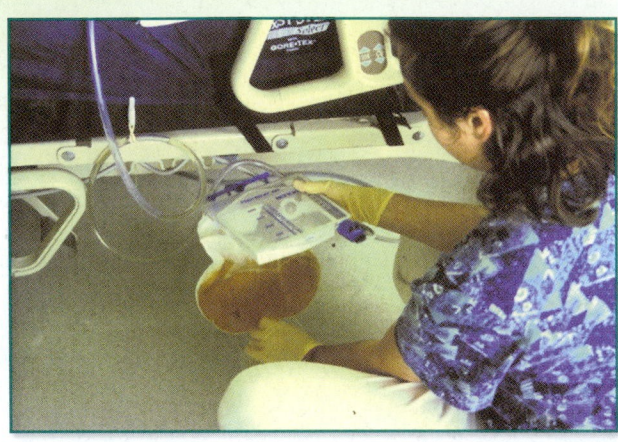

▶ OVERVIEW OF THE SKILL

One of the most basic methods of monitoring a client's health is measuring intake and output, commonly called "I and O" or "I&O." By monitoring the amount of fluids a client takes in and comparing this to the amount of fluid a client puts out (i.e. excretes or loses through vomiting or diarrhea), the health care team can gain valuable insights into the client's general health as well as monitor specific disease conditions.

To maintain good health, fluid intake should approximately equal fluid output. Intake that exceeds output can indicate medical conditions ranging from renal failure to congestive heart failure. Output that exceeds intake can be caused by things as serious as life-threatening diarrhea or as benign as diuretic medications. An accurate record of a client's fluid balance is an important nursing function.

Intake and output monitoring is often ordered by the health care provider but can also be initiated by the nurse. Some institutions have policies regarding conditions that require intake and output monitoring as well. Generally clients who are receiving fluids through any route other than oral or who are losing fluids through any route other than voiding are placed on intake and output measurement. Clients with conditions that affect fluid balance—for example, diabetes, renal failure, diuretic therapy, or anorexia—also require intake and output monitoring.

Ideally, intake and output should be monitored over several days to obtain an accurate record of the client's status. In critical situations, however, this may not be possible, and the client's intake and output may be monitored and reported on an hourly basis. A urine output of less than 30 mL per hour should be reported.

Daily weights are often performed in conjunction with intake and output. Daily weights can indicate fluid retention or loss. One gallon of water weighs 8 pounds. An 8-pound weight gain during a 24- to 48-hour period could indicate a life-threatening condition for the client. A significant change in a client's weight or a significant difference in a client's total intake and output should be reported to the client's health care provider.

Intake is considered to be any fluid consumed or infused, including water, juice, coffee, milk, ice cream, soup broth, and Jell-O®. Be sure to calculate the amount of water the client has consumed from the bedside water pitcher. Any fluids infused through intravenous (IV) lines, central lines, feeding tubes, or irrigant that is not returned is considered intake. Blood and blood products as well as the saline used to flush IV lines before and after the transfusion are also included in this count. IV piggybacks, fluids used to measure cardiac output, central line flushes, and TKO (to keep open) fluids are also considered in the intake total.

Urine is the largest component of output fluid volume, but there are a number of other fluid loss avenues that must be considered. Diarrhea, diaphoresis, wound drainage, gastric or other fluids removed by suction, and bleeding are all fluid losses as well. These losses should be measured or estimated and recorded in the total output.

Clients who are able to understand and cooperate with the intake and output measurement should be encouraged to keep track of their fluid balance. Particularly in clients who are on a fluid restriction, client understanding and participation can greatly increase cooperation.

▶ ASSESSMENT

1. Assess the client's risk factors for fluid overload, such as congestive heart failure, renal failure, or ascites **because edema can result from excess volume in extracellular fluid spaces and transferring of fluid into tissues.**
2. Determine whether the client is receiving fluids or medications that would predispose to fluid overload, such as large amounts of IV fluids or steroid therapy **because steroids cause sodium and water retention and excretion of potassium.**
3. Assess the client's risk factors for fluid loss such as diaphoresis, rapid respirations, diarrhea, gastric suction, blood loss, or wound drainage **because dehydration can result from reduction of fluid within the tissues and circulatory system.**
4. Determine whether the client's urine output is in excess of his fluid intake **because the kidneys excrete excess fluid during periods of overhydration and conserve body water during periods of dehydration.**
5. Assess the client's ability to understand and cooperate with intake and output measurement **because cooperation in these measurements will help ensure accuracy.**

▶ DIAGNOSIS

Excess Fluid Volume

Deficient Fluid Volume

Risk for Deficient Fluid Volume

▶ PLANNING

Expected Outcomes:

1. The client's fluid intake and output will be accurately measured and recorded.

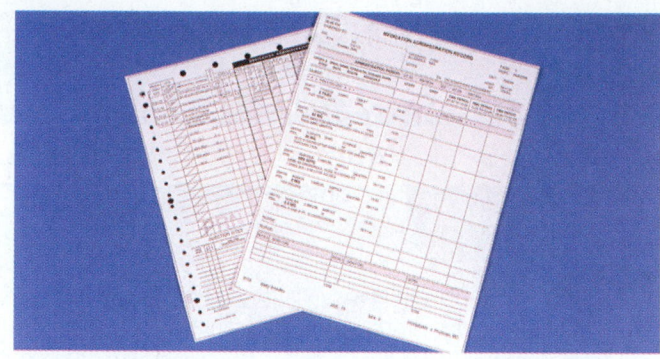

Figure 1-7-1 Intake and Output (I&O) forms.

2. The client will participate in the recording of fluid intake and output if possible.

Equipment Needed (see Figure 1-7-1):

- I&O form at bedside
- I&O graphic record in chart
- Glass or cup
- Bedpan or urinal bedside commode
- Graduated container for output
- Nonsterile gloves
- Sign at bedside stating client is on I&O

▶ CLIENT EDUCATION NEEDED:

1. Instruct the client how to measure fluid intake using standardized volumes of glassware and dishes.
2. Teach the client which intake is considered to be fluid and which is not. Remind the client what is considered fluid intake (e.g., coffee, tea, and soda pop, as well as gelatin, ice cream, and popsicles).
3. Teach the client to measure and record the amount of fluid standard utensils hold and then to use those utensils exclusively.
4. Instruct the client to void into a bedpan or urinal, not into a toilet.
5. Teach the client to dispose of toilet tissue in a plastic-lined container, not in the bedpan.

Estimated time to complete the skill: **5–10 minutes**

▶ DELEGATION TIPS

Intake and output measurement may be delegated to ancillary personnel who should be knowledgable regarding the following:
- Obtaining accurate measurements and reporting incontinence.
- Observing the amount, color, and any odor from the output.
- Protecting themselves from contamination from a body fluid and storing collection containers in designated areas.
- Recording measurements on proper clinical records.

IMPLEMENTATION—Action/Rationale

Action	Rationale

1. Wash hands.

1. Reduces transmission of microorganisms.

2. Explain the rules of the I&O record. All fluids taken orally must be recorded on the client's intake and output form (sometimes called a fluid balance flow sheet).
  - Client must void into bedpan or urinal, not into toilet (see Figures 1-7-2 and 1-7-3).
  - Toilet tissue should be disposed of in plastic-lined container, not in bedpan.

2. Elicits client support.

  - Fluid voided into the toilet cannot be measured.

  - Liquids absorbed into toilet tissue cannot be measured by volume.

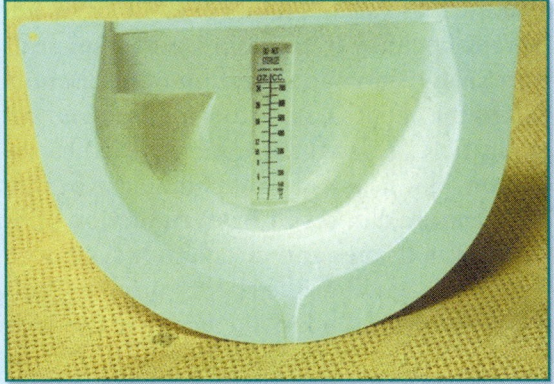

Figure 1-7-3 Graduated specimen container is used to measure urine, drainage, or other output.

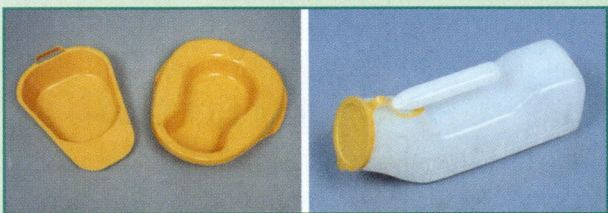

Figure 1-7-2 Bedpan and urinal, protective pad, and graduated specimen container.

Input

3. Measure all oral fluids in accord with institution policy; for example, cup: 5–150 mL, glass-5–240 mL.
  Record all IV fluids as they are infused (see Figure 1-7-4).

3. Provides for consistency of measurement.

4. Record time and amount of all fluid intake in the designated space on bedside form (oral, tube feedings, IV fluids).

4. Documents fluids.

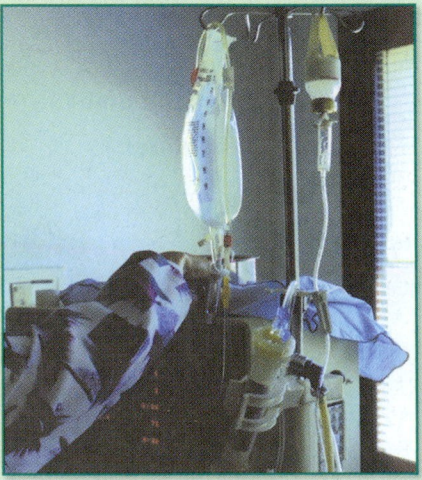

Figure 1-7-4 All IV infused fluids must be measured.

continues

Action	Rationale
5. Transfer 8-hour total fluid intake from bedside I&O record to graphic sheet or 24-hour I&O record on client's chart.	5. Provides for data analysis of the client's fluid status.
6. Record all fluid intake, in the appropriate column of the 24-hour record.	6. Documents intake by type and amount.
7. Complete 24-hour intake record by adding all 8-hour totals.	7. Provides consistent data for analysis of the client's fluid status over a 24-hour period.

Output

Action	Rationale
8. Apply nonsterile gloves.	8. Reduces potential for transmission of pathogens.
9. Empty urinal, bedpan, or Foley drainage bag (see Figure 1-7-5) into graduated container or commode "hat" (see Figure 1-7-6).	9. Provides accurate measurement of urine.
10. Remove gloves and wash hands.	10. Prevents cross-contamination.
11. Record time and amount of output (urine, drainage from nasogastric tube, drainage tube) on I&O record.	11. Documents output.
12. Transfer 8-hour output totals to graphic sheet or 24-hour I&O record on the client's chart.	12. Provides for data analysis of the client's fluid status.
13. Complete 24-hour output record by totaling all 8-hour totals.	13. Provides consistent data for analysis of the client's fluid status over a 24-hour period.
14. Wash hands.	14. Reduces transmission of microorganisms.

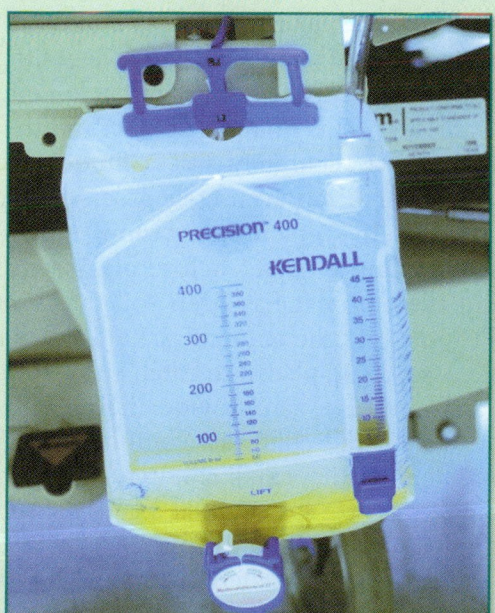

Figure 1-7-5   Urine in Foley drainage bag must be measured.

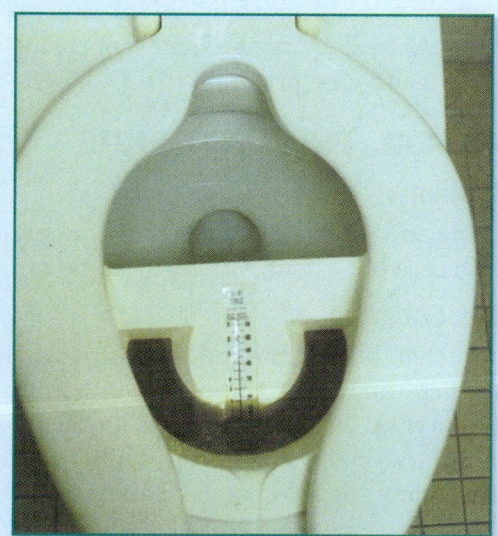

Figure 1-7-6   Empty urine into a graduated container for measurement.

▶ REAL WORLD ANECDOTES

Mr. Aguilar is a critically ill client in the coronary care unit. During the night, his nurse noted that his urinary output was 10 mL an hour for the past 2 hours. She called Mr. Aguilar's physician and received an order to give Mr. Aguilar an IV diuretic. While preparing to give Mr. Aguilar the diuretic, she took his vital signs and reassessed his condition. She noted that Mr. Aguilar's skin turgor was very poor and his skin was dry. He was complaining of thirst and his blood pressure was low. Mr. Aguilar's urine was dark and concentrated in appearance. The nurse called Mr. Aguilar's physician back with this information and voiced her concern that perhaps Mr. Aguilar's low urine output was caused by dehydration rather than fluid retention. Mr. Aguilar's physician ordered a urine-specific gravity test, which revealed that Mr. Aguilar was in fact dehydrated. An IV diuretic could have seriously harmed Mr. Aguilar in his dehydrated condition.

▶ EVALUATION

- The client's fluid intake and output was accurately measured and recorded.
- Note whether the client was able to participate in the recording of fluid intake and output to the best of his or her ability.
- Note and report any abnormal findings to the client's health care provider.

▶ DOCUMENTATION

Intake and Output Record

- Record all fluid I&O.
- Add totals at the end of every shift.
- Add totals for 24-hour period.

Nurses' Notes

- Any unusual findings, excessive intake, excessive output, or serious imbalance of intake and output should be documented and reported to the client's health care provider.

▶ CRITICAL THINKING SKILL

Introduction

Measuring and monitoring intake and output is critical to the care of a client, especially an infant.

Possible Scenario

An infant has been admitted to the pediatric unit. Her mother notes that she has been vomiting and having diarrhea. When asked, the mother was able to report how many times the infant had vomited and how many diaper changes she had performed, but she was unable to document how much fluid the infant had lost overall. The nurse admitting the infant was puzzled about how she was going to determine the fluid balance baseline and how she was going to measure the infant's output. The nurse chose to use the infant's admission weight and hydration status as the baseline, ignoring the infant's current hydration status.

Possible Outcome

The infant's admission dehydration and electrolyte imbalance went untreated. The infant's status rapidly worsened, resulting in coma.

Prevention

Small children, and especially infants, are at increased risk of fluid imbalance problems. Infants have very small fluid reserves; a tablespoon of liquid is a much larger proportion of an infant's body weight than it is of an adult's. Uncontrolled diarrhea can kill infants in a matter of days. This infant is at risk, and the nurse must be able to accurately assess fluid intake and output. The nurse can accurately assess incontinent fluid amounts by remembering how much water weighs. Weighing a diaper before placing it on the baby and then after it has been soiled can provide a good estimate of the amount of fluid the baby has lost. Likewise, a pad placed to catch emesis, weighed before and after use, can provide an estimate of the amount of fluid the child has vomited. It is important to remember that small children cannot tolerate fluid and electrolyte loss as well as adults. Accurate measurement and keeping the physician informed of the results are essential when caring for children.

▶ VARIATIONS

Geriatric Variations:
- *Elderly clients are sometimes incontinent. Measuring output in an incontinent client can be difficult. Weighing the client's linen or incontinence pad before use and then weighing it again after it has been soiled can help the caregiver keep track of the amount of fluid output the client is generating.*
- *Elderly clients need a caregiver to monitor their fluid intake, especially when they are taking diuretics, supplemental potassium, and cardiac medication.*
- *Elderly clients are at risk for fluid and electrolyte imbalances from prolonged fever or gastroenteritis.*

Pediatric Variations:
- *The amount of fluid loss a child can tolerate is much smaller than that of an adult because of the proportionately smaller size of the child. Small amounts of fluid loss can be serious or fatal for small children.*
- *Infants and young children are at risk for fluid and electrolyte imbalances from prolonged fever or gastroenteritis.*

Home Care Variations:
- *The nurse should help the caregiver use standard cups and other utensils to measure intake and output.*
- *Assess the client's and caregiver's ability and compliance to record I&O.*
- *Provide appropriate charts and equipment, and teach how to record I&O.*
- *Ask the client and caregiver to perform a return demonstration for the procedure.*

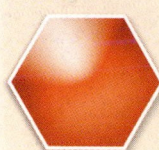

Long-Term Care Variations:
- *Clients may suffer from a loss of appetite, including fluids.*
- *Clients may need assistance from a dietitian to prepare fluids that are appealing to them.*

▶ COMMON ERRORS

Possible Error:
Not counting the water the client drinks from the bedside pitcher.

Prevention:
Be sure the client is aware of the reasons for measuring intake and output. Teach the client how to keep track of it. Be sure that any caregiver who is refilling water pitchers or providing juice understands the need to keep track of intake and how to do it. Teach the caregiver not to use the water in the pitcher to water flowers.

Establish a system to mark each new pitcher of water the client receives. Measure the water left in the pitcher at the end of each shift. Ask the client to help you keep track of the intake.

▶ NURSING TIPS

- Keep I&O flow sheet close to the bedside.
- Teach clients the necessity to keep accurate I&O records.
- Keep water fresh, encourage beverages as allowed.
- Record measurements immediately instead of waiting until the end of the shift.
- 240 mL of ice chips equal 120 mL of fluid.
- Pureed food is not considered to be fluid intake.
- Bottled nutrient tube feedings are liquid and must be considered in I&O.
- All postoperative clients are at risk for fluid loss through blood or plasma from their incision sites. Monitor the dressings.

- Remember that fluids taken to swallow pills must be recorded as intake (see Figure 1-7-7).
- Do not have visitors or family members empty bedpans, urinals, or catheter bags.

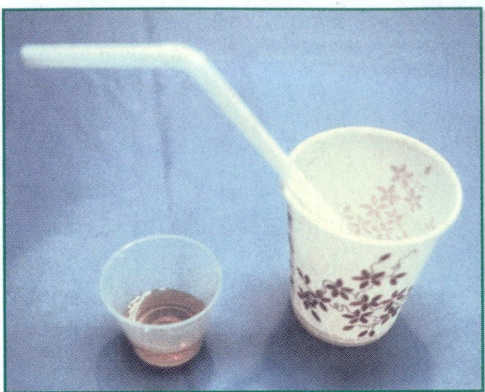

Figure 1-7-7 Even fluid used to swallow pills must be measured.

▶ SPECIAL CONSIDERATIONS

- *Proper aseptic technique should be taken when handling clients' body fluid output. Blood first, urine last. For example, if the drainage from the Hemovac and urine from the urine bag need to be emptied at the same time, the health care provider should empty the Hemovac first and then the urine bag and should change gloves between procedures.*
- *Infant diapers should be weighed. One gram of weight equals one mL of fluid.*

Breast Examination

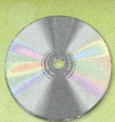
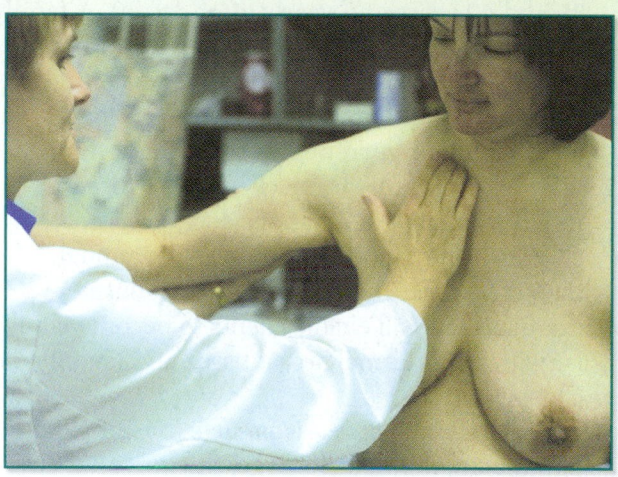

▶ OVERVIEW OF THE SKILL

Physical assessment of the breast and axillae is part of periodic health maintenance examinations for both men and women of all ages. Breast cancer cannot be prevented, but early detection offers more treatment options and a greater chance of cure. A breast examination performed by the nurse is accompanied by breast examination education whenever possible. Teaching the client to perform monthly breast examinations, discussing risk factors, and prompting the client to seek recommended mammograms are essential for early diagnosis and treatment of breast cancer.

▶ ASSESSMENT

1. Assess client's musculoskeletal and range of motion ability **to determine client's ability to participate and cooperate in examination.**
2. Assess demonstrated health-seeking behaviors specific to obtaining breast examination as well as Pap and pelvic examinations to **identify any education or health-seeking deficits.**
3. Assess client's knowledge of breast self-examination and health maintenance recommendations for clinical examination to **identify further education or health-seeking deficits.**
4. Assess personal and family history relevant to cancers as well as breast and cervical abnormalities **to assist in planning health management and screening schedules.**

5. Assess if the client's health history reveals past or present use of hormonal medications, because **a thorough follow-up may be necessary if any abnormalities are found as hormonal use is a known risk factor that may increase the risk for breast cancer.**
6. Assess if the client's family history includes breast cancer in first-degree (mother or sister) or second-degree (aunt or grandmother) relatives, **because a thorough follow-up may be necessary as this is a known risk factor.**
7. Assess whether the woman is postmenopausal **because breasts in postmenopausal women may show normal atrophy of glandular tissue and increased striations.**
8. Assess age for a male client with enlarged breasts **because breast enlargement in adolescent boys is usually normal for puberty and is common when a boy is overweight.**

▶ DIAGNOSIS

Potential for Impaired Tissue Integrity

Health-Seeking Behaviors

Deficient Knowledge

▶ PLANNING

Expected Outcomes:

1. Normal breast examination. No dimpling, nodules, masses, inflammation, lesions,

discharge, lymph node enlargement, or tenderness.

2. Client is able to demonstrate proper procedure for breast examination and offer a plan of when it will be performed monthly.

3. Client will identify when next screening should be performed.

Equipment Needed:

- Small pillow or towel
- Centimeter ruler
- Nonsterile gloves (sterile if open lesions or drainage)
- Drape/gown
- Teaching aid for breast self-examination

▶ CLIENT EDUCATION NEEDED:

1. Instruct clients not to use creams, lotions, or powders and not to shave underarms 48 hours before the scheduled assessment because these actions could alter the breast skin or cause folliculitis and lymph node enlargement.

2. Instruct clients how to prepare for and what to expect from the procedure to decrease unnecessary anxiety and to maximize cooperation.

3. Remind clients to inform you of any discomfort experienced during the procedure, because it should not be uncomfortable.

4. Teach clients to initiate breast examinations starting at puberty when they start noticing breast growth and generally are interested in their bodies at this stage of development. Subsequently, routine examinations should take place before the beginning of each menstrual cycle; this will help establish a routine time, and prior to menses when breast changes are most noticeable.

5. Teach clients to examine on an easy to remember monthly date (first day of the month, last day of the month, the 15th, or on the day of their birth, for instance a client born April 26 would examine on the 26th of every month) rather than in relationship to the menstrual cycle. Menses are not always regular.

6. Preventive mammograms, as recommended by age or medical history, should be scheduled as part of routine breast examination. Women need a mammogram once between the ages of 35 and 40 years and yearly after age 40. A family history of breast disease, previous abnormalities, and certain medical conditions require more frequent screening. Contact the American Cancer Society for current recommendations.

7. It is still necessary for the client to perform monthly breast examinations and have a yearly clinical examination even if receiving annual mammograms. The performance of routine examinations will enable clients to become familiar with their normal breast tissue and identify changes.

8. Instruct clients to assess breasts for lumps, dimpling, pain, nipple discharge, thickness, or any changes in breast tissue.

9. Persistent lumps should always be biopsied. Insist on a biopsy, if necessary.

10. Educate men to perform a monthly breast examination and obtain a clinical examination every 1 to 3 years, because 1% of all breast cancer is found in men.

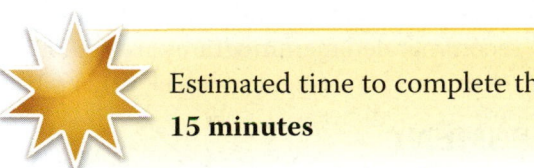

Estimated time to complete the skill:
15 minutes

▶ DELEGATION TIPS

Breast examination and the concomitant client education skills are within the realm of a nurse's role and licensure and require assessment and problem-solving behaviors in addition to client teaching responsibilities. These functions must not be delegated. Ancillary personnel may reinforce the importance of breast self-examination.

IMPLEMENTATION—Action/Rationale

Action	Rationale
1. Review personal history, medications, allergies, and family health history.	1. Identifies risk factors and previous baseline (or lack of). Identifies allergies to latex.
2. Ask the client to disrobe to the waist and to put on a gown with the opening in the front.	2. Provides easy access while maintaining maximum privacy.
3. Wash hands. Apply gloves if required by institutional policy.	3. Prevents microorganism transfer and possible contact with discharge when palpating nipples.
4. Assist the client to a sitting position facing you and expose chest and breasts (see Figure 1-8-1).	4. Allows comparison of breasts bilaterally.

5. Inspect breasts, areola, and nipples:
• With client's arms at sides
• With client's arms raised (see Figure 1-8-2)
• With client's hands pressed on hips (see Figure 1-8-3)
• With client's arms extended straight ahead as client leans forward (may omit this position for male unless gynecomastia is present)
	5. Observe for flesh color, slight inequities in size and symmetry, rounded shape, and smooth skin surface.
	    Redness, blue hue, retraction, dimpling, enlarged pores, edema, lumps, lesions, rashes, ulcers, and discharge are abnormal.
	    Supernumerary nipples along the milk line are a normal variant.

6. Palpate adjacent lymph nodes: supraclavicular, infraclavicular, and subclavian (see Figures 1-8-4 and 1-8-5).	6. Nodes should be less than 1 cm in diameter and nontender.
7. Palpate breast: Using the pads of the palmar surfaces of the fingertips, palpate the right breast by gently compressing the mammary tissues against the chest wall. Palpation may be performed from the periphery to the nipple, in either concentric circles or in wedge sections (see Figure 1-8-6). Explain the procedure to the client as you examine.	7. Observe the breast for warm temperature, elasticity, tenderness, pain, erythema, masses, or nodules, which are abnormal.

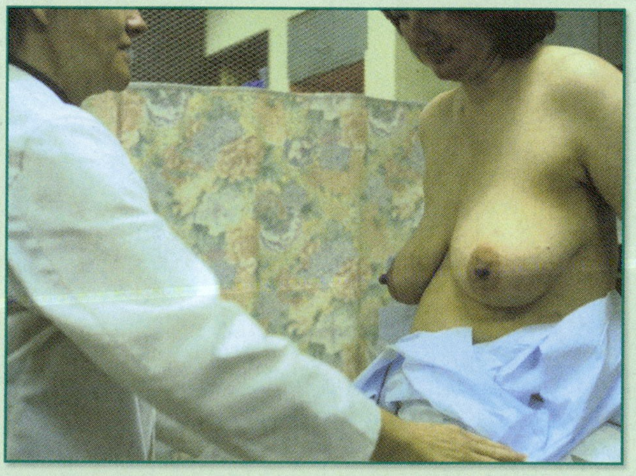

Figure 1-8-1   Assist the client to a sitting position facing the examiner.

continues

Action	Rationale

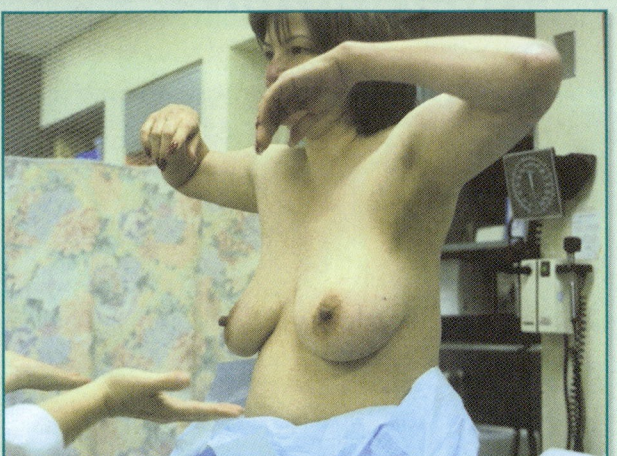

Figure 1-8-2   Inspect the breasts with the client's arms raised.

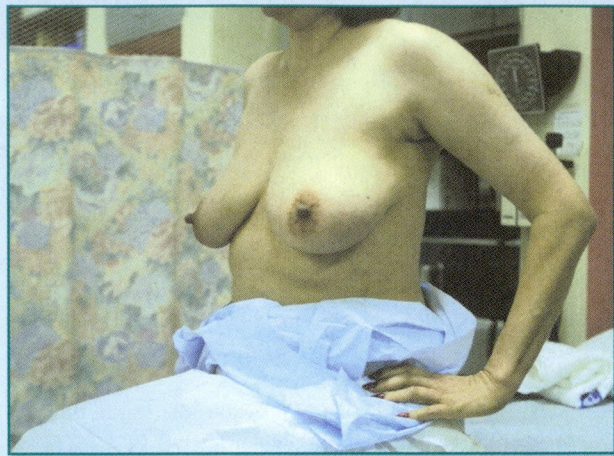

Figure 1-8-3   Inspect the breasts with the client's hands resting on hips.

8. Teach breast examination as you examine. Teach the client to use the right hand to palpate the left breast and the left hand to examine the right breast. During part of the exam, place the client's fingers under the practitioner's fingers.

9. Palpate areola and nipple by using a similar circular technique as with breast. Pay special attention to subareolar area and gently press the nipple between your fingers.

10. Palpate into axilla, starting at anterior axillary line and continuing at an angle to the midaxillary line and up into the axilla (using same circular fingertip motion). Have client place arm at side and palpate deep into the axilla.

8. Teaching the client during the examination reinforces the need for and understanding of breast exams and enables the client to identify normal breast tissue and abnormal tissue if present. Increases the client's confidence in performing breast examination.

9. Observe abnormalities such as inflammation discharge, nodules, fissuring, or lesions.

10. Identify posterior axillary, central axillary, anterior axillary, and lateral axillary node locations. Nodes should be less than 1 cm and nontender.

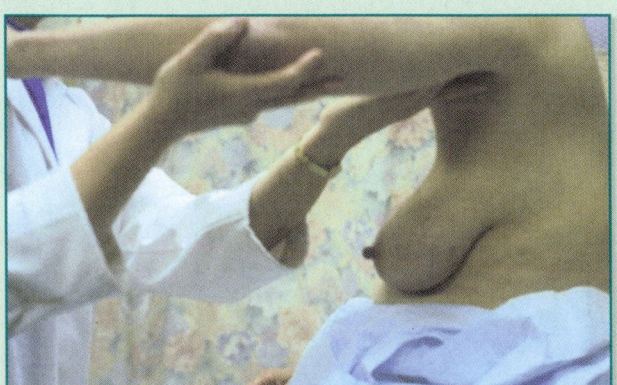

Figure 1-8-4   Palpate lymph nodes adjacent to breast tissue.

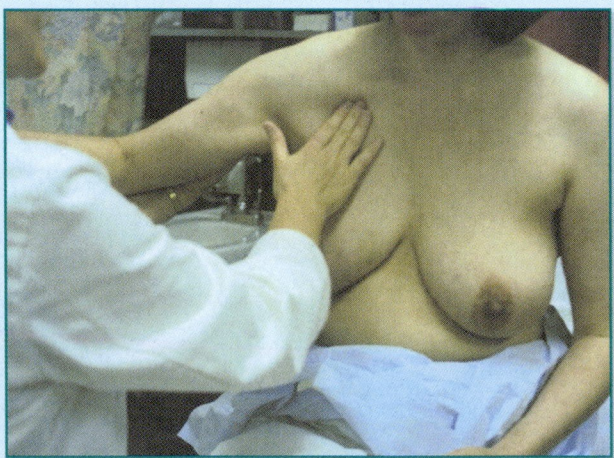

Figure 1-8-5   Palpate infraclavicular lymph nodes.

continues

Action	Rationale

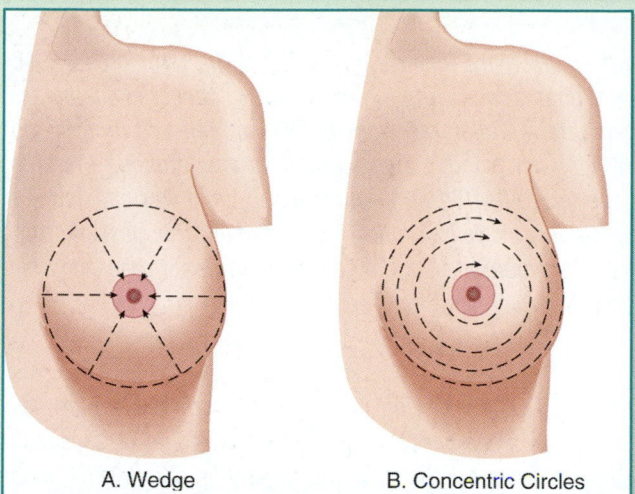

A. Wedge   B. Concentric Circles

Figure 1-8-6 Palpation methods.

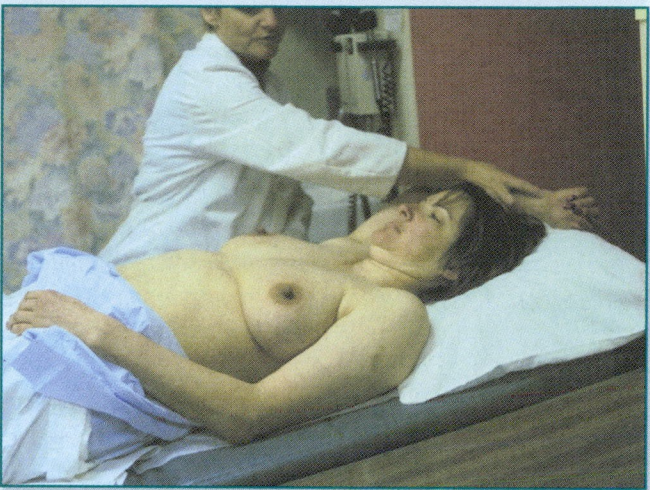

Figure 1-8-7 Place the client in a supine position.

11. Repeat Actions 7 to 9 on the left breast, areola, nipple, and axilla.

11. Identify normal versus abnormal as with the right breast. Compare breasts bilaterally.

12. Assist the client to the supine position. Place arm on examination side under head and place a small pillow under the same side scapula (see Figure 1-8-7).

12. Position spreads breast tissue over the chest wall, maximizing palpation accuracy.

13. Palpate breast, areola, and nipple as in Actions 7 to 10 (see Figures 1-8-8 and 1-8-9).

13. Reevaluate examination in second position.

14. Assist the client to a sitting position. Review the steps and ask the client to return-demonstrate breast self-examination.

14. Provides more comfort for client. Evaluates success of your teaching.

15. Allow the client to dress.

15. Provides for client's comfort.

16. Remove gloves and wash hands.

16. Reduces transmission of microorganisms.

17. Give the client written materials to reinforce teaching. Instruct the client when to schedule the next clinical examination.

17. Reinforces teaching. Provides a readily available form to client for reference when at home.

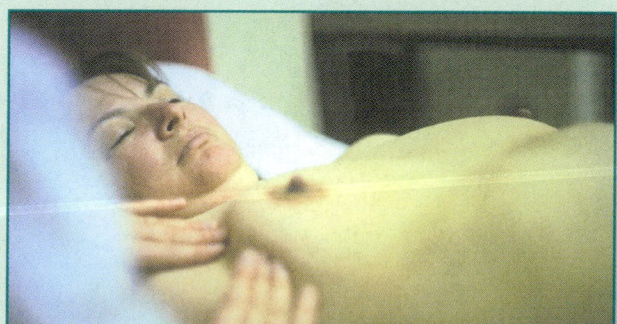

Figure 1-8-8 Palpate the breast.

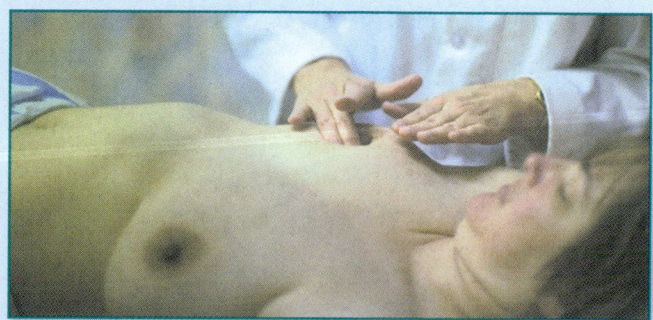

Figure 1-8-9 Palpate the areola and nipple.

► EVALUATION

- Client is able to perform monthly breast examination.
- Client returns for clinical breast examination at prescribed time.
- Any abnormalities are identified early for referral evaluation and possible treatment.

► DOCUMENTATION

Nurses' Notes

- Record the date and time.
- Document findings of abnormalities and absence of abnormalities.
- Record the client's response to findings and teaching.
- Record a follow-up plan, if necessary.

► CRITICAL THINKING SKILL

Introduction

Ms. Hernandez, who is 30 years old, asks whether she should worry about the lumps she frequently finds in her breasts. She has a history of polycystic disease.

Possible Scenario

She ignores the lumps, attributing them to polycystic disease.

Possible Outcome

One of the lumps is not just a cyst; it is malignant.

Prevention

Advise the client to never ignore lumps or diagnose them herself. She should continue to perform monthly breast examinations and, at a minimum, have a yearly clinical exam. She should report any new or changed lumps to her health care provider and ask for an assessment no matter how many times the tests show a lump is benign.

► **VARIATIONS**

Geriatric Variations:

- *Breasts are less firm, more pendulous, and often atrophied in elderly clients. The tissue is coarser and more nodular.*
- *Be sure to lift pendulous breasts to inspect the skin under the breasts. This is a frequent site of yeast infection and needs immediate treatment. Do not use cornstarch to dry this area because cornstarch promotes yeast growth.*
- *Striae are normal with aging.*

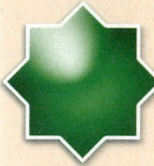

Pediatric Variations:

- *At puberty, when breast development starts, breasts are frequently asymmetric.*
- *Overweight adolescents often falsely appear to have gynecomastia, especially during the prepubescent increase in adipose tissue.*
- *Inverted nipples are "normal" variants.*
- *Infants may have nipple discharge and up to 2 cm breast tissue from maternal estrogens.*

Pregnancy Variations:

- *Striae are common during pregnancy and sometimes after pregnancy if breasts remain large.*
- *Enlargement, tingling, tenderness, increased vascularity, increased alveoli, nodularity, darkening of the areolae, and erect and sensitive nipples are common during pregnancy.*
- *Lactation may occur before delivery. Colostrum may be secreted beginning in the second trimester (week 16).*
- *Note whether nipples are inverted, because this requires additional client instruction if breast-feeding is planned.*

Home Care Variations:

- *Teach a caregiver or family member the breast examination procedure if the client is unable to perform her own examination.*
- *Omit certain positions, if necessary, for clients with medical conditions that limit movement or balance.*
- *If a client is rarely out of bed, teach the client or a caregiver to perform the breast examination when the client is both sitting up in a chair and lying in bed.*

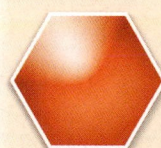

Long-Term Care Variations:

- *Omit certain positions, if necessary, for clients with medical conditions that limit movement or balance.*
- *If a client is rarely out of bed, the nurse or caregiver can perform the breast examination when the client is sitting up in a chair or lying in bed.*

► **COMMON ERRORS**

Possible Error:

Examination of a client's breast was stopped after no lumps were detected using the first two positions. An existing lump was not detected.

Prevention:

Never assume that no detection of lumps in the first few positions means you will find nothing in the remaining positions. Do not rush the examination.

Carefully explain each step and substep to the client. It is important for the client to understand the importance of every step so as to perform breast self-examinations and receive follow-up screening.

Possible Error:

Client does not understand how to correctly perform breast examination.

Prevention:

It is important for the client to understand the importance of every step so as to perform regular breast examinations and receive follow-up screening.

► **NURSING TIPS**

- Breast examinations vary. Many practitioners use the "roll" method, whereby the examiner's hands never leave the breast. Finger pads roll back and forth across the breast from the sternum to the axillae and advance an inch with each forward motion. When this method is used, all areas of the breast are examined.
- Special attention should be given to the area under and surrounding the nipple and in the upper outer quadrant because most lumps are found in these locations.
- Putting on gloves before palpation often makes the client more comfortable, because it adds an element of depersonalization.
- To reinforce self-examination, use the same circular examination techniques recommended for breast self-examination; however, a wedge or vertical pattern may be used as well. It is often helpful to use these alternate techniques to reexamine any abnormalities you find. It does not alarm the client as much.
- Use the flat pads of three fingers to palpate the breast tissue by compressing it gently against the breast wall.

- Use a bimanual palpation technique in large and/ or pendulous breasts.
- Usually, if you explain exactly what you are doing and what you are looking for as you examine, there are no misunderstandings. If you are at all uncomfortable performing an examination, ask a "witness" to assist you to be sure that the client does not misinterpret your actions as inappropriate. With children, have the parent witness your examination.
- Expose only the area(s) being examined without undue exposure of other areas. For example, expose both breasts for inspection to compare bilaterally and then cover one breast while you palpate the other.
- Breasts are not always symmetric. Always review breast development in light of Tanner's sexual maturity ratings (see Table 1-8-1). Correlate this with genital development whenever possible.
- Refer all abnormal or questionable findings. Describe nodules and masses as to number, shape, consistency, definition, mobility, tenderness, and skin retraction.

Table 1-8-1   **Sexual Maturity Rating for Female Breast Development**

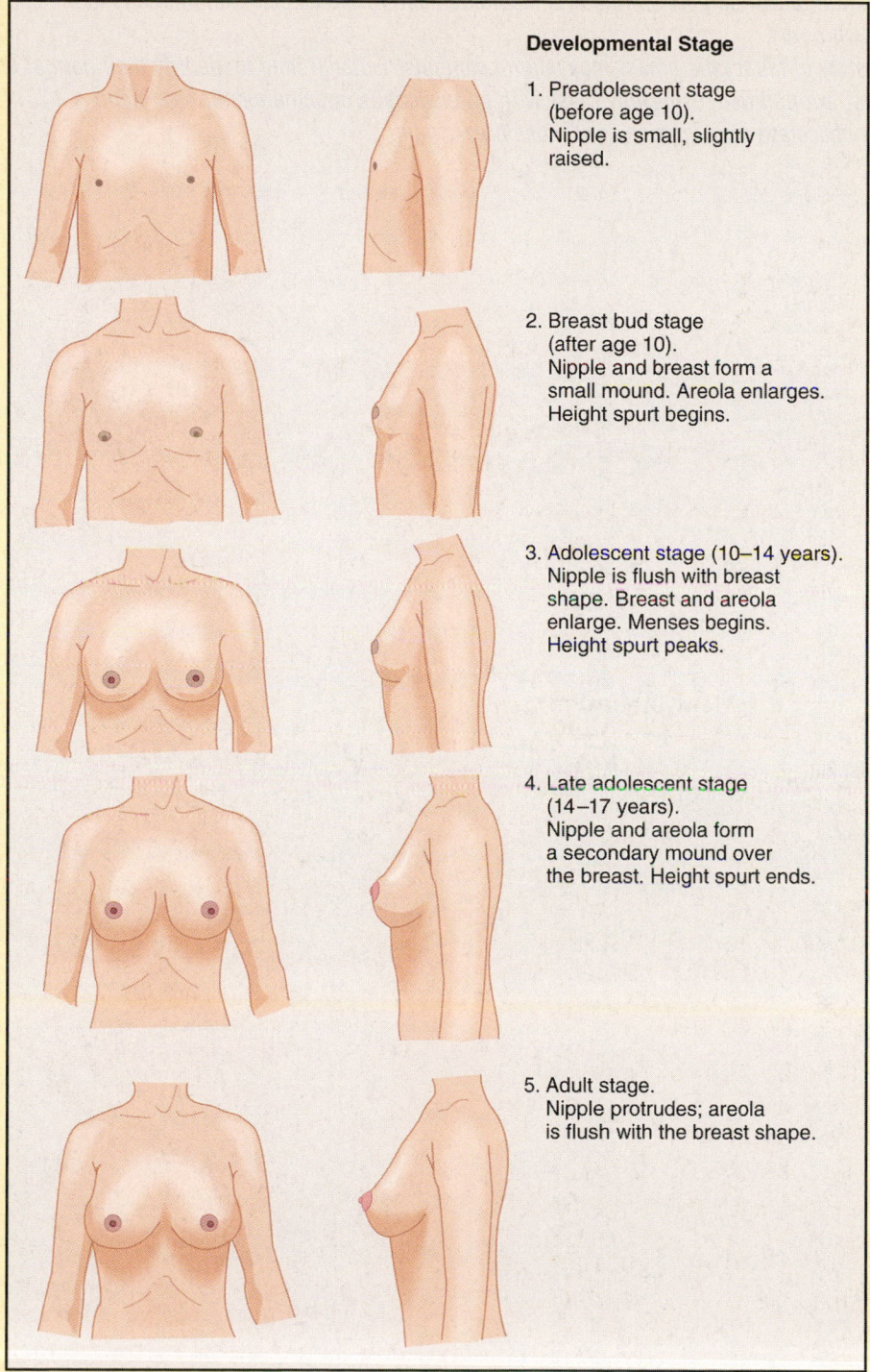

Developmental Stage

1. Preadolescent stage (before age 10). Nipple is small, slightly raised.

2. Breast bud stage (after age 10). Nipple and breast form a small mound. Areola enlarges. Height spurt begins.

3. Adolescent stage (10–14 years). Nipple is flush with breast shape. Breast and areola enlarge. Menses begins. Height spurt peaks.

4. Late adolescent stage (14–17 years). Nipple and areola form a secondary mound over the breast. Height spurt ends.

5. Adult stage. Nipple protrudes; areola is flush with the breast shape.

Data from *Health Assessment: Physical Examination,* Third Edition by M. E. Zator-Estes, 2006, Clifton Park, NY: Delmar Cengage Learning.

► **SPECIAL CONSIDERATIONS**

- *Women who have had breast surgery still need clinical and monthly breast self-examinations to the chest, clavicle, axillae, and incision areas.*
- *Women with a history of fibrocystic breast may require more instructional time to identify their normal breast tissue.*
- *Men require breast examination, especially those with gynecomastia or on hormonal treatment.*
- *Heavy caffeine or chocolate consumption may cause breast pain.*

Male Genitalia, Hernia, and Rectal Examination

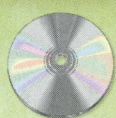

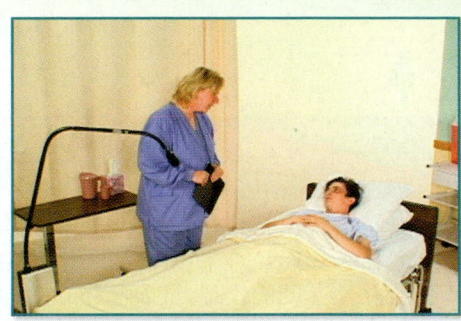

▶ OVERVIEW OF THE SKILL

Physical assessment of the male genitalia is an essential part of the physical examination. It is helpful to provide a private, warm examining area where the client is made to feel at ease. The novice examiner, as well as the client, is often anxious about the examination and will benefit greatly from a confident, professional approach by the provider. This is also a key time to educate the client about monthly testicular self-examination as a method to enhance health awareness and self-care. (Testicular cancer is the most common form of cancer in men between 20 and 35 years of age.) The best position for the examination is to have the gowned client stand and the examiner sit on a chair or stool. The examination includes inspection, palpation, and possibly transillumination of the scrotum. Areas examined are the penis, scrotum and its contents, testis, epididymis, spermatic cord, vas deferens within the cord, inguinal ring, inguinal areas, and the rectum. The genitalia and inguinal areas are exposed for the examination. The examiner should wear gloves.

▶ ASSESSMENT

1. Assess sexual maturation, the size and shape of the penis, the skin integrity to include erythema or discolorations, swelling, or lesions.
2. Note the color and texture of the scrotal skin as well as the character and distribution of pubic hair. Note size, contour, and symmetry.
3. Tanner stage for children and adolescents.
4. Assess testicular size and adnexal structures.
5. Inspect the inguinal areas and groin for nodules, swelling, or bulges.

6. Assess the cremaster reflex.
7. Assess the prostate gland for size, shape, consistency, sensitivity, and mobility of the prostate.
8. Assess the seminal vesicles for tenderness and masses.
9. Assess the sacrococcygeal and perianal areas for lumps, lesions, inflammation, excoriations, and tenderness.
10. Assess rectal sphincter tone and palpate for nodules, tenderness, induration, or irregularities of the rectal surface.

▶ DIAGNOSIS

Potential for Impaired Tissue Integrity

Health-Seeking Behaviors

Deficient Knowledge

Anxiety

▶ PLANNING

Expected Outcomes:
1. Normal penile exam. No erythema or discolorations, swelling, or lesions.
2. Normal exam of the scrotum, with normal size, contour, and symmetry.
3. Tanner stage is appropriate for age.
4. Testicular size and adnexal structures are within normal limits.
5. Inguinal areas and groin are free of nodules, swelling, and bulges.
6. The prostate gland is within normal limits for size, shape, consistency, sensitivity, and mobility.

Equipment Needed:

- Gloves
- Flashlight for transillumination
- Lubricant for rectal exam

▶ **CLIENT EDUCATION NEEDED:**

1. Instruct the client on how to prepare for the examination and what to expect to decrease unnecessary anxiety and to illicit cooperation.

2. Remind the client to inform you of any discomfort experienced during the exam.
3. Teach and encourage monthly testicular self-examination.

Estimated time to complete the skill:
15–20 minutes

▶ **DELEGATION TIPS**

Testicular examination and the concomitant client education are skills within the realm of the nurse's role and licensure and require assessment and problem-solving behaviors in addition to client teaching. These functions must not be delegated. The ancillary personnel may reinforce the importance of testicular self-examination. During the provision of personal hygiene to a male client, the ancillary personnel must note any abnormalities of the genitalia such as unusual odors, discharge, or edema.

IMPLEMENTATION—Action/Rationale

Action	Rationale
Penile Examination	
1. Ask the client to disrobe completely and to put on a gown.	1. Provides easy access for the exam.
2. Explain the procedure to the client (see Figure 1-9-1).	2. Decreases the client's anxiety level.
3. Wash hands and apply clean gloves.	3. To perform clean technique.
4. Have the client stand and hold up his gown to expose the genitalia.	4. Provides best exposure for examination.
5. Inspect the penis and pubic hair distribution. Check the skin at the base of the penis for rash, lesions, nits, or lice.	5. Tanner stage in boys; note size, color, integrity (lesions, rash, pustules).
6. Retract, or have the client retract, the prepuce (foreskin), if present.	6. The uncircumcised male client will have foreskin of the glans, which should be easily retracted. It is necessary to retract the prepuce to detect chancres or carcinoma. Smegma, a cheesy secretion, may accumulate normally under the foreskin.
7. Observe the glans penis and the urethral meatus (see Figure 1-9-2). Open the urethral meatus by compressing the glans gently between your index finger above and thumb below. Note the location of the urethral meatus as well as any discharge, ulcers, scars, nodules, lesions, or signs of inflammation.	7. The skin of the glans penis should be smooth and without ulceration. The urethral meatus is normally located ventrally on the end of the penis. There is normally no discharge. If discharge is present, obtain a culture for gonorrhea and *Chlamydia* (see Figure 1-9-2).

continues

Action	Rationale
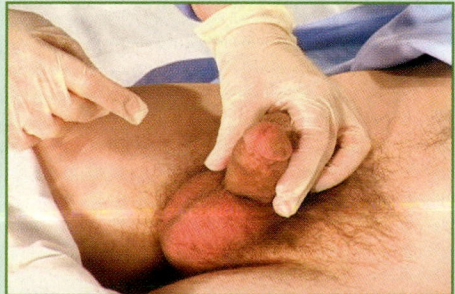 **Figure 1-9-1** Provide for the client's privacy and explain the procedure.	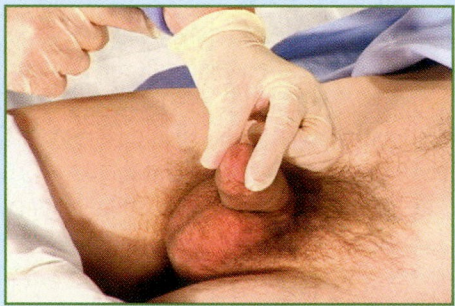 **Figure 1-9-2** Inspect the glans penis and urethral meatus.

Action	Rationale
8. Palpate the entire length of the penis between your thumb and the first two fingers (see Figure 1-9-3).	**8.** Note any tenderness, induration, or masses. Palpation of the shaft may be omitted in a young, asymptomatic client. Replace the foreskin, if retracted, before continuing with the exam.
Scrotal Examination	
9. Inspect the scrotum for erythema, discoloration, swelling, and skin integrity.	**9.** Abnormalities in the scrotum can be indicative of local trauma, inflammation, hernias, or systemic conditions, such as heart or renal failure.
10. Elicit the cremaster reflex on both sides (see Figure 1-9-4).	**10.** Absence of this reflex may be the most sensitive physical finding for torsion of the testicle. It is performed by gently stroking or pinching the superior medial aspect of the thigh, resulting in brisk ipsilateral testicular torsion or retraction.

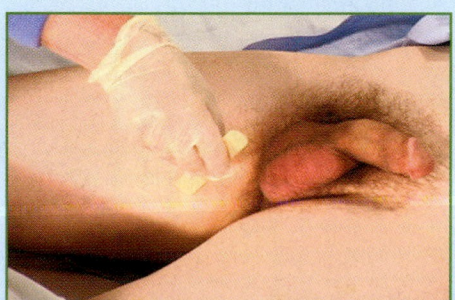

Figure 1-9-3   Use the thumb and first two fingers to palpate the entire length of the penis.

Figure 1-9-4   Elicit the cremaster reflex.

continues

Action	Rationale

Scrotal Examination *continued*

11. Palpate each testis and epididymis between the thumb and first two fingers. Note their size, lie (high or low within the scrotum), shape, consistency, and tenderness. The length of a normal testis should be greater than 4 cm and the volume greater than 20 mL.
NOTE: Testicular Torsion is a Surgical Emergency.

12. Palpate each spermatic cord, including the vas deferens within the cord, between your thumb and fingers from the epididymis to the inguinal ring. Note any nodules or swelling.

Hernia Examination

13. Inspect the inguinal and femoral areas. Ask the client to strain down or cough while you continue your observation.

14. Palpate for a **femoral** hernia by placing your fingers on the anterior thigh in the region of the femoral canal. Ask the client to bear down or cough as you note any palpable masses, tenderness, or swelling.

15. Palpate for an **inguinal** hernia. Using your right hand for the client's right side and your left hand for the client's left side, just above the testicle, invaginate the loose scrotal skin with your index finger. Follow the spermatic cord upward to find a triangular slit-like opening of the external inguinal ring. If the inguinal ring is enlarged enough to admit your finger, then gently follow the inguinal canal and ask the client to cough. Note any herniating mass felt against the finger.

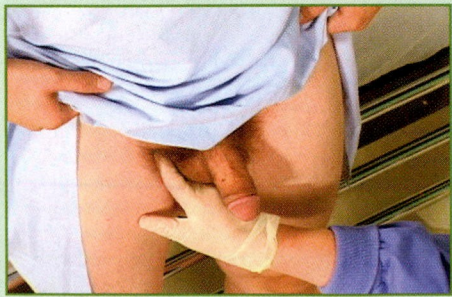

Figure 1-9-5 Palpate for a femoral hernia.

11. The left testicle normally sits slightly lower than the right testicle. The testicles are rubbery and approximately equal in size.
Pressure on the testis normally produces a deep visceral pain.
Twisting or torsion of the testis causes venous obstruction, edema, and eventually arterial obstruction (rarely seen in clients older than 20–30 years of age). It is a significant cause of sterility and morbidity in men.

12. Any swelling in the scrotum should be evaluated by transillumination. Shine a beam of light (flashlight) from behind the scrotum through the mass. Normal testes do not transilluminate. Look for transmission of light as a red glow: swellings that contain serious fluid (hydrocele, spermatocele) transilluminate.

13. A bulge that presents on straining suggests a hernia.

14. Small (1.0 cm), freely mobile lymph notes may normally be found in the inguinal area (see Figure 1-9-5).

15. If present, a herniating mass will generally be felt against the side of the finger (see Figure 1-9-6).

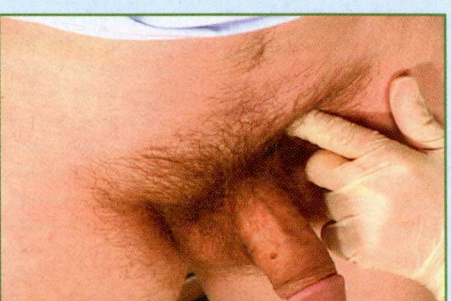

Figure 1-9-6 Palpate for an inguinal hernia.

continues

Action	Rationale

Rectal Examination

16. If the client is standing after the completion of the genital examination, have him bend and lean on the exam table, with legs slightly apart, exposing the rectum to the examiner. Or:
Ask the client to lie in a lateral decubitus position, on his left side, placing his buttocks close to the edge of the table nearest the examiner. Flex the client's hips and knees to stabilize the client and improve visibility.

16. Positions the client for ease of examination.

17. Provide a warm, quiet environment with appropriate lighting. Drape the client so that only his buttocks are exposed. Explain the procedure to the client.

17. Decreases the client's anxiety and provides privacy. Gentle, slow movement of the examiner's finger accompanied by explanation and a calm demeanor will ensure a successful exam.

18. Wash hands and apply clean gloves.

18. This is a clean procedure.

19. Spread apart the buttocks and examine the anus, perianal area, and sacral region for any scars, lesions, nodules, inflammation, ulcerations, or abnormalities. Ask the client to bear down as you assess for any bulges (see Figure 1-9-7).

19. Adult perianal skin is normally more pigmented and coarser than the skin over the buttocks.
As the client strains down, note any tissue protrusions or hemorrhoids. Reassure the client that sensations of urination and defecation are normal.

20. Lubricate the gloved index finger. As the client strains down, rest the pad of the finger over the anus. As the sphincter relaxes, slowly insert the finger into the anal canal, with the finger facing the umbilicus. Note sphincter tone and any masses, nodules, or tenderness.

20. The anal canal is approximately 2.5 cm long. It is bordered by the external and internal anal sphincters, which normally are firm and smooth.

21. Insert the finger as far as possible into the rectum. Rotate your hand to palpate the walls of the rectum laterally and posteriorly while rotating your index finger.

21. The wall of the rectum should be smooth and moist.

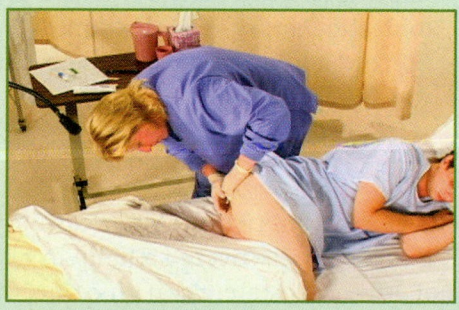

Figure 1-9-7 Left dorsal positioning for rectal examination.

continues

Action	Rationale
Rectal Examination *continued*	
22. Anteriorally palpate the two lobes of the prostate gland and its sulcus. Note the size, shape, and consistency of the prostate as you identify any irregularities such as nodules, masses, or tenderness.	22. Inform the client that he may feel the urge to urinate when you examine the prostate, that this is a normal sensation, and that he will not void. The male prostate gland is approximately 2.5 cm long. It is smooth, nonmovable, nontender, and rubbery to the touch.
23. If possible, extend your finger above the prostate region and palpate the superior portion of the lateral lobe to the region of the seminal vesicles and the peritoneal cavity.	23. The seminal vesicles are not normally palpable unless swollen. Note nodules, cysts, or tenderness.
24. Gently withdraw your finger. Note the color of any fecal material on your glove and test for occult blood.	24. There is normally no occult blood in the stools.
25. Offer the client tissues or wipe excess lubricant/stool from the anus.	25. Provide for client comfort.

▶ REAL WORLD ANECDOTES

Mr. Amin is a 35-year-old Somalian who presents to the clinic complaining of a swollen right testicle. It causes him pain when he turns his foot out to the side and when he bends over. He states that he is sexually active and usually uses condoms during coitus. On examination, his right testicle is enlarged and tender. His epididymis also is very tender on this side. You obtain a culture from the meatal opening and send it to the lab. Then you get a urine sample for culture and sensitivity testing. It is important to get the culture from the penis before you get the urine culture, because the urine will wash away the specimen needed for a diagnosis of Chlamydia. You treat Mr. Amin for Chlamydia and give him information about preventing sexually transmitted diseases.

▶ EVALUATION

• Any abnormalities are identified early for treatment and/or referral evaluation.
• The client is able to perform monthly testicular self-examinations.
• The client returns to his health care provider for regular checkups.

▶ DOCUMENTATION

Nurses' Notes

• Record the date and time of the examination.
• Include the client's physiologic findings of abnormalities and absence of abnormalities.

• Record the client's response to the findings.
• Document instruction and return demonstration of testicular self-examination.
• Record a follow-up plan, if necessary.

▶ CRITICAL THINKING SKILL

Introduction

Mr. Gomez, an African-American 50-year-old laborer, states he has discovered a lump in his testicle. He has not had a prostate exam since he was 40 years old, and he was fine at that time.

Possible Scenario

- He ignores the lump as a normal sign of aging.

Possible Outcome

- The lump may be a malignancy from prostate cancer.

Prevention

Advise Mr. Gomez never to disregard a lump. He should report it to his health care provider immediately.

Commend him for performing self-testicular exams and encourage him to have yearly clinical examinations. African-American men are at increased risk for prostate cancer and should be screened regularly with prostate-specific antigen (PSA) testing and digital rectal examination.

► VARIATIONS

Geriatric Variation:

- *The external genitalia reveals thinner, sometimes gray, pubic hair in elderly clients.*
- *The penis decreases in size, and the testicles may appear small or atrophied as they hang lower in the scrotum.*
- *Testosterone production and secretion decrease with age; however, serum levels may be in the low-normal range through the age of 80 years.*
- *The ability to attain an erection may be delayed, and full erection is not always possible.*
- *The elderly male might note a reduction or absence in pre-ejaculatory fluid emission. Advise sexually active older men that spermatogenesis may continue into advanced age.*

Pediatric Variation:

- *Check for sexual maturity rating in boys by using the Tanner Staging criteria. A noticeable increase in the size of the testes, usually between the ages of 9.5 and 13.5 years, is a sign of initiation of puberty. Next, pubic hair begins to grow and the penis increases in size. The change from preadolescent to adult takes about 3 years, with a range from less than 2 years to almost 5 years.*

Home Care Variations:

- *If a client is disabled, he may not be able to perform testicular self-examination. He may need a health care provider to do so and relay any significant findings to the physician.*

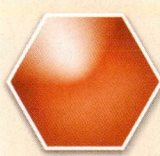

Long-Term Care Variations:

- *Urinary retention and incontinence may occur related to prostatic changes in the elderly. It is imperative to provide yearly checkups and testicular self-examination in this population.*

► COMMON ERRORS

Possible Errors:

The client presented with an enlarged scrotum and urinary frequency, and was asked for a urine sample.

Prevention:

With a male client, always obtain the urine specimen **after** the physical examination because a sample from the urinary meatus may be needed. When *Chlamydia* is suspected, the meatus must be swabbed for a culture. Urination washes away the sample and should be deferred until the culture is taken.

► **NURSING TIPS**

- If a large scrotal mass is found, ask the client to lie down for further examination. If the mass returns to the abdomen, a hernia is confirmed. If you can get your fingers above the mass in the scrotum, then a hydrocele is suspected. Listen to the mass with a stethoscope. Bowel sounds can be heard over a hernia but not over a hydrocele.
- When the uncircumcised male client is examined, the foreskin must be retracted for a thorough examination. This prepuce must be returned to its normal position after the examination to prevent injury to the client.

► **SPECIAL CONSIDERATIONS**

- *When a client presents with testicular torsion, the history may reveal a minor similar pain in the past that resolved spontaneously. Clients usually present with sudden onset of severe, unilateral scrotal pain that may be associated with nausea and vomiting. Scrotal edema and erythema as well as abdominal pain may occur.*
- *According to the American Urological Association, African-American men and men with a first-degree relative with prostate cancer should be evaluated with annual PSA testing and rectal examination beginning at 40 years of age. All other men should have an initial evaluation at 50 years of age.*
- *Use latex free gloves to avoid reaction to natural rubber latex.*

Collecting a Clean-Catch, Midstream Urine Specimen

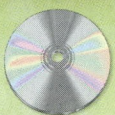

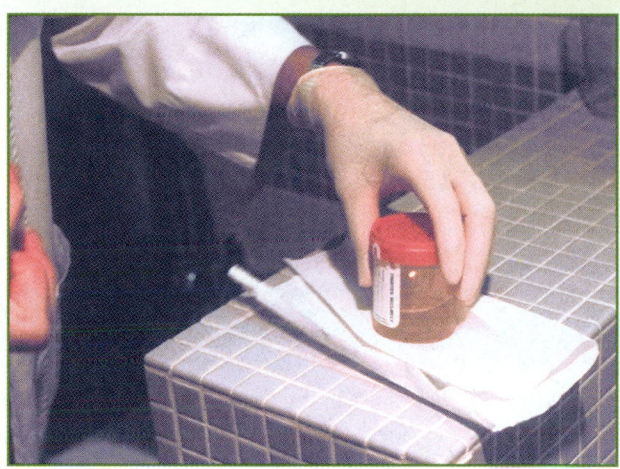

▶ OVERVIEW OF THE SKILL

A clean urine specimen to be used for culture and sensitivity can be collected without using an invasive method such as catheterization. This procedure is referred to as a clean-voided, clean-catch, or midstream urine specimen in that it is not a sterile procedure such as catheterization but, rather, a method of obtaining a clean specimen. This procedure is best accomplished with the client on the toilet because the use of a urinal or bedpan increases the risk of contamination. The client is asked to clean him-or herself and initiate urination. After the client starts voiding, a sterile collection cup is placed under the stream of urine and a specimen collected. Hence, it is called midstream collection. The initial urine is not collected because this portion of the stream flushes the urethral opening and meatus of any bacteria. The end urine is not collected because as the urine stream slows and increased dripping and contact with the meatus occurs, the chance of contamination increases. The clean-catch specimen is sent to a laboratory for analysis.

▶ ASSESSMENT

1. Evaluate the client's ability to obtain a clean-catch specimen **to determine whether the client is able to clean him-or herself appropriately and understands the need to obtain a midstream specimen.**

2. Assess the presence of signs and symptoms of urinary tract infections or other abnormalities **because burning or the inability to control urination may hamper the client's ability to obtain a clean specimen.**

▶ DIAGNOSIS

Impaired Urinary Elimination

Pain

Deficient Knowledge

Disturbed Body Image

▶ PLANNING

Expected Outcomes:

1. Client will be able to obtain a clean, midstream specimen.
2. Client will have absence of urinary abnormalities, such as burning, tingling, pain upon urination, or inability to control stream.
3. Client will understand the procedure.

Equipment Needed (see Figure 1-10-1):

- Sterile collection container with lid and label
- Sterile midstream kit, antiseptic towelettes, or cotton balls with antiseptic solution
- Toilet paper
- Nonsterile latex free gloves
- Sterile gauze (optional)

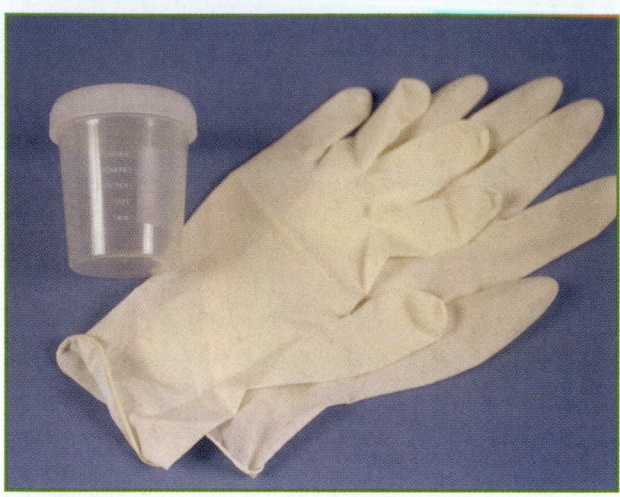

Figure 1-10-1   Sterile specimen cup and gloves

▶ **CLIENT EDUCATION NEEDED:**

1. Instruct clients regarding the need for a clean, noncontaminated specimen.
2. Instruct clients how to collect specimen, open kit or towelettes, and use antiseptic solutions.
3. Instruct clients regarding need for procedure.

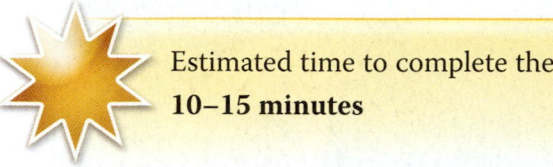

Estimated time to complete the skill:
10–15 minutes

▶ **DELEGATION TIPS**

Collection of a clean-catch specimen may be delegated to ancillary personnel properly trained in the technique of cleaning the client and obtaining the voided specimen.

IMPLEMENTATION—Action/Rationale

Action	Rationale
1. Check orders and assess need for the procedure.	1. Provides understanding of the purpose of the procedure.
2. Gather equipment.	2. Provides for organization.
3. Assess the client's ability to complete the procedure, including understanding, mobility, and balance.	3. Improves compliance and likelihood of obtaining sterile specimen.
4. Assess the client for signs and symptoms of urinary abnormalities.	4. Improves compliance and provides baseline data.
5. Check the client's identification.	5. Ensures accuracy.
6. If the client is to complete the procedure in privacy, explain the procedure, give equipment to the client, and wait for specimen. If the client has decreased personal hygiene, perform the procedure after a bath or have the client wash the perineal area before a procedure.	6. Increases compliance. Protects client from embarrassment.
7. If the nurse is to perform the procedure: wash hands and apply gloves. If the client is to perform the procedure, instruct the client to wash hands before and after the procedure. If the client is more comfortable, allow him or her to wear gloves.	7. Decreases transmission of microorganisms.
8. Provide privacy.	8. Decreases embarrassment.

continues

Action	Rationale

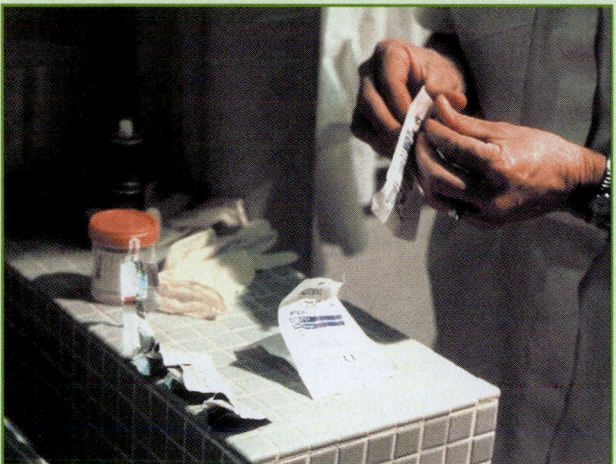

Figure 1-10-2   Open specimen cup and kit or cleansing towel packages prior to beginning the procedure.

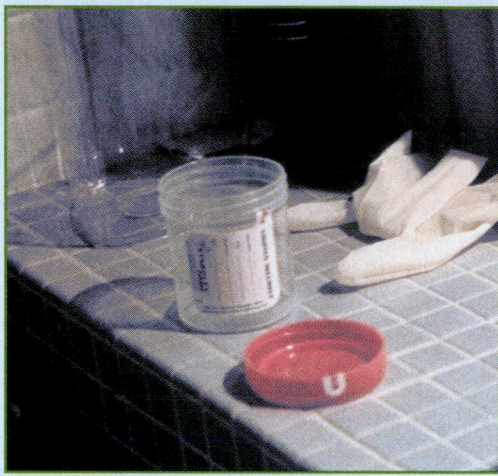

Figure 1-10-3   Place the lid on a firm surface, sterile side up. Do not touch the inside of the lid.

9. Instruct the client. Female client: Sit with legs separated on the toilet. Male client: Sit down to help control splashing.

9. Increases compliance and understanding.

10. Using sterile procedure, open kit or towelettes (see Figure 1-10-2). Open sterile container, placing the lid with sterile side up on a firm surface (see Figure 1-10-3).

10. Prevents contamination of the specimen.

11. Female client: Use the thumb and forefinger to separate the labia, or have the client separate the labia with fingers (see Figure 1-10-4).

With the labia separated, use a downward stroke (from the top of the labia down toward the rectal area), and cleanse one side of the labia with the towelette (see Figure 1-10-5).

Discard the towelette and repeat the procedure on the other side with another towelette, keeping the labia separated at all times. With a third towelette, use a downward stroke from the top of the urethral opening to the bottom. Discard the towelette.

11. Provides access for cleaning the labia.

Cleanses area and prevents contamination of clean area. Prevents contamination by feces. Keeping labia separated avoids contamination and decreases microorganisms in specimen.

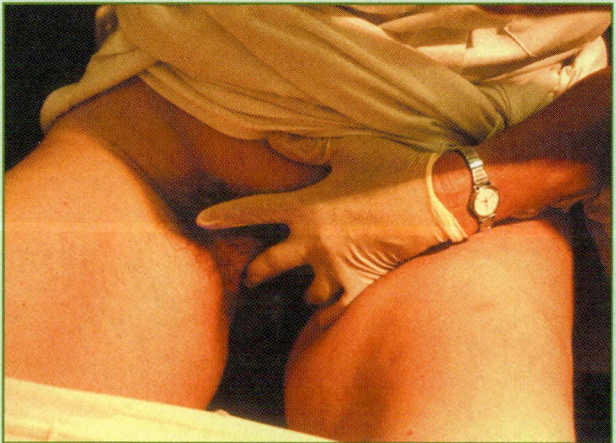

Figure 1-10-4   Separate the labia with the fingers of the nondominant hand.

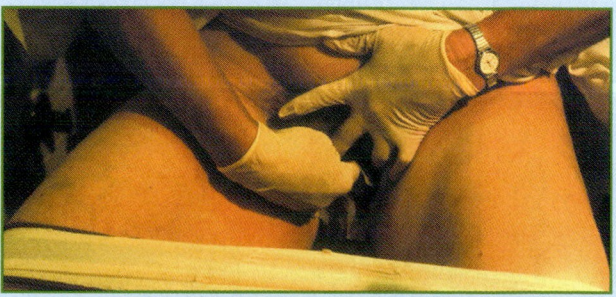

Figure 1-10-5   Cleanse each side and down the middle using a single downward stroke for each towelette. Keep the labia separated.

continues

Action	Rationale

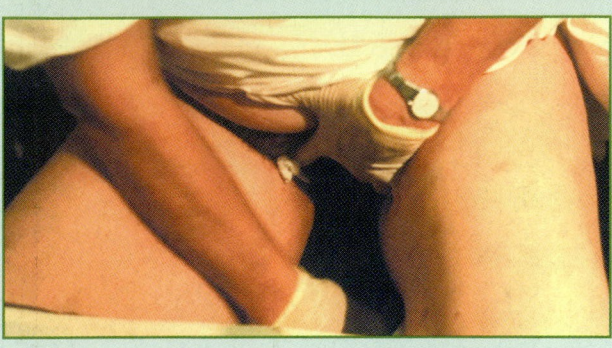

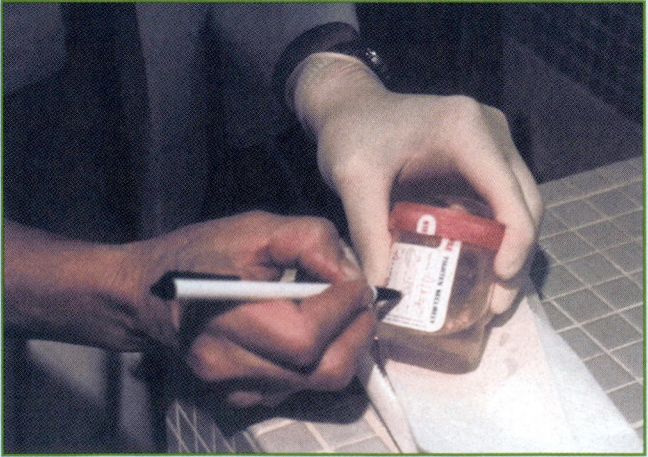

Figure 1-10-6 Place the specimen cup under the urine stream.

12. Male client: Pull back the foreskin (if present in uncircumcised male) and clean with a single stroke around meatus and glans.

Use a circular motion starting with the head of the penis at the urethral opening, moving down the glans shaft.

Discard the towelette and repeat the procedure with another towelette, keeping the foreskin retracted. Cleanse the head of the penis three times using a circular motion. Use a new towelette each time.

12. Prevents contamination of microorganisms from foreskin. Single strokes and moving away from the opening prevents contamination of the urethral opening.

13. Ask the client to begin to urinate into the toilet. After the stream starts with good flow, place the collection cup under the stream of urine. Avoid touching the skin with the container. Fill the container with 30 to 60 mL of urine and remove the container before urination ceases (see Figure 1-10-6). Wipe with toilet paper.

13. The specimen is collected midstream to avoid contamination of urine that touches the labia. The initial urine flushes bacteria from the orifice and the end urine may have contact with the meatus or labia and, hence, be contaminated.

14. Place the sterile lid back onto the container and close tightly (see Figure 1-10-7).

Clean and dry the outside of the container with a towelette. Wash hands. Label and enclose in a plastic biohazard bag (see Figure 1-10-8), and follow facility policy for transporting specimen to the laboratory.

14. Prevents contamination of sterile specimen, prevents spillage, and ensures accuracy.

15. Remove and dispose of gloves and wash hands.

15. Decreases transmission of microorganisms.

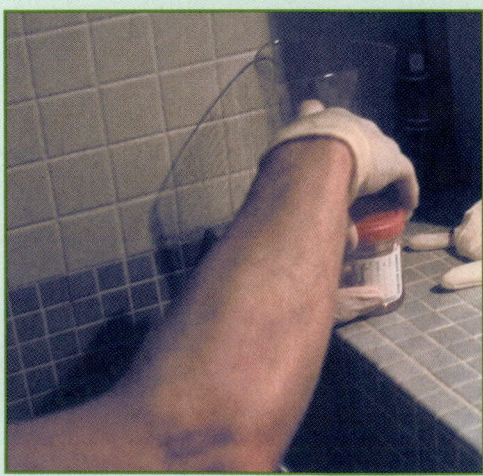

Figure 1-10-7 Replace the lid and close tightly.

Figure 1-10-8 Label the container with the client, date, and time the specimen was collected.

▶ EVALUATION

- Evaluate characteristics of urine.
- Evaluate client's compliance.
- Evaluate client's complaints associated with urination, such as burning, pain, or inability to initiate urination.

▶ DOCUMENTATION

Nurses' Notes

- Document procedure.
- Document characteristics of urine.
- Document client's signs and symptoms associated with urination.

▶ CRITICAL THINKING SKILL

Introduction

Helping a client overcome embarrassment can prevent an invasive procedure.

Possible Scenario

A client came into the emergency room at 2:30 a.m. with a fever of 102.3°F, complaining of bloody urine, dizziness, chills, and pelvic pain. The physician ordered a clean-catch urine specimen. The client was given a sterile specimen cup and ordered to go into the bathroom and return with the sample immediately, because the lab courier was waiting. At the front counter, with several staff and family members within earshot, the nurse gave the client instructions on how to clean herself and void.

Possible Outcome

Embarrassed by the request to void on demand, and the thought that several people knew she was in the bathroom, the client was not able to void. The nurse was unable to collect a specimen. After several attempts, the physician ordered the client catheterized to obtain a sterile sample.

Prevention

Increase fluids. Provide both visual and auditory privacy for client education. Assess the client for signs of anxiety and embarrassment, and plan the procedure to minimize embarrassment and provide support and education. If the client is having difficulty complying, obtain a specimen later, if possible. Plan ahead, if possible, and encourage fluids before it is time to collect the specimen. Do not stand over the client and do not stand immediately outside the door unless there is a risk of fainting or falling. If the client is embarrassed, leave the room after the explanation. Inform the client that you are leaving and when you will return. Point out the assistance call button before leaving. Instruct the client to call when the specimen is collected. Use techniques to encourage urination, such as running water, applying a moist compress over the abdomen or labia in women, pouring water over the labia, and placing hands under warm water.

▶ REAL WORLD ANECDOTES

Mr. Alvarez, 65 years old, is asked to provide a urine specimen. The nurse gives him a container and instructions on how to obtain a sterile clean-catch specimen. Mr. Alvarez is afraid he will not be able to produce enough urine if he waits for a midstream collection so he places the cup before beginning urination. When he returns the filled specimen cup, the nurse asks him if he followed her instructions. He admits that he did not get the sample midstream. The nurse explains the importance of following the procedure to obtain a sterile sample. Mr. Alvarez is asked to return after lunch.

▶ VARIATIONS

Geriatric Variations:

- *Elderly clients may have difficulty controlling stream and need assistance in cleaning and catching the urine midstream.*
- *If arthritis is present, the client may have difficulty holding labia apart.*
- *Labia are enlarged with age and can be difficult to keep separated.*

continues

► VARIATIONS *(continued)*

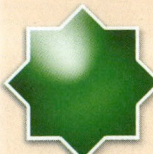

Pediatric Variations:
- *Explain the procedure to a family member.*
- *In young children, parents may prefer to obtain the specimen.*
- *Teenagers may be especially embarrassed by the request for a specimen and need control and privacy over the procedure when possible.*

Home Care Variations:
- *Ensure that client understands the need for the sterile specimen.*
- *Specimens must be fresh and transported to the laboratory shortly after collection. Plan a specimen collection time and a time when the specimen will be delivered to the laboratory.*
- *If specimens will be collected at home, ensure that the client has a sterile specimen cup and towelettes. Instruct clients to place container in a plastic bag with sealable top and refrigerate until it is delivered to a laboratory; this prevents the growth of bacteria and promotes accuracy of results.*

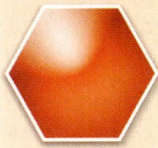

Long-Term Care Variations:
- *Ensure that client understands the need for the sterile specimen.*
- *Specimens must be fresh and transported to the laboratory shortly after collection. Plan a specimen collection time and a time when the specimen will be delivered to the laboratory.*
- *If specimens will be collected at home, ensure that the client has a sterile specimen cup and towelettes. Instruct clients to place container in a plastic bag with sealable top and to refrigerate it until it is delivered to a laboratory; this prevents the growth of bacteria and promotes accuracy of results.*

► COMMON ERRORS

Possible Error:
Specimen is contaminated because the client does not understand the cleaning procedure and need for the specimen to be collected midstream.

Prevention:
Explain to the client the importance of obtaining a clean specimen and the correct procedure. Ask the client to provide another sample.

Possible Error:
Specimen contaminated by labia not held apart during voiding.

Prevention:
Explain to the client the importance of obtaining a clean specimen and the correct procedure. Ask the client to provide another sample.

Possible Error:
The specimen container lid is placed upside down on a surface and contaminated.

Prevention:
Do not use the contaminated lid. Obtain a new one instead.

Possible Error:
The specimen is not labeled.

Prevention:
Always label the specimen immediately after it is obtained. There is no other way to identify the specimen.

► **NURSING TIPS**

- Labia may be slippery after cleansing; therefore, use sterile dry gauze to hold apart during urination.
- Clients often do not understand the need to remove the specimen container before completing urination; therefore, carefully explain the purpose for midstream collection.
- Encourage fluids before collecting specimen, if not contraindicated.

- If the client is unable to void, run tap water within hearing distance or place a warm compress over the bladder.
- Place the lid on a firm surface within close reach.
- Send the specimen to the laboratory immediately. It must be fresh for accurate analysis.
- Label the time of collection on the specimen.
- If a container touches the client's skin and is contaminated, obtain a new specimen cup. If necessary, arrange to have the client return to obtain another specimen.

► **SPECIAL CONSIDERATIONS**

- *Urine samples should be sent to the laboratory within 30 minutes. If this is not possible, the specimen may be refrigerated for 2 to 4 hours. Delaying the lab testing may alter the test results.*
- *Menstrual blood may alter the test results. In a menstruating client, perineal care should be performed before urine specimen collection, and a tampon or 4 × 4 gauze pad may be placed in the vaginal orifice to prevent contamination of urine by vaginal secretion or blood. Notify the lab of the possible presence of menstrual blood.*
- *When initiating a 24-hour urine sample, the client must void before starting the collection process to provide an accurate measurement.*
- *Clients with urinary tract infections may have difficulty controlling the stream of urine and may need assistance.*
- *Avoid using latex gloves when coming in contact with mucous membranes to avoid reaction to latex.*

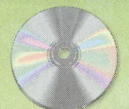

Testing Urine for Specific Gravity, Ketones, Glucose, and Occult Blood

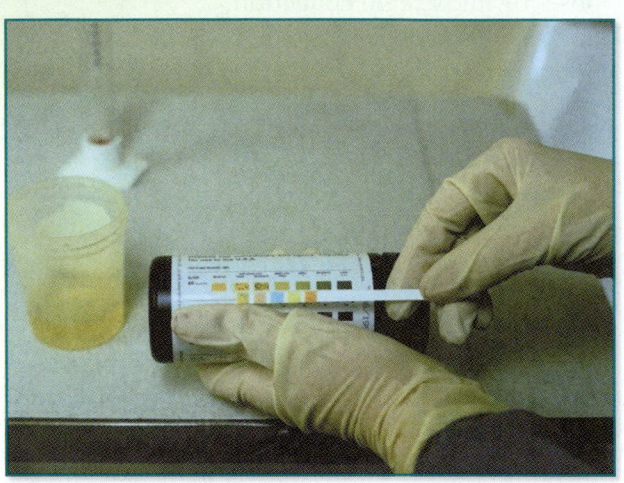

▶ OVERVIEW OF THE SKILL

Urine samples can be used to test specific gravity, ketones, glucose blood, pH, protein, nitrates, and bilirubin. Specific gravity is the concentration of dissolved substances in the urine compared with water. The normal range of specific gravity is between approximately 1.010 and 1.025 g/mL. If urine is dilute and less concentrated, the specific gravity will be closer to that of water with no substances, 1.000. Overhydration, or any disease that affects the ability of the body to concentrate substances in the urine, will cause a low specific gravity. Any condition that increases water reabsorption in the kidney will result in a high specific gravity.

Specific gravity testing takes only a few minutes. A rough screen can be done using a dipstick that measures specific gravity, such as a reagent strip. Reagent strips measure specific gravity through color changes, which are compared with a chart provided by the manufacturer. For greater precision, a urinometer or refractometer may be used. A urinometer measures specific gravity by displacement. Dissolved substances in the urine will push, or displace, the bulb upward. A reading is taken at the meniscus. The measurement revealed by the urinometer is a comparison of where the bulb would be floating in pure water. Concentrated particles in the urine push the bulb higher and yield a higher reading. A refractometer measures specific gravity using the refraction of light as it passes through a drop of urine on glass. A beam of light passing through the urine will bend and change direction. The amount of the bend, or refraction, is changed by the amount of dissolved substances in the urine. When frequent, exact measurements of specific gravity are required, refractometers are the best choice; however, refractometers are expensive compared with urinometers or dipsticks.

Test strips or dipsticks that are specific for ketones, glucose, blood, pH, proteins, nitrates, and bilirubin can be used to measure specific substances. These products use various names. Some examples and substances measured are Ketostix (ketones), Keto-Diastix (glucose, ketones), Clinistix and Diastix (glucose), Hemastix (blood), Hemacombistix (pH, protein, glucose, blood), Uristix (protein, glucose, nitrite, leukocytes), and Labstix (pH, protein, glucose, ketone, blood). Many other examples are available. Other products can also be used to measure bilirubin, phenylketones, and leukocytes.

Multistix can be used to measure many possible substances (glucose, ketones, specific gravity, blood, pH, protein, nitrite, leukocytes, urobilinogen, and bilirubin). Sticks that measure multiple substances are generally more expensive. Tablets are available to measure glucose; however, these products are rarely used because dipsticks are readily available and easy to use. Many different systemic changes can cause glucose, ketones, or blood in the urine. The presence of glucose usually indicates an increased blood glucose level (usually greater than 180 mg/dL); however, renal threshold can vary with each client. Most often, blood-glucose levels are used rather than urine-glucose levels; however, this does require a venipuncture or finger prick. Ketones are present in the urine in cases of starvation, dehydration, and diabetic acidosis. The presence of ketones in the urine indicates that the body is burning fats for energy. Ketones alter the pH of urine to acidic. Blood in the urine indicates bleeding in the renal system or erythrocyte breakdown elsewhere in the body, such as in trauma. Local bleeding such as that from menstruation, surgery or, in women, a recent birth may cause blood in the urine.

▶ ASSESSMENT

1. Assess the client's understanding of the urine test to be performed. **Determines what education should be provided.**
2. Assess the client's hydration, such as skin turgor, condition of the mucous membranes, fontanels (in infants), sunken eyes, intake, and output. **Provides information to help determine physical status in addition to urine tests.**
3. Assess the client's history for renal function (e.g., medical history and lab values, creatinine clearance). **Influences how the results of tests might be interpreted. Influences what tests might be performed.**
4. If measuring glucose, assess the client for signs and symptoms of increased glucose (polyuria, polydipsia, polyphagia, recent loss of weight, fatigue). **Provides information to help determine physical status in addition to urine tests.**
5. If the client is to perform long-term tests, assess the client's ability to perform the tests. **Determines what education should be provided.**

▶ DIAGNOSIS

Excess Fluid Volume

Deficient Fluid Volume

Imbalanced Nutrition: More Than Body Requirements

Imbalanced Nutrition: Less Than Body Requirements

Deficient Knowledge

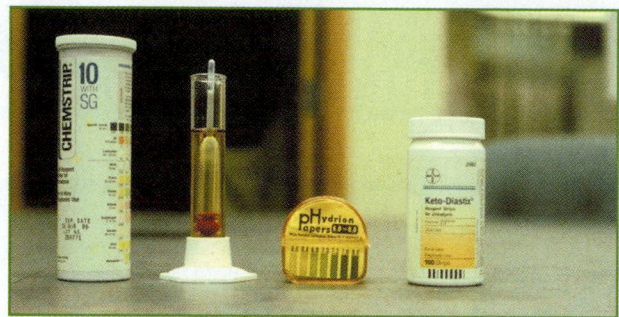

Figure 1-11-1 Reagent strips, pH papers, and urinometers are used to test urine for concentration, pH level, and specific substances, such as blood or ketones.

▶ PLANNING

Expected Outcomes:

1. Normal specific gravity.
2. Absence of glucose and ketones in the urine.
3. The client understands the purpose of the test.
4. The client understands how to perform the test (if it is needed on a long-term basis).

Equipment Needed (see Figure 1-11-1):

- Urine specimen container
- Urinometer or refractometer for specific gravity
- Dipstick specific to product to measure
- Nonsterile gloves
- Watch or clock

▶ CLIENT EDUCATION NEEDED:

1. Carefully explain the purpose of the test to the client.
2. Instruct the client on the need for an uncontaminated specimen.
3. Instruct the client on the need for a second voided specimen for accuracy.
4. If the test is abnormal, explain what changes are necessary, for example, increased glucose or dietary changes.

Estimated time to complete the skill:
5 minutes to collect urine;
5 minutes to perform test

▶ DELEGATION TIP

Testing urine is routinely delegated to properly trained ancillary personnel. The prompt reporting of abnormal results and the recording of all results on the correct clinical records are essential.

IMPLEMENTATION—Action/Rationale

Action	Rationale

Overview—Measuring Specific Gravity

1. Wash hands. Apply nonsterile gloves.

2. Obtain urine from the client either via clean-catch method (Skill 1-10) or from catheter.

3. Measure the specific gravity using equipment available in your facility.

4. Discard urine according to Standard Precautions.

5. Remove gloves and wash hands.

6. Clean the equipment with soap and water or according to the manufacturer's instructions.

7. Record the results and compare with the previous recording.

Using a Digital Clinical Refractometer to Measure Specific Gravity

8. To use a digital refractometer (see Figure 1-11-2), become familiar with the manufacturer's instructions.

9. Use an eye dropper to drip urine onto the prism at the center of the stainless steel stage until the prism is covered.

10. Press the start/off button, or the button designated by the manufacturer, to activate the meter. The specific gravity reading is displayed.

Rationale:

1. Reduces the transmission of microorganisms.

2. Acquires a pure sample for testing.

3. Obtains a measurement using equipment available in your facility.

4. Reduces the transmission of microorganisms.

5. Reduces the transmission of microorganisms.

6. Reduces the transmission of microorganisms and prepares equipment for the next use.

7. Allows for accuracy and monitoring of the client.

8. Ensures an accurate test.

9. Following the manufacturer's instructions ensures an accurate reading.

10. Following the manufacturer's instructions ensures an accurate reading.

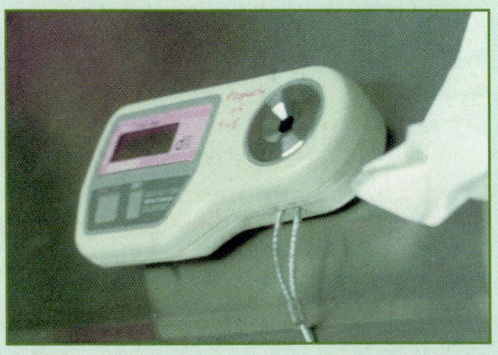

Figure 1-11-2 Digital refractometer is used to measure specific gravity of urine.

continues

Action	Rationale
Using a Nondigital Refractometer to Measure Specific Gravity	
11. For a urine refractometer: Collect a few drops of urine.	11. Refractometers require only a drop or two of urine to measure specific gravity.
12. Place a drop of urine on the horizontal glass slide at the top of the scope.	12. Following the manufacturer's instructions ensures an accurate reading.
13. Close the cover over the slide and turn on the light.	13. Following the manufacturer's instructions ensures an accurate reading.
14. Look through the scope with one eye while keeping both eyes open.	14. It is easier to visualize if both eyes are kept open.
15. Read the number at the line where the top black and lower white circles meet. Write down the number.	15. Following the manufacturer's instructions ensures an accurate reading. Records an accurate reading because refractors are often kept in the utility room away from charting area.
16. Clean the slide with a damp towel or gauze, or according to manufacturer's recommendations.	16. Ensures equipment is ready for next use.
Using a Urinometer to Measure Specific Gravity	
17. To measure specific gravity with a urinometer, at least 20 cc of urine are needed. Pour fresh urine specimen into glass cylinder to indicated line of urinometer, approximately two-thirds to three-quarters full (see Figure 1-11-3).	17. There must be enough time to make the bulb float, but it should not overfill the urinometer. The bulb should not touch the bottom of the urinometer. The meniscus of urine should be slightly below the top of the urinometer.
18. Place urinometer on flat surface and gently spin the top of the glass stem (see Figure 1-11-4).	18. Necessary to obtain an accurate reading.
19. Wait until the stem stops moving up and down, then visualize the urinometer scale at eye level. Read at lowest point of meniscus where the urine level touches the calibrated scale (see Figure 1-11-5).	19. Necessary to obtain accurate results.

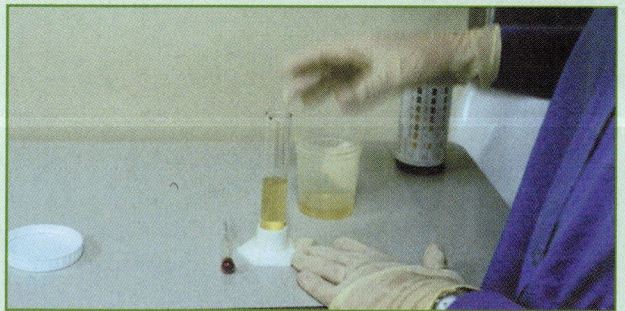

Figure 1-11-3   Fill the glass cylinder to the line with fresh urine.

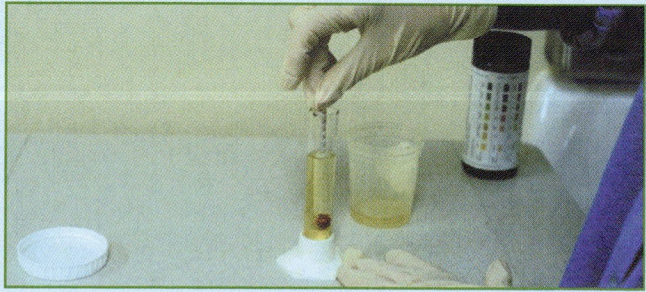

Figure 1-11-4   Spin the glass stem in the urine.

continues

Action	Rationale
Using a Dipstick to Test Urine for Glucose, Ketones, Occult Blood, or Specific Gravity	
20. Collect a clean voided specimen.	20. Ensures accurate results.
21. Obtain the correct product for testing. Check the expiration date.	21. Products vary according to what is being measured. An expired product may produce an inaccurate reading.
22. Review the instructions on the label. Visualize which color scale will be used.	22. Accurate timing of reading is necessary for accurate results. Different manufacturers and different products require different procedures.
23. Follow the directions. The dipstick will usually be dipped into the container of urine and read at a specified time interval and according to a color scale on the bottle or tape holder, as indicated by the manufacturer's instructions (see Figure 1-11-6).	23. Direction may vary according to the product used. Check manufacturer's accompanying instructions for color indicator scale and time to be read.
24. Record the results.	24. Because the procedure is generally done in the utility room, results should be written down so accurate information will be transferred to the chart.
25. Discard the urine and strip according to Standard Precautions.	25. Reduces the transmission of microorganisms.
26. Remove gloves and wash hands.	26. Reduces the transmission of microorganisms.

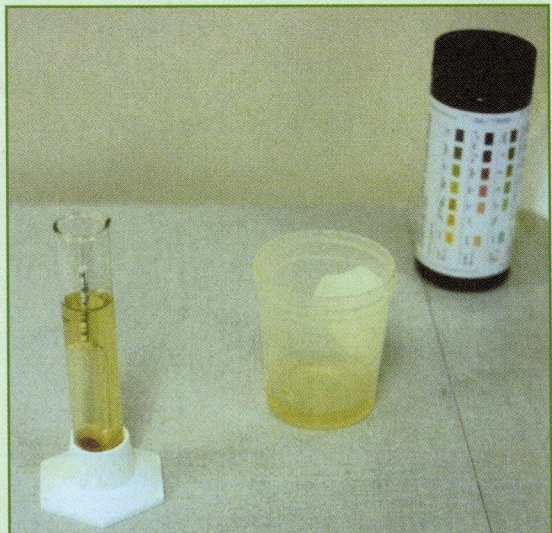

Figure 1-11-5   Read the calibrated scale when the stem stops spinning.

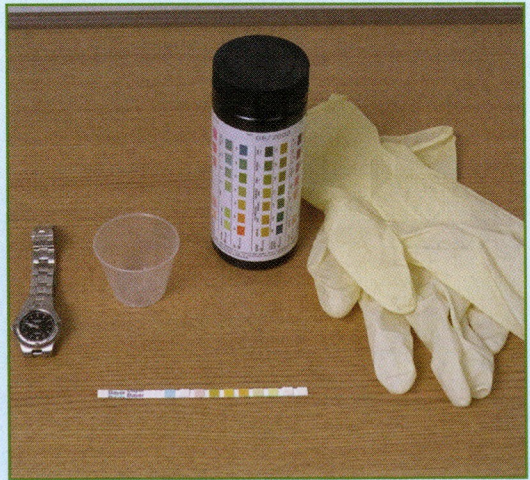

Figure 1-11-6   After dipping in fresh urine, wait the specified time interval before interpreting the results.

▶ REAL WORLD ANECDOTES

One nurse recalls her early nursing days and a particular learning curve. When she knew she needed to do a urine test using a dipstick, she would grab a strip from the bottle in the supply room and carry it down the hall to the client's room. She would then dip it in the sample in the client's bathroom and subsequently realize that she needed to compare it to the chart on the container that was sitting down the hall in the supply room.

▶ EVALUATION

- Evaluate the test results and compare them with the previous results.
- Evaluate the color of the urine and any abnormal changes.

▶ DOCUMENTATION

Nurses' Notes

- Document the procedure and results.
- Document any visual changes noted in the urine.

▶ CRITICAL THINKING SKILL

Introduction

Nurses should be able to evaluate visual changes in urine and the results of the test.

Possible Scenario

Your client comes in for a routine outpatient visit and physical exam. You need a urine sample, so you instruct the client on the procedure for obtaining a clean-catch urine specimen. The client returns from the bathroom with the specimen, which looks dark. You perform the test for occult blood, and the result is positive.

Possible Outcome

You question the client further and discover that prior to voiding she removed her tampon so that the string would not dangle in the cup. You determine that the urine has been contaminated with blood from menstruation. You make arrangements to have the client return later in the afternoon to provide a second specimen.

Prevention

Because you cannot cover every possible contingency when providing instruction on how to collect a clean-catch urine sample, teach the client the importance of the goal to obtain uncontaminated urine for accurate testing.

▶ VARIATIONS

Geriatric Variations:

- *Elderly clients may have a more difficult time collecting uncontaminated urine. Women especially may have difficulty because of labial changes that occur with age. They may need more careful assistance or instruction in collecting specimens.*
- *Elderly clients may have a difficult time reading the small print on the label or the color scale and may need assistance or a magnifying glass.*

Pediatric Variations:

- *A specific gravity can be obtained with a urine refractometer even with only a drop or two of urine from a wet diaper.*
- *Normal specific gravity values may vary slightly for children.*

continues

> **VARIATIONS** *(continued)*

Home Care Variations:
- *Contamination of the specimen may occur. Carefully instruct the client on the need for a clean-catch and second-voided specimen.*

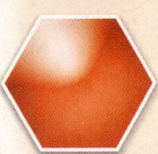

Long-Term Care Variations:
- *Instruct the client and caregiver on the need to use dipsticks or test tapes that are not past the expiration date. To save money, some clients may cut test tapes; doing so increases the risk for inaccurate readings.*

> **COMMON ERRORS**

Possible Error:

Overfilling the urinometer with urine.

Prevention:

Avoid pouring from a large container with a large volume of urine. It is more difficult to control. Note carefully how much urine is needed to fill the urinometer to the correct amount.

Possible Error:

Urine contaminated with feces.

Prevention:

Remind the client that the urine is being measured and tested when you place the bedpan, or commode, or escort the client to the bathroom.

Possible Error:

Inaccurate timing with test strip if instructions not read ahead of time.

Possible Error:

Read the instructions before testing the urine.

> **NURSING TIPS**

- Visualize urine before tests to look for contamination.
- Read instructions before dipping stick or test tape in urine.
- Have at least 20 mL of urine for urinometer.
- Verify that the urine is a second-voided specimen and explain this need to the client.

> ▶ **SPECIAL CONSIDERATIONS**

- Normally, ketones, blood, glucose, and protein are absent in the urine. However, consuming a high-carbohydrate meal may result in glucosuria. In female clients, blood may be present in the urine during menstruation. Blood may be present in the urine of clients on anticoagulants or high doses of aspirin.
- Conditions such as strenuous exercise and starvation that increase the fatty acid metabolism can cause ketoacidosis, resulting in ketone bodies in the urine.
- Secretions from the penis or vagina can cause false readings of proteinuria. Obtaining a thorough health history and a clean specimen is important for the diagnostic purpose.

Performing a Skin Puncture

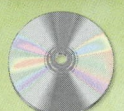

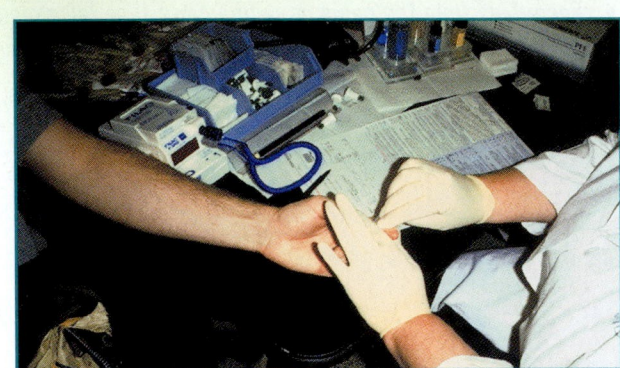

▶ OVERVIEW OF THE SKILL

Skin punctures are performed when small quantities of capillary blood are needed for analysis or when the client has poor veins. Capillary puncture commonly is performed for blood-glucose analysis. The common sites for capillary punctures follow:

• Heel—most common site for neonates and infants
• Fingertip—the inner aspect of palmar fingertip used most commonly in children and adults
• Earlobe—used when the client is in shock or the extremities are edematous.

▶ ASSESSMENT

1. Assess the condition of the client's skin at the potential puncture site **to determine whether it is intact, free of bruising, and can be used without causing undue trauma to the site.**
2. Assess the circulation at the potential puncture site **to determine whether it is a good site to obtain a sample, and to determine whether healing at the site might be compromised.**
3. Assess the client's comfort level regarding the procedure **to determine client education and support needed.**
4. Assess the cleanliness of the client's skin **to determine how much cleansing is needed before the skin puncture.**

▶ DIAGNOSIS

Risk for Impaired Skin Integrity

Pain

Anxiety

▶ PLANNING

Expected Outcomes:

1. An adequate blood specimen will be obtained.
2. The client will suffer minimal trauma during the specimen collection.
3. The specimen will be collected and stored in a manner compatible with the ordered tests.

Equipment Needed (see Figure 1-12-1):

• Antiseptic 70% isopropanol or povidone-iodine
• Microhematocrit tubes or micropipette (collection tubes)
• Sterile 2 × 2 gauze
• Sterile lancet
• Nonsterile gloves
• Hand towel or absorbent pad

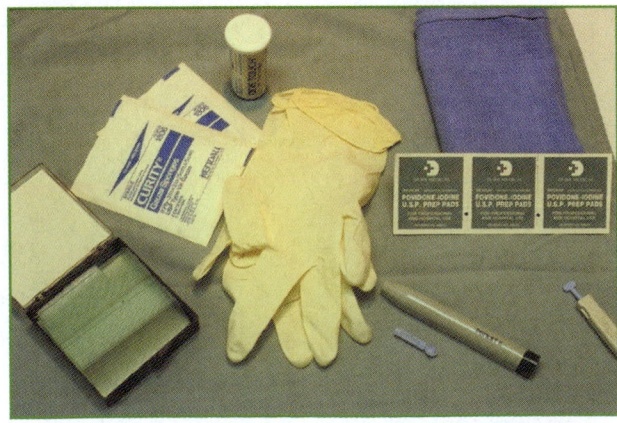

Figure 1-12-1 Various lancet devices, alcohol wipes, povidone-iodine, gauze, and gloves.

► **CLIENT EDUCATION NEEDED:**

1. Explain the reason that the lateral aspect of the finger is used to avoid the nerve endings at the tip of the finger.
2. Inform the client that a small sharp prick will occur.
3. Tell the client to hold pressure on the site for several minutes following the blood collection to prevent seepage of blood into the tissues.

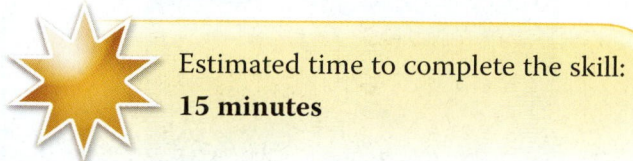

Estimated time to complete the skill:
15 minutes

► **DELEGATION TIPS**

Properly trained ancillary personnel may perform skin puncture. Agency policy usually dictates certification and recertification requirements for this skill. Proper client and specimen identification are of the utmost importance and must be consistently demonstrated by the ancillary personnel.

IMPLEMENTATION—Action/Rationale

Action	Rationale
1. Wash hands.	1. Reduces transmission of microorganisms.
2. Check the client's identification band if appropriate.	2. Ensures the correct client.
3. Explain the procedure to the client.	3. Allays anxiety and encourages cooperation.
4. Prepare supplies: • Open sterile packages. • Label specimen collection tubes. • Place in easy reach.	4. Ensures efficiency
5. Apply gloves.	5. Decreases the health care provider's exposure to blood-borne organisms.
6. Select site: lateral aspect of the fingertips in adults/children; heel for neonates and infants	6. Avoid damage to nerve endings and calloused areas of the skin.
7. Place the hand or heel in a dependent position; apply warm compresses if fingers or heel are cool to touch.	7. Increases the blood supply to the puncture site.
8. Place hand towel or absorbent pad under the extermity.	8. Prevents soiling the bed linen.
9. Cleanse puncture site with an antiseptic, and allow to dry. Use 70% isopropanol if the client is allergic to iodine (see Figure 1-12-2).	9. Reduces skin surface bacteria; povidone-iodine must dry to be effective.
10. With nondominant hand, apply gentle milking pressure above or around the puncture site. Do not touch the puncture site.	10. Increases blood to puncture site and maintains asepsis.

continues

Action	Rationale

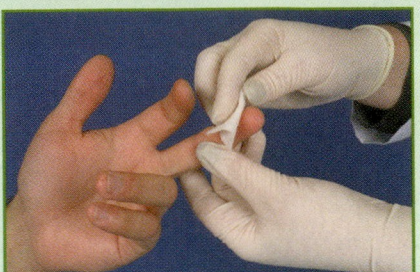

Figure 1-12-2 Cleanse the puncture site and allow it to dry.

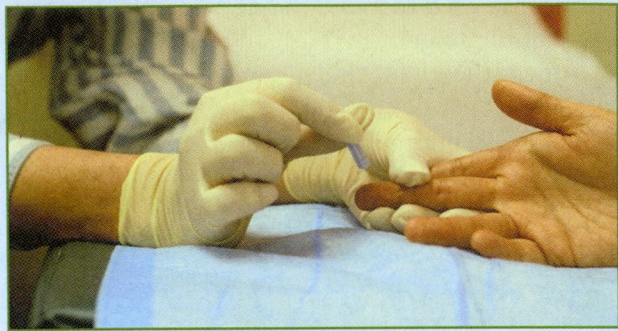

Figure 1-12-3 Use a quick stab to puncture the skin.

11. Read directions carefully before using the lancet.
    • With the sterile lancet at a 90-degree angle to the skin, use a quick stab to puncture the skin (about 2 mm deep) (see Figure 1-12-3).
    • With the automatic Unistik, push the lancet into the body of Unistik until it clicks. Hold the body of the Unistik and twist off the lancet cap. Place the end of the Unistik tightly against the client's finger and press the lever. The needle automatically retracts after use.

11. Provides a blood sample with minimal discomfort to the client.

12. Wipe off the first drop of blood with sterile 2 × 2 gauze; allow the blood to flow freely (see Figure 1-12-4).

12. The first drop may contain a large amount of serous fluid, which could affect the results. Pressure at the puncture site can cause hemolysis.

13. Collect the blood into the tube(s). If blood for a platelet count is to be collected, obtain this specimen first (see Figure 1-12-5).

13. Allows blood collection; avoids aggregation of platelets at the puncture site.

14. Apply pressure to the puncture site with a sterile 2 × 2 gauze (see Figure 1-12-6).

14. Controls bleeding.

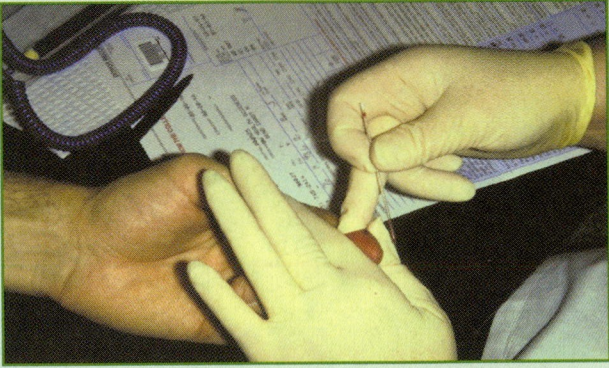

Figure 1-12-4 Allow the blood to flow from the puncture site to ensure an adequate amount can be obtained.

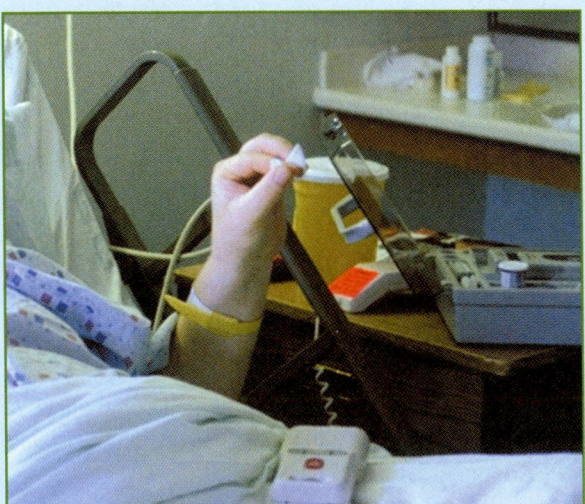

Figure 1-12-5 Collect a small sample of blood.

continues

Action	Rationale
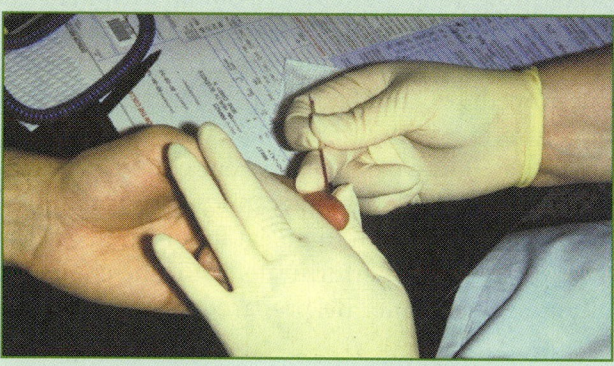	
	Figure 1-12-6 Apply pressure to the puncture site to stop further bleeding.
15. Place contaminated articles into a sharps container.	15. Reduces the risk of needle stick.
16. Remove gloves; wash hands.	16. Reduces transmission of microorganisms.
17. Position client for comfort with call light in reach.	17. Provides for comfort and communication.
18. Wash hands.	18. Reduces transmission of microorganisms.

▶ REAL WORLD ANECDOTES

While performing capillary puncture for blood-glucose monitoring, the nurse noted that despite what appeared to be an adequate puncture, the site was not bleeding. In an attempt to encourage a free flow of blood, the nurse gently squeezed the client's fingertip. Blood suddenly squirted from the puncture site, spraying the nurse's face. It is a good idea not to squeeze the area of a skin puncture but to let the blood flow freely.

▶ EVALUATION

* Determine that the specimen is adequate.
* Evaluate the client's finger for bruising or bleeding.

▶ DOCUMENTATION

Nurses' Notes

* Document the puncture site and the reason for the puncture.
* Report test results if the testing is performed at the time of the puncture.

▶ CRITICAL THINKING SKILL

Introduction

It is important to put the client at ease as much as possible.

Possible Scenario

A local company is offering free cholesterol tests. The sample is obtained by using skin puncture and a capillary tube. Because of an unexpectedly large turnout at lunchtime, some clients have been waiting in line for an hour. A heavy-set male client sits down to have his cholesterol tested. He is pale and diaphoretic. He notes that he has always been frightened of any kind of needles and has fainted in the past. His stomach is growling.

Possible Outcome

The nurse feels pressure to work quickly because of the long line. She ignores the client's words and fails to note his physical symptoms. As she begins, the client complains of "feeling queasy," then abruptly tumbles from the chair in a faint. Supplies and tubes tumble with him, and the chair is knocked over. The waiting line shortens considerably.

Prevention

Skin puncture is a frightening procedure to most people. Many people have unpleasant memories regarding this procedure. This client's apprehension regarding the procedure caused him to faint. Before performing a skin puncture to obtain a capillary sample, the nurse should have allowed the client to sit a few minutes and talk about his concerns regarding the procedure. He needed to be reassured that skin puncture is done with a much smaller and sharper blade than in the past. If the client continued to seem pale and perhaps hypoglycemic, the nurse should have encouraged him to go eat lunch and come back a little later. Only perform the test if the client's condition seems stable. Be prepared if the client faints or vomits.

► **VARIATIONS**

Geriatric Variations:
- *The elderly often have very thin, fragile skin. When performing capillary puncture, be careful not to tear the skin.*

Pediatric Variations:
- *The heel is the most frequently used site for infants and neonates. Placing a warm pack on the infant's heel often increases the blood flow from the puncture site.*

Home Care Variations:
- *The home care client should be encouraged to rotate sites even if this is awkward at first.*
- *Teach the home care client to maintain sharp lancets for capillary puncture by frequently changing lancets rather than using the same one repeatedly.*

Long-Term Care Variations:
- *Clients who require frequent capillary puncture for blood level monitoring should be encouraged to rotate the sites used for puncture. Using both lateral aspects of all fingers can help prevent soreness and bruising at any one site.*

▶ COMMON ERRORS

Possible Error:

The puncture is too shallow to obtain a sufficient specimen.

Prevention:

This problem is usually resolved with practice. Think to yourself, why wasn't the puncture deep enough to obtain enough blood? Could this be the result of poor equipment or poor technique? Is the puncture blade sharp enough? Is the lancet designed to enter skin to a measured depth and then retract? Did I use enough force to puncture the skin deeply enough? There are a number of devices on the market designed specifically for skin puncture. Try several types of devices until you find one you are comfortable using. Occasionally, the blade is not pressed tightly enough against the skin to obtain a deep, clean puncture. Be sure to use enough force to hold the puncture device tightly enough against the skin to obtain a deep, clean puncture.

▶ NURSING TIPS

- Have the client hold his or her hand in a dependent position while you are setting up the equipment to promote venous engorgement in the fingertips.
- Be sure the client's hands are warm.
- Use the client's nondominant hand, if possible.
- Avoid fingers with calluses or previous injury.

▶ SPECIAL CONSIDERATIONS

- *The puncture site may be cleaned with warm, soapy water instead of an alcohol swab. Constant alcohol prepping may result in thickening of the skin and make future fingersticks more painful. The warmth of the water helps to increase peripheral blood circulation.*
- *A less painful procedure can be achieved by choosing the sides of the client's fingertips, which have fewer nerve endings compared with the soft, central part of the fingertips.*
- *A stroking or milking technique toward the fingertip can facilitate obtaining a maximum amount of blood.*

Measuring Blood-Glucose Levels

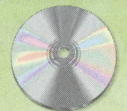

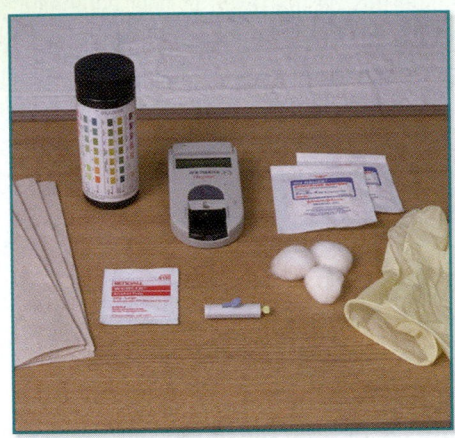

▶ OVERVIEW OF THE SKILL

Advances in technology have enabled the nurse, client, and/or caregiver to perform some laboratory tests at the bedside or in the home setting. Blood-glucose monitoring, using either reagent strips or glucose meters, combined with a skin puncture lancet, is an example of such technology. The convenience of this test has dramatically changed the ongoing management of many clients, particularly those with diabetes.

Testing of blood glucose can be done by obtaining a blood sample through venipuncture or by obtaining capillary blood with a skin puncture. In situations requiring frequent blood-glucose monitoring, the preferred method of blood sampling is the skin puncture technique.

There are primarily two methods used to measure blood glucose. Both methods require a large drop of blood obtained through skin puncture with a sterile lancet. The first method requires that the drop of blood be applied to a special chemical reagent strip. The participant visually compares the reagent strip to a color chart on the reagent container. Accuracy may be compromised if the result falls between two colors and the participant must estimate the blood-glucose level. Examples of reagent strips include Chemstrip BG, Glucostix, and Trendstrips.

A second method of blood-glucose monitoring replaces the visual comparison method with the use of a portable meter. Once the blood is placed on the reagent strip, the meter provides an accurate measurement of the blood glucose. There are a variety of meters available, including Accu-Check Advantage (Accu-Check), Accu-Check Active (Accu-Check), Bayer Elite (Bayer), Glucometer (Bayer), One Touch II (Lifescan), Sure Step Pro (Lifescan), InDuo (Lifescan), and Precision (Medisense). Because models vary and technology continues to evolve, it is essential that the nurse or client using the device review the specific manufacturer's operating guidelines and be familiar with the equipment. Failure to do so could compromise the test results.

▶ ASSESSMENT

1. Review the health care provider's order for glucose monitoring **to determine whether the order specifies the method (reagent strip versus meter).**
2. Identify which type of equipment is available at your facility. **It is imperative to be knowledgeable of the type of method used and specific meter that is available for use. Accurate test results depend on proper use of all equipment involved.**
3. Review the client's medical history for diabetes, visual impairment, or anticoagulant therapy. **A thorough knowledge of the client's medical history is important—even when the test performed is a relatively simple procedure.**

Visual impairment or other disabilities can hinder self-care and may affect test results. Anticoagulant therapy may result in prolonged bleeding at the skin puncture site and require pressure to the site.

4. Determine whether the test requires special timing, for example, before or after meals. **Blood-glucose levels are affected by diet, and the test may be scheduled at very specific intervals. Therapy orders are based on the assumption that the test results are accurate.**

5. Assess the client's or caregiver's ability to manage the equipment and perform the test accurately if the care will be provided at home. **Proper client/caregiver education is essential; clients/caregivers should return-demonstrate their ability to carry out the test and clean the equipment before they assume such a responsibility.**

6. Assess the client's understanding of the rationale for the test and the importance of accurate results. Determine the client's willingness to perform the test and identify if the client will incorporate the test schedule into his or her daily routine. **Compliance with the expected schedule and procedure is more likely to occur when the client is knowledgeable about the rationale for the procedure. Some clients may have difficulty with some aspects of the procedure, such as the finger stick, and may be unwilling to participate in self-care.**

7. Assess the client's sites for skin puncture. **Sites should have good skin integrity in order to minimize the risk of infection and promote healing.**

▶ DIAGNOSIS

Anxiety

Risk for Impaired Skin Integrity

Disturbed Sensory Perception

▶ PLANNING

Expected Outcomes:

1. Blood-glucose level is maintained within a normal range.
2. Client/caregiver demonstrates accurate performance of the procedure.
3. Client verbalizes an understanding of the importance of the test and the need for accurate results.
4. Client verbalizes minimal anxiety associated with the procedure.
5. Skin puncture sites remain free of signs and symptoms of infection.

Equipment Needed (see Figures 1-13-1 and 1-13-2):

- Reagent strips
- Disposable latex-free gloves
- Lancet or automatic lancing device
- Paper towels
- Alcohol wipe
- 2 × 2 gauze
- Cotton ball
- Blood-glucose meter

▶ CLIENT EDUCATION NEEDED:

1. Explain the purpose and schedule for the test.
2. Provide information related to how the test results will affect the client's disease state management.
3. Discuss the time it will take for the client to master the skill.
4. When possible, include the caregiver in the teaching session to provide backup for the client in the home setting. Provide written instructions.
5. Provide information to clients regarding providers who can supply equipment needed for their diabetes care.

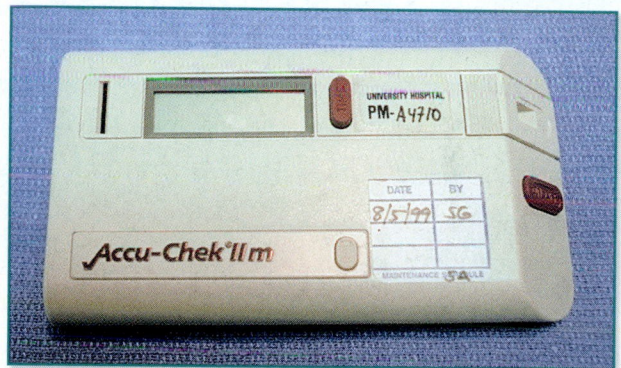

Figure 1-13-1 Blood-glucose meter. There are many types and brands of glucose meters available.

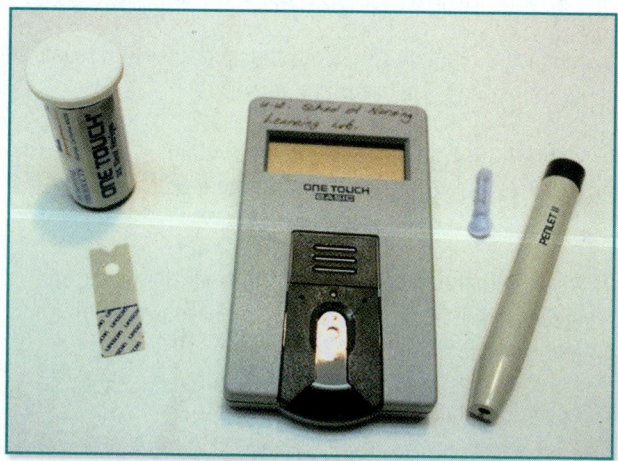

Figure 1-13-2 Test strips, blood-glucose meter, and penlette.

6. Require the learner to return-demonstrate the procedure—including proper management of the equipment (cleaning, storage).

7. Help clients determine resources available if the meter malfunctions.

8. Help clients determine what their insurance plan covers related to nursing care, equipment, and medication needs.

9. Offer information on local and national organizations that provide information or support to clients with diabetes.

10. Review Standard Precautions with the client/caregiver.

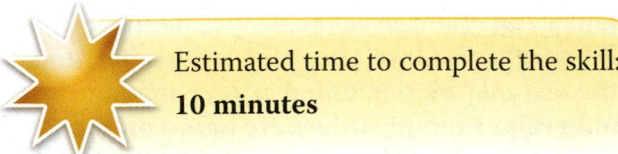

Estimated time to complete the skill:
10 minutes

▶ DELEGATION TIPS

Properly trained ancillary personnel may measure blood-glucose levels. Agency and state health department policies usually dictate certification and recertification requirements for this skill. Proper client and specimen identification are of the utmost importance and must be consistently demonstrated by the ancillary personnel. Proper recording of results and prompt reporting to the nurse of abnormal findings are essential.

IMPLEMENTATION—Action/Rationale

Action	Rationale
1. Review orders, identify the client, and review the manufacturer's instructions for meter usage.	**1.** Prevents performing an invasive procedure on the wrong client and promotes accuracy of results
2. Wash hands.	**2.** Reduces transmission of microorganisms.
3. Assemble the equipment at the bedside (see Figure 1-13-3).	**3.** Allows for a smooth procedure.
4. Have the client wash hands with soap and water, and position the client comfortably in a semi-Fowler's position or upright in a chair.	**4.** Reduces transmission of microorganisms and increases blood flow to the puncture site. Avoids having the client stand during the procedure, as some clients may be prone to fainting.
5. Remove a reagent strip from the container and reseal the container cap. Then, turn on meter.	**5.** Tight closure of the container keeps strips from discoloring from environmental factors. Activates meter for test.
6. Following the manufacturer's instructions, calibrate the meter by inserting the strip into the meter.	**6.** Some meters need to be calibrated; others require the timer to be adjusted; each meter has different requirements when setting it up for use.
7. Remove the unused reagent strip from the meter and place it on a clean, dry surface (paper towel) with the test pad facing up.	**7.** Moisture may alter the test results.
8. Apply disposable gloves	**8.** Protects from contamination by blood.
9. Select appropriate puncture site and perform skin puncture (see Figure 1-13-4)	**9.** Collects blood necessary for the test.

continues

Action	Rationale

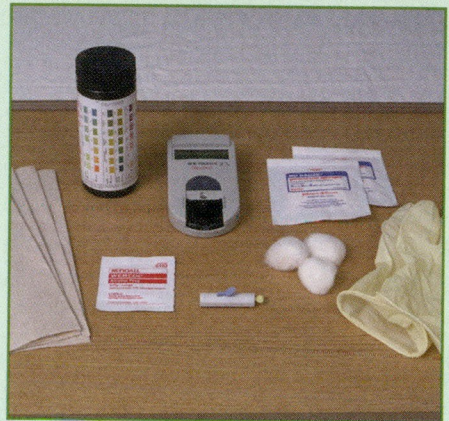

Figure 1-13-3   Supplies for blood-glucose testing.

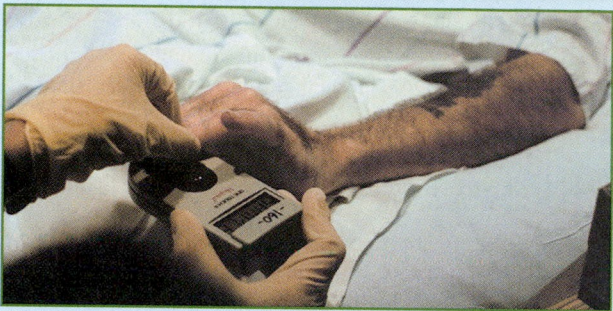

Figure 1-13-4   Perform the skin puncture.

10. Wipe away the first drop of blood from the site.

11. Gently squeeze the site to produce a large droplet of blood.

12. Transfer the drop of blood to the reagent strip by carefully moving the site over the strip. The droplet should transfer without smearing (see Figure 1-13-5). (Note: Some meters require that the blood droplet be applied to the strip that is already in the meter.) Follow instructions on monitor selected because they may vary.

13. Quickly press the timer on the meter and lay the strip next to the meter on a clean, dry surface.

14. Apply pressure to the puncture site (see Figure 1-13-6).

10. This drop may impede accurate results because it may contain a large amount of serous fluid.

11. Do not contaminate the site by touching it; the droplet of blood must be large enough to cover the test pad on the reagent strip.

12. The test pad must absorb the droplet of blood for accurate results. Smearing of the blood will alter results.

13. Timing is critical to produce accurate results. Always check the manufacturer's instructions because the technique varies between meters.

14. This will stop the bleeding at the site.

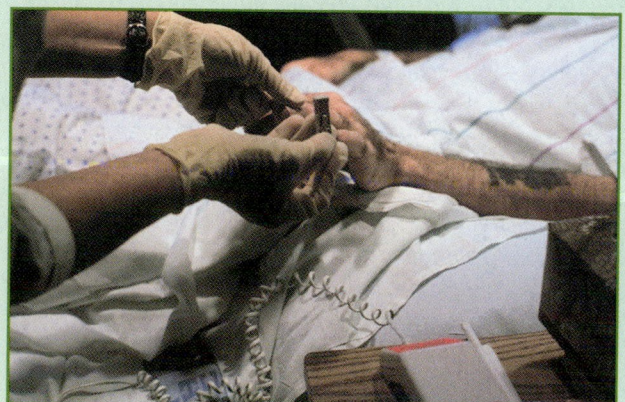

Figure 1-13-5   Transfer a drop of blood to the test strip.

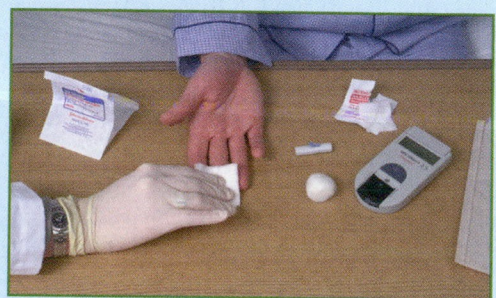

Figure 1-13-6   Apply pressure to the site.

continues

Action	Rationale
15. After 60 seconds, wipe the blood from the test pad with a cotton ball; place the strip into the meter. (Note: This step may vary with the type of meter.) Allow the timer to continue.	**15.** This step is specific to certain meters (e.g., Accu-Check III) that require the strip to enter the meter dry.
16. Read the meter for results found on the unit display.	**16.** Each meter has a specified time for the reading to occur.
17. Turn off the meter and properly dispose of the test strip, cotton ball, and lancet.	**17.** Reduces contamination by blood to other individuals; sharps must always be handled properly to protect others from accidental injury.
18. Remove disposable gloves and place them in the appropriate receptacle.	**18.** Reduces transmission of microorganisms.
19. Wash hands.	**19.** Reduces contamination by microorganisms.
20. Review tests results with the client.	**20.** Promotes participation in health care.
21. Notify the health care provider of the test results.	**21.** Results will be used to determine the client's treatment plan.
22. Wash hands.	**22.** Reduces transmission of microorganisms.

▶ REAL WORLD ANECDOTES

Scenario 1

Ms. Smith is an elderly woman, newly diagnosed with type II diabetes. The new diagnosis was overwhelming to her. She is fearful that she cannot remember all the material that she needs to learn to administer insulin and test her blood-glucose level. The nurse in the clinic scheduled her teaching appointments and began the process of client education. In the clinic setting, Ms. Smith gradually felt more competent with the blood-glucose monitoring technique. The next day at home, she tried the technique she had been taught. Her blood-glucose level was significantly lower than the results she had recorded when at the clinic. She called her clinic nurse, who in turn reported the low results to the physician, who decreased her next dose of insulin. Ms. Smith was later urgently admitted for symptoms of hyperglycemia. Apparently, when reviewing information with her nurse, Ms. Smith realized she had forgotten to wipe off the first drop of blood from her finger. She had used a blood sample that was diluted with serous fluid, making her blood glucose level abnormally low. In retrospect, it would have been more appropriate to have asked Ms. Smith to recheck her results at the clinic before changing her prescription, especially because the nurse was familiar with the client's usual blood-glucose levels.

Scenario 2

Kelly is a 5-year-old girl, newly diagnosed with type I diabetes, whose parents are becoming quite efficient in the care of their daughter. The mother demonstrated the procedure for blood-glucose monitoring and was comfortable performing the procedure. However, when it was time to test Kelly's blood glucose, Kelly refused to allow her mother to puncture her finger with the lancet. After much frustration, the nurse recommended that Kelly try the automated device. With her mother's help, Kelly and her favorite doll learned how to press the release button. Eventually, as Kelly became more comfortable with the "magic button," she allowed the device to be used for her blood-glucose monitoring. It is important to incorporate play into the medical care of young children and to allow them to actively participate in the process.

► **EVALUATION**

* Reinspect the puncture site for bleeding and tissue injury.
* Compare the glucose reading to the client's previous glucose results.
* Compare the client's results to normal blood-glucose levels.
* Ask the client to explain the importance of the results.
* Ask the client to return-demonstrate the procedure at the next scheduled test.

► **DOCUMENTATION**

Appropriate Flow Sheet or Electronic Medical Report (EMR)

Record:

* Glucose test results
* Procedure and site used
* Appearance of puncture site
* Client's response to the procedure (feelings of lightheadedness, nausea, etc.)
* Abnormal results reported to health care provider
* Client's understanding of the procedure and ability to demonstrate the technique
* Medications administered
* Date and time insulin administered

► **CRITICAL THINKING SKILL**

Introduction

Accurate test results for blood-glucose monitoring are critical because treatment decisions are based on those results. Documenting the results in a designated log/chart in the client's record is equally important.

Possible Scenario

Mr. Jones was admitted for symptoms of hyperglycemia associated with his long history of diabetes. His treatment plan included 6-hour management of his blood glucose. The nurse was very busy and neglected to document the meter reading on the flow chart. The physician asked Mr. Jones whether his test had been performed. He answered "yes" and stated what meter reading he had seen on the display. The physician ordered a dose of insulin based on those results.

Possible Outcome

The obvious concern is that the meter reading was not properly documented and only anecdotal. There is considerable risk to the client if the insulin dosage is based on inaccurate blood-glucose readings.

Prevention

Prompt documentation of all meter readings; notification of abnormal results to the health care provider; and informing the client of test results are actions that help prevent errors in this situation.

► **VARIATIONS**

Geriatric Variations:

* *Warming fingertips will facilitate vasodilatation and collection of the blood droplet.*
* *Older clients are at risk for visual impairment; care should be taken to verify that the client is able to read the meter results accurately.*
* *Involve a caregiver in the teaching to provide backup for the elderly client, particularly in the home setting.*

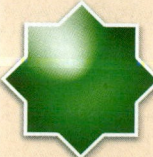

Pediatric Variations:

* *Painful procedures such as a skin puncture for a blood sample should be performed in a procedure room rather than the client's hospital room.*
* *Have assistance from staff to restrain the child or infant during the skin puncture.*
* *Topical numbing creams applied to the site prior to the puncture may reduce the discomfort associated with the test.*
* *Allow the child to choose the puncture site when possible.*
* *Allow the child and parent to demonstrate the procedure; incorporate play activity into the procedure as needed.*
* *When using the heel of an infant, warm the foot before the skin puncture.*

continues

▶ VARIATIONS *(continued)*

Home Care Variations:

- *Glucose-monitoring meters are common devices used for the home management of clients with diabetes. The nurse should note the manufacturer of the equipment and review proper maintenance and calibration of the device with the client. The nurse should also review proper disposal of equipment in the home environment.*

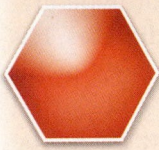

Long-Term Care Variations:

- *In long-term care facilities, employees performing blood-glucose monitoring should be familiar with the device used for the client to ensure accurate results.*

▶ COMMON ERRORS

Possible Error:

The manufacturer's requirements were not reviewed before testing, which resulted in an inaccurate result, or the wrong strips were used for the equipment selected.

Prevention:

Maintain information related to the meter in a place that is accessible to all nursing personnel. Review the specific technique required by the manufacturer.

Repeat the test using the correct technique. Select a different puncture site on the client. Be sure to match strip and code with equipment and follow the manufacturer's instructions.

▶ NURSING TIPS

- Clients admitted to the hospital who have been performing blood-glucose monitoring may choose to continue to perform the procedure themselves. The nurse has an opportunity to review information, assess accuracy of the client's techniques, and offer information on new equipment that may be available.
- Clients referred to home care may rent meters from those providers. It is important that the client teaching plan is consistent with the equipment delivered to the home.
- Understand the blood-glucose level "norms" for an individual client. If the new level is significantly different, suspect an error in administration of the procedure and determine other factors that may impair accurate results.

▶ **SPECIAL CONSIDERATIONS**

- *Avoid sharing lancet pen/holder (often supplied with glucose-monitoring devices) with others, because blood-borne disease can be transmitted through lancet devices.*
- *In clients such as those with diabetes who require regular blood-glucose monitoring, "shallow penetration" should be encouraged to avoid tissue damage. Milking toward the fingertip can facilitate obtaining a maximum amount of blood. Rotate sites to allow time for the penetrated site to heal. A less painful procedure can be achieved by choosing the side of the fingertips where fewer nerve endings are located compared with the soft, central part of the fingertips.*
- *In the home health setting or in clients who perform the fingertip puncture on a regular basis, hand-washing with warm, soapy water is recommended instead of using alcohol to clean the area to be punctured. Repeated cleaning of the fingerstick site with alcohol can result in thickening of the skin and make the fingerstick more painful. The warmth of the water helps increasing peripheral blood circulation.*

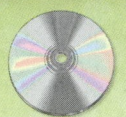

Collecting Nose, Throat, and Sputum Specimens

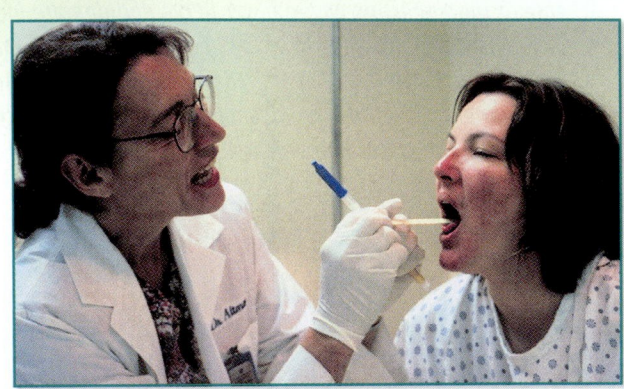

▶ OVERVIEW OF THE SKILL

A nose, throat, or sputum specimen is a simple diagnostic tool for clients with signs or symptoms of upper respiratory or sinus infections. Nose and throat specimens are collected from the client using a sterile swab. Sputum specimens are collected in a sterile cup. Sputum specimens also can be obtained via a specimen trap connected to suction. Specimens are sent to the laboratory and placed in a culture medium to allow pathogenic organisms to grow. The type of organism can be identified, thereby enabling diagnosis and appropriate antimicrobial therapy.

▶ ASSESSMENT

1. Assess the client's understanding of the purpose of the procedure **so the client will be able to cooperate.**
2. Assess the type of nasal or sinus drainage **to determine what kind of collection equipment will be needed.**
3. Review the health care provider's orders for the cultures requested **so repeat cultures are not done.**
4. Assess the client for postnasal drip, sinus headache or tenderness, nasal congestion, or sore throat **to know why the procedure is being done.**
5. Identify whether the client has received recent antimicrobials and obtain a specimen before treatment, if possible.

▶ DIAGNOSIS

Risk for Infection

Anxiety

Risk for Injury

Deficient Knowledge

▶ PLANNING

Expected Outcomes:

1. An adequate specimen will be obtained and sent to the laboratory.
2. The procedure will be performed with a minimum of trauma to the client.

Equipment Needed (see Figures 1-14-1, 1-14-2, and 1-14-3):

- Two sterile swabs in sterile culture tubes or a flexible wire sterile swab with cotton tip for nose or throat cultures (see Figure 1-14-2).
- Tongue blades
- Penlight
- Facial tissues
- Clean, disposable latex-free gloves
- Nasal speculum (optional)
- Emesis basin or clean container
- Sterile specimen cup, or sputum specimen collector

▶ CLIENT EDUCATION NEEDED:

1. Teach clients the rationale for the procedure.
2. Although the procedure is generally painless, alert clients that gagging may occur.

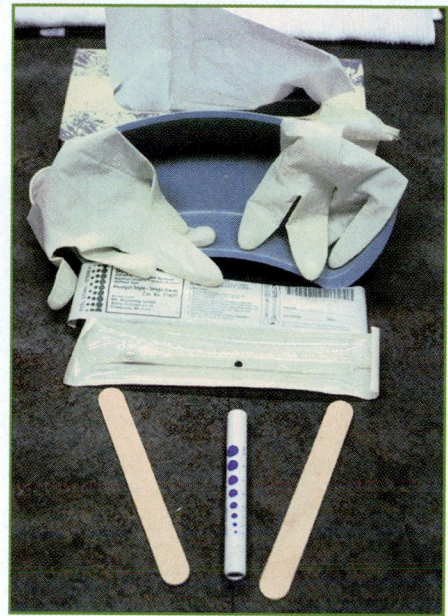

Figure 1-14-1   Penlight, tongue depressors, cotton swabs, culture medium, emesis basin, and gloves.

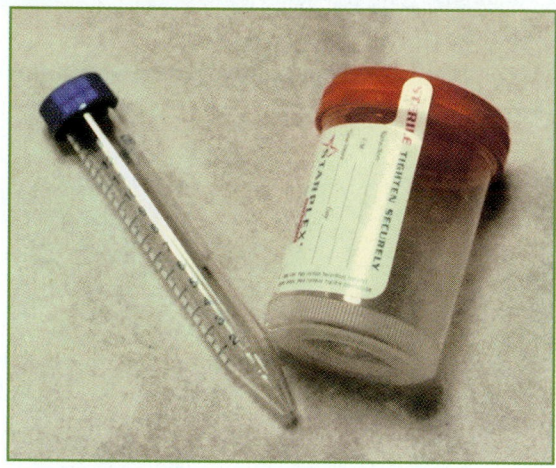

Figure 1-14-3   Sterile specimen tube and cup.

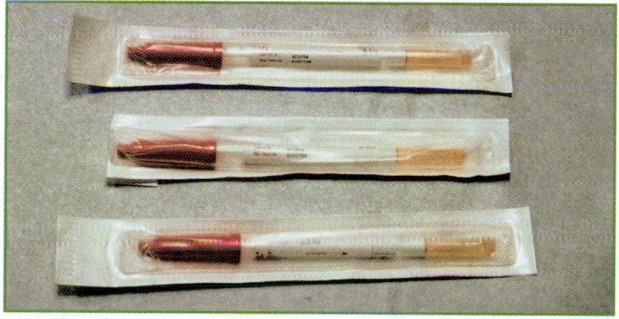

Figure 1-14-2   Prepackaged sterile swab and culture medium containers.

3. Discuss the rationale for obtaining the culture.
4. Discuss the time delay for the culture results.
5. Remind the client that the culture collection requires cooperation.

Estimated time to complete the skill:
5–10 minutes

► **DELEGATION TIPS**

Sputum specimens may be obtained by ancillary personnel. Avoiding specimen collection immediately after a client has eaten is important as is the use of Standard Precautions when handling the specimen. Obtaining nose and throat cultures requires problem-solving skills and techniques of a nurse, so obtaining these specimens may not be delegated.

IMPLEMENTATION—Action/Rationale

Action	Rationale
1. Wash hands and put on clean gloves.	1. Reduces transmission of microorganisms.
2. Ask the client to sit erect in the bed or on a chair facing the nurse.	2. Provides easy access to the nose or throat..
3. Prepare a sterile swab for use by loosening the top of the container (see Figure 1-14-4).	3. Prevents contamination of the swab.

continues

Action	Rationale

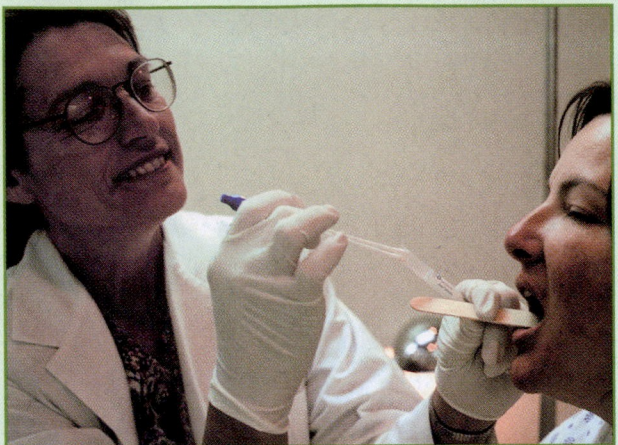

Figure 1-14-4   Loosen the swab top from container.

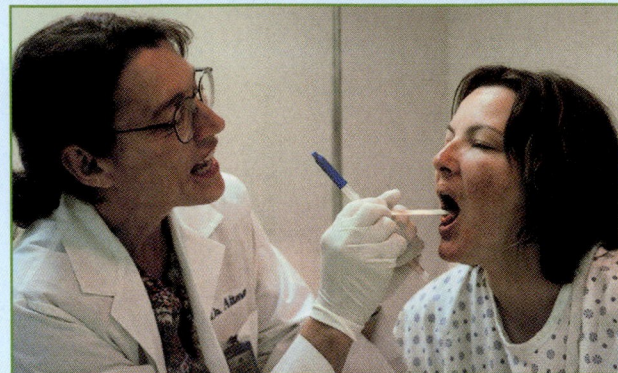

Figure 1-14-5   Depress the tongue with the tongue blade.

Collecting a Throat Culture

4. Ask the client to tilt the head backward, open the mouth, and say "ahh."

5. Depress the anterior one-third of the tongue with a tongue blade for better visualization (see Figure 1-14-5).

6. Insert the swab without touching the cheek, lips, teeth, or tongue.

7. Swab the tonsillar area from side to side in a quick, gentle motion (see Figure 1-14-6).

8. Withdraw the swab without touching adjacent structures and place in the culture tube. Crush ampule at bottom of tube and push swab into liquid medium (see Figure 1-14-7).

9. Secure the top to the culture tube and label with the client's name.

10. Discard the tongue depressor. Remove gloves and discard. Wash hands.

4. Promotes visualization of the pharynx, relaxes the throat muscles, and minimizes the gag reflex.

5. Promotes visualization of the pharynx, but may induce the gag reflex.

6. Prevents contamination of the specimen with oral flora.

7. Ensures collection of microorganisms. Retains microorganisms in the culture tube and ensures the life of bacteria for testing.

8. Prevents contamination from outside microorganisms and erroneous culture results.

9. Prevents identification mistakes.

10. Reduces transmission of microorganisms.

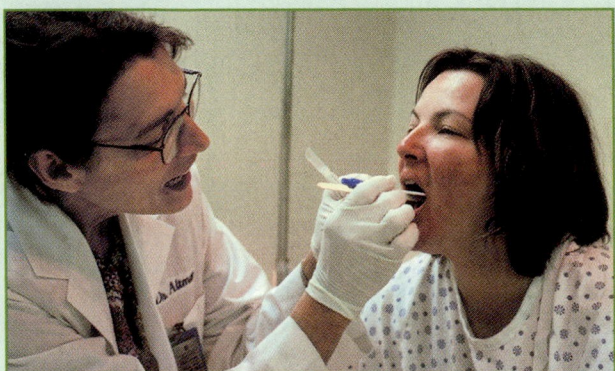

Figure 1-14-6   Swab the sample area using a quick, gentle motion.

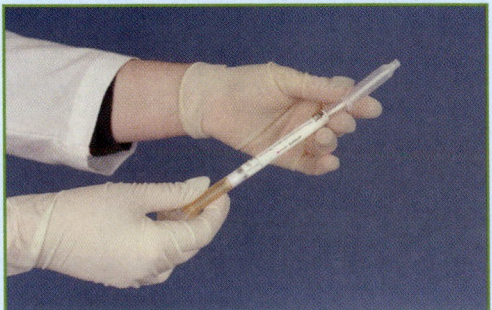

Figure 1-14-7   Crush ampule to release the culture medium.

continues

Action	Rationale
Collecting a Nasal Culture	
11. Instruct the client to blow nose as you check the client's nostrils for patency with penlight.	11. Clears nasal passages of mucus containing resident bacteria.
12. Ask the client to occlude one nostril, then the other, and exhale.	12. Determines the optimal nasal passage from which to obtain the specimen.
13. Ask the client to tilt the head back.	13. Promotes visualization of the sinuses.
14. Insert the swab into the nostril until it reaches the inflamed mucosa and rotate the swab.	14. Ensures the swab will be covered with the appropriate exudate.
15. Withdraw the swab without touching adjacent structures and place in culture tube. Crush ampule at bottom of tube and push swab into liquid medium.	15. Prevents contamination from normal nasal flora and erroneous culture results.
16. Secure the top to the culture tube and label with the client's name.	16. Prevents identification mistakes.
17. Remove gloves and discard. Wash hands.	17. Reduces transmission of microorganisms.
Collecting a Nasopharyngeal Culture	
18. Follow Actions 11 to 17 except use a swab on a flexible wire that can reach the nasopharynx via the nose.	18. Allows for access to the nasopharyngeal area.
Collecting a Sputum Culture	
19. Explain to the client that the specimen must be sputum, coughed up from the back of the throat or lungs.	19. Promotes client cooperation.
20. Have a sterile specimen cup ready for the sample and some tissue at hand.	20. The specimen must be collected in a sterile cup to prevent contamination.
21. Have the client take several deep breaths and then cough deeply (see Figure 1-14-8).	21. Helps to loosen secretions so the client will be able to provide a specimen.
22. Have the client expectorate the sputum into the sterile cup without touching the inside of the cup.	22. Prevents contamination of the specimen.
23. Place the lid on the specimen container without touching the inside of the lid or the container.	23. Prevents contamination of the specimen.
24. Provide the client with tissues and make him or her comfortable.	24. Promotes client comfort.
Alternative Sputum Collection Method	
This method is generally used if the client is unable to expectorate an adequate sample	
25. Obtain a sterile suction catheter and an in-line sputum collection container.	25. Prevents contamination of the specimen.

continues

Action	Rationale

Alternative Sputum Collection Method
continued

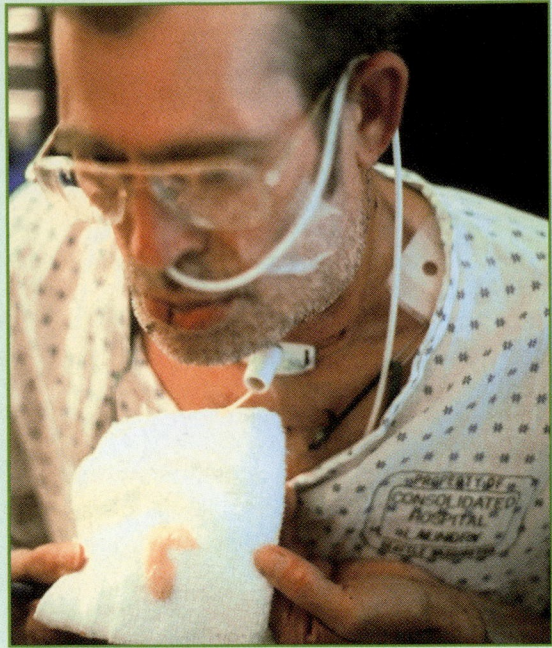

Figure 1-14-8   Have the client cough deeply.

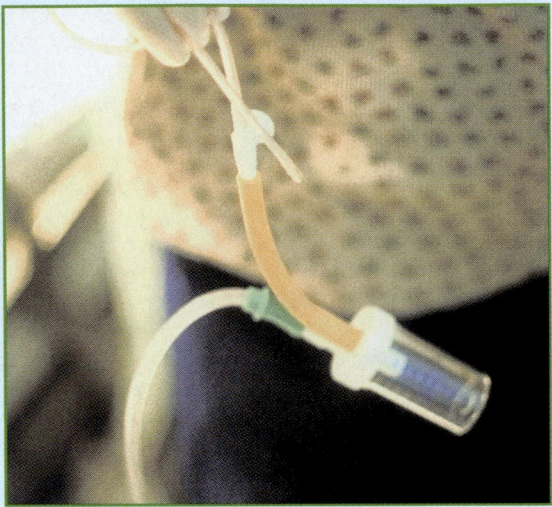

Figure 1-14-9   Sputum collector for use with suction.

26. Provide the client with warm humidified air for about 20 minutes if it is not contraindicated by the client's condition.

26. Helps to loosen secretions in the lungs.

27. Hook up the sputum collector to the suction tubing and a suction device (see Figure 1-14-9). Hook up the suction catheter to the sputum collector.

27. Prepare the equipment before having the client cough.

28. If the client is able to cooperate, have him or her take several deep breaths and cough.

28. Loosens the secretions and brings them up to the back of the throat.

29. As the client is coughing up sputum, carefully insert the catheter either orally or nasopharyngeally into the back of the throat and suction the sputum into the specimen container.

29. Obtains a sterile specimen that is not contaminated with saliva.

30. Safely dispose of the suction catheter.

30. Prevents the spread of microorganisms.

31. Close the specimen container.

31. Prevents contamination of the specimen.

32. Provide tissues or other measures for client comfort.

32. Promotes client comfort.

33. Wash hands.

33. Reduces transmission of microorganisms.

34. Label each specimen with the client's name.

34. Promotes the correct diagnosis for the client.

35. Send the specimen to the laboratory.

35. Provides the most accurate results.

▶ REAL WORLD ANECDOTES

When a respiratory syncytial virus epidemic broke out in the city, school children were lined up to have throat cultures taken. Many of the children were frightened, and their parents were impatient. Three nurses were taking the cultures, and the child at the head of the line was supposed to go to the next-available nurse. Danny was next in line and saw Nurse Prezbindowski. Danny was frightened, and his mother was angry about the long wait. Danny was crying, and his mother had to hold him and encourage him as the nurse took the throat culture. Danny's mother was obviously upset by the procedure and vented her frustrations to Nurse Prezbindowski. The culture was finally obtained, and Danny and his mother quickly left the room. After they left, Nurse Prezbindowski discovered that Danny's mother had not fully completed the laboratory form. She did not put an address or a phone number on the form. Nurse Prezbindowski was not able to contact Danny's mother to obtain the information and, without that information, Danny's culture could not be processed by the lab. Danny's long wait and fearful cooperation was jeopardized by the missing information. Complete paperwork was required before the sample could be submitted to the lab. Before Danny and his mother left, the nurse should have reviewed the paperwork.

▶ EVALUATION

- An adequate specimen was obtained.
- The procedure was performed with a minimum of trauma to the client.

▶ DOCUMENTATION

Nurses' Notes

- Record the date, time, and site from which the specimen was obtained.
- Note any bleeding or obvious trauma as a result of the procedure.
- Chart the description and time the specimen was collected. Note if the specimen is the first morning specimen, not pooled secretions.

▶ CRITICAL THINKING SKILL

Introduction

An accurate specimen is necessary so that appropriate treatment can be initiated.

Possible Scenario

Mr. Habakangus was admitted to the hospital with suspected pneumonia. His doctor had ordered a sputum specimen to confirm a diagnosis of pneumonia and determine the causative microorganism of the infection. You give Mr. Habakangus a sterile specimen cup and explain the procedure to him. Mr. Habakangus speaks very little English, but he seems to understand what you are asking him to do. He takes several deep breaths, coughs, and spits into the cup. The specimen is obviously saliva and you attempt to explain again that what is needed is sputum from his lungs. He tries to provide the needed specimen once more, but again he is able to provide only saliva.

Possible Outcome

You report to Mr. Habakangus' physician that you were unable to obtain a specimen. Without an accurate culture and sensitivity, his physician will have to prescribe a broad-spectrum antibiotic and hope it will work against the pneumonia. Mr. Habakangus may or may not get better quickly. His hospital stay and illness could be unnecessarily prolonged.

You reassure Mr. Habakangus and place a heated mist mask on him to help loosen the secretions. After about 15 minutes, you return with a sterile suction catheter, suction tubing, and an in-line specimen container. You explain to Mr. Habakangus that you will try to suction the sputum from the back of his throat. You assure him that the procedure is a little unpleasant but not painful. Once again you instruct him to take several deep breaths and cough, but you ask him to cough with his mouth open so you can insert the suction catheter. When you use the catheter to suction his airway, the specimen in the cup is green and thick and appears to be sputum. You dispose of the catheter, cap the specimen cup, and comfort Mr. Habakangus. Because a sterile sputum specimen was obtained, the doctor will be able to pinpoint what organism is causing the pneumonia and how best to treat it.

Prevention

Educate the client regarding the importance of obtaining an actual sputum specimen and not saliva. Sputum has diagnostic value; sending an inadequate specimen only delays appropriate treatment of the client.

▶ VARIATIONS

Geriatric Variations:
- *Older clients may have difficulty tilting their head back because of osteoarthritis.*

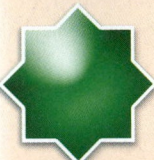

Pediatric Variations:
- *Showing the tongue blade and penlight to a child before inserting them into the mouth may decrease anxiety.*
- *Ask the parent to help gently hold a child's head while obtaining a nose or throat culture.*

Home Care Variations:
- *When obtaining a specimen that will not be sent to the lab right away, be sure to store it in a cool place to prevent growth of microorganisms.*

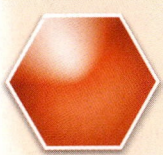

Long-Term Care Variations:
- *When obtaining a specimen that will not be sent to the lab right away, be sure to store it in a cool place to prevent growth of microorganisms.*

▶ COMMON ERRORS

Possible Error:

The agitated, confused client moves his head while a nasal culture is being obtained, thus contaminating the specimen and causing bleeding.

Prevention:

Assess the client's ability to hold still during the procedure.

Stop the bleeding by applying pressure to the bridge of the nose. Use a new culture swab and ask for assistance from a coworker to help stabilize the client's head while obtaining the culture.

Possible Error:

The client gags on the tongue blade and contaminates the swab with the tongue.

Prevention:

Instruct the client on how to obtain a throat culture.

Remove the tongue blade and swab. Obtain a new culture swab. Ask the client to relax and take deep breaths. Depress the tongue blade on only the anterior half of the tongue. Swab the throat.

▶ NURSING TIPS

- Ask the parent or caregiver for assistance in obtaining the culture.
- Have the appropriate culture media available.
- Reassure the client of the short time of the procedure.
- Loosen the swab in the tube before having the client open the mouth for obtaining the throat culture.

> ▶ **SPECIAL CONSIDERATIONS**

- *Sputum specimens are best collected right after the client awakens, before ingesting anything by mouth (including fluids), and before brushing teeth or rinsing the mouth. If the client has eaten or brushed teeth, rinse with water and wait from 15 to 30 minutes before collecting a throat specimen.*
- *It is essential to ensure an adequate specimen. Have the client use a deep cough to force out sputum. Nebulized saline solution may be necessary to facilitate adequate sputum production.*
- *If a specimen was collected and found unlabeled with the time collected, discard and obtain a new specimen.*
- *Copious amount of purulent sputum mixed with blood may be associated with bronchiectasis; pink sputum is suggestive of pulmonary edema fluid. Currant jelly sputum may be indicative of necrotizing pneumonia; putrid sputum, which is foul smelling, is found in lung abscesses.*
- *If the client is on antimicrobial therapy, specimen results will be of limited value because of suppression of microbials.*
- *Repeated sputum specimens may be of limited value in some conditions. For certain specimens, such as those for mycobacteria, three consecutive first morning specimens (not pooled) are optimal.*
- *If hemoptysis is present it is of diagnostic value. Chart the description and notify the appropriate staff.*
- *Sputum cytology may be used to identify certain cell types in cancer. A negative cytology result does not rule out disease.*

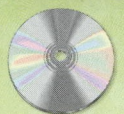

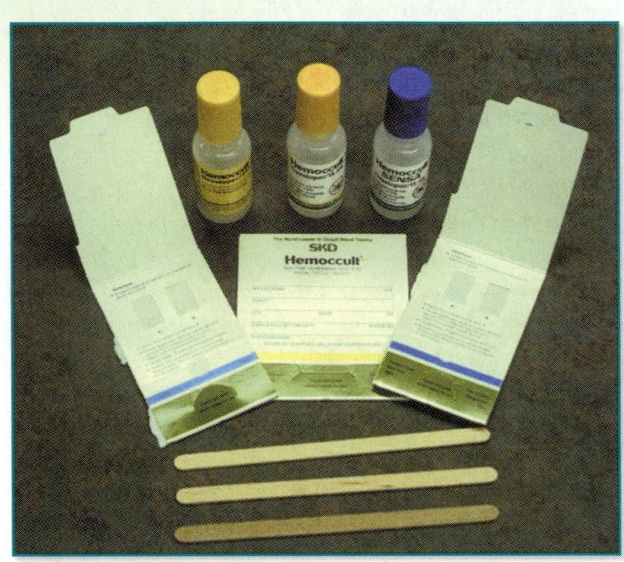

▶ OVERVIEW OF THE SKILL

Stool tests for occult blood in combination with rectal exams is the best simple screening procedure for detecting gastrointestinal (GI) bleeding that can originate from many causes, such as ulcers, varicies, colitis, tears, polyps, and cancer. The fecal occult blood test (FOBT), also known as the guaiac or guaiac-based test, detects microscopic amounts of blood in the stool. Usually this blood is *occult* (not grossly visible), although it may be observable. When blood is present in the stool, a color change is visualized by the use of hydrogen peroxidase on guaiac-impregnated paper. The test is useful in detecting GI bleeding that subsequently will lead to further evaluation of causation. When more than 50 mL of blood enters the feces from the upper GI tract, the stool becomes darker and is called *melena*.

Hemorrhoids, rectal fissures, or rectal trauma can lead to blood in the stool; however, blood can also appear in the stool as the result of more severe conditions, such as ulcers, chron's disease, ulcerative colitis, and, most importantly, cancer. When the blood originates from the upper GI tract, the stool is often black ("tarry"), whereas lower GI bleeding may still show unchanged blood and color the stool red. In the case of stool guaiac there is significant improvement in the detection rate when more than one specimen is obtained. This easy test requires only a small amount of stool, and the client can be instructed how to collect the specimen at home.

▶ ASSESSMENT

1. Assess the client's or family member's understanding of the need for this test **so the nurse can provide needed teaching.**
2. Assess the client's ability to cooperate with the procedure to collect the specimen **to maintain privacy while a sample is obtained.**
3. Assess the client's medical history for bleeding or GI disorders. **The nurse can initiate screening tests.**
4. Assess any medications the client receives that can cause GI bleeding, such as anticoagulants, steroids, or acetylsalicylic acid, **to help determine the need for the test and/or the possible source of bleeding.**

▶ DIAGNOSIS

Constipation

Diarrhea

Deficient Knowledge

▶ PLANNING

Expected Outcomes:

1. The client will understand the purpose of the test.

2. The client will be able to collect the specimen, or allow the specimen to be collected.
3. The test for occult blood will be conducted properly and results will be recorded.

Equipment Needed (see Figure 1-15-1):

- Paper towel
- Disposable gloves
- Wooden applicator
- Occult blood test kit: Hemoccult slide and Hemoccult developing solution or Hematest tablets with guaiac-impregnated paper

▶ CLIENT EDUCATION NEEDED:

1. Teach the client the rationale for the stool test.
2. Instruct the client to avoid red meat for 24 hours before the test because of the possibility of producing a false-positive result.
3. Reassure the client that a simple positive test does not confirm a diagnosis of rectal bleeding or colorectal cancer. Three tests need to be done as well as further testing such as a sigmoidoscopy.
4. Ask the client to list all medications he or she is taking to assess which ones the client should not take before the Hemoccult test.

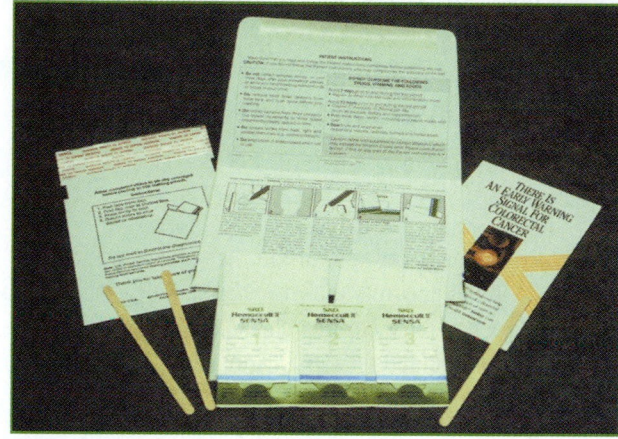

Figure 1-15-1   Hemoccult slide test kit to test for occult blood.

5. If the client is collecting the specimen, instruct the client how to collect the specimen from two different areas of the stool.
6. Instruct the client to keep the specimen free of urine and tissue.

 Estimated time to complete the skill: **5–10 minutes**

▶ DELEGATION TIPS

The collection and testing of stool for occult blood may be delegated. Ancillary personnel should be instructed to report the presence of red blood in the stool immediately to the nurse. Positive results indicated on the Hemoccult slide should be reported immediately to the nurse and recorded on the appropriate clinical record.

IMPLEMENTATION—Action/Rationale

Action	Rationale
1. Wash hands and apply clean gloves.	1. Reduces transmission of microorganisms from fecal specimen to nurse.
2. Obtain a stool specimen from the client, commode, specimen cup, or bedpan.	2. Uncontaminated specimen will be in a dry container without urine, water, or tissue.
3. Obtain a small portion of feces with a wooden applicator.	3. Test can be performed on a small specimen.
4. Read and follow the manufacturer's instructions.	4. Ensures accurate results.
Perform Occult Blood Slide Test	
5. Open the flap of the slide and smear a thin sample of feces on the paper in the first box.	5. Guaiac-impregnated paper is sensitive to fecal blood.

continues

Action	Rationale

Perform Occult Blood Slide Test *continued*

6. Apply feces from a different area of the specimen to the second box.

7. Close the slide cover and turn to the reverse side.
    Open the flap and apply two drops of developing solution on each sample box and on each control box according to the manufacturer's instructions (see Figure 1-15-2).

8. Note color change after 60 seconds or according to manufacturer's instructions.

9. Dispose of slide and applicator wrapped in a paper towel in the proper receptacle. Remove gloves and wash hands.

10. Apply a small amount of feces on guaiac-impregnated paper.

11. Place a Hematest tablet on top of the stool specimen.

12. Apply two to three drops of tap water to the tablet.

13. Note color change after 2 minutes.

14. Dispose of tablet, paper, and applicator wrapped in a paper towel in the proper receptacle.

15. Remove gloves and wash hands.

6. Occult blood from the upper GI tract is not always equally dispersed throughout the stool.

7. Developing solution penetrates the fecal specimen through the paper.

8. A bluish color indicates the presence of occult blood. Control box color can be used for comparison. No change in color is negative.

9. Reduces transfer of microorganisms.

10. Guaiac-impregnated paper is sensitive to fecal blood.

11. Tablet contains solid form of developing solution.

12. Tap water dissolves tablet, which releases solution over the specimen and paper.

13. A bluish color indicates the presence of occult blood. Results obtained after 2 minutes may be false.

14. Reduces transmission of microorganisms.

15. Reduces transmission of microorganisms.

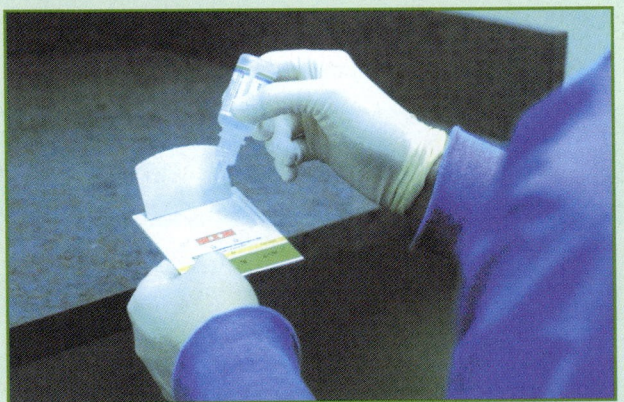

Figure 1-15-2 Apply the developing solution to the slide.

▶ REAL WORLD ANECDOTES

Martha had a family history of colorectal cancer so her physician recommended yearly screening for occult blood. The nurse taught her how to collect the specimen and how to apply a small sample of the stool onto the guaiac paper in the first box. Martha then showed the nurse how to take a sample from another part of the stool and apply it to the second box. Satisfied with the return-demonstration, the nurse gave Martha test kits for 3 days. The nurse told Martha to bring the kits to the office when she had completed them. The nurse would develop the test and tell her the results.

► EVALUATION

- Note presence or absence of color change in the guaiac paper.
- Note color, character, and consistency of stool.
- Ask the client to explain the rationale and procedure for the stool test.

► DOCUMENTATION

Nurses' Notes

- Record the date and time the collection was obtained and the test performed.
- Record the results of the test.
- Record the color, character, and consistency of the stool.
- Record when the results of the test were reported to the health care provider.

► CRITICAL THINKING SKILL

Introduction

There are several causes for a false-positive occult blood test. One is eating red meat or citrus fruit; another is taking medications such as iron preparations, aspirin, anticoagulants, ascorbic acid, steroids, or indomethacin. Hemorrhoids can cause bleeding and may be misinterpreted as upper or lower GI bleeding.

Possible Scenario

A client noticed small flecks of blood in his stool. He was instructed to collect a stool sample and apply it to an occult blood kit. When the nurse developed it, the results were strongly positive.

Possible Outcome

The nurse reviewed the client's history and found that he had received treatment for hemorrhoids in the past. The client also admitted he had failed to stop taking his daily aspirin prescribed by his cardiologist.

Prevention

A careful health assessment would have revealed these two common reasons for blood in the stool—hemorrhoids and taking aspirin.

► VARIATIONS

Geriatric Variations:

- *Some clients will need to bring the entire stool sample in a plastic specimen container if they are unable to use the occult blood test kit.*

Pediatric Variations:

- *Children may not be able to produce a specimen at a given time. Parents may need to assist them at home.*
- *Small children may be curious about what is done to the sample. They should be allowed to watch the test being done.*

Home Care Variations:

- *If the specimen is collected at home, the client should be instructed how to store it before it is taken to the laboratory.*

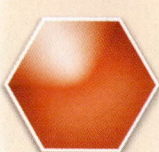

Long-Term Care Variations:

- *Review correct testing procedures with staff who may not be familiar with the test. If the test must be repeated periodically, encourage the client to be as independent as possible when collecting the sample.*

▶ COMMON ERRORS

Possible Error:

The stool becomes contaminated with urine.

Prevention:

Use a plastic insert in the toilet to facilitate collection of the stool (see Figure 1-15-3).

Discard the stool and wait for the next opportunity to collect a stool sample.

Possible Error:

The nurse opens the developing flap to apply the smear of stool.

Prevention:

Read the directions on the flap to choose the correct side to apply the sample.

Discard the Hemoccult slide and use a new one to apply the stool to the correct side. Proceed with the development of the test.

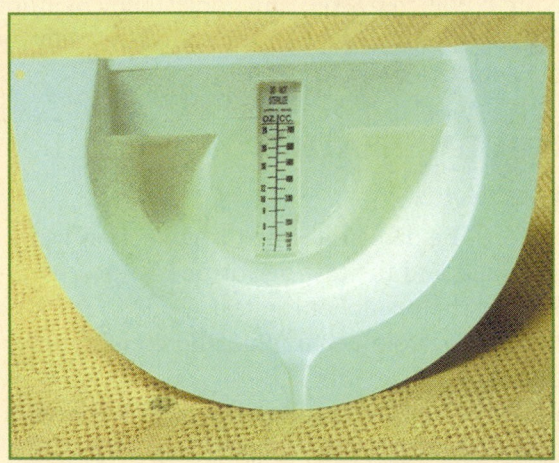

Figure 1-15-3   Use a graduated specimen container to collect a stool sample.

▶ NURSING TIPS

- Using a plastic insert in the toilet may facilitate obtaining a stool specimen.
- Occult blood should be tested regardless of the character or color of the stool, for example, bismuth (e.g., Pepto Bismol) produces black stool in the absence of bleeding. Black or tarry stools do not exclude a diagnosis of GI bleeding. Red, black, or melena stool may be an indication of GI bleeding.
- Check the lot number and brand name to ensure efficacy of the developing solution or slide. Mixing brand names can diminish the reliability of the reaction.
- Stool specimens should be tested within 48 hours after collection.

▶ SPECIAL CONSIDERATIONS

- *Stool tested for occult blood may have positive results up to 14 days after a single, major episode of upper GI bleeding.*
- *False-positive results are related to ingestion of red fruits and meats, methylene blue, chlorophyll, iodide, cupric sulfate, and bromide preparations.*
- *False-negative results are rare but may be caused by bile or from ingestion of magnesium-containing antacids.*
- *A Hemoccult test may be unreliable to evaluate gastric contents for occult blood.*
- *In newborns, maternal blood that is swallowed during delivery may cause bloody stools. The Apt test is used to differentiate maternal from neonatal blood.*

Safety and Infection Control

Proper Body Mechanics, Safe Lifting, and Transferring

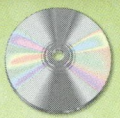

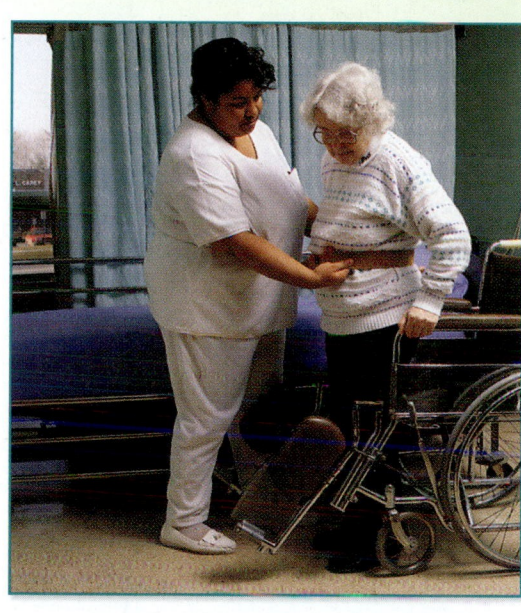

▶ OVERVIEW OF THE SKILL

Skills needed to care for clients often require that nurses/caregivers have the physical strength to provide individuals with the assistance that they require to remain mobile. Nurses/caregivers may need to carry, pull, push, or lift clients or equipment to accomplish daily care. It is imperative that nurses/caregivers know and use proper lifting techniques and seek assistance as needed to avoid injury to self and clients. Body mechanics is the term used when referring to lifting techniques. Correct body mechanics are essential to avoid work-related musculoskeletal injuries, diminish excessive strain and fatigue, and minimize the potential for injury (see Figure 2-1-1).

Body mechanics involve pushing, pulling, stooping, carrying, and lifting correctly. Knowledge of various client transfer techniques, the use of a team as needed, and the use of proper supportive equipment are included in this skill. Proper techniques of body mechanics, specialized lifting skills of transfer from bed to stretcher and from bed to chair or wheelchair, and the use of the bed transfer board and a hydraulic lift are reviewed. Specific tips for client and staff safety are highlighted. Promotion of client independence and self-help behavior as an intervention to reduce the risk of client and nurse injury is discussed. Warm-up exercises to avoid injury are reviewed (see Figure 2-1-2).

▶ ASSESSMENT

1. Assess the need and degree to which the client requires assistance to achieve physical movement. **Identifies client's ability to attain maximum level of self-help before initiating intervention.**
2. Identify the type of physical movement required **to assure the use of proper body mechanics such as pushing, pulling, or lifting.**
3. Identify the potential need for assistive equipment to accomplish the goal of safe lifting **to minimize the risk of client/nurse injury.**
4. Identify any unusual risks to safe lifting, such as an extra heavy client or a home care setting. **Allows nurse to plan modifications to ensure good body mechanics and reduce the risk of injury.**
5. Assess the client's vital signs, pain status, and need for pain medications before ambulating. Assess incisional areas and/or areas of injury.
6. Check equipment to ensure that it is in working order to facilitate a safe and uninterrupted transfer. Especially check locks on wheelchair.

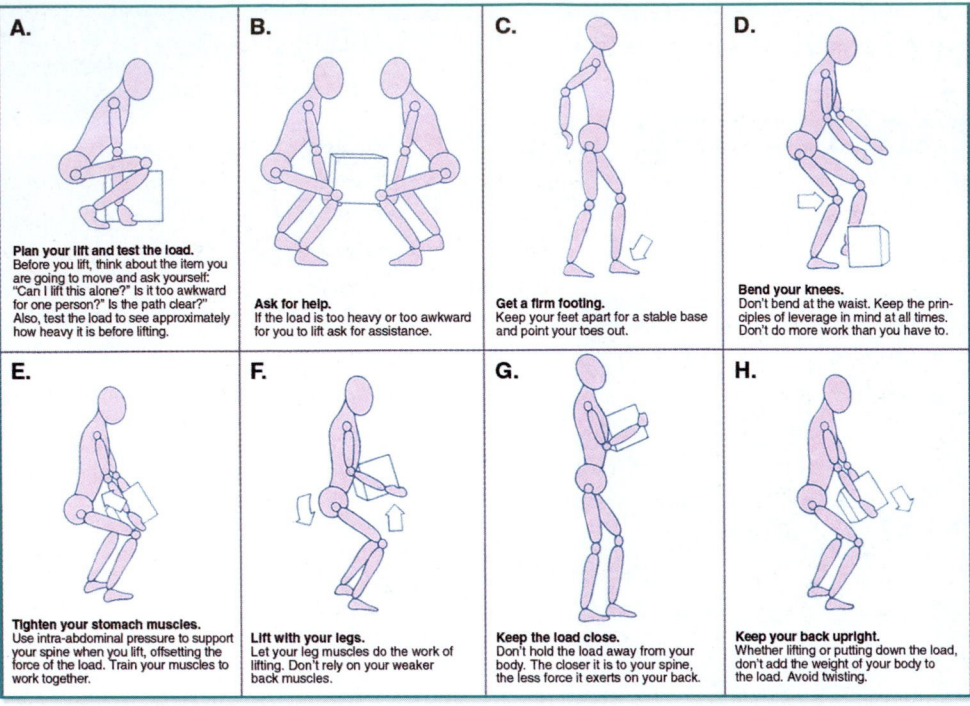

Figure 2-1-1 Always follow these eight rules for lifting. (Reprinted with permission from Ergodyne Corporation, St. Paul, MN.)

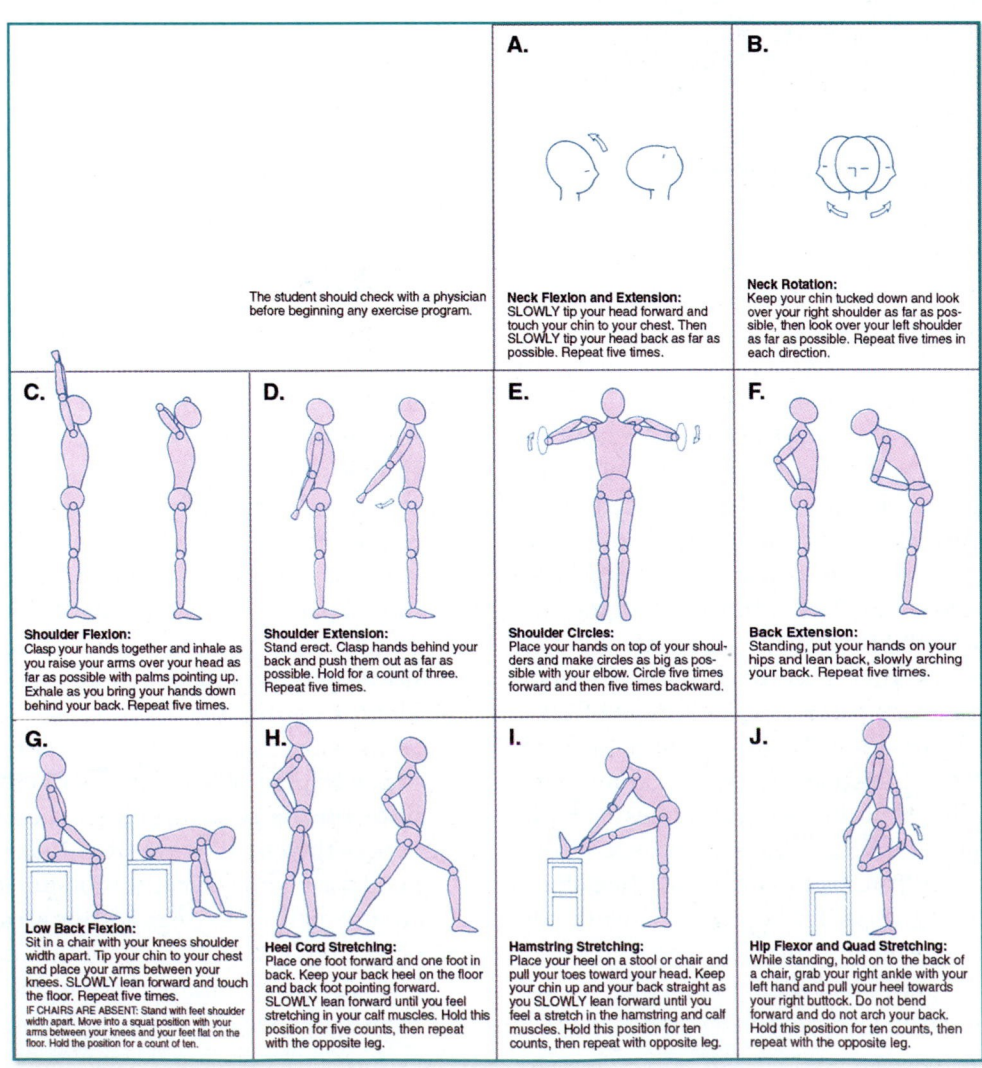

Figure 2-1-2 Follow these warm-up exercises to prepare for safe lifting. (Reprinted with permission from Ergodyne Corporation, St. Paul, MN.)

7. Identify all equipment and tubes connected to the client and take appropriate preventive measures. Frequently, clients that require lifting or transfer have intravenous tubing, other tubing, or orthopedic equipment.

8. Assess the client's understanding of the steps required to achieve the goal of a safe transfer and the ability to assist. Explanation of the steps in a clear, concise fashion will decrease anxiety, secure cooperation, and ease physical requirements for both the client and the nurse/caregiver.

▶ DIAGNOSIS

Risk for Injury

Impaired Physical Mobility

▶ PLANNING

Expected Outcomes:

1. Clients will be safely lifted/transferred by staff using appropriate equipment and correct body mechanics.

2. Accidents during lifting of clients will be avoided by using proper body alignment and mechanics.

3. Heavy lifting will be facilitated by mechanical devices and a team effort.

4. Clients and families will be taught safe lifting/transfer techniques to facilitate this process in home and extended-care environments.

5. The nurse will practice safe lifting and proper body mechanics when performing nursing care that requires bending or lifting.

Equipment Needed (see Figures 2-1-3A, B, C, and D):

- Transfer or gait belts
- Wheelchair equipped with working locks
- Transfer board
- Draw or lift sheet
- Nonslip shoes or slippers
- Safety or gait belt
- Stretcher equipped with working locks
- Hydraulic lift

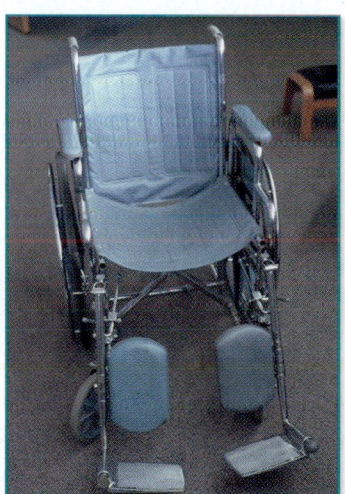

Figure 2-1-3A Wheelchair

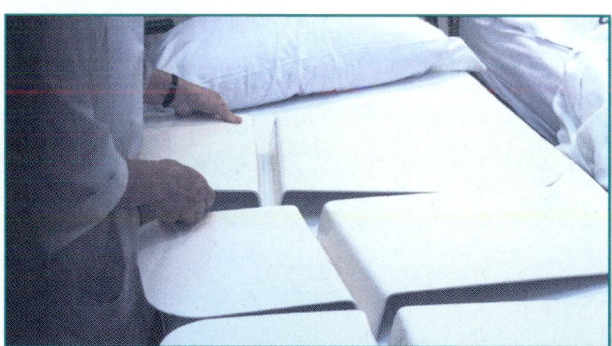

Figure 2-1-3B Transfer boards

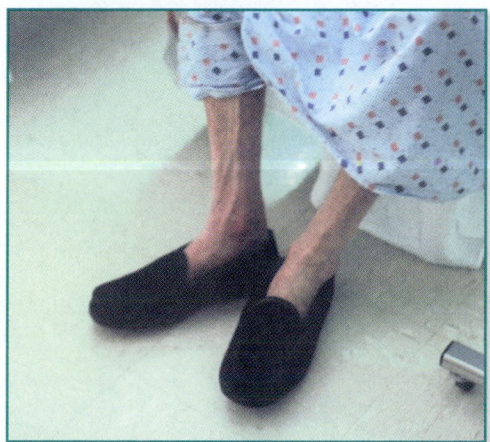

Figure 2-1-3C Nonskid footwear

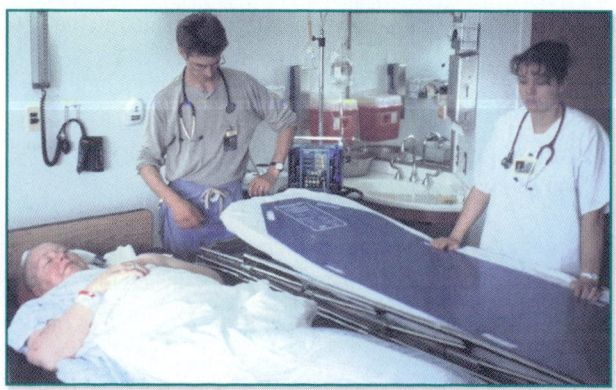

Figure 2-1-3D Stretcher

▶ CLIENT EDUCATION NEEDED:

1. Advise clients of the plan to transfer them from one position to another.
2. Explain the procedure, provide a demonstration, and describe the individual client's specific participation requirements.
3. Explain that the ultimate goals of safe lifting and transfers are to encourage independence and to facilitate self-achievement.
4. If lifting requires the use of equipment, demonstrate the equipment before the application occurs.
5. Reassure client that every effort will be made to maintain individual privacy and dignity and that his or her body will be covered throughout the move and upon completion.
6. Allay fear of falling, fear of isolation, and potential for the loss of well-being.
7. Encourage family member participation to facilitate safe lifting at sites external to the acute-care setting.
8. Advise client to inform the nurse immediately if he or she becomes dizzy or lightheaded and not to wait in the hope that it will go away.
9. Advise client to inform the nurse if more blankets are needed for warmth while being transported to other parts of the hospital.
10. Instruct client not to lean forward in the wheelchair because it may cause the wheelchair to tip.

Estimated time to complete the skill:
10–25 minutes for each variation of safe lifting

▶ DELEGATION TIPS

Delegation to ancillary personnel of the moving, transferring, and lifting of clients is an expectation of their role after proper instruction and/or certification. Ancillary personnel are routinely expected to place the bed at proper height, use a wide base of support, properly position the client, and safely use assistive devices. After repositioning the client, ancillary personnel are expected to evaluate the client's level of comfort. The client that requires complex turning or lifting devices needs the supervision of the professional nurse.

IMPLEMENTATION—Action/Rationale

Action	Rationale
1. Wash hands.	1. Reduces the transmission of microorganisms.
2. Assess the situation for obstacles, heavy clients, poor handholds, or equipment or objects in the way. Reduce or remove safety hazards prior to lifting the client or object. Assess for any tubing or equipment connected to the client.	2. Good planning helps prevent accidental injury.
3. Assess the situation for slippery surfaces, including wet floors; slippery shoes on client, helper, or nurse; and towels, linen, or paper on the floor. Resolve the slippery surface prior to lifting the client or object.	3. Removes the cause of many falls and slips.
4. Assess the situation for hidden risks, including client confusion, combativeness, orthostatic hypotension, drug effects, pain, or fear (see Figure 2-1-4).	4. Allows the nurse to anticipate and plan for unexpected events.

continues

Action	Rationale

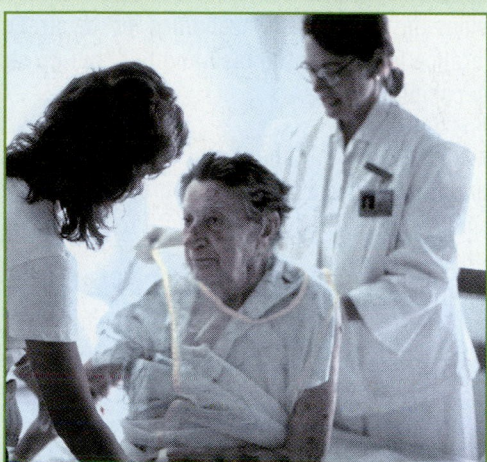

Figure 2-1-4   Assess the client and the setting for safety risks before moving, lifting, or transferring the client.

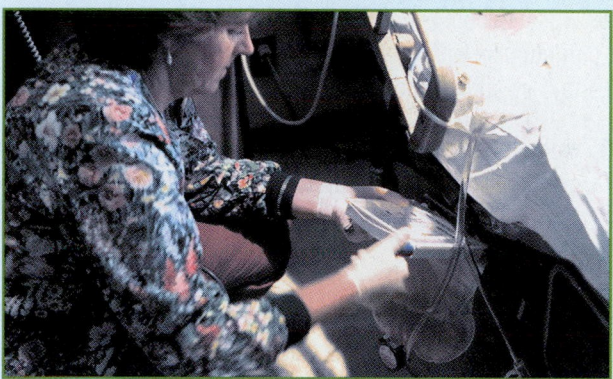

Figure 2-1-5   Squat, rather than bend, to maintain good posture.

5. Maintain low center of gravity by bending at the hips and knees, not the waist. Squat down rather than bend over to lift and lower (see Figure 2-1-5).

6. Establish a wide support base with feet spread apart (see Figure 2-1-6).

7. Use feet to move; do not engage in a twisting or bending motion from the waist.

8. When pushing or pulling, stand near the object and stagger one foot partially ahead of the other.

9. When pushing a client or an object, lean into the client or object and apply continuous light pressure (see Figure 2-1-7). When pulling a client or an object, lean away and grasp with light pressure. Never jerk or twist your body to force a weight to move.

5. Provides for the equal distribution of body weight and assists in maintaining safe balance.

6. Provides stability and lowers the center of gravity.

7. Assists in maintaining correct body alignment, which increases strength to lift, push, pull, and carry.

8. Provides a safety net for avoiding potential back injuries.

9. Firm pressure will provide continuous movement of the object and will avoid abrupt movements that require the expenditure of increased energy.

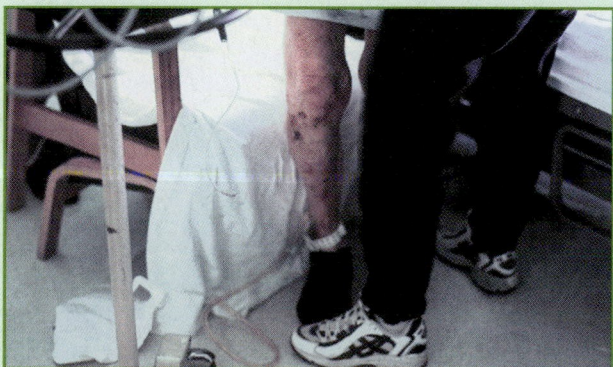

Figure 2-1-6   Spread feet apart to establish a wide base of support.

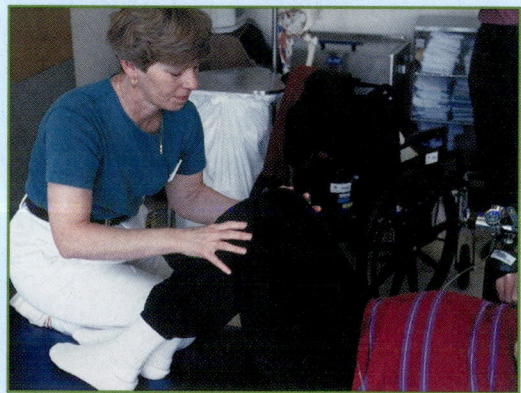

Figure 2-1-7   Lean into the client or object being pushed.

continues

Action	Rationale
10. When stooping to move an object, maintain a wide base of support with feet, flex knees to lower body, and maintain straight upper body.	**10.** Provides the appropriate mechanics for the strength and endurance to achieve the task and to stand up straight upon completion.
11. When lifting or carrying an object, bend the knees in front of the object, take a firm hold, and assume a standing position by using the leg muscles and keeping the back straight.	**11.** This stance will avoid the use of the back, diminish the potential for spinal twisting, and provide the lifter with a firm center of gravity and strength to lift the required weight.
12. When rising up from a squatting position, arch your back slightly. Keep the buttocks and abdomen tucked in and rise up with your head first.	**12.** Keeps the back from bowing and increasing the strain on the back muscles.
13. When lifting or carrying heavy objects, keep the weight as close to your center of gravity as possible (see Figure 2-1-8).	**13.** Reduces the strain on arm, leg, and back muscles.
14. When reaching for a client or an object, keep the back straight. If the client or object is heavy, do not try to lift the client or object without repositioning yourself closer to the weight (see Figure 2-1-9).	**14.** Avoids straining the back and arm muscles.
15. Use safety aids and equipment. Use gait belts (see Figure 2-1-10), lifts (see Figure 2-1-11), drawsheets, and other transfer assistance devices (see Figure 2-1-12). Encourage clients to use handrails and grab bars (see Figure 2-1-13). Wheelchair, cart, and stretcher wheels should be locked when they are not actually being moved.	**15.** Reduces the strain on the nurse and improves the safety for the client.

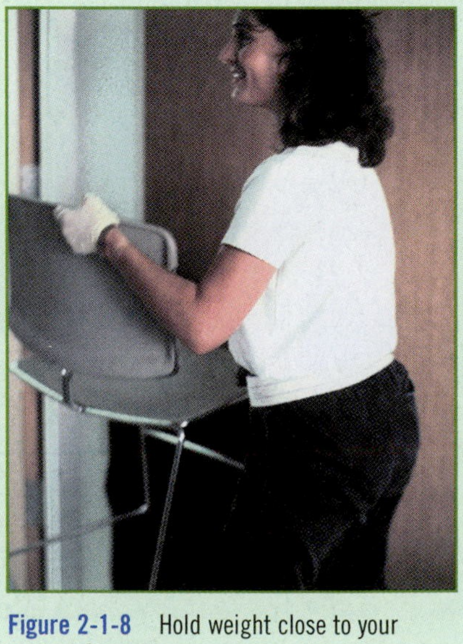

Figure 2-1-8 Hold weight close to your center of gravity.

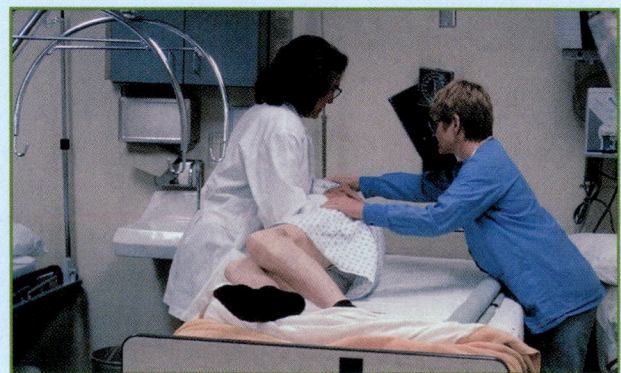

Figure 2-1-9 Keep your back straight when reaching.

continues

Action	Rationale

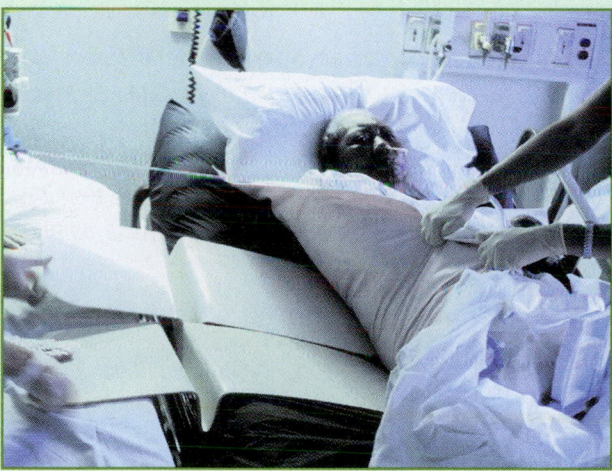

Figure 2-1-10 Use gait belts for better grip and control.

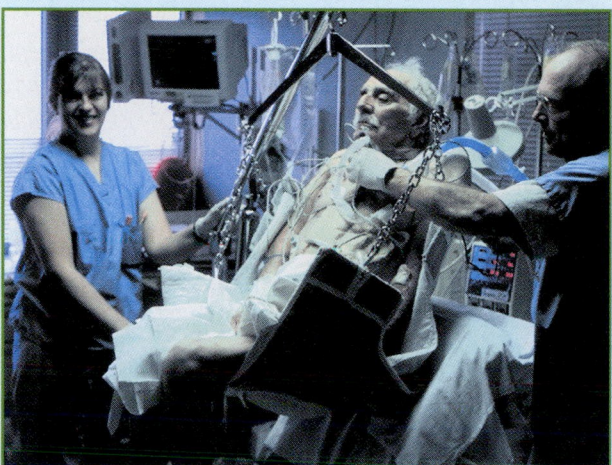

Figure 2-1-11 Use lifts to carry the weight of the client. Monitor equipment, lines, tubes, and drains and adjust as needed to prevent them from being dislodged.

Figure 2-1-12 Use transfer boards to reduce shearing forces and to reduce the effort needed to slide the client.

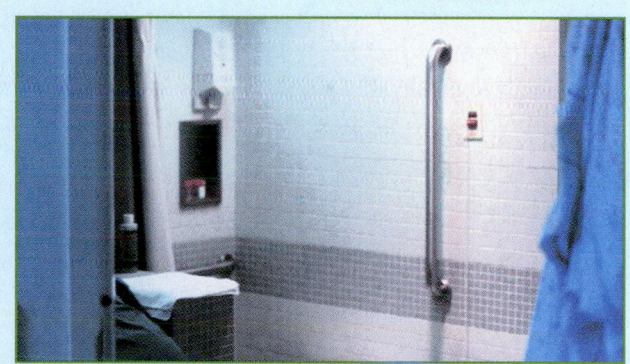

Figure 2-1-13 Encourage the client to use handrails and grab bars to reduce the risk of slipping or falling.

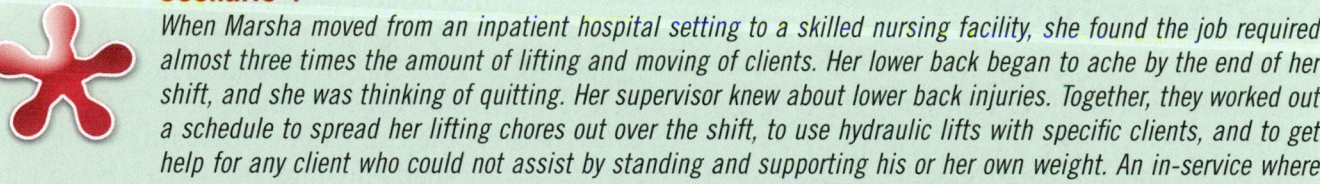

▶ **REAL WORLD ANECDOTES**

Scenario 1

When Marsha moved from an inpatient hospital setting to a skilled nursing facility, she found the job required almost three times the amount of lifting and moving of clients. Her lower back began to ache by the end of her shift, and she was thinking of quitting. Her supervisor knew about lower back injuries. Together, they worked out a schedule to spread her lifting chores out over the shift, to use hydraulic lifts with specific clients, and to get help for any client who could not assist by standing and supporting his or her own weight. An in-service where staff practiced lifting and moving techniques and exercising outside of work completed the intervention. Marsha stayed on the job with no further problems.

continues

▶ **REAL WORLD ANECDOTES** *(continued)*

Scenario 2

A nurse was working in the home setting. Her elderly client was taking a tub bath, which he generally did every evening. This evening, the client felt dizzy after getting into the tub and started to get out unassisted. The nurse was in the bathroom. She saw her client stand up, sway, and start to lose his balance. She stepped forward, placed one foot into the bathwater, set her feet wide, bent her knees, and started to assist her client to sit on the edge of the tub safely. The bathtub had nonslip protection, but her other foot, on the wet bathroom floor, slid out from under her. They both fell into the tub. Fortunately, neither was seriously hurt.

Scenario 3

Annabel, a client with breast cancer that has metastasized to her spine, is also hearing impaired. Although medicated with continuous opioids with a transdermal fentanyl patch, she has break-through pain. The health care team has planned to move her from her bed to undergo radiation palliation for her pain. The team decides to move Annabel from the bed to a stretcher using three assistants, one at the head of the bed, one at the side of the bed, and the third by the stretcher. Because Annabel is hearing impaired, her nurse writes the plan down for Annabel to read, thereby decreasing the client's anxiety and maximizing her ability to assist with the transfer. The nurse also plans to coordinate the transfer at a time when Annabel is pain-free and can help herself move onto the stretcher. Summoning adequate assistance and enabling the client to assist and cooperate reduces the risk of back injury for the staff.

Scenario 4

Bobby is a hefty 16-year-old client who has sustained a crushing injury to his leg and foot from a lawn mower accident. He is taken to the hospital, the extremity is cleaned, hematomas are drained, lacerations are sutured, and the wounds dressed. His dressings require changing every 24 hours, and he needs to be turned in bed to accomplish this task. The nurses caring for Bobby determine that their safety will require the use of two nurses and a draw sheet to turn and hold him. Bobby will be turned by both nurses. One nurse will hold and distract, and the other nurse will change the dressings. One nurse working alone would risk a twist or strain injury if she tried to hold, distract, restrain, and change a large dressing over a painful wound.

Scenario 5

A client is walking in the hall and becomes dizzy. She reaches out to grab onto the medication cart. The nurse had not locked the wheels of the cart. It rolls away, and the client falls to the floor.

▶ **EVALUATION**

- The client or object is lifted and/or moved without sustaining injury or damage.
- The nurse who is lifting and moving clients or objects is not injured.

▶ **DOCUMENTATION**

Nurses' Notes

- Document type of lift or transfer in the progress notes.
- Document client's tolerance of the lift or move in the progress notes.

▶ **CRITICAL THINKING SKILL**

Introduction

Plan ahead to avoid back strain.

Possible Scenario

Angela is 2 days status post a bilateral mastectomy and has been getting up to the bathroom alone for more than 24 hours. During the night, she puts on her call light to ask for assistance to the bathroom because she feels "groggy." She weighs 250 pounds. The nurse is concerned that the client seems confused. She checks the medication chart and notes that Angela was given chloral hydrate, a sleeping pill, at 10 PM.

Possible Outcome

The nurse notes that chloral hydrate can often cause clients to hallucinate or become confused. In addition, the client is obese. The nurse asks another nurse to come in and assist. Angela stands up and lurches forward. She grabs the intravenous line (IV) pole, thinking it is the bathroom door handle. Both nurses move into position to catch her before she falls, bracing their feet apart and bending at the knees. Injury to both nurses and the client is averted.

Prevention

In this case, the nurse realized there was an additional safety hazard and took the steps to prevent a fall and possible serious injury.

► VARIATIONS

Geriatric Variations:
- *Elderly clients often have reduced flexibility and muscle strength.*
- *Although frail-looking elderly are assumed to have lower muscle strength, obesity may hide poor muscle tone as well.*
- *Elderly clients often live alone and are very independent. They know what their bodies can and cannot do. When assessing an elderly client, ask about his or her normal routine. Assist, but follow his or her lead when possible to promote independence, control, and exercise.*

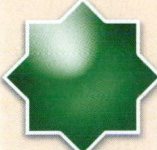

Pediatric Variations:
- *Younger children are often moved and carried by parents in the hospital setting. Make sure the parent is used to carrying the child and that the child has not grown too heavy for safe lifting and carrying by one adult.*

Home Care Variations:
- *The home care setting poses special challenges for safe lifting and moving. Often the nurse is the only person in the setting physically able to move and lift. Furniture, especially beds and chairs, may not be designed for client care.*
- *Know the policies and procedures for obtaining assistance and alternatives to lifting and moving heavy clients at home.*
- *Instruct home caregivers about the basics of good body mechanics. Practice and have the home caregiver demonstrate proper techniques.*
- *Many safety risks not considered in the hospital can be present in the home. Scatter rugs, slippery tile, older furniture in poor repair, narrow hallways, and confined spaces with reduced maneuverability must all be considered when planning to move or lift the client.*

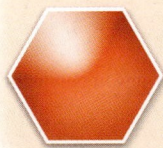

Long-Term Care Variations:
- *Workers in long-term care settings may have to do greater amounts of heavy lifting with less staffing, especially during night or evening shifts. Make sure lifting equipment is in good repair, gait belts are available, and personnel know how and when to use equipment safely.*

► COMMON ERRORS

Possible Error:

The client is moved but Foley catheters, pumps, drainage tubes, and IVs are not considered in the move and the client or nurse is injured by traumatic removal of or falling equipment.

continues

> ▶ **COMMON ERRORS** *(continued)*

Prevention:

Do a mental checklist of all tubes, drains, braces, and other devices. Mentally plan the move before you begin. Do not be in a hurry. If more than one nurse is involved in the move, do not assume that someone else has readied the tubes and equipment. Ensure that brakes are secured on wheelchairs, beds, and stretchers, reducing the client's risk for injury.

Possible Error:

Underestimating the strain or force required to assist a client.

Prevention:

Often nurses focus on the task and time schedule and consider how difficult it would be to summon help versus performing the task. Instead, consider the weight, level of consciousness, and physical impairment of the client. A good rule of thumb is not to lift or move any client by yourself who cannot bear his or her own weight.

Possible Error:

Slipping on spilled liquids on the floor.

Prevention:

Make sure none of your nursing techniques, such as priming IV tubing, wringing out wet dressings or wet compresses, and giving bed baths systematically, allows water to spill. Clean up spills immediately, and warn others of the spill.

▶ NURSING TIPS

- Lock elevator doors before entering and exiting with clients in wheelchairs or stretchers. This will help avoid twisting to prevent the door from closing on a client, and prevent injury.
- Use portable IV poles on stretchers and wheelchairs instead of independent IV poles. This will help you focus your attention on ambulating the client instead of the IV pole.
- All assistive devices used to facilitate safe lifting must receive periodic safety checks by the appropriate department assigned. It is imperative that staff oversee this effort and report equipment that may cause potential danger for clients and staff.

- Keep yourself strong and healthy. Nursing is a physical job. Nurses must have physical ability to avoid fatigue and injury associated with pushing, pulling, lifting, and carrying clients. Stay in shape and practice basic health habits. Poor eating habits, not enough sleep, stress, obesity, and inactivity all decrease strength, flexibility, and judgment, which increases the risk of injury.
- Be sure the bed is aligned to the same height as the stretcher.
- Be sure client is kept in alignment when lifting or transferring. Always seek help if in doubt.

> ▶ **SPECIAL CONSIDERATIONS**

- *If the client has an indwelling catheter, secure it and the drainage bag to the client. Do not disconnect or attach above the level of the bladder to avoid an increased risk of contamination.*
- *If the client is on oxygen, assure that the tubing is long enough or that portable oxygen is available.*
- *If the nurse/caregiver has experienced prior back pain, back injury, or other injuries that may lead to future disability, seek assistance. If the nurse/caregiver is pregnant, seek assistance for lifting.*
- *Certain clients with spinal injuries or spinal surgery may require "logrolling," a technique of moving or turning a client, whereby the body is kept in a protected straight alignment during the transfer.*
- *Hydraulic lifts will be necessary for large clients or for more difficult transfers.*
- *Special protocols are generally available for clients with orthopedic procedures, such as avoidance of adduction and internal rotation in clients with total hip replacement. Use pillow splints or trochanter roll as appropriate. Know the protocol for weight bearing on surgical hip. Clients with knee surgery generally require splinting before ambulation.*

Assisting with Ambulation and Safe Falling

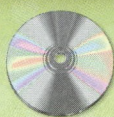

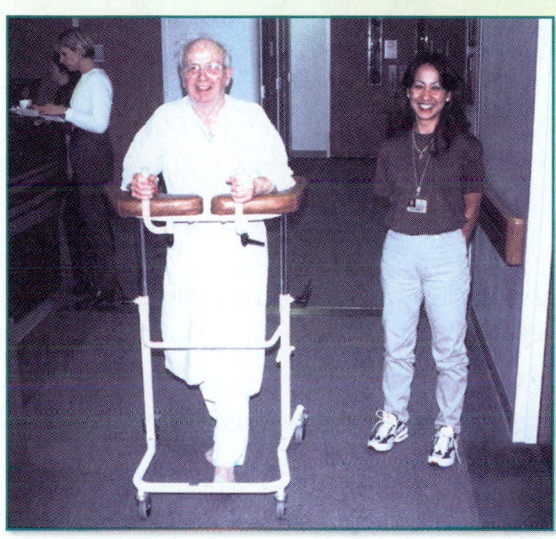

▶ OVERVIEW OF THE SKILL

Client ambulation (assisted or unassisted walking) is encouraged soon after the onset of illness or surgery to prevent the complications of immobility. First, the nurse assesses the strength, endurance, mobility, and orientation of the client. The nurse assists with client ambulation, especially if equipment (intravenous [IV] infusions, urinary catheters, closed chest drainage systems, drainage tubes) is present. Finally, the nurse must evaluate client ambulation to plan the progression of activity.

Clients at high risk for falls include those with prolonged hospitalization, those taking sedatives or tranquilizers, confused clients, or those with a history of physical restraint use. A great majority of falls:

- Occur in the evening
- Occur in the client's room
- Involve wheelchairs
- Involve confused clients
- Involve unattended clients
- Involve clients with poor footwear
- Occur with poor lighting
- Involve clients with poor vision
- Occur with clients experiencing neuromuscular impairment

Awareness of risk factors for falls allows the nurse to prevent many client injuries.

The nurse continually evaluates the client's strength and endurance during the entire ambulation process.

▶ ASSESSMENT

1. Determine the client's most recent activity level and tolerance **to evaluate the client's current ambulatory ability.**
2. Assess the client's current status, including vital signs, fatigue, pain, and medications **to identify conditions that might adversely affect ambulation.**
3. **To evaluate the client's environment for safety:** Check for handrails to help the client stand and to hold onto while walking. Check that the floor is level, clean, and not slippery or wet. Make sure there is adequate lighting so the client can see where he or she is going (see Figure 2-2-1).
4. Assess the client's ambulation equipment, including the use of a walker, cane, or other assistive device **to determine whether the equipment is in safe condition.**
5. Check the client's clothing **to determine that the client's shoes or slippers are safe to walk in and that he or she has adequate covering for warmth and privacy.**
6. While the client is ambulating, assess his or her gait and bearing. This assessment enables

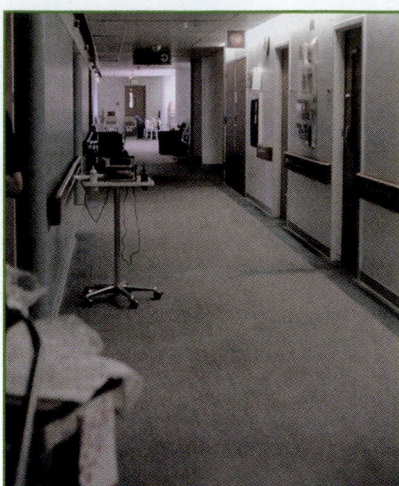

Figure 2-2-1 Before ambulating the client, check planned route for safety concerns. Check for good lighting, nonskid floors, accessible handrails, and possible barriers.

the nurse **to determine how well the client is tolerating the activity and also allows the detection of hypotension, diaphoresis, breathlessness, or weakness.**

7. After ambulation, assess the client's ability to recover from the activity, including exhaustion, energy, and recovery times. **Determine whether modifications need to be made in the distance, type of assistance, or length of time the client is ambulating.**

▶ DIAGNOSIS

Activity Intolerance

Impaired Physical Mobility

Impaired Transfer Ability

Impaired Walking

Risk for Falls

Risk for Injury

▶ PLANNING

Expected Outcomes:

1. The client will be able to walk a predetermined distance, with assistance as needed, and return to the starting point.
2. While walking, the client will not suffer any injury.
3. The client will be able to increase the distance he or she can walk, or will require less

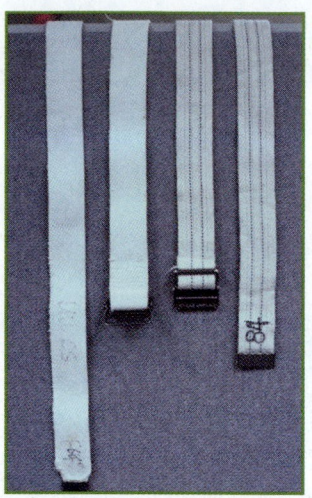

Figure 2-2-2 Gait or transfer belts.

assistance to accomplish the distance on a regular basis.

Equipment Needed:

- Gait belt (transfer) as needed (PRN) (see Figure 2-2-2)
- Assistive devices—walker, cane
- Shoes or nonslip footwear

▶ CLIENT EDUCATION NEEDED:

1. Explain to the client the importance of ambulation to recovery, including the role of early ambulation in increasing peristalsis and venous return from the lower legs.
2. Be sure the client understands the need to have assistance standing by the first few times ambulating.
3. Educate the client regarding the importance of proper gait and posture while ambulating.
4. Encourage the client to void before ambulating, especially with elderly clients, to prevent the need to interrupt ambulation.
5. Advise the client that even though ambulation may be uncomfortable or even painful, the activity will help the body produce endorphins and provide a natural form of pain relief.

Estimated time to complete the skill: **20–30 minutes**

▶ DELEGATION TIPS

The ambulation and safe movement of clients is routinely delegated after proper instruction regarding planning the move, arranging for adequate help, if necessary, and positioning oneself close to the client to prevent injury.

IMPLEMENTATION—Action/Rationale

Action	Rationale

Ambulation Safety

1. When assisting a client with an IV infusion, place the IV pole with wheels at the head of the bed before having the client dangle the legs, so that there is room to swing the legs from the bed to the floor. If orders allow, place a saline lock on the IV.

2. Transfer the IV infusion from the bed IV pole to the portable IV pole. The client or the nurse can guide the portable IV pole ahead during ambulation (see Figure 2-2-3).

3. When assisting the client with a urinary drainage bag, empty the drainage bag prior to ambulation. Have the client sit on the side of the bed with legs dangling.

    Remove the urinary drainage bag from the bed. The nurse or client can hold the urinary drainage bag during ambulation. Make sure the drainage bag remains below the level of the bladder (see Figure 2-2-4).

4. When the client has a drainage tube such as a T-tube, Hemovac, or Jackson–Pratt drainage system, be sure to secure the drainage tube and bag prior to ambulation. Place a rubber band around the drainage tube near the drainage bag. Secure the drainage tube and bag with a safety pin through the rubber band. Allow slack. The safety pin can be secured to the client's gown or robe (see Figure 2-2-5).

---

1. Prevents the client's legs from becoming tangled in the IV pole or tubing, causing a fall or causing the tubing to become dislodged. Provides more freedom of movement.

2. Supports the IV while the client ambulates.

3. Emptying the bag reduces the weight of the bag. An empty bag kept below the level of the bladder reduces the risk of urine flowing back into the bladder, and, hence, reduces risk of contamination.

    Having the nurse hold the drainage bag allows the client to concentrate on safe ambulation.

4. Prevents the tubing from becoming dislodged or tangled in clothing or other tubes.

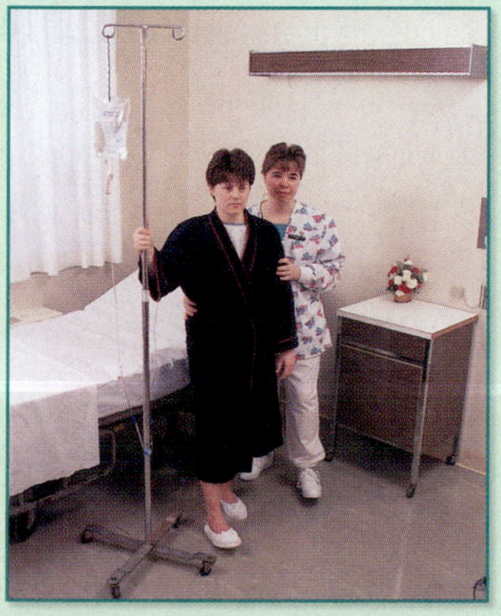

Figure 2-2-3 Ambulating a client who has an IV.

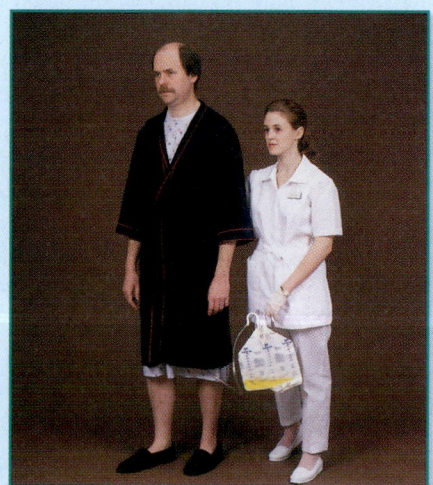

Figure 2-2-4 Ambulating a client who has a urinary drainage bag.

continues

Action	Rationale

Ambulation Safety *continued*

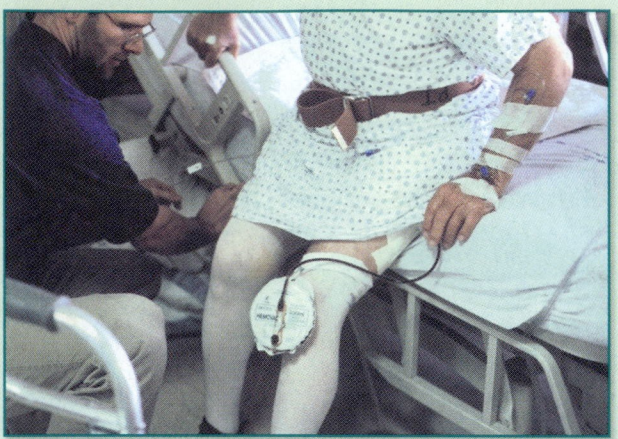

Figure 2-2-5 Secure tubes and drainage bags before ambulation so they do not become dislodged.

5. Ambulating the client with a closed chest tube drainage system often requires two nurses, one nurse assisting the client and one nurse managing the closed chest tube drainage system. While the client is sitting on the edge of the bed with feet dangling, remove the hangers from the drainage system. Hold the closed chest tube drainage system upright at all times to maintain the water seal. Make sure the closed chest tube drainage system remains below the level of the chest. Do not pull or tug on the chest tubes; they may not be sutured into place.

6. Use a transfer belt or gait belt when ambulating a client who is weak (see Figure 2-2-6). For additional safety, a wheelchair can be pushed alongside the client for ready access if the client feels weak, tired, or faint.

7. If a client feels faint or dizzy during leg-dangling, return the client to a supine position in bed and lower the head of the bed. Monitor the client's blood pressure and pulse.

8. If the client feels faint or dizzy during ambulation, allow the client to sit in a chair. Stay with the client for safety. Request another nurse to secure a wheelchair if not already available to return the client to bed.

9. If the client feels faint or dizzy during the ambulation and starts to fall, ease the client to the floor while supporting and protecting the client's head. Position yourself next to and slightly behind the ambulating client, thus being able to step behind the client and safely ease the client to the floor. Ask other personnel to assist you in returning the client to bed. Assess orthostatic blood pressures.

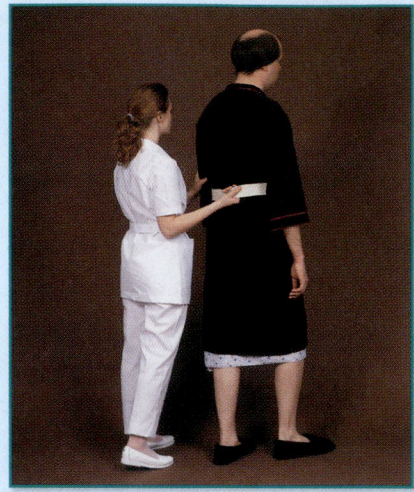

Figure 2-2-6 Ambulate the client by using a gait belt for better grip and control.

5. The presence of two nurses enables one nurse to focus on the client's safety and ambulation while the other nurse focuses on maintaining the chest drainage system and keeping the tubes from becoming dislodged

6. The transfer belt is a 2-inch-wide webbed belt worn by the client for the purposes of stabilization during transfers and ambulation. It provides more support for the client by having the nurse hold the back of the belt.

7. Keeps the client from falling from the bed. Lowering the head of the bed will allow gravity to support blood flow to the brain in the hypotensive client.

8. May stop the client from progressing to full syncope.

9. Easing the client to the floor prevents injury to the client.

continues

Action	Rationale
10. Encourage the client to void before ambulating, especially with elderly clients.	10. Prevents need to interrupt ambulation. Restroom may not be readily available.

Safe Walking

Action	Rationale
1. Inform client of the purposes and distance of the walking exercise (see Figure 2-2-7).	1. Reduces client anxiety and increases cooperation.
2. Elevate the head of the bed and wait several minutes.	2. Prevents orthostatic hypotension.
3. Lower the bed height.	3. Reduces distance client has to step down, thus decreasing risk of injury.
4. With one arm on the client's back and one arm under the client's upper legs, move the client into the dangling position.	4. Provides client support and reduces risk of fall.
5. Encourage client to dangle at side of bed for several minutes.	5. Prevents orthostatic hypotension. Allows for assessing tolerance for the sitting position.
6. Place gait belt around client's waist; secure the buckle in front.	6. Provides handholds for the caregiver to support the client.
7. Stand in front of client with your knees touching client's knees.	7. Prevents client from sliding forward if dizziness or faintness occurs.
8. Place arms under client's axilla.	8. Supports client's trunk.
9. Assist client to a standing position, allowing client time to balance (see Figure 2-2-8).	9. Reduces risk of fall.

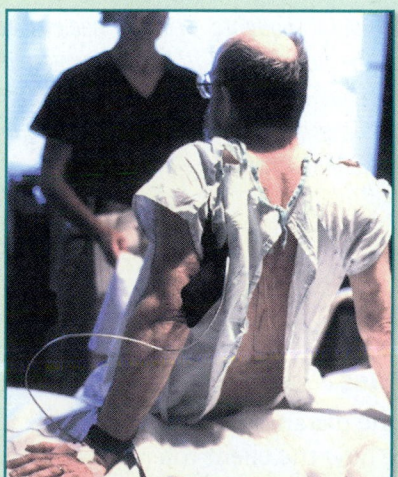

Figure 2-2-7 Discuss the planned walking exercise with the client prior to ambulation.

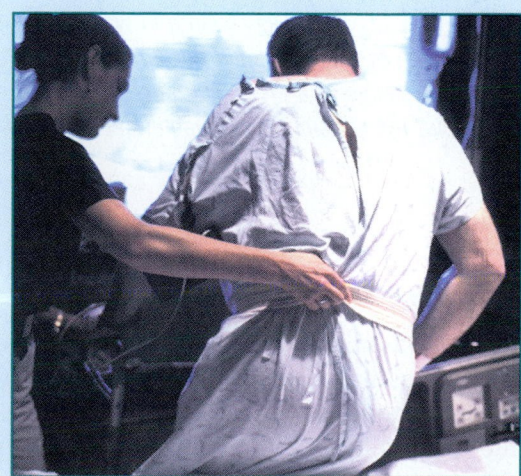

Figure 2-2-8 Assist the client to stand.

continues

Action	Rationale
Safe Walking *continued*	
10. Help the client ambulate the desired distance or distance of tolerance by placing your hand under the client's forearm and ambulating close to the client. Alternatively, place a gait belt around the client's waist and walk to the client's side and slightly behind with one hand grasping the belt at the center back.	10. Provides assistance in achieving ambulatory goals.
11. Help the client back to the bed or chair. Make the client comfortable, and make sure all lines and tubes are secure.	11. Promotes safety and comfort.
12. Wash hands.	12. Reduces the transmission of microorganisms.

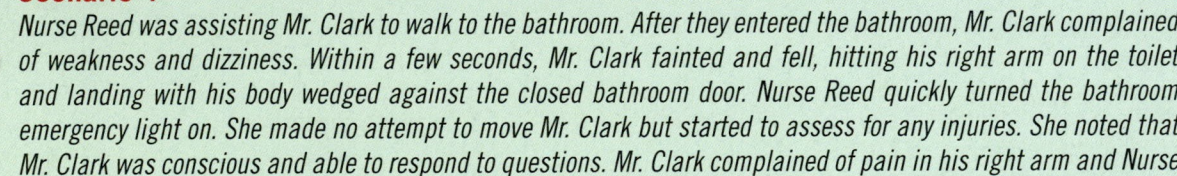

► REAL WORLD ANECDOTES

Scenario 1

Nurse Reed was assisting Mr. Clark to walk to the bathroom. After they entered the bathroom, Mr. Clark complained of weakness and dizziness. Within a few seconds, Mr. Clark fainted and fell, hitting his right arm on the toilet and landing with his body wedged against the closed bathroom door. Nurse Reed quickly turned the bathroom emergency light on. She made no attempt to move Mr. Clark but started to assess for any injuries. She noted that Mr. Clark was conscious and able to respond to questions. Mr. Clark complained of pain in his right arm and Nurse Reed noted that Mr. Clark's right arm was deformed and discolored. As she was talking to Mr. Clark, other staff members arrived to assist Nurse Reed and Mr. Clark. Nurse Reed had to move Mr. Clark in order to get the door open and she did this while making sure to maintain Mr. Clark's head and neck alignment and without further injuring Mr. Clark's arm. The other staff members were able to assist Nurse Reed and Mr. Clark. Mr. Clark's right arm was found to be broken at the point where it had hit the toilet.

Scenario 2

Cindy was an adolescent client in an open psychiatric ward for evaluation of suicidal thoughts. She had been given an initial dose of Haldol 5 mg IM for agitation and was resting on the bed in her room. The nurse stood in the doorway and asked her to come down to the meeting room for an afternoon group session. Cindy made it as far as the hall when she fainted and hit her head on the edge of a chair. The nurse was not used to psychiatric clients experiencing mobility problems. He needed to remember that hypotension is one side effect of Haldol and be extra alert for the client's safety.

► EVALUATION

- The client was able to walk a predetermined distance, with assistance as needed, and return to the starting point.
- While walking, the client did not suffer any injury.
- The client was able to increase the distance walked and/or required less assistance to accomplish the distance on a regular basis.

► DOCUMENTATION

Nurses' Notes

- Record the distance the client was able to ambulate and note how the client tolerated the ambulation.
- List any assistive devices the client required and any teaching done regarding using the device.
- Document any special concerns or unusual findings noted while ambulating the client.

▶ **CRITICAL THINKING SKILL**

Introduction

Be prepared to take rapid and decisive action to avoid injury to the client.

Possible Scenario

Mr. Hayes had abdominal surgery several days ago. You have been assigned his care, which includes ambulating him in the hallway. While walking with Mr. Hayes, you note that he has become pale and sweaty. His skin is clammy, and he complains of dizziness and spots in front of his eyes. There are no chairs nearby to seat Mr. Hayes in and you are concerned that he is going to fall if you do not do something.

Possible Outcome

Without intervention Mr. Hayes will probably faint or simply fall because of hypotension. He could injure himself in the fall or possibly tear open his surgical site.

Prevention

The best thing to do as soon as this happens is to gently lower Mr. Hayes to the floor before he falls. You can then call for assistance to get Mr. Hayes into a wheelchair or onto a gurney and back to bed.

To prevent this from happening, be aware of good locations to seat a client before ambulation. Place a chair at a midway point if needed. Clients who are prone to dizziness can sometimes ambulate while using a wheelchair as a modified walker. The chair is available should the client become dizzy or need to rest. Also be sure to take into account that the distance walked from the bed is only half the distance the client will have to walk. If the client is to ambulate 10 feet it is 5 feet away from the bed and 5 feet back.

▶ **VARIATIONS**

Geriatric Variations:

- *Elderly clients are more likely to use ambulatory aids such as walkers or canes. Proper gait is even more important when one is using an assistive device. Encourage urination before walking.*

Pediatric Variations:

- *If ambulation is difficult or painful, children may give up and refuse to try. Offering a reward or treat for accomplishing the task may help motivate a child.*
- *Small children may not be as coordinated when walking and may require additional care and attention to safety.*

Home Care Variations:

- *Home care environments vary widely. Be sure the environment in which the client ambulates is safe. Remove throw rugs and eliminate clutter on floors.*
- *Do not let barriers keep the client from moving about. Think of creative ways to overcome obstacles. Being able to go outdoors or to move to the living room from the bedroom can offer an uplifting change of scenery and improve feelings of independence.*

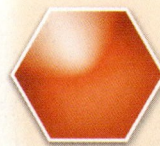

Long-Term Care Variation:

- *Clients with long-term ambulatory problems may become careless regarding their gait and their equipment. Be sure to check their equipment and reinforce proper gait.*

► **COMMON ERRORS**

Possible Error:

Providing too much or too little support for the client during ambulation.

Prevention:

When assisting with ambulation, place your hand under the client's forearm and ambulate close to the client. Another way to provide firm yet minimal support is with a gait belt around the client's waist.

► **NURSING TIPS**

- Be sure to take into account that the distance walked from the bed is only half the distance the client will have to walk. If the client is to ambulate 10 feet, it is 5 feet away from the bed and 5 feet back.
- Be aware of the surrounding environment. Think ahead regarding the client's activity tolerance and be aware of places the client might stop to sit or rest.
- Do not allow the client to place an arm around your shoulders for support. If the client falls, the weight of the client could cause twisting injuries to your back.

- Try to match your gait to the client's to provide a more even support.
- Remember to assess if the client can see and hear (i.e., glasses and hearing aids) before ambulation.
- Elderly clients are generally less stable with gait, have more vertigo, and may need to dangle for longer periods of time to stabilize the vascular system. Encourage enough fluids to avoid orthostatic hypotension; however, be aware that elderly clients may need to void more often. Elderly clients may require a slow, patient pace in ambulating.

► **SPECIAL CONSIDERATIONS**

- *If the client requires oxygen, secure a portable canister of oxygen; have adequate length of tubing.*
- *When ambulating clients who have had a total hip surgery, avoid adduction and internal rotation when moving a client from lying, to sitting, to standing. Use trochanter or pillow splint as appropriate. Be aware of weight-bearing protocol.*
- *When ambulating clients who have had knee surgery apply appropriate splint before ambulating.*
- *Once client is returned to bed secure equipment (tubings, sequential stockings, orthopedic equipment) and replace call light.*

Applying Restraints

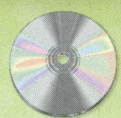

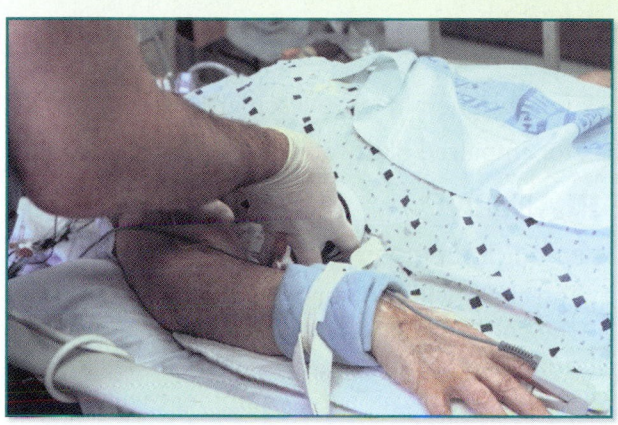

▶ OVERVIEW OF THE SKILL

Restraint devices are used to limit movements that could be harmful to clients who are confused, agitated, or disoriented. A restraint is a physical or mechanical method of involuntarily restricting movement and physical activity so that the client is protected from causing harm to self and/or to others.

Restraints may be used to prevent movement during a procedure. When clients cannot support their posture or balance, a restraint may be used to provide the needed support or to prevent the client from falling. If a client is restless or confused, a restraint may be used to prevent the client from damaging therapeutic equipment.

The procedure to restrain a client is fairly simple. The legal, emotional, and ethical considerations that accompany this procedure are complex. State and federal laws as well as hospital policies govern the use of restraints. The use of restraints encompasses restrictions and cautions that can include verbal, medical, and physical restrains. Restrains can include managing clients with anything from firm words, use of medications, physical restraints, and/or the use of gown, bed, or chair alarms to alert the nurse of a client's movements. Nursing judgments need to be made based upon the danger to the client and danger to the health care workers. In psychiatric settings where clients may be dangerous, interventions such as strong verbal commands, confinement, isolation, medications, or physical restraints may be used. For the purpose of this skill, restraint devices are in reference to those used in hospitals or skilled nursing facilities.

Nurses or caregivers may not restrain or confine clients without documented necessity. Nonetheless, the nurse or caregiver can be liable if a confused client sustains injury without appropriate protection, which may include restraints. Staff in a medical facility may restrain, confine, or monitor (by an electronic device) a client if it is necessary to prevent serious bodily harm to the client or another person. Clients and caregivers often have strong opinions regarding the use of restraints. Many people see the use of restraints as demeaning and dehumanizing. Others feel that restraints are used to replace nursing contact in understaffed environments. Confused clients often feel that they are being imprisoned. While trying to balance these considerations, the nurse has a legal and ethical duty to keep his or her clients safe. The decision to restrain a client and by how much is a delicate balancing act of nursing judgment.

The uses of physical restraints are controlled by state and federal regulations. Hospitals must have a policy and procedure that address the use of restraints. Restraints are used as a last resort, never as a convenience, and the use of restraints are to protect the client from self-harm or protect the staff from harm. Hospitals must establish a plan of care based upon the client's need, interventions and treatments, and goals and have a standarized format for consistency of care and documentation. A written physician order must be obtained within 24 hours of initiating a restraint. The order must be renewed every 24 hours if the restraint is continuous. The client is to be monitored every 2 hours during the time of his or her restraint. Accrediting organizations and the Center for Medicare and Medicaid Services (CMS) may have similar policies.

There are a number of different types of restraints. They range from a simple armboard to prevent movement of a wrist or elbow to more complex locked restraints. The restraints most commonly used are soft restraints. They are made of mesh or soft canvas. They are designed to gently restrain the client without damaging the skin. Chest restraints, cloth wrist restraints, mitten restraints, and "posey" restraints fall into this category. Other types of restraints include locked web belt restraints, locked leather restraints, and full-body restraints. These are more often used in settings in which clients are extremely agitated and belligerent.

▶ ASSESSMENT

1. Assess the client's level of consciousness. **This will help you determine the client's ability to protect him- or herself from potential harm.**
2. Assess the client's degree of orientation. **A client who is confused regarding time, place, or person is more likely to be at risk of injuring him or herself. A client who is agitated or angry may be at risk of injuring others.**
3. Assess the client's physical condition. **A client who has weakness, paralysis, or impaired balance or mobility is at increased risk of injury. Impaired vision or hearing also increases the client's risk of injury.**
4. Assess the client's history for falls, accidents, confusion, agitation, or self-inflicted injury. **A client who has a history of this type is at increased risk for injury.**
5. Assess the client's intent. **A client who is verbalizing threats to harm self or others is at increased risk of injury.**
6. Assess the need for restraints. Determine whether the client's treatment plan requires and allows restraints, if orders are in place, and hospital policies and laws are specified. **This will prevent the inappropriate use of restraints and is necessary for legal protection in the event of an injury.**
7. Assess client and family knowledge regarding the use of and rationale for restraints or protective devices. **The more the client and family understand regarding the reason for restraints, the more cooperative and understanding they will be.**

▶ DIAGNOSIS

Risk for Injury

Low Self-Esteem

Powerlessness

Deficient Knowledge

Impaired Physical Mobility

Risk for Falls

Acute Confusion

Risk for Peripheral Neurovascular Dysfunction

Risk for Impaired Skin Integrity

▶ PLANNING

Expected Outcomes:
1. The client will remain uninjured.
2. The client will not suffer injury or impairment from the restraints.
3. The client's therapeutic equipment will remain intact and functional.
4. Others will not be harmed by the client.
5. The client will be restrained just enough to prevent injury.

Equipment Needed (see Figures 2-3-1, 2-3-2, and 2-3-3):
- Restraints appropriate to the client's condition and type of restraint required
- Cotton batting or foam padding

▶ CLIENT EDUCATION NEEDED:

1. Explain the reason for the need to use restraints/protective devices. Reassure the client and family that the restraint is not a punitive device but is intended to ensure the client's safety.

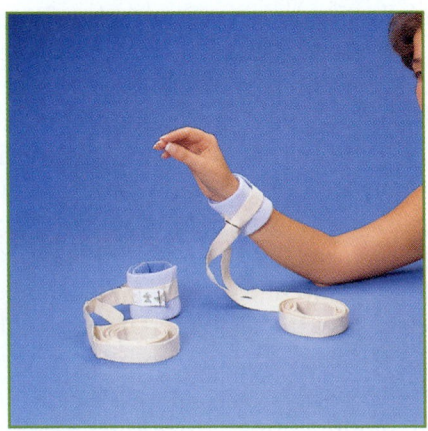

Figure 2-3-1 Wrist restraints

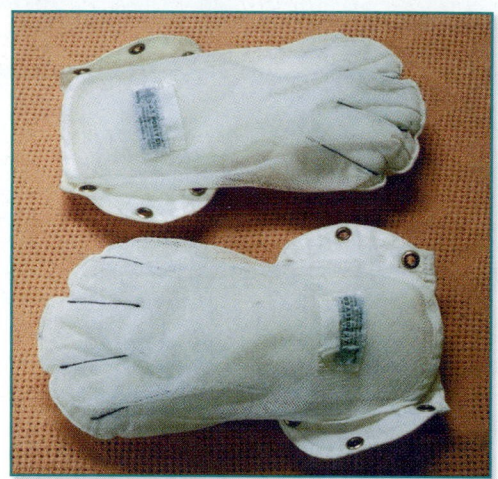

Figure 2-3-2 Mitten restraints

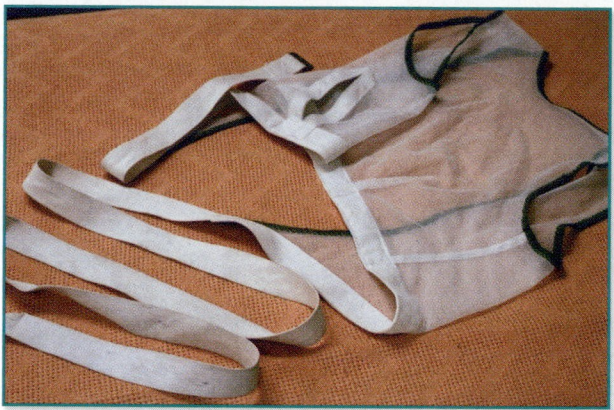

Figure 2-3-3 Jacket restraint

2. Show the client the equipment to be used and provide a simple explanation of how it is applied.

3. Reassure the client and family that the client will be monitored constantly and that assistance for personal care will be provided.

4. Allay fear of isolation and potential loss of well-being.

5. Teach the client how to communicate with the staff for needs to be identified and attended. Ensure that the client's call bell or the nurse's cellular telephone number is available.

6. Help clients develop an awareness regarding what is a comfortable application of the restraint and encourage them to report discomfort associated with the application.

Estimated time to complete the skill: **10–20 minutes. The time may vary depending upon the type of restraint, the physical and emotional condition of the client, and staff availability.**

▶ **DELEGATION TIPS**

Delegation of the application of restraints to ancillary personnel is acceptable if appropriate orders are in place and proper training has occurred. The assessment of the need for and the type of restraints required and their proper application and maintenance requires the professional nurse's observation and documentation per facility policy.

IMPLEMENTATION—Action/Rationale

Action	Rationale
Chest Restraint	
Follow the manufacturer's instructions when applying any restraint.	
1. Obtain written or verbal order from a physician. If an emergency, apply the restraint then contact the physician for an order	1. A physician's order is required for restraints.

continues

Action	Rationale
Chest Restraint *continued*	
2. Choose an appropriately sized vest or jacket restraint for client.	**2.** Vest fits client correctly.
3. Explain to the client that, for safety reasons, he or she will be wearing a restraint.	**3.** Promotes client cooperation.
4. Wash hands.	**4.** Prevents the spread of microorganisms.
5. Place the restraint on the client For a vest restraint: a. Place the restraint with the opening in front (see Figure 2-3-4). b. Overlap the front pieces, threading the ties through the slot/loop in front of the vest. For a jacket restraint: a. Place the restraint on the client with the opening in the back (see Figure 2-3-5). b. Zip jacket, if jacket has a zipper.	**5.** Secures the vest restraint.
6. If the client is in bed, secure the ties to the movable part of the bed frame with a slip (easy-release) knot (see Figure 2-3-6). Slip knot (easy release): a. Wrap the tie once around the moveable part of the bed frame. b. Make a loop with the loose tail of the tie. c. Place the loop underneath where the ties cross each other. d. Pull on loop to secure the tie.	**6.** Allows the restraint to move with the bed if the head of the bed is raised or lowered. A slip knot (easy release) allows the restraint to be easily removed in case of client emergency.
7. If the client is in a chair, cross the straps behind the seat of the chair and secure the straps to the chair's lower legs, out of the client's reach. If the client is in a wheelchair, thread the straps through the armrests and seat. Once the straps are threaded through the back, you may loop one strap over another in the center. Tie each strap in a slip knot to the kick-spur on the opposite side (see Figure 2-3-7).	**7.** Proper procedure for securing restraint.

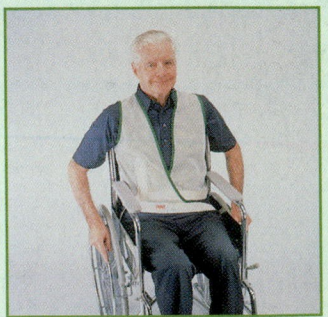

Figure 2-3-4   Vest restraint must be applied with the straps crossed in front of the client.

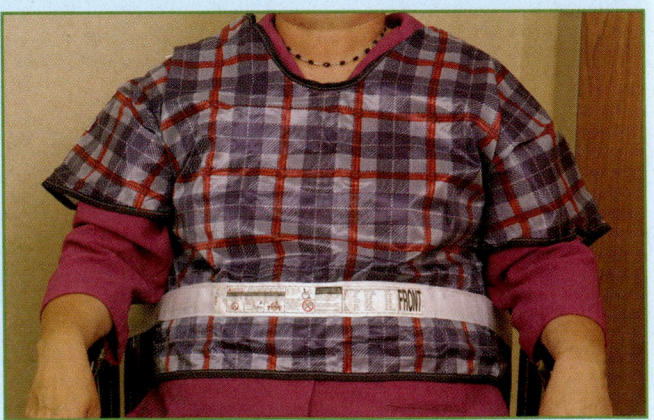

Figure 2-3-5   Jacket restraint applied with opening in the back.

continues

Action	Rationale
8. Slip two fingers under the restraint to check for tightness. Be sure that the restraint is tight enough so that the client cannot slip it off and that it restricts the client from getting up, but loose enough that it does not compromise the client's respirations.	8. Respirations can be compromised if the vest is too tight.
9. Step back and assess the client's overall safety.	9. Assessing the client can allow you to see dangers you might have missed.
10. Place the call light within the client's reach.	10. Allows the client to contact the nurse to have any needs met. Provides client with an increased sense of safety.
11. Assess the client every 2 hours (it may be more frequent; follow the institution and state guidelines) while in restraint. Assess the safety of the restraint placement and the client's respiratory status.	11. Assures that the client remains safe. Clients may try to escape from the restraint and injure themselves in the attempt. Follow the instructions and state regulations on the frequency of client checks while the client is in a restraint.
12. Wash hands.	12. Prevents the spread of microorganisms.

Applying Wrist or Ankle Restraints

Follow the manufacturer's instructions when applying any restraint.

Action	Rationale
13. Obtain written or verbal order from a physician. If an emergency, apply the restraint then contact the physician for an order.	13. A physician's order is required for restraints.
14. Explain to the client that you will be placing a wrist or ankle restraint that will restrict movement.	14. Promotes client cooperation.

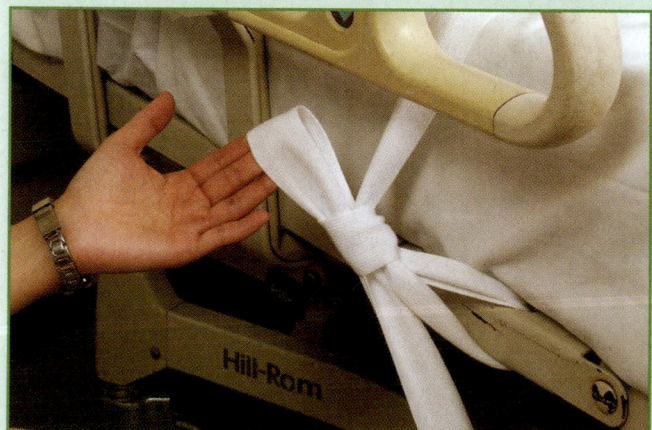

Figure 2-3-6 Slip (easy release) knot

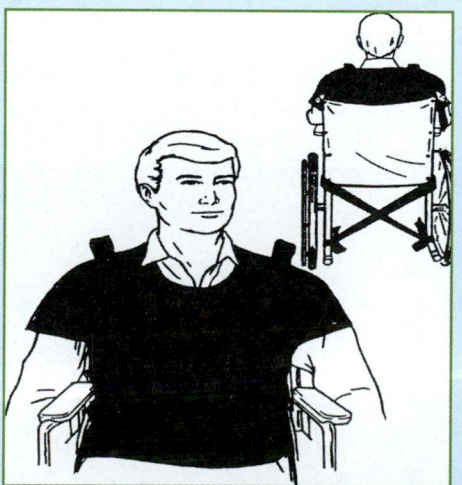

Figure 2-3-7 Secure chest restraint to a wheelchair. Tie each strap in a slip (easy release) knot to the kick-spur on the opposite side.

continues

Action	Rationale

Applying Wrist or Ankle Restraints *continued*

15. Wash hands.

15. Prevents the spread of microorganisms.

16. Wrap the restraint around the client's wrist/ankle. If the restraint does not have foam padding, pad the client's wrist/ankle before applying restraint.

16. Prevents the restraint from chafing the client's skin.

17. Secure restraint by pulling a tie through the loop in the restraint (see Figure 2-3-1). If the restraint uses Velcro, secure the restraint with the Velcro closure (see Figure 2-3-8).

17. Secures the restraint.

18. Slip two fingers under the restraint to check for tightness. Be sure the restraint is tight enough that the client cannot slip it off but loose enough that the neurovascular status of the client's extremity is not impaired (see Figure 2-3-9).

18. If the restraint is too tight, the client's neurovascular status may be impaired, causing injury to the client.

19. Tie restraints to the moveable part of the bed using a slip (easy-release) knot (see Figure 2-3-6 and Figure 2-3-10). Slip knot (easy release):
   a. Wrap the tie once around the moveable part of the bed frame.
   b. Make a loop with the loose tail of the tie.
   c. Place the loop underneath where the ties cross each other.
   d. Pull on loop to secure the tie.

19. Allows the restraint to move with the bed if the head of the bed is raised or lowered. A slip knot (easy release) allows the restraint to be easily removed in case of a client emergency.

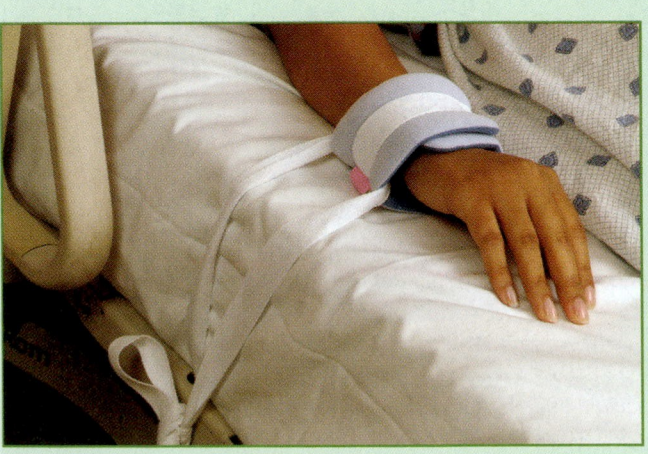

Figure 2-3-8   Wrist restraints with Velcro

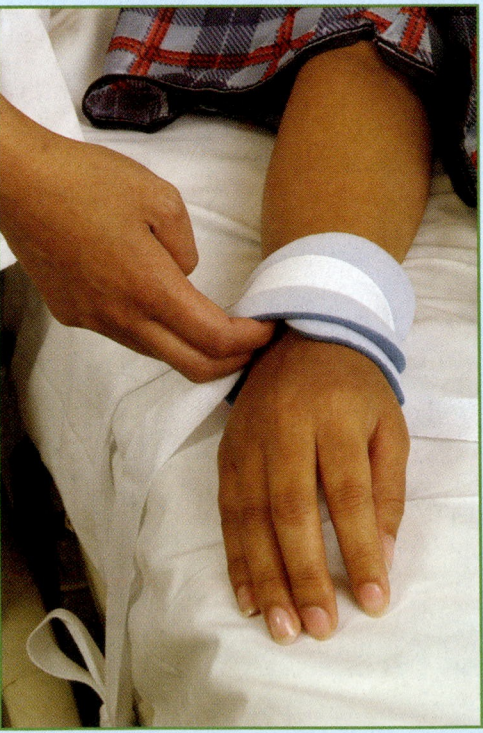

Figure 2-3-9   Slip two fingers under restraint to check for tightness.

continues

Action	Rationale

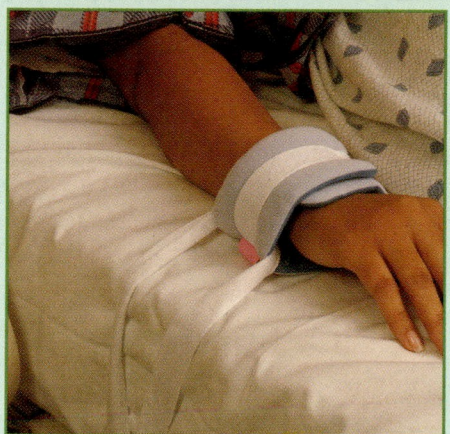

Figure 2-3-10 Wrist restraint with slip (easy release) knot

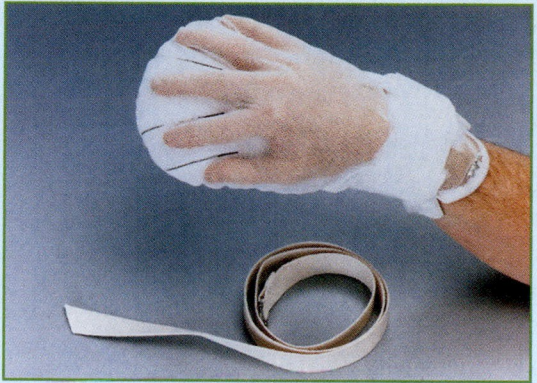

Figure 2-3-11 Hand mitts

20. Step back and assess the client's overall safety.

21. Place the call light within the client's reach.

22. Assess the client every 2 hours (it may be more frequent; follow the institution and state guidelines) while in restraint. Assess the safety of the restraint placement and the client's neurovascular status and the status of the extremity.

23. Wash hands.

Applying Mitten Restraints (follow manufacturer's instructions when applying a restraint)

24. Obtain written or verbal order from a physician. If an emergency, apply the restraint then contact the physician for an order.

25. Explain to the client that, for safety reasons, he or she will be wearing a mitten restraint.

26. Wash hands.

27. Place the mitten restraint on client's hand, securing the strap around the wrist (see Figure 2-3-11).

20. Assessing the client can allow you to see dangers you might have missed.

21. Allows the client to contact the nurse to have any needs met. Provides the client with an increased sense of safety.

22. Assures that the client remains safe. Clients may try to escape from restraint and injure themselves in the attempt. Follow the institutional and state regulations on the frequency of client checks if the client is in restraint.

23. Prevents the spread of microorganisms.

24. A physician's order is required for restraints.

25. Promotes client cooperation.

26. Prevents the spread of microorganisms.

27. Secures restraint.

continues

Action	Rationale

Applying Mitten Restraints (follow manufacturer's instructions when applying a restraint) *continued*

28. Secure the ties to the moveable part of the bed using a slip (easy-release) knot (see Figure 2-3-6).
    Slip knot (easy release):
    a. Wrap the tie once around the moveable part of the bed frame.
    b. Make a loop with the loose tail of the tie.
    c. Place the loop underneath where the ties cross each other.
    d. Pull on loop to secure the tie.

28. Allows the restraint to move with the bed if the head of the bed is raised or lowered. A slip knot (easy release) allows the restraint to be easily removed in case of a client emergency.

29. Slip two fingers under the restraint to check for tightness. Be sure the restraint is tight enough that the client cannot slip it off but loose enough that it does not compromise the client's circulation.

29. If the mitten restraint is too tight, the client's neurovascular status may be impaired, causing injury to the client.

30. Step back and assess the client's overall safety.

30. Assessing the client can allow you to see dangers you might have missed.

31. Place the call light within the client's reach.

31. Allows the client to contact the nurse to have any needs met. Provides the client with an increased sense of safety.

32. Assess the client every 2 hours (it may be more frequent; follow the institution and state guidelines) while in restraint. Assess the safety of the restraint placement and the client's neurovascular status and the status of the extremity.

32. Ensures that the client remains safe. Clients may try to escape from restraint and injure themselves in the attempt. Follow the institutional and state regulations on the frequency of client checks if the client is in restraint.

33. Wash hands.

33. Prevents the spread of microorganisms.

▶ REAL WORLD ANECDOTES

Scenario 1

Bertha was an 80-year-old woman admitted to the oncology unit with a diagnosis of lung cancer metastatic to her brain. She was confused, agitated, and unable to safely transfer from her bed without assistance. The plan was for her to begin radiation treatments and IV Decadron to diminish the side effects associated with the brain metastases. Bertha had a peripheral IV inserted in her left forearm. The nursing plan was to restrain her at night for safety precautions using soft limb restraints. The morning of day 2 of the hospitalization, while on rounds, the nurse assessed that the IV bag still contained half of the solution and that the left arm at the site of the IV was infiltrated and the surrounding tissue was swollen. The nursing staff was reminded never to apply a limb restraint above an IV site because of the strong possibility of occluding the infusion or infiltrating the surrounding tissue. Additionally, the nursing team was told that half-hour checks are a requirement every shift, especially for elderly restrained clients.

continues

► **REAL WORLD ANECDOTES** *(continued)*

Scenario 2

A busy medical-surgical floor of an urban hospital admitted a 20-year-old man to the unit from the emergency room at 4 AM. The client was admitted because of multiple injuries sustained in a car accident. His blood alcohol level was double the normal limit upon admission, and head trauma was documented. The client was restrained with a vest in the emergency room because of combative behavior. When he was transferred from the stretcher to his bed, someone retied the vest restraints to the side rails of the bed. On early morning rounds the nurse lowered the side rail to administer care and the client's leg and arm were caught in between the side rail and he suffered a sprained wrist and ankle. The nursing staff was in-serviced on the seriousness of tying restraints to the side rails. All staff were told that, in order to avoid injury, restraints must be secured to a movable part of the bed frame only (i.e., those parts that move with the client), not parts that move independently of a client's position, such as side rails.

► **EVALUATION**

- The client remains uninjured.
- The client has not suffered injury or impairment from the restraints.
- The client's therapeutic equipment has remained intact and functional.
- Others have not been harmed by the client.
- The client is restrained just enough to prevent injury.

► **DOCUMENTATION**

Nurses' Notes

- Document the use of restraints. Include the reason the client was restrained, the type of restraint placed, the time the restraints were placed, the condition of the client's skin at the site of restraint at the time of placement, and any unusual findings at the time the client was restrained.
- Nurses' notes should be made at least every 2 hours even if a flow sheet is used.
- Be sure to document the ongoing need for restraints.
- If the client's status changes, restraints may no longer be necessary.

Document on appropriate flow sheet or electronic medical record (EMR).

Flow Sheet

- Some institutions have flow sheets that are used when a client is restrained. These flow sheets document the frequency of client checks, the client's condition, and how often the restraints are released.

► **CRITICAL THINKING SKILL**

Introduction

Look at an example in which the clinical nurse specialist mobilizes the staff by using expert educational strategies and teaches the ethics of using restraints. This effort helps to avoid communication problems and conflict and ultimately ensures that safe and appropriate client care is provided.

Possible Scenario

A 30-year-old woman was admitted to the psychiatric unit of a large institution with a diagnosis of chemical dependency withdrawal. She was severely agitated, confused, and combative upon admission. A psychiatrist's order was written for four-point leather restraints. The use of this type of restraint is approved in this institution and sanctioned by state regulation. The medical order to use four-point restraint on this client created immediate staff dissension. Part of the staff felt that it was an extreme request and far too restrictive for the clinical management of this case. Several staff members felt that they could manage this client using soft restraints on an as-needed basis. They also felt that they would be able to maintain vigilant watch, including half-hour checks for safety. A portion of the staff felt that if they chose not to restrain the client, it would help to establish a trusting relationship and hasten her recovery.

This client, while restrained, began to strongly resist the restraints. She began kicking, biting, and banging her head in an attempt to resist the restraints. The staff remained divided about the need to restrain. The psychiatric clinical nurse specialist was consulted to meet with the professional nursing staff, the attending physician, and the client's family in an attempt to reach agreement concerning the use of restraints in this clinical situation. The clinical nurse specialist (CNS) arranged a meeting with the nursing staff, attending psychiatrist, client, and family (if possible). Through the use of expert facilitation and profound knowledge regarding the clinical use and ethical application of restraints, the CNS was able to educate the involved parties by providing information on the appropriate use of four-point restraints. A compromise among the parties was reached, and it was agreed that the restraints would be used during the acute phase of clinical management. A specific schedule would be prepared to allow the client time off of the restraints with staff providing one-to-one supervision during times when the restraints would be removed.

Possible Outcome

If the CNS had not intervened, staff dissension would have escalated and client care would have been compromised. Channels of communication would have been blocked, misinformation would have led to lack of evidence-based practice, and mistrust among colleagues could have resulted.

Prevention

The CNS prevented compromised care delivery and enhanced client comfort and safety while maintaining the individual's dignity along the continuum of care. Additionally, relationships between the client, the client's family, the attending psychiatrist, and staff all solidified because of access to accurate knowledge and the opportunity for all parties to partake actively in the plan of care.

▶ VARIATIONS

Geriatric Variations:

- *Older clients may require repetitive explanations about the rationale for using restraints.*
- *Older clients may have less body mass and require more protection of bony prominences.*
- *Older clients may have involuntary tremors and may require the assistance of more than one person to restrain them.*
- *Older clients may have compromised hearing and seeing and may require additional information about the type of restraint.*
- *Older clients may be more prone to aspiration and may require to be restrained on their sides.*

Pediatric Variations:

- *Children require simple, clear, and brief explanations to reassure them and minimize fear.*
- *Children need to be constantly monitored and intensely observed.*
- *It is vital that the child's family understands the need for the restraint.*
- *Reassurance to family members of the rationale for the restraint use and that it will not harm the child or be uncomfortable.*
- *Ties and safety pins, if used, must not be within the child's reach.*
- *Always align the infant/child's body properly when using restraints in order to avoid dislocation of body joints.*
- *Children and their families should be reassured that the restraint is not a punitive measure.*

Home Care Variations:

- *Family members and other caregivers must be taught the safe application of restraints.*
- *The home environment must be thoroughly assessed for safety and appropriate use of restraints.*
- *A visiting nurse must prepare a schedule for the home caregivers to follow regarding all aspects of care required for the client at home who requires restraints.*

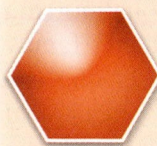

Long-Term Care Variations:

- *Vigilant provision of the client's nutrition, elimination, and positioning must occur in long-term care settings.*
- *Prevention of pressure ulcers must occur by frequent repositioning, massaging, and protecting bony prominences with padding.*
- *Assess for pneumonia, urine retention, constipation, and sensory deprivation caused by long-term restraint use.*

▶ COMMON ERRORS

Possible Error:

Nurse waits for order from the physician to apply restraints during acute emergency.

Prevention:

Know hospital policy regarding application of emergency restraints without physician's or qualified practitioner's immediate order. Know hospital policy to provide safe, effective, and prompt client care. In an emergency, apply restraints (know what constitutes an emergency situation), then seek medical order within reasonable time frame.

Possible Error:

Client at high risk for aspiration is restrained in supine position.

Prevention:

Clients at high risk for aspiration must be restrained on their side or in a high Fowler's position. Assess client's condition: Know that status may change and warrant different clinical interventions.

Possible Error:

Client has had four-point restraints applied and secured to same side of the bed.

Prevention:

Assess client; know that restraints secured to one side of the bed will place the client at a greater risk of falling. Careful, continuous assessment when using four-point restraints; always apply to all four sides of bed frame to minimize risk of injury caused by falls.

Possible Error:

Restraint is applied above an IV site.

Prevention:

Assess restraint placement carefully, relative to IV sites; this will prevent infiltration. Assess for IV sites, sites of shunts, or implanted ports. Always place restraints strategically below these sites.

Possible Error:

Restraints are secured to side rail of the bed.

Prevention:

Always assess location of restraints and check for permanence of site. Always secure restraints to parts of the bed that move with the client because caregivers may lower the rail, an independent part, not realizing that the client's restraints are attached to it. This action can cause harm to the client.

Possible Error:

Restraining a client in the prone position.

Prevention:

Never restrain someone in the prone position. This can cause limited vision and intensified sense of loss of control and may decrease respirations if the person has been sedated.

Possible Error:

Restraints applied too tight.

Prevention:

Cautiously apply restraints comfortably. Avoid tight and constrictive securing methods. Tight restraints can decrease peripheral circulation and impair respirations. Apply carefully; pad bony prominences; reposition and check client frequently.

▶ NURSING TIPS

- Know facility policies and state laws that govern the use of restraints. Determine whether the treatment plan authorizes a client to be restrained or monitored in accordance with medical orders and regulations. Know the laws regarding specified person to prescribe restraints. Reassess according to regulations.
- Become familiar with restraint equipment: vest, limb, mitt, belt, body (posey), and leather restraints.
- Be safe and efficient when applying restraints. Always have organized and available assistance when placing restraints on a client. A team effort can provide simultaneous client teaching by one health care professional while another applies the restraint.
- Ensure that client comfort is not compromised. Provide frequent checks. Assess need for padding bony prominences to avoid pressure ulcers. Provide assistance with nutrition, elimination, repositioning, and general care.
- Always keep the client and family well informed regarding the rationale for restraints and the associated care required.
- Continuously assess client need for restraints. Allow changes in condition to dictate withdrawing or maintaining restraints.

- Restraints must be sized properly and according to the client's body build and weight. If restraints are loose, and smaller ones are unavailable, use gauze pads or soft towels to build them up and then tape securely.
- If leather restraints are used, have a key that fits the locks readily available.
- Pad the client's bony prominences before applying a protective device.
- Attach the device to the movable bed frame, not the side rails.
- Check client's respiratory status if a chest device is used.
- Check position of chest device so it is not constricting the client's neck.
- Restrain clients on their side if risk of aspiration is assessed.
- Do not secure four restraints to one side of the bed.
- When applying two-point restraints, restrain one arm and the opposite leg.
- Never apply restraint above an IV site.
- Provide frequent repositioning, massage, and surveillance of bony prominences.
- Be sure to place the client's call light within reach.

▶ SPECIAL CONSIDERATIONS

- *Nursing care for clients with restraints should include frequent checks and a release of restraints every 2 hours to facilitate peripheral circulation and provide extremity range of motion. Exceptions to this rule are clients with combative behavior or violent tendency. In these situations additional help should be summoned when restraints are released or other measures taken to ensure adequate circulation and range of motion.*
- *Chemical restraint, using sedative type medications, may be prescribed in situations with combative clients.*
- *Restraints that are tied incorrectly can cause injury or asphyxiation. Restraint related injuries and deaths occur every year.*
- *Clients experiencing alcohol withdrawal may have a tendency to exert increased force and fracture bones. Appropriate observation is essential.*

Handwashing/Hand Hygiene

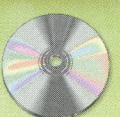

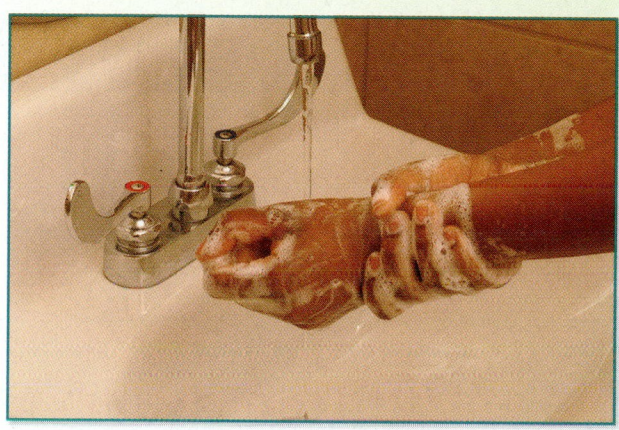

▶ OVERVIEW OF THE SKILL

Handwashing is the rubbing together of all surfaces and crevices of the hands using a soap or chemical and water. Handwashing is a component of all types of isolation precautions and is the most basic and effective infection control measure to prevent and control the transmission of infectious agents.

The three essential elements of handwashing are soap or chemical, water, and friction. Soaps that contain antimicrobial agents frequently are used in high-risk areas such as emergency departments and nurseries. Friction is the most important element of the trio because it physically removes soil and transient flora.

Handwashing should be performed after arriving at work, before leaving work, between client contacts, before donning gloves, after removing gloves, when hands are visibly soiled, before eating, after excretion of body waste (urination and defecation), after contact with body fluids, before and after performing invasive procedures, and after handling contaminated equipment. The exact duration of time required for handwashing depends on the circumstances. A washing time of 10 to 15 seconds is recommended to remove transient flora from the hands. High-risk areas, such as nurseries, usually require about a minimum 2-minute hand-wash. An alcohol-based hand rub may be used if hands are not visibly soiled (Centers for Disease Control and Preventions, 2002).

▶ ASSESSMENT

1. Assess the environment **to establish whether facilities are adequate for cleansing the hands.** Is the water clean? Is soap available? Is there a clean towel to dry hands?
2. Assess your hands **to determine whether they have open cuts, hangnails, broken skin, or heavily soiled areas.**

▶ DIAGNOSIS

Risk for Infection

▶ PLANNING

Expected Outcomes:

1. The caregiver's hands will be cleansed adequately to remove microorganisms, transient flora, and soiling from the skin.

Equipment Needed:

- Soap
- Paper towels
- Sink
- Running water

▶ CLIENT EDUCATION NEEDED:

1. Teach clients to wash their hands when they are visibly soiled, before eating, after excretion of body waste, and after contact with body fluids.

2. Teach clients to wash their hands from the least to the most contaminated areas.
3. Teach clients to turn off the water with a paper towel to prevent recontamination of their hands.

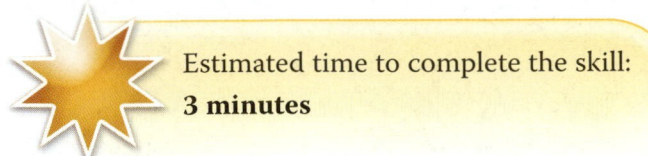

Estimated time to complete the skill:
3 minutes

▶ **DELEGATION TIPS**

All hospital personnel are expected to maintain proper handwashing technique and routinely apply Standard Precautions.

IMPLEMENTATION—Action/Rationale

Action	Rationale
Handwashing/Hand Hygiene	
1. Remove jewelry. Wristwatch may be pushed up above the wrist (midforearm). Push sleeves of uniform or shirt up above the wrist at midforearm level.	1. Provides access to skin surfaces for cleaning. Facilitates cleaning of fingers, hands, and forearms.
2. Assess hands for hangnails, cuts, or breaks in the skin, and areas that are heavily soiled.	2. Intact skin acts as a barrier to microorganisms. Breaks in skin integrity facilitate development of infection and should receive extra attention during cleaning. Hands that are visibly soiled or contaminated with blood or body fluids require washing the hands with soap and water. (Centers for Disease Control, 2002)
3. Turn on the water. Adjust the flow and temperature. Temperature of the water should be warm.	3. Running water removes microorganisms. Warm water removes less of the natural skin oils.
4. Wet hands and lower forearms thoroughly by holding under running water. Keep hands and forearms in the down position with elbows straight. Avoid splashing water and touching the sides of the sink.	4. Water should flow from the least contaminated to the most contaminated areas of the skin. Hands are considered more contaminated than arms. Splashing of water facilitates transfer of microorganisms. Touching of any surface during cleaning contaminates the skin.
5. Apply approximately 5 mL (1 teaspoon) of liquid soap. Lather thoroughly.	5. Lather facilitates removal of microorganisms. Liquid soap harbors less bacteria than bar soap.
6. Thoroughly rub hands together for about 10 to 15 seconds. Interlace fingers and thumbs and move back and forth to wash between digits. Rub palms and back of hands with circular motion (see Figure 2-4-1). Special attention should be provided to areas such as the knuckles and fingernails, which are known to harbor organisms (see Figure 2-4-2).	6. Friction mechanically removes microorganisms from the skin surface. Friction loosens dirt from soiled areas.

continues

Action	Rationale

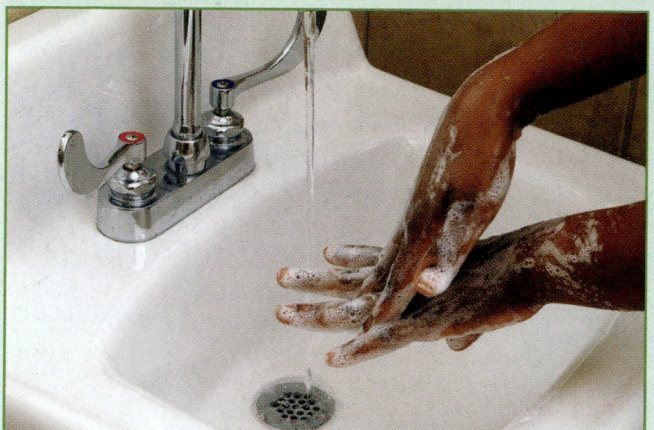

Figure 2-4-1   Lather thoroughly and rub hands together.

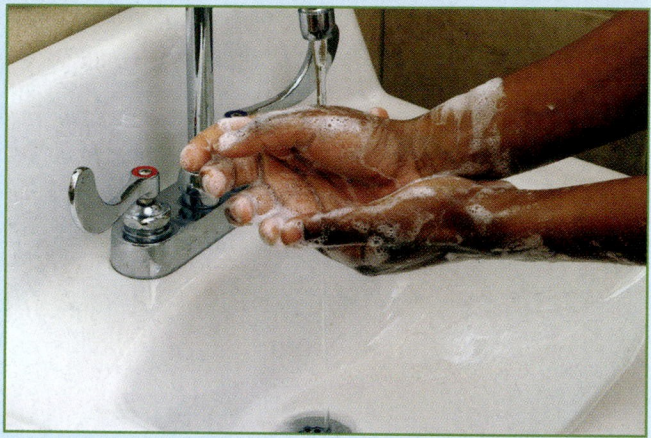

Figure 2-4-2   Give special attention to fingernails and knuckles.

7. Rinse with hands in the down position, elbows straight. Rinse in the direction of forearm to wrist to fingers.

8. Blot hands and forearms to dry thoroughly. Dry in the direction of fingers to wrist and forearms. Discard the paper towels in the proper receptacle.

9. Turn off the water faucet with a clean, dry paper towel (see Figure 2-4-3).

7. Flow of water rinses away dirt and microorganisms.

8. Blotting reduces chapping of skin. Drying from cleanest (hand) to least clean area (forearms) prevents transfer of microorganisms to cleanest area.

9. Prevents contamination of clean hands by a less clean faucet.

Alcohol-based Hand Rub

Performed if hands are not visibly soiled.

10. Apply product to palm of one hand. Rub hands together, covering all surfaces of hands, until hands are dry. Follow the manufacturer's recommendation for the amount of product to use.

10. Alcohol-based hand rubs remove or destroy transient microorganisms and reduce resident flora. (Centers for Disease Control, 2002).

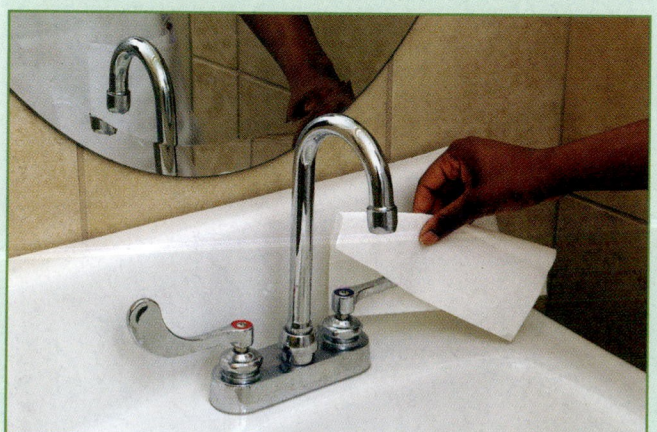

Figure 2-4-3   Turn of faucet with a clean, dry paper towel.

▶ REAL WORLD ANECDOTES

Nurse Wilkerson has been asked to assist with repositioning a client. She is very busy with her own assignments but agrees to help for a minute. The only gloves available in the room are a small size. While she is putting the gloves on, one tears. Nurse Wilkerson proceeds to assist with the client without changing gloves. The repositioning takes longer than expected and Nurse Wilkerson hurries out of the room without washing her hands. The next day Nurse Wilkerson discovers that the client she had helped to reposition was diagnosed with hepatitis. Through her carelessness, Nurse Wilkerson has endangered herself, her coworkers, and her clients. She has violated the Nightingale Pledge, taken during graduation from nursing school, to "devote myself to the welfare of those committed to my care." She has also placed herself in danger of litigation if any of her clients should contract the same strain of hepatitis.

▶ EVALUATION

- The handwashing was adequate to control topical flora and infectious agents on the hands.
- The hands were not recontaminated during or shortly after the handwashing.

▶ DOCUMENTATION

No documentation is needed for routine handwashing by the nurse.

Nurses' Notes

- Document handwashing teaching provided to clients, visitors, or caregivers.

▶ CRITICAL THINKING SKILL

Introduction

It is important that you are always aware of situations when handwashing is necessary.

Possible Scenario

While working as a visiting nurse, you are assigned to perform a dressing change on Mrs. Abercrombie's open leg ulcer. The ulcer is known to be contaminated with multiple antibiotic-resistant *Staphylococcus aureus*, and you are careful to wear gloves while performing the procedure. As you are leaving, Mrs. Abercrombie takes your hands in hers and kisses them, thanking you for your help. You have just enough time to get to your next appointment. It is past lunch time and you are hungry, so you detour via the fast food drive-through and eat while driving to see your next client.

Possible Outcome

Mrs. Abercrombie recontaminated your hands with highly resistant *Staphylococcus aureus* when she kissed them. You have touched the steering wheel of your car, handled money, and eaten lunch without washing your hands. You review the symptoms of a *Staphylococcus* infection.

Prevention

Try to think ahead in situations in which handwashing facilities may not be readily available. Be sure to keep antiseptic wipes or hand disinfectant close by if you are not sure you will be able to wash your hands when necessary.

▶ VARIATIONS

Geriatric Variations:

- *The geriatric home care client may not have the fine motor skills or grip strength to operate a faucet. They may avoid washing their hands for this reason. Make modifications as needed.*

continues

▶ VARIATIONS (continued)

Pediatric Variations:

- *Encourage parents to incorporate the handwashing routine into toilet training.*
- *Young children who are actively exploring their environment cannot tell the difference between "clean" and "dirty" things to explore with their hands and mouths.*
- *Infants, toddlers, and young children have runny noses and saliva and do not have bowel and bladder control over feces and urine. When working with young children, be sure to wash your hands frequently to reduce the transmission of microorganisms.*
- *Encourage parents to carry prepackaged wet-wipes or disinfectant to clean contact surfaces that might have been contaminated by unwashed hands.*

Home Care Variations:

- *You may need to carry hand disinfectant or bactericidal soap and clean towels with you.*
- *Assess the home for adequate handwashing facilities. Does the sink drain adequately? Can the faucet be operated without too much torque?*
- *The bathroom sink may not be the best place to wash hands when caring for the client. Be flexible in setting up a handwashing station that is easy and accessible.*

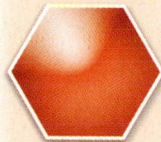

Long-Term Care Variations:

- *Encourage independence in handwashing. Modify the faucet or sink height or provide alternative handwashing facilities as needed.*
- *It is easy to remember to wash when working with visible dirt, bodily wastes, or contaminants. It is harder to remember to wash when the sources of infection cannot be seen. Reinforce the principles of asepsis and the transmission of microorganisms on a regular basis.*
- *Consider the sink area contaminated. Do not touch the sides of the sink or lean against the sink.*
- *Correct handwashing technique specifies that the hands always remain lower than the elbows. This is easy if the caregiver or client is an adult able to stand at the sink. For clients or caregivers in wheelchairs or children, modify the handwashing facilities where possible to allow proper technique.*

▶ COMMON ERRORS

Possible Error:

After washing his or her hands, the nurse picks up the IVAC thermometer that has been carried from room to room while taking vital signs.

Prevention:

Be aware of the environment. Be conscious of the differences between a clean and dirty environment. Think about who or what has previously come in contact with equipment.

▶ NURSING TIPS

- If in doubt, it is dirty.
- Wash hands *before* and *after every* client contact. The most common cause of nosocomial infections is contaminated hands of health care providers.
- When you turn on the faucet of a sink with which you are unfamiliar (especially in the home care setting), you might get wet! Be a little tentative the first time until you investigate the water pressure and the faucet.

▶ **SPECIAL CONSIDERATIONS**

- *Teaching kits with ultraviolet lamp and ultraviolet glow/activated potion and powder are available to assess the effectiveness of handwashing and to provide a visual demonstration to show when improper cleaning or handwashing has taken place.*
- *Frequent daily handwashing with soap and detergent could result in increasing resident flora and sometimes increasing bacteria over baseline count of clean hand. Plain soap helps to remove the transient microorganism and bacteria but does not necessary kill the bacteria. Antiseptic solution should be used if there is a concern.*
- *Topical foam or alcohol-based antiseptic products are sometimes used in areas where frequent handwashing is required and soap and water are not available at the bedside (newborn nurseries, intensive care units). If you find yourself using a foam/without-water product, make sure that you are familiar with the manufacturer's instructions for use. Most application requires a specified amount of product and time for contact duration.*
- *A variety of methods, warm-air, paper towel, and cloth towel drying, are available for drying hands after handwashing. The warm-air drying and the paper towel drying provide a more optimal result than cloth drying. The warm-air drying produces the greatest result in further reduction of flora, and cloth drying the least. However, because of the feasibility and the noise produced by warm-air drying machine, paper towel drying method is adopted by most health care settings.*
- *Neonatal units usually require handwashing with a designated length of time, scrubbing with a brush, and cleaning under the fingernails. Check the hospital protocol.*

Donning and Removing Clean and Contaminated Gloves and Mask

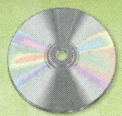

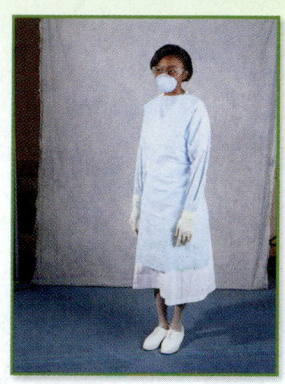

▶ OVERVIEW OF THE SKILL

Infection control is an essential area of concern for the nurse in any setting. Effective implementation serves to prevent or reduce the incidence of nosocomial infections. A nosocomial infection is defined as an infection acquired at least 72 hours after hospitalization or a hospital-acquired infection. The hospitalized client is at increased risk for infection because of added exposure to pathogens, compromised immunologic state, and potential invasive procedures. Development of infection can delay healing, prolong the hospital stay, and cause permanent disability or even loss of life. To prevent complications, it is important to understand the principles of infectious disease with regard to how a pathogen can enter the body and develop into an infection. The following criteria, or chain of events, must be present for a pathogen to develop into an infection: a pathogen (infectious agent); a reservoir for the pathogen to grow; a portal of exit from the source; a mode of transmission; a portal of entry to the host; and a susceptible host. A break in the chain will prevent infection. Medical asepsis is the process of reducing microorganisms and preventing their spread. Handwashing (hand hygiene) remains the single most important technique for infection control. Surgical asepsis, or sterile technique, consists of those practices that eliminate all microorganisms and spores from an object or area. Sterile technique is practiced in the surgical arena to reduce the risk for infection. Surgical scrub and applying sterile gown and gloves is discussed in Skills 9-8 and 9-9.

Standard precautions: consider all clients and their body fluids (except sweat) to be potentially infectious, thereby replacing the term Universal Precautions, which applied only to blood and visibly bloody fluids (CDC, 2002). Standard precautions are to be used on all clients regardless of their condition or diagnosis. Standard precautions require the use of personal protective equipment to prevent the transmission of microorganisms. Personal protective equipment includes the following:

- Gloves are required when hand contact with any body fluid is anticipated, including touching mucous membranes and nonintact skin. Latex- and powder-free gloves are recommended. Hands should be washed before and after the gloves are removed.
- Impervious gowns must be worn by heath care workers to prevent soiling of clothing by splashes of blood or body fluids.
- Masks are worn when caring for clients who are on airborne and droplet precautions and when splashes toward the face are anticipated. They may also be worn when caring for the immuno-compromised client as you may present a threat to his or her ability to fight infection.
- Eye protection (goggles) or face shields should be worn during care activities that may be associated with splashes or sprays of blood or body fluids.

▶ ASSESSMENT

1. Assess the specific isolation precautions needed for the client's condition. **The type of**

microorganism and mode of transmission determine the degree of precautions.

2. Assess the client's laboratory results **to learn which organism the client is infected with and the client's immune responses.**

3. Assess what nursing measures are required before entering the room **to have all the necessary equipment ready.**

4. Assess the client's knowledge for the need to wear a cap, gown, and mask during care **to direct client teaching.**

5. Assess whether the isolation is airborne, droplet, or contact and which isolation attire is necessary, **as not all sterile procedures require a cap, gown, and mask.**

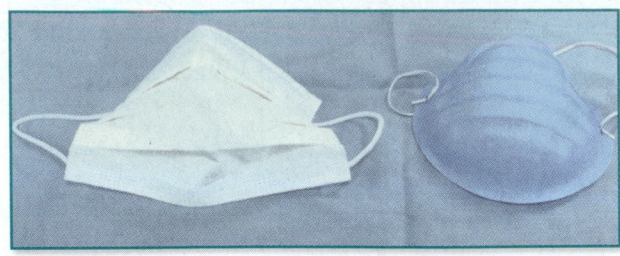

Figure 2-5-1A   Masks

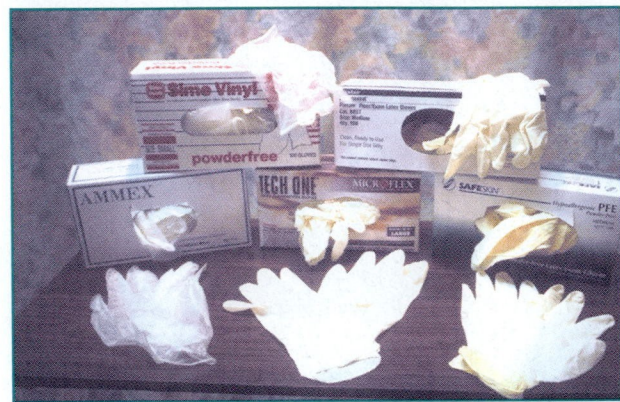

Figure 2-5-1B   Clean gloves

▶ DIAGNOSIS

Risk for Infection

Ineffective Protection

Social Isolation

Situational Low Self-Esteem

▶ PLANNING

Expected Outcomes:

1. The client and staff will remain free of nosocomial infection.

2. The health care provider and staff will be protected from infection when caring for the client.

3. The staff will avoid transmitting microorganisms to others.

4. The client will interact on a social level with nurse, staff, family members, and other visitors.

Equipment Needed (see Figure 2-5-1A and B):

• Gloves, clean
• Gown
• Cap
• Mask

▶ CLIENT EDUCATION NEEDED:

1. Explain the rationale for isolation to the client.

2. The client should be assured that the isolation attire (gown, mask, cap) will be discontinued when possible; however, gloves will be worn, when appropriate, to ensure standard precautions.

3. The client and caregiver should be taught to identify signs and symptoms of infection and encouraged to report these upon occurrence.

4. The client should be encouraged to assist the staff in maintaining isolation standards and may monitor others for any breaks in technique.

Estimated time to complete the skill:
5 minutes

▶ DELEGATION TIPS

Donning and removing gloves, caps, and masks is a skill that is required of all personnel, including ancillary personnel. Proper technique should be monitored by the nursing staff.

IMPLEMENTATION—Action/Rationale

Action	Rationale
1. Wash hands.	1. Reduces the transmission of microorganisms.
2. Assemble supplies that will be needed before entering client's room.	2. Facilitates organization of client care.
3. Apply gown. Unfold gown, slip arms into sleeves, and pull up to shoulders. Tie the neck ties. Reach behind and overlap the edges of the gown so your uniforms are completely covered and then tie waist ties.	3. Gowns act as a protective barrier to protect the nurse's uniform. Gowns also reduce exposure to blood, body fluid, or other potentially infectious material.
4. Apply a mask around mouth and nose and secure in a manner that prevents venting. For masks with strings (see Figure 2-5-2): a. Hold mask by top and pinch center (metal strip) over bridge of nose. b. Adjust mask to cover nose and mouth. c. Pull top two strings over ears and secure at top, back of head. d. Tie two lower ties around back or nape of neck so bottom of mask fits snugly under chin (see Figure 2-5-2). For masks with elastic bands: • Hold the mask in one hand and the elastic band in another. Place and hold mask over your nose and mouth, then stretch the band over your head (see Figure 2-5-3).	4. Masks are worn to contain and filter droplets of microorganisms that are expelled when talking, sneezing, or coughing. Masks prevent the transmission of oral and nasopharyngeal organisms between the nurse and client.
5. Protective eyewear (goggles or faceshield) should be worn whenever the health care provider is at risk for splash and contamination. These are applied as goggles/glasses or face shields, which have elastic ties for around the ears.	5. Protective eyewear reduces the incidence of contamination to the eyes. If eyewear or face shields become contaminated they should be discarded immediately and replaced with a clean barrier.

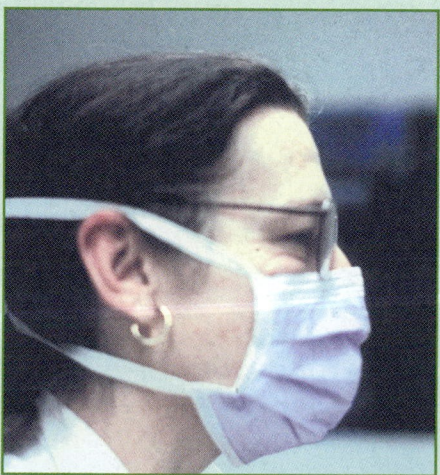

Figure 2-5-2 Bottom of the mask should fit snugly under the chin.

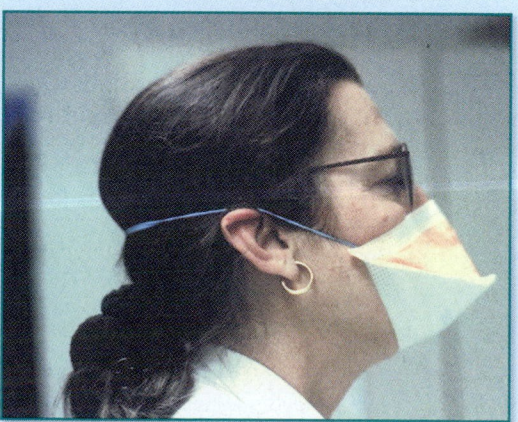

Figure 2-5-3 Secure mask around mouth and nose.

continues

Action	Rationale
6. Don clean gloves. Stretch the glove cuff over the gown sleeves at the wrist.	**6.** Gloves protect the hands and wrists from microorganisms.
7. Enter the client's room and explain the rationale for wearing isolation attire.	**7.** Minimizes anxiety and feelings of isolation.
8. After performing necessary tasks, remove personal protective equipment:	**8.**
a. Remove gloves	a.
• Grasp the outside cuff of one glove and pull off, turning inside out. (see Figure 2-5-4). Hold removed glove in palm of gloved hand.	• Prevents the transmission of microorganisms. Contaminated glove does not come in contact with skin.
• Slide fingers of ungloved hand inside the wrist of the gloved hand (see Figure 2-5-5). Pull the glove off turning it inside out and over the other glove. Dispose into receptacle.	• Ungloved hand is clean and should not come in contact with contaminated glove.
b. Remove protective eyewear	b.
• Remove by handling the ear pieces and dispose into receptacle.	• Front of eye wear is considered contaminated.
c. Remove gown	c.
• Untie gown at neck and waist. Remove from each shoulder. Fold and roll gown down in front into a ball, so contaminated area is rolled onto center of gown. Dispose into receptacle.	• Outside of gown is considered contaminated. Prevents transmission of microorganisms.
d. Remove mask	d.
• Untie bottom strings of mask first, then top strings. Hold mask by strings and lift off face. Do not touch the outside of mask. Dispose into receptacle.	• Outside of mask is considered contaminated.
9. Wash hands.	**9.** Prevents transmission of microorganisms.

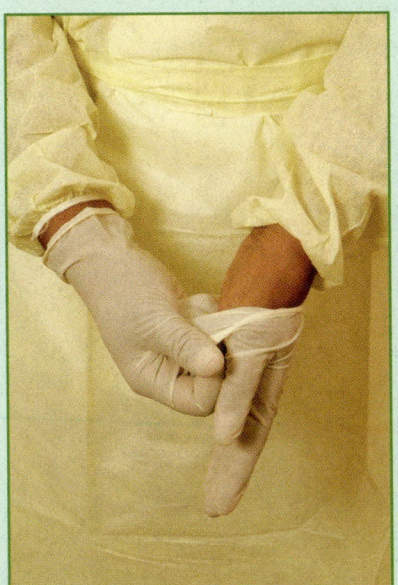

Figure 2-5-4 Grasp the outside cuff and turn the glove inside out.

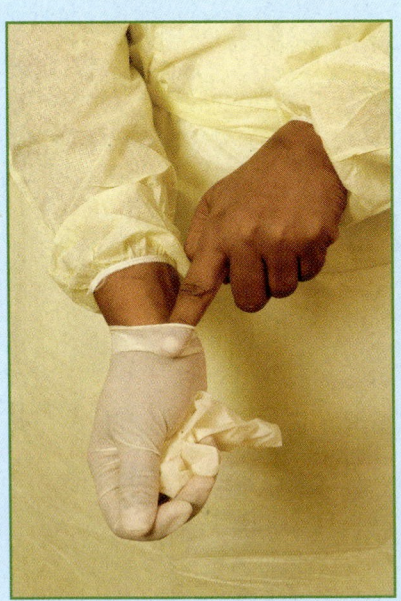

Figure 2-5-5 Turn the second glove over the first glove.

► REAL WORLD ANECDOTES

Scenario 1

Andrea was only 4 years old when she was admitted to the hospital with respiratory symptoms. After diagnostic tests, she was found to have pneumonia caused by an antibiotic-resistant organism. She was immediately placed in isolation. Andrea cried when the nurse came in with gown, gloves, cap, and a mask covering her face. She did not recognize her favorite nurse until she heard her say her name and laugh as she sat down beside Andrea. The nurse assured her that she would get better and then everyone who came into her room would not have to wear the masks, caps, and gloves anymore. The nurse also used a marker to make a smiley face on her mask the next time she came in. This pleased Andrea and she didn't feel so isolated.

Scenario 2

A doctor is in a client's room properly gowned and gloved and working with a wound debridement at the bedside. His pager goes off, and he quickly lifts the gown aside to silence it with his gloved hand. His pager is now contaminated and he has increased the chance of transmitting microorganisms to other clients. The assisting nurse takes the pager and uses disinfectant before returning it to the ungloved physician after the procedure.

► EVALUATION

- The client and staff remained free of nosocomial infection.
- The health care provider and staff were protected from infection when caring for the client.
- The staff avoided transmitting microorganisms to others.
- The client interacted on a social level with nurse, staff, family members, and other visitors.

► DOCUMENTATION

Nurses' Notes

- Document the type of protective barriers used and any breaks in isolation technique.
- Record the client's compliance with and verbalization of understanding and adjustment to isolation.
- Record family members' compliance of isolation procedures.

Document on appropriate flow sheet or electronic medical record (EMR).

► CRITICAL THINKING SKILL

Introduction

Standard precautions are used when handling any body fluid other than sweat, including handling blood, body fluids, and tissues and fluids, such as pericardial, peritoneal, amniotic, semen, synovial, vaginal, cerebrospinal, and pleural space. Standard precautions include wearing a mask with goggles, or a mask with face shield, when a splash is possible.

Possible Scenario

The nurse is caring for a client with a gastrointestinal bleed. The client has been vomiting bright red blood since he was admitted from the emergency room. The nurse steps out of the room to get some clean towels and medication. When she returns, the client has a bloody projectile emesis that splashes in her face as she approaches the client to assist him.

Possible Outcome 1

The nurse, anxious to help the client, uses one of the clean towels to wipe the emesis off her face. She proceeds to help the client get cleaned up, medicated, and comfortable. Once she has seen to her client's comfort, she proceeds to the sink by the door and washes her face with antiseptic soap. She later reports the incident to her supervisor.

Possible Outcome 2

The nurse observes that the client is not in any immediate danger so she washes her face with antiseptic soap at the sink by the door, puts on her mask with protective eyewear, and continues to care for the client. She later reports the incident to her supervisor.

Prevention

Don the mask and protective eyewear before approaching the client. With a gastrointestinal bleed, there is always the potential for splash. Fresh supplies of gowns, masks, and goggles should always be kept outside the closed door of an isolation room. Unless the client is in grave danger, you must don the appropriate isolation apparel prior to entering the room.

► VARIATIONS

Geriatric Variations:

- *The older client can feel depressed and shunned when in isolation. Provide the client with as much stimulation and company as possible.*
- *Reassure client that isolation is for a limited time only.*
- *Older clients who are confused may become more confused or agitated if they are unable to identify their caregiver. Reorient the client as needed.*
- *Older clients should be assured that they will not be left alone any longer than necessary.*
- *Older clients who lip-read may have difficulty understanding a person wearing a mask. Make sure alternative communication devices are available, such as a pad and pencil. If the client wears a hearing device, make sure it is in place.*

Pediatric Variations:

- *Younger children may feel that they are being punished for being sick. Be sure to regularly reinforce your reason for isolation techniques.*
- *Showing the gown and gloves to the child will help him or her understand why they are being used and will help the child to recognize that there is a real person under the isolation attire.*
- *Allow the child to play with the cap and mask so he or she will become more familiar with them.*
- *The nurse should show her face from the doorway before donning the cap and mask.*
- *Provide a cap for the child's stuffed toy to wear as well.*

Home Care Variations:

- *A safe receptacle for contaminated items needs to be identified and used properly. Review agency policy and determine how this receptacle will be emptied and the items disposed of or cleaned properly.*
- *Promote compliance by reducing the inconvenience with good assessment and planning.*
- *There are several possible drawbacks to the caregiver maintaining precautions at home, including the cost of supplies, the difficulty involved, and the low perceived benefit. This is a situation where careful, supportive education of the caregiver and client is essential to help caregivers understand the need to consistently implement the procedures.*

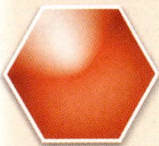

Long-Term Care Variations:

- *A safe receptacle for the contaminated items needs to be identified and used properly.*
- *In long-term care settings, the clients and caregivers can get careless regarding precautions. Be sure to reinforce the ongoing need for following strict guidelines regarding isolation and Standard Precautions.*
- *Make sure that the workers who are not normally exposed to barrier methods in the facility understand the need and procedures for the specific precaution for the client.*

► COMMON ERRORS

Possible Error:

You do not remove your mask when leaving one room and wear it into the next room.

Prevention:

Always remove contaminated items when leaving a room. Return to the room where you wore the mask and cap. Remove them and leave them in the receptacle there. Wash your hands.

continues

▶ **COMMON ERRORS** (continued)

Possible Error:

A nurse observes a visitor go into an isolation room without putting on a gown and gloves.

Prevention:

A sign at the door of the isolation room might include a caution to check with the nurse before entering the room, or the client in isolation might be near the nurses' station so visitors can be monitored.

▶ **NURSING TIPS**

- Post signs on the doors of clients who require specific barrier methods using words and/or pictures that are clear and understandable.
- Review isolation procedures regularly.
- Provide a supply of the appropriate barrier at the doorway of the client's room.
- If you need equipment, such as an item you are carrying in your pocket, you will not be able to reach your pocket after you don your gown. You will not be able to touch needed items if your gloves and gown are contaminated. Think ahead. Plan.
- Remember masks become ineffective if worn too long, become wet, or are not changed between clients.
- Remember that anything you touch with a contaminated glove will be contaminated. Think: sterile can touch sterile, clean can touch clean.

▶ **SPECIAL CONSIDERATIONS**

- *A nurse is required to have a surgical conscience when working with isolation or when using aseptic technique. Surgical conscience is an individual's inner awareness of aseptic principles and adherence to aseptic technique in all situations. It is professional honesty.*
- *Latex allergy poses a threat to workers and clients in health care settings. Latex allergy can range from skin irritation to anaphylaxis and death. Those at greatest risk are workers (nurses) frequently using latex products, clients with multiple surgeries, and individuals with a history of atopy (genetic predisposition to allergies). Latex allergy should be elicited with the history. Those with latex allergy need to be informed of risk, signs and symptoms, treatment, the multiplicity of products that contain latex, the cross-reactivity with food products, and the risk of aerosolized latex. Avoidance of latex is the most effective treatment and mandatory for staff and clients with latex allergy. Many latex-free alternative products are available, and facilities should aim for a latex-safe environment by using latex-free and powder-free gloves. Avoid surgical caps and masks with elastic straps or bands if client has latex allergy.*

Removing Contaminated Items

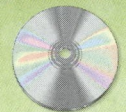

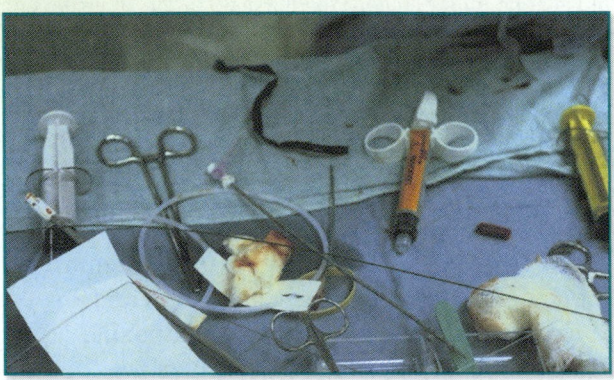

▶ OVERVIEW OF THE SKILL

Infection control measures are used for all clients, regardless of the settings. Careful handling and removal of contaminated items from the client's environment are the responsibility of all personnel involved in the care of the client with an infection. Bagging these items properly prevents cross-contamination within the client's environment as well as accidental contamination of other individuals within the surrounding area. Items require bagging if they are contaminated with infective materials such as blood, pus, body fluids, feces, or respiratory secretions. This step is especially important in any setting where medical personnel may be working with several clients throughout the day and risk spreading microorganisms from client to nurse, from nurse to nurse, or to other clients (see Figure 2-6-1).

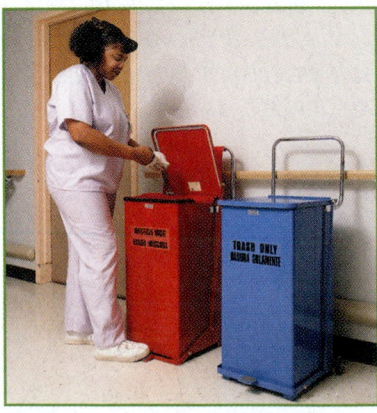

Figure 2-6-1 Proper handling and disposal of client care items reduces the risk of contamination.

▶ ASSESSMENT

1. Assess the client's disease process and medical condition. **Understanding the disease process and client's current status will help the nurse plan and organize care appropriately and institute appropriate infection control measures.**
2. Assess the client's level of understanding regarding infection precautions. **Determine whether the client understands basic infection prevention measures. The client may be confused or anxious if isolation measures are initiated.**

▶ DIAGNOSIS

Risk for Infection

Social Isolation

Situational Low Self-Esteem

▶ PLANNING

Expected Outcomes:

1. Client will demonstrate an understanding regarding infection control procedures.
2. Client will demonstrate self-care measures related to preventing infections.
3. All contaminated items within the client's environment will be disposed of in an appropriate manner.
4. Personnel caring for the client will use appropriate infection prevention measures as determined by the client's condition and Standard Precautions guidelines.

Equipment Needed (see Figure 2-6-2):

• Disposable gloves.

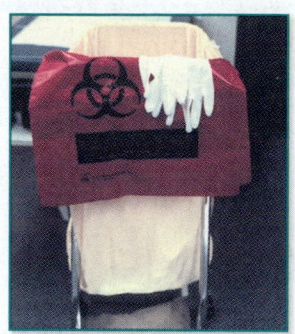

Figure 2-6-2 Biohazard bags and gloves are used to handle and dispose of contaminated items.

- Self-supporting stand for the linen bag.
- Labeled bag for disposal of soiled linen. Bag should be hot-water soluble; the bag may also be colored (red) for easy identification. (*Note:* Some agencies may require that linen be double bagged for removal.)
- Second linen bag if the double-bagging technique is used.

▶ CLIENT EDUCATION NEEDED:

1. Educate client on the infection prevention measures that apply. An informed client can

monitor staff/visitor compliance to Standard Precautions.
2. Explain to the client the rationale for the infection prevention measures.
3. Explain to the client the purpose of any related equipment, that is, specially designated linen or trash bags.
4. Demonstrate the technique of proper hand-washing for visitors and client.
5. Ask clients to remind visitors to wash their hands when entering and leaving the room and to dispose of soiled client items appropriately. This is especially important if the visitor participates in the care of the client.
6. Encourage the client and caregiver to comply with Standard Precautions. This applies to the client cared for in the home as well as in the hospital setting.

 Estimated time to complete the skill: **15 minutes**

▶ DELEGATION TIPS

Infection control measures are used for all clients. Careful handling of all contaminated items from the client's environment is the responsibility of all personnel involved in the client's care. The professional nurse may delegate these activities but is responsible to monitor the adherence to Standard Precautions.

IMPLEMENTATION—Action/Rationale

Action	Rationale
Removal of Soiled Linen	
1. Wash hands when entering the client's room.	1. Proper handwashing reduces transmission of microorganisms.
2. Wear disposable gloves; wear other protective items (gowns, goggles) as determined by the situation and agency policies.	2. Protects the nurse from contamination from blood and body fluids.
3. Place labeled linen bag in stand.	3. Proper labeling or identification of the linen bag ensures proper handling by other agency personnel. Check agency policy for issues of confidentiality with regard to labeling.
4. Gather linen and separate from disposable items.	4. Prevents waste from being placed in linen bag.

continues

Action	Rationale
Removal of Soiled Linen *continued*	
5. Do not allow any linen to touch the floor.	5. The floor is always considered a contaminated area.
6. Place soiled linen in the linen bag; keep clean linen in a different area (see Figure 2-6-3).	6. It is important to prevent cross-contamination to clean supplies and linen.
7. Take care not to shake the linen when removing items from the bed or bathroom.	7. Minimizing movement through the air of the linens helps to reduce the risk of transmission of microorganisms.
8. Do not allow the soiled linen to contact your clothing. Carry linens with arms extended in front of you.	8. Prevents contamination of the nurse and cross-contamination to other clients.
9. Do not overfill the bag.	9. Ensures proper closure of bag.
10. Tie ends of the bag securely.	10. Prevents linen from spilling out of the bag.
11. Check for any punctures or tears in the bag.	11. The linen bag must be intact to prevent transmission of microorganisms.
12. Double bag items if there is concern that the outside of the bag is contaminated or is torn.	12. This is necessary to prevent cross-contamination and transmission of microorganisms to other personnel or other areas.
13. Remove gloves and wash hands.	13. Reduces transmission of microorganisms.
Double-Bagging Technique	
14. With double bagging of linens, follow Actions 1–11. Then place the first bag into a second bag. Either a second nurse holds the second bag or it is in a stand immediately outside of the room.	14. Some agencies require the double bagging of linens as a measure to reduce the possibility of transmission of microorganisms. In most situations, it is not necessary unless the single bag is not sturdy enough to hold the items or if the outside of the single bag has become contaminated.
15. The second bag is properly labeled and secured.	15. Proper labeling or identification of the linen bag ensures proper handling by other agency personnel. Most agencies will have bags marked as biohazardous.
16. The linens are then ready for the laundry.	16. Linens should be disposed of as soon as possible per agency policy.

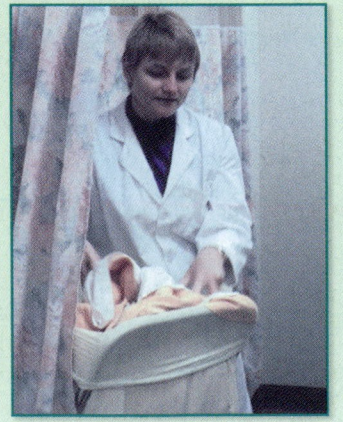

Figure 2-6-3   Place soiled linen in a bag.

continues

Action	Rationale
17. Remove gloves and wash hands thoroughly upon leaving the room.	17. Proper handwashing reduces transmission of microorganisms.

Removal of Other Contaminated Items

Action	Rationale
18. Removal and bagging of trash bag follow the same procedure as for linens (see Figure 2-6-4).	18. Check agency policy to determine if double bagging is required.
19. Sharps containers need to be removed when they are three-quarters full or if the outside of the container becomes contaminated. Lock down the lid if available, and follow hospital policy for removal (see Figure 2-6-5). Never reach into a container with your hand.	19. Overfilling a sharp container can lead to injuries to staff members.
20. Use disposable equipment when able (see Figure 2-6-6).	20. Reduces the possibility of transmission of microorganisms.

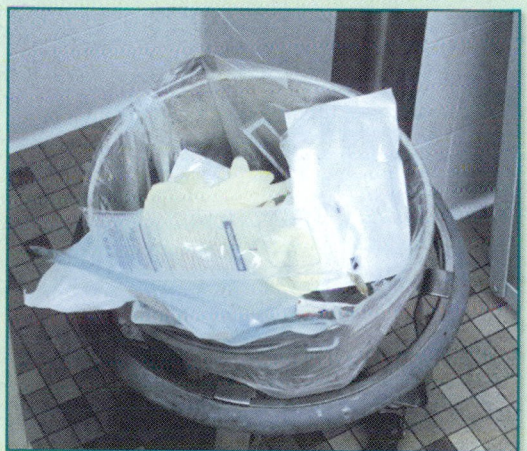

Figure 2-6-4   Bag all trash prior to removal.

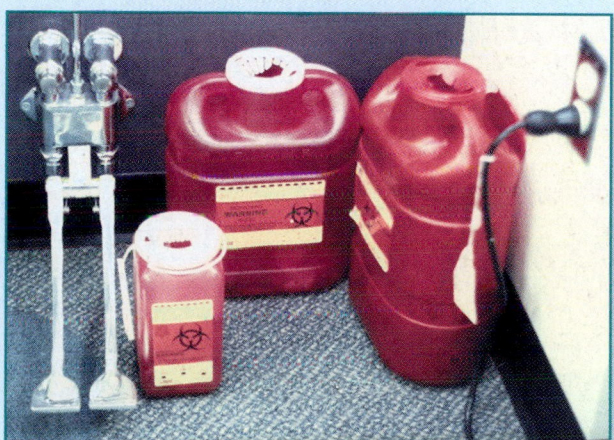

Figure 2-6-5   Remove and replace full sharps containers to avoid needlestick injuries from pushing sharp items into a full container.

Action	Rationale
21. Properly bag, label, and remove any nondisposable equipment that will require special cleaning (disinfection and sterilization).	21. Proper handling and labeling of the items ensures proper handling by other agency personnel.
22. Disassemble special procedure trays into disposable and nondisposable parts. Send nondisposable items (after proper bagging) to central services for decontamination.	22. Some agencies require that items that can be sterilized by autoclave (glass, metal) be separated from rubber and plastic items.
23. Laboratory specimens should be placed in a leak-proof container and require no other precautions. Check to see that containers are not visibly contaminated on the outside (see Figure 2-6-7).	23. Personnel handling laboratory specimens should use Standard Precautions.

continues

Action	Rationale

Removal of Other Contaminated Items *continued*

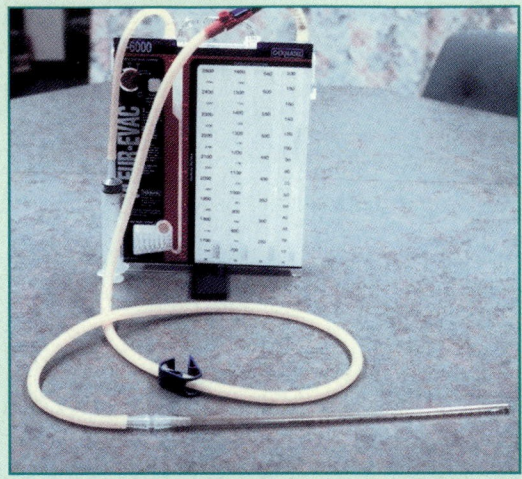

Figure 2-6-6   Using disposable equipment reduces contamination risks.

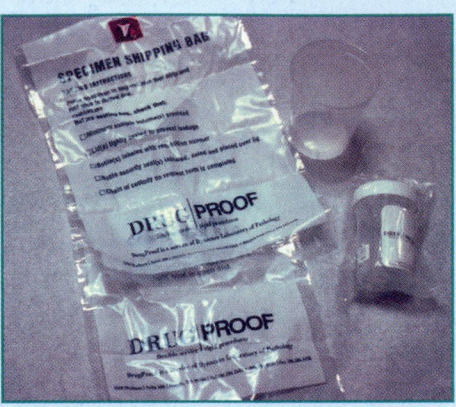

Figure 2-6-7   Place specimens in leak-proof containers to avoid contamination.

24. Remove gloves and wash hands.

24. Reduces transmission of microorganisms.

▶ REAL WORLD ANECDOTES

Scenario 1

Mrs. Jones regularly participated in the care of her child. Her child was a frequent client at the medical center because of a diagnosis of cystic fibrosis and frequent bouts of pulmonary infections. Mrs. Jones was very aware of the importance of managing her child's secretions and was very upset when the nurse did not supply bags for disposal of trash (tissues) in the room. Mrs. Jones also noticed that the housekeeping personnel did not wear gloves when handling the trash. Her observations were reported to the nurse manager who instituted the appropriate infection prevention measures.

Scenario 2

Mr. Smith was admitted to a medical surgical unit with a possible diagnosis of tuberculosis (TB) during a very busy evening shift. The admitting nurse failed to initiate orders for pulmonary infection precautions. The error was discovered in the morning report. Unfortunately, several nurses and other personnel had been exposed to Mr. Smith's secretions. The diagnosis of TB was confirmed and the exposed personnel were subsequently tested at expense to the agency, and disciplinary action was taken.

► EVALUATION

- Client demonstrates an understanding regarding infection control procedures.
- Client demonstrates self-care measures related to infection prevention.
- All contaminated items within the client's environment were disposed of in an appropriate manner.
- Personnel caring for the client used appropriate infection prevention measures as determined by the client's condition.

► DOCUMENTATION

Nurses' Notes

- Note specific isolation precautions that were followed.
- Document any specific breaches of isolation noted.

► CRITICAL THINKING SKILL

Introduction

The importance of properly bagging linens should not be minimized. Prevention of transmission of microorganisms is everyone's responsibility.

Possible Scenario

Mr. Kelley was transferred from a local nursing home with a wound infection. The microbiology results indicated the client had vancomycin-resistant enterococcus (VRE). The nurse was changing the bed of Mr. Kelley, whose linens were contaminated with exudate from a recent dressing change. The nurse removed the linens from the bed and tucked them under her arm as she reached to pick up the call light that had fallen on the floor. She then placed the soiled linens in the proper bag in the room.

Possible Outcome 1

After changing Mr. Kelley's linens, the nurse answered a call light. The client who called wanted to be helped from the bed to the commode. During the transfer, the client grasped the nurse under the arms, placing her hand directly on the now contaminated area. This client was later found to have the same strain of VRE.

Possible Outcome 2

After changing Mr. Kelley's linen, the nurse started to answer a call light. While walking to the client's room, the nurse remembered that she had placed linen contaminated with an antibiotic-resistant bacteria against her uniform. She did not see any obvious contamination, but as a precaution she decided to wear an isolation gown over her uniform. There were no other cases of VRE in the facility.

Prevention

Microorganisms on the linens can be transmitted to the nurse's clothing with direct contact. This may cause possible risk of infection to other personnel and clients. Carry linens at arm's length when removing them from the bed and placing them in the appropriate container.

► VARIATIONS

Geriatric Variations:

- *Some older adults may lack the dexterity to assist in the bagging or labeling of soiled items and may need assistance from a health care worker.*
- *Some older clients with impairment of memory may have difficulty in understanding the importance of infection prevention measures or may be confused as to the purpose of such measures.*

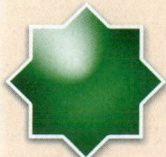

Pediatric Variations:

- *Children's toys and books that are contaminated should be disinfected or destroyed.*
- *Teach the child and caregiver not to share toys with other children or siblings if the child has an illness that may be transmitted to others.*
- *It is also important to keep all bagging supplies (plastic bags) away from the reach of very young children as these items may pose a risk for suffocation.*

continues

▶ VARIATIONS *(continued)*

Home Care Variations:
- *In the home setting, the client and caregivers should be instructed to wash linens and clothing in a separate load of laundry if these items are considered contaminated. Laundry soap and a hot-water cycle should be used.*

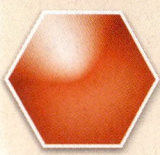

Long-Term Care Variations:
- *Clients with impaired cognitive function will be unable to assist with bagging and removal of items in accordance with infection prevention measures.*

▶ COMMON ERRORS

Possible Error:

Overfilled linen bag that cannot be secured properly.

Prevention:

Use caution in handling soiled linens. Keep spare bagging supplies in a convenient location for use. Allow room at the top of each bag for proper closure. Put on gloves; set up an additional linen bag on stand; remove some of the linen from the first bag (take care not to contaminate the outside of the bag) until there is room for proper closure of the first bag. Place soiled linens in the second bag as appropriate.

Possible Error:

Placement of improper items in the bag.

Prevention:

Separate disposable from nondisposable items when bagging for removal. Put on gloves. Carefully sort the items and separately bag the nondisposable items for sterilization and chemical disinfection.

▶ NURSING TIPS

- Check supplies (bags, labels) before beginning bagging of items for removal.
- Always wash your hands before and after entering a room and bagging soiled items, even when wearing gloves.
- Use disposable equipment and supplies when possible.
- Do not take items such as your stethoscope into another client's room for use without proper cleaning when there is risk of transmission of infection.
- Review your agency's policies for specific guidelines, that is, some institutions may require double bagging for some items.
- Recheck labels and restock special bags as needed so that supplies are readily available for other caregivers and personnel.

▶ **SPECIAL CONSIDERATIONS**

- *Avoid using a label with a client's name on biohazardous bags. These labeled items may be seen and the client's right to confidentiality violated.*
- *When separating disposable from nondisposable items after a procedure, make sure that all sharps are accounted for and disposed of properly. Those handling the trash may be inadvertently stuck with a contaminated needle if the nurse is not prudent about sharp safety.*

Applying Sterile Gloves via the Open Method

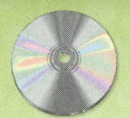

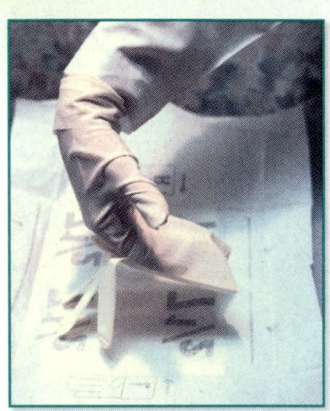

▶ OVERVIEW OF THE SKILL

Asepsis, or sterile technique, consists of those practices that eliminate all microorganisms and spores from an object or area. The use of sterile gloves is at the heart of aseptic technique. The ability to manipulate sterile items without contaminating them is critical to many diagnostic and therapeutic interventions. Common nursing procedures that require sterile technique are:

- All invasive procedures, either intentional perforation of the skin (injection, insertion of intravenous [IV] needles or catheters) or entry into a body orifice (tracheobronchial suctioning, insertion of a urinary catheter)
- Nursing measures for clients with disruption of skin surfaces (changing a surgical wound or IV site dressing) or destruction of skin layers (trauma and burns)

There are two methods for applying sterile gloves: open and closed. The open method is used most frequently when performing procedures that require the sterile technique, such as dressing changes, but that do not require donning a sterile gown.

▶ ASSESSMENT

1. Assess the glove package. Is it intact? Is it wet or otherwise contaminated? **Assesses the sterility of the glove.**
2. Assess the local environment. Is there an area suitable for opening the package and applying the gloves? Is the area dry? Is it reasonably stable and horizontal? Are there obvious airborne contaminants? **A flat, clear workspace is necessary to successfully carry out the procedure.**
3. Assess the correct glove size for proper fit. Gloves come in many sizes and proper fit is conducive to maintaining asepsis.

▶ DIAGNOSIS

Risk for Infection

▶ PLANNING

Expected Outcomes:

1. Sterility of the gloves will be maintained while they are being applied.
2. Sterility of the procedure will be maintained.

Equipment Needed (see Figure 2-7-1):

Package of proper-sized sterile gloves

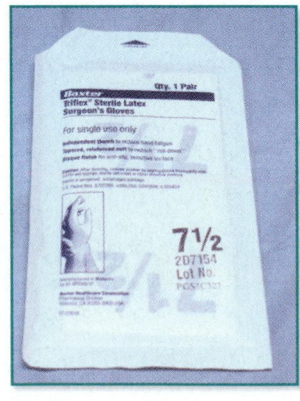

Figure 2-7-1 Sterile gloves

▶ **CLIENT EDUCATION NEEDED:**

1. Inform the client that you are establishing a sterile field and request cooperation in not touching the sterile gloves or other sterile objects.

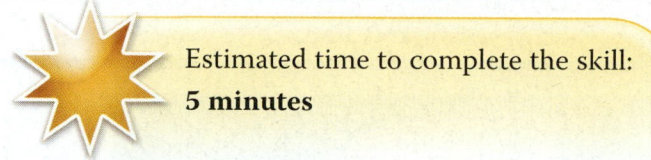

Estimated time to complete the skill: **5 minutes**

▶ **DELEGATION TIPS**

Sterile gloving is only delegated if the personnel are specifically trained such as in a surgical suite or a testing laboratory setting.

IMPLEMENTATION—Action/Rationale

Action	Rationale
1. Wash hands.	1. Reduces the transmission of microorganisms.
2. Read the manufacturer's instructions on the package of sterile gloves; proceed as directed in removing the outer wrapper from the package (see Figure 2-7-2), placing the inner wrapper onto a clean, dry surface (see Figure 2-7-3). Open inner wrapper to expose gloves (see Figure 2-7-4).	2. Different manufacturers package gloves differently; the instructions will tell you how to open properly to avoid contamination of the inner wrapper; any moisture on the surface will contaminate the gloves.
3. Identify right and left hand; glove dominant hand first.	3. Dominant hand should facilitate motor dexterity during gloving.
4. Grasp the 2-inch- (5-cm) wide cuff with the thumb and first two fingers of the nondominant hand, touching only the inside of the cuff (see Figure 2-7-5).	4. Maintains sterility of the outer surfaces of the sterile glove.
5. Gently pull the glove over the dominant hand, making sure the thumb and fingers fit into the proper spaces of the glove (see Figure 2-7-6).	5. Prevents tearing the glove material; guiding the fingers into proper places facilitates gloving.

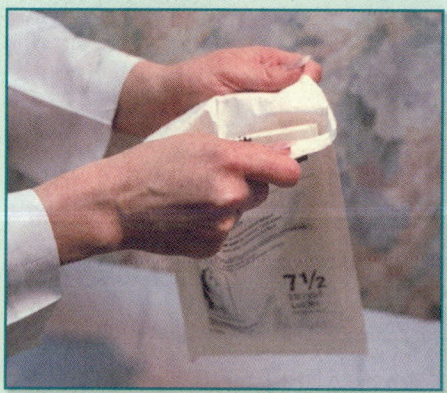

Figure 2-7-2 Remove the outer wrapper of the sterile glove package.

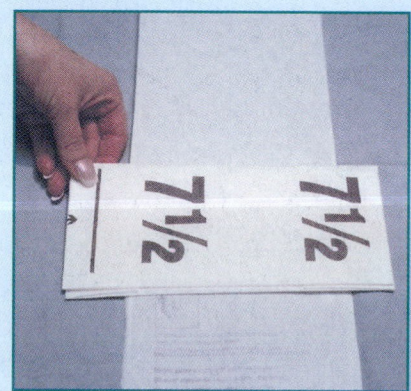

Figure 2-7-3 Place the gloves in the inner wrapper on clean, dry surface.

continues

Action	Rationale

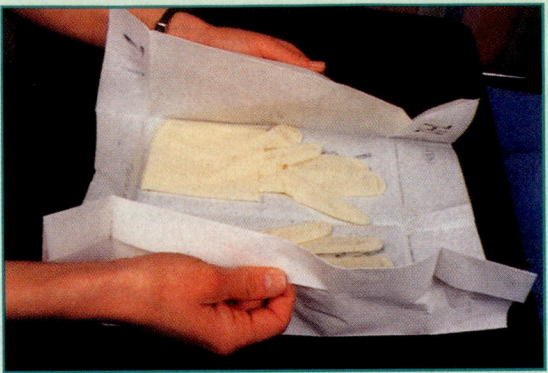

Figure 2-7-4 Open the inner wrapper to expose glove.

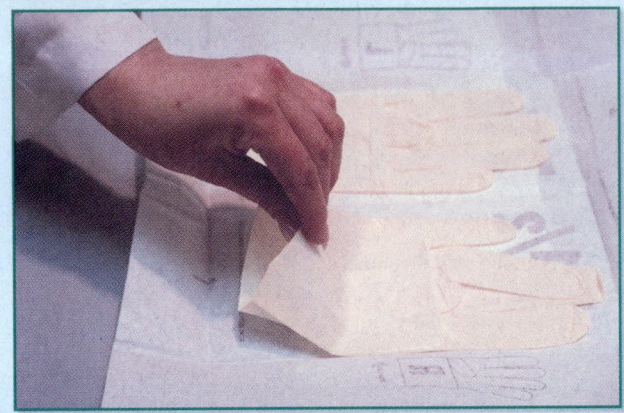

Figure 2-7-5 Grasp first cuff with the nondominant hand.

6. With the gloved dominant hand, slip your fingers under the cuff of the other glove, gloved thumb abducted, making sure it does not touch any part on your nondominant hand (see Figure 2-7-7).

6. Cuff protects gloved fingers, maintaining sterility.

7. Gently slip the glove onto your nondominant hand, making sure the fingers slip into the proper spaces (see Figures 2-7-8 and 2-7-9).

7. Contact is made with two sterile gloves.

8. With gloved hands, interlock fingers to fit the gloves onto each finger.

8. Promotes proper fit over the fingers.

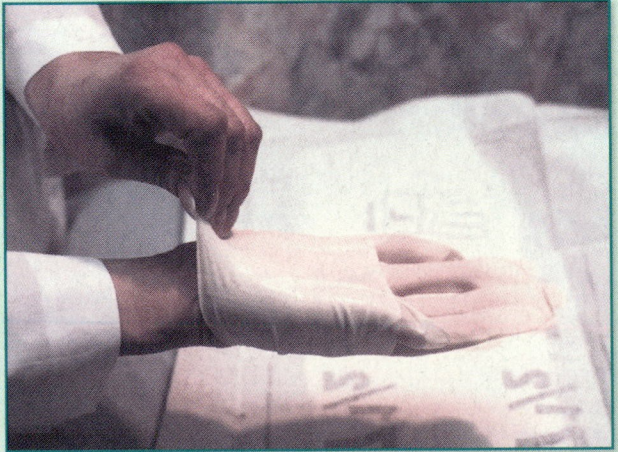

Figure 2-7-6 Pull the glove over the dominant hand.

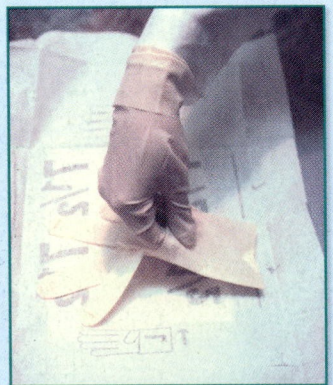

Figure 2-7-7 Slip fingers under the cuff of the second glove.

continues

Action	Rationale

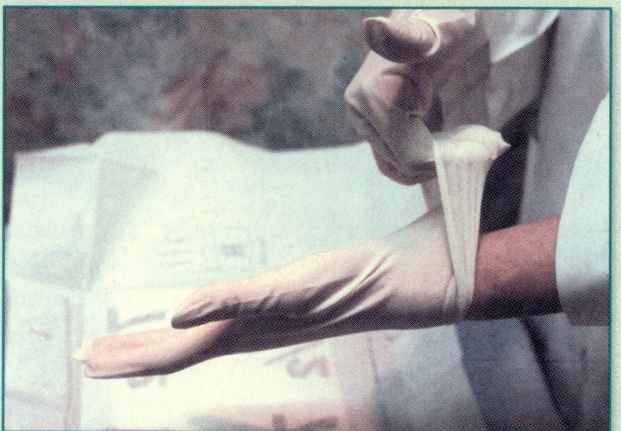

Figure 2-7-8 Pull on the second glove.

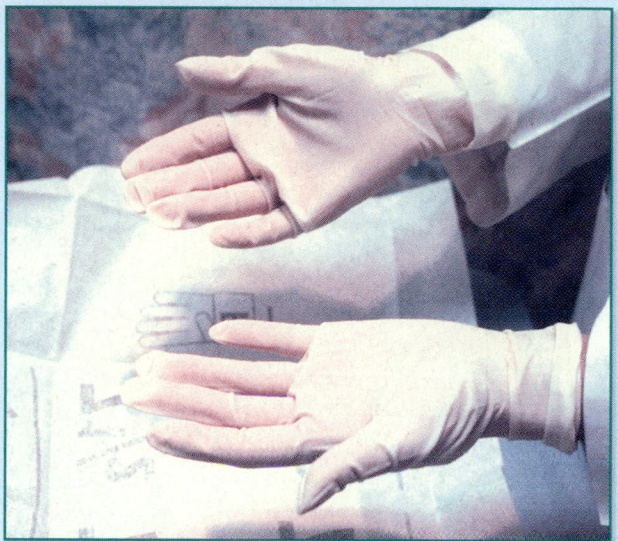

Figure 2-7-9 Make sure all fingers are in the proper spaces.

To remove the gloves:

9. With your dominant hand, grasp the other glove at the wrist. Avoid touching the skin of your wrist with the fingers of the glove. Pull the glove off turning it inside out. (see Figure 2-7-10).

10. Place removed glove in palm of gloved hand.

11. Place thumb of ungloved hand inside the cuff of the gloved hand touching only the inside of the glove (see Figure 2-7-11).

9. Prevents the transfer of microorganisms. Contaminated glove does not contact skin.

10. Prevents the transmission of microorganisms.

11. Reduces the transmission of microorganisms.

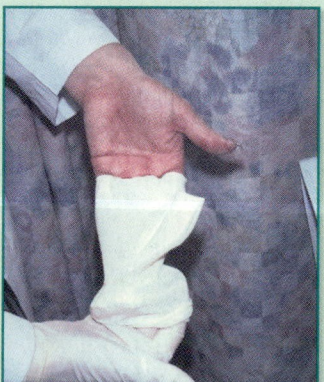

Figure 2-7-10 Pull off glove, turning it inside out.

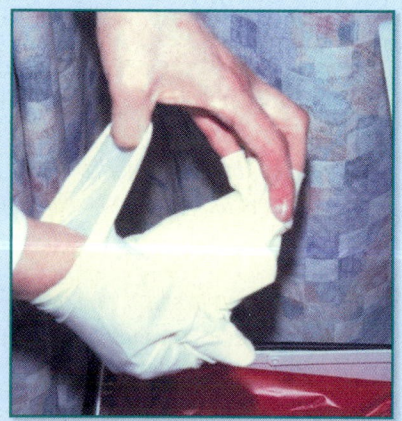

Figure 2-7-11 Slip uncovered thumb into the opposite glove.

continues

Action	Rationale
12. Pull the glove off, turning it inside out and over the other glove (see Figure 2-7-12).	**12.** Reduces the transmission of microorganisms.
13. Dispose of soiled gloves according to institutional policy and wash hands (see Figure 2-7-13).	**13.** Prevents the transfer of microorganisms.

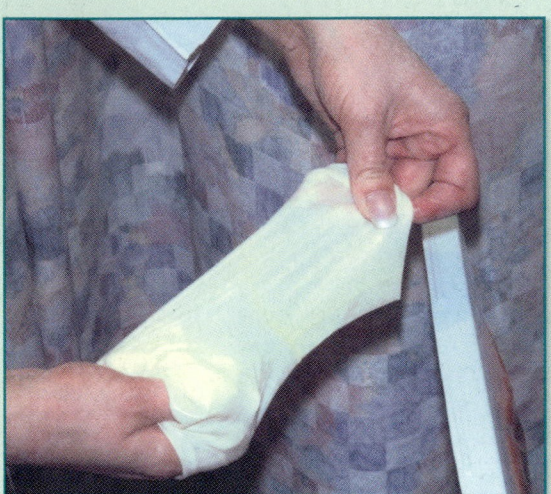

Figure 2-7-12 When soiled gloves are removed correctly, only the inside, clean surface of one glove is exposed.

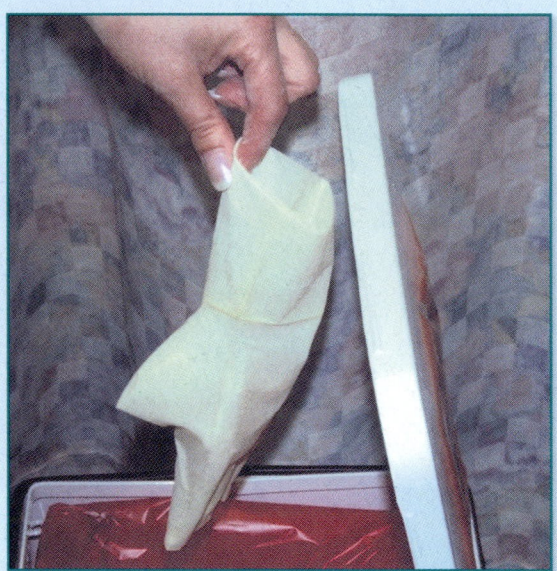

Figure 2-7-13 Dispose of gloves in appropriate receptacle.

▶ REAL WORLD ANECDOTES

Scenario 1

A nurse is preparing a sterile field for a central-line insertion. She has the field established and puts on the sterile gloves. It is only after applying the sterile gloves that the nurse remembers that she has not opened the outer, contaminated wrapper on the prepackaged central-line kit. In order to add the central-line kit to the sterile field, the nurse must break the sterility of her gloves, open the outer, contaminated wrapper and then apply new, sterile gloves. The nurse is reminded to be sure she has everything in order and ready to use before applying her sterile gloves.

Scenario 2

While working in a teaching hospital, a nurse has the opportunity to assist a new intern in the insertion of a central line. The nurse has gathered the necessary equipment and established a sterile field. While applying the sterile gloves, the intern slides her bare, contaminated hand under the cuff of the glove to apply it to her dominant hand. The nurse, noting that the intern has contaminated the glove, hands her a fresh set of gloves. As the intern is about to contaminate a second set of gloves, the nurse gently points out the correct method of putting on sterile gloves.

▶ EVALUATION

- Sterility of the gloves and sterile field was maintained without breaks.
- Sterility of the procedure was maintained.

▶ DOCUMENTATION

Nurses' Notes

- Document that the procedure was performed using sterile technique.

Document on appropriate flow sheet or electronic medical record (EMR).

▶ CRITICAL THINKING SKILL

Introduction

Environment is an important consideration in maintaining sterility.

Possible Scenario

You are getting ready to change a client's dressing. This is a sterile dressing change and you gather the equipment to establish a sterile field. The client's bedside table is the handiest place to set up the sterile field, and you clear the client's personal effects and water pitcher off the table. You lay out the supplies and start to establish a sterile field. As you are working, you do not notice that the sterile gloves are lying in a pool of water that has collected under the client's bedside pitcher.

Possible Outcome

The package of sterile gloves has become contaminated by getting wet. You infect this client's wound with transient flora off the bedside table.

Prevention

When establishing sterility, you must be aware of the environment and possible means of compromising the sterile field and gloves. Especially in hospital settings, everything is dirty unless it has been specifically cleaned and maintained otherwise.

▶ VARIATIONS

Geriatric Variations:
- *When gloving to care for a confused or restless client, make sure you open the gloves away from the client, so accidental contamination does not occur.*
- *Seek assistance restraining or holding a client in position prior to applying sterile gloves.*

Pediatric Variations:
- *Create a play set of sterile gloves using clean gloves in a small size, cuffed, and wrapped in paper. Use play therapy to let a younger child go through the motions of gloving along with you. Teach the basics of clean versus dirty, and reinforce how handwashing is the first and last step to fight germs.*
- *Seek assistance restraining or holding a client in position prior to applying sterile gloves.*

Home Care Variations:
- *Caregivers may shy away from the cost of sterile gloves and be tempted to perform procedures at home with clean gloves or find other ways to "cut corners." Be supportive as you listen to their concerns. Even with insurance, the costs associated with illness are often overwhelming to a caregiver on a limited budget. Make sure an adequate supply of gloves is available, and educate the caregiver on the need for proper technique to prevent infection.*
- *Uncluttered table-top space is often at a premium in the home care setting. If you need space to lay out supplies or open your glove package, bring along a TV tray or stand. You can quickly set it up and take it down in the client care area.*

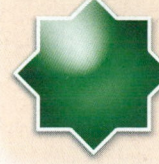

Long-Term Care Variations:
- *Make sure care providers not familiar with putting on sterile gloves have an opportunity to review the technique prior to caring for the client.*

▶ **COMMON ERRORS**

Possible Error:

While putting on sterile gloves the nurse puts her fingers in the wrong fingerholes. In an attempt to straighten this out, the nurse reaches up with her ungloved hand to adjust the position of the glove's fingers.

Prevention:

Be careful to slide your hand into the sterile gloves in a way that the fingers will not become tangled and confused. If they do, do not try to adjust them. Put the second glove on touching only the sterile portion of the glove with the sterile portion of your gloved hand. Only after both hands have sterile gloves on can you adjust the fingers and the fit of the gloves. If you cannot adjust the fingers, get another pair of gloves and start over.

▶ **NURSING TIPS**

- Only touch dirty to dirty, clean to clean, and sterile to sterile.
- Be aware of the immediate environment when applying sterile gloves to avoid accidental contamination.
- Be sure to have everything that you need ready before putting on sterile gloves.

▶ **SPECIAL CONSIDERATIONS**

- *Latex allergy is an increasing concern for health care providers. When performing tasks that require nonsterile gloves, wearing vinyl or latex-free gloves is recommended. It is important to use powder-free gloves because the latex protein may adhere to the powder and become an airborne contaminant. Latex-free sterile gloves are also available.*

Surgical Scrub

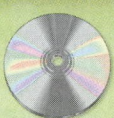

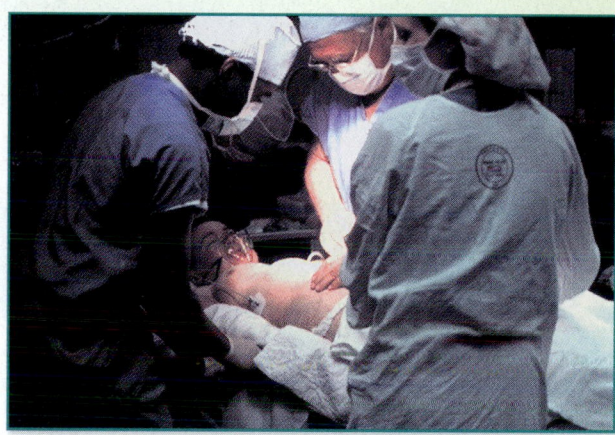

▶ OVERVIEW OF THE SKILL

Surgical hand washing or scrub is used to remove debris from nails, hands, and forearms; reduce the numbers of transient and colonizing microorganisms on the skin; and inhibit rapid rebound growth of microorganisms. Nurses working in the operating room perform surgical handwashing to decrease the client's risk for an infection should a sterile glove tear or break. The skin on the nurse's hands and arms should be intact (free of lesions), and the nails should be kept short, clean, and healthy. Agency policy determines how to perform the scrub with regard to method and timing. The Association for Operating Room Nurses (AORN) recommends that all personnel be in surgical attire before beginning the surgical hand scrub; that an effective antimicrobial surgical hand scrub be used; and that the scrub procedure be standardized for all personnel according to institutional policy and procedure (AORN Standards, Recommended Practices and Guidelines, 2003). This procedure describes the basic principles in performing surgical handwashing.

▶ ASSESSMENT

1. Assess the scrub environment for equipment and cleanliness **to reduce the risk of infection.**
2. Assess your preparedness. **Are you prepared with the sterile towels and gown?** Have you already changed into scrub clothes and applied shoe covers? **Preparedness helps prevent**

infection by reducing the risk of recontamination following the surgical scrub.

▶ DIAGNOSIS

Risk for Infection

▶ PLANNING

Expected Outcomes:

1. Hands and forearms will be adequately cleansed for applying sterile gloves and gown.
2. The hands and forearms will not be recontaminated following the scrub by touching contaminated surfaces.

Equipment Needed (see Figure 2-8-1):

- Surgical scrub items (antimicrobial soap, two brushes, and nail file)

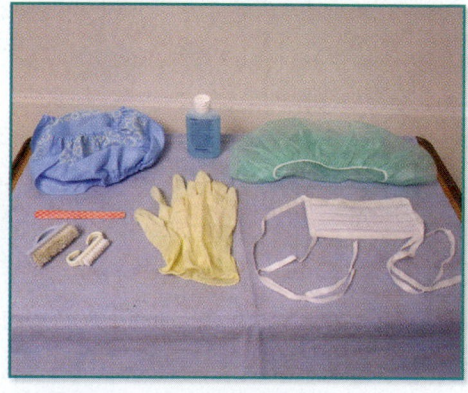

Figure 2-8-1 Surgical scrub items

- Surgical shoe covers (booties) and cap, face mask, sterile gown, and proper-size gloves
- Sterile towel

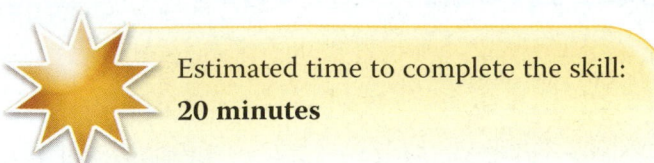

Estimated time to complete the skill:
20 minutes

▶ **CLIENT EDUCATION NEEDED:**

Client education occurs during preoperative care.

▶ **DELEGATION TIPS**

Surgical scrubbing is only delegated if the personnel are specifically trained, such as in a surgical suite or a testing laboratory.

IMPLEMENTATION—Action/Rationale

Action	Rationale
Preparing for Surgical Handwashing	
1. A nurse's rings, watches, and bracelets should be removed before beginning the surgical scrub. AORN recommends washing and rinsing moistened hands and forearms with an approved surgical scrub agent before beginning the surgical scrub procedure.	1. Decreases resident and transient microorganisms.
2. Use a deep sink with side or foot pedal to dispense anti-microbial soap and control water temperature and flow.	2. Prevents hands and forearms from touching a soiled surface.
3. Have two surgical scrub brushes and nail file.	3. Enhances mechanical friction during the scrub.
4. Apply surgical shoe covers and cap to cover hair and ears completely.	4. Prevents introduction of contaminants into environment.
5. Apply mask (see Figure 2-8-2).	5. Provides a respiratory barrier.

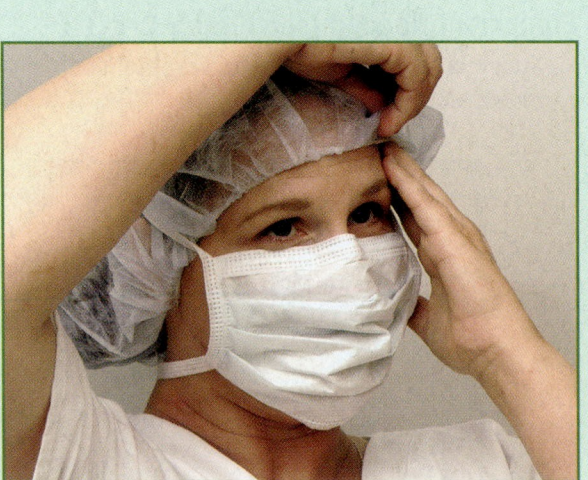

Figure 2-8-2   Apply cap and mask.

continues

Action	Rationale

6. Before beginning the surgical scrub:
  a. Open the sterile package containing the gown; using aseptic technique, make a sterile field with the inside of the gown's wrapper.
  b. Open the sterile towel and dropt it onto the center of field.
  c. Open the outer wrapper from the sterile gloves and drop the inner package of gloves onto the sterile field beside the folded gown and towel.
	6. Preparing the sterile items prior to the scrub decreases the risk of contaminating scrubbed hands.

7. At a deep sink with foot or knee controls (see Figure 2-8-3), turn on warm water; under flowing water, wet hands, beginning at tips of fingers, to forearms—keeping hands at level above elbows. Prewash hands and forearms to 2 inches above the elbows.	7. Water should flow from the hands to the elbow to promote taking contaminants away from the hands.
8. Apply a liberal amount of soap onto hands and rub hands and arms to 2 inches above elbows (see Figures 2-8-4 and 2-8-5).	8. Reduces number of microorganisms on hands.
9. Use nail file under running water, clean under each nail of both hands, and drop file into sink when finished (see Figure 2-8-6).	9. Removes dirt that harbors microorganisms.

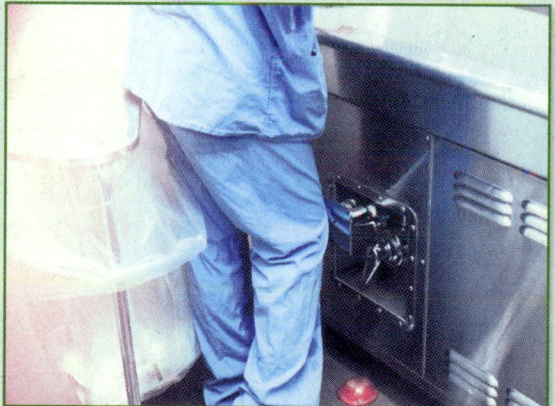

Figure 2-8-3 Handwashing sink with knee controls.

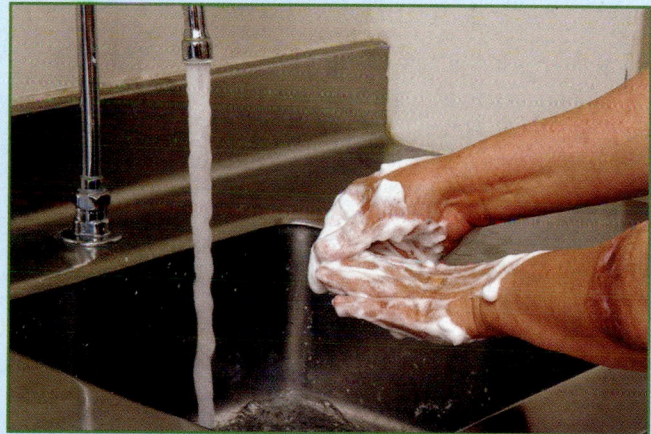

Figure 2-8-4 Apply a liberal amount of soap.

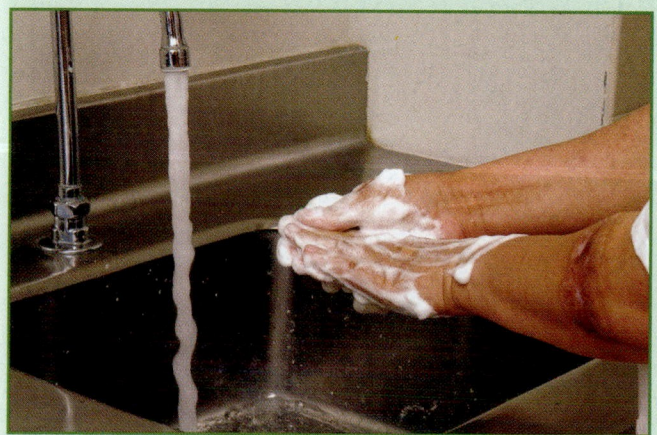

Figure 2-8-5 Scrub hands and arms.

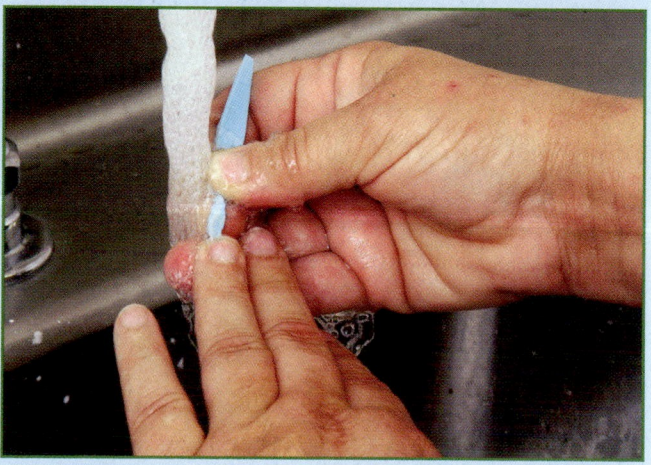

Figure 2-8-6 Use a nail file under running water to clean fingernails.

continues

Action	Rationale

Preparing for Surgical Handwashing *continued*

10. Wet and apply soap to scrub brush, if needed. Open prepackaged scrub brush if available. With brush in your dominant hand and using a circular motion, scrub nails and all skin areas of nondominant hand and arm (10 strokes to each of the following area; see Figure 2-8-7):
   a. Nails
   b. Palm of hand and anterior side of fingers

10. Removes resident bacteria from the skin's surfaces; the circular motion mechanically removes microorganisms. Scrubbing the nondominant hand first sets a routine you can remember if you should get interrupted during the scrub.

11. Rinse brush thoroughly; reapply soap.

11. Decreases transfer of microorganisms.

12. Continue with scrub on nondominant arm with a circular motion for 10 strokes each to the lower, middle, and upper arm; drop brush into the sink.

12. Decreases transfer of microorganisms from the arm; dropping the brush avoids contamination.

13. Maintaining the hands and arms above elbow level, place the fingertips under running water and thoroughly rinse the fingers, hands, and arms (allow the water to run off your elbow into the sink); take care not to get your uniform wet (see Figure 2-8-8).

13. Allows flow of water to cleanse from the area of least contamination to the area of most contamination. Water conducts microorganisms, and keeping the uniform dry aids in maintaining sterility of the gown.

14. Take the second scrub brush and repeat Actions 10–13 on your dominant hand and arm.

14. See Rationales 10–13.

15. Keep arms flexed and proceed to area (operating or procedure room) with sterile items (see Figure 2-8-9).

15. Prevents water from flowing from least (elbows) to most (hands) clean area.

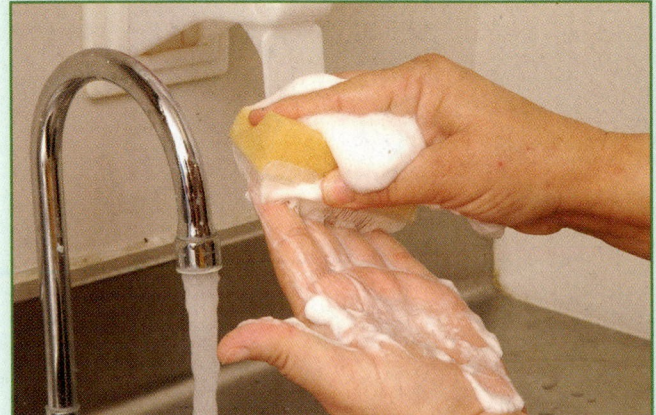

Figure 2-8-7 With brush, scrub nails, hands, and arm.

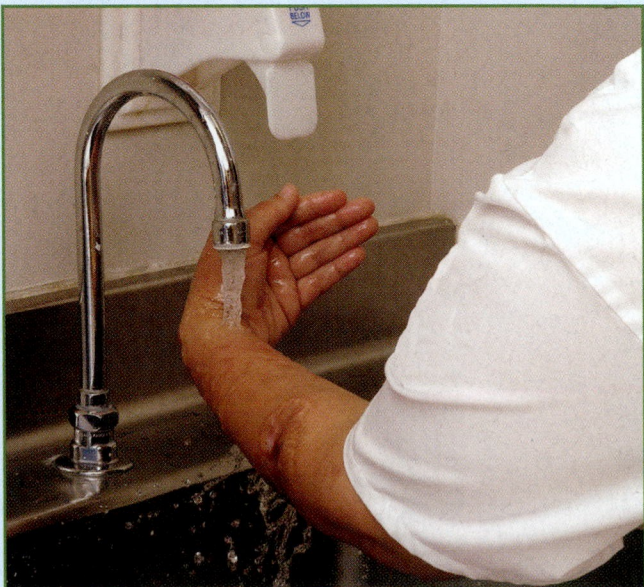

Figure 2-8-8 Thoroughly rinse fingers, hands, and arms.

continues

Action	Rationale

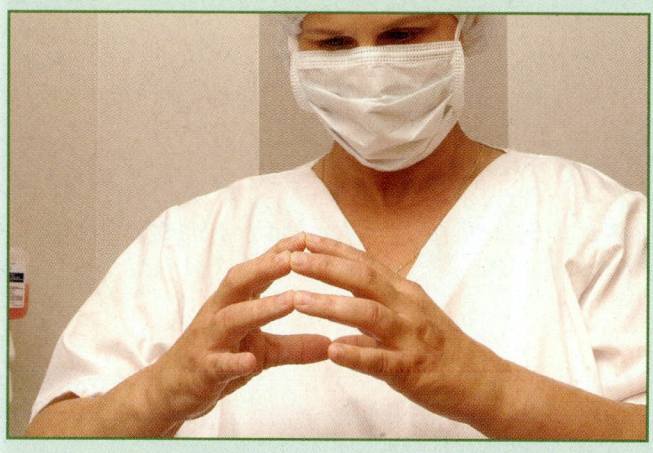

Figure 2-8-9   Keep arms flexed and proceed to area.

16. Secure sterile towel by grasping it on one edge, opening the towel, full length, making sure it does not touch your uniform.

17. Dry each hand and arm separately; extend one side of the towel around fingers and hand and dry in a circular motion up to the elbow (see Figures 2-8-10 and 2-8-11).

18. Reverse the towel and repeat the same action on the other hand and arm, thoroughly drying the skin.

19. Discard the towel into a linen hamper.

16. Maintains the sterility of the towel.

17. Prevents contamination by drying from cleanest to least clean area.

18. Prevents contamination of the gown.

19. Keeps the environment clean.

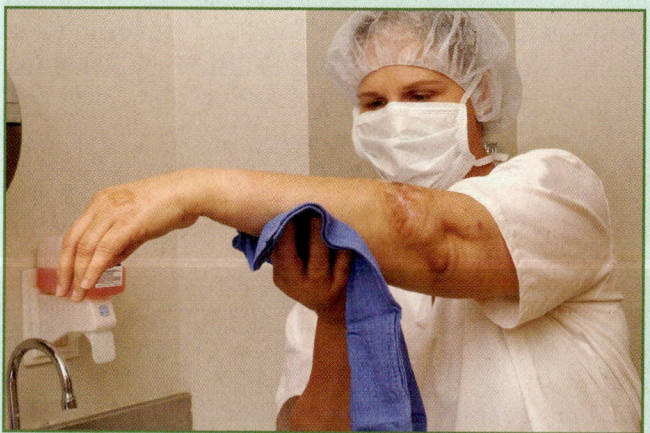

Figure 2-8-10   Dry arms using a circular motion.

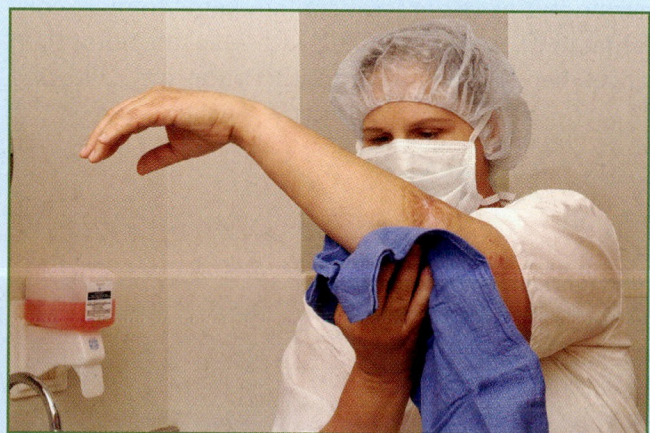

Figure 2-8-11   Dry arms up to the elbows.

▶ **REAL WORLD ANECDOTES**

Scenario 1
The nurse was well into her surgical scrub when she realized she forgot to take off her rings. She stopped, removed and stored her rings, and started over. This nurse usually followed a mental checklist, but she had been distracted that day and had not followed her normal routine.

Scenario 2
Charles found that singing the lyrics to a popular song either out loud or in his head kept him from rushing his scrub session. Scrubbing to the beat of the music helped him stay focused on the repetitive task.

▶ **EVALUATION**

• The nurse's hands and forearms were adequately cleansed for applying sterile gown and gloves.
• The hands or forearms were not recontaminated following the scrub by touching contaminated surfaces.

▶ **DOCUMENTATION**

• No documentation of surgical scrub is required.

▶ **CRITICAL THINKING SKILL**

Introduction
Least contaminated to most contaminated.

Possible Scenario
During a surgical scrub, the nurse wets her hands and arms, allowing the water to flow from her elbows to her fingertips (from least contaminated to most contaminated). After scrubbing with soap, the nurse then rinses her hands and arms the same way, allowing the rinse water to flow from her elbows to her fingertips.

Possible Outcome
The nurse's hands, the portion of her body that most comes in contact with the client and the instruments, remain the most contaminated portion of her lower arms. This could potentially compromise surgical sterility and the client's health.

Prevention
The nurse should understand the reasoning involved in the surgical scrub procedure. During the scrub, the nurse holds her arms flexed upward to allow contaminated water and soap to flow off her elbows, thus making her elbows the most contaminated portion of her lower arms. The rinse water is also allowed to flow from fingertips to elbows to maintain the hands as the least contaminated portion of the lower arm. It is preferable to keep the hands least contaminated as this is the portion of the body that comes in most contact with the client and the surgical implements.

▶ **COMMON ERRORS**

Possible Error:
Not scrubbing long enough.

Prevention:
Friction is the most important component of handwashing for the removal of soil and transient flora. Be sure to take the time to use plenty of friction and wash at least 10 strokes per area washed.

► **NURSING TIPS**

- Be sure to keep your hands and forearms above elbow level.

- Avoid products with iodine if allergy is present.
- Make sure you are not splashed by another person washing his or her hands.

► **SPECIAL CONSIDERATIONS**

- Topical foam products are sometimes used in areas where frequent handwashing is required or soap and water are not available (newborn nurseries, intensive care units). If you find yourself using a foam/without-water product, make sure that you are familiar with the manufacturer's instructions for use. Most applications require a specified amount of product and time for contact duration.

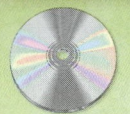

Applying Sterile Gloves and Gown via the Closed Method

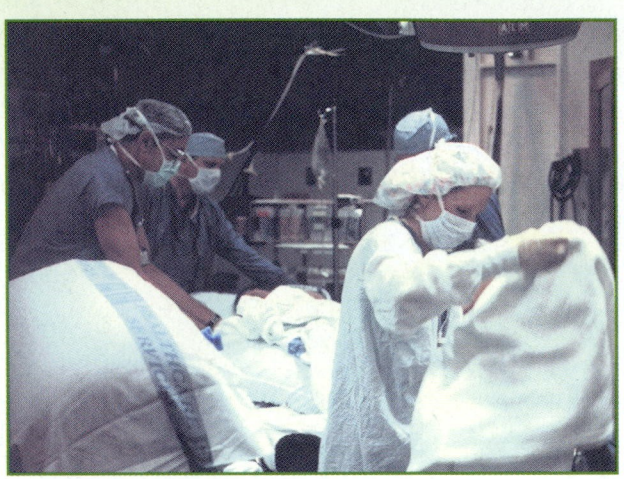

▶ OVERVIEW OF THE SKILL

Nurses in the operating room and special procedure areas such as cardiac catheter labs use the gown and closed glove method to don these protective items. "Closed glove" refers to a technique where, after the surgical scrub, the gown is put on first; then the gloves are put on by *grasping the gloves with the hands still in the sleeves of the gown*. The sterile gown and gloves serve as a barrier to decrease the risk of wound contamination. They also allow the nurse to move more freely in the environment with sterile drapes and objects.

▶ ASSESSMENT

1. Before applying gown and gloves, assess the surrounding environment. Where is the sterile field? Are both the gown and gloves dry and intact? **Maintains the sterility of the gown and gloves.**
2. Assess the condition of your hands. Have they remained uncontaminated since you scrubbed? **Prevents any breaks in sterile technique that could compromise the procedure.**

▶ DIAGNOSIS

Risk for Infection

▶ PLANNING

Expected Outcomes:

1. The caregiver will don a sterile gown and gloves without compromising their sterility.

▶ Equipment Needed (see Figure 2-9-1):

- Sterile gown
- Sterile and proper-sized gloves

▶ CLIENT EDUCATION NEEDED:

Client education occurs during preoperative care.

Estimated time to complete the skill:
15 minutes

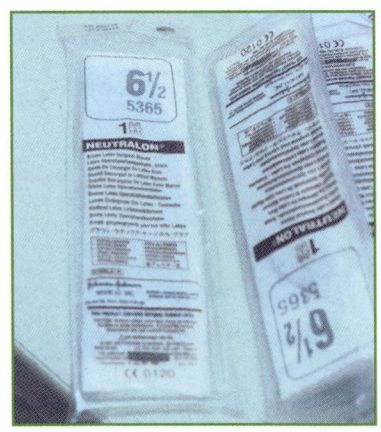

Figure 2-9-1   Sterile gloves

▶ **DELEGATION TIPS**

Sterile gloving and gowning is delegated only if the personnel are specifically trained, such as in a surgical suite or a testing laboratory setting.

IMPLEMENTATION—Action/Rationale

Action	Rationale
Gowning	
1. Note that the sterile gown is folded inside out.	1. Allows ungloved hands to touch only the inside.
2. Grasp the gown inside the neckline, step back, and allow the gown to open in front of you; keep the inside of the gown toward you; do not allow it to touch anything (see Figure 2-9-2).	2. Keeps the outside of the gown sterile.
3. With hands at shoulder level, slip both arms into the gown; keep your hands inside the sleeves of the gown (see Figure 2-9-3).	3. Prevents the gown from touching nonsterile objects; allows sterile items to come in contact only with other sterile items.
4. The circulating nurse will step up behind you and grasp the inside of the gown, bring it over your shoulders, and secure the ties at the neck and waist.	4. Prevents any part of the gown from touching a nonsterile object; provides complete coverage of undergarments.

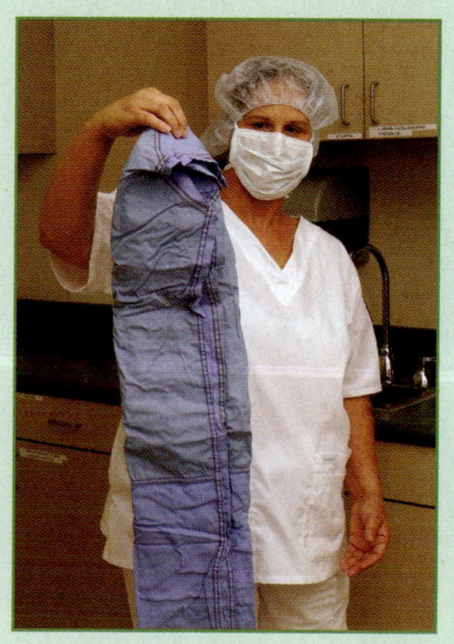

Figure 2-9-2 Allow the gown to fall open.

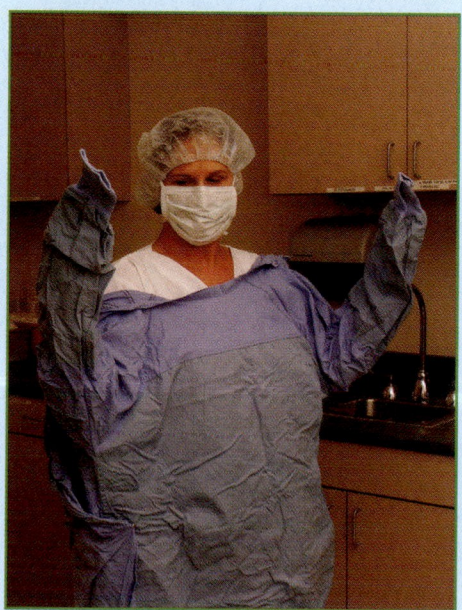

Figure 2-9-3 Slip both arms into the gown.

continues

Action	Rationale
Closed Gloving	
5. With hands still inside the gown sleeves, open the inner wrapper of the gloves on the sterile gown field (see Figure 2-9-4).	**5.** Maintains sterility of the gloves.
6. With your nondominant sleeved hand, grasp the cuff of the glove for the dominant hand and lay it on the extended dominant forearm (see Figure 2-9-5); with palm up; place the palm of the glove against the sleeved palm, with fingers of the glove pointing toward the elbow (see Figure 2-9-6).	**6.** Only sterile items come in contact with each other.
7. Manipulate the glove so that the sleeved thumb of your dominant hand is grasping the cuff; with your nondominant hand, turn the cuff over the end of dominant hand and gown's cuff.	**7.** Prevents the hands from contaminating the sterile glove.
8 With sleeved nondominant hand, grasp the cuff of the glove and the gown's sleeve of the dominant hand; slowly extend the fingers into the glove, making sure the cuff of the glove remains above the cuff of the gown's sleeve (see Figure 2-9-7).	**8.** Provides a closed sterile method for gloving; the glove cuff over the gown prevents contamination of the operative field with microorganisms.
9. With the gloved dominant hand, repeat Actions 7 and 8 (see Figures 2-9-8 and 2-9-9).	**9.** Only sterile items can touch each other.
10. Interlock gloved fingers; secure fit.	**10.** Promotes dexterity of gloved hands.

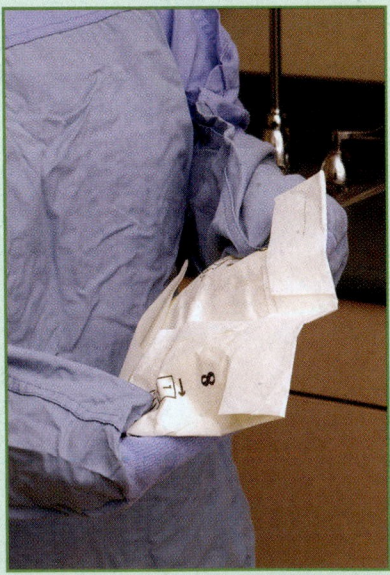

Figure 2-9-4 Keep hands inside the gown sleeves when opening gloves. Handle the gloves through the fabric of the gown.

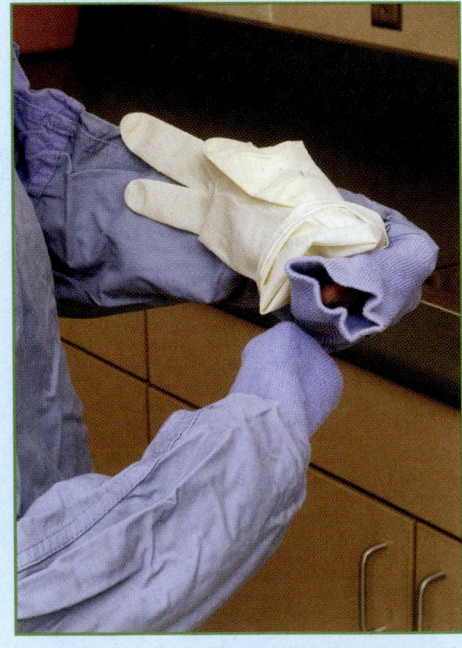

Figure 2-9-5 Grasp the cuff of the glove.

continues

Action	Rationale

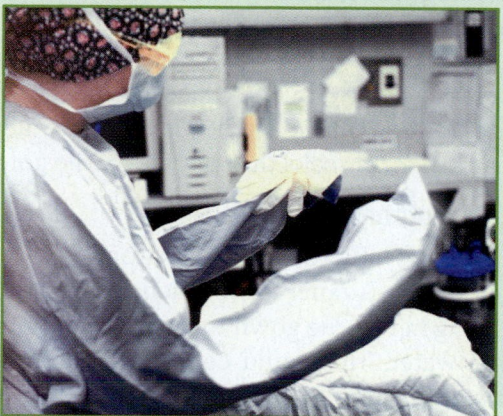

Figure 2-9-6 Keep the fingers of the glove facing the elbow.

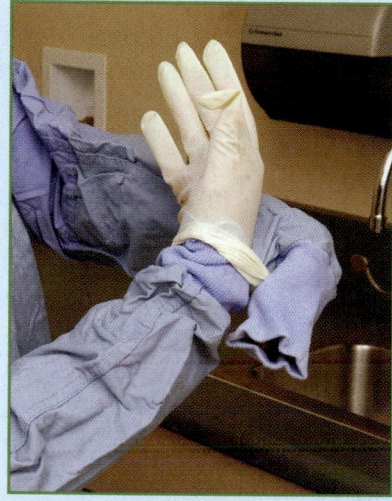

Figure 2-9-7 Extend fingers into the glove.

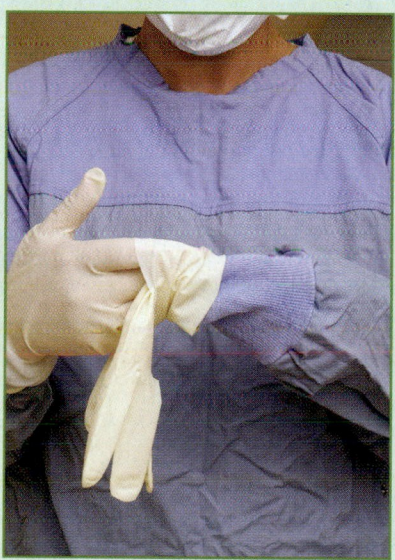

Figure 2-9-8 Place the second glove on the gown.

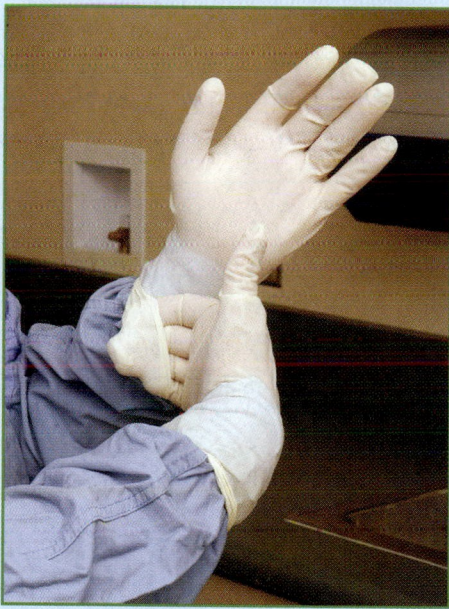

Figure 2-9-9 Extend the fingers into the second glove.

▶ REAL WORLD ANECDOTES

Scenario 1

It is lunchtime for the operating room nurses. They carefully cover their scrub uniforms with gowns to prevent contaminating them and walk down to the cafeteria. They sit and eat lunch, in their gowns, surgical caps, and shoe covers, their masks dangling around their necks. After lunch, they return to the changing area to go back to work. They remove the gowns, adjust their masks, and go to the scrub area to wash their hands. Nobody thinks to replace their now-contaminated shoe covers, masks, and caps before they scrub for the next surgical case.

Scenario 2

The nurse has finished her surgical scrub. She is about to don the gown when she realizes she left her watch on the counter. She picks it up with her fingernails and drops it in her pocket. She proceeds to gown and glove. Touching a contaminated object after scrubbing and before gloving allows microorganisms to contaminate her fingernails. The fingernail is a likely spot for a glove tear and could contaminate the surgical site.

▶ EVALUATION

- Sterility of the gown and gloves was maintained while the caregiver applied them.
- Sterility of the environment was maintained while the caregiver applied the gown and gloves.

▶ DOCUMENTATION

- Document in nurses' notes or an incident report only if an incident occurred that could affect the care of the client or increase the risk of transmission of microorganisms.

Document on appropriate flow sheet or electronic medical record (EMR).

▶ CRITICAL THINKING SKILL

Introduction

Neatness counts.

Possible Scenario

Nurse Adams reports for work in the operating room as usual. She changes out of her street clothes and into scrubs. She places protective covers on her shoes and dons a surgical mask and cap. She then proceeds to the scrub area and scrubs her hands and forearms, using liberal amounts of water. Happily talking with other workers in the scrub area, she does not notice water splashing onto the front of her scrubs. She continues to the operating theater to don a sterile gown and gloves. As she is putting on the sterile gloves, the water from her scrub uniform soaks through her sterile gown.

Possible Outcome

Water carries microorganisms from one site to another. Nurse Adams has broken sterile technique by allowing her sterile gown to become contaminated with the water. This could compromise the sterility of the entire operation and present a danger to the client. She returns to the changing area, changes into a new scrub uniform, returns to the scrub area, and rescrubs her hands. She then returns to the operating theater to regown and reglove. The surgery is delayed 15 minutes.

Prevention

Be aware of possible contaminants and avoid anything that might compromise sterile technique.

▶ COMMON ERRORS

Possible Error:

Reaching behind yourself to adjust the sterile gown on your shoulders and free the ties.

Prevention:

Wait for the circulating nurse to adjust the gown and tie it. Do not be in a hurry to be too helpful.

▶ NURSING TIPS

- Only touch sterile to sterile.

- Be careful not to get your scrub uniform wet. This will contaminate the sterile gown.
- Do not lean against the scrub sink.

▶ SPECIAL CONSIDERATIONS

- *Topical foam products are sometimes used in areas where frequent handwashing is required or soap and water are not available (newborn nurseries, intensive care units). If you find yourself using a foam/without-water product, make sure that you are familiar with the manufacturer's instructions for use. Most applications require a specified amount of product and designated time for contact.*

Emergency Airway Management

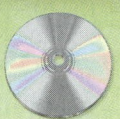

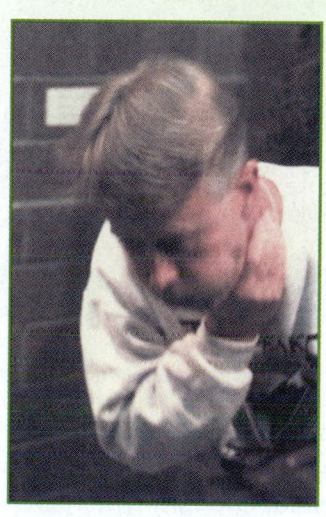

▶ OVERVIEW OF THE SKILL

An open airway is essential for oxygenation of the body. In an emergency situation, providing a patent airway is the top priority. If the client cannot get oxygen, the function of any other body system is superfluous. Maintaining an open airway for the client is a critical nursing function.

There are several causes of airway obstruction. The tongue may fall back into the pharyngeal cavity and obstruct the airway in an unconscious client. This is sometimes seen after grand mal seizures. Thickened secretions may obstruct or narrow the airway. This can be seen in clients with chronic obstructive pulmonary disease. Their ability to clear their airway is decreased, and the secretions thicken and pool, blocking airflow. Soft-tissue edema may narrow or obstruct the airway. This is more often observed in children, whose airways are much smaller and more easily obstructed by a small amount of swelling. Aspiration of a foreign object can narrow or obstruct the airway. This is often caused by food or fluids entering the airway while eating.

If the airway is not patent, with air not being moved in and out of the lungs, the client is at risk for injury or death. This can be the result of a partially or fully obstructed airway. Rescue breathing with an Ambu®-bag and the insertion of an oral airway may be necessary until intubation can be accomplished.

When performing an initial assessment on a client, use the acronym ABC. This stands for Airway, Breathing, Circulation.

Airway emergency management is the prime initial step as the airway must be patent for air to enter the lungs. Without this initial step, administering breaths will either be ineffective or push the foreign object farther into the respiratory system.

▶ ASSESSMENT

1. Assess the client for any visible respirations **to determine whether the airway is open.**
2. Assess the client's mental status. Determine whether the client can respond to verbal or tactile stimulus. This action will help **determine whether the client is conscious and receiving adequate oxygen to the brain.**
3. Assess for stridor, ability to speak or cough effectively, or clutching of the throat **to determine whether the client's respirations are partially obstructed.**
4. Assess for the presence of obstruction, such as thick secretions, food, or other foreign bodies **to avoid advancing the obstruction deeper into the respiratory system.**

▶ DIAGNOSIS

Ineffective Airway Clearance

Ineffective Breathing Pattern

Impaired Spontaneous Ventilation

Ineffective Tissue Perfusion

Risk for Aspiration

Risk for Suffocation

▶ PLANNING

Expected Outcomes:

1. The client will breathe effectively through an open airway.
2. The client will maintain adequate color and oxygen saturation within normal limits as assessed by pulse oximeter (refer to Skill 7-5).

Equipment Needed (see Figure 2-10-1):

The following may be needed:

- Supplemental oxygen
- Gloves
- Oropharyngeal airway
- Yankauer suction
- Pocket mask
- Ambu®-bag and mask

▶ CLIENT EDUCATION NEEDED:

1. Caregivers of clients at risk for airway obstruction should be instructed regarding the steps to take in case of obstruction. They should have the necessary equipment available and know how to use it.
2. Explain to the client what is happening and the steps you are taking to establish a patent airway.
3. Explain to the family what is happening. Update the explanations as the airway is

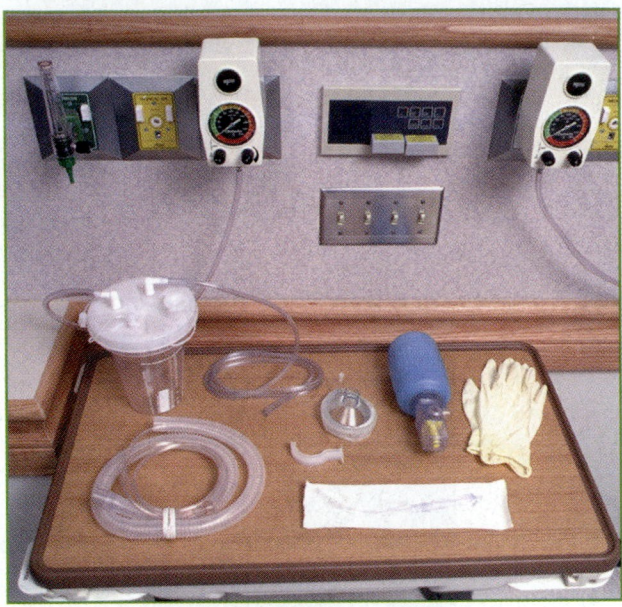

Figure 2-10-1   Equipment used to establish an emergency airway includes pocket masks, oropharyngeal airways, suction equipment and extra tubing, and oxygen-delivery equipment.

reestablished and supportive measures are implemented. Often, in emergency situations, the family and client are never informed of exactly what occurred.

Estimated time to complete the skill: **Time is of the essence and, thus, the skill should be completed within minutes, depending upon the situation.**

▶ DELEGATION TIPS

The skill of reestablishing an open airway in adults and children using techniques such as the head-tilt/chin-lift method, suctioning, and oral airway insertion are skills that may not be delegated to ancillary personnel.

IMPLEMENTATION—Action/Rationale

Action	Rationale
1. Wash hands and apply gloves if available.	1. Reduces the transmission of microorganisms.
2. Assess airway. Call for assistance.	2. If airway is not open, the client is at risk for injury or death.

continues

Action	Rationale

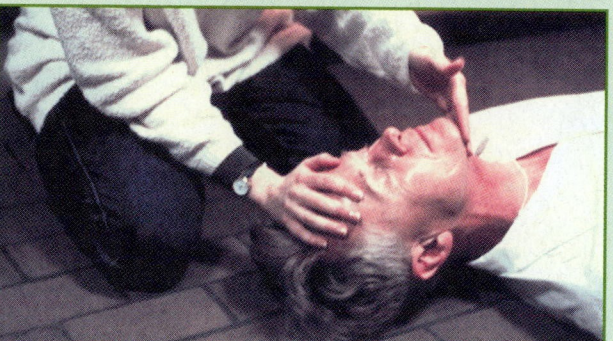

Figure 2-10-2 Tilt the jaw forward and the forehead back.

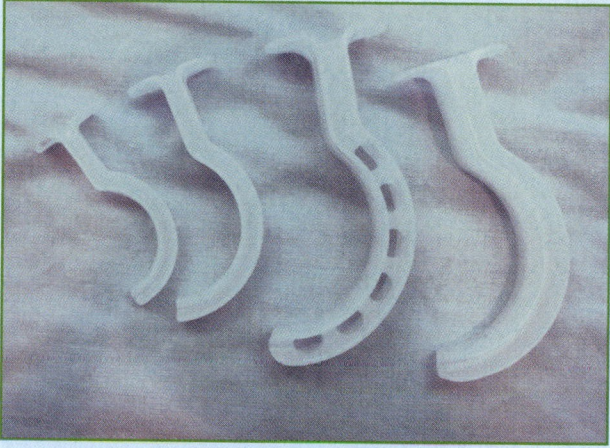

Figure 2-10-3 Oropharyngeal airways come in different sizes.

3. Open the airway. Head tilt/chin lift: place one hand on the forehead and two fingers of the other hand under the bony part of the lower jaw. Tilt head back and the jaw forward. (see Figure 2-10-2).

4. Assess for spontaneous respirations.

5. If spontaneous respirations occur, maintain head in proper position.
   - Insert oropharyngeal airway if available (see Figure 2-10-3) (refer to Skill 7-15).

6. If respirations do not resume, initiate artificial respiration. Give one breath every 5-6 seconds; each breath given over 1 second (see Figures 2-10-4 and 2-10-5).
   - If unable to ventilate, open mouth. If you see an object, remove it using the finger-sweep method (see Figure 2-10-6).

3. If the tongue is blocking the airway, the head tilt will reposition the tongue, allowing air to pass freely into the lungs.

4. If spontaneous respirations are present, no other interventions may be required. If client is still not breathing, continue with interventions.

5. Head must still be positioned correctly once respirations resume to maintain a patent airway.
   - Keeps the tongue from slipping into the pharyngeal area and blocking the airway.

6. Hypoxia can cause irreversible brain and tissue damage after 4 to 6 minutes.
   - Removing the object may cause spontaneous respiration to occur.

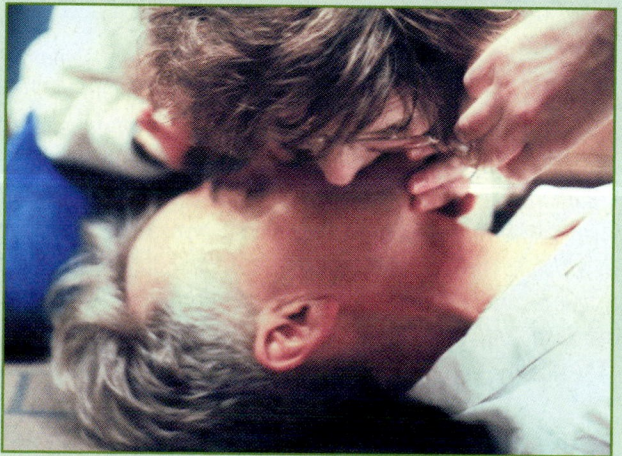

Figure 2-10-4 Initiate artificial respiration.

continues

Action	Rationale

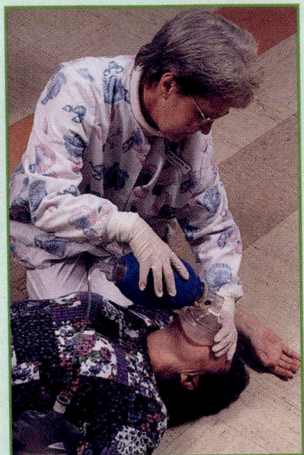

Figure 2-10-5   To initiate artificial respiration, seal the client's mouth and nose before attempting to ventilate.

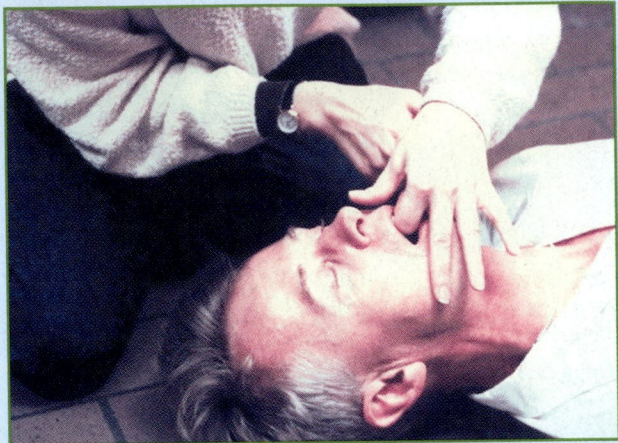

Figure 2-10-6   Clear the mouth of obstructions.

7. Check for pulse every 2 minutes. If no pulse, initiate CPR (see Skill 2-11).

8. Continue efforts until assistance arrives.

9. When client is stable or other assistance has arrived, remove gloves if you are wearing them and wash hands.

10. If in an institutional setting, document the incident on the appropriate forms. If the incident occurred in a noninstitutional setting, provide information to the aid personnel.

7. Often respiratory arrest progresses to cardiac arrest.

8. Assures that every effort has been made.

9. Reduces the risk of transferring microorganisms.

10. Provides for continuity of care.

▶ REAL WORLD ANECDOTES

Susan was doing her initial rounds on her clients; upon entering John's room, she saw immediately that something was wrong. The 55-year-old man was lying in his bed, and his skin was a dusky color. He did not respond to Susan calling his name. Susan immediately called for assistance, at the same time assessing his airway. It appeared to be open, but there was no air movement. She performed the head-tilt/chin-lift on John and, again, assessed for breathing, but there was no air movement. Assessing for circulation, she felt no carotid pulse. A code was called. The code team was able to resuscitate John, and it was found that he had experienced a myocardial infarction. John's airway had not been blocked. However, assessing the patency of John's airway was the appropriate first step in assessing his condition. Note: In the immediacy of the moment, Susan did not follow correct cardiopulmonary resuscitation (CPR) protocol, which is to provide two rescue breaths before assessing for a pulse. Susan did, however, review and study the CPR skill so she would be better prepared for future episodes. (Reference: 2005 American Heart Association Guidelines for Cardiopulmonary Resuscitation.)

▶ EVALUATION

- The client is breathing effectively through an open airway.
- The client is maintaining adequate color and oxygen saturation within normal limits as assessed by pulse oximeter (refer to Skill 7-5).

▶ DOCUMENTATION

Nurses' Notes/Code Record

- Note the time and condition in which the client was found.
- Record interventions that were implemented, including accurate times, results of the implementations, orders received from the physicians, vital signs of the client, timing of the incident, and status of the client afterward.

Document on appropriate flow sheet or electronic medical record (EMR).

Medication Administration Record

- Record any medications the client received, including time and route, during the procedure.

▶ CRITICAL THINKING SKILL

Introduction

Keeping a client's airway patent may require problem solving by the nurse.

Possible Scenario

Mrs. Koski was intubated and being mechanically ventilated. You hear the ventilator alarms and check on her condition. The alarms indicate that there is increased airway pressure occurring. You note that Mrs. Koski is agitated and biting on the endotracheal tube. Her physician has indicated that he does not want to sedate Mrs. Koski so he can monitor her neurologic status.

Possible Outcome

You attempt to calm Mrs. Koski by talking to her soothingly and reassuring her that she is fine. You turn down the lights and reduce the extraneous stimulation. The high-pressure alarm continues to sound frequently and you return to the room often to assure Mrs. Koski that everything is fine. Toward the end of your shift, the alarm sounds yet again. You return to Mrs. Koski's room to find her extremely agitated. The ventilator tubing is on the floor and the upper half of the endotracheal tube is still attached to the tubing. You immediately determine that Mrs. Koski has bitten through her endotracheal tube and that the other half of the tube is probably still in her trachea, choking her. You call for emergency assistance and attempt to open Mrs. Koski's airway.

Prevention

You attempt to calm Mrs. Koski by talking to her soothingly and reassuring her that she is fine. You turn down the lights and reduce the extraneous stimulation. Despite these measures, Mrs. Koski continues to agitatedly bite the endotracheal tube. You obtain a bite block or oropharyngeal airway and tape it in place to protect the tube from the pressure of Mrs. Koski's teeth, being careful to secure it. If it is not properly secured, the bite block could slip into Mrs. Koski's throat, causing trauma and possible airway obstruction. You also notify Mrs. Koski's physician of her agitated state.

▶ VARIATIONS

Geriatric Variations:
- When assessing an elderly client's airway, bear in mind that the client may have dentures and a dental plate may be the source of airway obstruction.
- Care must also be taken with the elderly population as they have a high possibility of osteoporosis and spinal injuries. If clients are suspected of having neck injuries, the airway should be opened without tilting the head, using the jaw thrust method.

continues

▶ VARIATIONS *(continued)*

Pediatric Variations:

- *Respiratory arrest is a major cause of death in children; thus careful, continuous assessment of the pediatric client's respiratory status should be performed.*
- *The normal respiratory rate changes with age. Be aware of what is normal for the age of the client you are assessing. In newborns, the average rate is 40 breaths/min in the 1-year-old child, it is 24 breaths/min; and in the 18-year-old it is 18 breaths/min.*
- *The child's upper airway is smaller and more flexible than an adult's and more easily blocked by over-tilting the head. An infant's head should only be tilted slightly to open the airway.*
- *Noninvasive methods of opening the airway should be attempted prior to using invasive methods.*
- *If there is a large pediatric population to be served, be sure to have properly sized equipment. If you will be caring for infants and children, it is imperative to have oropharyngeal airways and endotracheal tubes of the proper size. Using adult-sized equipment on children can injure a child, potentially causing severe, permanent damage.*

Home Care Variations:

- *If a home care client is at risk for respiratory distress or failure at home, the client and his or her caregivers should be well educated on the risk factors for their particular situation and how to effectively deal with this potential problem.*
- *If the client will be traveling in a car, respiratory support equipment should be available in the car.*

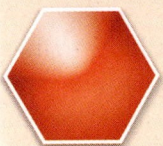

Long-Term Care Variations:

- *All caregivers in long-term care facilities should know how to assess and respond to the ABCs.*
- *Emergency equipment should be available at long-term care facilities and within easy access to personnel.*

▶ COMMON ERRORS

Possible Error:

Assessing circulation before assessing the client's airway. In the excitement of finding a client in respiratory distress or collapse, it is common for health care team members to check for a pulse prior to assessing the airway.

Prevention:

Think of the ABCs—Airway, Breathing, Circulation.

Possible Error:

With a trauma victim use the jaw-thrust method of opening the airway, as the client may have a neck injury. If the victim has a neck injury, tilting the head may cause more injury, such as possibly permanent spinal cord injury.

Prevention:

The jaw-thrust is preferable to the head-tilt method. This is especially true when clients are suspected of having a neck injury.

► NURSING TIPS

- Always know the location of airway equipment on your unit.
- Do not forget the ABCs—Airway, Breathing, and Circulation—and initiate complete CPR as necessary.
- Practice until you are comfortable with initiating oxygen at the bedside. The equipment can be awkward to manipulate.
- Have mock codes on your unit to practice what should happen if a nurse finds a client in respiratory and/or cardiac arrest.
- Use latex-free and powder-free gloves.

► SPECIAL CONSIDERATIONS

- *Avoid head-tilt in victims of trauma, especially if there is the possibility of neck injury. Cervical spine injury is often occult; therefore, a cervical spine injury should be considered in all cases of blunt trauma, major falls, and motor vehicle accidents.*
- *Conditions that may be associated with difficult airway management are facial trauma, oral infections, congenital abnormalities, burns to the face or neck, radiation to the face or neck, neck or oral cavity tumors, obesity, or arthritis.*
- *Anesthetic/anti-inflammatory oral sprays may be part of standing orders in postoperative recovery rooms and helpful in clients with increased oral swelling. A swollen uvula may partially block the airway.*
- *Assessment for aspiration pneumonia should be considered after obstruction of the airway.*
- *A nasopharyngeal airway may be necessary in clients with oral swelling.*
- *Use latex-free gloves and equipment to avoid latex allergy reaction.*

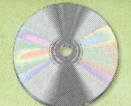

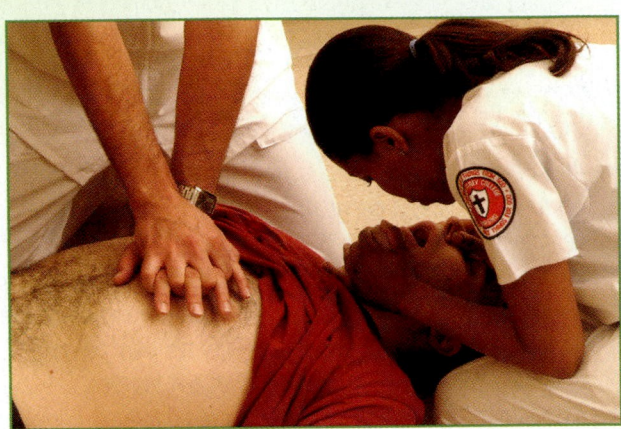

Administering Cardiopulmonary Resuscitation (CPR)

▶ OVERVIEW OF THE SKILL

Cardiac or respiratory arrest can occur at any time to individuals of all ages. It is a crisis event that can be the result of an accident (e.g., foreign body aspiration, motor vehicle accident, drowning) or a disease process (e.g., cardiac arrhythmia, epiglottis). Cardiopulmonary resuscitation (CPR) is the basic life-saving skill that is used in the event of cardiac, respiratory, or cardiopulmonary arrest to maintain tissue oxygenation by providing external cardiac compressions and/or artificial respiration.

This life-saving skill is initiated in the event that an individual is found with or develops the absence of a pulse or respiration or both. The basic goals of CPR, which are often referred to as the ABCD of emergency resuscitation, follow:

A: Establish **A**irway

B: Initiate **B**reathing

C: Maintain **C**irculation

D: **D**efibrillate

Cardiopulmonary resuscitation must be initiated immediately once it is determined that a cardiac or pulmonary arrest has occurred. Lack of oxygen to the tissues can result in permanent cardiac and brain damage within 4-6 minutes.

Cardiopulmonary resuscitation is a basic life-saving skill that nurses are expected to be able to perform not only in the hospital and other clinical settings but in the outside environments as well. It is expected that nurses maintain certification in the administration of CPR to individuals of all ages and participate in annual review or recertification courses. In addition, this skill is frequently taught to the lay public and caregivers of medically fragile individuals. This skill will review CPR for health care providers.

Do Not Resuscitate Orders

Sudden death from a cardiac arrest requires the initiation of CPR by competent persons. In a health care facility, caregivers, often a nurse, perform CPR and other life-saving measures in accord with agency policy unless the primary physician has written an order in the client's medical record: *do not resuscitate (DNR)*. The physician's DNR order provides an exception to the universal standing order to resuscitate.

Health care agencies are required to have policies in place that provide a mechanism for reaching a DNR decision as well as for resolving conflicts in decision making. The principles of informed consent must be respected by the physician who writes a DNR order. When the client is either comatose or near death, there should be knowledgeable concurrence by the physician and the client's family or guardian about the actions that should be implemented concerning prolonging the client's life. It is the responsibility of the nurse to know and follow the client's wishes relative to resuscitation and the application of life-support systems. This information should be documented in the client's medical record.

► **AMERICAN HEART ASSOCIATION GUIDELINES UPDATE**

In March 2008, the American Heart Asociation (AHA) recommended hands-only CPR (compressions only), for use by bystanders who witness an adult suddenly collapse outside of he hospital setting. Hands-only CPR is a two-step process:

1. Acivate the emergency response system (call 911, or send someone else to call).

2. Begin providing high-quality chest compressions by pushing hard and fast in the center of the chest, with minimal interruptions.

Hands-only CPR should be continued until an automated external defibrillator (AED) arrives and is ready for use or until the EMS providers take over care of the victim. According to the AHA, an adult who suddenly collapses from a cardiac arrest has "enough oxygen in their lungs and blood to keep vital organs healthy for the first few minutes, as long as someone provides high-quality chest compressions with minimal interruptions" (AHA, 2008). It is important to note that hands-only CPR is recommended only for adults who suddenly collapse. Conventional CPR (CPR with a combination of breaths and compressions) continues to be the recommendation for unresponsive infants and children, adult victims who are found already unconscious and not breathing normally, and victims of drowning or collapse due to breathing problems.

► **ASSESSMENT**

1. Assess responsiveness and level of consciousness by gently shaking or tapping the client while shouting, "Are you OK?" **It is important to differentiate an unconscious individual from someone who is intoxicated, hypoglycemic, sleeping, or in shock. In addition, it is important to touch the clients in case they are hearing impaired.**

2. Assess the amount and abilities of any available assistance. **CPR cannot be performed indefinitely by a single individual. If in the hospital or a clinical setting, activate the appropriate "code" to signify there is an emergency situation. If outside of the hospital, call for help to activate emergency assistance (e.g., call 911 or the local emergency medical service).**

3. Assess the client's position. **Proper positioning, in a supine position (flat) on a hard surface, is essential to assess respiratory and cardiac status and to adequately perform cardiopulmonary resuscitation. Care must be taken when positioning a client with a suspected neck injury.**

4. Assess respiratory status by looking for the client's chest rising and falling, listening for air exchange, and feeling for the presence of air movement. **Presence of respirations contraindicates the initiation of artificial respiration. In addition, assessment of the respiratory status will uncover complicating factors, including foreign body obstruction and vomit or other excessive airway secretions. These complicating factors will need to be resolved in order to open the airway prior to the initiation of artificial respiration.**

5. Assess circulatory status by using the carotid or brachial pulse points. **The presence of pulse contraindicates the initiation of external chest compressions.**

► **DIAGNOSIS**

Ineffective Breathing Pattern

Impaired Gas Exchange

Impaired Spontaneous Ventilation

Decreased Cardiac Output

► **PLANNING**

Expected Outcomes:

1. Client will experience improved clinical status, as evident by:
   - Patent airway with spontaneous respirations
   - Return of cardiac circulation

2. Client does not experience negative sequela related to hypoxic event.

3. Client does not have damage inflicted by incorrect positioning for CPR (e.g., paralysis from manipulation of neck injury, cracked ribs, or sternum).

4. Cardiopulmonary resuscitation will be terminated only in the following situations:
   - Cardiopulmonary resuscitation was successful in reestablishing respirations and circulation.
   - The client is placed on advanced life support (e.g., intubated and transferred to the intensive care unit).
   - The rescuer is unassisted, fatigued, and unable to continue.
   - The physician or qualified practitioner pronounces the client dead and orders CPR to be discontinued.

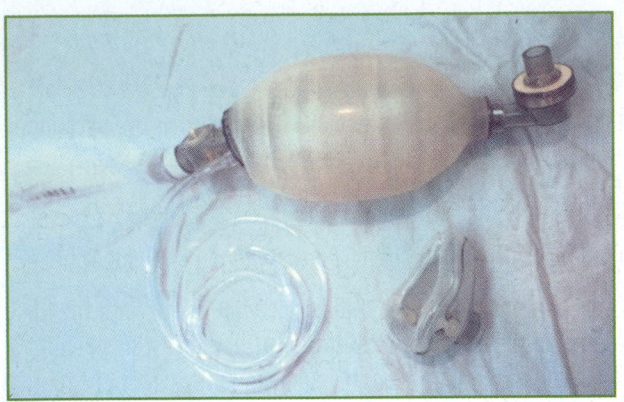

Figure 2-11-1   Ambu®-bag

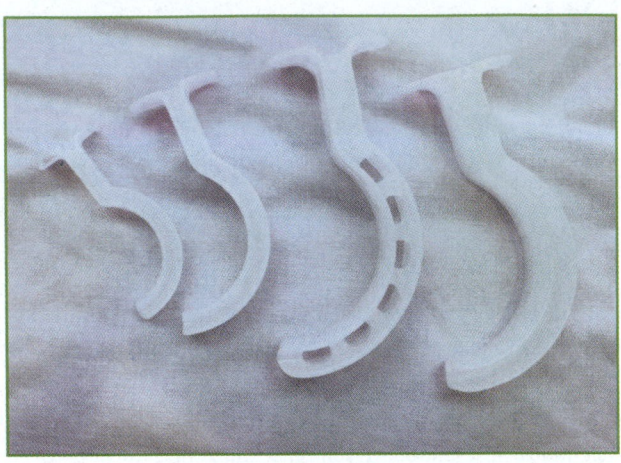

Figure 2-11-2   Oropharyngeal airways

Equipment Needed (see Figures 2-11-1, 2-11-2, and 2-11-3):

Hospital or Clinical Setting

- Hard, flat surface (e.g., chest compression board)
- Body substance isolation items:
  Gloves
  Face shield
  Mask/CPR oral barrier device
- Ambu®-bag
- Oral airway
- Emergency resuscitation cart (including defibrillator)
- Documentation forms

Outside: Public Environment

- Hard, flat surface (e.g., floor)
- Body substance isolation items, if available:
  Gloves
  Face shield
  Mask/CPR oral barrier device
- Automated external defibrillator (AED)

▶ CLIENT EDUCATION NEEDED:

Frequently, CPR is taught to caregivers and family members of clients who are at an increased risk for cardiopulmonary arrest (e.g., infant with a near sudden infant death experience). A certified instructor from either the hospital ambulatory clinical setting or the American Heart Association should provide this instruction.

1. Family members or caregivers of individuals at risk for cardiopulmonary arrest should be taught CPR. The client and family should take a refresher course on an annual basis.

Estimated time to complete the skill:

This skill must be initiated as soon as possible and continues indefinitely until one of the following occurs:

1. **CPR is successful and there is a return of spontaneous respirations and circulation.**
2. **Advanced life support measures are implemented (in the hospital) or the client is transferred to a facility to provide advanced life support.**
3. **A rescuer is alone and unable to continue CPR because of fatigue.**
4. **A physician or qualified practitioner declares the client dead and discontinues CPR.**

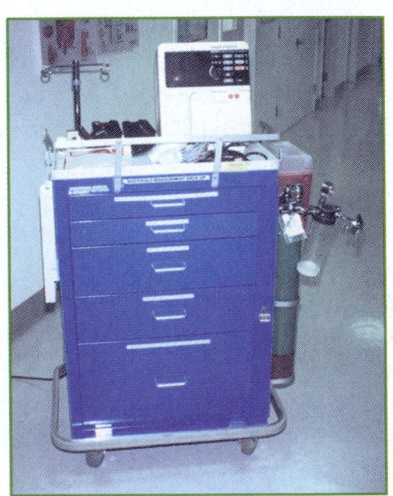

Figure 2-11-3   Emergency resuscitation cart.

2. The pediatric client usually experiences respiratory arrest more frequently than cardiopulmonary arrest.

3. The client and family members should keep pertinent information such as current medications easily accessible at home and when traveling.

4. Rescuers who perform CPR without body substance isolation are at an increased risk for contagious or communicable disease transmission.

These risks must be evaluated against the risk of client death.

5. Lay learners in the community are frequently taught one-person CPR because of the complexity of sequencing with two-rescuer CPR. Good Samaritan laws usually protect lay individuals who participate in emergency resuscitation from any lawsuits in the event that the client is injured during rescue efforts.

▶ DELEGATION TIPS

The administration of CPR to adults and children is a skill that may be delegated to ancillary personnel and caregivers after proper instruction and CPR certification.

IMPLEMENTATION—Action/Rationale

Action	Rationale
CPR: One Rescuer—Adult (Adolescent and older), 1. Assess responsiveness by tapping or gently shaking client while shouting, "Are you OK?" (see Figure 2-11-4).	1. Prevents injury to a client who is not experiencing cardiac or respiratory arrest. Also assists in assessing level of consciousness and possible etiology of crisis.

2. Activate emergency medical system (EMS). In the hospital or clinical setting, follow institutional protocol. In the community, for a witnessed sudden collapse of a client of any age, and unresponsiveness has been determined, activate the local emergency response system (e.g., 911), and get AED (if available). Send second rescuer (if available) to do this while you stay with the client.
  • If you are the lone rescuer for an unresponsive client of any age, most likely due to an asphyxial cause (drowning), provide 5 cycles of CPR, then activate the emergency response system and get the AED (if available). Return to the client, begin CPR and use AED.
	2. Activates assistance from personnel trained in advanced life support.
	  • Provide oxygenation and circulation prior to going for help.
	
	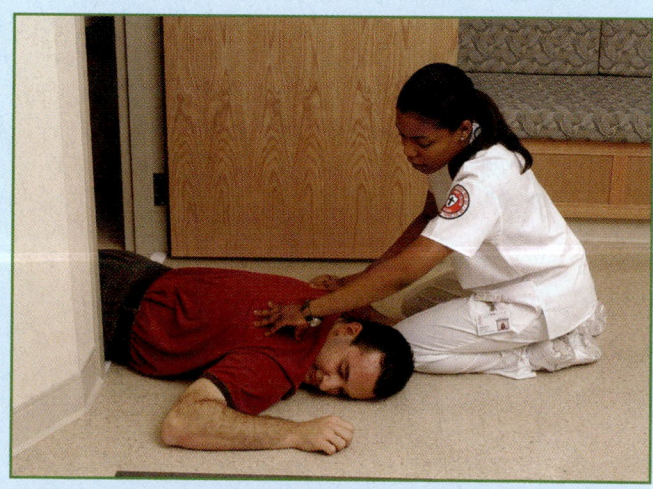

Figure 2-11-4 Assess the client's responsiveness.

continues

Action	Rationale
CPR: One Rescuer—Adult (Adolescent and older), *continued*	
3. Position client in a supine position on a hard, flat surface (e.g., floor or cardiac board). Use caution when positioning a client with a possible head or neck injury.	3. Proper positioning facilitates assessment of the cardiac and respiratory status and successful external cardiac massage. Care must be taken in positioning a client with a potential head or neck injury to prevent further damage.
4. Apply appropriate body substance isolation items (e.g., gloves, face shield), if available.	4. Prevents transmission of disease.
5. Kneel parallel to the client, next to the head, to begin to assess the airway and breathing status.	5. Proper positioning prevents rescuer fatigue and facilitates CPR by allowing the rescuer to move from chest compressions to artificial breathing with minimal movement.
6. Open airway. The most commonly used method is the head-tilt/chin-lift method. This is accomplished by placing one hand on the client's forehead and applying a steady backward pressure to tilt the head back while placing the fingers of the other hand below the jaw at the location of the chin and lifting the chin (see Figure 2-11-5). • In the event of a suspected head or neck injury, this lift is modified and the jaw thrust is used. To perform the jaw thrust, place hands at the angles of the lower jaw. Rest your elbows on the surface on which the client is laying, and lift lower jaw with both hands, displacing the jaw forward.	6. A patent airway is essential for successful artificial respirations. The head-tilt/chin-lift assists in preventing the tongue from obstructing the airway. • The jaw thrust is used when a head or neck injury is suspected because it prevents extension of the neck and decreases the potential of further injury.
7. Assess for breathing. Look, listen, and feel for air movement (5-10 seconds).	7. Cardiopulmonary resuscitation should not be administered to a client with spontaneous respirations or pulse because of the potential risk of injury.
8. If the client is not breathing, give rescue breaths: • Occlude nostrils with the thumb and index finger of the hand on the forehead that is tilting the head back (see Figure 2-11-6). • Form a seal over the client's mouth using either your mouth or the appropriate respiratory assist device (e.g., Ambu®-bag and mask) and give two breaths that make the chest rise. Each breath is given over 1 second. If chest does not rise, reposition the head and repeat the breaths. (see Figure 2-11-7). • In the event of a serious mouth or jaw injury that prevents mouth-to-mouth ventilation, mouth-to-nose ventilation may be used by tilting the head as described earlier with one hand and using the other hand to lift the jaw and close the mouth.	8. Occluding the nostrils and forming a seal over the client's mouth will prevent air leakage and provide full inflation of the lungs. Visual assessment of chest movement helps to confirm open airway. • Lifting the jaw and closing the mouth will prevent air leakage and provide full inflation of the lungs.

continues

Action	Rationale

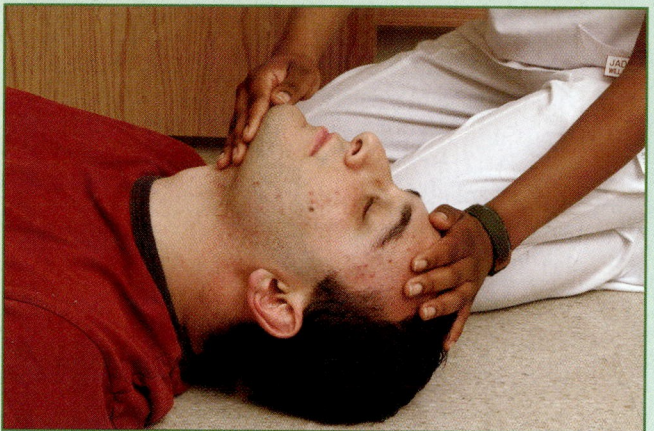

Figure 2-11-5   Use the head-tilt/chin-lift method to open airway.

9. Palpate the carotid pulse (no longer than 10 seconds):
   - If present, continue rescue breathing, at the rate of 10-12 breaths/minute (one breath every 5-6 seconds). Recheck pulse every 2 minutes.
   - If absent, begin external cardiac compressions.

10. External cardiac compressions are performed as follows (see Figure 2-11-8):
   - Kneel at client's side, parallel to client's sternum.
   - Remove clothing to visualize chest.
   - Place heel of one hand on the center of client's sternum at the nipple line.
   - Put heel of other hand on top of the first hand.
   - Keep arms straight with shoulders directly over your hands.
   - Compress chest 11/2 to 2 inches at a rate of 100 compressions per minute.
   - Allow chest to recoil completely after each compression.

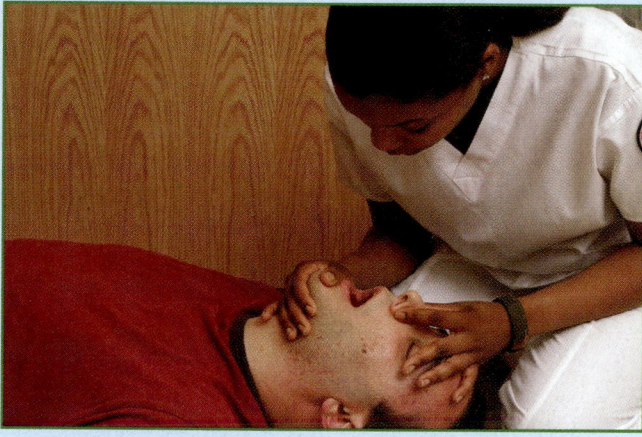

Figure 2-11-6   Occlude both nostrils with thumb and forefinger.

9. Performing chest compressions on an individual with a pulse could result in injury. Additionally, the carotid pulse may persist when peripheral pulses are no longer palpable. Hyperventilation assists in maintaining blood oxygen levels. Additionally, a pulse may be present for about 6 minutes after respirations have ceased.

10. Irreversible brain and tissue damage can occur if a client is hypoxic for longer than 4-6 minutes. Proper positioning and technique is essential for the following reasons:
   - Allows for maximum compression of the heart between the sternum and vertebrae.
   - Keeping fingers off the chest during compressions reduces the risk of rib fracture.
   - Incomplete chest recoil is associated with decreased coronary and cerebral perfusion.

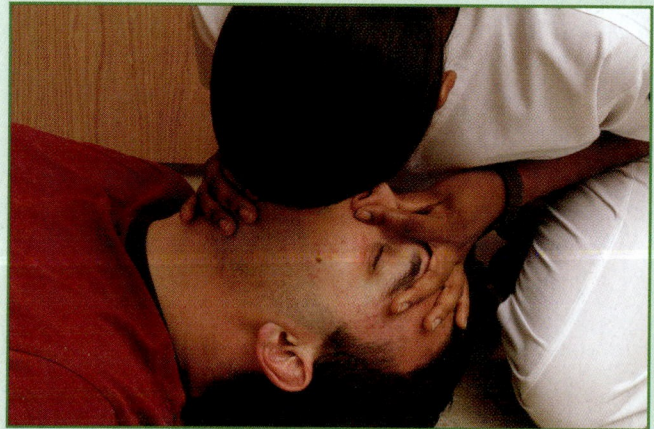

Figure 2-11-7   Give two breaths.

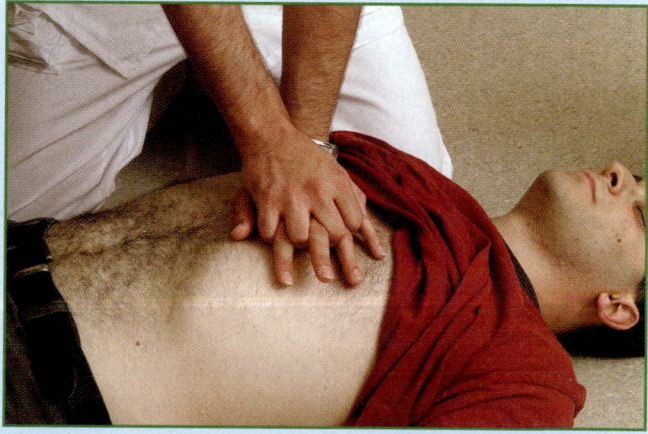

Figure 2-11-8   Place heel of one hand on the center of client's breastbone between the nipples. Put heel of other hand on top of the first hand.

continues

Action	Rationale
CPR: One Rescuer—Adult (Adolescent and older), *continued*	
11. Give cycles of 30 compressions and 2 ventilations until AED arrives.	11. Provides blood to coronary arteries and brain.

12. AED and Defibrillation
• Power on the AED.
• Attach electrodes to client's chest.
  a. Choose correct size, adult pads (for adults and children 8 years of age or older).
  b. Wipe sweat or water off of skin, if present.
  c. Place one electrode pad on upper right side of the chest, to the right of the breastbone and below the collar bone.
  d. Place other electrode pad on the left side, below the left axilla and to the left of the nipple.
  e. Do not place electrode pad directly on top of transdermal medication patches. Remove the patch and wipe the area before applying the electrode pad.
  f. If an implantable medical device is located where an electrode pad is to be placed, position electrode pad at least 1 inch away from device.
  g. Attach AED connecting cables to the AED box, if not preconnected
  h. Analyze the rhythm; some AEDs require you to push a button to analyze the rhythm. Be sure no one is touching client during analysis.
  i. If shock needs to be delivered, loudly state "Clear the client!" so that no one is touching client, and press shock button.
  j. After shock delivered, resume CPR.
	12. Early defibrillation increases survival of client. Electrode pads placed directly on medication patch may block the energy from the electrode pad to the heart and may cause small burns.

13. After every 5 cycles of CPR (30 compressions: 2 ventilations), approximately 2 minutes, allow AED to analyze the rhythm. If AED does not detect a rhythm that needs shock, continue chest compressions and ventilations.	13. Irreversible brain and tissue damage can occur if a client is hypoxic longer than 4-6 minutes.
14. Continue CPR and rhythm analysis until emergency response providers arrive or the client begins to move.	14. Irreversible brain and tissue damage can occur if client is hypoxic longer than 4-6 minutes.
CPR: Two Rescuers—Adult (Adolescent and Older)	
15. **Follow the steps above with the following changes:** Position of two rescuers (Figure 2-11-9): • The rescuer positioned at the client's trunk is responsible for performing cardiac compressions of 100 per minute and counting out loud (see Step 10). This is rescuer 1.	15. Proper positioning allows one rescuer to perform rescue breathing while the other administers chest compressions without getting in each other's way. In addition, this facilitates ease in changing positions when one becomes fatigued. When rescuer becomes fatigued, chest compressions become ineffective, decreasing the volume of oxygenated blood circulating to organs and tissue.

continues

Action	Rationale

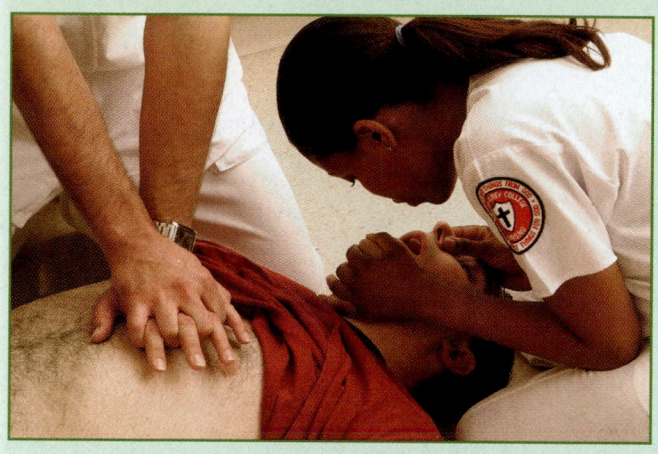

Figure 2-11-9 Two-rescuer positioning. One person kneels on each side of the client.

- The rescuer positioned at the client's head is responsible for maintaining an open airway, and giving breaths 2 breaths after 30 compressions. This is rescuer 2.
- Rescuer 2 is responsible for palpating the carotid pulse.
- The rescuers switch roles after 5 cycles of compressions and ventilations.
- Use AED when it arrives (see step 12). Rescuer 2 is responsible for setting up AED.

16. Follow steps 13-14.

16. See rationale steps 13-14.

CPR: One Rescuer—Child (1 Year of Age to Onset of Adolescence)

17. Assess responsiveness by tapping or gently shaking client while shouting, "Are you OK?"

17. Prevents injury to client who is not experiencing cardiac or respiratory arrest. Also, assists in assessing level of consciousness and possible etiology of crisis.

18. For a witnessed sudden collapse of a child, and child is unresponsive, activate the local emergency response system (e.g., 911) and get AED if available. Send second rescuer (if available) to do this, while you stay with the child.
    - If unresponsiveness is most likely due to an asphyxial cause (drowning), perform five cycles of CPR (about 2 minutes) before leaving to activate the emergency response system (e.g., 911) and getting the AED, if available.

18. Respiratory arrest is more common in children than cardiac arrest. The child is more likely to benefit from the initiation of CPR.

    - Provide oxygenation and circulation prior to going for help.

19. Position client in a supine position on a hard surface (floor or cardiac board). Use caution when positioning a client with a possible head or neck injury.

19. Proper positioning facilitates assessment of the cardiac and respiratory status and successful external cardiac massage. Care must be taken in positioning a client with a potential head or neck injury to prevent further damage.

continues

Action	Rationale
CPR: One Rescuer—Child (1 Year of Age to Onset of Adolescence) *continued*	
20. Apply appropriate body substance isolation items (e.g., gloves, face shield), if available.	20. Prevents the transmission of disease.
21. Open airway. See step 6.	21. See Rationale step 6.
22. Assess for breathing: look, listen, and feel for air movement (5-10 seconds).	22. Cardiopulmonary resuscitation should not be administered to a client with spontaneous respirations or pulse because of the potential of further injury.
23. If client not breathing, give rescue breaths (see step 8)	23. See Rationale step 9.
24. Palpate the carotid pulse (no longer than 10 seconds) • If present, continue rescue breathing at a rate of 12-20 breaths/minute. • If absent, begin external cardiac compressions.	24. Performing chest compression on an individual with a pulse could result in injury.
25. External cardiac compressions are as follows: • Kneel at client's side, parallel to client's sternum. • Place heel of one hand on the center of client's sternum at the nipple line. (Heel of other hand may be placed on top of the first hand or you may use only one hand for compressions). • Keep arms straight with shoulders directly over your hands. • Compress chest 1/3 to ½ the depth of the chest at a rate of 100 compressions/minute. • Allow chest to recoil completely after each compression.	25. Irreversible brain and tissue damage can occur if client is hypoxic for longer that 4-6 minutes. Proper positioning and technique is essential to allow for maximum compression of the heart and to reduce the risk of rib fractures. Incomplete chest recoil is associated with decreased coronary and cerebral perfusion.
26. After 5 cycles of 30 compressions and 2 ventilations, attach AED. • If sudden collapse of child was witnessed, use AED as soon as available.	26. Provides blood to coronary arteries and brain.
27. AED and Defibrillation • Use a pediatric dose-attenuating system for children 1 to 8 years of age. Use conventional AED if pediatric dose-attenuating system is not available. If using adult electrode pads, do not allow pads to touch each other. • If conventional AED has child shock dose, follow directions on AED to deliver shock. • See step 12 for AED set up and delivering shock.	27. Early defibrillation increases client's survival.

continues

Action	Rationale
28. After every 5 cycles of CPR (30 compressions : 2 ventilations), approximately 2 minutes, allow AED to analyze the rhythm. If AED does not detect a rhythm that needs shock, continue chest compressions.	28. Irreversible brain and tissue damage can occur if a client is hypoxic for longer than 4-6 minutes.
29. Continue CPR and rhythm analysis until emergency response providers arrive or the client begins to move.	29. Irreversible brain and tissue damage can occur if a client is hypoxic for longer than 4-6 minutes.
CPR: Two Rescuers—Children (1 Year of Age to Onset of Adolescence	
30. Follow actions for one-rescuer CPR for a child with the following changes: • Give cycles of 15 compressions and 2 rescue breaths. • Use AED after five cycles of compressions and breaths. • If witnessed collapse, use AED as soon as it is available.	30. Etiology of cardiac arrest for children is different than adults and requires modification of CPR.
CPR: One Rescuer—Infant (Under 1 year of age)	
31. Assess responsiveness, activate emergency medical system, position the child on a flat surface, apply appropriate body substance isolation, position self, open airway, and assess for respirations as described in Actions 1–7. Remember, respiratory arrest is more common in the pediatric population.	31. See Rationales 1–7.
32. For a witnessed sudden collapse of an infant, and the infant is unresponsive, activate the local emergency response system (e.g., 911) and get AED if available. Send second rescuer (if available) to do this, while you stay with the infant. • If unresponsiveness is most likely due to an asphyxial cause (drowning), perform five cycles of CPR (about 2 minutes) before leaving to activate the emergency response system (e.g., 911) and getting the AED, if available	32. Activates assistance from personnel trained in advanced life support. • Provides oxygenation and circulation prior to going for help.
33. If respirations are absent, begin rescue breathing: • Avoid overextension of the infant's neck. • Make a tight seal over both the infant's nose and mouth and gently administer artificial respirations. • Give two breaths (1 second each) with visible chest rise.	33. Irreversible brain and tissue damage can occur if a client is hypoxic for longer than 4–6 minutes. Proper positioning is essential for the following reasons: • It is believed that overextension of an infant's head can cause a closing or narrowing of the airway. • Making a complete seal over the infant's mouth and nose prevents air leakage.

continues

Action	Rationale

CPR: One Rescuer—Infant (Under 1 year of age)
continued

34. Assess circulatory status using the brachial pulse:
    - Locate the brachial pulse on the inside of the upper arm between the elbow and shoulder by placing your thumb on the outside of the arm and palpating the proximal side of the arm with the index finger and middle fingers.
    - If a pulse is palpated, continue rescue breathing 12-20 breaths/minute.
    - Recheck pulses every 2 minutes.
    - If no pulse, perform external cardiac compressions.

35. External cardiac compressions (infant under 1 year of age):
    - Maintain a position parallel to the infant. Infants can easily be placed on a table or other hard surface.
    - Position the hands for compressions:
        a. Draw an imaginary line between nipples. Place 2 fingers on breastbone, just below this line.
        b. Press breastbone down 1/3 to 1/2 the depth of the chest. Deliver 100 compressions per minute. Allow chest to recoil after each compression.

36. After 5 cycles of CPR (30 compressions: 2 ventilations) activate the EMS.

37. Resume CPR until emergency response providers arrive or the infant begins to move.

CPR: Two Rescuers—Infant (Under 1 year of age)

38. Follow actions for CPR: One Rescuer—Infant with the following changes
    - Provide 15 compressions to 2 ventilations.
    - Use two thumb-encircling hands technique for compressions:
        a. Place both thumbs side by side in the center of infant's breast bone, just below the nipple line
        b. Encircle infants back with both hands
        c. Use thumbs to depress the breastbone one third to one half the depth of infant's chest.

Rationale

34. The carotid pulse is often difficult to locate in the infant; therefore the brachial artery is the recommended site.

35. Irreversible brain and tissue damage can occur if a client is hypoxic for longer than 4-6 minutes. Proper positioning is essential for the following reasons:
    - Allows for maximum compression of the heart between the sternum and vertebrae.
    - Compressions over the xiphoid process can lacerate the liver.
    - Keeping other fingers and hands off the chest during compressions reduces risk of rib fracture.
    - Keeping one hand on the infant's forehead helps maintain an open airway.

36. Respiratory arrest is more common in children than cardiac arrest. The child is more likely to benefit from the initiation of CPR.

37. Irreversible brain and tissue damage can occur if a client is hypoxic for longer than 4-6 minutes.

38. Etiology of respiratory and cardiac arrest is different for infants and requires modification of CPR sequence.
    Table 2-11-1 provides a quick overview of the various cardiopulmonary standards.

Table 2-11-1   Cardiopulmonary Standards

CLIENT	HAND POSITION	CHEST COMPRESSION DEPTH	CHEST COMPRESSION RATE	CHEST COMPRESSION TO VENTILATION RATION	ACTIVATE EMERGENCY RESPONSE	USE AED
Adult (Adolescent and older)	Center of breastbone between nipples	1.5 to 2 inches	100 per minute	30:2 (1 or 2-rescuer CPR)	For a witnessed sudden collapse, after verifying the adult is unresponsive. If asphyxial cause of arrest (drowning), after providing 5 cycles of CPR	Give cycles of 30 compressions and 2 ventilations; use AED when it arrives.
Child (1 year of age to onset of adolescence)	Center of breastbone between nipples	One third to one half depth of chest	100 per minute	30:2 for 1-rescuer CPR 15:2 for 2-rescuer CPR	For a witnessed sudden collapse, after verifying that the child is unresponsive If asphyxial cause of arrest (drowning), after providing 5 cycles of CPR	After 5 cycles of CPR (out of hospital) For sudden collapse use AED as soon as available
Infant (Under 1 year of age)	Just below nipple line on breastbone	One third to one half depth of chest	100 per minute	30:2 for 1-rescuer CPR 15:2 for 2-rescuer CPR	For a witnessed sudden collapse of an infant, after verifying that the infant is unresponsive. If asphyxial cause of arrest (drowning), after providing, 5 cycles of CPR	No recommendations for infants < 1 year of age

▶ **REAL WORLD ANECDOTES**

Scenario 1

A child was found unconscious in a pool. One neighbor called 911 while another neighbor immediately yelled, "I know CPR," and positioned the child supine on the walkway. He assessed for respirations and found no air movement, opened the airway, and began mouth-to-mouth resuscitation. After two breaths, he proceeded to check the child's carotid pulse, but could not locate it. The time was ticking, he could feel his own heart beating, his head was pounding, and he could feel his hands were shaking slightly; all these nervous symptoms made his assessment of the child difficult. Luckily, another neighbor who knew CPR came to help right away. The two neighbors supported and coached each other. They were able to calmly assess the child's condition; the child's pulse was felt within the next 15 seconds. They then moved back into position to continue rescue breathing until the emergency medical team arrived. In an emergency situation, victim's pulsation may be weak and hard to locate; both health care professionals and the lay public must remember to assess for both respiratory and circulatory status of a victim when performing CPR.

continues

> ► **REAL WORLD ANECDOTES** *(continued)*

Scenario 2

One trauma nurse mentally practiced CPR skills in a very effective way. Once or twice a month, she would set the alarm on her wrist watch to sound at some point in the day. When the alarm sounded, she would look at the first person she saw—the man in the cafeteria line or the driver in the car ahead, for example—and imagine the person collapsing in front of her. She would then mentally "go through the steps" of CPR, including who to call and how to position the client in this setting. This exercise gave her "mental experience" and kept the CPR techniques fresh in her mind.

► EVALUATION

- Client experienced improved clinical status, as evident by patent airway with spontaneous respirations and return of cardiac circulation.
- Client did not experience negative sequela related to hypoxic event.
- Client does not have damage inflicted by incorrect positioning for CPR (e.g., paralysis from manipulation of neck injury, cracked ribs, or sternum)
- Cardiopulmonary resuscitation was terminated only in the following situations:

  Cardiopulmonary resuscitation was successful in reestablishing respirations and circulation.

  The client is placed on advanced life support (e.g., intubated and transferred to the intensive care unit).

  The rescuer is unassisted, fatigued, and unable to continue.

  The physician or qualified practitioner pronounces the client dead and orders CPR to be discontinued.

- There should be a constant evaluation for the return of spontaneous pulse and respirations.
- Successful intervention with CPR is illustrated as follows:
  The nurse maintains an open airway, as evident by the chest rise and fall.

  The nurse is able to feel the resistance and compliance of the client's lungs.

The nurse feels and hears airway movement during expiration.

The indicators of circulation, such as color, improved.

The client has return of spontaneous pulse and respirations, as evidenced by a palpable carotid or brachial pulse and the presence of respiratory effort.

Assist with transfer to hospital/advanced life-support unit.

- If CPR was unsuccessful, assist in notifying next of kin and providing psychosocial support.

► DOCUMENTATION

Nurses' Notes/Code Record

- Note the time and condition in which the client was found.
- Record interventions that were implemented, including accurate times, results of the implementations, orders received from the physicians, vital signs of the client, timing of the incident, and status of the client afterward.

Document on appropriate flow sheet or electronic medical record (EMR).

Medication Administration Record

- Record any medications the client received, including time and route, during the procedure.
- If the incident occurs in a noninstitutional setting, the nurse should report her findings and interventions to aid personnel when they arrive.

▶ CRITICAL THINKING SKILL

Introduction

Cardiopulmonary resuscitation is an emergency life-support intervention that is used in both the clinical and outside community settings. For a nurse working in a hospital or other acute-care setting, it is not unusual to encounter an individual in respiratory or cardiac arrest. This is especially true in the emergency room or other high-acuity settings.

Possible Scenario

A client presented to the emergency room and had a rapid deterioration of clinical status leading to a cardiopulmonary arrest. The first nurse on the scene immediately began resuscitative efforts without putting on the appropriate body substance isolation apparel.

Possible Outcome

This nurse could potentially develop a contagious disease, transmitted by improper utilization of body substance isolation garb during CPR.

Prevention

Body substance isolation should be practiced whenever possible during CPR, especially in a clinical setting where the equipment is readily available.

▶ VARIATIONS

Geriatric Variations:

- *It is important to remember that the older adult is at risk for rib or cartilage fractures, which may result from improper hand positioning.*
- *Age-related changes in the muscle skeletal system (e.g., osteoporosis) might limit positioning of the geriatric client.*
- *Many older adults may be wearing dentures, which should be removed during emergency resuscitation.*

Pediatric Variations:

- *Parents and caregivers should be taught the proper hand positions, ventilation-to-compression ratio, and breathing techniques for use in the pediatric population.*
- *It is important to reinforce that respiratory arrest is more common than a cardiopulmonary arrest in the pediatric population.*
- *Safety education with a focus on accident prevention should also be included in CPR instructional sessions. Refresher courses should be encouraged on an annual basis.*

Home Care Variations:

- *Caregivers and family members of clients requiring home care should be assessed for their educational level and ability to learn and retain the principles of CPR.*
- *It is important to have a working phone in the home and the client/family member/caregiver should know how to assess the emergency medical response system in the community.*
- *The home care nurse is ideally in a position to assess the home environment and the ability of the caregiver/family members to return-demonstrate CPR skills. Referrals to the community resources may be useful (e.g., the American Red Cross, the American Heart Association, or the local hospital).*

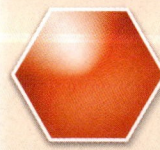

Long-Term Care Variations:

- *In a long-term care facility, it should be expected that all health care providers have certification in CPR.*
- *Special attention should be made for individuals wearing dentures, those at risk for choking (e.g., stroke victims), and clients with impaired cognitive function who may be at risk for falls or accidents.*
- *A complete evaluation should be made on all clients, and care plans should include choking prevention measures as well as reinforcement of safety measures.*

▶ COMMON ERRORS

Possible Error:

Incorrect hand placement during cardiac compressions.

Prevention:

Be sure to review, on an annual basis, (at minimum) the proper methods of administering chest compressions. In addition, always remember to think, "What do I have to do differently for a child or infant?" Immediately correct anyone that you see performing chest compressions incorrectly. If you realize that your hand placement is wrong, take immediate action to correct placement and continue with the emergency resuscitation.

Possible Error:

Incorrect placement of client for CPR.

Prevention:

Be sure to place anyone receiving CPR on a hard, firm surface. If a client is not placed on a hard, firm surface, the cardiac compressions will be ineffective and the rescuer will not be able to palpate a carotid pulse. Immediately move the client to a hard, firm surface.

▶ NURSING TIPS

- Maintain a current and valid CPR/emergency resuscitation certification.
- Differentiate between emergency resuscitations that occur in the hospital setting-versus those occurring in the nonclinical environment.
- Understand the differences in lay public CPR teaching versus what is taught to health professionals.
- Maintain an ongoing assessment of the cardiac and respiratory status throughout emergency resuscitation efforts.
- Be aware of the emergency response systems available in each new environment.

▶ SPECIAL CONSIDERATIONS

- *The American Heart Association (AHA) and the Centers for Disease Control and Prevention (CDC) recommendation for health care workers: Face masks with one-way valves are recommended for trained rescuers who give CPR to people.*
- *Use a pediatric dose-attenuating system for children 1 to 8 years of age. If not available, and child is in cardiac arrest, a standard AED may be used.*
- *There is no recommendation for or against the use of an AED in infants less than 1 year of age (AHA, 2005).*

Performing the Heimlich Maneuver

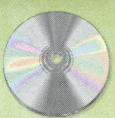

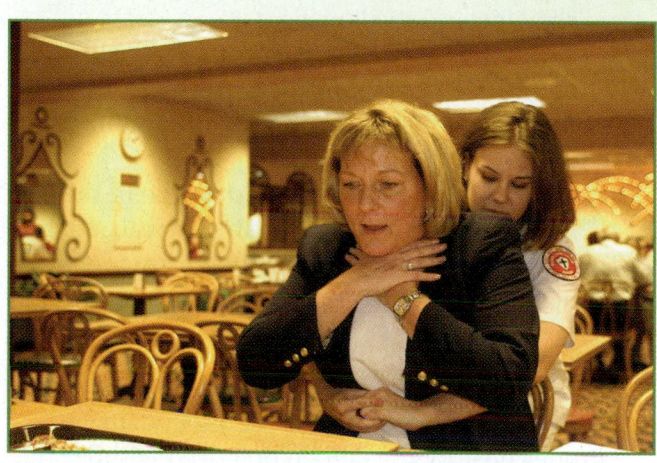

▶ OVERVIEW OF THE SKILL

Foreign body obstruction of the breathing passages has consistently ranked as one of the top ten causes of accidental deaths in the United States. Complete or partial airway obstruction by a foreign body can occur in numerous settings. In adults, large, poorly chewed pieces of food are most frequently the cause of airway obstruction, but in other situations an elevated blood alcohol level or dentures may be the culprit. Pediatric clients are at risk for choking, especially the infant and young child, and in this population food (e.g., grapes, hot dogs, raisins, and peanuts) as well as foreign bodies (e.g., coins, beads, marbles, thumbtacks, and paper clips) can cause airway obstruction. The Heimlich maneuver or subdiaphragmatic abdominal thrusts can assist a health care provider in successfully treating airway obstruction. It is important in the pediatric population to differentiate airway obstruction as a result of infection (e.g., epiglottis) versus a foreign body aspiration.

Health professionals frequently teach the Heimlich maneuver to the general public as most food/foreign body obstructions occur outside the hospital/clinic settings. It is important for the nurse to have a good comfort level with this skill as well as have the ability to disseminate this information in an easily understood manner to the public.

▶ ASSESSMENT

1. Assess air exchange. A foreign body obstruction can be complete or partial. Partial airway obstruction will have some air exchange. If the client can cough, this should be encouraged and the nurse should not interfere with the client's efforts. In the event of partial airway obstruction, the client will usually be able to cough but may wheeze between coughs. **If the client has complete airway obstruction as indicated by a weak, ineffective cough, high-pitched inspiratory noises (stridor), and signs of respiratory distress (cyanosis, loss of consciousness), intervention is necessary.**
2. Establish airway obstruction. The universal sign of airway obstruction is clutching the neck with hands. In addition, the inability to talk or breathe as well as cyanosis and the progression to an unconscious state are indicative of airway obstruction. **Determine the problem.**
3. In the pediatric client differentiate between infection and airway obstruction. Fevers,

gradually increasing respiratory distress, retractions, stridor, and drooling are all signs of infection. **In this situation it is important to maintain an upright position, keep the child as calm as possible, and seek immediate medical attention.** The Heimlich maneuver is not appropriate in these cases.

▶ DIAGNOSIS

Impaired Gas Exchange

Ineffective Airway Clearance

Ineffective Breathing Pattern

Risk for Suffocation

Risk for Aspiration

Fear

▶ PLANNING

Expected Outcomes:

1. The client will demonstrate improved clinical status as evident by airway clearance or establishment of a patent airway.
2. The client will demonstrate improved gas exchange as evident by absence of signs and symptoms of partial or complete airway obstruction (e.g., cough, wheezing, stridor, loss of consciousness, cyanosis).
3. The client will experience minimal discomfort during the Heimlich maneuver or other method of airway clearance.
4. The client will not experience complications related to airway obstruction/hypoxia.

Equipment Needed:

- An individual with the training to perform this procedure

▶ CLIENT EDUCATION NEEDED:

1. The prevention of food or foreign body obstruction is a key element of client teaching. Educate clients on the conditions under which airway obstruction occurs as well as prevention activities (e.g., childproofing a home). Sample prevention activities include:
   - Food should be cut into small pieces and thoroughly chewed, and individuals wearing dentures should be particularly careful.
   - Avoid physical activity during the process of chewing and swallowing.
   - Avoid excess intake of alcohol, especially before and during meals.
   - Avoid laughing and talking with food in the mouth.
   - Gum and hard candy should not be in the mouth of anyone engaged in physical activity.
   - Restrict children from walking, running, or playing while they are eating.

2. The actual Heimlich maneuver or chest thrusts should not be practiced on human subjects because of the risk of internal organ damage. Proper positioning can be practiced without the actual thrusts. "Dummy" models are available in the adult, child, and infant sizes.
3. Provide an opportunity for the clients to practice the positions and actions to be utilized in the event of an actual choking.
4. Encourage ongoing parent/public education on the risks of accidental choking and methods of prevention or steps to follow if an obstruction should occur. In addition, teach the signs of airway distress and the need for immediate medical intervention.

Estimated time to complete the skill: **1–4 minutes**

▶ DELEGATION TIPS

The Heimlich maneuver may be performed by any trained individual. A technique adjustment may need to be demonstrated in pregnant women.

IMPLEMENTATION—Action/Rationale

Action	Rationale
1. Ask the client "Are you choking?" Assess airway for severe airway obstruction. Hands around the neck is the universal choking sign. (see Figure 2-12-1).	1. If there is good air exchange and the client is able to forcefully cough, you should not intervene or interfere with the client's attempts to expel the foreign body. Encourage attempts to cough and breathe, as attempts to cough will provide a more forceful effort. If severe airway obstruction is apparent, the Heimlich maneuver or alternative method of subdiaphragmatic thrust should be performed immediately.
2. Activate emergency response assistance if there is respiratory distress or complete blockage, for example, ask a bystander to call 911.	2. Provides follow-up care by professionally trained personnel.

Conscious Client—Adult and Children Older Than 1 Year of Age (Heimlich Maneuver) Sitting or Standing

Action	Rationale
3. Stand behind the client.	3. Proper positioning is necessary to provide an effective subdiaphragmatic thrust.
4. Wrap your arms around the client's waist (see Figure 2-12-2).	4. Proper positioning is necessary to provide an effective subdiaphragmatic thrust.
5. Make a fist with one hand. Place the thumb side of your fist against the client's abdomen. The fist should be placed midline, above the navel and below the xiphoid process. Grasp fist with other hand (see Figure 2-12-3).	5. Correct hand placement is important to prevent internal organ damage.
6. Press fist into abdomen with a quick upward thrust; each thrust should be separate and distinct.	6. This subdiaphragmatic thrust can produce an artificial cough by forcing air from the lungs.

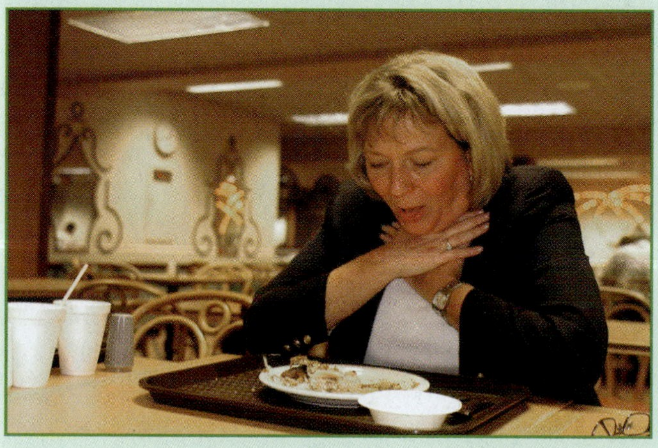

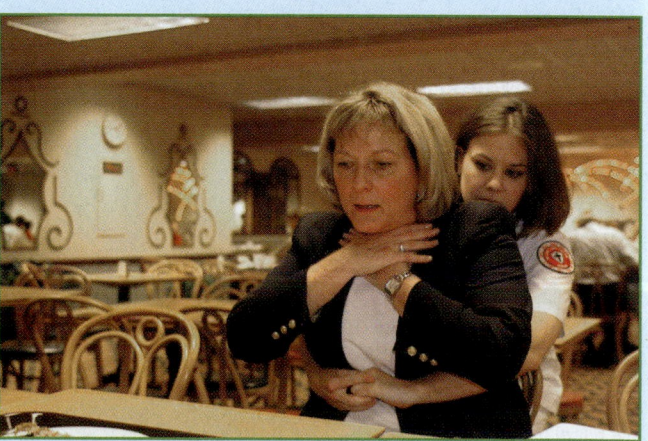

Figure 2-12-1 Universal choking sign is hands around the neck.

Figure 2-12-2 Wrap both arms around the client's waist.

continues

Action	Rationale
Conscious Client—Adult and Children Older Than 1 Year of Age (Heimlich Maneuver) Sitting or Standing *continued*	
7. Repeat this process until the client either expels the foreign body or loses consciousness.	7. Attempts to dislodge food or a foreign body to relieve airway obstruction should be continued as long as necessary because of the serious consequences of hypoxia.
8. If client is obese or in later stages of pregnancy, perform chest thrusts: • Stand behind the client. • Wrap your arms under arm pits and around the client's chest. • Make a fist with one hand. Place thumb side of fist in the middle of the sternum. Grasp fist with other hand • Press fist into chest and deliver thrusts back and upward. • Repeat this process until the client either expels the foreign body or loses consciousness	8. Rescuer may not be able to wrap arms around client's waist. Peforming abdominal thrusts in late stages of pregnancy can cause injury. • Proper positioning is necessary to provide effective thrusts. • Proper positioning is necessary to provide effective thrusts. • Proper hand placement is necessary to avoid damage to internal organs. • Creates pressure to force object out. • Chest thrusts may not be effective on the first attempts.
Unconscious Client—Adult and Children ≥ 1 Year of Age	
9. When the client becomes unconscious, lower client to floor. Protect the client's head. Place in supine position	9. Avoids injury to the head. Places the client in the most effective position to apply interventions.
10. Activate the emergency response assistance (call 911), if not previously done.	10. Activates assistance from personnel trained in advanced life support.
11. Open client's mouth. Use one hand to grasp the lower jaw and tongue between your thumb and finger. Lift the jaw. If you see an object remove it (see Figure 2-12-4).	11. Draws the tongue away from any foreign body lodged in the back of the throat.

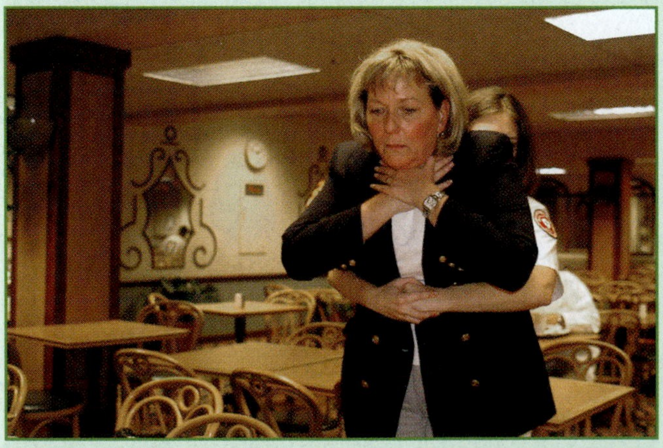

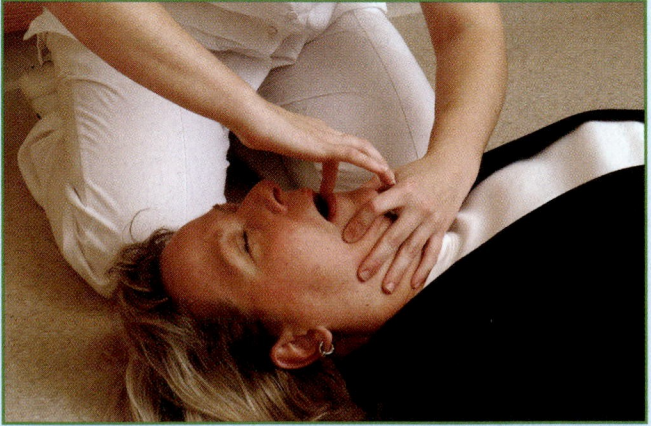

Figure 2-12-3   Place thumb side of fist below the xiphoid process and above the naval.

Figure 2-12-4   Use a sweeping motion to remove obstruction.

continues

Action	Rationale
12. Open the airway and provide 2 breaths and look for chest to rise. If chest does not rise, reposition client's head, reopen the airway and provide 2 breaths.	12. The brain can suffer irreversible damage if it is without oxygen for 4-6 minutes.
13. If unable to ventilate, begin CPR (see Skill 2-11).	13. Performs life-saving procedure.
14. Every time you give breaths, open the mouth. If you see an object, remove it.	14. Removes object blocking the airway.
15. Continue to provide CPR until emergency response arrives or the client begins to move.	15. Performs life-saving procedure.

Infant Airway Obstruction—Under 1 Year of Age

Action	Rationale
16. Differentiate between infection and airway obstruction	16. Infectious complications that lead to airway obstruction require immediate medical attention, establishment of a patent airway (intubation or emergency tracheotomy), and treatment of the underlying infection. Food/foreign body airway obstruction also needs immediate attention; however, airway management differs between each scenario.
17. Straddle infant over forearm in the prone position with the head lower than the trunk. Support the infant's head, positioning a hand around the jaw and chest.	17. Proper positioning is essential for success of the maneuver and prevention of other organ damage.
18. Place the heel of your hand between the infant's shoulder blades and deliver 5 back blows. (see Figure 2-12-5).	18. Technique for dislodging the obstruction.
19. Keeping the infant's head down, place the free hand on the infant's back and turn the infant over, supporting the back of the child with your hand and thigh.	19. Safely rotates the infant's position to continue life-saving procedures.
20. With your free hand, place 2 fingers in the middle of the breast bone, just below the nipple line. Deliver 5 thrusts, compressing 1/3 to 1/2 the depth of the chest. Deliver chest thrusts at a rate of 1 per second (see Figure 2-12-6).	20. Technique for dislodging the obstruction.

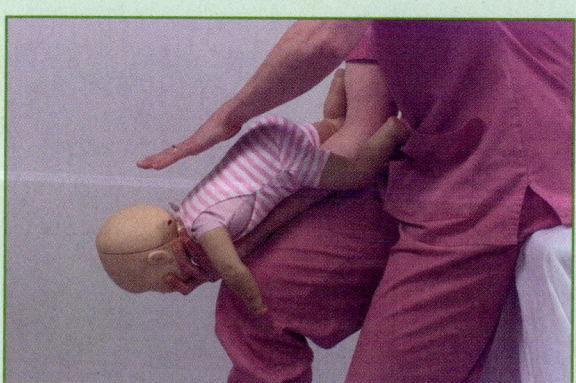

Figure 2-12-5 Place the infant face down, with face lower than trunk. Deliver 5 back blows.

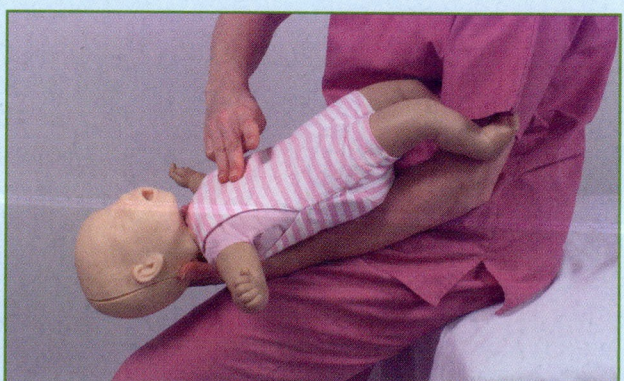

Figure 2-12-6 Turn the infant face up and deliver chest thrusts. Fingers are placed just below the nipple line.

continues

Action	Rationale
Infant Airway Obstruction—Under 1 Year of Age *continued*	
21. Repeat the sequence of 5 back blows and 5 chest thrusts until the object is removed or until the infant becomes unresponsive.	21. Technique for dislodging obstruction.
22. Place unresponsive infant on a flat surface.	22. Proper positioning is necessary to provide life-saving procedure.
23. Open the airway; if you see an object, remove it.	23. The brain can suffer irreversible damage if it is without oxygen for 4-6 minutes.
24. Begin CPR (see Skill 2-11); every time you open the airway, look for an obstruction. If you see it, remove it.	24. The brain can suffer irreversible damage if it is without oxygen for 4-6 minutes.
25. After 5 cycles of CPR, activate the emergency response system, if not previously done.	25. Provides needed assistance.
26. Continue with CPR until emergency response arrives or the infant begins to move.	26. Provides life-saving procedure.

► REAL WORLD ANECDOTES

Scenario 1

An infant was brought into the emergency room in respiratory distress, with audible stridor and visible drooling. Before the parents could report that the child had a fever and had been sick, a new emergency room nurse turned the child over and began the procedure for removal of a foreign body obstruction. The infant's respiratory distress worsened immediately. Other emergency room personnel intervened, and it became immediately apparent that the child had an infection with epiglottis and required an emergency tracheotomy. Failure to quickly differentiate the cause of respiratory distress in an infant or child can result in incorrect interventions and exacerbation of symptoms.

Scenario 2

A very obese gentleman was eating dinner in a restaurant. He stopped talking and grabbed his neck, and his tablemates began to yell for help. Someone began to deliver hard slaps to his back while another person attempted the Heimlich maneuver while the client sat in his chair. The client soon became unconscious before a nurse in the restaurant came over and yelled for someone to activate the local emergency response system and performed chest thrusts, dislodging a piece of meat. She then used a finger sweep to remove the meat and began rescue breathing. Luckily, the gentleman regained consciousness and had no adverse sequela from the event. This illustrates the need for health care professionals to be leaders in providing both emergency support to individuals with airway obstruction and education of the general public on the appropriate interventions to utilize in the event of an airway obstruction. In this case chest thrusts were the appropriate intervention.

▶ EVALUATION

- The client demonstrates improved clinical status as evident by airway clearance or establishment of a patent airway.
- The client demonstrates improved gas exchange as evident by absence of signs and symptoms of partial or complete airway obstruction (e.g., cough, wheezing, stridor, loss of consciousness, cyanosis).
- The client experienced minimal discomfort during the Heimlich maneuver or other method of airway clearance.
- The client did not experience complications related to airway obstruction/hypoxia.

▶ DOCUMENTATION

- If the airway obstruction occurs in the health care setting, document the following in the narrative notes and in the emergency procedure notes if needed:

  Time and date of onset of symptoms

  Presentation including onset and type of symptoms

  Type (complete or partial) and cause of obstruction, if known

  Interventions used to alleviate obstruction

  Results of interventions

  Other emergency support needed (e.g., emergency tracheotomy)

- If the airway obstruction occurs in an alternate setting (e.g., restaurant, home), provide the following information to the responding health care providers for documentation:

  Presentation including onset and type of symptoms

  Type (complete or partial) and cause of obstruction, if known

  Interventions used to alleviate obstruction

  Length of time with airway obstruction

  Results of interventions

Document on appropriate flow sheet or electronic medical record (EMR).

▶ CRITICAL THINKING SKILL

Introduction

The Heimlich maneuver and alternative methods to relieve airway obstruction are basic nursing skills. The choking on food or a foreign body resulting in the lack of oxygen is a significant and life-threatening event that requires emergency management.

Possible Scenario

A woman begins choking on some food in a restaurant. She is alone, panics, grabs her throat, and runs toward the restroom.

Possible Outcome

Failure to follow this individual into the restroom could result in her death. The universal sign of choking is hands clutching the throat. This individual is alone with no tablemates to assist her. Anyone with the knowledge of the Heimlich maneuver, especially health care professionals and restaurant employees, should follow her into the bathroom to provide interventions if needed. This is not a time to be embarrassed about entering a women's restroom if you are a male or entering a men's restroom if you are a female.

Prevention

The best prevention is nursing education to the general public about the dangers of accidental choking, emergency interventions, and the need to chew food thoroughly and eat slowly. In addition, restaurant workers are key individuals to target with this health education.

▶ VARIATIONS

Geriatric Variations:
- *The older adult is at risk for rib or cartilage fractures, which may result from forceful thrusts or improper hand positioning.*
- *Age-related changes in the muscle skeletal system (e.g., osteoporosis) might limit positioning of the geriatric client.*
- *Many older adults may be at risk of choking because of dentures, and appropriate education should take place when such devices are fitted on an individual and should be reinforced by all other health care professionals working with the client.*

continues

▶ **VARIATIONS** *(continued)*

Pediatric Variations:

- All individuals in health care and daycare settings should be educated in the hand placement and methods to remove food or foreign bodies from a child with an airway obstruction and in how they differ from treating an adult.
- In addition, how to access emergency medical assistance as well as prevention should be a key educational piece for all new parents and any facility that has infants and young children under its care.
- Infants and toddlers should not be given foods that they can choke on, especially children who do not have the ability to properly chew yet. These foods include peanuts, round hard candies, and cut-up hot dogs.

Home Care Variations:

- Both the caregivers and the clients requiring home care should be assessed for their educational level on interventions to take if someone is choking.
- Identify a working phone in the home; the client/caregiver should know how to access the emergency medical assistance available in his or her area.
- Referrals to community resources may be necessary (e.g., classes held at the local American Red Cross or the local hospital).
- Clients in the home care setting may have impaired swallowing abilities and are at higher risk of choking. They and their caregivers should be made aware of the proper feeding techniques to decrease the possibility of choking on food.

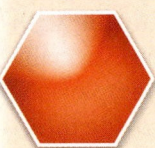

Long-Term Care Variation:

- In a long-term care facility, all employees should be educated in emergency resuscitation measures.
- Special attention should be made for individuals wearing dentures and those at higher risk for choking, for example, stroke victims.
- Foods may have to be pureed and liquids may need to be thickened.

▶ **COMMON ERRORS**

Possible Error:

Not assessing for full versus partial airway obstruction.

Prevention:

Make airway assessment and questions to the client (e.g., "Are you choking?") the first priority when a suspected airway obstruction occurs. If clients are able to cough forcefully and breathe, assist them in relaxation and coach them to cough. Reassure clients that you will not leave them. If there is total airway obstruction, follow the appropriate protocol outlined earlier.

Possible Error:

Not using the correct technique for obstructed airway on an obese individual or a woman in the advanced stages of pregnancy.

Prevention:

Evaluate the situation and use chest thrusts for obese individuals or women in the advanced stages of pregnancy. Maintain regular recertification for cardiopulmonary resuscitation, which includes a review of managing airway obstruction.

▶ **NURSING TIPS**

- Maintain a current and valid cardiopulmonary resuscitation/emergency resuscitation certification.
- Differentiate between emergency resuscitations that occur in the hospital settings versus those occurring in the nonclinical environment.
- Approach clients with confidence and reassure clients that you will remain with them throughout the procedure.
- Maintain an ongoing assessment of the respiratory status as well as the need to progress to full cardiopulmonary resuscitation.
- Be aware of the emergency response systems in each new environment.

▶ **SPECIAL CONSIDERATIONS**

- *If a choking victim is pregnant or extremely obese, place your fist in the middle of the breast b instead of the abdomen for the thrusts.*
- *It is important to wrap your fingers around your thumb when performing the Heimlich maneuver so as not to perforate the spleen with an extended thumb. Although unlikely, it is important to perform the maneuver in the safest way possible.*

Responding to Accidental Poisoning

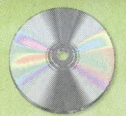

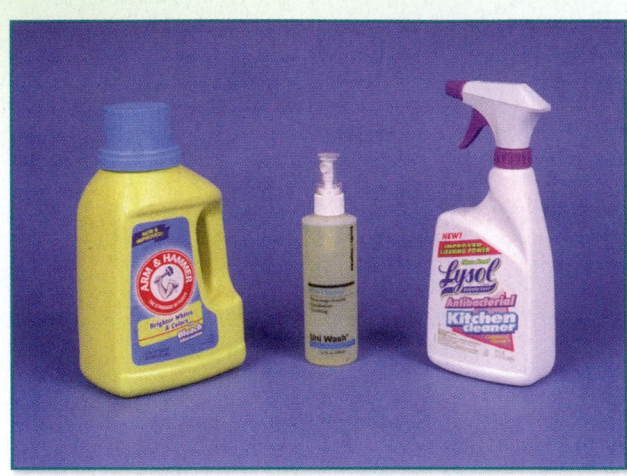

▶ OVERVIEW OF THE SKILL

Accidental poisonings result from the ingestion of cleaning products, household chemicals, and medications. Often, these items are stored in cupboards that are easily accessible to young children. Prevention is the best way to reduce the two million accidental poisonings that occur each year. However, if an accidental poisoning does occur, it is critical to act quickly and calmly to prevent or slow damaging effects. Poisoning may cause many physical reactions, including sleepiness, pneumonia, organ damage, and death. A quick response is your best chance to reduce the harmful effects of an accidental poisoning.

▶ ASSESSMENT

Preventing an Accidental Poisoning

1. Assess the environment to establish ways to keep all medications out of reach: use child-resistant caps and label medicine and household chemicals with poison symbols or "Mr. Yuk" stickers. Once children start crawling, use safety locks on all cabinets. It is best to secure toxic chemicals and household cleaning products in tall cabinets to avoid the risk of cabinets accidentally being unsecured. **These precautions help decrease the likelihood of an accidental poisoning.**
2. Assess whether the client is able to read medicine labels accurately. **An inability to read**

medicine labels can lead to overdose of medication and accidental poisoning.

Responding to an Accidental Poisoning

1. Assess for signs of poisoning, such as congestion, crankiness, drowsiness, abdominal pain, nausea, and vomiting. These symptoms may indicate poisoning as well as the severity of the situation.
2. Assess what, when, and how much of the harmful substance was taken. This information is important to identify actions to be taken.

▶ DIAGNOSIS

Risk for Poisoning

▶ PLANNING

Expected Outcomes:

1. Accidental poisoning will be prevented.
2. If accidental poisoning occurs, the client will experience a minimum of trauma.

Equipment Needed:

- Phone number for Poison Control Center
- Ipecac syrup or activated charcoal

▶ CLIENT EDUCATION NEEDED:

1. Explain intervention before initiated. For example, ipecac syrup induces vomiting by

irritating the stomach lining and triggers a vomiting response. Activated charcoal absorbs poisons from the stomach and intestines until the poisons can be excreted during a bowel movement.

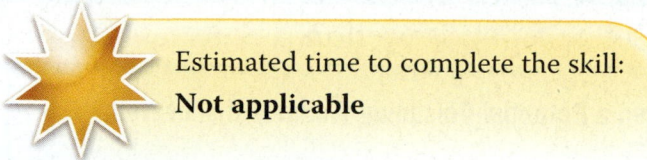

Estimated time to complete the skill: **Not applicable**

► **DELEGATION TIPS**

Any individual or adult may initiate an emergency response to an accidentally poisoned victim. A rapid response is the best chance to reduce harmful effects of accidental poisoning.

IMPLEMENTATION—Action/Rationale

Action	Rationale
When a Potential Poisoning Victim Is Discovered	
1. Be familiar with the emergency procedures at your facility (see Figure 2-13-1).	1. Allows a quick and accurate response when the need arises.
2. Call for help. Assess the client. If the client does not have a pulse or is not breathing, call 911 for assistance with life-saving measures. Intervene to clear airway, reestablish breathing, and restore circulation as required.	2. Institute cardiopulmonary resuscitation (CPR) and life-saving measures immediately. First aid is only a stopgap measure until professional help is available.
3. If the client is conscious and breathing, call 911 or poison control for assistance with the poisoning.	3. First aid is only a stopgap measure until professional help is available.
4. Determine what substance was ingested and how much was ingested. Keep the container if it is available.	4. Helps determine the course of treatment.
5. If you are talking to poison control, have them determine what treatment is appropriate.	5. Different poisons have different treatments. Do not induce vomiting unless it has been specifically authorized. Inducing vomiting when a caustic substance has been ingested results in reexposure of the esophagus and mouth to the caustic substance.

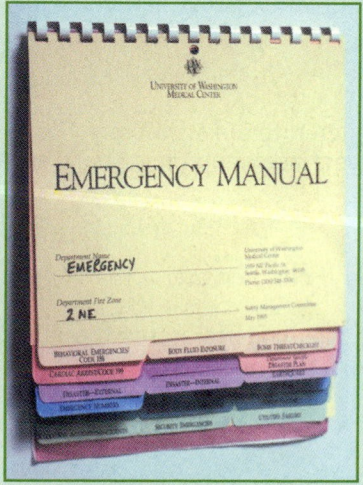

Figure 2-13-1 Know emergency procedures for accidental poisoning.

continues

Action	Rationale
When a Potential Poisoning Victim Is Discovered *continued* 6. If appropriate, give syrup of ipecac or activated charcoal. 7. Follow the instructions of the emergency providers. Instructions may range from transport to the emergency room, taking the victim to a physician, or simple observation. 8. Wash hands.	6. Ipecac will induce vomiting. Activated charcoal will bind with the poison so it can be excreted in the stool. 7. Even if the victim seems to have recovered, a physician or nurse practitioner should examine the victim for damage or residual effects. 8. Reduces transmission of microorganisms. Steps to prevent poisoning are presented in Table 2-13-1.

Table 2-13-1   Steps to Prevent Poisoning

SAFETY WITH DOSAGES
- Do not take or give medicines meant for someone else.
- Take or give medicines according to clear directions from health care professionals. Request these directions in writing. This prevents ingestion of medication at incorrect dosage.
- Do not take or give medicines unless the container labels can be read accurately to prevent ingestion of wrong medication or incorrect dosage.

SAFETY WITH LABELS
- Keep medicine labels attached to medicine containers for quick reference in case of accidental ingestion.
- Do not keep medicines beyond the time of directed use or beyond a year if there are no expiration dates.
- Label medicine and household chemical containers with poison symbols to alert people that the substance is dangerous. Do not store household chemicals in soda bottles or cans.
- Return unused or expired prescription medications to a pharmacy that participates in a medication recycling program.

SAFETY WITH CHILDREN
- Refer to medicines by their proper names in front of children to alert children that medicine is not candy.
- Do not take medicines in front of a child. This may prevent accidental ingestion, especially when the child is imitating adult activity, behavior, and expressions.
- Store medicines out of a child's reach, in a cabinet with a safety lock, to prevent accidental ingestion by a child.
- Use child-resistant caps and keep in the locked position if children are in the home or visit occasionally. This may prevent accidental ingestion by a child.
- Post the number for the Poison Control Center near the telephone to assure the number is available in an emergency.

► **REAL WORLD ANECDOTES**

Jane was sent home with a prescription for dexamethasone and was instructed to take 2 mg b.i.d. When she got home, she forgot the dose she was to take and called her doctor's office to clarify. By this time, the office was closed. Jane thought the nurse had said to take 2 pills b.i.d. instead of 2 mg b.i.d., and she took two pills twice a day for 3 days. By the third day, she was having difficulty sleeping at night and was drowsy all day. She went back to see her doctor and the overdose was discovered. The nurse was reminded to always give the client written instructions in addition to verbal instructions regarding new medications.

► **EVALUATION**

- Accidental poisoning was prevented.
- If accidental poisoning occurred, the victim experienced a minimum of trauma.

► **DOCUMENTATION**

Nurses' Notes

- Document time and date of accidental poisoning incident.
- Document client's condition on arrival.
- Indicate the harmful substance and how much may have been ingested.
- Document circumstances of the accidental poisoning.
- Record the names of people with the client or those who accompanied the client.
- Document interventions used and the client's response.

Document on appropriate flow sheet or electronic medical record (EMR).

Incident Report (if poisoning occurred within an institution)

- Follow the institution's guidelines for accident reports.
- Document all of the items noted in the Nurses' Notes, as required.

► **CRITICAL THINKING SKILL**

Introduction

When a potentially poisonous substance is ingested, action must be taken quickly. If poisoning is suspected, do not wait to see what effect the substance may have; obtain help from emergency services (911) or the Poison Control Center.

Possible Scenario

Jimmy is a 3-year-old boy who was at his grandmother's house when he was found sitting on the floor playing with pills from a container.

Possible Outcome 1

Jimmy's grandmother scolded him for getting into her things and checked the bottle. Upon discovering that he was holding a bottle of her pain pills, she checked to see how many were left. There did not seem to be any missing. Jimmy's grandmother remembered that these pain pills had not been very strong and she decided to watch Jimmy for any symptoms. Shortly afterward, the phone rang. As his grandmother talked on the phone, Jimmy fell asleep on the carpet. When his grandmother hung up, she found Jimmy lying on the carpet breathing stertorously. She quickly scooped him up, ran to the car, and rushed him to the hospital. As a result of Jimmy's grandmother's delay in getting him to the hospital, he was found to have suffered hypoxic brain damage.

Possible Outcome 2

Jimmy's grandmother checked the bottle of pain medication. Although she did not notice any missing, she suspected that Jimmy might have ingested some of the pills. She immediately called 911 for assistance. The emergency service team induced vomiting using ipecac syrup. Jimmy vomited immediately and was admitted to the hospital to be observed overnight.

Prevention

All medications, cleaners, and any other potentially poisonous substances must be kept out of reach, especially when young children are present. Clients should be cautioned when given potentially poisonous medications. Children are curious and inventive. They will explore everything and everywhere and can get into things adults cannot imagine. Advise clients, when childproofing a house, to get down on the floor at a child's eye level and look around. Have them ask themselves what a child would find interesting from the lower angle. If it is something dangerous, put it away.

► **VARIATIONS**

Geriatric Variations:
- *Elderly clients may have difficulty hearing instructions or reading medication bottles.*
- *Elderly clients may be forgetful regarding when they actually took their last dose of medication. Be sure to establish a dosing system that will help prevent an accidental overdose.*
- *Elderly clients may have grandchildren or neighbor children in their homes. Many elderly clients choose to remove medications from child-resistant bottles, especially if children are rarely in the home. Caution them to secure medications when children are present.*

Pediatric Variations:
- *Children can mistake medication for candy and chemicals for soda or juice.*
- *When giving potentially poisonous medications to clients, always stress the possible dangers. Have them use poison stickers or "Mr. Yuk" stickers to emphasize things that should not be touched. Then put those things well out of the child's reach.*
- *It is critical that child-resistant safety locks be placed on any cabinets where dangerous chemicals are stored, especially once children start crawling. Secure all cabinets within reach, or, better yet, move all chemicals to tall, secured cabinets.*
- *Cosmetics and personal care items are common products ingested by children, as are vitamins, cold remedies, and mouthwash (contains alcohol). Drain cleaners are especially dangerous and can scar children for life, and/or damage the esophagus. Do not leave any medicines on countertops, and always use safety caps. Note that certain houseplants are poisonous.*
- *Some Poison Control Centers recommend ipecac. Be aware that ipecac should not be used when oil, hydrocarbons, or caustics solutions have been ingested in that the risk for aspiration and extreme tissue damage to the lungs exists. If seizures are present avoid ipecac or induced vomiting. Replacement fluid will be needed.*

Home Care Variations:
- *Chemicals and other potentially poisonous materials are often present in the home. In suspected poisonings, do not assume the poison came from the medicine cabinet or the kitchen. Consider other sources, including the garage, shed, workshop, and basement.*
- *In a home with young children, common potential poisons may be placed safely out of reach. When leaving medications at the home, be sure to follow the same safety procedures for these potential poisons.*

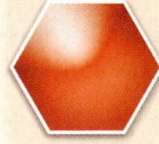

Long-Term Care Variation:
- *Safety precautions can become lax in the long-term setting. For example, pouring a cleaning solution in a drinking cup and then leaving it at the bedside can increase the risk of accidental poisoning.*
- *Clients may be confused and have less supervision than in other settings.*

► **COMMON ERRORS**

Possible Error:

Client misunderstands instructions regarding medication ingestion.

Prevention:

Provide both verbal and written instructions to the client. Ask the client to repeat the correct name, dosage, and frequency of the medication.

► **NURSING TIPS**

- Have poison prevention pamphlets and stickers with the phone number of the local poison control center available for clients.
- Remind clients to keep medication and chemicals in a safe location, especially if they have young children.
- Review dosage schedules with elderly clients, especially if the schedule has changed recently.

► **SPECIAL CONSIDERATIONS**

- *Information is available from the American Association of Poison Control Centers (aapcc.org). The most common overdoses are cleaning products and medications from overdose, misidentification, or accidental misuse. Examples are analgesics, cold medications, topical creams, vitamins, and antidepressants. Other common calls to Poison Control Centers include foreign body ingestion, dangerous plants, mushrooms, and insecticides.*
- *Contact the Poison Control Center before the need arises and know routine procedure; for example, some centers recommend keeping one ipecac antidote for each child, others may not recommend ipecac or may use charcoal.*
- *When calling a Poison Control Center, bring the container to the telephone to be able to exactly identify the substance and ingredients. Carefully assess history, especially with children. Ascertain how much of the item is missing and how much should be in the container.*
- *Bee stings can cause anaphylactic reactions. If a history of any bee sting reactions exists be alert to symptoms of a reaction (difficulty breathing, vomiting, diarrhea, or headache). Call 911 when symptoms are present or if a client with a positive history is stung. Teach clients with a positive history to avoid areas with increased risk of exposure, carry an epi-pen, wear a medical alert bracelet, and seek immediate medical care if stung.*

Emergency Client Transport

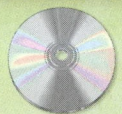

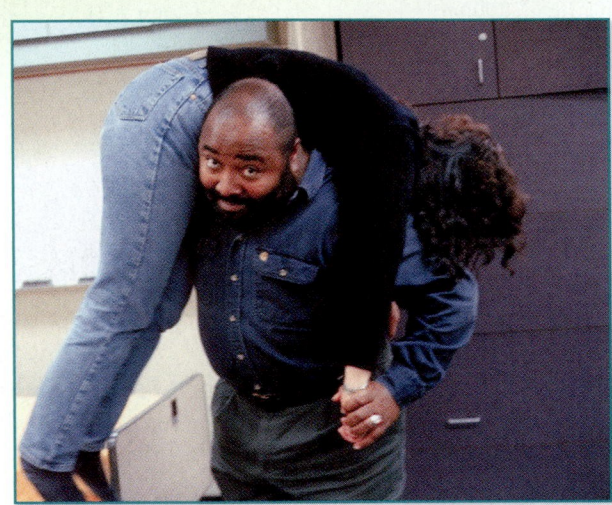

▶ OVERVIEW OF THE SKILL

A disaster is an emergency incident with destructive potential. Some examples of a disaster are a fire, a bombing, a tornado, an earthquake, a storm, or a chemical spill. In the event of a disaster, your quick action in safely evacuating clients may save their lives. Quickly and safely moving a client in an emergency situation is an essential nursing skill.

Planning ahead, or disaster preparedness, is the first step in safely moving a client. Assess the situation as much as possible before a disaster occurs. Read the emergency or disaster manual (see Figure 2-14-1). Think about potential obstacles, such as stairs to navigate, equipment to move, and the physical conditions of your clients. Know the location and availability of portable equipment, the location and condition of emergency supplies, and how much help will probably be available in the immediate area.

During the disaster, it is critical to communicate clearly to send and receive important information. It is important to know and use the emergency evacuation plan for the disaster you encounter. Use the safest means of transport available or if the clients must be moved. After you have moved everyone to a safe place, reassess the situation. Make sure all clients were moved, and that all clients and staff are accounted for.

After the clients have been evacuated, their needs may still be critical. Check the clients' conditions and determine what additional equipment or supplies are needed immediately, such as portable oxygen, a crash cart, IV poles, or Ambu®-bag.

Check whether any clients, rescuers, or other staff members have sustained additional injury from the move or the disaster. Determine whether the client, other staff members, or you yourself need any decontamination or have suffered inhalation exposure. Check for the onset of shock.

From the beginning to the end, safety is the number one concern. Good body mechanics can help you

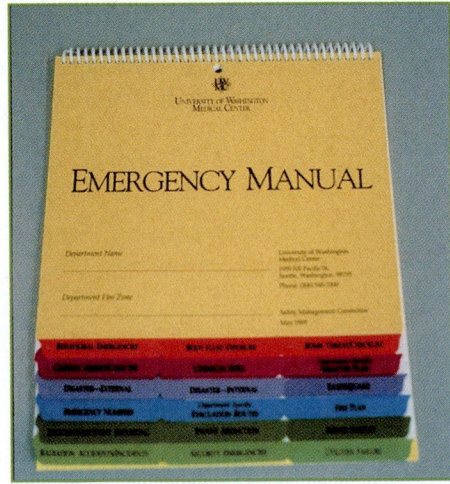

Figure 2-14-1 Read the emergency manual to know the procedures that may be required in a disaster.

avoid injury and fatigue, as well as reduce the risk of injuring a client.

Types of emergency transportation include ambulation, ambulation with assistance, wheelchairs, stretchers, the bed, and one or more people carrying or dragging the client. Using a manual carry may cause injury or increase the severity of an existing condition or injury. It can be exhausting to the rescuer; however, it may be the only option to save a life. If a manual carry is necessary, use two rescuers whenever possible. This will reduce the fatigue and risk of injury to the rescuers and is less traumatic to the client.

Select the best mode of manual carry. For example, the fireman's carry is one of the easiest ways for one person to carry a client. A support carry can be used when the client can use only one leg or can walk weakly.

▶ ASSESSMENT

1. Determine the nature of the disaster and where the danger is located. **Helps determine the extent and urgency of the evacuation.**
2. Determine who is in charge of the evacuation, both overall and in your part of the facility. **Defines who to locate to obtain orders and report information.**
3. Determine obstacles to the evacuation, including stairs, structural damage, darkness, or smoke. **Helps to determine the type of evacuation used.**
4. Determine your current client's medical needs, activity level, and tolerance. **Helps determine which clients are evacuated using which method.**
5. Review what equipment and supplies will be needed immediately to ensure client stability and safety. **Helps determine which equipment is gathered along with the evacuation, or obtained from other sources immediately.**

▶ DIAGNOSIS

Risk for Injury

Impaired Physical Mobility

Fear

Deficient Knowledge

▶ PLANNING

Expected Outcomes:

1. Client will be evacuated to a safe environment without injury to the client or the staff member.
2. Client will have essential medical support restored after the evacuation.

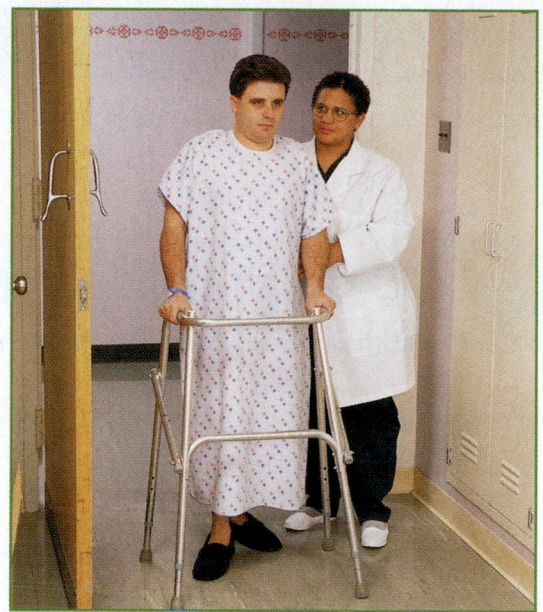

Figure 2-14-2 Client using a walker

Equipment Needed (see Figure 2-14-2):
- Flashlight, if needed

Equipment required for evacuation choice may include:
- Stretcher
- Wheelchair
- Walker
- Mattress
- Sheets

Support equipment needed to maintain client:
- Portable oxygen
- Occlusive dressing
- Bandages
- Sterile syringes
- Portable suction

▶ CLIENT EDUCATION NEEDED:

1. Calmly explain to the client the emergency situation, including the type of disaster and the need to evacuate.
2. Explain to the client the method that will be used to transport him or her to safety.
3. Give the client specific instructions on how to assist you, if the client is able.
4. Give visitors or family specific instructions on how to assist you.
5. Reassure the client that his or her medical needs will continue to be met in the safe area.

Estimated time to complete the skill:
30 seconds to 6 minutes per client

► **DELEGATION TIPS**

All ancillary personnel should be instructed in emergency client evacuation.

IMPLEMENTATION—Action/Rationale

Action	Rationale
1. Remain calm; do not panic.	1. Enables you to receive and process information about the disaster and the evacuation. Enables you to think and plan more clearly; helps your clients to remain calm.
2. Assess the source of the danger.	2. Helps you plan the evacuation route.
3. Assess for the increasing risk of danger from secondary source (fire after an earthquake, for example).	3. Helps you assess the total risk for the client. Helps anticipate unexpected emergency situations.
4. Determine the immediate risk to yourself and your ability to handle the situation. Intervene to reduce the risk to your safety and to get help, if needed.	4. Reduces the risk of the rescuer becoming an additional victim.
5. Check the condition of the clients and staff who may have been injured. Assess airway, breathing, and circulation.	5. Allows emergency life-saving responses.
6. Determine who is in charge of the evacuation, as per the emergency manual. Locate that person. Listen to and follow his or her instructions.	6. Ensures an orderly and safe evacuation.
7. Determine a safe location where clients will be transported.	7. Allows you to evacuate in the proper direction.

8. Determine who needs to be transported. Clients in the most physical danger from the disaster need to be transported first.
 	
    If the physical danger is the same for all and your rescuing resources are limited, evacuate those who can be quickly moved first, then those trapped under debris or those who require moderate time to move.
 	
    Finally, move those trapped behind walls, those who need to be extricated, or those who require intensive time and assistance.
	8. Allows you to prioritize the evacuation.

9. Determine what mode of transport will be used.	9. Allows you to plan the evacuation and assemble the equipment.
10. Inform the client what is happening and how he or she will be transported.	10. Elicits client cooperation and provides information.
11. Gather equipment and personnel.	11. Allows for a smooth procedure.

continues

Action	Rationale

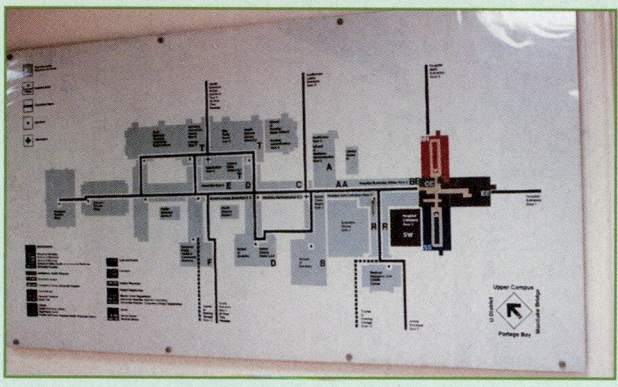

Figure 2-14-3 It is important to have a clear understanding of possible escape routes.

12. Make sure the escape route is clear and you or the assistant knows where to go (see Figure 2-14-3).

13. Make sure you have a light source if you will be passing through areas that are dark.

14. Transport the client as predetermined.

15. Recheck the client after evacuation, and provide immediate intervention to treat injuries, shock, or immediate medical needs.

16. If the evacuation location is outdoors, protect the client from the elements.

17. Continue to monitor the situation. If you need to return to the disaster site to evacuate additional clients, assign someone to remain with the present client.

18. Continue with the disaster protocol as outlined in the facility's disaster manual.

Emergency Transfer from Bed to Wheelchair, Walker, or Ambulation for Evacuation

19. Put the head of the bed up.

20. Pull covers down past the feet.

21. Put slippers or shoes on feet if readily available and if time permits.

22. Put on robe, coat, or blanket if client will be going outside, or if heat or electricity has been cut off.

---

12. Decreases the risk of leading a client into greater danger.

13. Decreases the risk of falls or injury from unknown hazards while transporting the client.

14. Allows the client to be moved to a safe location.

15. Continues to provide client care.

16. Protects the client from the additional trauma of cold, heat, rain, or other weather.

17. Ensures that the client will not be alone. Allows you to return to where you are needed most.

18. Ensures smooth and efficient disaster response.

19. Prepares the client to sit.

20. Allows you to check for tubes or drains. Prevents the feet from getting tangled in the bedding.

21. Provides traction and warmth.

22. Provides warmth and protection.

continues

Action	Rationale
Emergency Transfer from Bed to Wheelchair, Walker, or Ambulation for Evacuation *continued*	
23. Disconnect IV pumps, suction, oxygen, or other devices from the wall. Reconnect to portable devices if available, and if time permits.	23. Prevents trauma to the body. Continues essential therapy.
24. Assist the client to stand and help with wheelchair or walker, if needed.	24. Prepares the client to move safely.
25. Walk with the client to the safe location, or assign an assistant to walk with the client.	25. Allows the client to be moved to a safe location.
Emergency One-Person and Two-Person Evacuations	
26. *Support-walk with the client.* Use this technique if the client is conscious, can walk, walk with difficulty, or hop on one foot. **Use only if the client has no suspected neck injuries.**	26. Allows evacuation with minimal fatigue to the rescuer.
27. *One person.* Assist the client to a standing position. Firmly grasp the client's wrist and wrap the client's arm around the back of your neck. Place your arm around the client's waist, and walk with the client, supporting and stabilizing him or her.	27. Safe evacuation technique.
28. *Two people.* Each person firmly grasps one of the client's wrists and wraps the client's arm around the back of the rescuer's neck. Each person places an arm around the client's waist, and together the rescuers walk the client, supporting and stabilizing him or her.	28. Safe evacuation technique.
29. *Piggyback carry (one person).* Use this technique if the client is conscious and has no suspected neck or arm injuries. • Have the client stand or sit, or lift to a standing position. Turn your back to the client. Bend your knees and have the client place his or her hands on your shoulders. Lift the client, shifting the weight of the client onto your back, and grab his or her legs behind the knees with your hands or forearms. Instruct the client to "hang on" with his or her arms and hands. Make sure the client does not position hands or arms to block your vision or hearing or to choke you.	29. Safe evacuation technique.

continues

Action	Rationale
30. *Cradle/arms carry (one person).* Have the client stand, or lift to a standing position. Place one arm under the client's knees and the other arm around the client's back and lift, taking the weight with your knees.	**30.** Safe evacuation technique.
31. *Drag (one or two people).* Place the client on his or her back, and kneel at his or her head. Slide your hands under the client's shoulders and grasp the rib cage under the armpits. Rise and drag the client backwards. Support the client's head on one or both forearms. • *Using clothing as a handhold.* A variation of this technique is to grasp the clothing on each side of the client, under the armpits, and drag. • *Using a blanket or mattress.* Another variation is to quickly place a blanket or mattress under the client and use this to support the client as you drag him or her to safety (see Figure 2-14-4). • *Using this technique on stairs.* With the client in a semi-sitting position, rise and drag backwards. Then back down or climb up the steps. Support the client's head and body. Let the hips and legs slide and drop from step to step.	**31.** Safe evacuation technique. • Safe evacuation technique. • Safe evacuation technique. • Safe evacuation technique.
32. *Chair drag (one or two people).* Place the client in a chair (secure hands across chest, if necessary). Secure the person in the chair if the client is confused or unconscious. Drag the chair and the client to safety.	**32.** Safe evacuation technique.

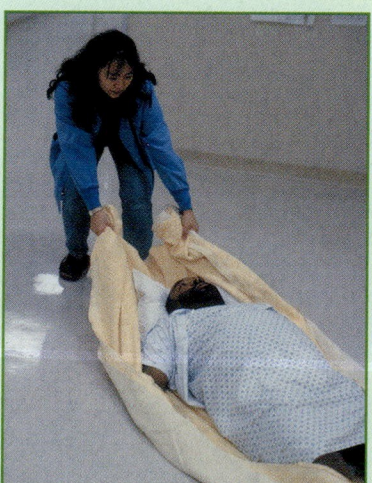

Figure 2-14-4   Use a blanket to drag the nonambulatory client to safety.

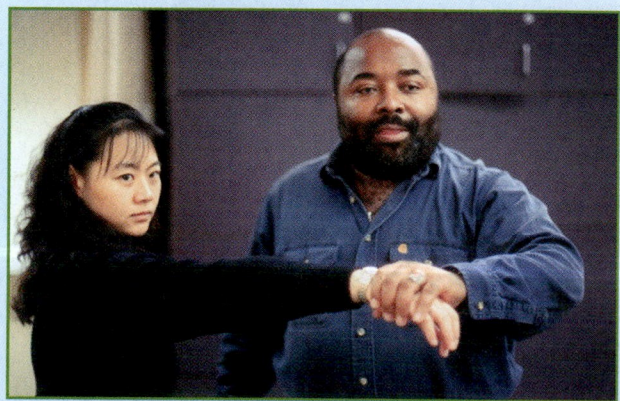

Figure 2-14-5   Grab the client's wrist farthest from you with your hand.

continues

Action	Rationale

Emergency One-Person and Two-Person Evacuations
continued

33. *Fireman's carry (one person).* Hoist, lift, or have the client stand facing you. Grab the client's wrist farthest from you with your hand (see Figure 2-14-5). Squat/lean and grab the client's thigh closest to your body (see Figure 2-14-6). Hoist the weight of the client over your shoulder closest to the client, and lift with your legs (see Figure 2-14-7). Balance the weight of the client (see Figure 2-14-8), keeping a firm grip on the client's wrist and thigh (see Figure 2-14-9). You may briefly let go of the client's wrist, if necessary, to open doors or grab railings.

33. Safe evacuation technique.

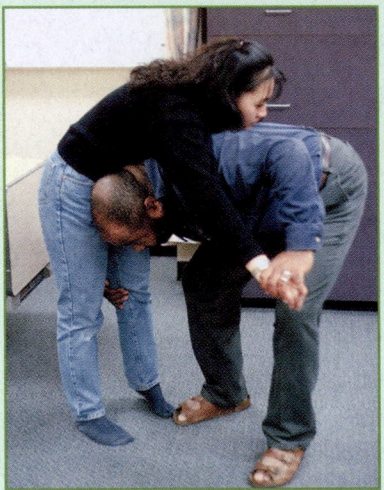

Figure 2-14-6 Grab the client's thigh closest to your body.

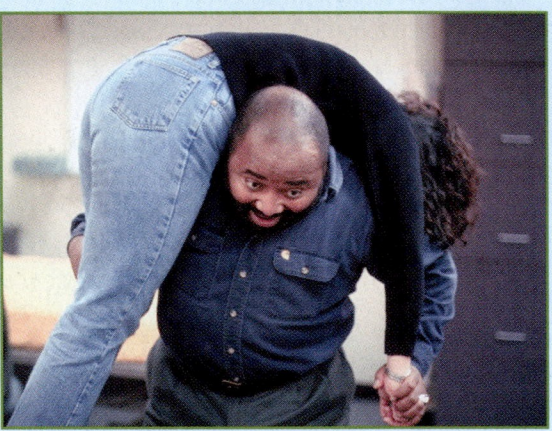

Figure 2-14-7 Hoist the client's weight over your shoulder, lift the client, and rise up to a walking position using your legs to avoid back strain.

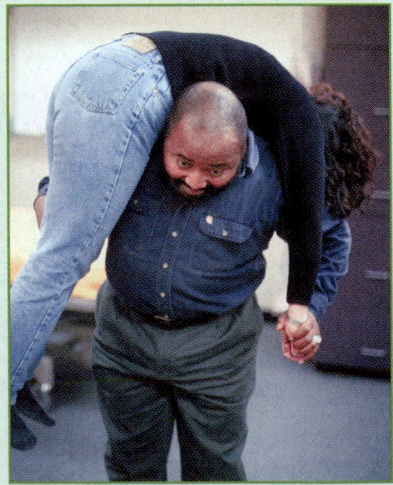

Figure 2-14-8 Balance the weight of the client prior to walking.

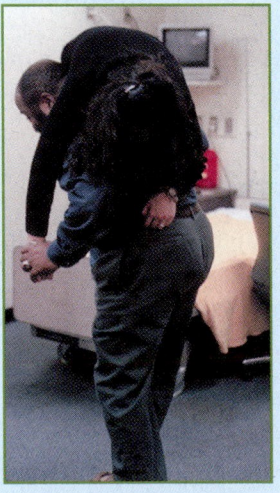

Figure 2-14-9 Keep a firm grip on the client's wrist and thigh.

continues

Action	Rationale
34. *Two-person packsaddle carry (two people).* Each rescuer grasps his or her own wrist and the other bearer's wrist, forming a seat. Bend your knees and lower the seat. Have the client sit, and wrap each of his or her arms around a rescuer for support. Rescuers must communicate clearly with each other when starting, stopping, turning, and changing direction.	**34.** Safe evacuation technique.
35. *Cradle carry (two people).* Lay client on his or her back and have one rescuer kneel on each side. Each rescuer slides one arm under the client's thighs and the other under the client's back. Each rescuer grasps the other's wrists. On a signal, they rise together, using their legs to lift the client.	**35.** Safe evacuation technique.

▶ REAL WORLD ANECDOTES

Maria has always considered disaster drills an interesting, if far-fetched, diversion from the normal workday. Her feelings changed in one quick moment. It was evening, and she was on her way home from work. Waiting at an intersection, she was startled to see two cars collide in a rainy, dark intersection. One car immediately caught fire. Then, she watched a motorcycle rider, unable to stop in time, lose control and slide under the burning cars. There was hardly time to think, and little time to react, as Maria ran to the rider and pulled him from under the car. Using a modified drag carry, she supported the rider's helmeted head and cervical spine between her forearms, grabbed his motorcycle jacket, and pulled him away from the fire.

▶ EVALUATION
- Client was evacuated to a safe environment without injury to the client or staff member.
- Client had essential medical support restored after the evacuation.

▶ DOCUMENTATION

Nurses' Notes
- Document date and time the disaster occurred.
- Document time of the evacuation.
- Document method used to evacuate the client.
- Document how the client tolerated the evacuation.
- Document postevacuation vital signs.
- Document injuries sustained during the disaster or evacuation.

- Document visitors or family present during or after the disaster and evacuation.

Document on appropriate flow sheet or electronic medical record (EMR).

▶ CRITICAL THINKING SKILL

Introduction
In real life, the client who goes down may need to come back up.

Possible Scenario
A large electrical fire has started somewhere in your outpatient clinic. You are with a client in a treatment room on the third floor when you hear the fire alarm go off. You step out into the hall and immediately see smoke, three feet deep, acrid, thick, and choking, pouring through the vents, rolling along the ceiling

tiles, and swirling around the lights. You hear someone down the hall yelling, "It's on the fourth floor! Get out now!" Your client is in a long-leg cast and crutches. You assist her over to the nearest stairwell, push open the door, check that the stairwell is free of smoke, and tell her to go down quickly. You remain in the clinic, looking for other clients, following the facility's disaster drill protocol.

Possible Outcome

Your client works her way down the stairs. At the first floor, she opens the fire door right into the heart of the fire. A wall of heat and smoke rushes into the stairwell, sucking away the oxygen. Your client turns to make her way back up the stairs, but her heavy cast and crutches slow her down. She gasps for air, breathing in the thick, caustic smoke. Her life is saved by another coworker, who also mistakenly came down the same stairs. He grabs her in a support-walk carry and quickly helps her back up the stairs to another evacuation route. She is hospitalized for smoke inhalation and shock.

Prevention

In your panic, you misunderstood a critical piece of information. The person yelling down the hall actually said, "It's on the *first* floor! Get out now!" While you were not hysterical, you did panic. You should have taken a little more time to assess the information and determine the source of the danger. You needed to assess what evacuation routes were available, then try to determine the source of the fire prior to selecting a route. You should have considered the limited mobility of the client. There were many able-bodied people evacuating at the same time. You should have enlisted one of them to accompany the client if you could not go with her yourself.

► **VARIATIONS**

Geriatric Variations:

- *Older clients may be mobile but may not have the strength or stamina to climb or descend stairs or walk fast.*
- *Older clients may have respiratory deficits that make breathing more difficult with panic or exertion.*
- *Older clients may have hearing or vision difficulties that make it more difficult to navigate in a disaster situation or to hear critical instructions.*

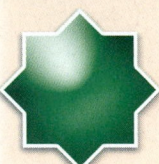

Pediatric Variations:

- *Children should always be accompanied by a parent or rescuer, even if they are physically able to evacuate themselves.*
- *If possible, quickly grab a favorite stuffed animal for the child to hold during and after the evacuation.*
- *If the parent is not with the child at the time of the disaster, keep watch for the parent arriving at the evacuation location. Make it as easy for the parent to locate the child as possible.*
- *Make sure someone remains with the child in the evacuation location.*

Home Care Variations:

- *Take a moment during the home health visit to mentally locate emergency stairwells and evacuation routes in case of a fire, earthquake, or explosion.*
- *Take a moment to check smoke alarms in the home, and know where the fire extinguishers are. Keep a fire extinguisher in your car.*
- *You may need to improvise a stretcher in the home setting. Enlist neighbors and home caregivers to help evacuate the client.*
- *Remember that in the home setting you are more or less on your own to follow an evacuation plan. If the setting is in a high-rise, for example, you may need to carry the client a long distance or down narrow stairs. Keep the principles of safe evacuation in mind, and do not be afraid to recruit help from bystanders.*
- *When possible, grab essential supplies as you evacuate. Equipment or materials will not likely be available nearby in the community setting. If it is a large disaster, help may be delayed.*

continues

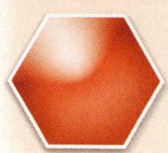

► **VARIATIONS** *(continued)*

Long-Term Care Variation:
• *Study evacuation procedures in the facility, and participate in disaster drills when available.*

► **COMMON ERRORS**

Possible Error:
The client was not disconnected from all tubes, monitors, or intravenous equipment prior to moving.

Prevention:
Mentally review the condition of each client to recall what tubes or equipment are currently in use. Perform a head to toe check for tubes and lines. In an emergency or urgent situation, don't be afraid to move the bed linen away from the body to check for equipment. Be especially careful if the client is unfamiliar to you, or if you are assisting in the evacuation of another floor or area of the facility. If the error occurred, apply pressure to bleeding sites. Clamp tubing. Clamp chest tube (only with physician or qualified practitioner's order) or apply occlusive dressings if needed. Cover sterile sites or tubes with sterile dressings. Take disconnected equipment and new sterile supplies with you to reconnect the client after the evacuation.

► **NURSING TIPS**

• Learn the disaster plan for each facility where you work. Read the manual on your break periodically to refresh your memory.
• Use blankets, sheets, or even privacy curtains to place under the client. Roll up the sides of the material to the client and use as a stretcher or drag the client along on the material.
• Never use the elevator to evacuate clients in an emergency, unless the fire or rescue team in charge of the evacuation gives the "OK" and supervises the elevator use.
• Remove contaminated clothing that may have metal or glass fragments, spilled medications, or liquids that could potentially cause injury to a caregiver or the client.
• Doors, short ladders, and backboards can all be used to improvise stretchers. Keep an eye out for suitable materials.

• Make sure any improvised stretcher will clear passageways and doorways.
• When evacuating any client with a chest tube, remember to toss clamps and occlusive dressings in your pocket for emergency use. Monitor the client for respiratory distress frequently as you evacuate, especially if the environment is chaotic and noisy. There is increased risk that the chest tube might become dislodged and that you will not hear clients in distress in the confusion.
• Support and immobilize the neck whenever possible prior to evacuation, especially if there is the possibility the client has been injured in the disaster. Use tape, sandbags, pillows, towels, full IV bags, or whatever is available.

► **SPECIAL CONSIDERATIONS**

- *In a disaster situation such as earthquake or fire, in order to provide safe and sufficient care, the health care providers need to ensure personal safety first so that the most optimal level of care can be delivered.*
- *If a client has a chest tube in place, be alert for signs and symptoms or tension pneumothorax (shortness of breath, deviation of trachea, changes in mentation).*
- *If clients are on oxygen, IV tubes, or other tubes, be prepared with emergency transport oxygen and other equipment.*

Client Care and Comfort

The Effective Communication Process

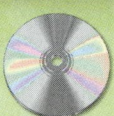

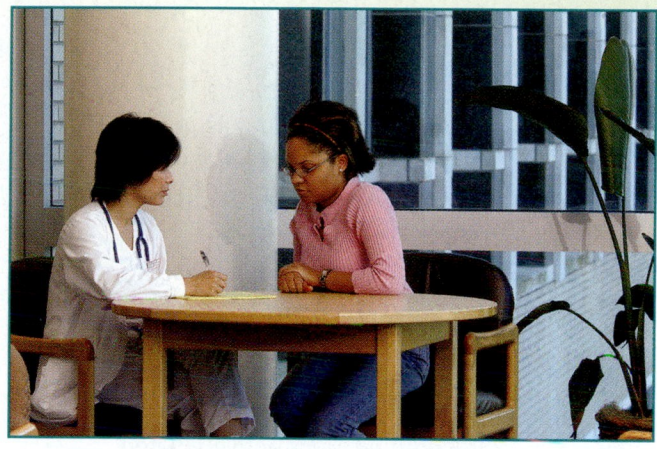

▶ OVERVIEW OF THE SKILL

Communication is a foundation of nursing care. Effective nursing requires clear communication with the client, the family, and other members of the health care team. Communication is a basic ingredient of the nursing process. Assessing, mediating, problem solving, teaching, planning, implementing care, receiving feedback, and many other nursing tasks require clear communication.

The essential components of communication include the sender, the receiver, the message, the message channel, and the feedback to the message (see Figure 3-1-1). The sender is the individual who generates and communicates the message. The sender senses a need to communicate—to express a feeling, to relate to another, to seek to understand, or to request information from another person. The message is generated mentally, then encoded into a form that can be communicated. Eye movements, gestures, words, sounds, facial expressions, and body postures are all forms of communication. The receiver is the person who receives and interprets the message. The message is heard, seen, or felt, then mentally interpreted, or decoded, as the individual decides what is being communicated. How messages are received and interpreted depends on many factors, including the receiver's vision, hearing, level of anxiety, mood, beliefs, values, expectations, and previous experiences.

The message is defined as the package of information being transferred from the sender to the receiver via one or more communication channels. Although messages are often thought of as written or spoken words, a message can be verbal, nonverbal, written, drawn, or sculpted. Verbal messages can be words, language, sounds, songs, or noises. Nonverbal messages include hand and body gestures, facial expressions, and postures. Written and artistic messages include the written word, drawings, photos, and models.

Most messages are packets of information communicated via multiple channels. A verbal message, for example, is a selection of spoken words of certain loudness, pitch, and rate, communicated via the auditory channel, accompanied by facial expressions, posture, and gestures communicated via the visual channel.

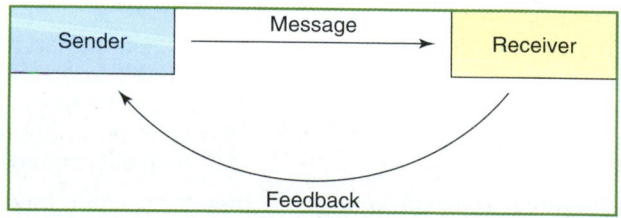

Figure 3-1-1 The nurse and client each act as a sender and receiver, comminicating messages and feedback.

Therapeutic communication is the use of purposeful dialogue directed toward an outcome to improve a client's insight into his or her condition, to manage symptoms and promote healing. The two basic goals of therapeutic communication are: 1) to formulate and send clear messages and 2) to receive, interpret, clarify, and respond to messages sent by the client and other members of the health care team. Two key elements of this process are active listening and communication barriers.

Active listening is the dynamic process individuals engage in when they desire to receive accurate messages.

Table 3-1-1	Therapeutic Communications Techniques	
COMMUNICATION TECHNIQUE	**PURPOSE**	**EXAMPLE**
Broad openings or general leading statements	Initiate conversation, seek information	"Tell me how your day is going." Or, "What brings you in today?"
Restating	Let the client know what the nurse understood	"Are you saying you are angry at the care you have received?"
Clarification/Validation	Seek clear understanding to what client meant	"Let me understand, are you saying that you are upset by my bedside manner? Can you be more specific?"
Reflection	Provide feedback on ideas that emerge from dialogue	"You feel hurt that your wife didn't visit you today."
Listening	Keep eye contact, remain fully attentive	Say nothing. Just actively listen.
Silence	Be completely quiet	Allows client and nurse to reflect and gather thoughts.
Informing or explanation	Educate client by providing facts or recommendations	"This medication is to be taken daily to help lower your cholesterol level."
Suggesting	Present new ideas or alternatives in a nonthreatening manner	"Have you considered increasing your walk by 5 minutes each day to increase your stamina?"
Focusing	Direct dialogue to important topics and further exploration	"Let's go back to discuss the discomfort you mentioned that you had in your abdomen."
Confronting	Redirect client by presenting inconsistencies	"You say you're not upset by your wife's illness; however, when you visit her you cry often." Or, "You say you have minimal pain; however, when I touch your abdomen you jump and grimace."
Share observations	Help to clarify direction	"I noticed that you limp when you put weight on your right leg."
Use of empathy	Respond to client's feeling to demonstrate concern	"It must be difficult to have lost such a dear friend."
Acknowledge client's feelings	Provide feedback	"I recognize that you are upset. How can I help you?"
Open-ended questions	Direct general narrative information, not limited by specific, directed questions. Enables client to lead conversation in the direction desired and may elicit more information.	"You mentioned that you don't sleep well at night. Can you tell me more about this?"
Closed or direct questions	Ask for specific information	"Can you tell me if your chest pain is worse when you exercise?"

It consists of hearing and interpreting words; watching for and interpreting gestures and postures; and identifying and surfacing feelings, undercurrents, or themes in a communication sequence. The goal of active listening is to accurately hear the complete message being sent. Other examples of therapeutic communication skills are listed in Table 3-1-1.

Barriers to communication block or distort communication. Some examples include gender and sociocultural differences, language differences, pain, and cognitive or sensory deficits. More subtle barriers include differences in knowledge, daydreaming, environmental noise, privacy, fatigue, fear, or the use of jargon. Individuals can introduce barriers to communication as they communicate. Blaming or belittling, pressuring, being defensive, using clichés, changing the topic to a more comfortable one, or using "yes or no" questions are all examples of communication blocks. Other examples are given in Table 3-1-2.

▶ **ASSESSMENT**

1. Assess the client's ability to send clear messages. Check for physical barriers such as mental confusion, sedation, or the restricted ability to speak or gesture. Check for emotional or social barriers such as the fear of communicating certain messages, doubts about the appropriateness of when and how to communicate with health care members, or embarrassment over the content of the message. **Determines how to intervene to remove barriers to communication.**

2. Check the ability to receive messages. Look for hearing or vision difficulties. Check for confusion, anxiety, dizziness, or sedation. Check for emotions that may block or skew incoming messages, such as anger, frustration, depression, or doubt. **Determines how to intervene to remove or decrease barriers to communication.**

3. Assess for the amount of information that may effectively be delivered or received and processed in a time block. Sedation, pain, anxiety, and distractions all reduce the amount of information the client can process at one time. Difficult concepts or complicated or detailed information must be delivered at a rate and clarity level that the client can absorb. The nurse must be able to focus on the communication process without distraction. Competing demands may necessitate moving the communication to a different time. **Allows the nurse to select the most appropriate time and amount of information to send and receive.**

4. Check for impediments to communication in the surrounding environment. Ambient noise, bright or dim lighting, the presence of strangers or family members, the lack of privacy, task-oriented "busy" staff, and isolation precautions such as masks and goggles can all impede effective communication. **Allows interventions and modifications to the environment to reduce barriers to communication.**

5. Assess your own ability to receive and send messages. Check for internal biases or beliefs

Table 3-1-2	Barriers to Communication
Lack of eye contact	Use of light-hearted reassurance
Not actively listening	Lack of patience in allowing clients to finish story
Change the subject matter	Previous promises not kept
Posture that reflects impatience	Negative nonverbal clues
Inappropriate use of authority	Use of "why" in an accusatory manner
Avoid answering questions	Unkempt physical appearance
Give your opinion	Talking too much, interrupting
Disagree with client or express disapproval	Using professional jargon
Make stereotyped or culturally insensitive comments	Giving too much "advice"
Use biased questions, such as, "You don't drink, do you?"	Uncomfortable environment—noise or temperature
Become defensive	Use of age-insensitive communication

about clients that may cause you to skew or distort your interpretation of the messages they are sending. Check for your openness to receive messages, including your focus on other tasks, priorities, comfort level with the subject matter, and ability to understand the words and gestures of the client. **Determines how to interpret or seek additional communication.**

▶ DIAGNOSIS

Acute Confusion

Anxiety

Chronic Confusion

Disturbed Sensory Perception

Disturbed Thought Processes

Fear

Hopelessness

Impaired Verbal Communication

Knowledge Deficit

Readiness for Enhanced Communication

Risk for Acute Confusion

▶ PLANNING

Expected Outcomes:

1. The client's environment will be as free from barriers to communication as is possible given the client's physical condition and immediate environment.
2. The nurse will communicate internally generated messages successfully as evident by feedback that confirms the intended message was received by the client or health care team member.
3. The client or health care team member will communicate internally generated messages successfully as evident by feedback that confirms the intended message was received by the nurse.

Equipment Needed:

- Quiet, private area free of distractions or interruptions

- Aids to communication as necessary, including glasses, hearing aids, pencil and paper, computer, sign board, or interpreters
- Comfortable chair or bed for the client and chair for the nurse that places him or her at eye level with the client

▶ CLIENT EDUCATION NEEDED:

1. Explain the need to communicate and the nature of the messages to the client such as assessment, counseling, teaching, delivering or receiving information, or planning.
2. Arrive at mutually agreed upon goals for the communication session: understanding the nature and level of client distress, understanding teaching needs, understanding postoperative exercises, open-ended discussion about client frustrations, and so on.
3. Assure the clients that they are in control of the situation and that they may stop or modify the communication session at any time.
4. Inform the client of the need to provide feedback for messages sent by the nurse. Discuss the nature of feedback, and inform the client how you will signal the need for feedback from the client.
5. Remind clients that even though it is often easier to let a family member communicate for them, it is OK to speak up directly.
6. Teach clients that it is normal to forget information about their care and condition in the stressful hospital setting. Let them know it is OK to ask questions.
7. Remind clients that there are no "dumb" questions.

Estimated time to complete the skill: **1–60 minutes, depending on the nature and content of the communication.**

▶ DELEGATION TIPS

Therapeutic communication is the goal of all professional interactions with clients. Ancillary personnel can greatly facilitate communication with the client if they are properly prepared to do so. To maintain confidentiality, client problems and issues and concerns should be communicated to the nurse for evaluation. All communication should be culturally sensitive, caring, and respectful.

IMPLEMENTATION—Action/Rationale

Action	Rationale
1. Wash hands.	1. Reduces the transmission of microorganisms.
2. Arrange for an uninterrupted time block.	2. Interruptions disrupt the process.
3. Prepare to be an effective communicator: • Decide what information you wish to communicate or solicit. • Determine the appropriate difficulty level for your language and how much information you should attempt to communicate at any one time. • Decide how long the session will be and at what pace to provide messages. • Review the tenants of active listening. • Do a quick internal check for beliefs or prejudices that might affect the ability to communicate.	3. Facilitates successful communication.
4. Assess the environment for barriers to communication. Adjust the environment to facilitate the communication process. Close doors for privacy and move sources of noise away (see Figure 3-1-2) or turn them off if possible. Provide glasses or hearing aids, turn off the TV, remove visual distractions, and so on. Adjust lighting so the client can see you (see Figure 3-1-3), and do not stand with your back to a sunlit window or a bright light (see Figure 3-1-4).	4. Facilitates the transmission of messages.

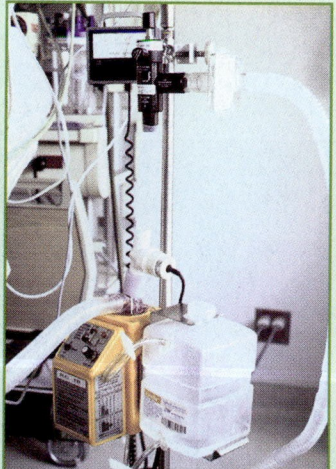

Figure 3-1-2 Noisy equipment or environments can interfere with verbal communication.

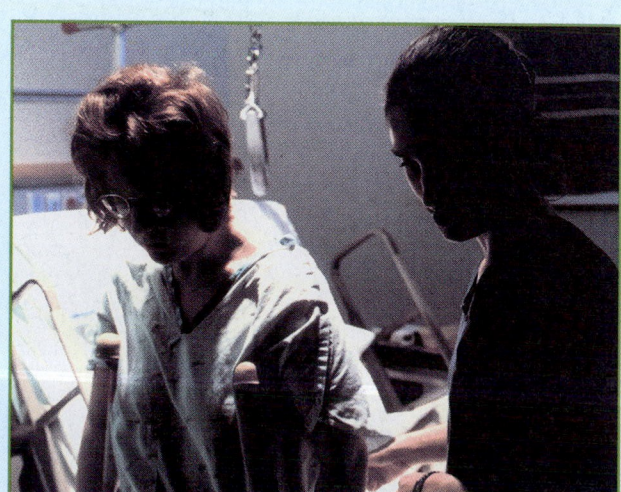

Figure 3-1-3 Poor lighting can interfere with nonverbal communication.

continues

Action	Rationale

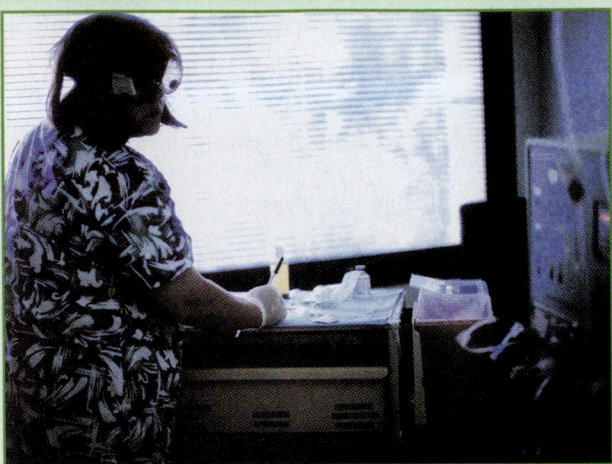

Figure 3-1-4   Standing in front of a bright window or light can prevent the client from seeing the nurse's face or gestures.

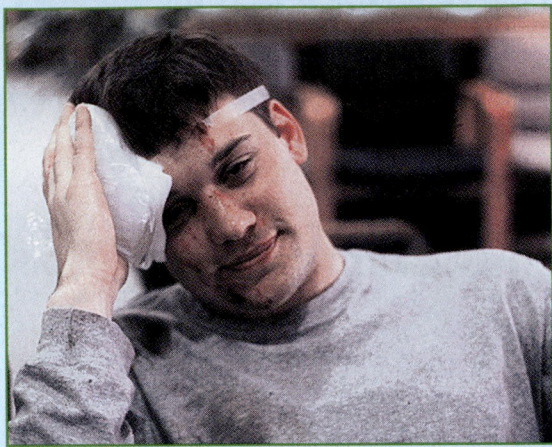

Figure 3-1-5   Pain or anxiety can distract the client from sending and receiving clear messages.

5. Assess the client for barriers to communication, and intervene where possible. Intervene for pain (see Figure 3-1-5), nausea, anxiety, or chills. If appropriate, select a time when the client is feeling alert, awake, and ready and willing to communicate.

5. Establishes the best available environment for the type of communication desired.

6. Sit in a comfortable chair, or squat close to the client (see Figure 3-1-6). You should be at eye level to allow eye contact, to hear and be heard, and to use touch if appropriate (see Figure 3-1-7). Make sure the client is warm and comfortable.

6. Increases client comfort.

7. Provide similar seating to an interpreter or other person participating in the communication.

7. Allows messages to be clearly transmitted.

8. Introduce yourself, and state the purpose of your communication.

8. Reduces confusion.

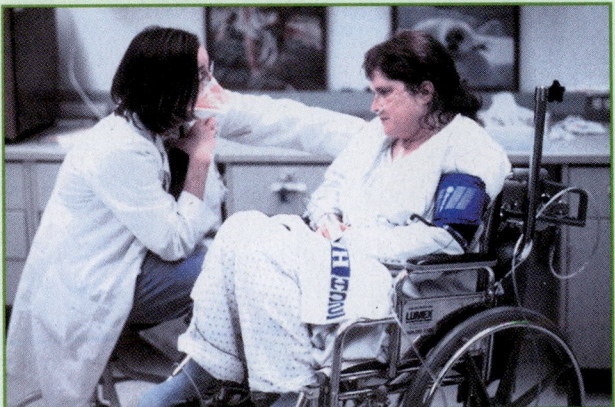

Figure 3-1-6   Squat or sit close to the client to facilitate seeing and hearing messages.

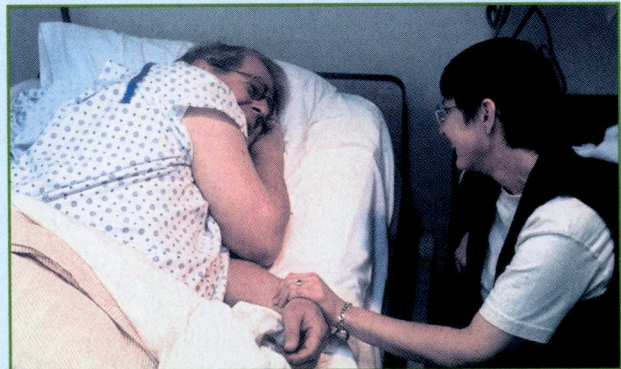

Figure 3-1-7   Position yourself at eye level so both of you can hear, read lips, and observe facial expressions.

continues

Action	Rationale
9. Using the purpose of the communication as a guide, draw the client into the communication session with you. Use techniques that allow the client to set the pace, encourage spontaneity, focus on the client, and encourage the expression of feelings.	9. Initiates the process of communication.
10. At regular intervals during the communication session, request feedback from the client to assess if your communication is being received as you intended it.	10. Gathering feedback enables the nurse to modify the communication and detect barriers.
11. At regular intervals during the session, provide feedback to the client that states what you are hearing the client communicate, both verbally and nonverbally. Request clarification when needed.	11. Providing feedback helps clients assess if they are communicating the message intended. Providing feedback allows the nurse to communicate active listening. The focus of the feedback helps the nurse direct the conversation toward areas not completely understood or communicated.
12. Monitor yourself and your client for nonverbal messages (see Figures 3-1-8 and 3-1-9).	12. Allows further clarification of the messages being communicated. Allows detection of thoughts or emotions that you or the client may be reluctant to verbalize.
13. Assess for signs of boredom, distraction, confusion, or emotional responses. Ask for feedback and clarification. Adjust your communication or terminate the session, if needed.	13. Allows early detection of barriers that might reduce the quality of or end the communication.
14. If the communication session is interrupted, terminate the session if the interruption is a higher priority, or at the client's request. Identify a time and place to resume.	14. Reduces confusion and establishes the importance of the communication.
15. When the information has been communicated by the client, nurse, or family and adequate feedback has been obtained on both sides, terminate the communication session. • Review information if appropriate. • Schedule follow-up communication if appropriate. • Confirm follow-up actions or third-party communications as planned. If information to be passed along is confidential, verify the client's consent.	15. Provides closure to the communication session.

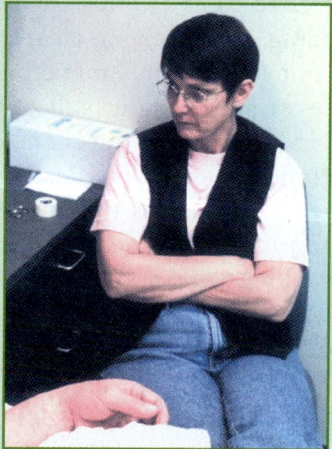

Figure 3-1-8 Crossed arms can communicate a defensive nonverbal message.

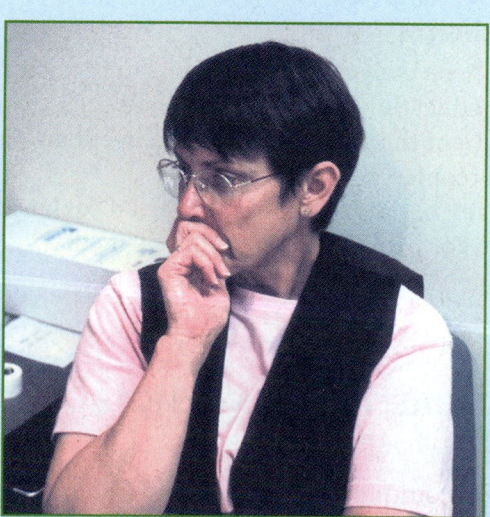

Figure 3-1-9 A hand covering your mouth can interfere with verbal communication.

► REAL WORLD ANECDOTES

David was a newly hired night-shift nurse who abused drugs. Bad days consisted of wild mood swings punctuated by angry outbursts and long silent stares. Other nurses on the lightly staffed unit were afraid of David and concerned about the care he was providing. One nurse who had worked with David in another facility went to the supervisor with her concerns. The supervisor did not keep the information confidential, and the nurse was so harassed by David for "squealing" on him that she requested a transfer.

Things came to a head one night when David restrained an alert and conscious elderly client who was on the unit for telemetry. David would not let him up, and he became more and more agitated. Another nurse intervened. The client called family members who reported the incident to the hospital administrator. David was fired on the spot, and the nurses were reprimanded for not reporting the situation.

Communication about this potentially dangerous situation was suppressed by a barrier of fear. The nurses feared that the supervisor would "tattle," yet "do nothing," and they feared reprisals from David. The nurses needed to communicate with each other to define the problem, identify the barriers, and plan a solution. In this case, putting their concerns in writing and going to the supervisor as a group may have been effective ways to overcome these potentially disastrous communication barriers.

► EVALUATION

- If the communication was about a client concern, have the client evaluate, on a 1–10 rating scale how well the client feels the message was heard and how satisfied the client is with the response.
- Review the discussion. Determine what worked well and whether any distractions were evident. Identify the emotions that arose during the session and describe any nonverbal gestures that were noted.
- Evaluate the outcome of the communication. Determine whether behaviors or nonverbal communications have changed and whether learning has occurred.

► DOCUMENTATION

Nurses' Notes

- Document the type of communication such as client education, support, and planning.
- Document the subject matter, the feedback, and the outcomes, if any.
- Note any barriers to communication such as pain, anxiety, or hearing or visual impairments.

Document on appropriate flow sheet or electronic medical record (EMR).

► CRITICAL THINKING SKILL

Introduction

Nonverbal communication can be ambiguous. Clarify with verbal communication when possible.

Possible Scenario

Joy is on your unit recovering from a hysterectomy. She is not on client-controlled analgesia (PCA) and has requested pain medication. You enter her room about 10 minutes after her request, and she is resting in bed with her eyes closed.

Possible Outcome

Assuming that she has fallen asleep, you pause in the doorway. After a few seconds, you conclude that she is not in pain and leave the room. A half-hour later, she calls again. When you arrive and ask how her nap was, she bursts into tears. "I can't sleep! I hurt so much and you forgot to bring me a pain shot! I keep trying to doze off to escape the pain, but it is no use! Where have you been?"

Prevention

The nurse needed to assess this client for pain. This requires sending and receiving clear messages, both verbal and nonverbal. The nonverbal messages of closing the eyes and holding still were misread by the nurse as indicating that the client was asleep and that she no longer desired medication for the pain. The nurse needed to assess the nonverbal messages while standing at the bedside, then send a quiet verbal message, along with nonverbal touch, announcing her presence and confirming the request for pain medication.

▶ VARIATIONS

Geriatric Variations:

- *Geriatric clients are much more likely to have hearing and visual difficulties that make communication more difficult. Be sure to assess the cognitive and sensory abilities.*
- *Geriatric clients may not be as familiar with the "jargon" used by younger generations. This could lead to confusing messages.*
- *Geriatric clients with sensory deficits may have more stress and anxiety caused by the difficulty of maintaining good communication and feedback about unfamiliar procedures and environments.*
- *If elderly clients are hard-of-hearing, remember to stand in front of them at eye level so they can see your lips. Keep your hands away from your mouth. Speak slowly and distinctly. Do not shout.*

Pediatric Variations:

- *Match the difficulty of the words you choose with the age of the child.*
- *Remember that younger children will more likely take what you say literally.*
- *Ask the parent to tell you special words or phrases that have meaning for the child.*
- *The parent can often help interpret complex nonverbal behaviors that indicate the child is afraid, tired, or in pain.*
- *Assessing the needs of the preverbal, nonverbal, or sensory-impaired child can be a challenge. Do not assume needs are not present just because they are not communicated verbally.*

Home Care Variations:

- *Remember that as a caregiver, you are a guest in the client's home. The client may need some time to evaluate you and establish trust before communicating important messages. Facilitate this by using nonjudgmental, open, and friendly words or gestures. Keep communication short and friendly, and select nonthreatening topics while trust is being established.*
- *Communications and education in the stressful hospital environment are often poorly received. A post-hospitalization home visit is a good time to review and clarify education and information received in the hospital.*

Long-Term Care Variations:

- *Smaller staffing in long-term facilities may limit the communication a staff member can engage in with a client. Staff members need to take every opportunity to communicate while other tasks are being performed such as eating or bathing.*
- *Staff members in task-oriented positions may find it difficult to practice active listening, especially with clients who have physical or mental communication restrictions. Setting aside time for one-on-one communication is important nursing care.*

▶ COMMON ERRORS

Possible Error:

Reassuring the client before completely listening to the concern.

Prevention:

Recognize your desire to make the client feel better. Recognize that the real concerns may not come up in the first few sentences. Use open-ended questions to gently explore the concern.

Possible Error:

Avoiding an uncomfortable message: "Nurse, I think I am dying."

continues

▶ COMMON ERRORS *(continued)*

Prevention:

Learn to recognize your internal reactions to a threatening or uncomfortable message. Learn to recognize ways of dealing with uncomfortable messages. Set a priority on communication over tasks, especially when the message is important.

Respond by stopping the task and expressing the desire to hear more. Communicate quietly and gently to the client the message heard, and ask for feedback and confirmation. Ask open-ended questions, and ask if the client wishes to discuss the message further. If necessary, schedule a time to return to the client later. Do not forget.

Possible Error:

The client cannot hear your words.

Prevention:

Position yourself close to the client. Speak clearly but do not yell. Speak into the client's ear if helpful. Make sure your voice does not lower in volume at the end of a sentence.

▶ NURSING TIPS

- As a rule of thumb, when soliciting information, ask two to three open-ended questions for every statement you make.
- As a rule of thumb, when providing education, try to ask one open-ended question for every three points you make.
- When practicing active listening, restate what you have heard in your own words. Rather than saying, "I hear you," say, "This is what I am hearing . . . is this correct?"
- Understand that angry messages often hide fear and vulnerability. Find and respond to the underlying messages as well as the communicated one.

- Communication is a complex subject. To truly learn therapeutic communication, seek out additional learning resources. Practice your skills in a variety of settings, then apply what you have learned to your nursing care.
- Drawing pictures as you speak, or having the client draw or point to pictures to illustrate concepts, helps minimize daydreaming and provides another avenue of communication.
- Remember that a client can speak the same language but be from a different culture or country. Words may have different meanings.
- Maintain eye contact when speaking with clients.

▶ SPECIAL CONSIDERATIONS

- *When interviewing a cognitively capable client whose spouse or significant other answers all or many of the questions, the nurse should suspect that the client may be a victim of domestic abuse. The client might look at the partner before answering questions as well. The nurse should find a way to isolate the client from the spouse or significant other and tactfully ask if the client feels safe at home, or feels threatened in any way. This can be done by developing a policy where part of the exam is always done with only the client in the room or you can request, if the client is a woman, that she go to the bathroom for a urine sample (if appropriate) where you might assist her and talk with her.*
- *When a child presents with injuries inconsistent with the history given by the parent, the nurse should suspect child abuse and would be remiss not to follow up. Abusive parents are usually overly attentive when they have injured a child, and this communication should be noted as well.*

Guided Imagery

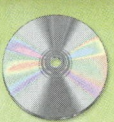

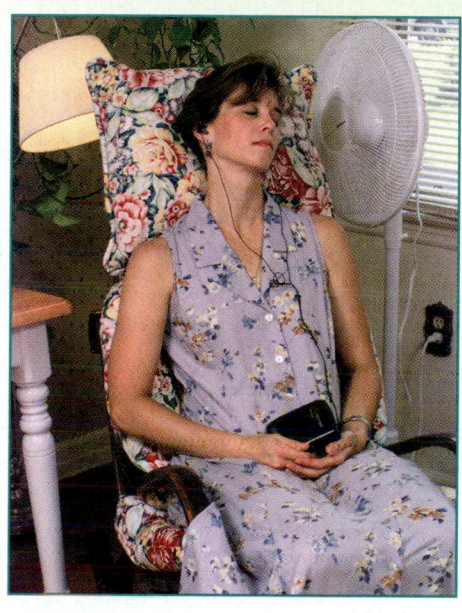

▶ OVERVIEW OF THE SKILL

Guided imagery or visualization is a technique that uses an individual's imagination to elicit positive images to reduce stress, decrease pain, or promote healing. Imagery has been used effectively in a wide variety of situations: symptom management of cancer and chemotherapy, chronic pain management and stress reduction, substance abuse counseling, sleep disorders, allergies and asthma, labor and delivery, headaches, migraines, hypertension, and a myriad of other conditions.

There are many types of visualization techniques. Clients will sometimes listen to a prerecorded audiotape guiding them through the imagery process. Common to all techniques is a positive mental image that encompasses all the senses in a very comfortable atmosphere free of interruption (see Figure 3-2-1). With practice, nurses can guide clients through this process using a variety of scripts that elicit positive images from the client. There are several resources available offering scripts and tapes for using imagery.

▶ ASSESSMENT

The procedure should first be explained to the client, then assess the client for the following:

1. Assess the client's mental status **to determine whether the client has signs of active psychosis or has a tenuous hold on reality. Such clients should not take part in guided imagery.**

2. Assess the client's sensory or cognitive deficits **to establish whether any hearing,**

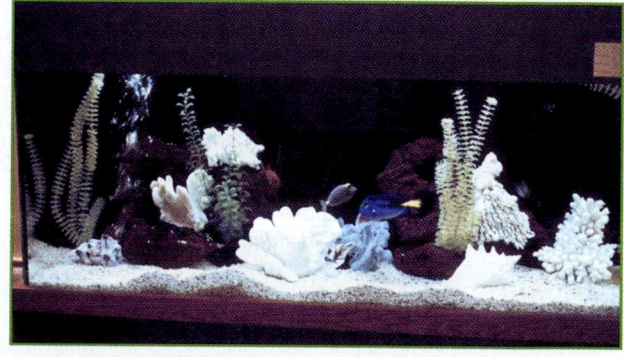

Figure 3-2-1   Help the client visualize a calming place or scene.

vision, or neurologic deficits will influence the procedure.

3. Discuss the procedure with the client **to determine his or her willingness to participate in the imagery exercise.** The intervention will be more beneficial with a willing client.

4. Have clients describe their current problem; identify key words in their description such as "sharp, stabbing pain," "throbbing headache," or "agitated and jumpy." **Identifying key descriptors both before and after the session will help to determine whether there has been improvement in the client's condition.**

5. Identify your own feelings regarding imagery's effectiveness. **Confidence in imagery as an intervention will increase the effectiveness of the session.**

▶ DIAGNOSIS

Acute Pain

Chronic Pain

Anxiety

Disturbed Sleep Pattern

▶ PLANNING

Expected Outcomes:

1. The client will experience a decrease in pain.
2. The client will experience a decrease in anxiety.

3. The client will verbalize an increase in coping methods.
4. The client will experience an increased sense of self-control.

Equipment Needed:

- Quiet, comfortable environment free of distractions
- Music or other material for client's comfort
- Prerecorded script if not providing your own
- Blankets, pillows, and a comfortable bed or recliner

▶ CLIENT EDUCATION NEEDED:

1. Explain the procedure and potential benefits to the client.
2. Arrive at a mutually agreed upon goal and positive expectation for the session: reduced anxiety, pain, and so on.
3. Assure clients that they are in control of the situation and may stop at any time if they wish.
4. Let the client know that it is not uncommon for pent-up emotions to surface. Unexplained feelings of sadness, anger, or joy are common.

Estimated time to complete the skill:
10–20 minutes

▶ DELEGATION TIPS

Guided imagery techniques may be delegated to any individual prepared to teach the technique.

IMPLEMENTATION—Action/Rationale

Action	Rationale
1. Wash hands	1. Reduces the transmission of microorganisms.
2. Explain the procedure to the client.	2. The client must have an understanding of the procedure to gain the most benefit.
3. Select a comfortable quiet environment that will be free of distraction for approximately 20 minutes. Ensure that the room temperature is comfortable.	3. The client must be comfortable and the session uninterrupted for maximum effectiveness.

continues

Action	Rationale

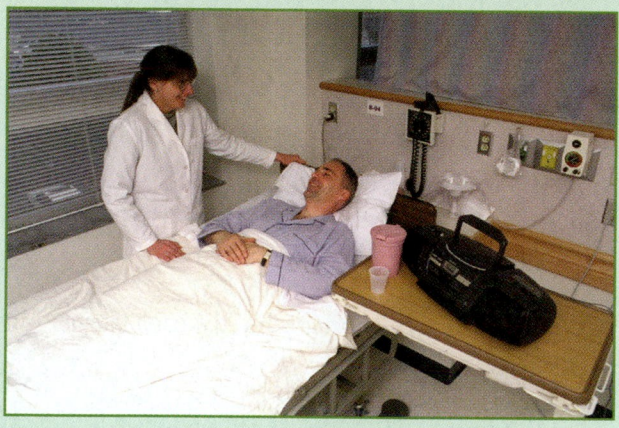

Figure 3-2-2 Place the client in a comfortable position prior to beginning the session.

4. Ensure that the client is in a comfortable position and turn on either the relaxing background music or prerecorded audiotape (see Figure 3-2-2).

4. This maximizes the client's comfort.

5. If you are using your own script, begin the session with a few relaxing breaths, then proceed to guide the client to a pleasing, restful place. Use a soft, relaxed voice. Use pauses in your script for maximum effectiveness.
Example:

"Relax with each breath." Ask the client to focus on feeling inspiration and expiration, and allow for a prolonged cleansing expiration.

"Let your imagination take you to a place where you are comfortable and safe. Go deeper into your thoughts with each breath."

Help guide clients to their special place. It may be a mountain meadow, a spot in the forest, a garden, the beach, or a special room. "This is your safe and special place. Any time that you're stressed, you can go to this place."

There are many options from here, depending on what the client has selected as the special place.

"Imagine yourself walking along your mountain path. Listen to the sounds of your feet on the path . . . smell the air . . . the trees . . . the flowers . . . feel the cool breeze."

"You are nearing a spot next to a creek . . . listen to the water splash off the rocks."

"Sit down next to the creek and relax."

"Dip your feet into the cool water . . . feel the shiver up your spine . . . the refreshing coolness on your feet."

"Relax next to the creek . . .you're cooled from your dip . . . lie down and listen to the birds . . . the creek."

5. A relaxing breath is an inhalation followed by a slow exhalation with a conscious relaxation of the whole body with each breath.

Briefly discuss the client's special place so that you can help to guide the client and tailor the imagery to the special place.

Pause between statements to help clients concentrate on their visions.

You can vary your script as needed for the situation. Feel free to ask the client about his feelings about the experience and whether the imagery is effective.

Bring as many of the senses as possible into the image.

Allows the client to relax.

continues

Action	Rationale
"Feel the warmth of the sun coming through the trees. See the white clouds against the blue sky." "You don't have to go anywhere, just relax by the creek for awhile." Trust your intuition and watch for signs of relaxation, tension, and emotion. Watch for changes in body language, facial expressions, and signs of sadness such as tears.	
6. Slowly bring the client back to the present. Have the client begin moving the hands, arms, and feet while taking some deep breaths. Assure the client that he or she is safe and can go to this special place whenever needed.	**6.** Brings the client back to reality in a calm manner and reenergizes him or her.

▶ REAL WORLD ANECDOTES

Mrs. Fung was going through her second round of chemotherapy. She had suffered from extreme mucositis during her first chemotherapy round and expected the same during her second course. She was approached about trying some guided imagery this time and was open to the suggestion. The imagery technique was introduced early in her regimen before the chemotherapy's effects. Her image included imagining that the skin in her mouth was growing together, closing the sores with the aid of small helping hands reaching toward one another. She also worked with imagining the pain of her mouth sores as a light bulb that she could control using a dimmer switch. Mrs. Fung still needed a client-controlled analgesic of morphine to help control her pain but required less morphine and felt more in control of her situation than during her first course of chemotherapy.

▶ EVALUATION

- The client experienced a decrease in pain.
- The client experienced a decrease in anxiety.
- The client verbalized an increase in coping methods.
- The client experienced an increased sense of self-control.

▶ DOCUMENTATION

Nurses' Notes

- Document the session according to institutional policy.
- Include date, time, and length of the session.
- Identify the client's specific complaint and key descriptors from both before and after the session.
- Note any emotional or physiologic changes that the client experiences, especially statements of satisfaction with the experience.

Document on appropriate flow sheet or electronic medical record (EMR).

▶ CRITICAL THINKING SKILL

Introduction

Guided imagery can be used in many situations. Imagery can be used to promote healing, increase self-control, and decrease recovery time.

Possible Scenario

A client has been admitted to the oncology floor for an autologous stem cell transplant. There will be a prolonged period of neutropenia while she is waiting for engraftment. The client is taught guided imagery early in her regimen. Her image is one of the "baby" stem cells being infused into her empty marrow, growing and rapidly dividing, filling up her marrow. As they are growing they are getting more and more defensive, protecting her from invaders. As her neutrophil counts increase, she imagines them as large troops of soldiers protecting her.

Possible Outcome

The client will still be covered with prophylactic antibiotics during her regimen and time of neutropenia. The imagery will give her a sense of self-control during a period of otherwise helplessness and vulnerability to infection.

Prevention

Anxiety and the fear of infection are substantial factors during the period of neutropenia after stem cell or bone marrow transplant. By giving people a sense of self-control, this anxiety can be reduced, decreasing the amount of anti-anxiety medications normally required. This can increase client activity and ambulation, decreasing problems such as respiratory compromise and venostasis, which are caused by inactivity, and also decreasing recovery time.

► VARIATIONS

Geriatric Variations:
- *Often senior adults will enjoy remembering back to times of their youth. This can be a time of recollection for them.*
- *Be sure to assess for cognitive and sensory deficits. The session may need to be altered to accommodate them.*
- *Stay alert for signs of sleeping or loss of interest.*

Pediatric Variations:
- *Children have very active imaginations and are adept at guided imagery.*
- *Children may be more comfortable with a parent or guardian with them.*
- *If appropriate, teach a parent or guardian how to guide the child through the process.*
- *Encourage children to use their safe spot on their own during times of stress.*
- *Watch for signs of distraction—children have shorter attention spans.*

Home Care Variations:
- *Make sure the area is free of distraction. You may want to take the phone off the hook.*
- *Train caregivers or loved ones how to use or assist with imagery techniques, if appropriate.*
- *Encourage clients to try the technique on their own.*

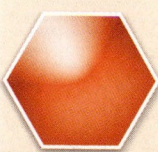

Long-Term Care Variations:
- *Arrange for a quiet area free of distraction.*
- *Be sure to assess cognitive and sensory abilities, you may need to speak louder or keep sessions shorter.*
- *Sessions may be performed with small groups on a regular basis to increase socialization and discussion.*

► COMMON ERRORS

Possible Error:
Client did not relax or enjoy the session because the setting and scenario were not conducive to relaxation and imagery.

Prevention:
Prepare for each session. Some ways to prepare include:
If you are not using a prerecorded tape, practice your script's general flow.

continues

► **COMMON ERRORS** (continued)

Do not read your script. Let the script flow naturally, following your intuition.
Use pauses in your script for maximum effectiveness.
Do not talk too much; let the imagination work.
Encourage the client to suggest effective imagery. The image of an ocean beach may be empty and relaxing for one client but crowded with people and energizing for another.
Choose a quiet time of the day and eliminate distractions as much as possible. A knock on the door can abruptly terminate the most focused imagery session.

► **NURSING TIPS**

- Introduce guided imagery as early as possible in the client's regimen. Research shows that the earlier it is introduced the more effective it is.
- Know your own feelings toward imagery. You must believe in its effectiveness to maximize its benefits.
- This is the client's experience; you are only the guide. Do not be disappointed if the client does not report a positive experience. It is not a sign of failure on your part. Explore other relaxation options with the client.
- Do not prejudge whether a client will be receptive to guided imagery. Offer it to anyone who may benefit from its results.
- Some clients twitch and fidget and send nonverbal cues of throat clearing and hand motions. They cannot seem to relax and concentrate. Allow this to happen, especially at the start of the session. If it continues and you feel the client is not able to follow the process, gently inquire. Stop if necessary and talk with the client about possible solutions.

- Make sure your nonverbal communication is not stressful. If you are feeling rushed or uncomfortable, your respiratory rate might be increased, your muscles might be tense, and you may fidget and be a distraction to the client. Make it a habit to quiet and calm yourself before interacting with the client. One way to do this is to imagine that your tension is like a tightly wound spring. Take a deep breath and "unhook" each end of the spring, and allow 10 seconds of visualization as you "watch" it unwind into a flat line. Take another deep breath. Relax your shoulders. Continue to breathe slowly and deeply, and stay relaxed as you approach the client.
- Warm compresses, used in conjunction with imagery, may enhance relaxation.
- Breathing techniques, with varying patterns, require concentration and can be used to enhance imagery. Information is available through childbirth educators.

► **SPECIAL CONSIDERATIONS**

- *Gather as much information as you can about the client before conducting the relaxation session. The client may have a history of posttraumatic stress, fear of certain objects, phobias, or past unpleasant experiences associated with certain scenes or objects. Avoid those experiences from the imagery script.*
- *For clients with posttraumatic stress or a history of sexual assault or abuse, be aware of the professional therapeutic relationship. Avoid conducting the imagery session in an isolated environment. Avoid using an opposite sex therapist if sexual assault was involved. Stimulation that is related to the event may trigger the memory of the past unpleasant or stressful experience.*
- *Guided imagery and visualization can be an effective tool in relaxation and distraction during labor and delivery. If the client has not received instruction previously in the use of these techniques, practice it in the early stages of labor. Help create an image or use an actual picture that can be placed on the wall or ceiling if the client is in a recumbent position.*

Progressive Muscle Relaxation

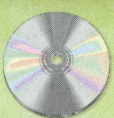

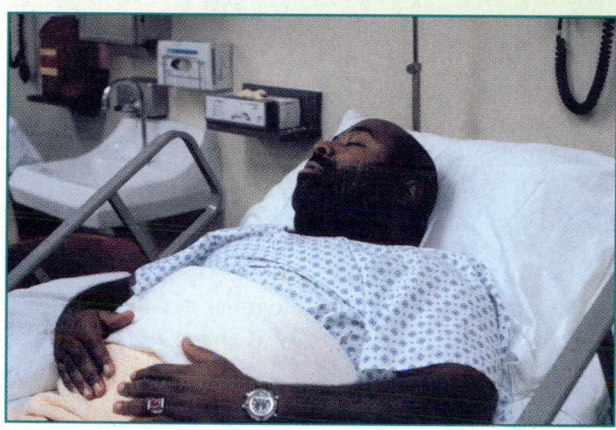

▶ OVERVIEW OF THE SKILL

Developed by Dr. Edmund Jacobsen in 1927, progressive relaxation is based on the theory that muscle tension is the body's response to anxiety-provoking thoughts, whereas deep muscle relaxation decreases physiologic tension and blocks anxiety. Clients tightly tense, then completely relax, muscle groups in a systematic manner. Progressive relaxation can reduce pulse and respiratory rates and has provided positive results for those with muscle spasms, lower-back pain, migraines, hypertension, irritable bowel, and mild phobias. It has also been used as an adjunct to traditional therapies for chemotherapy-induced nausea and vomiting. Progressive muscle relaxation is a procedure that is easily learned, easy to teach, and can be beneficial in a wide variety of situations.

Each muscle group is tightly tensed for 5 to 7 seconds, then relaxed for 20 to 30 seconds. Respirations can be coordinated with these actions, inhaling while tensing, then slowly exhaling while relaxing the muscle group. The major muscle groups are covered: face, neck, and shoulders; hands, forearms, and biceps; chest, abdomen, and lower back; and buttocks, thighs, calves, and feet.

When clients enter a state of deep relaxation, they may experience a release of blocked emotional issues both at a conscious and unconscious level. It is not unusual for a client to experience unexplained sadness or tears or for unexplained physiologic changes to take place, for example, rapid breathing, change in heart rate, and so forth. Many clients report a feeling of release with these experiences, often invoking thoughts of long-buried emotional experiences. Other common sensations are feelings of floating, drifting, or moving, and a feeling that limbs and joints are disconnected from the body.

▶ ASSESSMENT

1. Check the client's mental status. **Clients with active psychosis or those with a tenuous hold on reality are contraindicated for this procedure.**
2. Check for any sensory deficits. **Hearing, vision, or other neurologic deficits affect how you administer the procedure.**
3. Determine that the client is willing to participate in the relaxation exercise. **The procedure is more beneficial with a willing client.**
4. Check the nature of the medical or emotional problem. **Areas that are injured should not be actively tensed. Knowing the problem will help assess the intervention's effectiveness.**
5. Have the client quantify the problem, such as using a 1- to 10-point pain scale. Quantifying results provides more validity to the intervention.

▶ DIAGNOSIS

Disturbed Energy Field

Acute Pain

Anxiety

Insomnia

▶ PLANNING

Expected Outcomes:

1. The client will experience a decrease in anxiety.
2. The client will experience a decrease in pain.
3. The client will experience a decrease in nausea.
4. The client will experience a decrease in insomnia.
5. The client will report an increase sense of self-control.

Equipment Needed:

- Quiet environment, without distraction or interruptions
- Music or ambient noise recordings
- Blankets
- Pillows
- Recliner (see Figure 3-3-1)
- Bed

▶ CLIENT EDUCATION NEEDED:

1. Explain procedure and the potential benefits to the client.
2. Arrive at mutually agreed upon goals for the session: reduced tension, decreased pain, anxiety, and so forth.
3. Practice relaxed breathing and its timing with alternating tensing and relaxation.
4. Assure the client that he or she is in control of the situation and may stop the procedure at any time.
5. Encourage the client to listen to his or her own body and not to tense or overtighten an injured or sore muscle.
6. Let the client know that it is normal to get distracted but, with practice, he or she will be able to stay better focused.

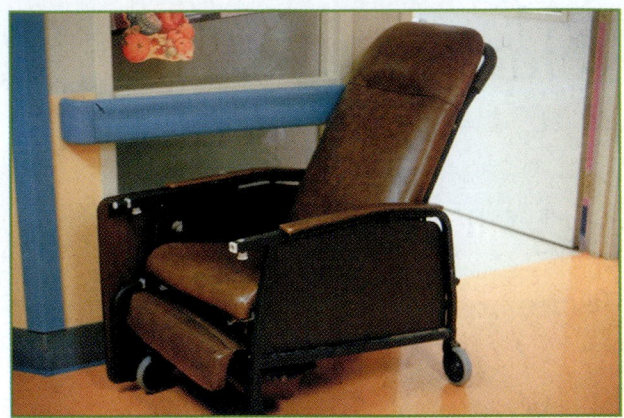

Figure 3-3-1   Recliner

7. Assure the client that feelings of floating, warmth, spinning, or heaviness are all natural experiences of relaxation. If these sensations become uncomfortable, the client can open the eyes to reorient self.
8. Let the client know that he or she should do a session 1 hour before or 2 hours after meals. Relaxation with a full stomach can lead to sleep.
9. Make sure that the client knows that you are only a guide. Any benefits received from the session are the result of the client's own efforts.
10. Make sure that the clients knows that they can perform the procedure any time on their own and that it is beneficial for a variety of problems.
11. Help the client to distinguish between a tense and a relaxed muscle state. Encourage client to assess the degree of tension at regular intervals during the day, and to relax the muscles in between sessions.

Estimated time to complete the skill:
15–30 minutes

▶ DELEGATION TIPS

Progressive muscle relaxation techniques may be delegated to any individual prepared to teach the technique.

IMPLEMENTATION—Action/Rationale

Action	Rationale

Action

1. Wash hands.

2. Arrange for an uninterrupted 15–30 minute time block.

3. Decrease lighting level and turn on music to desirable level.

4. Seat client in comfortable recliner, or in bed if necessary, using pillows to prop up arms at the sides (see Figure 3-3-2). Make sure that client is warm.

5. Have client take 3–6 breaths, relaxing deeply with each breath (see Figure 3-3-3).

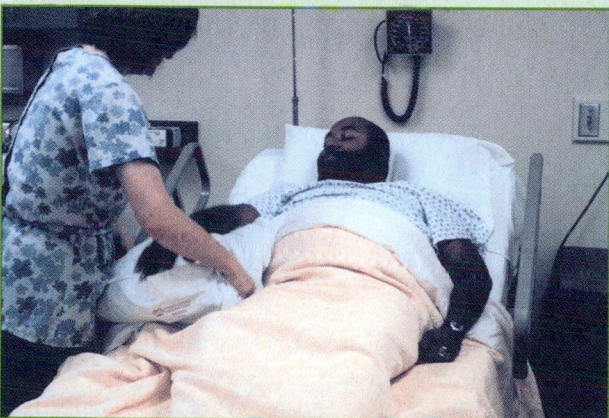

Figure 3-3-2 Use pillows to prop up the client's arms for comfort prior to beginning the session.

6. As you instruct the client, keep your voice calm and smooth. Gently correct positioning and tensing if needed, but then move smoothly on to the next segment (see Figure 3-3-4).

7. Begin the tensing–relaxation process in the following order, coordinating inhalation, and slow exhalation with relaxation:
- Face, jaw, mouth (squint eyes and grimace)
- Neck (pull chin to neck)
- Right hand (make a fist) and then relax (see Figures 3-3-5 and 3-3-6)
- Right arm (bend elbow in tightly and then relax)
- Left hand (make a fist and then relax)
- Left arm (bend elbow in tightly then relax)
- Back, shoulders, chest (shrug shoulders up tightly then relax them)
- Abdomen (pull abdomen in strongly then relax)
- Right upper leg (push upper leg down strongly then relax leg (see Figure 3-3-7)

Rationale

1. Reduces the transmission of microorganisms.

2. Interruptions disrupt the process.

3. Heightens relaxation.

4. Increases client comfort.

5. Allows client to center thoughts.

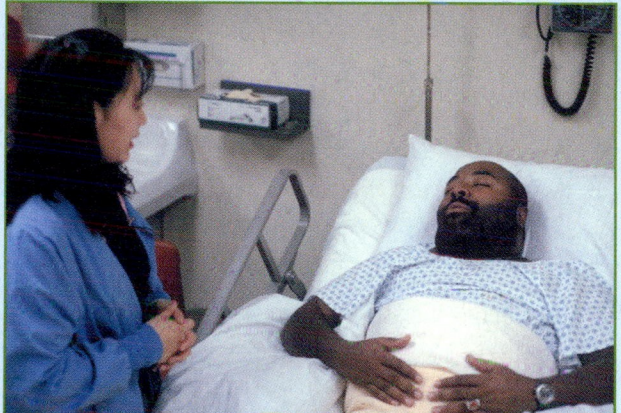

Figure 3-3-3 Have the client take 3–6 slow, deep breaths.

6. Allows the client to focus on the content of your voice and not be distracted.

continues

Action	Rationale

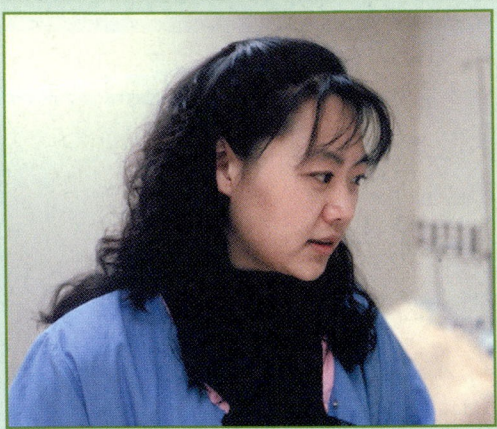

Figure 3-3-4 Keep your voice calm and smooth when guiding the client through progressive relaxation stages.

- Right lower leg (point toes toward body then relax leg)
- Left upper leg (push upper leg down strongly then relax leg)
- Left lower leg (point toes toward body then relax leg)

8. Have client finish with 3–6 additional relaxation breaths (see Figure 3-3-8).

9. Have client slowly move feet, hands, arms, legs, reopen eyes, and reorient himself or herself (see Figure 3-3-9).

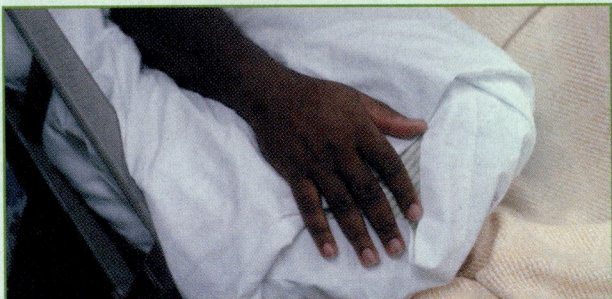

Figure 3-3-6 Have the client relax hand completely.

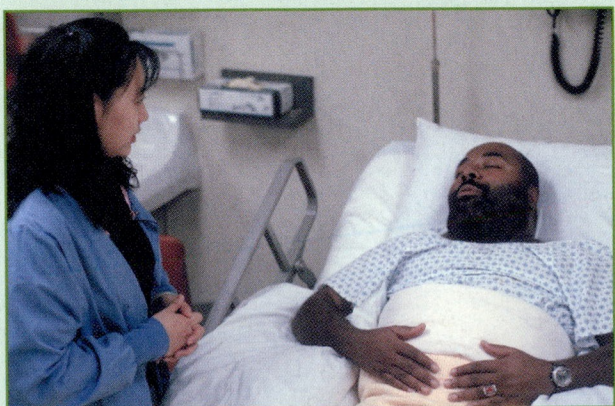

Figure 3-3-8 Finish the session by instructing the client to take 3–6 deep relaxation breaths.

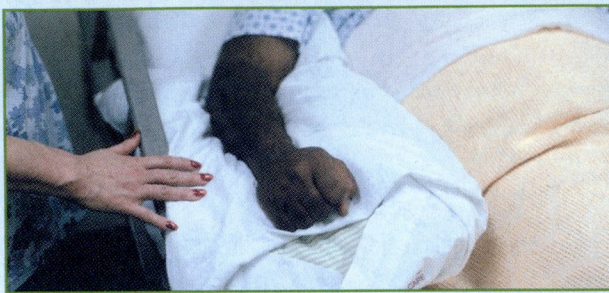

Figure 3-3-5 Have the client tense each hand by making a fist.

7. Coordinating the breathing increases relaxation.

8. Provides a sense of closure to the procedure.

9. Slowly reenergizes the client.

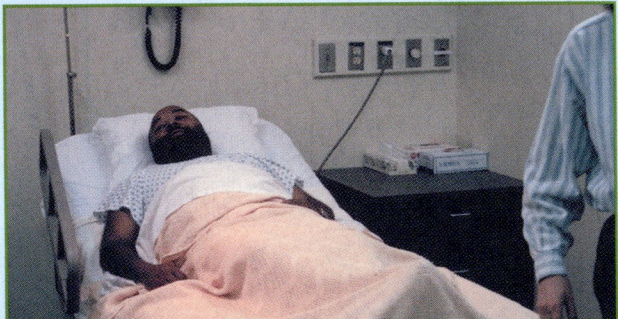

Figure 3-3-7 Have the client tense and relax one leg at a time.

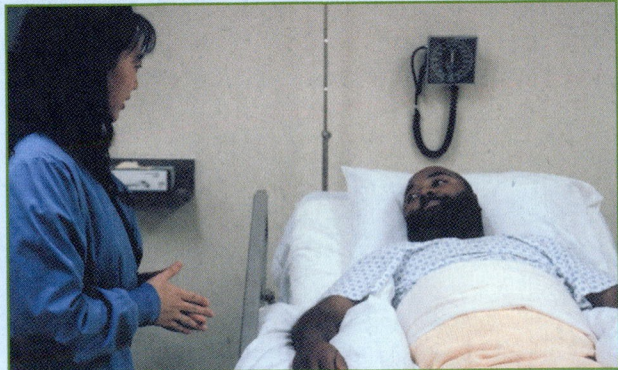

Figure 3-3-9 Allow the client time to open his or her eyes and reorient to the surrounding environment.

▶ REAL WORLD ANECDOTES

Mrs. Smith, a high-dose chemotherapy client with breast cancer, reported a very uncomfortable sadness during the first two sessions of progressive muscle relaxation. She stated that the sessions were improving her nausea, but she couldn't shake the uneasy feelings she was experiencing. After the third session, she mentioned that she was experiencing flashbacks to her adolescence in the early 1970s, when her aunt died of breast cancer, and the circumstances surrounding that experience. The nurse discussed the differences between the treatments her aunt received back in the 1970s and what she was receiving, and also what a better prognosis she had because her cancer was caught much earlier than her aunt's cancer. Mrs. Smith reported that the following session was much nicer, and much more relaxing. She was able to continue the relaxation sessions on her own after a few more sessions.

▶ EVALUATION

- The client experienced a decrease in anxiety.
- The client experienced a decrease in pain.
- The client experienced a decrease in nausea.
- The client experienced a decrease in insomnia.
- The client reported an increased sense of self-control.

▶ DOCUMENTATION

Nurses' Notes

- Record intervention and outcomes.
- Record the specific complaint, pain, and so forth, with a quantitative rating, both before and after the intervention.
- Note emotional or physiologic changes that the client experiences, such as reduced pain or anxiety, and especially statements of satisfaction with the experience.

Document on appropriate flow sheet or electronic medical record (EMR).

▶ CRITICAL THINKING SKILL

Introduction

In this situation, a nurse introduces progressive muscle relaxation to a client who has been experiencing anticipatory nausea and vomiting before her daily chemotherapy sessions.

Possible Scenario

Mrs. Jones has been receiving daily doses of oral busulfan in preparation for peripheral stem cell transplantation. She has had a problem with gagging and retching before she begins taking the large capsules. She does not like the "loopy" feeling that she gets from Aptiva, and none of the antiemetics she has been taking has been helping. The nurse suggests that she might want to try some progressive muscle relaxation before taking her medication. Mrs. Jones is a little hesitant but willing to try anything at this point.

Possible Outcome

Mrs. Jones's nurse contacts the psychosocial nurse practitioner, who arranges a session in the hour before the medication is due. With Mrs. Jones's permission, the nurse practitioner explains the treatment, lowers the lights, turns off the ringer on the phone, and turns off her pager. She plays some low-key music on a portable CD player she has brought. She helps Mrs. Jones lower the head of the bed and get comfortable with pillows under her arms and her head. She places a "Do Not Disturb" sign on the door. After 20 minutes of progressive relaxation, Mrs. Jones is relaxed and drowsy. She is breathing slowly, deeply, and evenly while lying quietly with her eyes closed. The nurse comes in and quietly administers the busulfan. Mrs. Jones has no difficulty swallowing the capsules and returns to her restful state almost immediately.

Prevention

Without control of her nausea, Mrs. Jones may vomit her medication, leading to inaccurate dosing. Anticipation of each treatment can cause significant nausea. Without some measure of control, Mrs. Jones's nausea could decrease her compliance with the regimen and lead to nutritional deficits and potential electrolyte imbalances. Introducing progressive muscle relaxation early in Mrs. Jones's treatment gives her a sense of self-control. It also gives her an alternative to the sedative qualities of many of the antiemetics such as Compazine. By avoiding the use of antianxiety medications, the client was able to stay more alert and oriented during her treatments. She felt more active and ambulatory. Her increased activity helped her to avoid respiratory and circulatory stasis.

► VARIATIONS

Geriatric Variations:

- *If the client has problems with chronic joint pain or arthritis, passive muscle relaxation may be substituted for the active tension–relaxing of progressive muscle relaxation. The procedure is done in the same order as progressive muscle relaxation. The client brings his or her awareness to the muscle group of focus and, using a deep relaxing breath, relaxes the muscle group a little more with each exhalation.*
- *Be sure to assess the client's cognitive and sensory abilities. You may need to speak louder, or make the session a little shorter.*

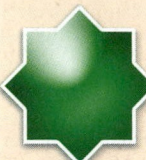

Pediatric Variations:

- *Children generally enjoy the experience.*
- *Be certain that the child feels comfortable and safe.*
- *If appropriate, include the child's parents in the session and teach them how to guide the child through the procedure.*

Home Care Variations:

- *Make sure there will be no distractions. The client may want to take the phone off the hook and put a note on the door requesting quiet.*
- *Encourage any caregivers in the home to take part in the session so they can help guide the clients with future sessions.*

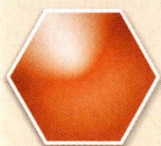

Long-Term Care Variations:

- *Arrange for a quiet area without interruptions.*
- *The sessions can be performed with small groups of 2 to 4 people encouraging socialization and discussion.*
- *Be sure to assess cognitive and sensory abilities. You may need to speak louder, or keep sessions shorter.*

► COMMON ERRORS

Possible Error:

Having the session interrupted by a pager beeping or the telephone ringing.

Prevention:

Set your pager to vibrate before the session. Turn your pager off, if that is an option. Turn off the phone.

Possible Error:

The client cannot hear the instructions.

Prevention:

Position yourself close to the client. Make sure your voice does not lower in volume as you become more relaxed.

▶ NURSING TIPS

- Introduce progressive muscle relaxation as early as possible when you anticipate that a client's treatment has the potential for pain, anxiety, nausea, and so forth.
- Do not prejudge whether a client will be receptive to treatments. Offer it to anyone who may benefit from treatments.
- This is the client's experience; you are only the guide. Do not be disappointed if the client does not enjoy or get any benefit from the session.
- Use a variety of expressions to describe the relaxation of the muscles: melting away, letting go, loosen and soften, drift away, smooth out, and so forth.
- Give examples to help the client relax: "Make yourself feel like a warm, limp washcloth," or "Let your fingertips feel warm and feel the warmth move up your fingers to the wrist, to the arms," and so forth.
- Some clients may benefit from the use of pictures to start the relaxation process. Examples of relaxing pictures are scenes from beaches, oceans, and mountains.
- As clients start to relax give suggestions such as: "Think of your favorite place," or "Feel the warm ocean breeze blow through your hair."

- Practice the procedure yourself; not only does it help you memorize the steps, but in the stressful job of nursing you can also benefit.
- Documenting progressive relaxation can be very subjective. An example of good documentation follows: Progressive muscle relaxation session performed. Client rated lower-back pain as 6 out of 10 before the session and 4 of 10 after the session. Client states that he was distracted by call lights going off in the hall, and his mind wandered to thoughts other than the task at hand. Client reports some unexplained feelings of sadness during the session. Client states he would like to try another session, and feels that he will be able to continue the practice on his own.
- Be prepared for the session. If you do not have the order of progression memorized, prepare a "cheat-sheet."
- Do not talk too much.
- Ask simple yes or no questions when checking for the correct music volume, comfort level, and so forth.
- A lack of environmental disruptions is essential.
- Clients who are unable to relax may respond to the practitioner's relaxation and breathing in conjunction with their own.
- Back rubs or other touching techniques may be beneficial in conjunctions with relaxation techniques. Assess the client's acceptance of touching.

▶ SPECIAL CONSIDERATIONS

- *Allow clients to pace breathing at their own rate. People who have learned or were trained to compensate their respiratory patterns, such as athletes, may have lower rates than normal. To breathe at a rapid rate with deep volume may induce hyperventilation, a situation in which the client may progress to feeling light-headed and/or numbness in the fingertips. In this situation, breathe with the client to slow the respiratory rate or have the client breathe into a bag (to allow for rebreathing of carbon dioxide). In contrast, some clients may breathe at a slower rate and induce hypoventilation, whereby they appear agitated and anxious.*
- *Relaxation techniques can be beneficial to clients with excessive pain as well as clients in labor and delivery. Many clients may have practiced with a coach before labor. Encourage practice in the early stages of labor. If the client has no previous experience with relaxation techniques, instruct client during the early stages of labor. As labor progresses and the client's pain increases, the practitioner may need to have the client focus directly on the practitioner's face and breathe with the client with very direct instructions, "Look at me, breathe with me." Clients may feel they are losing control and may need encouragement and praise.*
- *Effleurage, a smooth brush-like touching on the abdomen, can be used in conjunction with relaxation techniques during labor and delivery or with clients undergoing a painful procedure.*

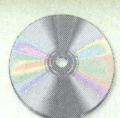

Therapeutic Massage

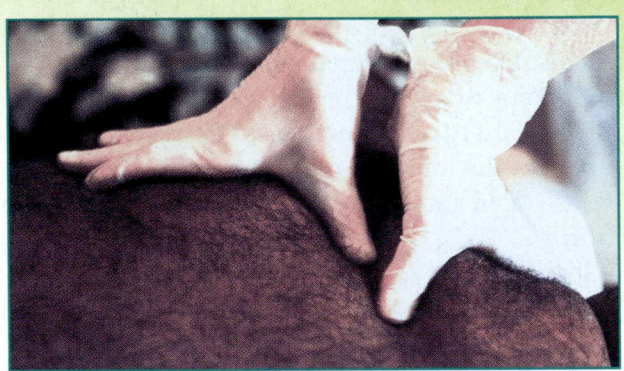

► OVERVIEW OF THE SKILL

Therapeutic massage is the application of pressure and motion by the hands with the intent of improving the recipient's well-being. It involves kneading, rubbing, and using friction or light touch. Massage therapy is now recognized as a highly beneficial modality and is prescribed by a number of physicians and qualified practitioners. Back rubs traditionally have been administered by nurses to provide comfort and relaxation to hospitalized clients. Today, they are considered standard practice.

Massage techniques can be used with all age groups and are especially beneficial to those who are immobilized. A back rub or massage can promote relaxation; increase circulation of the blood and lymph nodes; and provide relief from musculoskeletal stiffness, pain, and spasms (see Table 3-4-1). Massage can significantly reduce the anxiety, heart rate, blood pressure, and perception of pain in hospitalized clients with cancer.

► ASSESSMENT

1. Assess the client's current emotional and physical condition to determine if the client is anxious, tense, or in pain. **Determines what benefits the client would receive from therapeutic massage.**
2. Review the client's current diagnosis. **Determines precautions to use, particularly for clients with heart disease, diabetes,** hypertension, or kidney disease. **Massage should never be attempted in areas of circulatory abnormalities such as aneurysm, varicose veins, necrosis, phlebitis, or thrombus or in areas of soft-tissue injury, open wounds, inflammation, joint or bone injury, dermatitis, recent surgery, or sciatica. Increased circulation and physical pressure could be harmful in these conditions.**
3. Assess the client's current physical surroundings. **Determines the best way to provide the client with privacy and a restful environment.**
4. Assess the client's acceptance of touch and past experience with touch. Some clients may be uncomfortable with touch, or various forms of light or deep touch. The use of touch varies with cultural backgrounds. **Determines whether the client will respond to therapeutic massage and the type of touch that will be most effective.**
5. Assess for allergies **to lotion to avoid skin reactions or irritation.**

► DIAGNOSIS

Anxiety

Ineffective Tissue Perfusion

Deficient Knowledge

Acute Pain

Table 3-4-1	Massage Techniques
EFFLEURAGE:	Gliding and long rhythmic strokes are used. The whole hand is used. Firm, even-pressured strokes are directed toward the heart to assist blood return. Lighter pressure is used when moving away from the heart.
PÉTRISSAGE:	Pressing, squeezing, kneading, and rolling movements by both hands (use entire hand) are used. Deep circulation is enhanced. C-shaped motions stimulate the muscle body. Promotes muscle relaxation.
FRICTION:	Focused, deep, circular motions are used. Thumb pads, heel of hand, or fingertips are used. Penetrates deeper muscle layers. Done after effleurage and pétrissage.
TAPOTEMENT:	Brisk vigorous, rhythmic, percussive movements are used. Hands alternately tap, cup, slap, and pummel muscles. Palms, fingertips, and knuckles are used. Invigorates and stimulates tired muscles.
VIBRATION:	Very fine, rapid, shaking movements are administered by the entire hand. Stimulates or relaxes muscles.

▶ PLANNING

Expected Outcomes:

1. Client's relaxation will be increased, and muscle stiffness, pain, and spasms will be decreased.
2. Circulation to the massaged area will be increased.

Equipment Needed (see Figure 3-4-1):

- Flat sheet
- One or two pillows
- Lotion or oil
- Bath blanket or light coverlet

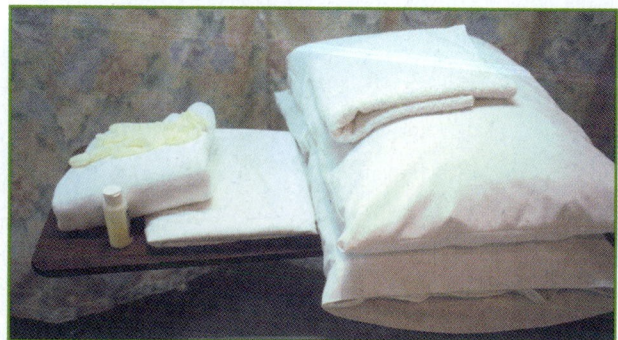

Figure 3-4-1   Lotion or oil is used to reduce friction. Towels and light blankets are used to keep the client warm and comfortable.

- Towel
- Tape or CD player

▶ CLIENT EDUCATION NEEDED:

1. Explain to the client how you will perform the procedure to ensure that the client is comfortable and to reduce stress over the unknown of the procedure.
2. Explain what kind of oil or lotion you will be using so the client can approve its use and to check for allergies.
3. Educate the client on ways to prolong the effects of the procedure.
4. Encourage the client to relax and enjoy the procedure and to advise of any part that is uncomfortable.

Estimated time to complete the skill:
15–25 minutes

► **DELEGATION TIPS**

Therapeutic massage techniques may be delegated to any individual properly trained in the technique.

IMPLEMENTATION—Action/Rationale

Action	Rationale
1. Set room temperature at approximately 75° F. Provide low or indirect lighting, privacy, and background music.	1. Maintains client's body heat, protects privacy, and promotes relaxation.
2. Prepare the massage table or hospital bed by placing a clean sheet on the surface. Adjust the surface height.	2. Both the massage table and hospital bed can be adjusted so that the height of the work surface can be raised or lowered as necessary.
3. Remove your rings and watches. Wash hands.	3. Avoids scratching the client and reduces the transmission of microorganisms.
4. Explain the procedure to the client.	4. Prepares the client for the treatment.
5. Help the client assume either a prone, supine, or sitting position, depending on client's condition (see Figure 3-4-2).	5. Appropriate position enables the nurse to apply the necessary amount of pressure to the back without causing discomfort to the client.
6. Loosen or remove clothing from the client's back and arms. Drape the client with a sheet to cover areas not being treated directly.	6. Exposes parts of the back on which the massage will be performed. Draping untreated parts of the back helps keep the client warm.
7. Squeeze a small amount of lotion or oil into the palm of the hand to warm before applying to the client.	7. Cold lotion or oil can cause discomfort to the client.

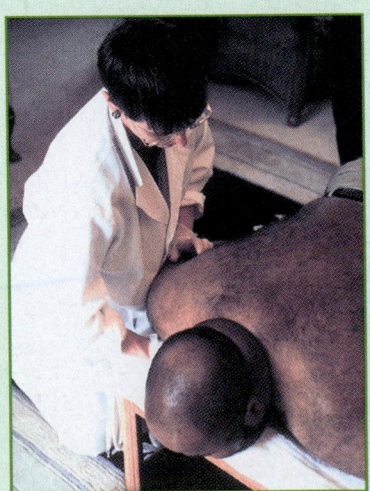

Figure 3-4-2 Position the client either sitting or prone. Assess for comfort before beginning the procedure.

continu

Action	Rationale

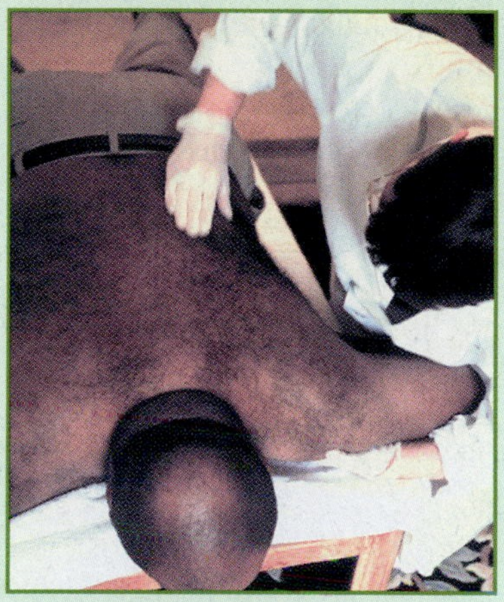

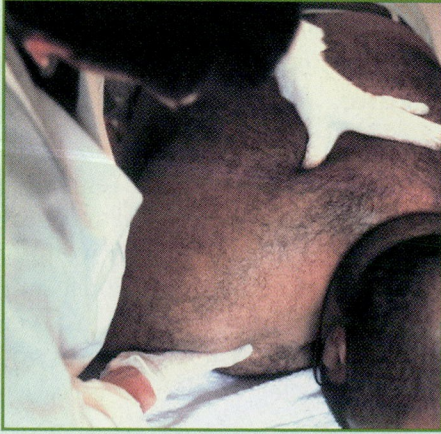

Figure 3-4-3   Massage gently but firmly, keeping your hands in contact with the client's skin.

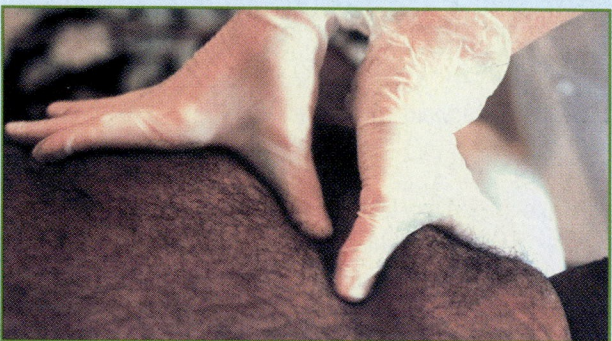

Figure 3-4-4   Pétrissage involves pressing, squeezing, kneading, and rolling hand movements.

8. Begin with light-to-medium effleurage at lower back and continue upward following muscle groups, being careful to avoid the spine and spinal processes. Move hands up toward the base of the neck and continue outward over the trapezius muscles with circular motions, over and around shoulders and upper arms, and return with lighter downward strokes laterally over the latissimus dorsi to the upper gluteals. Use slow, rhythmic movements, keeping in contact with the skin at all times. Check pressure. Continue the effleurage for approximately 3 minutes (see Figure 3-4-3).

8. Prevents damage to internal structures, stimulates circulation, and promotes relaxation.

9. Continue treatment, if appropriate, with gentle pétrissage (see explanation in text; also see Figure 3-4-4) to major muscle groups in the back, shoulders, and upper arms (see Figure 3-4-5).

9. Enhances circulation, stimulates muscles, and promotes relaxation.

10. Use friction on particular muscle groups where tension is being held.

10. Penetrates deeper muscle layers, thus promoting further relaxation.

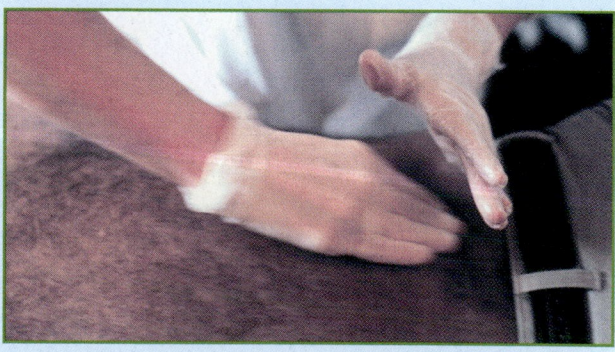

Figure 3-4-5   As the massage continues, move outward from the neck to the upper back and shoulders.

Figure 3-4-6   Use hands to tap, cup, slap, and pummel muscles to stimulate fatigued muscle groups.

continues

Action	Rationale
11. Use tapotement to stimulate any muscle groups that may be fatigued (see Figure 3-4-6).	11. Invigorates and stimulates tired muscles.
12. Finish treatment with effleurage.	12. Assists with relaxation and provides a sense of completion.
13. Wipe any excess lotion or oil from skin with a towel, or use a small amount of warm soap and water to clean the client's skin, taking care to dry it completely.	13. Promotes and maintains skin integrity.
14. Assist client into a comfortable position for a period of rest or sleep.	14. Allows client to fully experience the therapeutic benefit of massage.
15. Document treatment, client's response, and skin assessment data.	15. Communicates pertinent data to other members of treatment team; promotes continuity of care.
16. Wash hands.	16. Reduces the transmission of microorganisms.

► REAL WORLD ANECDOTES

Mrs. Nguyen, a 94-year-old client, is admitted to the hospital with two broken ankles. She is on bed rest preoperatively. Her nurse, Tom, is aware that therapeutic massage would benefit Mrs. Nguyen, as her mobility level is decreased. He explains the procedure and the potential benefits to Mrs. Nguyen, who adamantly refuses therapeutic massage. Tom is sensitive to the possibility that Mrs. Nguyen is concerned about the gender difference and offers to have a female nurse perform the massage. Mrs. Nguyen happily accepts the offer. This nurse was sensitive to differences in cultural and social perceptions.

► EVALUATION

- The client's relaxation was increased, and muscle stiffness, pain, and spasms were decreased
- The circulation to the massaged area was increased.

► DOCUMENTATION

Nurses' Notes

- Record the date and time.
- Document the client's response to the treatment.

Document on appropriate flow sheet or electronic medical record (EMR).

► CRITICAL THINKING SKILL

Introduction

Massage is not always appropriate.

Possible Scenario

Carl is a client recovering from abdominal surgery yesterday. He asks you to massage his left calf. He is complaining of pain and cramping in the area. When you uncover his left leg, you note that his left calf is slightly reddened and is painful when you apply light pressure to the area.

Possible Outcome

You do not massage this client. You remember that massage should never be attempted in areas of circulatory abnormalities. Areas with open wounds, redness or inflammation, necrosis, or obviously impaired circulation should not be massaged. You contact Carl's physician and report the signs and symptoms of a blood clot in Carl's leg.

Prevention

Therapeutic massage is a valuable tool to help clients relax and feel more comfortable, especially if their mobility is impaired. As in any modality, however, it is not universally appropriate. Clients who have recently had surgery are at risk of thrombus (clot) formation. The left leg is frequently the site of the clot. Massage to this site could cause the clot to break free from the vessel wall. The clot could then lodge in the lungs (pulmonary embolism), causing potentially fatal complications.

▶ VARIATIONS

Geriatric Variations:

- *Geriatric clients are more likely to be confused and may misinterpret the intent of the therapeutic massage. They may become combative or react in other inappropriate ways.*
- *Geriatric clients are more likely to be immobilized. Therapeutic massage is especially beneficial for these clients*
- *Massage over bony prominences in an elderly person with thin skin may increase the potential of developing a pressure sore. Massage the skin around these areas.*

Pediatric Variations:

- *Pediatric clients are often fearful of strange situations and strange people. Therapeutic massage is contraindicated in these clients.*
- *Pediatric clients who have been neglected or abused may respond negatively to therapeutic massage.*

Home Care Variations:

- *The home care setting is often more relaxing for the client and can increase the effectiveness of therapeutic massage. Provide for privacy.*

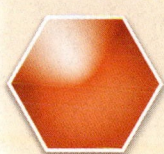

Long-Term Care Variations:

- *Clients in long-term care are sometimes in the position of receiving decreased contact and human touch. Therapeutic massage is one method of increasing the clients' level of awareness and involvement in the world around them.*

▶ COMMON ERRORS

Possible Error:

The client requests a back rub because his back itches from lying in bed. When he rolls over so the nurse can rub his back, the nurse notes a large raised red rash on the client's back.

Prevention:

Before beginning the massage, ask the client about the history of this rash. Check to see whether any medications have changed. Ask the client whether he has other symptoms that might indicate an allergic reaction to medications, the sheets, or the lotion used for back rubs. Do not perform the back rub. Check with the client and in his chart regarding a history of rash and/or allergies. If this is a new symptom, notify the client's physician. Document the client's symptoms and any other findings.

▶ **NURSING TIPS**

• Be sure the client is comfortable with the procedure. Cultural and personal beliefs regarding touch must be respected.

• To warm the lotion before use, place the lotion bottle in a pan of warm water while preparing the table and the client.

• Use this opportunity to assess the client's skin integrity and condition.

▶ **SPECIAL CONSIDERATIONS**

• *Past experiences with touch may interfere with therapeutic effects. If a client has posttraumatic stress, a history of sexual assault, or past experiences with pain from therapeutic massage, this intervention may not be useful.*

• *Consider other tools used in therapeutic massage, such as heated rocks or back rollers. Assess the client's experience with other measures.*

• *If the client has a history of sexual assault use same-sex therapist.*

Applying Moist Heat

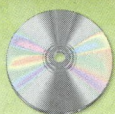

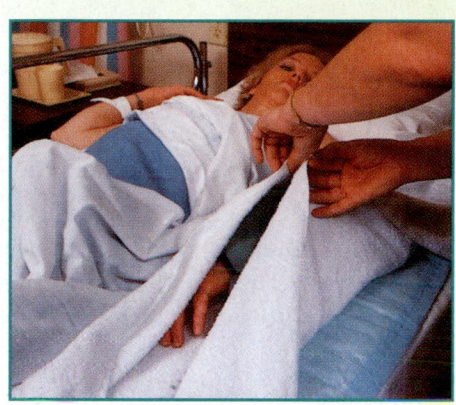

▶ OVERVIEW OF THE SKILL

Heat application is used to promote vasodilatation, increase capillary permeability, decrease blood viscosity, increase tissue metabolism, and reduce muscle tension. Moist heat can be in the form of immersion of a body part in a warmed solution or water. It can also be accomplished by wrapping body parts in dressings that are saturated with warmed solution.

▶ ASSESSMENT

1. Assess the area to receive heat treatment for circulation. **Heat increases circulation; adequate vasculature must be present to be effective.**
2. Assess the skin sensation and integrity around the area to be treated. **Heat treatment cannot be used over areas of blisters, burns, or redness indicative of burning.**
3. Assess for open wounds that may be affected by the treatment. **Moist heat provides an ideal climate for the growth of microorganisms. Moist heat should be applied to open wounds only with orders from a physician or qualified practitioner.**

▶ DIAGNOSIS

Ineffective Tissue Perfusion

Acute Pain

Risk for Impaired Skin Integrity

▶ PLANNING

Expected Outcomes:

1. If heat treatment is being used to decrease muscle tension or alleviate pain, then the client will experience a decrease in pain and tension.
2. If heat treatment is being used to increase circulation, then circulation will improve as demonstrated by color or assessment for blanching.
3. If heat treatment is being used to decrease edema, then the client will experience a decrease in swelling in the area being treated.
4. The skin will not have signs of heat sensitivity such as excessive redness, swelling, or blistering.

Equipment Needed (see Figure 3-5-1):

- Aquathermia pad
- Commercial heat pack
- Solution for heat treatment

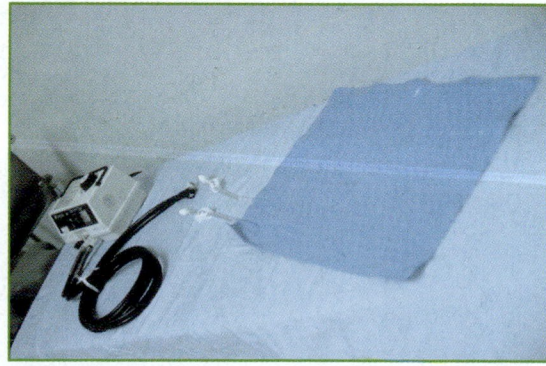

Figure 3-5-1 Aquathermia pad

- 4 × 4 gauze and waterproof pads
- Examination gloves
- Sterile gloves if open wounds
- Towel

▶ CLIENT EDUCATION NEEDED:

1. Teach client that overuse of heat can cause tissue damage and burn the skin.
2. The application of heat longer than the prescribed time can cause reflex vascular constriction.
3. Moist heat can cause damage faster than dry heat.
4. Do not use moist heat over scarred or exposed tissue unless treatment is specifically for those areas.
5. If electric heating systems are used, avoid high settings. Teach the caregiver to watch so that

the client at home does not fall asleep with the unit in place. Warn the client to stay awake when a heating unit is in place.

6. Teach the client not to use the wrong heat source—placing lower legs on a space heater for warmth, for example.

Estimated time to complete the skill: **Depends on condition and use. Usually heat is applied for 20 minutes, but the nurse may not need to be in attendance the entire time.**

▶ DELEGATION TIPS

This skill is routinely delegated to properly trained ancillary personnel. Reassessment of the client after application to maintain proper temperature and to evaluate the client response is essential.

IMPLEMENTATION—Action/Rationale

Action	Rationale
1. Check the physician's order and the reason for the warm compress.	1. A physician's or nurse practitioner's order is generally required.
2. Wash hands.	2. Reduces the transmission of microorganisms.
3. Assess the client's skin for areas of redness, breakdown, or scar tissue. If open wounds are involved, carefully assess the open wounds. Explain the reason for compresses.	3. Provides baseline information for comparison assessments. Because scar tissue may be heat sensitive or insensitive, this area should be avoided, if possible, when the compress is applied. Any open wounds should be avoided unless the treatment is specific for these areas, such as body immersion for debridement. The client's understanding of reasons for compresses will improve compliance.

continues

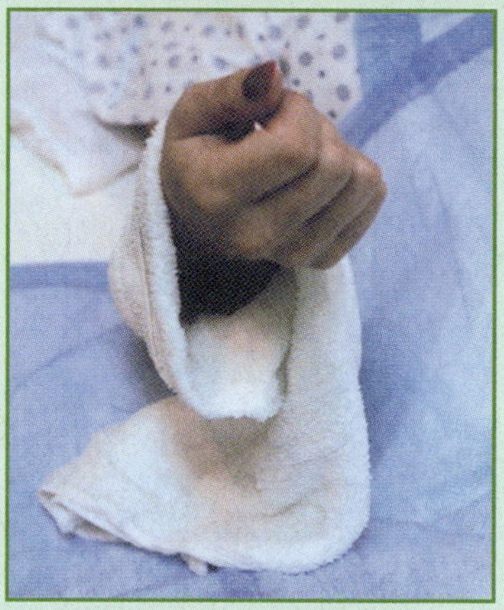

Action	Rationale

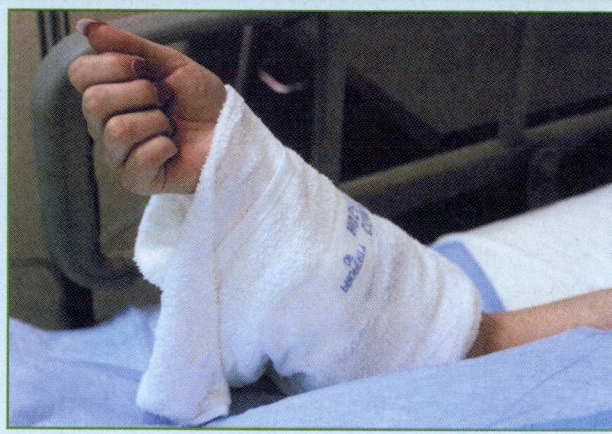

Figure 3-5-2 Use a waterproof pad to protect the client's bed and clothing.

Figure 3-5-3 Place the moist towel on the area being treated.

4. Determine the client's condition, medical diagnosis, and any history of diabetes mellitus or impairments in sensation.

4. Sensation is often impaired in clients with peripheral vascular disease, diabetes, and especially in peripheral neuropathy. People with impairments in sensation may not be able to identify when the compresses are too hot. The risk of burns is greater with moist heat than with dry heat. The client's history and medical diagnosis may alert you to other problems.

5. Warm the container of sterile saline or water by placing it in a bath basin filled with hot tap water. Sterile saline should be warmed to 105°–113° F. If you are using a commercial compress, follow the manufacturer's directions for heating the compress.

5. Sterile saline is used to prevent any contamination of the wound. A temperature greater than 113° F will cause further injury.

6. Place a waterproof pad under the body area that needs the warm compress (see Figure 3-5-2).

6. Protects the client's bed and clothing.

7. Pour the sterile saline into the sterile basin. Soak an appropriate-size piece of gauze or a towel, wring out the excess saline, and place it on the affected area (see Figure 3-5-3). Wear gloves if there is any drainage of the client's body fluids. Wear sterile gloves if there is an open wound.

7. A sterile basin is used to prevent further contamination. Excess saline may increase the chance of burns.

8. Wrap the area with a waterproof pad or apply a disposable heat or aquathermia pad (see Figure 3-5-4).

8. Maintains or holds in the heat.

9. Check the client's skin periodically for signs of heat intolerance. Tell the client to report any signs of discomfort immediately.

9. Signs of intolerance may include redness or further swelling.

continues

Action	Rationale

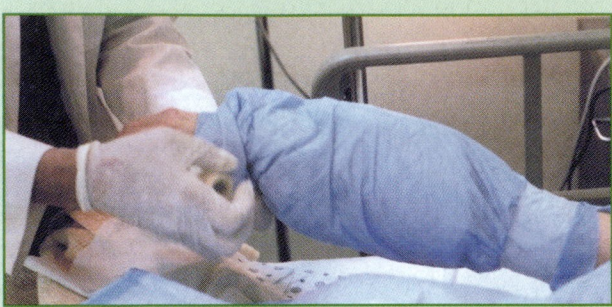

Figure 3-5-4   Wrap the hot, moist towel with a waterproof pad and secure.

10. If it is tolerated, leave the compress in place for approximately 20 minutes and then remove it.

10. Application of moist heat for a longer period of time may damage the client's skin and may predispose the client to edema formation from circulatory congestion.

11. Dry the affected area with sterile towels if there is an open wound and with clean towels if there is no open wound. Apply dressing to open wound.

11. The client may feel chilled when the warm compress is removed. Dry the area completely to prevent chilling.

12. Properly dispose of all single-use equipment according to hospital protocol.

12. Proper disposal of all other equipment reduces the transmission of microorganisms.

13. Remove gloves, if they were worn, and wash your hands.

13. Reduces the transmission of microorganisms.

14. Reassess the condition of the client's skin.

14. The condition of the client's skin and any signs of heat sensitivity should be assessed and documented.

15. Record the procedure. Note the condition of the client's skin and the length of the application. Report any abnormal findings to the physician.

15. Communicates the findings to the other members of the health care team and contributes to the legal record by documenting the care given to the client.

▶ REAL WORLD ANECDOTES

The IV in Mr. Kowalski's right forearm infiltrated, and the area was swollen and painful. Chen, the nurse on duty, offered to place warm, moist heat on the area to help reduce the swelling and ease the pain. Chen first tried running a washcloth under hot tap water, but she was unable to get the tap water hot enough for her satisfaction. In an attempt to get the wet cloth hot enough, Chen wrapped it in a waterproof pad and placed it in the microwave oven for one minute. When she opened the waterproof pad, the washcloth was hot and steamy. Carrying the cloth in the waterproof pad, she returned to Mr. Kowalski's room and placed the pad-covered cloth on Mr. Kowalski's right forearm. He initially complained that it was a little warm, but he soon adjusted to the temperature. By the time Chen left the room, Mr. Kowalski was resting comfortably with the hot pack on his arm. After about half an hour, Chen returned to check on Mr. Kowalski and remove the hot pack. As she removed the wet cloth, she noticed that Mr. Kowalski's arm was quite red and inflamed. To Chen's dismay, Mr. Kowalski sustained first-degree burns on his right forearm that required extra treatment and increased his suffering.

► EVALUATION

- If the heat treatment was used to decrease muscle tension or alleviate pain, then the client experienced a decrease in muscle tension or pain.
- If heat treatment was used to increase circulation, then the circulation was improved as demonstrated by color and assessment of blanching.
- If heat treatment was being used to decrease edema, then the client experienced a decrease in swelling in the area being treated.
- The skin did not have signs of heat sensitivity such as excessive redness, swelling or blistering.
- Evaluate posttreatment for decreased swelling, decreased edema, decreased muscle tension, and improved circulation depending on the purpose of the treatment.
- Evaluate skin posttreatment for any heat damage such as excess redness, swelling, or blistering.

► DOCUMENTATION

Nurses' Notes

- Document the treatment and the results of treatment.
- Document the condition of the skin.
- Document the purpose and type of moist heat application.
- Record the results of the treatment and the client's tolerance.
- Document client teaching.

Document on appropriate flow sheet or electronic medical record (EMR).

► CRITICAL THINKING SKILL

Introduction

Remind outpatient or home care clients to monitor water temperature carefully.

Possible Scenario

A diabetic client being seen in the diabetic clinic reports that he soaks his feet in hot water to decrease swelling. The nurse notes this in her record. She also notes that this client has peripheral vascular disease and peripheral neuropathy.

Possible Outcome

The nurse does not connect the two related pieces of information. She recalls it as she is performing a dressing change on this client, who could not sense the temperature of the water on his feet and suffered second-degree burns when his water heater malfunctioned.

Prevention

Burns can occur readily in clients with poor circulation and are extremely difficult to heal. The client is not able to gauge the water temperature and should, therefore either use the back of his hand or have someone else check the water temperature. If a household thermometer is available, have the client check the temperature with the thermometer. Make sure the client is not visually impaired and can read the thermometer correctly.

► VARIATIONS

Geriatric Variations:

- *Elderly clients have thin skin and decreased sensation and can be burned easily.*
- *Teach elderly clients not to use the "high" setting on their heating pad. Use a more moderate setting, even if it takes a little longer to achieve the desired warmth.*

Pediatric Variations:

- *Children have increased sensitivity to heat and a thin epidermis.*
- *Age-appropriate activities can be provided to distract and entertain the child during the treatment.*
- *Go over types of feedback children will give to tell you how comfortable they are with the heat treatment. "Cold, warm, hot, red hot" or "green, yellow, red" are ways to receive feedback from children.*

continues

► **VARIATIONS** (continued)

Home Care Variations:
- If pain continues and no relief is achieved from home heat treatment, further assessment of the cause of the pain should be performed. Make sure the client knows whom to contact.
- Make sure cords and electrical outlets are in good condition when assessing home heat therapies that use electric heating pads or other electric heat sources.
- Microwavable forms of heat are commonly available for home use. Make sure the client does not over-heat items in the microwave. Liquid packets can explode and cause burns.

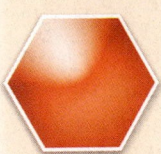

Long-Term Care Variations:
- Reusable sources of heat will wear out when used periodically over time. Check and replace as needed.

► **COMMON ERRORS**

Possible Error:

Redness, irritation, or burns occur.

Prevention:

Use protective cloth or padding between heat source and client. Do not leave heat on too long.

Possible Error:

Client assessment, history, and education regarding home heat treatments are not performed.

Prevention:

Remember to ask clients during assessment what heat treatments they are using at home. Ask how frequently they use heat, how they determine what temperature to make the treatment, and what effects they notice from the treatments.

► **NURSING TIPS**

- Do not use heat treatment more than 20 minutes.
- If a large area of the body is exposed to heat treatment, the client's systemic temperature may be affected. Dizziness or hypotension may occur from vasodilatation.
- Assess client's fluid status if large parts of the body are immersed in heat, and take vital signs before and after treatment.

► **SPECIAL CONSIDERATIONS**

- The use of hot tubs is associated with male infertility. If suggesting hot tubs as a means of moist heat therapy, then advise the client of this possible outcome.
- It is recommended that pregnant women should not use hot tubs or Jacuzzis.
- Heat therapy should not be used over scarred areas as sensation may be decreased.
- Warm, moist heat via a whirlpool bath may be suggested therapy after childbirth. The warm circulating water increases the circulation to the episiotomy site and offers pain relief for the new mother.
- A warm, moist cloth may be placed on an extremity when trying to visualize vessels for venipuncture. The heat encourages circulation to the area treated and the vessel is easier to visualize.

Warm Soaks and Sitz Baths

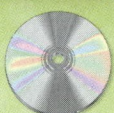

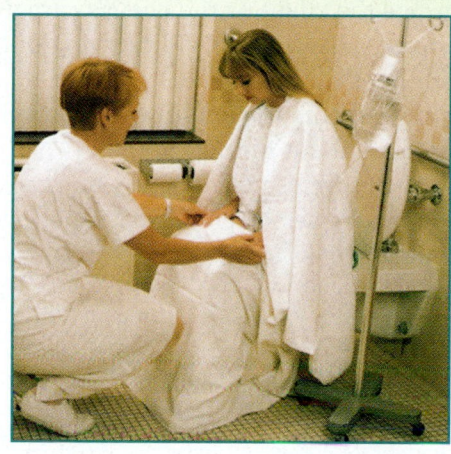

▶ OVERVIEW OF THE SKILL

The application of warm soaks promotes increased circulation and helps distribute the body's healing elements to a specific area. In addition to encouraging healing, warm soaks also provide nonpharmacologic pain relief and help to localize infection. Sitz baths are a method used to apply warm soaks to the perineum.

▶ ASSESSMENT

1. Assess the client for conditions such as circulatory problems, decreased sensation, age, or diagnosis that may require alteration to the treatment plan.
2. Assess the ability of the client to participate in treatment. For example, ascertain whether a client will be able to maintain a position for 15–20 minutes **to determine if any alterations to the procedure are necessary.**
3. Assess the area of injury for drainage, edema, or redness. The injured area should not have increasing edema at the time of heat application. **Determines the appropriateness of the procedure.**
4. Assess the availability of appropriate equipment and clean hot water **to determine whether changes to the procedure will be necessary.**
5. Warm soaks are used frequently in many people's homes. Assess each client's experience of using warm soaks before teaching **to determine the type and amount of client teaching needed.**

▶ DIAGNOSIS

Acute Pain

Ineffective Tissue Perfusion

Risk for Impaired Skin Integrity

▶ PLANNING

Expected Outcomes:

1. Client will experience decrease in pain.
2. Affected area will heal.

Equipment Needed:

Sitz Bath: Portable

- Portable sitz bath (see Figure 3-6-1)
- Towels
- Peri-care equipment

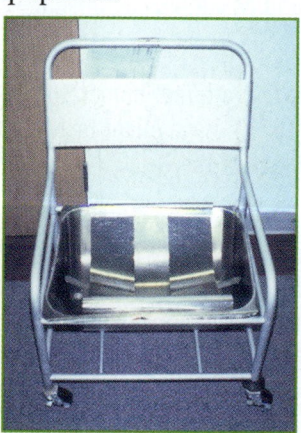

Figure 3-6-1   Portable sitz bath

► CLIENT EDUCATION NEEDED:

1. Do not begin using warm soaks until the initial injury phase is over, usually the first 12–24 hours after the injury. Some injuries may require up to 72 hours to stabilize. Warm soaks will add to posttrauma swelling in the first hours after injury, which could lead to more damage.

2. If there is no thermometer to measure the water temperature, water should be as warm as can be comfortably tolerated. Also, the client may become used to the temperature quickly, creating the feeling that the soak is not hot enough. Warn the client that this does not signal the need to increase the temperature.

3. Soak about 15–20 minutes (or as directed by health care provider). After this much time, the vessels may "rebound" and constrict, creating a situation opposite of the desired effect.

4. After the soak, elevate the affected area.

5. A sitz bath can be a time for a new mother to have a few minutes to herself. Ensure that the baby is cared for by others during this time. Encourage the mother to rest either flat or with hips elevated for 15–20 minutes (or longer if possible) after a sitz bath. This will help prevent unnecessary swelling or pressure. Sitz baths may be taken two to four times per day. Also, women should be encouraged to use a peri-bottle with warm or cool water to cleanse the perineal area after each void or defecation for the first week after childbirth.

6. If the client is to perform warm soaks at home, encourage the client or the client's caregiver to participate in setting up and carrying out the procedure as they are able.

7. Encourage clients to plan how this procedure will be carried out in their home.

8. Warm soaks are used frequently in many people's homes. Assess each client's experience of using warm soaks before teaching.

Estimated time to complete the skill:

30 minutes

This does not include time for assisting with perineal care.

► DELEGATION TIPS

This skill is routinely delegated to properly trained ancillary personnel. Reassessment of the client after application to maintain proper temperature and to evaluate the client response is essential.

IMPLEMENTATION—Action/Rationale

Action	Rationale
1. Wash hands and assemble equipment.	1. Reduces the transmission of microorganisms and organizes time.
2. Run tap water to preferred temperature (between 100° F and 110° F). Have client test the temperature on the dorsal surface of the wrist.	2. Prevents burn injury.
3. For toilet insert model, raise the seat of the toilet. Set the basin on the rim of the toilet bowel (see Figure 3-6-2). Fill water bag and prime tubing. Close the clamp. Hang the water bag above the toilet. Thread the tubing through the front of the basin. Secure the tubing in the notch in the bottom of the basin.	3. Basin will rest on the bowl. Water bag will create a gentle swirling of water. The higher the bag, the more forceful the flow and the faster the water will run out.

continues

Action	Rationale

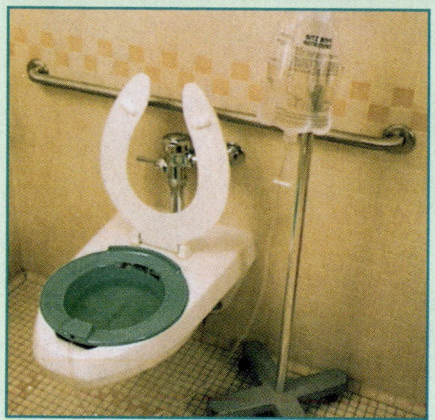

Figure 3-6-2 A portable sitz bath is placed on the rim of the toilet.

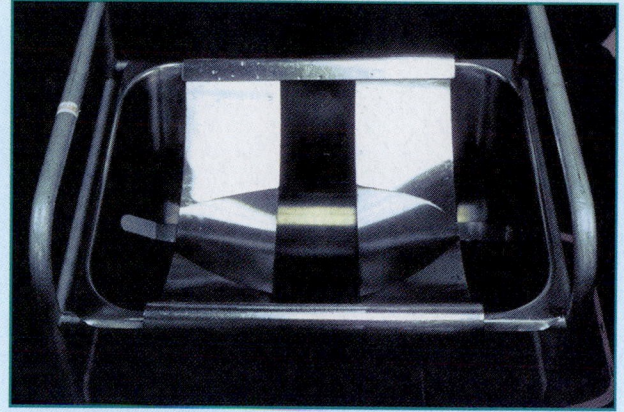

Figure 3-6-3 Fill the sitz bath basin with warm water.

4. For stand-alone model, fill basin with water (see Figure 3-6-3).

5. Pad the seat with a towel (see Figure 3-6-4).

6. Always use Standard Precautions when assisting with perineal care treatments.
   Have client remove and dispose of peri-pad in a biohazard receptacle.

7. Ensure that the floor is dry. Assist client to the bathroom if necessary.

8. Have client sit in the basin (see Figure 3-6-5). For toilet insert model, demonstrate how to unclamp the tubing to start the water flow.

9. Cover the client's lap for warmth and modesty (see Figure 3-6-6).

4. Allows client to sit in the water.

5. Provides client comfort.

6. Prevents infection. Dressings that contain blood are to be disposed in a biohazard container to prevent the spread of microorganisms

7. Prevents injury from falling.

8. Water flow is soothing and helps cleanse the area.

9. Provides client comfort and privacy.

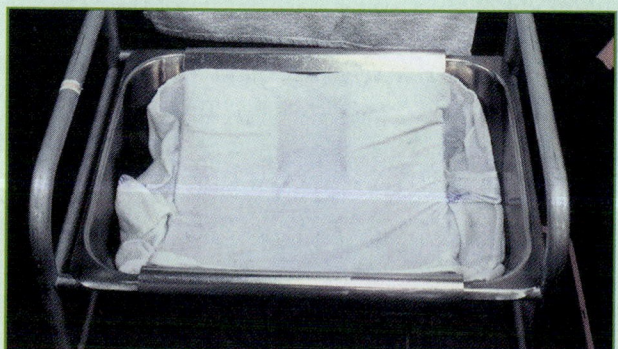

Figure 3-6-4 Pad the seat of the sitz bath with a towel for comfort.

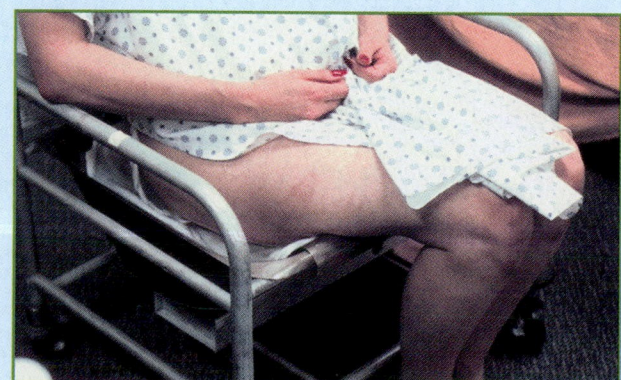

Figure 3-6-5 Have the client sit in the basin.

continues

Action	Rationale

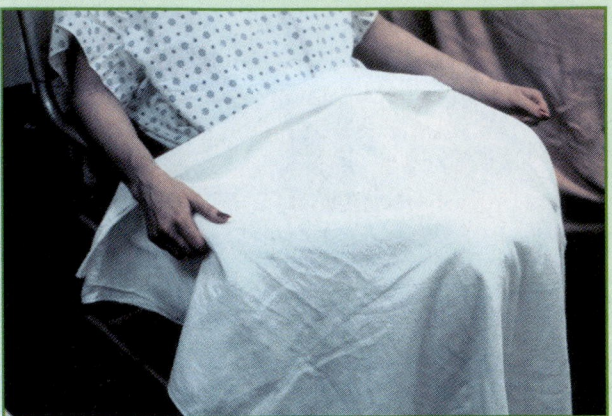

Figure 3-6-6 Cover the client's lap with a towel or blanket for warmth and modesty.

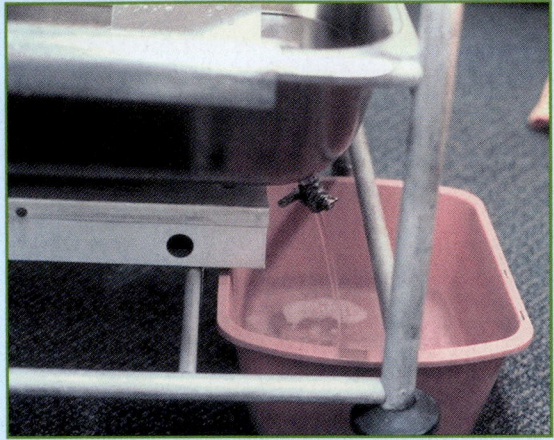

Figure 3-6-7 Open the drainage tap to allow waste water to empty into a basin for disposal.

10. Ensure that the client can reach the call button. Instruct the client to call before standing up.

10. Water may splash over the floor, creating a slipping hazard.

11. After 20 minutes (or sooner if client is finished), help the client dry the area by gently patting with clean towels.

11. Warm soaks should last no longer than 20 minutes to prevent rebound vasoconstriction.

12. Assist client to bed. Encourage client to lie flat or elevate hips for 20 minutes.

12. Prevents congestion and decreases swelling.

13. For toilet insert model, empty remaining water into toilet. Rinse basin and bag. Clean according to institutional policy. For stand-alone model, empty water from drain tap into basin (see Figure 3-6-7). Clean according to institutional policy.

13. Prepares equipment for the next use.

▶ REAL WORLD ANECDOTES

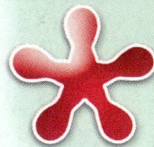

Patty had her first baby 24 hours ago and had an episiotomy. She had been taking codeine pills for perineal pain but complained that she did not like the way they made her feel. Her nurse suggested that she try a sitz bath to see whether she could reduce the amount of codeine she needed to relieve her pain. After using the sitz bath, Patty was able to reduce her use of codeine.

▶ EVALUATION

1. Client experienced decrease in pain.
2. Affected area is healing as indicated by improved appearance of the injured area.

▶ DOCUMENTATION

Nurses' Notes

• Record the date and time of each warm soak.

- Document any variation from expected, individual needs and preferences.
- Document improvement or decline in the client's condition.

Document on appropriate flow sheet or electronic medical record (EMR).

▶ CRITICAL THINKING SKILL

Introduction

Client teaching is an important part of the treatment.

Possible Scenario

Mr. Simpson presented to his nurse practitioner with a boil on his right buttock. The nurse practitioner lanced the boil. She prescribed twice daily sitz baths for Mr. Simpson to keep the area clean and to help the healing process.

Possible Outcome

Mr. Simpson did not know what a sitz bath was and was too embarrassed to ask the nurse practitioner.

As a result, he did not treat the area and the boil recurred, requiring more treatment and more discomfort for Mr. Simpson. The second time she lanced the boil, the nurse practitioner asked Mr. Simpson about his at-home care of the site. Once she realized that Mr. Simpson did not understand her previous instructions, she carefully explained how to set up and use a sitz bath.

Prevention

Do not assume the client is familiar with the process of a sitz bath. Because this treatment is generally used to treat the perineal area, clients may be embarrassed to ask questions regarding the procedure. The nurse may be embarrassed regarding this procedure as well, skimping on the instructions and relaying her discomfort to the client. Assess the client's level of comfort with the procedure and determine whether the client understands how to perform a sitz bath.

▶ VARIATIONS

Geriatric Variations:
- *As skin ages, it becomes more vulnerable to heat and maceration. If sitz baths are to be administered, consider decreasing the length of the procedure and be cautious about the temperature of the soak.*

Pediatric Variations:
- *Not all children will be able to cooperate with the length of time needed for a sitz bath.*
- *Children are susceptible to burns from water that is too hot. It is imperative to warn parents that a child's skin is much more sensitive to heat and burns than an adult's.*

Home Care Variations:
- *Do not assume that all homes have adequate water and heat. If your client will be performing sitz baths at home, these utilities must be evaluated.*

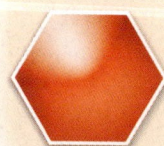

Long-Term Care Variations:
- *A client's need for a sitz bath must be reevaluated periodically.*
- *Check progress of healing on a regular basis.*

► **COMMON ERRORS**

Possible Error:

The nurse fills the sitz bath with water that is too hot.

Prevention:

Use a bath thermometer or test the water temperature with your forearm. It is better to have the water temperature a little too cool than too warm.

► **NURSING TIPS**

- Ensure that your client is comfortable and able to cooperate with the treatment.
- If it is appropriate to leave your clients during treatment, check on them periodically and ensure they have the call bell in reach.
- If a portable sitz bath is not available, disinfect the tub and wrap a towel in a horseshoe shape. The client sits on the round side of the horseshoe-shaped towel with the knees bent to keep the perineum off the tub floor. Do not use inflatable donuts for the sitz bath because these may prevent the warm water from giving the most benefit and cause undue pressure on the perineal area, preventing increased circulation. Fill the tub to about the top of the hip. This allows a regional vasodilation instead of a generalized increase in blood flow.
- A sitz bath can be a time for a new mother to have a few minutes to herself. Ensure that the baby is cared for by others during this time.
- Encourage the client to rest either flat or with hips elevated for 15 to 20 minutes (or longer if possible) after a sitz bath. This will help prevent unnecessary swelling or pressure.
- Sitz baths may be taken two to four times per day.
- If the client is to perform warm soaks at home, encourage the client or the client's caregiver to participate in setting up and carrying out the procedure.
- Encourage clients to plan how this procedure will be carried out in their home.

► **SPECIAL CONSIDERATIONS**

- *Special precautions to avoid burns should be implemented when providing warm soaks and sitz baths to clients with diabetes, peripheral vascular disease, or those who have had an epidural as peripheral sensory function is impaired.*
- *For the postpartum client, both cold sitz baths and warm sitz baths are effective for relieving perineal pain in the postpartum period after an episiotomy and for the treatment of hemorrhoids. However, if the client has received epidural anesthesia, be sure that complete sensation has returned before using a warm sitz bath. Kegel exercises after warm sitz baths are recommended.*

Applying Dry Heat

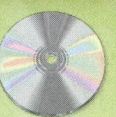

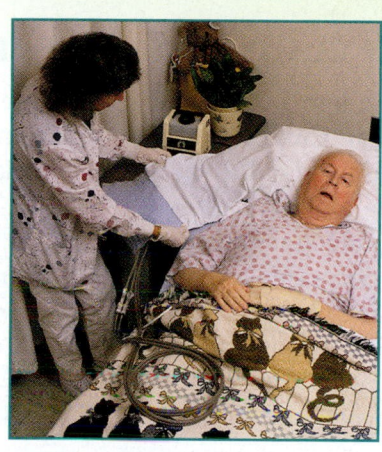

▶ OVERVIEW OF THE SKILL

Dry heat can be used to enhance circulation, promote healing, reduce swelling and inflammation, reduce pain, reduce muscle spasms, and increase systemic temperature. Different types of equipment are used to apply dry heat to body surfaces, specific areas, and the entire body. These can be divided into the following categories:

1. *Body surfaces.* Equipment used to apply heat to any body surface includes disposable instant hot packs, gel-filled hot packs, Aquathermia pads, electric heating pads, and hot water bags or bottles. Aquathermia pads are water-flow rubber heating pads with tubing and a reservoir control unit, sometimes called aqua pads, k-pads, t-pump, or hydroculator. Hot water bags or bottles should be used only by clients at home because bags and bottles cannot be cleaned properly to meet universal standards.

2. *Entire body.* Equipment used to heat the entire body to treat cases such as hypothermia includes thermal blankets and infant radiant warmers, which are discussed in Skill 3-8. The principles and precautions are similar in most types of heat application.

▶ ASSESSMENT

1. Assess the skin integrity in the area where heat is to be applied. If the client has preexisting skin breakdown, redness, or scar tissue, carefully evaluate before applying heat. Assess the level of pain or swelling in the area where heat is to be applied. **Heat treatment cannot be used over areas of blisters, burns, or redness indicative of burning.**

2. Assess the client's tolerance of heat. If there is scar tissue or any decreased sensitivity in the area of treatment, the client will not be able to feel the sensation of burning. Assess the client's ability to perceive and report pain and sensation of burning. If sedated, confused, or agitated, the client should not be left alone with heat treatment in place. **Ensures client safety.**

3. Assess the client's vascular status. Dry heat should be used only with a physician's or qualified practitioner's orders and then cautiously in clients with diabetes or vascular disease. **Because heat increases circulation, adequate vasculature must be present to be effective and not cause further tissue and vessel damage.**

4. Assess the client's condition, medical diagnosis, and any history of diabetes mellitus, peripheral neuropathy, or impairments in sensation. **Sensation is often impaired in peripheral vascular disease, diabetes, and peripheral neuropathy. The client may not be able to feel the sensation of burning.**

5. Assess the skin for the presence of any lotion or ointments. **Heat can be retained with the presence of these products and lead to increased risk of heat intolerance and burning.**

▶ DIAGNOSIS

Ineffective Tissue Perfusion

Acute Pain

Risk for Injury

Ineffective Thermoregulation

Risk for Impaired Skin Integrity

▶ PLANNING

Expected Outcomes:

1. The client will derive the benefits of the heat treatment such as increased circulation and healing; decreased swelling, inflammation, pain, or muscle spasms; or thermoregulation.
2. The client will not experience any injury to skin integrity.

Equipment Needed:

- Equipment determined by type of heat treatment: disposable gel-filled packs (see Figure 3-7-1), Aquathermia pad, heating pad, hot water bottle (generally used only in home setting if at all), hot blankets (see Figure 3-7-2), or hot air client warming system (see Figures 3-7-3 and 3-7-4)
- Protective cover to be used between heat source and client
- Electrical source for pads
- Timer or clock

▶ CLIENT EDUCATION NEEDED:

1. Client understands the need to report any increase in pain or sensation of burning.
2. Client understands the purpose and desired outcome of the treatment.
3. Client understands that if heat source is over area of decreased sensitivity that this must be monitored closely.
4. Client understands that the temperature of the heating device should not be changed without the knowledge of the nurse or qualified practitioner.

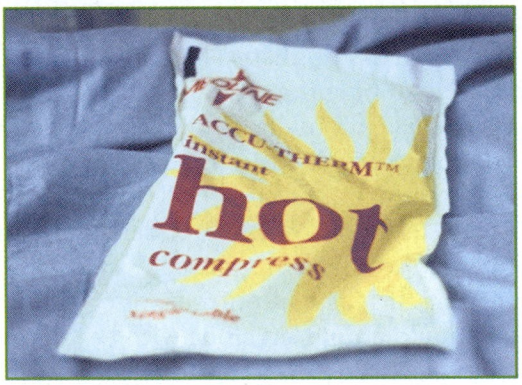

Figure 3-7-1   Disposable hot pack

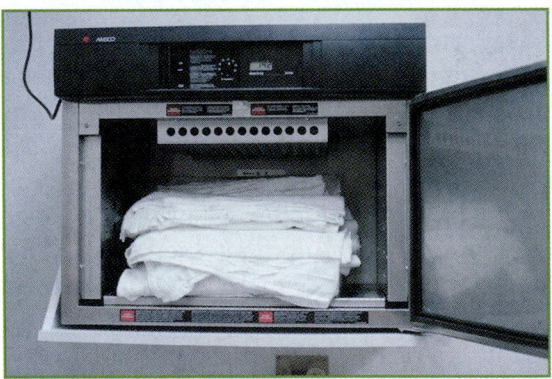

Figure 3-7-2   Blanket warmer

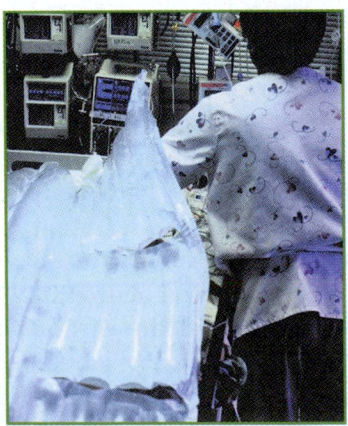

Figure 3-7-3   Forced-air warming blanket

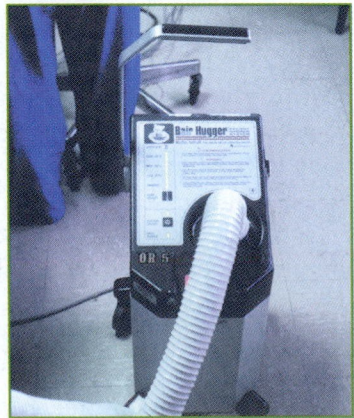

Figure 3-7-4   Forced-air warming blanket control unit

5. Client understands that heat treatment must be discontinued if symptoms of heat intolerance are present.

6. Client understands that heat treatment should not be used beyond the recommended time, which is usually no longer than 20 minutes.

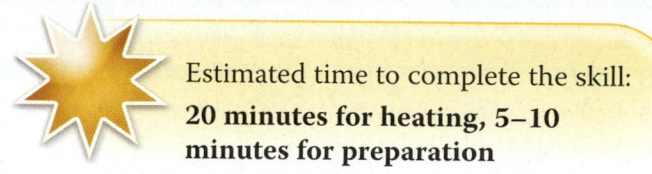

Estimated time to complete the skill: **20 minutes for heating, 5–10 minutes for preparation**

▶ DELEGATION TIPS

This skill is routinely delegated to properly trained ancillary personnel. Reassessment of the client after application is essential to maintain proper temperature and to evaluate the client response.

IMPLEMENTATION—Action/Rationale

Action	Rationale
1. Check the physician's or qualified practitioner's order and the purpose of the heat treatment.	1. An order is required. Because there are many purposes of heat treatment, it is helpful to know what outcomes are expected and the site/sites to be treated.
2. Determine whether there are any underlying problems that may affect the use of heat treatment such as decreased sensation; decreased mentation; or a history of diabetes mellitus, bleeding disorders, peripheral vascular disease, or peripheral neuropathy. Heat should not be used over areas of scarring.	2. If the client has decreased sensation or mental status, heat treatment should be used only if the client can be observed closely. Heat should not be applied over areas where the client cannot alert the nurse of sensation of burning.
3. Wash hands.	3. Reduces the transmission of microorganisms.
4. Check the skin for lotions or ointments and remove if present.	4. Lotions and ointments retain heat and can lead to an increased risk of burning.
5. Explain the reasons for heat treatment, the expected outcomes, any potential complications, and the necessity to alert the nurse of heat intolerance.	5. The client who understands the purpose of treatments will more likely comply, report any adverse responses (for example, sensations of burning) and, therefore, avoid any complications.

continues

Action	Rationale
6. Gather equipment and complete as follows: For a disposable heat pack: • Activate the pack according to the manufacturer's directions. Some packs must be heated in boiling water, others can be heated by microwave, and some require bending and chemical activation. • Wrap the pack in a towel or protective covering (some manufacturers include cover). Do not use pins. Use tape if needed to secure the towel. • Discard after use.	**6.** • Manufacturer's directions should be followed because activation differs. If a microwave is used to heat a pack that should be heated in boiling water, the bag might break. • A barrier between the client's skin and the heat source is necessary to avoid burns. • Chemically activated packs will not reactivate once activated. In medical facilities, gel packs cannot be reheated in common areas without causing the transmission of microorganisms. In the home setting, packs that are activated by boiling or the use of the microwave can be used on the same clients again.
For a heating pad: • Note: Heating pads are generally not used in hospital facilities. • Place a formed cover, usually a flannel, over the pad. Towels should not be used. Pins should never be used. If it is necessary to secure the cover, use tape. • Instruct the client not to lie on the heating pad. • Turn on the switch to low and place the heating pad on the affected area. The nurse may increase heat after the client adjusts to the heat. Instruct the client not to adjust the heat level. Generally, the highest setting is not used and is blocked from use by taping the control in place. • Set a timer and remove the pad after 20 minutes. • Clean appropriately after use.	• Generally, a heating pad is not used in medical facilities unless it belongs to an individual client because the pad cannot be cleaned appropriately to prevent the spread of microorganisms. • A protective cover is necessary between the client's skin and the pad to prevent burning. If the pad is not fitted, it may slip out of place and cause direct exposure of the skin to the heating pad and cause burning. Pins may puncture the electric wires and shock the client. • The heat will be excessive if the client lies directly on the heating pad. • Burning can occur when high levels of heat are used. The client's skin may be sensitive to higher levels of heat. • If a client falls asleep with the heating pad in place, heat administered for longer than 20 minutes can cause burning and rebound vascular changes. • Reduces the transmission of microorganisms.
For an Aquathermia pad: • Follow manufacturer's directions. • Fill the control unit with distilled water or as indicated by manufacturer's directions.	• There are various brands of Aquathermia pads and each one may have slight differences in operating instructions. • Distilled water prevents the accumulation of mineral deposits that will damage equipment.

continues

Action	Rationale
• Check the control unit and tubing for leaks. Turn on the unit and check the temperature of the water. The proper temperature of the water is 105° F. Some units require that the control unit is level with the pad to function because overcoming gravity can put undue strain on the motor.	• This step will ensure that the control unit is properly functioning. If there is a leak in the tubing, another pad should be obtained because this presents an electrical danger to the client and the staff.
For a hot water bottle: • Hot water bottles are usually used only in home care settings. • Fill the bottle with tap water, tighten the cap, turn the bottle upside down, then open the cap and empty. • Fill the bottle or bag with hot water (40.5–46° C or 105–115° F). Fill bag only two-thirds full, expel any air from top, and secure cap. Wipe off excess moisture. • Cover with protective cover or towel. Never use pins. Tape may be used. • Keep the bottle in place for 20 minutes.	• Hot water bottles and bags cannot be cleaned appropriately between client use to follow Standard Precautions. • The bottle is first filled with tepid water to ensure that there are no leaks. • The water temperature should be hot but not boiling so the client is not burned. The bag is not totally filled so that it will mold to the surface area to be treated. • A protective cover helps prevent burns. Pins can puncture the bottle or bag. • Heat that is applied longer than 20 minutes can lead to burns.

For diathermy:
   Diathermy is usually used in a physical therapy department for deep treatment.
   Prepare clients by informing them that the procedure is not dangerously invasive. Remove metal objects such as pins, rings, or watches. If clients have metal objects in the body such as a prosthesis or a pacemaker, diathermy should not be used. Clients are generally transported to a physical therapy department for the treatment.
	Diathermy works by electrical activation and deep heat; metal that is bombarded with diathermy waves becomes intensely hot and can burn the client.

7. Wash hands.	7. Reduces the transmission of microorganisms.

► REAL WORLD ANECDOTES

Mrs. Piukkula is an 82-year-old client in an acute care facility. Her practitioner has ordered an Aquathermia k-pad treatment for an infiltrated IV site in her right forearm. Just after the nurse placed the k-pad on Mrs. Piukkula's arm, he was called away to care for another client. The nurse dealt with several issues and forgot about the k-pad on Mrs. Piukkula's arm. About an hour later, the nurses' aid assigned to Mrs. Piukkula asked the nurse about the k-pad. He went to Mrs. Piukkula's room, removed the k-pad and assessed Mrs. Piukkula's skin for possible damage from the prolonged heat treatment. Mrs. Piukkula skin was reddened, but fortunately she did not have any other damage or blisters to the skin.

▶ EVALUATION

1. The client derived the benefits of the heat treatment such as increased circulation and healing; decreased swelling, inflammation, pain, or muscle spasm.
2. The client did not experience any injury to the skin.

▶ DOCUMENTATION

Nurses' Notes

- Document the time and date of the treatment.
- Document the procedure and the equipment used.
- Record the client's response to the procedure as determined in the evaluation.
- Document the length of time the heat treatment was in place.

Document on appropriate flow sheet or electronic medical record (EMR).

▶ CRITICAL THINKING SKILL

Introduction

Application of heat should always follow a plan from a nurse or qualified practitioner.

Possible Scenario

Mrs. Sullivan, a 72-year-old woman with a history of total hip prosthesis 3 years ago, turns on her call light. She informs the nurse that she brought her own heating pad and has had it on her hip set on high for 40 minutes. She has used an anesthetic cream, but she reports an increase of pain.

The nurse assesses the client's skin and asks her about pain before the heating pad was placed, if she has fallen recently, or if she has any underlying condition that may be causing the pain. Mrs. Sullivan may have been lying directly on the heating pad.

Possible Outcome

The client may have burned her skin or developed heat intolerance because of the cream on the skin in combination with the heat. It is also possible some underlying problems may be associated with the pain such as difficulty with the prosthesis or fractures.

Prevention

Inform the client that a heating pad requires an order from a physician or qualified practitioner and that she should have informed you that she had brought her own heating pad. Explain that it is important for the nurse and physician or qualified practitioner to know that she has pain and that she is using heat. Alert her that heating pads should have protective covers and not be turned on high. Let the client know that you will inform the physician or qualified practitioner of the pain and the use of the heating pad.

▶ VARIATIONS

Geriatric Variations:
- *Elderly clients have thin skin and sometimes decreased sensitivity and usually develop heat intolerance more rapidly than younger clients.*

Pediatric Variations:
- *Gel packs should be used with children because heating pads can pose more dangers of electrical hazards and misuse.*

Home Care Variations:
- *Some clients may prefer to use hot water bottles at home because they have used these in the past. These should be washed carefully with soap and water and dried out when stored.*

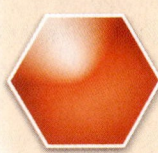

Long-Term Care Variations:
- *If heat is required on a long-term basis, the client should be evaluated for other underlying problems or seek adjunct therapy.*

▶ COMMON ERRORS

Possible Error:

Heat is applied for longer than 20 minutes.

Prevention:

Set a timer or find another way to remind yourself to remove the heat treatment after 20 minutes. It is easy to get busy and forget, so develop a method of reminding yourself when time is up.

Possible Error:

Gel packs are placed in the microwave and rupture.

Prevention:

If the microwave is the only way to heat a gel pack, set the oven for 10- or 15-second periods and check the gel pack between periods. Microwave ovens vary in intensity. Do not assume that a setting that works in one microwave oven works in all microwave ovens.

▶ NURSING TIPS

- Check the client frequently to avoid adverse reactions; especially check in the first 5 minutes.

- Set time to avoid heat treatment that is longer than 20 minutes, especially if using an electrical system.
- Tell the client to alert the nurse if there is increased pain or burning with the treatment.

▶ SPECIAL CONSIDERATIONS

- *The client's temperature may be elevated from the dry heat application. In this case, frequently monitor the vital signs and chart the measured readings until they return to normal.*
- *Creams or ointments on the skin increase the risk for burn in the heat application. Remove creams or ointments from the skin before the dry heat intervention. If the burn has occurred, notify the physician or qualified practitioner and assess skin for damage; a cooling device such as an ice bag may be applied to the area with the order.*
- *Avoid using a safety pin with a heating pad. Shock may occur if the electric wire were hit or punctured.*
- *Heating pads should only be used if the client is awake and alert.*
- *Some K-thermia pads or aqua-pads, which are used for both heating and cooling purposes, require alcohol and water to operate effectively. The nurse must be especially vigilant to ensure that the client is not lying in a pool of fluid containing alcohol and water. This would impair the skin integrity. Avoid safety pins or sharp objects when using K-thermia pads.*

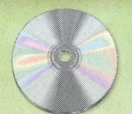

Using a Thermal Blanket and an Infant Radiant Heat Warmer

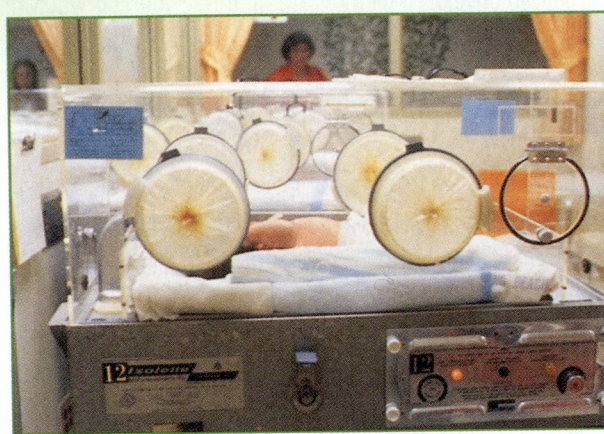

▶ OVERVIEW OF THE SKILL

A thermal blanket is a fluid-filled blanket that can be used to heat or cool a client who is hypothermic or hyperthermic. For hyperthermia, the physician or qualified practitioner will order a cooling blanket. If a client is hypothermic, a warming blanket can be used to gradually raise the client's core temperature to a normal range. Some thermal blankets have a rectal probe, which monitors the client's core temperature and regulates the blanket temperature according to set parameters. Some types of warmers use warm air instead of warm water to increase the client's core temperature. The Bair Hugger, a plastic convective warming blanket that inflates, uses circulating warm air to warm the client (see Figures 3-8-1 and 3-8-2).

Infants have specialized body-warming needs, and there are several types of appliances available to help infants maintain a healthy body temperature. Isolette incubators keep infants warm by providing a heated pad for the infant to lie on. Overhead radiant warmers heat the infant with overhead lights (see Figure 3-8-3). These and other products can be used to help maintain optimal body temperature when the infant cannot self-regulate temperature.

▶ ASSESSMENT

1. Assess the client's temperature. **Establishes a baseline measurement.**
2. Assess the client's skin condition and integrity. **If skin integrity is disrupted, protection**

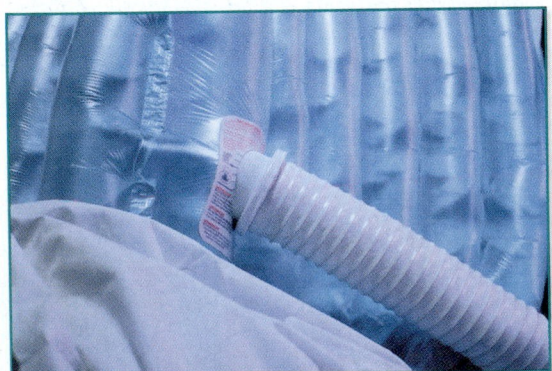

Figure 3-8-1 Circulating, warm air inflates the blanket and convection moves heat to the client.

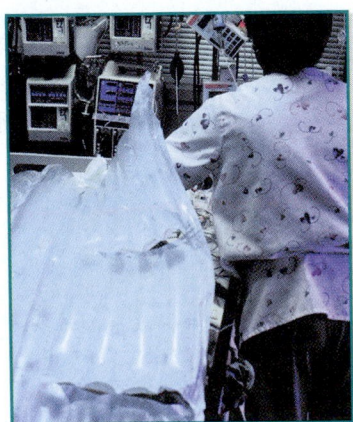

Figure 3-8-2 The warm, inflated blanket is placed on the client.

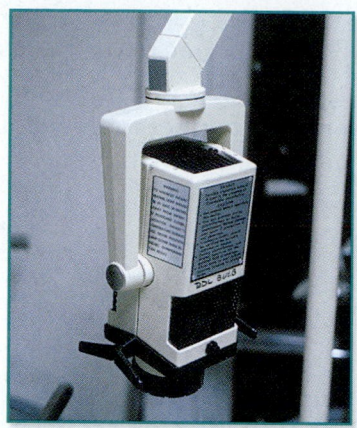

Figure 3-8-3 Overhead radiant warmer

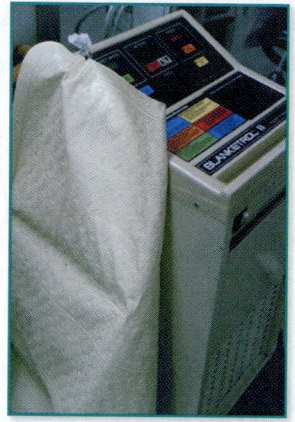

Figure 3-8-4 Blanketrol® circulating water hyper-hypothermia blanket

must be applied to that area. Applications of extreme cold to already compromised vascular areas can cause injury. **Heat or cold can injure areas of decreased sensitivity.**

3. Assess client's knowledge regarding treatment. **Determines client teaching needed.**

4. Assess the client's mental status. **Temperature extremes can cause confusion and agitation, and the client may not be able to cooperate with the treatment regime.**

▶ DIAGNOSIS

Risk for Imbalanced Body Temperature

Hypothermia

Hyperthermia

Risk for Impaired Skin Integrity

▶ PLANNING

Expected Outcomes:

1. The client's core temperature will be maintained within the desired range.

2. The client will not incur any skin or tissue damage as a result of the hypothermia/hyperthermia treatment.

3. The client will be as comfortable as possible during the treatment.

4. The client's core temperature will not change rapidly enough to cause chilling or diaphoresis.

Equipment Needed:

• Warming/cooling blanket with machine and temperature probe (see Figures 3-8-4 and 3-8-5)

• Thermometer, if not provided with blanket, to do comparison checks

• Blanket or sheet to protect skin from direct contact with warming/cooling blanket if not provided with commercial setup

• Lubricating solution for rectal temperature probe

• If an infant warmer is to be used, radiant warmer with accompanying skin or rectal probe and bedding for warmer (see Figure 3-8-6)

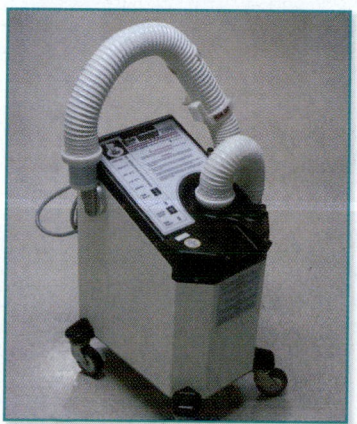

Figure 3-8-5 Bair Hugger® forced-air warming blanket control unit

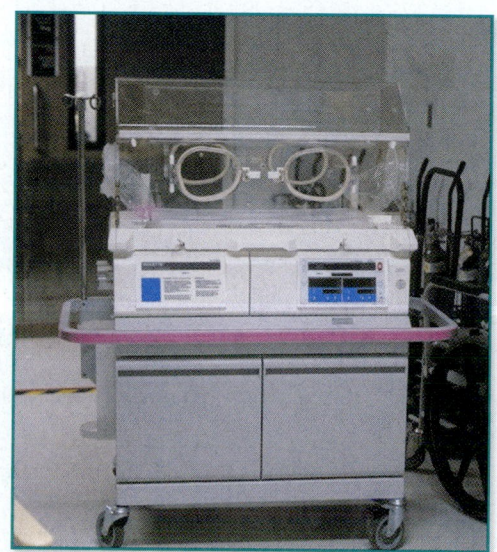

Figure 3-8-6 Isolette

► **CLIENT EDUCATION NEEDED:**

1. Instruct clients to alert the nurse if they feel chilled or overheated.
2. Teach the purpose of the blanket.
3. Instruct clients to alert the nurse if the temperature probe comes out.
4. If an infant warmer is used, instruct the parents of the goal of the warmer and the need for the infant to remain in the isolette.

Estimated time to complete the skill:
15 minutes for setup; time to reach optimal temperature will depend on the client's situation

► **DELEGATION TIPS**

Thermal blanket application is a skill routinely delegated to properly trained ancillary personnel. Reassessment of the client after application to maintain proper temperature and to evaluate the client response is essential. The application of a specialized body warmer for infants requires the supervision of a nurse, although it may be delegated to specially trained technicians in the nursery.

IMPLEMENTATION—Action/Rationale

Action	Rationale
1. Wash hands.	1. Reduces the transmission of microorganisms.
2. Assemble equipment and read manufacturer's directions. Check that equipment is functioning and that plug is grounded.	2. Prepares and ensures client's safety.
3. Check orders to ascertain desired systemic temperature to be attained.	3. Achieves desired outcome.
4. Check the client's vital signs, especially temperature.	4. Provides baseline data for future comparisons.
5. Explain the procedure to the client.	5. Explanations help decrease anxiety.
6. If necessary, add solution to the machine. Follow manufacturer's directions.	6. Cooling blanket equipment varies and some require the addition of solutions. Allows for proper function of equipment.

Hypothermia/Hyperthermia Blanket

Action	Rationale
7. Place the blanket over or under the client, according to the manufacturer's instructions. Place a sheet between the blanket and the client, and connect the machine. Protect any areas of disrupted skin integrity. Cover the client for privacy.	7. Sheet protects client from tissue injury. If clients have wounds, heel breakdown, frostbite, or areas of decreased sensitivity, these areas should be protected from further tissue injury.
8. Insert the temperature probe rectally and tape it in place.	8. Necessary for control of equipment to avoid overcooling or overheating. Securing the thermometer in place will help avert the danger of overheating or overcooling if the thermometer falls out of place.

continues

Action	Rationale
9. Set the machine on the desired temperature and turn on (see Figure 3-8-7). The temperature control should be set to gradually change the client's temperature. Some blankets will automatically make the adjustment.	9. Provides for appropriate effect from cooling blanket. The temperature should not be changed too rapidly so as to avoid chilling, or increasing metabolism.
10. Check the client's temperature every 15 minutes (see Figure 3-8-8) and vital signs every 30 minutes (see Figure 3-8-9). Observe for any chilling or overheating effect.	10. If the client is cooled too quickly, chilling, increased metabolism, and adverse reaction may occur.
11. Perform comparison check with another thermometer periodically (see Figure 3-8-10).	11. Avoids problems associated with equipment failure.
12. When the client's temperature is within close range of the desired temperature, turn off the machine and assess the client. Leave the blanket in place until the client is stabilized.	12. The blanket will not immediately return to room temperature and will continue to cool or heat the client even after it is turned off. Turning it off shortly before the goal temperature is achieved will prevent altering the client's core temperature beyond the desired outcome. Avoids the need to reposition blanket until the client is stabilized.
13. While the blanket is on, turn the client every hour and assess the skin condition (see Figure 3-8-11). Remove the blanket after the client is stabilized.	13. For cooling treatments, extended periods of cooling can cause areas of decreased perfusion, skin burns, and tissue injury. For heat treatments, extended periods of heat can cause skin irritation and burns.

Infant Radiant Warmer

Action	Rationale
14. Check the manufacturer's operating instructions. Check equipment, including caster locks, window seals, and heating system.	14. There are many different manufacturers of infant warmers and heaters. Each warmer may vary, so it is important to check instructions for operation and safety. It is important that the warmer function properly before placing the infant in the warmer.
15. Prepare the parents and inform them of the purpose of the warmer.	15. Decreases anxiety. Ensures that infant will be safe in enclosed environment.

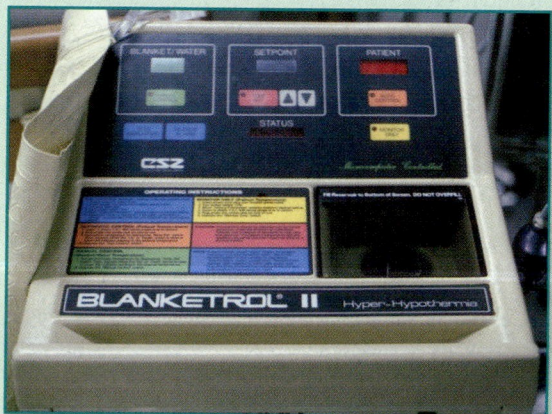

Figure 3-8-7   Set the machine on the desired temperature and start.

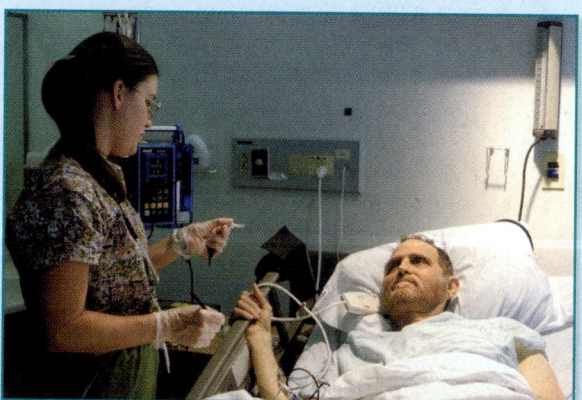

Figure 3-8-8   Check the client's temperature every 15 minutes.

continues

Action	Rationale

Infant Radiant Warmer *continued*

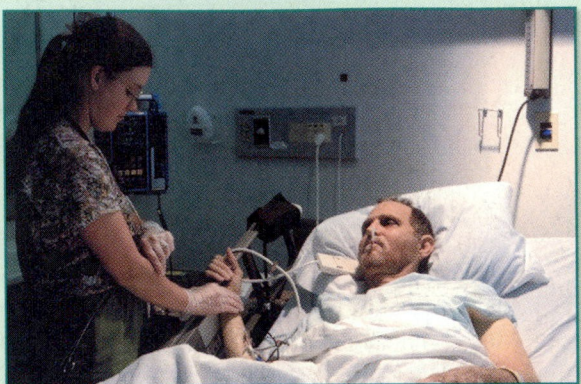

Figure 3-8-9   Check the client's vital signs every 30 minutes.

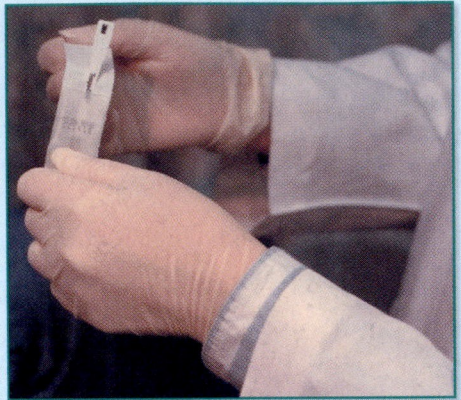

Figure 3-8-10   Comparison check the client's temperature using a different thermometer periodically to verify temperature readings.

16. Position the equipment in the room and plug electrical cord in a three-wire grounded receptacle. Turn on the equipment. Usually a red indicator light will glow.

16. Ensures client and staff safety and ensures equipment is properly functioning.

17. Turn on alarm switch and test alarm system. Turn on automatic temperature settings.

17. An alarm is necessary for the protection of the infant to avoid overheating.

18. Prewarm the isolette to the prescribed temperature.

18. If the unit is prewarmed, the infant will not be at risk for a decrease in body temperature in an unheated isolette.

19. Put on nonsterile gloves.

19. Reduces the transmission of microorganisms.

20. Place infant in warmer. Remove clothing, except diaper. Attach a skin temperature probe or insert rectal probe. Activate an audible alarm.

20. Alarm protects infant from overheating and adverse reactions.

21. For skin probe: Clean the skin surface and allow skin to dry. Place probe on skin, in right upper quadrant immediately below the right intercostal margin.

21. Oils on the skin may adversely affect adherence of the probe. Irritation can occur easily on the delicate skin of an infant, so careful assessment of the skin is necessary. Allergic or skin reactions can occur.

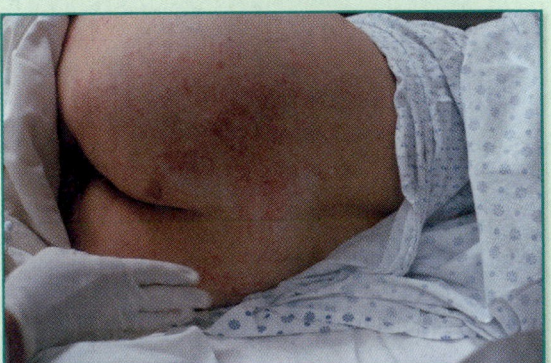

Figure 3-8-11   Assess the client's skin condition every hour.

continues

Action	Rationale
22. For rectal probe: Use lubricant and insert according to manufacturer's recommendations.	22. Lubricant adds comfort for insertion of probe.
23. Check the infant's temperature with another thermometer. Inspect probe at regular intervals.	23. Double-checking with another thermometer ensures that the equipment is functioning properly.
24. When the infant's optimal temperature is reached, the infant may be kept in the warmer until the core temperature is stabilized.	24. The infant should be gradually heated. If heated too rapidly, the metabolism will be increased and body fluids lost.
25. After the infant is removed from the warmer, the equipment should be cleaned following Standard Precautions, and preventive maintenance of the warmer should be performed, with inspection of all parts.	25. Reduces the transmission of microorganisms and provides for proper equipment function for future use.
26. Remove gloves and wash hands.	26. Reduces the transmission of microorganisms.

▶ **EVALUATION**

- The client's core temperature is stable within the desired range.
- The client did not incur any skin or tissue damage as a result of the hypothermia/hyperthermia treatment.
- The client was as comfortable as possible during the treatment.
- The client's core temperature did not change rapidly enough to cause chilling or diaphoresis.

▶ **DOCUMENTATION**

Nurses' Notes

- Document the procedure and results of the procedure.

- Document the client's temperature every 15 minutes, vital signs every 30 minutes, and the settings on the hypothermia/hyperthermia machine.
- Document any adverse outcomes such as chilling or tissue injury, and document any follow-up actions, such as notification of the physician or the administration of medication.

Document on appropriate flow sheet or electronic medical record (EMR).

Vital Signs Flow Sheet

- Note the client's core temperature according to the rectal probe, the core temperature according to the independent thermometer, and the client's other vital signs.

▶ **REAL WORLD ANECDOTES**

Carlos was brought to the emergency room by his wife. Carlos presented with complaints of chills. He was intermittently confused and belligerent. When the emergency room nurse took Carlos's oral temperature, she noted that it was 104.1° F. She took his temperature again using the aural thermometer. This reading was 104.2° F. The nurse reported her findings to the physician, and Carlos was admitted to the hospital. The physician ordered a hypothermia blanket to keep Carlos's core temperature below 100° F. When the hypothermia blanket was started, however, Carlos became quite agitated and insisted that he was lying in a puddle of ice water. Despite the staff and family efforts to calm and reorient him, Carlos remained agitated and combative. Carlos's physician ordered sedation and Carlos was finally able to rest easily and allow the blanket to work.

▶ CRITICAL THINKING SKILL

Introduction

Consider what to do if the client's temperature does not change.

Possible Scenario

Samuel is working in the trauma unit. His 42-year-old client has a fever of 103.3° F. A hypothermia blanket has been ordered. Samuel sets up the blanket. Fifteen minutes later, the client's temperature is 103.7° F.

Possible Outcome

Samuel increases the cooling rate of the blanket and sets the goal temperature lower than normal body temperature to increase the rate of cooling in the blanket. When he returns 15 minutes later, his client's core temperature is 104.0° F.

Prevention

When setting up a cooling/warming blanket, be sure it is working properly before placing it underneath the client. Know how much fluid is supposed to be in the machine and be sure that all of the hoses are patent. Check the connections for tightness and make sure that the mattress itself is intact and without holes or cracks. If the equipment does not seem to be working properly, have it replaced before using it on a client. If the blanket is working properly and the client's temperature is not decreasing, notify a physician or qualified practitioner.

▶ VARIATIONS

Geriatric Variations:

- *Temperature changes that are too rapid may cause chilling in elderly clients.*
- *Elderly clients have thin skin and subsequently can receive tissue injury more rapidly.*
- *Elderly clients may be less sensitive to heat and cold and may not be as aware of temperature changes or extremes.*

Pediatric Variations:

- *Children may be fussy when their temperature is increased and may resist a blanket.*
- *Children may move frequently, decreasing the amount of skin exposed to the cooling surface.*
- *If a rectal temperature probe is used, this may be embarrassing or uncomfortable.*
- *Infant radiant warmers or isolettes are especially useful for premature infants who are unable to regulate their systemic temperature. Isolettes, which confine infants and require viewing through plastic, can be very frightening for a parent. Nurses should provide ways for parents to touch or feed the infant to assist with maternal/paternal attachment.*

Home Care Variations:

- *Cooling blankets generally are not used in home care because of cost. Cool baths are more suited to the home setting. The client should be evaluated for long periods of increased temperature and the underlying cause treated.*

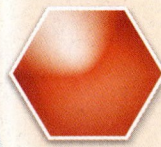

Long-Term Care Variations:

- *Make sure the equipment is kept in good condition and worn-out parts are repaired or replaced.*

▶ COMMON ERRORS

Possible Error:

The temperature probe falls out and the probe reports that the client's core temperature is within parameters but the client still feels hot.

Prevention:

Check the position of the probe frequently. Check the client's temperature with a thermometer that is not attached to the thermal blanket to verify the probe readings.

Possible Error:

The sheet comes off of the cooling blanket, and the client suffers areas of skin burn from lying directly on chilled plastic.

Prevention:

Check the cover sheet often for placement. With restless clients it may be necessary to tape the cover sheet to the blanket. Do not use pins on or near the thermal blanket. Pins can puncture or tear the blanket, rendering it useless.

▶ NURSING TIPS

- Assess the client every 15 minutes after the cooling blanket is put in place.
- Be sure to check the functioning of the temperature probe by cross-checking with other systems.
- Protect clients from tissue injury.
- Protect any open wound areas and areas of decreased perfusion.
- Clean the rectal probe every 4 hours.

▶ SPECIAL CONSIDERATIONS

- *In the operating room, the circulating nurse must be aware that instruments can penetrate thermal blankets and lead to electric shock or blanket dysfunction. As the client is covered with drapes, special precautions should be taken to protect the equipment. Because the client cannot respond to overheating, the thermostat and client's core temperature must be monitored carefully.*
- *Infants' core temperature can change rapidly; therefore, when infant radiant warmers are in use, carefully and frequently monitor core temperature. A probe should be in place.*
- *Warm compresses may retain heat, and, therefore caution should be used when thermal blankets or radiant infant warmers are used in conjunction with moist heat or compresses.*

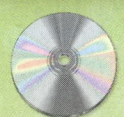

SKILL 3-9

Applying Cold Treatment

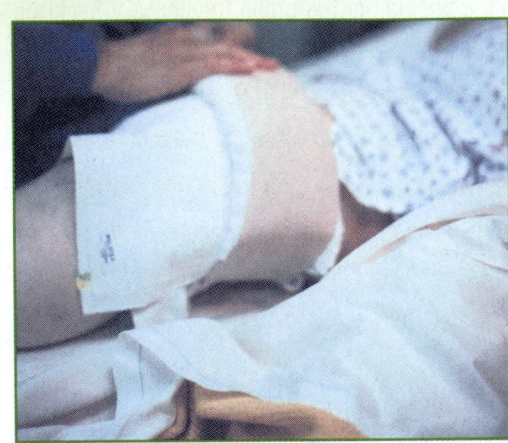

▶ OVERVIEW OF THE SKILL

Cold therapy is used to decrease blood flow to an area by promoting vasoconstriction and increased blood viscosity. These changes facilitate clotting and control bleeding. Cold decreases tissue metabolism, reduces oxygen consumption, and decreases inflammation and edema formation. Cold therapy has a local anesthetic effect by raising the threshold of pain receptors. It causes a decrease in muscle tension. Cold is used to reduce fever.

Sources of cold include ice packs, ice bags, cold collars, or commercial cold packs. If the client's systemic temperature is increased, cooling blankets or cooling tepid sponge baths can be used. Moist cold compresses or immersion of a body part can be used for large areas of acute inflammation or swelling. Cooling the extremity decreases blood flow and may also decrease pain and suppress inflammation.

▶ ASSESSMENT

1. Ascertain the client's sensation of hot and cold changes at the site where cold therapy is to be administered. **Certain areas of the skin have sensitivity to temperature variations, whereas other areas may not be as sensitive; the perineal areas are very sensitive.**

2. Assess whether decreased circulation is present at the site where cold therapy will be applied such as areas with wounds and damaged tissue

present **because cold application may cause further tissue damage.**

3. Check the client's systemic temperature. **If larger areas are exposed to cold, the total body temperature may be decreased. If the client is cooled too rapidly with extreme cold, a reverse chilling effect may occur, increasing body metabolism and defeating the cooling effect.**

4. Assess age. **Tolerance to cold varies with individuals and is related to age, thinner layers of skin, or general sensitivity to cold.**

▶ DIAGNOSIS

Ineffective Tissue Perfusion

Risk for Imbalanced Body Temperature

Risk for Injury

Risk for Impaired Skin Integrity

▶ PLANNING

Expected Outcomes:

1. The client will experience decreased bleeding.
2. The client will have decreased inflammation and/or edema.
3. The client will experience decreased pain or discomfort.

Equipment Needed:

- (Select equipment depending on the treatment chosen and supplies available.)

- Pan for cold soak
- Ice or ice bag
- Gauze or towel
- Water bottles or reusable containers if used for one client only
- Compresses (if moist cold) consisting of gauze dressing, iced or chilled solution, and a container of the appropriate size for the body part
- Commercially prepared ice pack (see Figure 3-9-1)
- Disposable ice pack
- Tape, elastic wrap, or bandage (see Figure 3-9-2)

▶ **CLIENT EDUCATION NEEDED:**

1. Report any pain or lack of sensation (if cold is being used as local anesthetic, then decreased sensation is expected).
2. Report chilling from overexposure since this would increase general metabolism. This can especially happen if the client has a large area of the body exposed to cold; therefore, it may be necessary to add increased covers to the rest of the body.

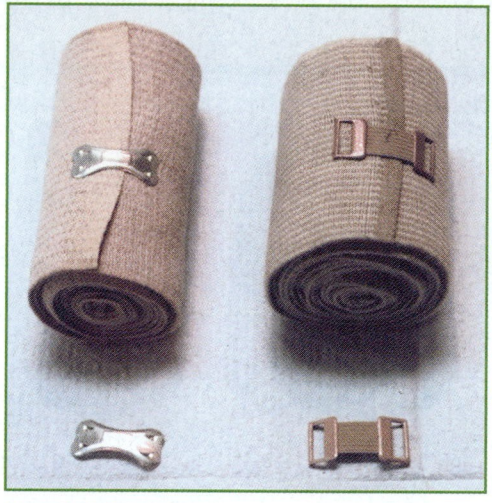

Figure 3-9-2 Elastic wrap

3. Teach the client the basics of cold application, why it is used, and how long the treatment will remain in place (20 minutes). Modify the therapy for home use, and teach the client how to apply the treatment at home, if applicable.
4. Teach clients the reason for cold therapy versus hot therapy.

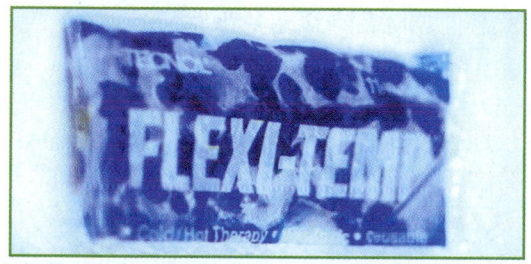

Figure 3-9-1 Ice pack

 Estimated time to complete the skill: **20 minutes for application plus preparation time of 5–10 minutes**

▶ **DELEGATION TIPS**

This skill is routinely delegated to properly trained ancillary personnel. Reassessment of the client after application to maintain proper temperature and to evaluate the client response is essential.

IMPLEMENTATION—Action/Rationale

Action	Rationale
1. Wash hands.	1. Reduces the transmission of microorganisms.
2. Assess the client's sensation and skin color at the site of planned application. Determine whether any tissue damage is present. Assess for bleeding or wound drainage (see Figure 3-9-3).	2. Provides baseline data for post-treatment comparison.

continues

Action	Rationale

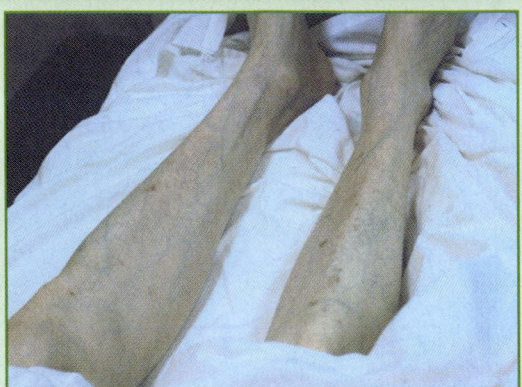

Figure 3-9-3   Assess the skin at the site of planned application for color, sensation, wounds, or skin irritation.

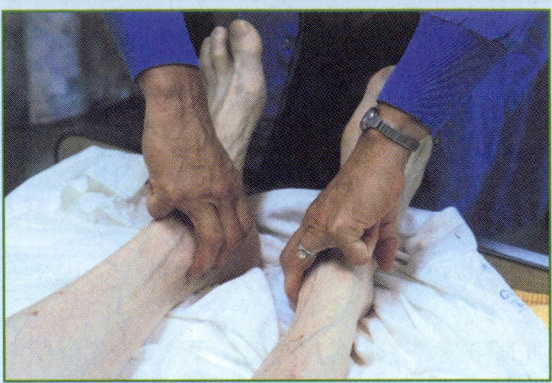

Figure 3-9-4   Assess for circulatory impairment or neuropathy before beginning treatment.

3. Determine the diagnosis. Identify whether the client has a history of circulatory impairment or neuropathy (see Figure 3-9-4).

4. Check the physician's or qualified practitioner's order and the reason for the application of cold.

5. If using an ice bag with moist gauze or towels, fill the bag three-fourths full with ice and remove the remaining air from the bag. Close the bag. Check for leaks. Wrap the bag in a towel or protective cover and place it on the affected area. If cold soaks are being applied, use the appropriate-size basin for the body part to be soaked.

6. If an ice collar is used, fill the collar three-fourths full with ice and remove the remaining air from the collar before closing the collar. Check for leaks. Place the collar in a protective cover and around the client's neck.

7. If a disposable cold pack is used, activate the pack according to the manufacturer's directions, wrap the pack in a towel (see Figure 3-9-5), and place it on the affected area (see Figure 3-9-6). Some packs come with covers. Secure pack in place with tape, elastic wrap, or bandage (see Figures 3-9-7, 3-9-8, and 3-9-9). Dispose of the pack after the treatment.

8. Assess the client's skin periodically for signs of cold intolerance or tissue damage.

9. If the client can tolerate the cold, leave the cold application in place for approximately 20 minutes at approximately 15° C (59° F).

3. Cold causes vasoconstriction and decreased metabolism and can cause tissue damage in people with impaired circulation and sensation.

4. A physician's or qualified practitioner's order is needed in most situations of cold treatment, and the client should be informed of the reason for the application of cold.

5. If air is removed from the bag, the bag will be easier to mold to the client's body. The bag is wrapped to prevent injury to the client's skin or exposed tissue because direct cold can cause damage.

6. Easier to mold to the client's body. The collar is wrapped to prevent injury to the client's skin.

7. When the pack is squeezed or kneaded, an alcohol-based solution is released, creating the cold temperature. The pack cannot be used again.

8. Signs of intolerance to cold are pallor, blanching, mottling, or numbness of the skin.

9. Longer application can cause tissue damage, especially because the client's pain sensation is decreased in the presence of cold. A reflex vasodilatation occurs after 20 minutes, thereby negating the therapeutic effect of the cold treatment.

continues

Action	Rationale

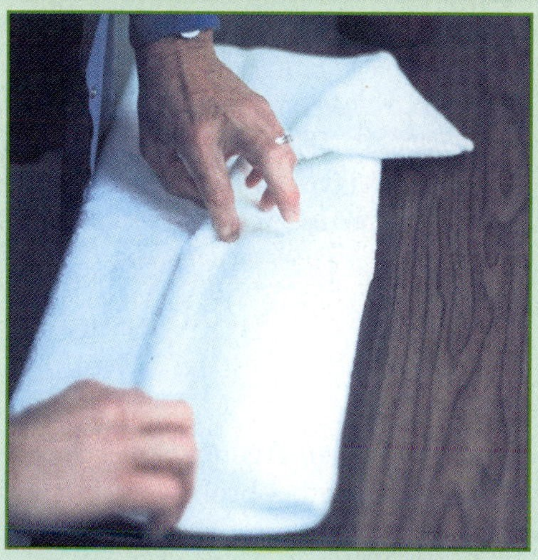

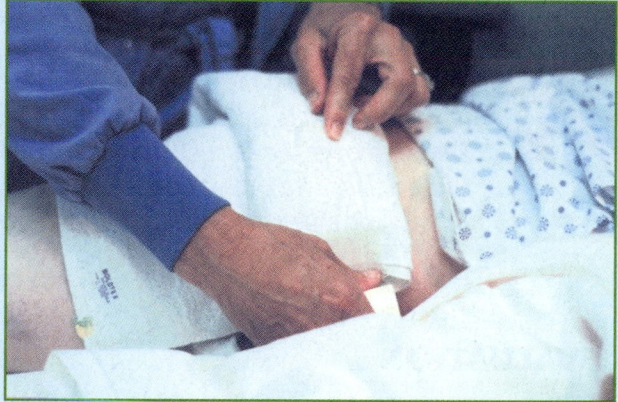

Figure 3-9-6   Place the cold pack on the affected area.

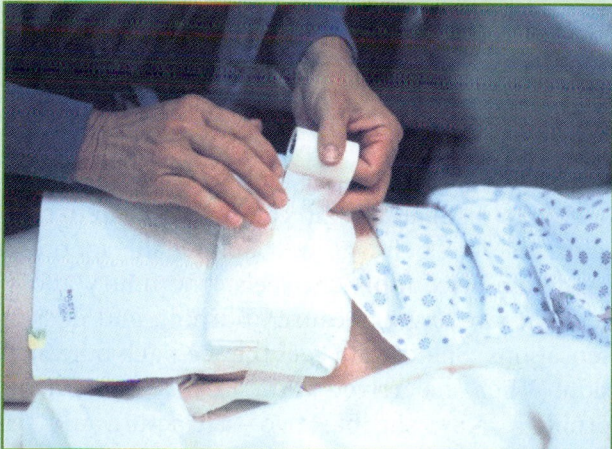

Figure 3-9-5   Wrap the cold pack in a towel.

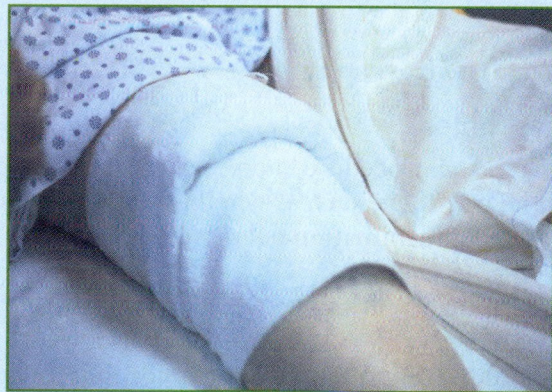

Figure 3-9-8   This cold pack is properly wrapped in a towel and secured with tape.

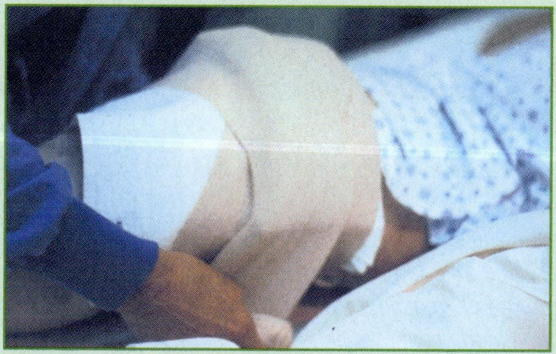

Figure 3-9-7   Use tape to secure the cold pack to the affected area.

10. Reassess the condition of the client's skin or exposed tissue.

11. Wash hands.

10. The client's skin should be assessed, and any signs of cold changes and intolerance should be documented.

11. Reduces the transmission of microorganisms.

Figure 3-9-9   Elastic wrap may be used to hold bulky cold packs in place.

> **REAL WORLD ANECDOTES**

Brittany just gave birth to her first child. She had an epidural and is in the recovery area waiting to return to her room. The recovery nurse placed a latex glove filled with ice over the site of Brittany's episiotomy. Brittany is recovering well and the nurse is called away to help with a second new mother. Brittany's nurse is gone longer than she had anticipated. Brittany cannot feel the ice pack or the numbness that is developing in her perineal area because of the epidural anesthesia. By the time Brittany's nurse returns, Brittany has started to experience tissue damage from the prolonged exposure to the cold. She cannot feel it now, but when the epidural wears off, Brittany will experience more than the expected amount of perineal pain and a longer healing time.

▶ EVALUATION

- The client's bleeding was decreased.
- The client had a decrease in inflammation and/or edema.
- The client verbalized a decrease in pain or discomfort.

▶ DOCUMENTATION

Nurses' Notes

- Record the procedure and the client's response to the treatment such as whether bleeding was stopped, inflammation decreased, or edema decreased.
- Record the client's skin condition after the procedure.
- Record the length of time of application.

Document on appropriate flow sheet or electronic medical record (EMR).

▶ CRITICAL THINKING SKILLS

Introduction

When applying cold treatment, it is important to check your client and assess treated sites to prevent tissue damage.

Possible Scenario

You are working in the emergency department (ED). A teenage girl arrives with a broken wrist from a fall at a roller rink. She is nauseous and shaking. She complains of pain, burning, and numbness from her elbow to her fingers, with particular numbness in her wrist area. You grab a splint, an ice pack, and an Ace bandage to hold it in place. The ED becomes really busy, and you leave her in an exam room with her companion.

Possible Outcome

Trying to rest and remain calm, and afraid to tamper with the Ace bandage and splint, she ignores the moderate discomfort she feels. The injury and subsequent swelling has caused burning and decreased sensations. She cannot feel the ice pack burning her skin. When she arrived at the ED, the client had one problem. Now she has two—a fracture and tissue damage from the ice pack.

Prevention

If the client has swelling, it still is appropriate to apply cold treatment to reduce the swelling. You must, however, assess the injured site 10 minutes after cold application to check for sensation and tingling.

> **VARIATIONS**

Geriatric Variations:

- *Older clients generally have reduced circulation, reduced sensation, and thin skin and are candidates for increased tissue damage from cold therapy.*
- *Older clients usually become cold more easily than the younger population and, therefore, may require covers on other parts of their body or they may not be able to tolerate treatment as long.*
- *Older clients may have peripheral nerve damage and decreased sensation.*
- *Commercial ice packs may be appropriate for the elderly because ice is not directly on the skin.*

continues

► VARIATIONS *(continued)*

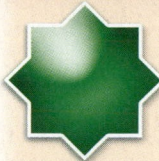

Pediatric Variations:

- *Children may dislike cold application and refuse to keep compresses in place. Holding an ice pack in place with a colorful scarf or cloth may help the child keep it in place. Allow the child to help place the pack. Placing crushed ice in a glove and drawing a face on the glove may increase acceptance of the treatment.*
- *Adolescents can take responsibility for their own cold therapy. Educate them to observe for signs of overexposure to cold and to limit their exposure. In this case, more is not necessarily better.*
- *Try to find a way to make cold therapy fun. A young child needing cold therapy on the fingers, for example, could play with "submarines" in a basin of ice water with "icebergs."*

Home Care Variations:

- *Clients may not watch time carefully and extend cold treatment beyond 20 minutes.*
- *In the home setting, clients may use their own equipment; however, these should be cleaned with soap and water and should not be used directly on open wounds.*
- *If the client will be breaking up ice cubes to use in home-based cold therapy, make sure they have a plan to do so safely. Instruct the home caregiver to keep fingers away from ice and not to use knifes or other sharp instruments to break ice.*
- *One effective way to break ice cubes is to place them in a plastic bag, then in an old pillowcase or other heavy cloth bag. Take the bag outdoors to a smooth cement surface and crush the ice with the side of a hammer, a heavy metal pot, or a rolling pin. Do not hold the bag while crushing the ice.*
- *Think of creative sources of cold for appropriate applications. Frozen peas, frozen orange juice cans, or frozen French fries can be used in an emergency. Always wrap the cold source in a protective cloth before placing it next to the skin.*
- *Soak several hand towels or bath towels in a basin of water, wring them out, and place them in the freezer. After they are frozen, they make a flexible, comfortable source of cold. Always wrap the cold source in a protective cloth before placing it next to the skin.*

Long-Term Care Variations:

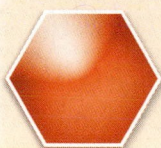

- *Make sure cold therapies used with multiple clients in the long-term setting are cleaned properly between clients to reduce the transmission of microorganisms.*
- *Allow clients to institute and monitor their own cold treatments when possible to improve a sense of control over pain, comfort, and healing.*

► COMMON ERRORS

Possible Error:

Cold application is left in place beyond 20 minutes and reflex vasodialation occurs.

Prevention:

Check the pack after 5 minutes. Teach the client to remove the ice pack when the allotted time is up.

Possible Error:

Cold application remains on longer than 20 minutes and tissue damage occurs.

Prevention:

Watch for signs and symptoms of burning or numbness, mottling of the skin, extreme paleness, redness, or bluish discoloration.

continues

► **COMMON ERRORS** (continued)

Possible Error:

The client may fall asleep and forget about cold application, and tissue damage occurs.

Prevention:

Choose a size or type of cold application that will warm up within the allotted period of time. Make sure another person is available to check the cold therapy, and remove it when necessary.

► **NURSING TIPS**

- Avoid cold therapy to extremities in clients with peripheral neuropathy.
- Take special precautions when cold application is used in elderly clients.
- Take precautions to avoid chilling effects in clients.
- If a large area of the body receives cold application, watch the time carefully and assess body temperature.

► **SPECIAL CONSIDERATIONS**

- *For the client receiving physical therapy, cold applications may be used to reduce pain and inflammation before exercise. At this point in therapy, it is generally the client's choice whether warm, moist heat, or cold therapy is used.*
- *Cold therapy is often implemented after orthopedic surgery. Make sure that it is monitored closely as clients may not notice injury because of postoperative pain or postoperative medications being used.*

Assisting with a Transcutaneous Electrical Nerve Stimulation (TENS) Unit

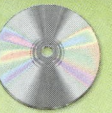

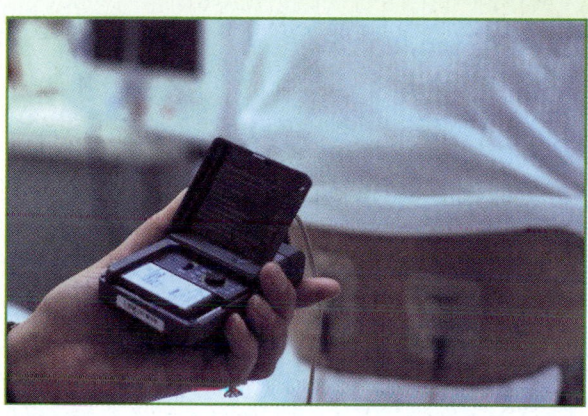

▶ OVERVIEW OF THE SKILL

The overall purpose of transcutaneous electrical nerve stimulation (TENS) is to manage acute and chronic pain. Pain is the body's warning system that protects from injury or damage. Without this mechanism, our bodies would be injured or harmed without us knowing. There are two categories of pain. Acute pain is limited in duration and related to specific causes such as muscle sprains and strains, traumas, and postoperative pain. Chronic pain is longer in duration and very persistent. It can last a few months to many years. At this point, the pain center in the brain has ceased to serve as a warning sign to the body and has become the problem itself. Chronic pain can be caused by such disorders as low back pain, arthritis, migraine headaches, or phantom limb pain. Sometimes the cause of the pain cannot be determined. The TENS unit, attached to electrodes placed on the skin's surface over the painful area, applies doses of low-voltage electricity to the electrodes to help relieve some types of acute and chronic pain by electrical stimulation on the large cutaneous axons.

There are two theories, gate control theory and pattern theory, that explain how electrical stimulation relieves pain. Gate control theory suggests that pain and nonpain impulses are sent to the brain from the local nervous system. These impulses travel through the skin's superficial cutaneous nerves to the deeper afferent nerves. Next, the impulses travel to the spinal cord and then to the brain stem. When these impulses reach a certain level, "gates" open, allowing the impulses to travel to higher brain centers. These "gates" control which impulses continue on to the brain. Because the same nerve cannot carry a pain impulse and a nonpain impulse simultaneously, the stronger, nonpain impulse (TENS unit in this case) controls the gate. TENS provides continuous mild electrical stimulation, blocking the pain signals traveling along the nerves to the brain cells. It is thought that if the pain signals do not reach the brain, by using electrical stimulation as a distraction, the pain will be decreased or not felt. TENS works by sending these small electrical impulses through the skin's cutaneous layer to the body's deeper afferent nervous system.

In pattern theory, the effectiveness of TENS is thought to work by stimulating the body's own natural pain control mechanism. The theory suggests that the intensity of the impulses creates a pattern that the brain senses as pain. The body then creates natural pain relievers, enkephalins and endorphins. The TENS unit, which provides a short burst of mild electrical activity, is thought to stimulate the body's natural pain relievers, which interact with receptors, thus decreasing pain sensation.

Assisting with the application of TENS involves the correct placement of electrodes on peripheral nerves, exhausting the area of pain. Identification of trigger and acupressure points is crucial for determining correct placement of the electrodes. Moreover, an understanding of the TENS apparatus and its mechanical functions is essential. TENS is not a cure for pain and should be used in conjunction with other therapies such as massage and relaxation.

▶ ASSESSMENT

1. Consider the appropriateness of applying TENS to the client. For example, clients with cardiac pacemakers or cardiac defibrillators are contraindicated. **TENS is considered electrical equipment and therefore has potential for electrical current leakage. This may interfere with the proper functioning of a pacemaker or a defibrillator**.

2. Assess the client's knowledge regarding the TENS device. **Positive preparation and understanding before a procedure promotes psychological safety by reducing fear and anxiety of the unknown. Safety feelings arise from familiar and predictable situations.**

3. Assess the client's skin condition. Do not place electrodes on areas with skin irritation or breakdown. **Application in these areas may affect the safety of clients, predisposing them to further skin problems or skin burns.**

▶ DIAGNOSIS

Acute Pain

Impaired Physical Mobility

Ineffective Coping

Chronic Pain

Deficient Knowledge

▶ PLANNING

Expected Outcomes:

1. The client will have a decrease in pain.
2. The client will have an increase in mobility.
3. The client will increase the activities of daily living.
4. The client will demonstrate how to operate TENS unit.

Equipment Needed (see Figure 3-10-1):

- Cutaneous stimulator (TENS)
- Appropriate electrodes (leads)
- Electrode gel for lead placement
- 9-volt battery with charger
- Cordset (2)
- Soap and water or recommended cleanser to clean the skin if needed

▶ CLIENT EDUCATION NEEDED:

1. Explain the reason for the TENS device prescribed by the physician or qualified practitioner.

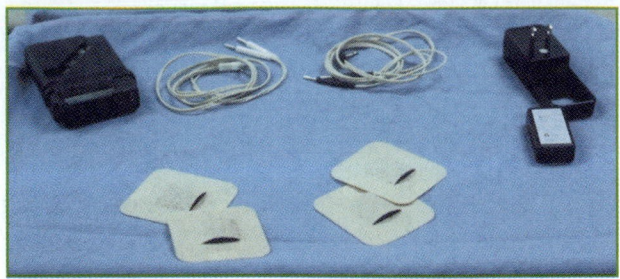

Figure 3-10-1 TENS unit, electrodes, cordsets, battery, and charger

2. Explain the procedure step-by-step and allow the client to view the equipment being used.

3. Instruct the client on skin care for long-term application.

4. Instruct the client to call a health care professional if skin irritation is noted at the electrode site.

5. Explain necessary positioning to access certain areas.

6. Do not use TENS while operating potentially dangerous equipment such as automobiles, power mowers, and power tools.

7. Do not use while bathing. Clients may shower with TENS electrodes on but should not stand with the spray directly on them for long periods of time. This will cause the electrodes to come off.

8. Do not carry batteries in a pocket or purse or where battery terminals could be short-circuited.

9. Inform the client that TENS devices should be kept out of the reach of children.

10. Do not use for other than condition of pain.

11. Use only appropriate battery rechargers.

12. Do not submerge the battery charger in water or other liquids.

13. The use of heat or cold applications affects the electrode or client circulation.

14. Instruct the client to turn the TENS device off before connecting the electrodes.

15. Instruct the client on usage frequency per physician's or qualified practitioner's orders, usually 30–40 minutes 3–4 times every day.

Estimated time to complete the skill: **30–40 minutes**

▶ **DELEGATION TIPS**

This skill is routinely delegated to properly trained ancillary personnel. Reassessment of the client after application is essential. Ancillary personnel, the client, or family members need to be instructed to report any changes in response to the treatment or a change in the client's condition to the nurse.

IMPLEMENTATION—Action/Rationale

Action	Rationale
1. Obtain order from a physician or qualified practitioner.	1. TENS units require an order from a physician or qualified practitioner.
2. Identify client through nurse/client verbalization and chart documentation.	2. Provides positive identification of client.

3. Verify that the internal controls are correct. The physician, qualified practitioner, or nurse presets internal controls prior to the procedure. The internal controls (pulse duration, rate, and mode) are located under the sliding cover of the stimulator and work together with the intensity setting to provide the correct stimulation sensation necessary for maximum pain control.
 	
    Pulse duration dial controls the width of each electrical pulse.
 	
    Rate indicates the number of electrical pulses that will be sent through the skin each second.
 	
    Modes indicate the different modes of stimulation. This will vary depending on type of unit (see Figure 3-10-2).
	3. Ensures proper electrical stimulation to client.

4. Introduce yourself and the procedure you will be doing.	4. Builds trust and decreases anxiety and fear.
5. Wash hands.	5. Reduces the transmission of microorganisms.
6. Explain actions of application throughout the procedure. Provide a clear description of the procedure confronting the client and verbally illustrate what can be expected to occur. Let the client view the equipment to be used.	6. Verbal communication provides comfort and psychological safety to the client, reducing fear and anxiety of the unknown.
7. Cleanse skin area gently where electrodes will be applied. Use mild soap and water (see Figure 3-10-3).	7. Prevents bacterial growth, prevents infection, and promotes cleanliness and comfort.
8. Rinse and dry skin in the area thoroughly.	8. Ensures adequate preparation of skin to allow proper adhesion of electrodes.
9. Apply conductive skin preparation product (electrode gel) to the skin.	9. Decreases potential for skin irritation such as redness, small pimple-like lesions, or blisters.

continues

Action	Rationale

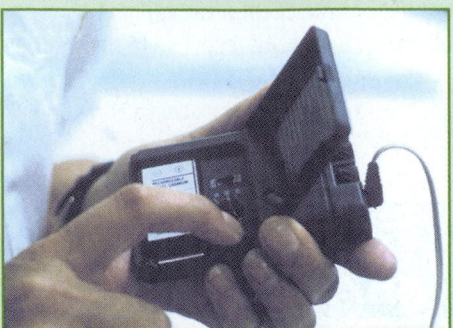

Figure 3-10-2   The internal controls for pulse duration, rate, and mode are located under the sliding cover of the stimulator.

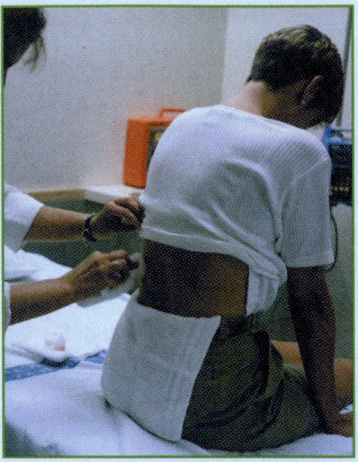

Figure 3-10-3   Using soap and water, gently cleanse the skin where the electrodes will be applied.

10. Connect the cordset to the electrodes before applying the electrodes to the skin.

10. Reduces the possibility of dislodging the electrodes.

11. Follow manufacturer's directions for electrode placement.
    Place electrode on skin over or near the area of pain.
    Identify trigger points—those specific areas that are more sensitive when stimulated. Identify acupressure points (see Figure 3-10-4).
    Place electrode on peripheral nerves around the area of pain. Allow the client to assist with placement and adjustments to produce the sensation that is most pleasant and best relieves pain.

11. Ensures correct application and safety of client.

12. Apply electrodes to the prepared skin area.

12. Prepares affected area for stimulation.

13. Hold the insulated connector portion of the cordset and insert into the corresponding jack, marked by channel numbers.

13. Ensures proper connection for device to function properly.

14. Set the stimulator controls to the appropriate configurations. There are usually two dials located at the top of the stimulator. They are used to increase or decrease the strength of stimulation (see Figure 3-10-5).

14. Provides electrical stimulation to relieve client's pain.

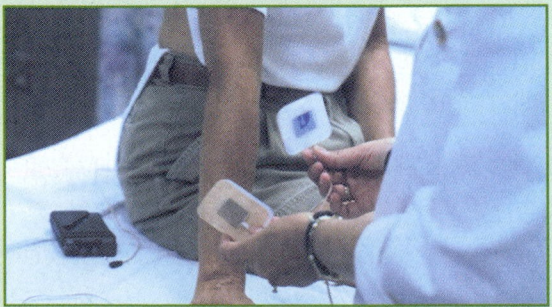

Figure 3-10-4   Assess trigger and acupressure points prior to electrode placement. Let the client guide placement for the most effective pain relief.

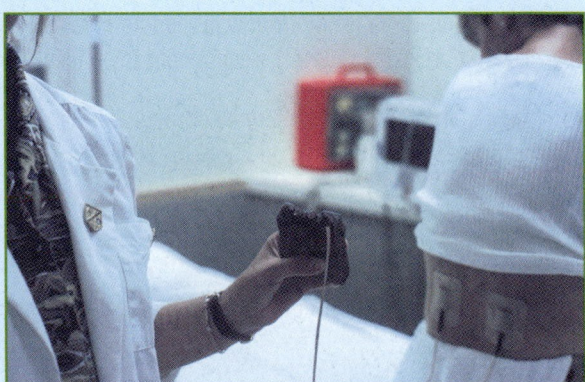

Figure 3-10-5   Set the stimulator controls to the appropriate strength of stimulation.

continues

Action	Rationale
15. Place the protective cap over the intensity controls.	**15.** Prevents accidental bumping of the dials and ensures safety of client.
16. Turn the machine on and instruct the client to adjust the level of intensity. Ensure that the green on/off indicator light is on. The green light indicates that the TENS unit is working. As intensity increases, the intensity of the light increases. The light flashes each time the unit stimulates the client. Ensure that the yellow battery status light is not on. A flashing yellow light indicates that the battery voltage is low and battery replacement is needed.	**16.** Ensures that the TENS unit is on and the proper intensity level is set for each individual. Ensures that the battery is functioning.
17. Wash hands.	**17.** Reduces the transmission of microorganisms.
18. Record the application and outcomes of TENS in the progress notes.	**18.** Provides documentation of event.

► **EVALUATION**

1. The client verbalized a decrease in pain.
2. The client's mobility increased.
3. The client increased the activities of daily living.
4. The client was able to demonstrate how to operate the TENS unit.

► **DOCUMENTATION**

Nurses' Notes

- Indicate the type of TENS unit. Give the manufacturer's information for tracking purposes.

- Record the TENS unit settings, rate, intensity, and frequency.
- Document the length of time the TENS unit was used by the client.
- Document any complications the client experienced during procedure, such as skin irritation, weakness, redness, and skin burns. Document if no complications occurred.
- Document the client's understanding of the TENS procedure.

Document on appropriate flow sheet or electronic medical record (EMR).

► **REAL WORLD ANECDOTES**

Mr. Dyer was sent home with a TENS unit. He was instructed on how to turn the stimulator on and off, viewing the channel light indicator. The unit was working perfectly until one day Mr. Dyer saw a yellow light flashing and the unit stopped working. He called the physician's office in a panic and asked to speak with the nurse. He told the nurse that he was no longer getting pain relief because his stimulator wasn't working and he didn't know why. He explained to the nurse that he had done nothing differently than before. The nurse troubleshot the problem and determined that the TENS unit had a dead battery. She then realized that she probably forgot to communicate to Mr. Dyer that a flashing yellow light means the battery is getting low and should be replaced.

If the nurse had instructed Mr. Dyer about the yellow battery status light or reviewed the troubleshooting literature in the manufacturer's booklet before discharge, Mr. Dyer would not have called the office in such a panic. In addition, Mr. Dyer would not have had to suffer during the resolution of this problem if he had been better instructed on how to operate the TENS device.

The nurse was reminded that clear, proper instruction to clients using TENS is necessary to ensure proper functioning. Moreover, providing educational information will increase a client's knowledge regarding the functions of the TENS unit. It will also decrease anxiety and frustration if the unit should malfunction as a result of battery failure.

▶ CRITICAL THINKING SKILL

Introduction

Clarify orders with the physician or qualified practitioner for the maximum benefit to the client

Possible Scenario

A physician ordered the application of a TENS unit for thoracic spine pain. Before applying the TENS, the nurse reviews the client's chart and notices that the primary diagnosis is low back (lumbar) pain, with a secondary diagnosis of mild thoracic pain. The physician may have written the order thinking it was the client's midspine that hurt most, instead of the lumbar region.

The nurse notifies the physician and questions the order for verification. The physician acknowledges the written error and informs the nurse that the correct area is the lumbar spine, which is where he wants the TENS to be applied.

Possible Outcome

If the nurse had not questioned and verified the order for the correct placement of TENS, the pads could have been placed on an improper area. The client may not have known that the TENS should have been placed farther down the spine, thus not communicating this to the nurse during application. The severity of this error would not be life-threatening, but improper placement of TENS would not have been beneficial for the client's low back pain. In addition, the client may have experienced unpleasant sensations in the area less affected by pain.

Prevention

The nurse prevented improper placement by checking the order through review of the chart and notifying the physician through verbal verification before applying the TENS unit. The nurse should also confirm the area of pain with the client.

▶ VARIATIONS

Geriatric Variations:

- *Elderly clients may have difficulty hearing and understanding information about the TENS unit instructions.*
- *Elderly clients may have trouble seeing the dial settings on the TENS unit.*
- *Elderly clients may be more sensitive to higher intensity settings.*
- *Elderly clients are more prone to falls and caution should be taken to ensure that lead placement remains secure.*
- *Elderly clients may have unsteady hand movements or arthritic conditions making it difficult for them to adjust the dials on the stimulator.*

Pediatric Variations:

- *Different age groups will have different levels of educational needs.*
- *An adult must supervise children at all times.*
- *Children may be more sensitive to sensory stimulation. Caution should be taken when setting intensity parameters.*
- *Child activities should be limited during usage of TENS therapy. Falling or rough play may dislodge lead placement or accidentally change parameter settings.*

Home Care Variations:

- *Home usage requires continuous monitoring by a physician or qualified practitioner.*
- *All previous instructions for usage and functioning on TENS apply.*

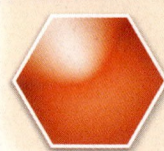

Long-Term Care Variations:

- *There is a potential for skin irritation. The client's skin may not be accustomed to long-term exposure to electrode gels and adhesives used with TENS units. Skin must be assessed and cared for to avoid problems.*
- *Long-term usage requires cleaning and maintenance instructions on TENS components.*

▶ **COMMON ERRORS**

Possible Error:

Stimulator does not seem to be working.

Prevention:

If stimulator does not seem to be working properly and replacing the battery does not help, try troubleshooting the unit. First, check the dial setting to make sure unit is on.

Possible Error:

Battery is installed improperly.

Prevention:

To avoid this error, be sure to observe proper polarity markings when installing or replacing the battery.

Possible Error:

Improper placement of electrodes.

Prevention:

Be sure electrodes are making contact with skin and stimulator.

Possible Error:

Worn-out electrodes.

Prevention:

Replace both electrodes, following the instructions on the package.

Possible Error:

Malfunctioning cordset.

Prevention:

Check and replace as necessary.

▶ **NURSING TIPS**

- Do not stimulate over the carotid sinus or its associated nerves, especially when sinus reflex sensitivity exists. Laryngeal or pharyngeal spasm may occur when electrodes are placed across the throat or in the mouth.
- Use caution in applying electrical stimulation to people suspected of having heart disease. There is scant clinical data on possible adverse results.
- Because of the risk of burns, areas of skin with reduced response to normal sensory stimuli should not be electrically simulated.
- To prevent skin burns, be sure metal electrode inserts and pins are fully inserted into electrodes and not lying directly on the client's skin.
- Be aware that some people find the electrical sensation extremely unpleasant and use should probably be discontinued in these cases.

- If the TENS unit is turned on, it may interfere with other electric monitoring such as cardiograph alarm systems, electrocautery equipment, or ECG machines.
- Defibrillation of a person wearing a TENS stimulator can damage the stimulator whether it is turned on or off. Also the client may be at risk of burns under the electrode site during defibrillation. To eliminate risk, remove the TENS electrode before defibrillation signals are applied. Consider having the client wear a Medic-Alert bracelet to identify the potential problem.
- TENS devices should not be used for undiagnosed pain syndromes for which etiology has not be determined.
- The safety of TENS units has not been clinically established during pregnancy or delivery.

▶ **SPECIAL CONSIDERATIONS**

- *Sometimes individuals react to the tape used to secure the electrodes of the TENS unit. Skin irritation is minimized by using self-adhesive disposable electrodes or hypoallergenic tape. It helps to reposition electrodes slightly for repeated applications.*

Basic Care

Changing Linens in an Unoccupied Bed

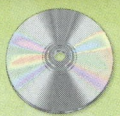

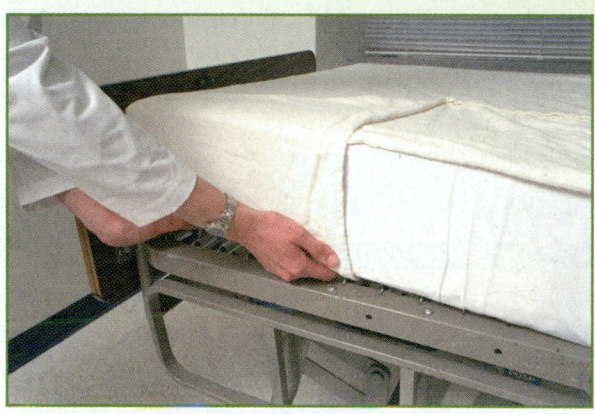

▶ OVERVIEW OF THE SKILL

After a bath, clean linens are placed on the bed to promote comfort and decrease transmission of microorganisms. When the client is able to get out of bed, assist the client to a chair and proceed with making the bed. After surgery, the client should be returned to a clean bed with the linens folded to the foot of the bed to promote easy client transfer.

▶ ASSESSMENT

1. Assess the equipment. Check for all linens necessary to change the bed. Check for a dirty linen hamper. **Facilitates a smooth procedure.**
2. Assess whether the bed itself needs cleaning before placing clean sheets on it. **Reduces the transmission of microorganisms.**
3. Assess the client's needs in the bed. Check for profuse drainage, incontinence, or special needs for comfort or skin integrity. **Determines how the procedure will be performed.**
4. Assess the client's ability to be out of bed in a safe place while changing linens.

▶ DIAGNOSIS

Risk for Impaired Skin Integrity

▶ PLANNING

Expected Outcomes:

1. The client will have clean linens on the bed.

2. The clean linens will be appropriate to the client's needs and condition.

Equipment Needed (see Figure 4-1-1):

- Bottom sheet (fitted, if available)
- Top sheet
- Draw sheet (regular top sheet may be used)
- Pillowcase (each pillow on the bed)
- Mattress pad
- Antiseptic solution, washcloth, and towel
- Linen bag hamper
- Nonsterile gloves

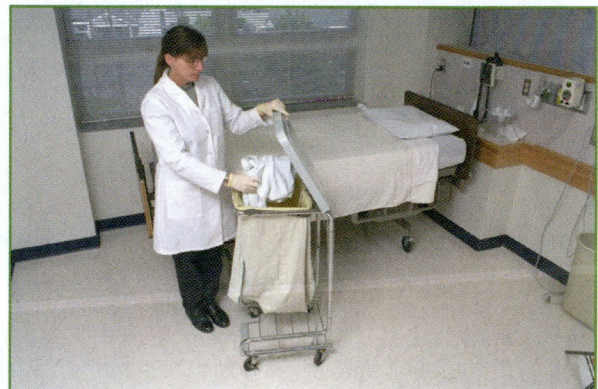

Figure 4-1-1 Clean linens and a laundry hamper for used linens are brought to the bedside to make the unoccupied bed. Gloves help reduce the transmission of microorganisms.

▶ **CLIENT EDUCATION NEEDED:**

Educate the client about the need for clean linens to increase comfort and to help prevent skin complications.

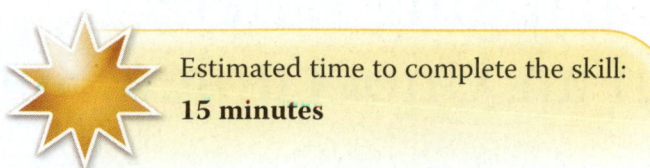

Estimated time to complete the skill:
15 minutes

▶ **DELEGATION TIPS**

Bed making is usually delegated to ancillary personnel. Their instruction should include safety precautions for themselves and the client, and understanding the appropriate use of Standard Precautions.

IMPLEMENTATION—Action/Rationale

Action	Rationale
1. Place hamper by client's door if linen bags are not available. Explain procedure to client. Assess condition of blanket and/or bedspread.	1. Provides for proper disposal of soiled linens. Encourages client cooperation. Allows for organization of supplies.
2. Gather linens and gloves. Place linens on a clean, dry surface in reverse order of usage at the client's bedside (pillowcases, top sheet, draw sheet, bottom sheet).	2. Provides easy access to items.
3. Apply gloves.	3. Reduces risk of infection from soiled, contaminated linens.
4. Inquire about the client's toileting needs and attend as necessary.	4. Provides for client comfort and prevents interruptions during bed making.
5. Assist client to a safe, comfortable chair.	5. Increases client's comfort and decreases risk of falls.
6. Position bed: flat, side rails down, adjust height to waist level.	6. Promotes good body mechanics and decreases back strain.
7. Remove and fold blanket and/or bedspread. If clean and reusable, place on clean work area.	7. Keeps reusable bed linens clean.
8. Remove soiled pillowcases by grasping the closed end with one hand and slipping the pillow out with the other. Place the soiled cases on top of the soiled sheet, and place the pillows on clean work area.	8. Allows easy removal of the pillowcases without contamination of uniform by soiled linens and keeps pillows clean.
9. Remove soiled linens: Start on the side of the bed closest to you; free the bottom sheet and mattress pad by lifting the mattress and rolling soiled linens to the middle of the bed. Go to the other side of the bed, repeat action.	9. Prevents tearing and fanning of linens. Linens are folded from cleanest area to most soiled to prevent contamination.
10. Fold (do not fan or flap) soiled linens: head of bed to middle, foot of bed to middle. Place in linen bag or hamper, keeping soiled linens away from uniform.	10. Fanning or flapping linens increases the number of microorganisms in the air. Folding linens reduces the risk of transmission of infection to others.

continues

Action	Rationale
11. Check mattress. If the mattress is soiled, clean it with an antiseptic solution and dry it thoroughly.	11. Reduces the transmission of microorganisms.
12. Remove gloves, wash hands, and apply a second pair of clean gloves (when appropriate).	12. Reduces the transmission of microorganisms to clean linens.
13. Open the clean mattress pad lengthwise onto the bed with the seamed side of the sheet toward the mattress. Unfold half the pad's width to the center crease and smooth the pad flat. If there are elastic bands to hold the pad in place, slide them under the corners of the mattress.	13. Facilitates making the bed in an organized, time-saving manner by not having to go from one side of the bed to the other.
14. Proceed with placing the bottom sheet onto the mattress. Linens differ from facility to facility. Bottom sheets may be fitted or they may be flat. Proceed to the appropriate Action for the linen available.	14. Use linens available at the facility.

Fitted Bottom Sheet

Action	Rationale
15. Position yourself diagonally toward the head of the bed.	15. Ensures good body mechanics and efficient procedure.
16. Start at the head with seamed side of the fitted sheet toward the mattress.	16. Placement of seamed side toward mattress prevents irritation to the client's skin.
17. Lift the mattress corner with your hand closest to the bed; with your other hand, pull and tuck the fitted sheet over the mattress corner; secure at the head of the bed.	17. Prevents straining of back muscles; decreases the chance that the sheet will pull out from under the mattress.
18. Pull and tuck the fitted sheet over the mattress corners at the foot of the bed.	18. Prevents straining of back muscles; decreases the chance that the sheet will pull out from under the mattress.

Flat Regular

Action	Rationale
19. Unfold the bottom sheet with the seamed side toward the mattress. Align the bottom edge of the sheet with the edge of the mattress at the foot of the bed.	19. Placement of the seamed side toward the mattress prevents irritation to the client's skin. Ensure proper placement of the sheet so that it can be tightly secured at the top and on both sides of the bed.
20. Allow the sheet to hang 10 inches (25 cm) over the mattress on the side and at the top of the bed.	20. Proper placement of linens ensures adequate sheeting for all sides of the bed.
21. Position yourself diagonally toward the head of the bed. Lift the top of the mattress corner with the hand closest to the bed and smoothly tuck the sheet under the mattress.	21. Prevents straining of back muscles; decreases the chance that the sheet will pull out from under the mattress.
22. Miter the corner at the head of the bed using the following technique.	22. Secures sheet tightly to the mattress, with the triangular fold providing a smooth tuck to keep the linen in place.
23. Face the side of bed and lift and lay the top edge of the sheet onto the bed to form a triangular fold.	23. Forms the base for the tuck.

continues

Action	Rationale
Flat Regular *continued*	
24. With your palms down, tuck the lower edge of sheet (hanging free at the side of the mattress) under the mattress.	24. Forms the first half of the tuck.
25. Grasp the triangular fold, bring it down over the side of the mattress. Allow the sheet to hang free at the side of the mattress.	25. Will form the final portion of the mitered corner when tucked in.
26. Place the draw sheet on the bottom sheet and unfold it to the middle crease (see Figure 4-1-2).	26. Provides a sheet to lift and move the client in bed without having to use the bottom sheet and remake the bed. Helps to keep the bottom sheet clean.
27. Face the side of the bed, palms of hands down. Tuck both the bottom and draw sheets under the mattress. Ensure that the bottom sheet is tucked smoothly under the mattress all the way to the foot of the bed.	27. Keeps sheet taut, in place, and wrinkle-free, thereby decreasing the risk of skin irritation.
28. Go to the other side of the bed, unfold the bottom sheet, and repeat the actions used to apply the mattress pad and bottom sheet.	28. Unfolding decreases air current; air currents can spread microorganisms.
29. Unfold the draw sheet, if used, and grasp the free-hanging sides of both the bottom and draw sheets. Pull toward you, keeping your back straight, and with a firm grasp (sheets taut) tuck both sheets under the mattress. Use your arms and open palms to extend the linen under the mattress. Place the protective pad on the bottom sheet.	29. Uses your body's weight in pulling the sheet taut and prevents strain on your back muscles.
30. Place the top sheet on the bed and unfold lengthwise, placing the center crease (width) of the sheet in the middle of the bed. Place the top edge of the sheet (seam up) even with the top of the mattress at the head of the bed. Pull the remaining length toward the bottom of the bed.	30. Saves time and movement, making one side of the bed at a time. Seam will be folded down to prevent contact with the client's skin, which can result in irritation.
31. Unfold and apply the blanket or spread. Follow the same technique as used in applying the top sheet (see Figure 4-1-3).	31. Provides warmth.

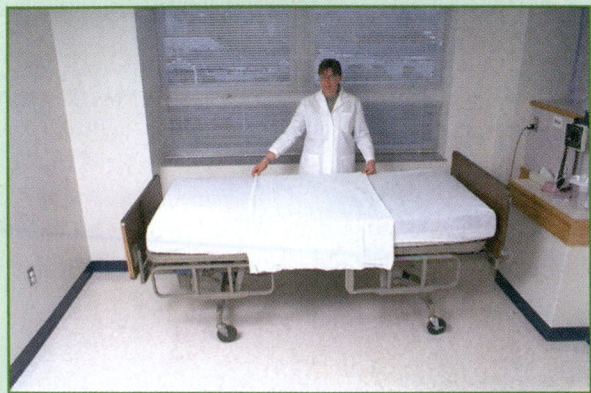

Figure 4-1-2   The clean draw sheet is placed on top of the bottom sheet.

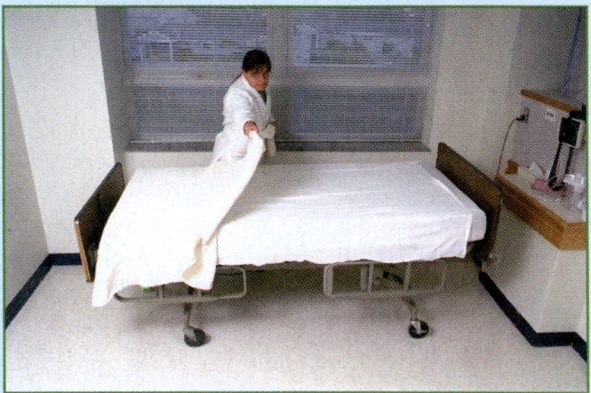

Figure 4-1-3   Place the blanket or spread over the top sheet.

continues

Action	Rationale

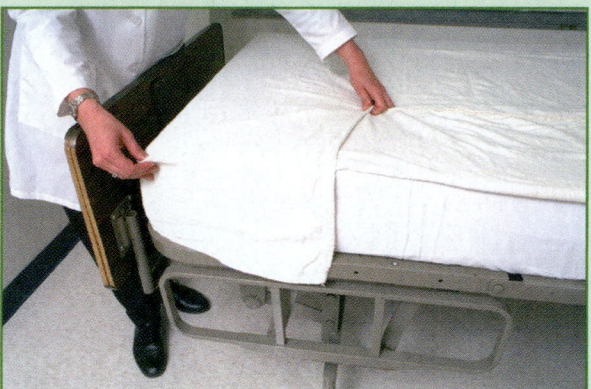

Figure 4-1-4 Lift and lay the hem of the sheet and blanket on the bed to form a triangular fold.

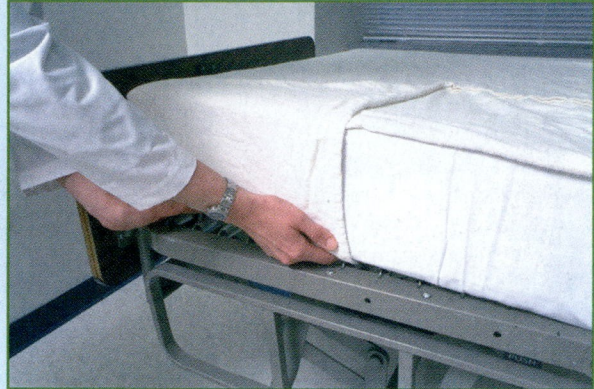

Figure 4-1-5 Tuck the lower edge of the sheet and blanket under the mattress.

32. Miter the bottom corners. With your palms down, tuck the lower edge of the sheet under the mattress. Grasp the triangular fold and bring it down over the side of the mattress. Allow the sheet to hang free at the side of the mattress (see Figures 4-1-4, 4-1-5, and 4-1-6).

32. Secures linen at the foot of the bed.

33. Face the head of the bed and fold the top sheet and blanket over 6 inches (15 cm). Fan-fold the sheet and blanket (from the foot to the middle of the bed) (see Figure 4-1-7).

33. Allows the client easy access to the bed.

34. Apply a clean pillowcase on each pillow (see Figure 4-1-8). With one hand, grasp the closed end of the pillowcase. Gather the pillowcase and turn it inside out over hand. With same hand, grasp the middle of one end of the pillow. With the other hand, pull the case over the length of the pillow. The corners of the pillow should fit snugly into the corners of the case.

34. Keeps clean pillowcase away from your uniform.

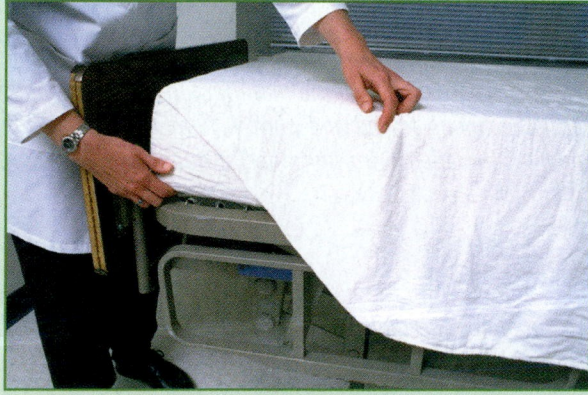

Figure 4-1-6 Bring the triangular fold down and let it hang freely at the side of the mattress.

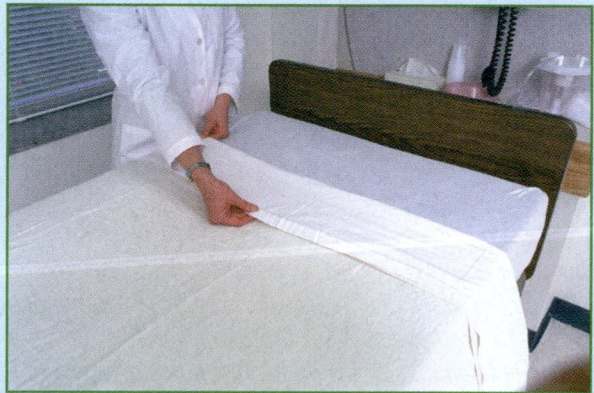

Figure 4-1-7 Fold the top sheet and blanket 6 inches.

continues

Action	Rationale

Flat Regular *continued*

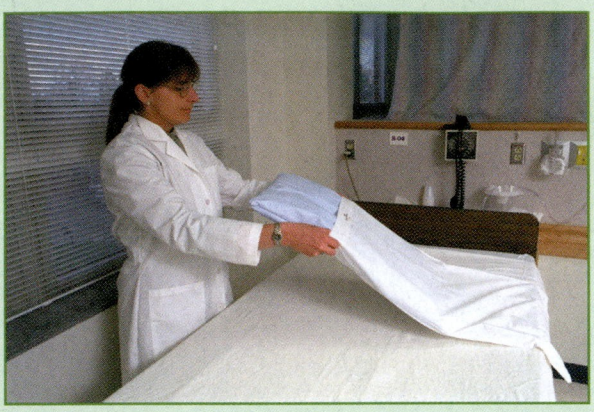

Figure 4-1-8   Place a clean pillowcase on each pillow while keeping the clean pillowcase away from your uniform.

Action	Rationale
35. Return the bed to the lowest position and elevate the head of the bed 30° to 45°. Put side rails up on side, farthest from client.	**35.** Provides for client safety.
36. Inquire about toileting needs of the client; assist as necessary.	**36.** Saves client energy and provides time to care for the client's needs.
37. Assist the client back into the bed and pull up the side rails; place call light in reach; take vital signs.	**37.** Promotes client safety and a means to call for assistance. Sitting up in a chair and movement may cause changes in the client's vital signs.
38. Remove gloves and wash hands.	**38.** Reduces the transmission of microorganisms.
39. Document your actions and the client's response during the procedure and to sitting up in a chair.	**39.** Documents completion of procedure and assessment findings of client's tolerance.

▶ REAL WORLD ANECDOTES

Scenario 1

An elderly woman in a long-term care facility is using a silicone sand bed. The nurse's aides change her bed linens daily. The linens are simply laid on top of the sand mattress in accordance with the manufacturer's recommendations. Unnoticed by the aide, the fabric covering the sand is becoming frayed and worn. It finally tears, releasing sand into the client area of the bed. The sand slowly engulfs the client, drowning her in quicksand. The nurse needed to be aware of new equipment requirements and hazards.

Scenario 2

The nurse has just finished removing soiled linen from an incontinent client's bed and replacing it with clean linen. She then picks up the soiled linen, tucks it under her arm, and takes it out to the dirty linen hamper in the hallway. As she is washing her hands afterward, she notices that the stool from the client's sheets has smeared her arm and uniform. She washes her arm but is unable to change her uniform. This nurse learned not to carry dirty linen too close to herself or her uniform.

▶ EVALUATION

- Confirm that fresh linens were placed on the bed in a manner appropriate to the client's needs.

▶ DOCUMENTATION

Nurses' Notes

- Document the linen change and the client's tolerance to being out of bed.

▶ CRITICAL THINKING SKILL

Introduction

Throwing dirty linen on the floors endangers the nurse.

Possible Scenario

You have gotten Mr. Nelson out of bed and into a chair. You are changing the soiled linen on his bed. As you strip the dirty linens off the bed, you realize that you do not have a dirty linen hamper nearby.

Mr. Nelson is confused and cannot be trusted to stay in the chair if you leave the room. You are not comfortable leaving the soiled linen on his bedside table or other clean surface, so you put the dirty linens on the floor. You finish changing the bed linens, return Mr. Nelson to bed, and then take the soiled linen to a dirty linen hamper.

Possible Outcome

Dirty linen on the floor can be a safety hazard to the nurse as she or he moves about the room or to clients if they are moving around the room. Putting dirty linen on the floor is also a violation of the health code in most states and can lead to infraction citations if discovered by a health inspector.

Prevention

Be prepared with everything you will need before you start a procedure. If you discover you need something and cannot leave the room, request assistance. Turn on the call light or call out the door for some help.

▶ VARIATIONS

Geriatric Variation:
- *Geriatric clients often have thin, easily damaged skin. Be sure to use linen that does not have jagged tags or rough edges.*

Pediatric Variation:
- *Be aware that children put things in their mouths and use only linens that a child could safely chew on. Also be sure that there are no decorations or patches that a child could chew off and swallow.*

Home Care Variations:
- *In home care situations, a nurse does not usually make the bed. It is part of the nurse's function to examine the conditions, including the bed, and make suggestions regarding the safety and comfort of the client. The nurse should check for bed rails, linens that the client could become entangled in, or a bed that is structurally unsafe.*

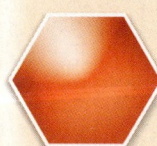

Long-Term Care Variations:
- *Be sure to keep the linen smooth and fairly unwrinkled to prevent unwanted pressure areas in long-term clients.*

► COMMON ERRORS

Possible Error:

While making a client's bed, the nurse flaps the linen to unfold it and to cover the bed.

Prevention:

Think about what you may be stirring up with the flapping linen. Remember you are possibly spreading bacteria around the room as well as into the air you are breathing. Gently unfold linen on the bed. Do not flap the bed linens around while making the bed.

Possible Error:

While making the bed, the nurse tucks the pillow under her chin to apply the pillowcase.

Prevention:

Think about where this pillow has been and if you may be infecting yourself by placing this pillow under your chin. Consider the possibility that you may be infecting pillows from different rooms using this technique. Put the pillowcase on by grasping the closed end of the pillowcase with one hand. Gather the case and turn it inside out over your hand. With the same hand, grasp the middle of one end of the pillow. With the other hand, pull the case over the length of the pillow (see Figure 4-1-8).

► NURSING TIPS

- If the bed raises and lowers, raise it up to a comfortable height to prevent back strain (see Figure 4-1-9).
- Make one side of the bed completely and then move to the other side to save time and steps.
- Be careful not to carry the dirty linen close to your uniform to prevent contamination.

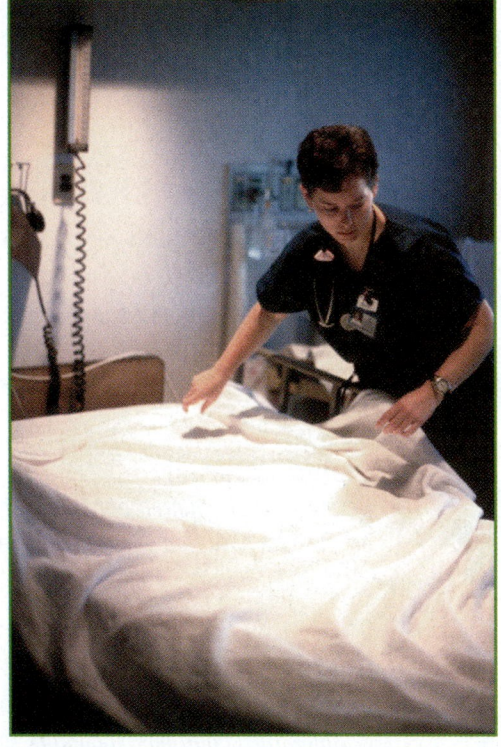

Figure 4-1-9 Raise bed to a comfortable height to prevent back strain.

► SPECIAL CONSIDERATIONS

- *Some facilities do not change clients' sheets daily. Know your hospital's policy and be comfortable with explaining it to clients if asked.*
- *Institution-laundered linen may be coarse on the client's skin (especially for elderly clients). Some institutions allow clients to bring linen from home to make their stay more comfortable.*

Changing Linens in an Occupied Bed

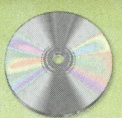

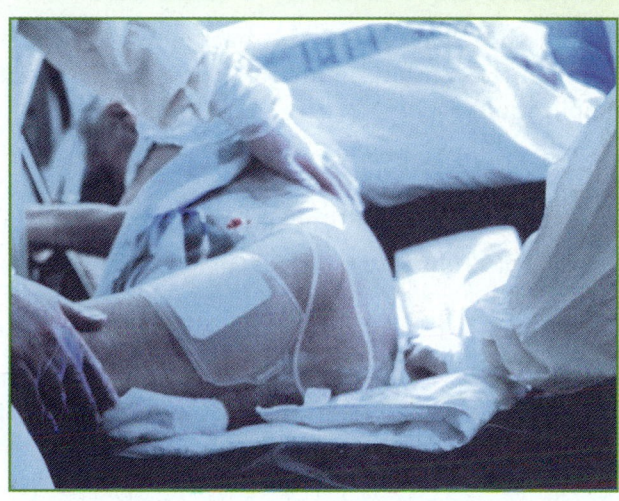

▶ OVERVIEW OF THE SKILL

After a bath, clean linens are placed on the bed to promote comfort and decrease the transmission of microorganisms. If the client is able to get out of bed, assist the client to a chair and proceed to make the bed. If the client is unable to get out of bed, the linens must be changed around the client. Assistance will be needed if the client is in traction or cannot be turned. Care must be taken to avoid disturbing the traction weights. If the client cannot be turned, change the linens from head to toe. Place a waterproof draw sheet on the beds of clients who are incontinent or have profuse drainage. The type and amount of linens placed on the bed will vary based on the type of bed the client is using. Air beds and Clinitron beds, for example, use only minimal linens under the client.

▶ ASSESSMENT

1. Assess your equipment. Check for all the linens necessary to change the bed. Check for a dirty linen hamper. **Facilitates an uneventful procedure.**
2. Assess whether the bed itself needs cleaning prior to placing clean sheets on it. **Reduces the transmission of microorganisms.**
3. Assess the client's needs in the bed. Check for profuse drainage, incontinence, or special needs for comfort or skin integrity. **Determines how the procedure will be performed.**
4. Assess the client's ability to assist with the procedure, including mobility, mental status, and muscle strength. **Determines whether assistance will be needed to change the client's linens.**
5. Assess for the presence of dressings, IV lines, tubes, or any equipment that may be attached to the client.

▶ DIAGNOSIS

Risk for Impaired Skin Integrity

Impaired Bed Mobility

▶ PLANNING

Expected Outcomes:

1. The client will have clean linens on the bed.
2. The clean linens will be appropriate to the client's needs and condition.
3. The linens will be changed with a minimum of trauma to the client.

Equipment Needed (see Figure 4-2-1):

- Linen hamper
- Top sheet, draw sheet, bottom sheet
- Pillowcase

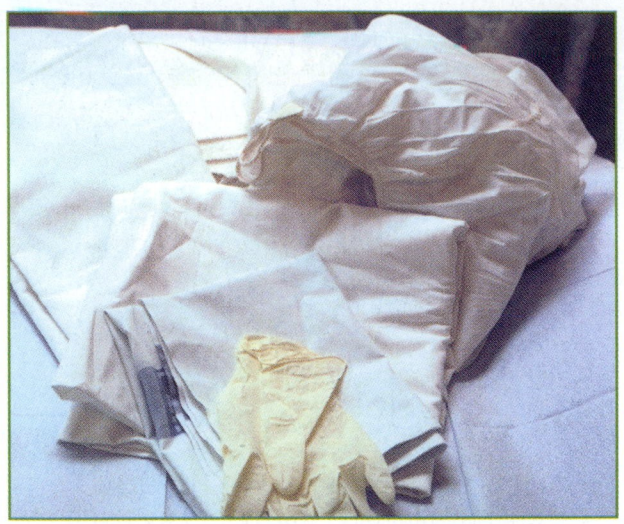

Figure 4-2-1   Top and bottom sheets, draw sheet, and pillowcase are used to make the occupied bed. Gloves reduce the transmission of microorganisms.

- Blanket
- Bath blanket

▶ **CLIENT EDUCATION NEEDED:**

Educate the client about the need for clean linen to increase comfort and to help prevent skin complications.

Estimated time to complete the skill:
20 minutes

▶ **DELEGATION TIPS**

Bed making is usually delegated to ancillary personnel. Their instruction should include the appropriate use of Standard Precautions and safety precautions for themselves and the client, such as the proper movement of the client in bed, how to manage drains and dressings, and the use of proper body mechanics. In certain situations where the client is in critical condition and multiple tubes, especially chest tubes, are present, the nurse should assist.

IMPLEMENTATION—Action/Rationale

Action	Rationale
1. Explain procedure to client.	1. Promotes client cooperation.
2. Bring equipment to the bedside (see Figure 4-2-2).	2. Facilitates a smooth procedure.

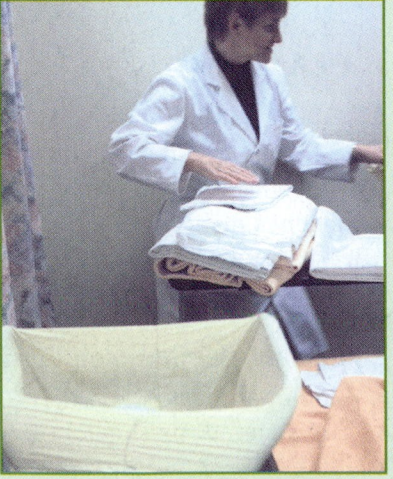

Figure 4-2-2   Bring clean linen and empty linen hamper to the bedside.

continues

Action	Rationale
3. Remove top sheet and blanket. Loosen bottom sheet at foot and sides of bed. Lower side rail nearest the nurse, if necessary for access. Client may be covered with a bath blanket (see Figure 4-2-3).	3. Facilitates easy removal of linens. Lowering only side rail close to nurse reduces client's risk of falls. Bath blanket prevents exposure and chills.
4. Position client on side, facing away from you. Reposition pillow under his or her head.	4. Provides space to place clean linens.
5. Fanfold or roll bottom linens close to client toward the center of the bed (see Figure 4-2-4).	5. Keeps soiled linen together. Promotes comfort when client later rolls to other side.
6. Smooth wrinkles out of mattress. Place clean bottom linens with the center fold nearest the client. Fanfold or roll clean bottom linens nearest client and tuck under soiled linen (see Figure 4-2-5). Maintain an adequate amount of sheet at head and foot of bed for tucking.	6. Provides for maximum fit of sheets and decreases chance of wrinkles.
7. Miter bottom sheet at head of bed, then at foot of bed. To miter, lift the mattress and tuck the sheet over the edge of the mattress, lift edge of sheet that is hanging to form a triangle, and lay upper part of sheet back onto bed; tuck the lower hanging section under the mattress. Repeat for each corner. Tuck the sides of the sheet under the mattress.	7. Holds linens firmly in place.
8. Fold the draw sheet in half. Identify the center of the draw sheet and place it close to the client. Fanfold or roll draw sheet closest to client and tuck under soiled linen. Smooth linen. Add protective padding if needed. Tuck draw sheet under mattress, working from the center to the edges (see Figure 4-2-6). Draw sheet should be positioned under the lower back and buttocks.	8. Draw sheet facilitates moving and lifting clients while in bed.
9. Logroll client over onto side facing you. Raise side rail.	9. Positions client off soiled linen. Protects client from falling.

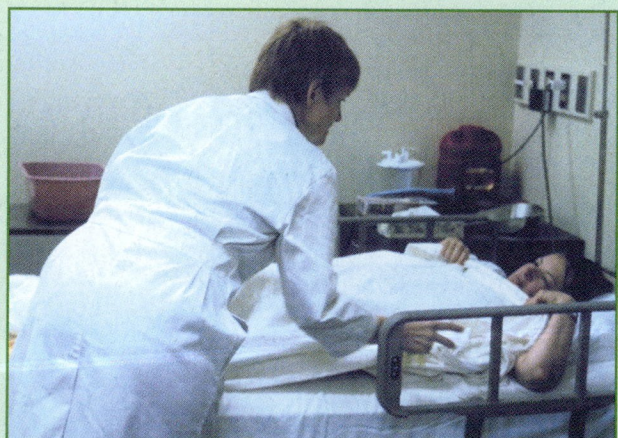

Figure 4-2-3   Client may be covered with a bath blanket for warmth and modesty while top sheet and blanket are removed.

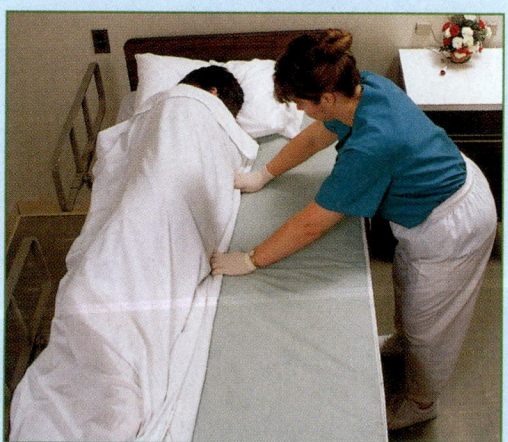

Figure 4-2-4   Fanfold the bottom linens close to the client toward the center of the bed.

continues

Action	Rationale

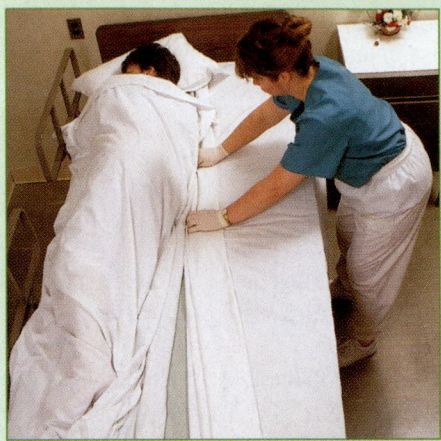

Figure 4-2-5 Fanfold the clean bottom linens nearest the client and tuck under the soiled linens.

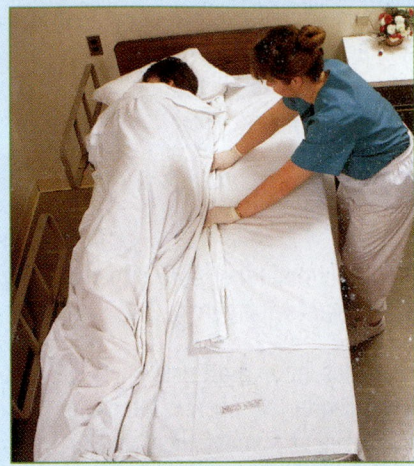

Figure 4-2-6 Fanfold the draw sheet close to the client and tuck under the soiled linens.

10. Move to other side of bed. Remove soiled linens by rolling into a bundle and place in linen hamper without touching uniform.

10. Prevents cross-contamination.

11. Unfold/unroll bottom sheet, then draw sheet. Look for objects left in the bed. Grasp each sheet with knuckles up and over the sheet and pull tightly while leaning back with your body weight. Client may be positioned supine (see Figure 4-2-7).

11. Tight sheets keep linens wrinkle-free and decrease the risk of skin irritation. Leaning back uses body weight for good body mechanics.

12. Place top sheet over client with center of sheet in middle of bed. Unfold top of sheet over client. Remove bath blankets left on client to prevent exposure during bed making. Place top blanket over client, same as the top sheet (see Figure 4-2-8).

12. Provides client with top sheet and blanket to prevent chilling.

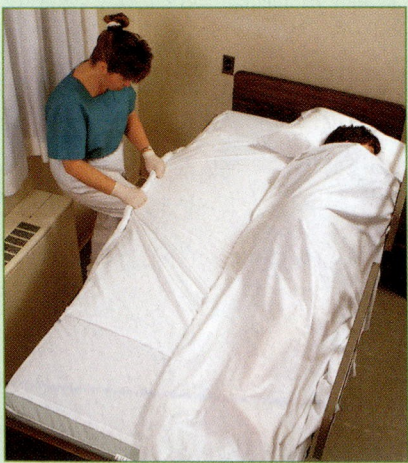

Figure 4-2-7 Grasp the bottom and draw sheet and pull tightly.

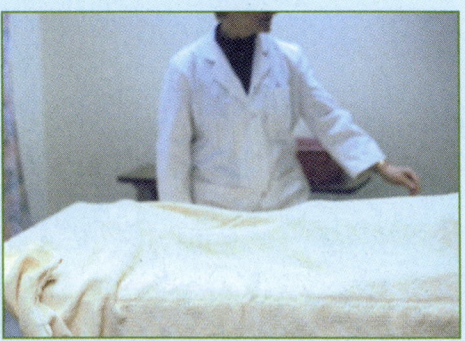

Figure 4-2-8 Place the top blanket over the client.

continues

Action	Rationale
13. Raise foot of mattress and tuck the corner of the top sheet and blanket under. Miter the corner. Repeat with other side of mattress (see Figure 4-2-9). Bend knees and not the back for proper mechanics.	**13.** Secures top sheet and blanket in place.
14. Grasp top sheet and blanket over client's toes and pull upward, then make a small fanfold in the sheet.	**14.** Permits client to move feet under the sheets. Provides room under the tight top sheet and blanket. Prevents toe decubitus and sheet burns from pressure.
15. Remove soiled pillowcase. Grasp center of clean pillowcase and invert pillowcase over hand/arm. Maintain grasp of pillowcase while grasping center of pillow. Use other hand to pull pillowcase down over pillow. Place pillow under client's head. While changing pillowcase, client can be instructed to rest head on bed, or place a blanket under client's head (see Figure 4-2-10).	**15.** Provides clean pillowcase without shaking pillow or pillowcase. Promotes comfort.
16. Document procedure used to change linens and client's condition during the procedure.	**16.** Provides documentation of nursing care and assessment of client's status.
17. Wash hands.	**17.** Reduces the transmission of microorganisms.

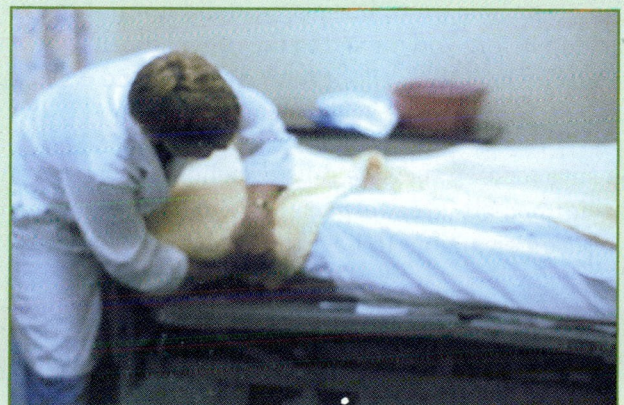

Figure 4-2-9   Raise the foot of the mattress and tuck in the corner of the top sheet and blanket. Note: The nurse has moved to the side for demonstration purposes.

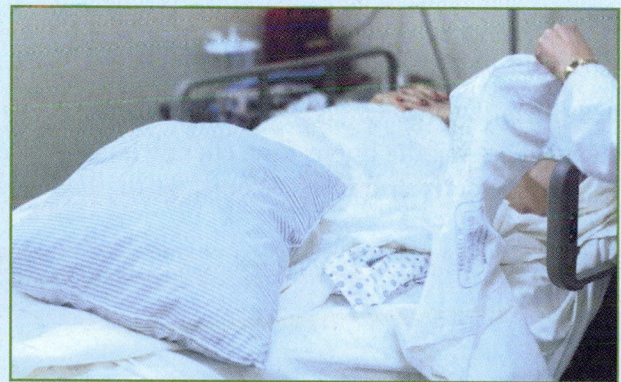

Figure 4-2-10   Changing the pillowcase is the final step in making the occupied bed.

▶ **REAL WORLD ANECDOTES**

Nurse Simmons changed Mr. Trumbull's linens. Because Mr. Trumbull was not able to get out of bed, she used the occupied bed technique. She dutifully rolled up the soiled linen and placed it in the linen hamper while placing the clean linens on the bed and unrolling them under the client. By the time she was finished with Mr. Trumbull's care, it was breakfast time and Nurse Simmons started to prepare Mr. Trumbull for breakfast. As she was raising the head of his bed and arranging the bedside table, Mr. Trumbull reached under his pillow for his dentures. He was unable to find them and became disturbed and agitated. He noted to Nurse Simmons that he always kept his

continues

► **EVALUATION**

- The client has clean, unwrinkled linen.
- The linen placed on the bed is suitable for the client's special needs.
- The linen was changed with a minimum of pain and trauma to the client.

► **DOCUMENTATION**

Nurses' Notes

- Document the bed change, how the client tolerated it, and any unusual findings.

Document on appropriate flow sheet or electronic medical record (EMR).

► **CRITICAL THINKING SKILL**

Introduction

Remember to consider safety at all times.

Possible Scenario

You are changing the linens for a client who is on bed rest. He is elderly and obese. You raise the bed to a comfortable height to work, put down the side rail, and have the client roll to the opposite side of the bed. You remove and roll the soiled linens so they are underneath the client and place clean linens on the vacant side of the bed. You then proceed to the opposite side of the bed, put down the side rail, and have the client roll over the rolled-up linens to the now clean side of the bed. As you are trying to pull the rolled up linens from under the client, you push him a little farther away from you and off the roll of linen.

Possible Outcome

That little extra nudge from you as well as the rocking effect of pulling the linen out from under him has unbalanced the client. He does not have a side rail to lean on or hold on to because you did not put the rail back up before you moved to the other side of the bed, and so he falls to the floor with a thump and a groan.

Prevention

Be sure to keep the side rails up when you are not in the immediate area, especially with clients who are confused or unable to help themselves.

► **VARIATIONS**

Geriatric Variations:

- *Geriatric clients often have thin, tender skin. Be careful not to tear it while pulling linens underneath the client.*
- *Be aware of wrinkles in the bed linens under the client to prevent damage to thin, tender skin.*
- *Provide towels, tissues, or washcloths within reach of clients to help them catch spills and keep their own linen clean.*
- *Elderly clients are prone to skin breakdown. Be sure to keep linens loose over the feet as sheet burns and toe decubitus can readily occur.*
- *Elderly clients may have a certain way they "like" the bed linen to be most comfortable such as untucked at the bottom, top sheet at the chin or at the armpits, or with an extra blanket. Give choices and seek advice on how to make them most comfortable whenever possible.*

Pediatric Variations:

- *Small children can be moved physically from one side of the bed to another to avoid pulling linens underneath them.*
- *Children may be most comfortable with a familiar blanket or cover brought from home for the bed. Do not forget to put it back on when you have finished changing the linen.*

continues

► VARIATIONS *(continued)*

Home Care Variations:

- *The nurse may be called upon to teach a caregiver how to change the linens in an occupied bed.*
- *If a hospital bed is not in use, enlist the aid of a caregiver, neighbor, or friend to improvise side rails to use at night or when making an occupied bed. An L-shaped device of wood or PVC tubing could be anchored under the mattress for support, then come up the side of the bed for safety. Make sure rough surfaces are smoothed or padded.*
- *Provide towels or washcloths within reach of clients to help them catch spills and keep their own linen clean.*

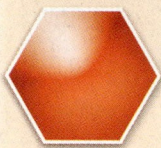

Long-Term Care Variations:

- *Long-term care clients often have special padding in the bed for increased comfort. Be aware whether they have a sheepskin or egg-crate mattress and adjust your bed-making technique accordingly. Wash and replace special padding regularly.*
- *Provide towels, absorbent pads, or washcloths within reach of clients to help them catch spills and keep their own linen clean.*
- *Remember to mark a client's personal linens, blankets, sheets, or protective padding so they can be returned if lost in the laundry. A family member may take these items home to launder.*

► COMMON ERRORS

Possible Error:

While making an occupied bed, the nurse pushes all the linens under the client (wadding up) rather than folding or rolling them up.

Prevention:

Using this technique may make it harder to make the bed and could be harmful to the client's skin. Roll or fold linens under the client. If the linens are just stuffed under the client, they are more difficult to pull through to the other side. It also increases the possibility of damaging clients' skin as the wad of linen is pulled out from under them.

► NURSING TIPS

- Roll or fold the linens under the client. Do not put them underneath the client.
- Be aware of wrinkles and seams that the client may be lying on. They can cause pressure areas in the client's skin.

- Check for personal belongings in the client's bed when changing the linens. Clients may keep important items near them in bed.
- Be sure to keep the side rails up on the opposite side of the bed.
- Get help from another caregiver if the client is combative or difficult to move.

► SPECIAL CONSIDERATIONS

- *Always inform the client of each step as you proceed. This will help gain the client's cooperation and will also avoid unnecessary client anxiety.*
- *If there is a risk for disease transmission, gloves and/or isolation gown should be worn when handling linens. Follow Standard Precautions for the type of isolation protocol. The soiled linen should be handled with care according to institutional policy.*
- *If clients have poor peripheral circulation, use a foot cradle to protect the feet from sheet burns and decubitus. Assess feet routinely for pressure sores, especially tips of toes. Heel protectors may be necessary.*

SKILL 4-3

Turning and Positioning a Client

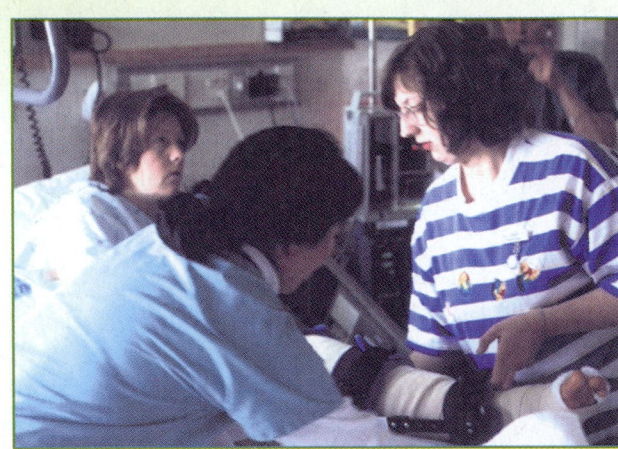

▶ OVERVIEW OF THE SKILL

Clients are not always able to independently move and position themselves in bed. Therefore, health care providers often use proper turning and positioning techniques. Proper turning and positioning allows the health care provider to make clients as comfortable as possible, prevent contractures and pressure sores, make portions of the client's body available for treatment or procedures, and allows clients greater access to their environment. There are three key concepts to remember when positioning a client: pressure, friction, and skin shear.

Any area that contacts the surface the client is lying on is a pressure site. Because of circulatory compromise, the pressure sites over bony prominences are at the highest risk of skin breakdown and ulceration. Always assess the blood flow to skin and tissue areas you are putting under increased pressure when placing a client in a given position. When repositioning a client, be sure the sheets under the client are smooth. This will help prevent increased areas of pressure that could contribute to pressure sores (see Figure 4-3-1).

Skin shear is caused when the skin is dragged across a hard surface. The deep layers of skin are torn by the resistance of being dragged. This damage to the skin can lead to skin breakdown and ulceration. To prevent skin shear, or friction burn from the sheets, do not drag a client across the bed. Lift the client into proper position or use a turning sheet.

Friction is caused when the skin is dragged across a rough surface, thereby causing heat and damaging the skin's surface. Any damage to the skin's integrity can lead to infection and skin breakdown.

If clients cannot reposition themselves, they must be repositioned at least every 2 hours and more frequently if they are uncomfortable, incontinent, or have poor circulation, fragile skin, decreased cognition, decreased sensation, or poor nutritional status. When repositioning a client, assess the skin for redness and integrity. Areas of redness should be resolved before the client is repositioned on that area. Areas of redness that do not resolve within 30 minutes after pressure relief should be documented (see Table 4-3-1, Pressure Sore Concerns).

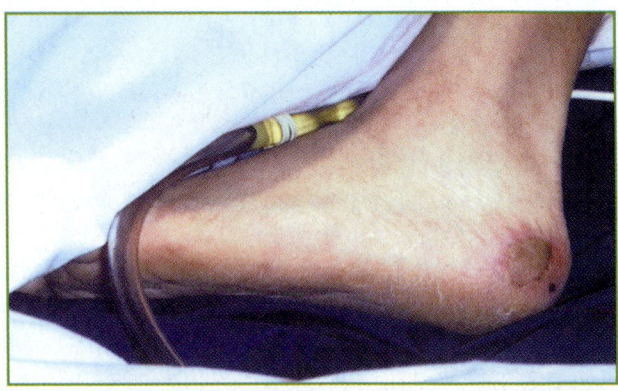

Figure 4-3-1 Any part of the body that contacts the surface the client is lying on is a pressure site and is at risk for skin ulceration.

Table 4-3-1 Pressure Sore Concerns		
SIDE-LYING POSITION	**PRONE POSITION**	**SUPINE POSITION**
Base of 5th metatarsal	Distal phalanges and metatarsals	Calcaneus
Lateral malleolus	Knee	Coccyx
Fibular head	Anterior superior and inferior iliac spines	Sacrum
Greater trochanter	Xiphoid process	Spinous processes
Iliac crest	Sternum	Ribs
Greater tubercle	Ear and side of face and scalp	Scapula
Lateral epicondyle		Occiput
Ear and side of face and scalp		

A plan to reposition the client more frequently may need to be instituted. Areas of prolonged redness are more likely to sustain tissue damage, as are tissue areas covering bony prominences. Finally, remember that proper body mechanics are essential to protect the caregiver's back and to ensure client safety.

▶ ASSESSMENT

1. Assess the client's ability to move independently. **Determine whether the client can assist with turning and repositioning.**
2. Assess the client's flexibility. **If clients have contractures or other flexibility limitations, their positions may need to be modified to allow for the restrictions.**
3. Assess the client's age, medical diagnosis, cognitive status, skin integrity, nutritional status, continence, altered sensation, as well as the overall condition of the musculoskeletal system. **Helps determine the client's potential for pressure sore development.**
4. Assess the physician's or qualified practitioner's orders for specific restrictions regarding client positioning **to ensure the correct positioning is implemented.**

▶ DIAGNOSIS

Risk for Impaired Skin Integrity

Impaired Physical Mobility

Activity Intolerance

Pain

Impaired Bed Mobility

▶ PLANNING

Expected Outcomes:

1. The client will maintain skin integrity without skin burns, pressure areas, or pressure ulcers.
2. The client will be comfortable as evident by verbal and nonverbal cues.

Equipment Needed:

- Pillows
- Rolled blankets or towels
- Footboard
- Heel protectors
- Hand rolls

▶ CLIENT EDUCATION NEEDED:

1. Explain the reason for and importance of frequent turning and positioning.
2. Educate the client and the client's caregiver regarding the signs and symptoms of pressure sore development.
3. Teach the client and the caregiver about the areas most at risk for skin breakdown and what to do if breakdown does occur.
4. Teach the client's family how to inspect the client's skin and how to turn and position the client before the client is discharged.

Estimated time to complete the skill:
5–10 minutes

IMPLEMENTATION—Action/Rationale

Action	Rationale
1. Wash hands.	1. Reduces the transmission of microorganisms.
2. Explain procedure to client. Elicit client cooperation and participation.	2. Decreases anxiety. Improves client compliance and cooperation.
3. Gather all necessary equipment. Provide for client privacy.	3. Ensures client dignity and allows for a smooth procedure.
4. Secure adequate assistance to safely complete task.	4. Prevents caregiver back and muscle strain as well as provides for client safety.
5. Adjust bed to comfortable working height. Lower side rail on side of bed from which you are assisting client.	5. Prevents caregiver back and muscle strain.
6. Follow proper body mechanics guidelines: When moving a client in bed, position the bed so that your legs are slightly bent at the knees and hips. Maintain the natural curves in your back while lifting. Position one foot slightly in front of the other and spread feet apart to create a wide base for balance. When your arms are placed under the client, slowly lean backward onto your back leg using your body weight to help you lift the client to one side of the bed. Do not extend or rotate your back to move a client in bed. If you cannot move the client easily, always ask for and obtain assistance for both your and the client's safety (see Figure 4-3-2). Be sure the floor is not slippery and that the bed is locked. Always use a turning sheet when rolling a client as this gives you better support and control of the client (see Figure 4-3-3).	6. Prevents caregiver back injury and muscle strain and promotes client safety. Spreading feet to create a wide base helps prevent loss of balance.
7. Position drains, tubes, and IVs to accommodate new client position.	7. Prevents accidental dislodgment and/or discomfort from movement by reduced mechanical tension.
8. Place or assist client into appropriate starting position. Monitor client status, and provide adequate rest breaks or support as necessary.	8. Prevents client injury.

continues

Action	Rationale

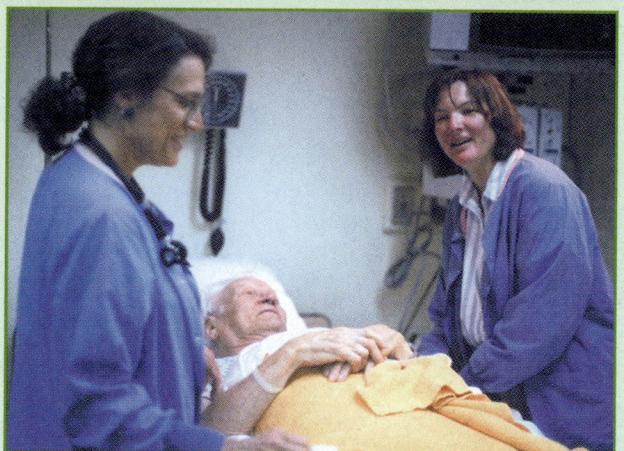

Figure 4-3-2 If the client is heavy or hard to move, always obtain assistance for both the client's and your safety.

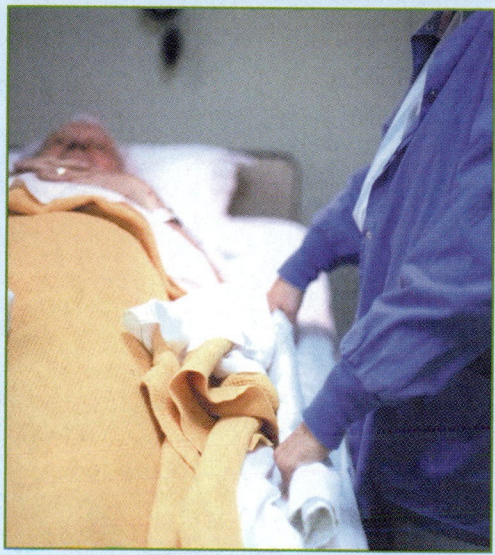

Figure 4-3-3 When rolling a client, use a turning sheet for better support and control.

Moving from Supine to Side-Lying Position

9. Slide your hands underneath the client. Move the client to one side of the bed by lifting the client's body toward you in stages—first the upper trunk, then the lower trunk, and finally the legs. Lift the client's body; do not drag the client across the sheets.

   Roll the client to side-lying position by placing the client's inside arm next to the client's body with the palm of the hand against the hip. Cross the client's outside arm and leg toward midline and log roll the client toward you using the client's outside shoulder and hip for leverage while maintaining stability and control of top arm and leg.

9. Prevents shearing of skin tissue. Maintains client body alignment. Protects caregiver's back and prevents muscle strain. Prevents client injury.

Maintaining Side-Lying Position

10. Repeat Actions 1–8.

10. See Rationales 1–8.

11. Pillows may be placed to support the client's head and arms (see Figure 4-3-4). An additional pillow may be used to support the topside leg, and fully and equally support the thigh, knee, ankle, and foot (see Figure 4-3-5). Move the lower arm forward slightly at the shoulder and bend the elbow for comfort. If the client is unstable, a pillow placed against the back will provide additional support and keep the client from rolling supine (see Figure 4-3-6).

11. Provides support and comfort.

continues

Action	Rationale

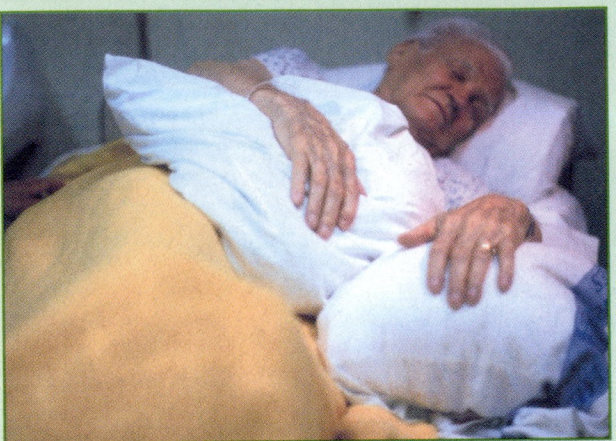

Figure 4-3-4   Place pillows to support the head and arms.

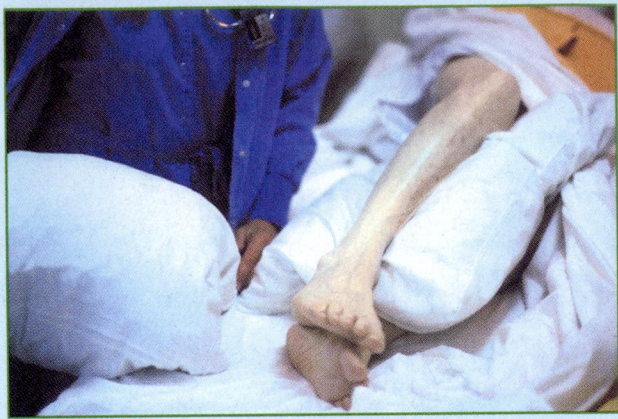

Figure 4-3-5   Place pillows to support the leg, ankle, and foot.

Moving from Side-Lying to Prone Position

12. Repeat Actions 1–8.

13. Remove positioning towels, pillows, or other support devices. Assess whether the client's position in bed needs to be adjusted to accommodate the continued movement into prone. Move the client's inside arm next to the client's body with palm against hip. Roll the client onto the stomach using the shoulder and hip as key points of control. The head must be placed in a comfortable position to one side without excessive pressure to sensitive areas. Pillows under the trunk are placed as needed to relieve pressure and increase comfort. The client's arms are placed comfortably at the client's side and the legs are uncrossed with the feet approximately a foot apart.

12. See Rationales 1–8.

13. Ensures comfort and safety in movement.

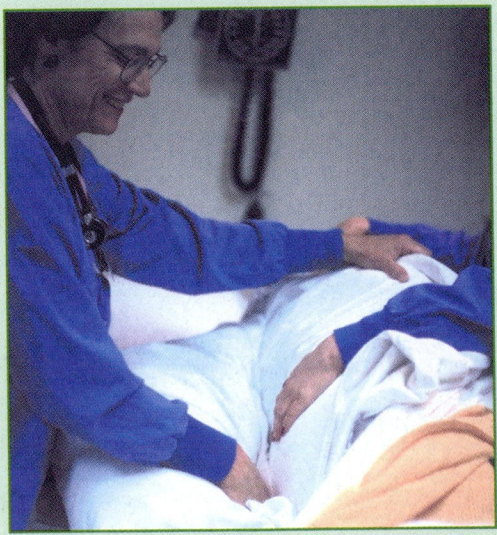

Figure 4-3-6   A pillow against the back will prevent a side-lying client from rolling into a supine position.

continues

Action	Rationale
Maintaining Prone Position 14. A shallow pillow or a folded towel may be used to support the client's head comfortably as well as a pillow placed under the abdomen to support the back. An additional pillow may be placed under the lower leg to reduce the pressure of the toes and forefoot against the bed.	14. Provides support and comfort.
Moving from Prone to Supine Position 15. Repeat Actions 1–8.	15. See Rationales 1–8.
16. Remove positioning towels, pillows, or other supporting devices. Slide your hands underneath the client. Move the client segmentally to one side of the bed to accommodate the new position. Position the inside arm next to the client's body with the client's palm next to the hip. Roll the client to supine by logrolling the client toward you using the client's outside shoulder and hip for leverage. Have the client's face positioned away from the direction of the roll to prevent undue pressure to the face or neck. When the client reaches supine, uncross the client's arms and legs and place them comfortably into anatomic positions.	16. Provides support and comfort.
Maintaining Supine Position 17. A footboard may be used to support the foot as well as heel protectors or a pillow placed between the heel and gastrocnemius muscle to reduce the pressure on the heels (see Figures 4-3-7 and 4-3-8). Assess and compare warmth, sensation, color, and movement of feet. To prevent excessive external rotation of the lower extremity, a trochanter roll may be used. For comfort, additional pillows may be used to support the client's head, arms, or lower back.	17. Provides support and comfort. Heel protectors and routine assessment of the feet help to prevent pressure sores. Trochanter rolls and pillows help to prevent displacement of the acetabulum (hip joint).

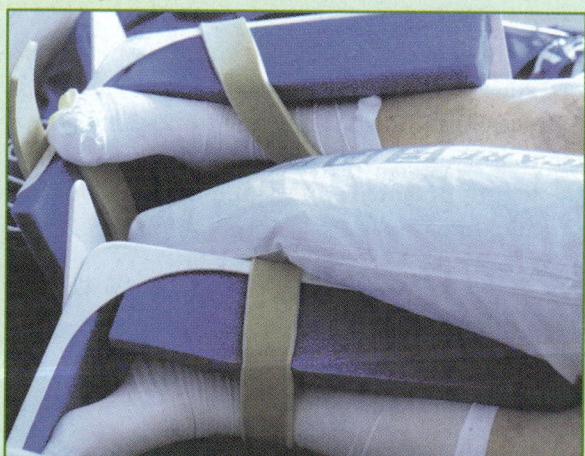

Figure 4-3-7   Heel protectors are placed on the foot to provide support and comfort.

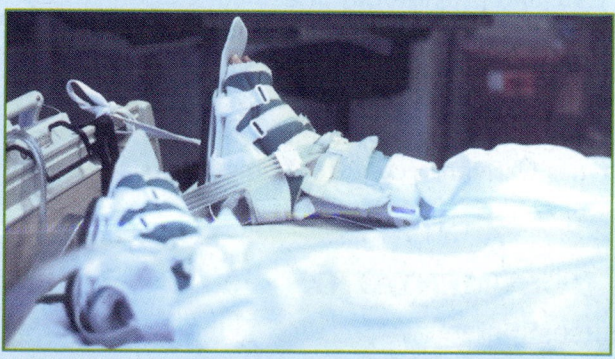

Figure 4-3-8   Heel protectors also provide padding to reduce the risk of skin breakdown where the heel rests on the mattress.

continues

Action	Rationale
Maintaining Supine Position *continued*	
18. Be sure to replace side rails to upright position as well as to lower bed to beginning position.	18. Provides for client safety.
19. Place call light within reach of the client.	19. Provides for client safety.
20. Move bedside table close to bed and place items of frequent use within reach of the client.	20. Provides for client safety.
21. Wash hands.	21. Reduces the transmission of microorganisms.

▶ REAL WORLD ANECDOTES

Scenario 1
A nurse on a home care visit notes the wife, who weighs approximately 130 lbs, is caring for a very weak husband, who weighs 220 lbs. To move him in bed, she places a leather belt around his waist and uses it to drag the heaviest part of his body toward her. This client is at a risk for skin breakdown because of skin shear and friction from the dragging. The nurse teaches the client's wife how to use a draw sheet to move her husband in bed as well as makes recommendations regarding the wife's body mechanics. The nurse also recommends that a home health aide come to the house to assist the client's wife with his care.

Scenario 2
A nurse caring for a client in a skilled nursing facility was repositioning a client in the middle of the night. To avoid disturbing the client, she turned on the bathroom light and worked in the semidarkness. Placing a pillow under the client's head, the nurse did not realize that the pillow tag had escaped from the case and that the edge of the tag was abrading the client's eye. The client suffered a scratched cornea. Although the nurse was right to be concerned about her client's comfort, client safety should never be sacrificed for client comfort.

▶ EVALUATION

- Safe and proper body alignment and movement were achieved for both client and caregiver.
- The client is comfortable in the new position as evident by verbal and nonverbal cues.
- The client's skin and underlying organs and tissues were protected from pressure, friction, and shear.

- Note any report or observation of pain, discomfort, or dyspnea.
- Note the findings of your integumentary assessment, including color and integrity of skin and the length of time redness persists over bony prominences.

Document on appropriate flow sheet or electronic medical record (EMR).

▶ DOCUMENTATION

Nurses' Notes
- Note the client's new position and the time of the position change.

▶ CRITICAL THINKING SKILL

Introduction
The nurse strains her back by not calling for assistance when needed.

Possible Scenario

A heavily sedated obese man has just been returned to his room from the special procedures lab. As the nurse is walking down the hall, she hears the sounds of retching and realizes he is vomiting. As she hurries into the room, she notes that vomitus has covered the floor and bedside railing. She quickly turns the client on his side and holds him in position with her left hand and forearm. She reaches behind her for a basin. As she reaches for the basin, her foot slips in the vomitus on the floor.

Possible Outcome

The nurse's body alignment is twisted and off balance. She falls hard and wrenches her back.

Prevention

Immediately turning the client to his side to clear his airway was appropriate. The nurse could have grabbed a pillow and placed it at his back to support his side-lying position and free her hands. She could have summoned assistance.

▶ VARIATIONS

Geriatric Variations:
- *Elderly clients may have more compromised body systems such as delicate skin, a more brittle skeletal system, cardiovascular shifts, more difficulty with balance, and less muscle strength to assist during positioning.*

Pediatric Variations:
- *Take care not to place babies in the prone position to sleep because this may contribute to sudden infant death. Infants should be propped in a side-lying position to sleep.*

Home Care Variations:
- *Assess the ability of the primary caregiver to adequately turn and position the client in the home care setting. Does the caregiver know proper body alignment technique, as well as basic information on the prevention and detection of pressure sores?*
- *Assess whether the home caregiver has enough support and help (friends, neighbors, or family) to turn the client as often as needed to avoid prolonged pressure over bony prominences.*
- *Examine the bed or chair where the client spends most of the day and night. Can the sheets be tucked tight? Is the upholstery on the chair a rough fabric or plastic? Could the fabric on the bed or the chair contribute to friction or shearing forces when the client is moved?*

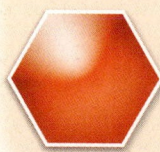

Long-Term Care Variation:
- *Long-term clients may have a "favorite" position and may shift back to this position, even if turned at regular intervals. Such a client needs to be assessed more frequently than every 2 hours.*

▶ COMMON ERRORS

Possible Error:

The nurse leaves the client's arm under his torso when turning him to a side-lying position.

Prevention:

Be aware of the client's position and relative comfort. After repositioning a client, step back and look. Does this position look comfortable? Could you lie this way for 2 hours? Does the client appear to be in pain?

▶ **NURSING TIPS**

• If client is assessed as a candidate for skin care precautions, post a turning schedule for the client in an easy-to-locate area in the client's room.

• Have all equipment necessary for proper positioning readily available in the client's room.

• Regularly check status of all splints and other devices to make sure they fit properly.

• Safe, proper body alignment for the nurse includes back aligned and straight, knees bent, and a wide base with feet apart.

• Have the client assist as much as possible to reduce the risk of injury for the caregiver.

▶ **SPECIAL CONSIDERATIONS**

• *Supports should be used when turning and positioning a client, especially a client who has a history of joint replacement surgery. Proper use of supports can help prevent joint dislocation from overextension/flexion.*

• *For immobile clients, turning and positioning should be implemented on a regular basis, usually every 2 hours. Skin breakdown, especially over the bony prominences, can easily form from prolonged positioning. Be aware that a red spot on the skin could be the first sign of a pressure sore. Document and establish a follow-up plan to prevent skin breakdown.*

• *Special devices such as a roller or sliding board may be used to facilitate positioning a client. Refer to the instruction manual or ask for assistance if not familiar with the device.*

Moving a Client in Bed

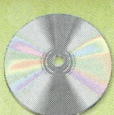

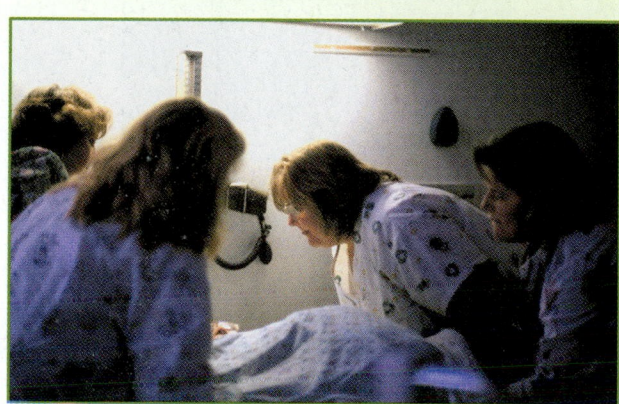

▶ OVERVIEW OF THE SKILL

Prolonged immobility is uncomfortable and presents an increased risk of many complications. Muscle wasting, clot formation, and skin breakdown are the most common risks associated with immobility. Clients who are unable to move themselves in bed or are only able to assist with moving in bed are at risk for discomfort and complications related to immobility. Often, clients' restlessness in bed will cause them to slide down toward the foot of the bed. This is especially true in beds in which the head raises up to a Fowler's or semi-Fowler's position. If the client slides down toward the foot of the bed while the head is elevated, it can lead to reduced respiratory effort, reduced lung capacity, and skin breakdown, thus impairing the client's recovery.

The nurse is often called upon to move a client to a more comfortable position. Repositioning a client can sometimes be done by a single staff member, but often it requires two or more people to do this procedure safely.

▶ ASSESSMENT

1. Assess the client's ability to assist with repositioning. Determine whether the client can move with the aid of an overhead trapeze or the side rail. Judge how much assistance will be needed. **Determines safety for the client and the nurse and good body mechanics for the nurse.**

2. Assess the client's ability to understand and follow directions and assist and cooperate with the move. **Affects how the procedure will be carried out. Affects client teaching.**

3. Assess the client's environment. Check the bed for cleanliness. Has the client been restless, sweaty, or incontinent? Check to see if the sheets have been turned or twisted. Tubes, lines, wires, traction, casts, or splints must be moved carefully (see Figure 4-4-1). **Affects how the procedure will be carried out. Affects what additional procedures will be performed. Prepares the caregivers to keep tubes and equipment from becoming dislodged or tipping or pulling.**

▶ DIAGNOSIS

Impaired Physical Mobility

Activity Intolerance

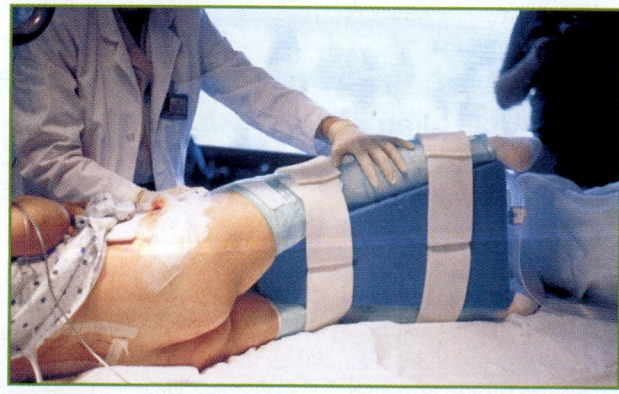

Figure 4-4-1 Before repositioning the client, assess the environment for items that could become dislodged or tip or pull.

Risk for Impaired Skin Integrity

Impaired Bed Mobility

▶ **PLANNING**

Expected Outcomes:

1. The client will be moved in bed without injury to self.
2. The client will be moved in bed without injury to the staff.
3. The client will report an increase in comfort following the move.
4. All tubes, lines, and drains will remain patent and intact.

Equipment Needed:

- Hospital bed with side rails
- Trapeze if required (see Figure 4-4-2)
- Turn sheet or draw sheet

▶ **CLIENT EDUCATION NEEDED:**

1. Explain to the client the need to move in bed to maintain circulation and lung capacity.
2. Teach clients "1-2-3 go" so they will be able to cooperate with the move.
3. Teach clients not to use their elbows to help push themselves up in bed. The elbows quickly

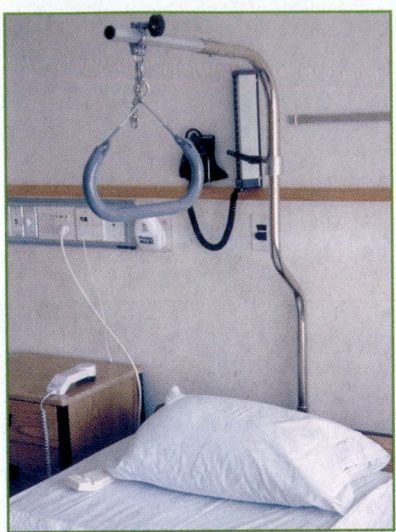

Figure 4-4-2   Overhead trapeze

become sore and abraded when the client moves this way. Instead, encourage use of an overhead trapeze.

 Estimated time to complete the skill: **5–10 minutes**

▶ **DELEGATION TIPS**

Turning and positioning is routinely delegated to ancillary personnel who have received appropriate training. The caregiver must protect him- or herself and the client from injury and report the client's response to the activity to the nurse.

IMPLEMENTATION—Action/Rationale

Action	Rationale
Moving Up a Client in Bed with One Nurse	
1. Wash hands and apply gloves.	1. Reduces the transmission of microorganisms.
2. Inform client of reason for the move and how to assist (if able).	2. Reduces anxiety; helps increase comprehension and cooperation; promotes client autonomy.
3. Elevate bed to just below waist height. Lower head of bed if tolerated by client. Lower side rails on the side where you are standing.	3. Lessens strain on nurse's back muscles.

continues

Action	Rationale

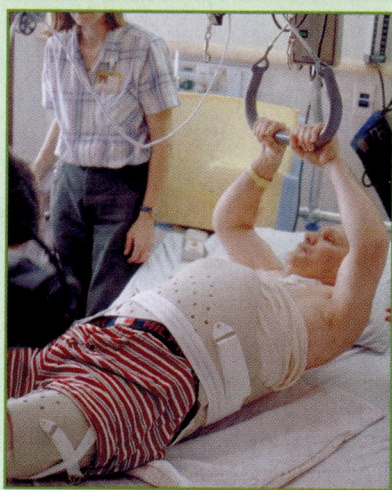

Figure 4-4-3 Have the client hold on to the overhead trapeze, if one is available, to assist in the move.

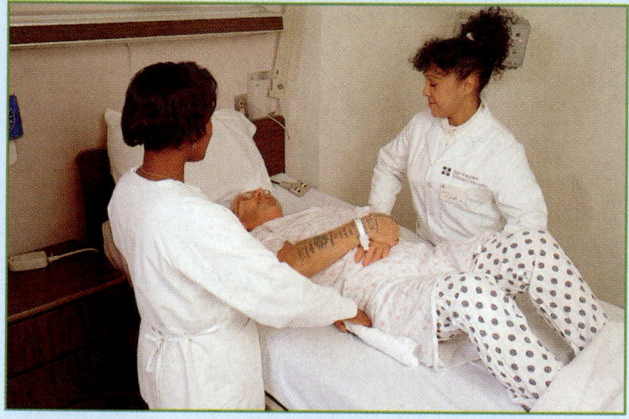

Figure 4-4-4 Have the client bend the knees and place feet flat on the bed.

4. Remove the pillow and place it against the headboard.

4. Prevents having to move against the pillow. Provides padding of the headboard if the client should be moved too high in the bed.

5. Have the client fold arms across the chest.

5. Prevents getting the client's arms trapped or injured during the move.

6. Have the client hold on to the overhead trapeze, if available (see Figure 4-4-3).

6. Promotes client autonomy by allowing the client to assist with the move.

7. Have the client bend the knees and place the feet flat on the bed if able (see Figure 4-4-4).

7. Allows the client to assist in the move; promotes client autonomy.

8. Stand at an angle to the head of the bed, feet apart, knees bent, feet toward the head of the bed.

8. Promotes good body mechanics.

9. Slide one hand and arm under the client's shoulder, the other under the client's thigh.

9. Distributes the client's weight more evenly. Promotes good lifting technique.

10. Rock forward toward the head of the bed, lifting the client with you. Simultaneously have the client push with the legs.

10. Allows a smooth motion to lift the client. Client assistance lessens strain on nurse's back muscles; promotes client autonomy.

11. If the client has a trapeze, have the client pull up holding onto the trapeze as you move the client upward in bed.

11. Client assistance lessens strain on nurse's back muscles; promotes client autonomy.

12. Repeat these steps until the client is moved up high enough in bed.

12. Large or very immobile clients are often not moved far enough in one step.

13. Return the client's pillow under the head.

13. Promotes client comfort.

14. Elevate head of bed, if tolerated by client.

14. Promotes comfort; facilitates eating and drinking; facilitates communication.

15. Assess client for comfort.

15. Comfort is subjective.

continues

Action	Rationale

Moving Up a Client in Bed with One Nurse *continued*

16. Adjust the client's bedclothes as needed for comfort.

17. Lower bed and elevate side rails.

18. Wash hands.

Moving Up a Client in Bed with Two or More Nurses

19. Wash hands and apply gloves if needed (see Figure 4-4-5).

20. Inform client of reason for the move and how to assist (if able).

21. Elevate bed to just below waist height. Lower head of bed if tolerated by client. Lower side rails (see Figure 4-4-6).

16. Comfort is subjective.

17. Promotes client safety.

18. Reduces the transmission of microorganisms.

19. Reduces the transmission of microorganisms.

20. Reduces anxiety; helps increase comprehension and cooperation; promotes client autonomy.

21. Lessens strain on nurse's back muscles.

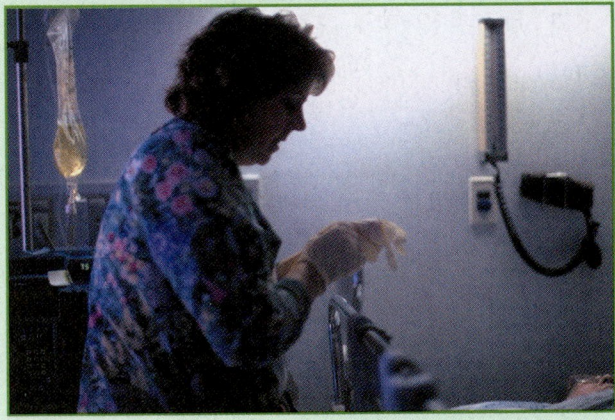

Figure 4-4-5   Apply gloves before repositioning the client, if needed.

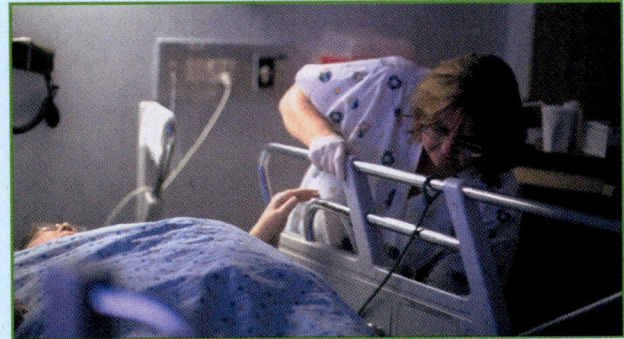

Figure 4-4-6   Lower the side rails to allow the nurse to use good body mechanics.

22. With two nurses, place turn/draw sheet under client's back and head.

23. Roll up the draw sheet on each side until it is next to the client (see Figures 4-4-7 and 4-4-8).

24. Follow Actions 4–7.

25. The nurses stand on either side of the bed, at an angle to the head of the bed. They stand with knees flexed, feet apart in a wide stance.

26. The nurses hold their elbows as close as possible to their bodies.

22. Reduces shearing force, which can precipitate skin breakdown.

23. Provides support under the heavy parts of the body and places the nurse's hands close to the weight to be moved.

24. See Rationales 4–7.

25. Promotes good body mechanics.

26. Allows the muscles of the torso to assist the arm muscles in bearing and moving the weight of the client.

continues

Action	Rationale

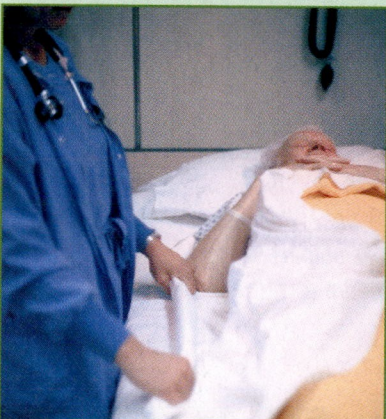

Figure 4-4-7 Roll up the draw sheet tightly on each side of the client.

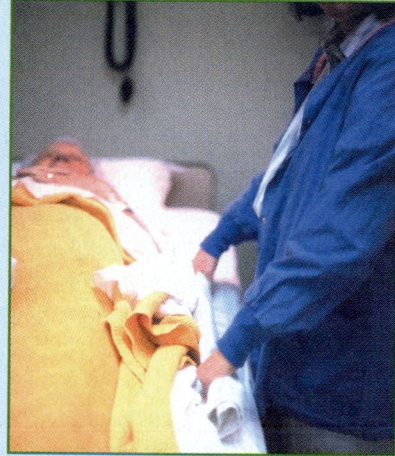

Figure 4-4-8 Rolling the draw sheet up tightly next to the client places the nurse's hands close to the weight of the client.

27. The lead nurse will give the signal to move: 1-2-3 go. The nurses will lift up (off the bed) on the turn/draw sheet and forward (toward the head of the bed) in one smooth motion (see Figure 4-4-9). The move is coordinated to transfer the client toward the head of the bed. Simultaneously, have the client push with the legs or pull using the trapeze

27. Allows a smooth motion to lift the client. Client assistance lessens strain on the nurse's back muscles; promotes client autonomy.

28. Repeat until the client is moved up high enough in bed to be comfortable.

28. Large or very immobile clients are often not moved far enough in one step.

29. Return the client's pillow under the head.

29. Promotes client comfort.

30. Elevate head of bed, if tolerated by client.

30. Promotes comfort; facilitates eating and drinking; facilitates communication.

31. Assess client for comfort.

31. Promotes comfort.

32. Adjust the client's bedclothes for comfort.

32. Promotes comfort.

33. Lower bed and elevate side rails.

33. Promotes client safety.

34. Wash hands.

34. Reduces the transmission of microorganisms.

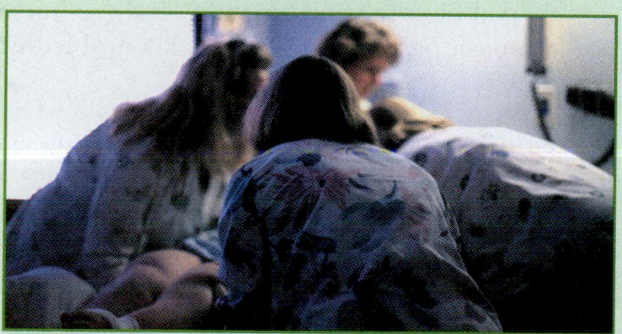

Figure 4-4-9 At the signal from the lead nurse, lift and pull in one smooth motion.

► REAL WORLD ANECDOTES

Scenario 1

Mrs. Jovanovich was 2 days postsurgery. She was receiving analgesia through an epidural catheter. Her nurse noted that Mrs. Jovanovich had slid down in bed and was now hunched over and appeared to be uncomfortable. Mrs. Jovanovich did not have a turn sheet, but she was able to assist the nurse with moving up in bed. As the nurse slid her up, Mrs. Jovanovich pushed with her heels. Mrs. Jovanovich was successfully moved up in bed and the nurse elevated the head of the bed and made the client comfortable. As the nurse started to leave the room, Mrs. Jovanovich asked the nurse about a wet spot she had suddenly found in the bed. While searching for the source of the liquid, the nurse discovered that the move up in bed had dislodged Mrs. Jovanovich's epidural catheter. Without an intact epidural catheter, Mrs. Jovanovich will have to either risk another lumbar puncture procedure or settle for less effective pain relief. It is important to always check the client before moving to avoid injury.

Scenario 2

A new nurse on the floor was accustomed to moving the client on the count of three, when the word "three" was spoken. The nurses on the floor were used to moving the client 1 second after the word "three" was spoken. The first few "moves" were not well-coordinated and resulted in some confusion and, in one case, peals of laughter by the nurses and the client. Finally, the nurses found that shaking their heads "no" on each count and "yes" on the actual move helped the new nurse wait the extra beat, and coordination was restored.

► EVALUATION

- The client was moved without injury to self or staff.
- The client reported an increase in comfort following the move.
- All tubes, lines, and drains remained intact.

► DOCUMENTATION

Nurses' Notes

- Note the time and position the client was moved.
- Document any unusual findings.

Document on appropriate flow sheet or electronic medical record (EMR).

► CRITICAL THINKING SKILL

Introduction

Consider all factors that could affect the safety and effectiveness of the procedure.

Possible Scenario

You have been asked to help move Mr. Miller in bed. Mr. Miller is an elderly client with a large, foul-smelling, open abdominal wound. The nurse who has requested your help is repelled by the odor. As you prepare to pull up the client in bed, the other nurse stands back from the bed, grasping the very edge of the turn sheet.

Possible Outcome

Because of the lack of leverage, pulling this client up will be more difficult and will require more energy from the nurse who is standing close to the client and using good body mechanics.

By standing too far back, the nurse risks injuring herself by having to use poor body mechanics to actually move the client.

By standing too far back, the nurse risks injuring the client by not having control of the motion being initiated. The client could fall against the side rails or pull on a tube accidentally, and the nurse is not in a position to be able to quickly deal with the situation.

Prevention

Part of good body mechanics is standing close to the object you are trying to move. Standing too far away makes the weaker lower back muscles take too much of the load. By standing close to the object to be lifted with feet apart, the bigger, stronger leg muscles can do most of the work.

▶ VARIATIONS

Geriatric Variations:
- *Older clients often have thin, fragile skin. Be sure not to drag clients across the sheets because this could tear their skin.*

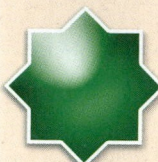

Pediatric Variations:
- *Children may be small enough to lift bodily in bed.*
- *Children tend to be more active in bed and may need to be repositioned more often.*

Home Care Variations:
- *Often a family member is caring for the home care client. The family member should be taught proper body mechanics to prevent injury to the caregiver.*
- *Very often, beds in the home care setting, even rented hospital beds, are in small rooms, positioned against the wall, or wedged in by furniture. Enlist the assistance of a family member or caregiver to assess whether the nurse has good access to the bed or if the care area should be rearranged. Consider moving the sick room to another part of the home such as the dining room.*
- *When using the home linens, remember they are often old and worn or not as strong as hospital linen. Bring a draw sheet with you, if needed. Check the linen to see whether it is strong enough to hold and pull without tearing.*
- *The family member should be encouraged to demonstrate and use proper lifting skills to become more comfortable with them.*
- *If the home bed is a regular double, queen, or king-size bed, think how you will modify the moving technique to maintain good body alignment. For example, extra care and thought will be needed to move a client in a waterbed.*

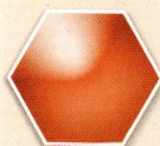

Long-Term Care Variations:
- *Long-term care clients are pulled up in bed fairly often. They are at increased risk for pressure ulcers on their coccyx and heels. Check these areas often and be sure they are not dragged across the sheets during the move. Make sure clients' heels have protectors on them before moving a client. Use draw sheets as much as possible to avoid shearing fragile skin.*
- *Encourage independence as much as possible. Give clients "something to grab on to" to help them move up in bed. A trapeze, a cloth tied to the headboard, or something to brace against may help. Make sure clients are able to move themselves without tearing or shearing the skin and that they are able to assess this.*

▶ COMMON ERRORS

Possible Error:
The nurse does not get enough help to safely and adequately move the client.

Prevention:
Think about what could happen if you do not have enough help to perform this procedure. You could injure yourself trying to lift too much. You could injure the client by trying to lift too much and dropping or inadequately supporting the client. Be sure to assess the client's ability to help and the complexity of the move. If in doubt, get help. Too much help is always better than too little.

▶ **NURSING TIPS**

- Position in bed can be maintained using bed Gatch, if tolerated by client.

- Have client take a deep breath and then breathe out as he or she is moved to prevent client from performing a Valsalva's maneuver, which can cause hypotension.

▶ **SPECIAL CONSIDERATIONS**

- *Avoid dragging the client against the bed linen when moving. This dragging friction may result in skin tearing and unnecessary injury to the client.*
- *To prevent occupational injury, use proper body mechanics when moving a client and do not hesitate to ask for help from the team. For heavy clients use mechanical devices and/or seek additional help as appropriate.*
- *If clients have complex wounds, IV lines, or tubes in place, ensure that appropriate assessment occurs prior to the move. Be sure all lines and tubes have appropriate length and are not tangled in bed linens. Drainage receptacles may need to be moved to the other side of the bed.*

Assisting with a Bedpan or Urinal

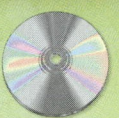

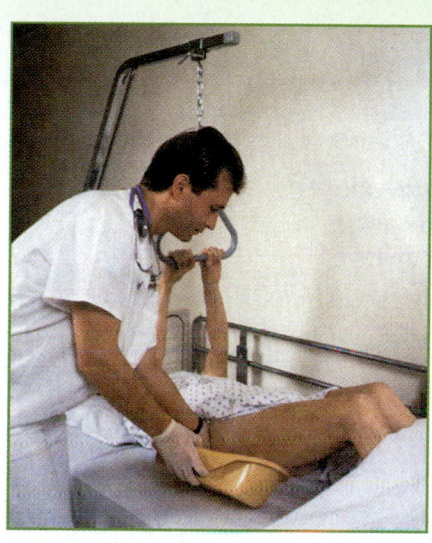

▶ OVERVIEW OF THE SKILL

Voiding and bowel elimination for the client confined to bed require a bedpan or a urinal. The bedridden client may have altered elimination patterns. Reduced mobility, pain, privacy issues, the need for assistance, delays in getting assistance when needed, and the fear of interruption can all alter normal elimination patterns. Fear of creating embarrassing noises, sights, or odors may compel the client to reduce fluid intake or avoid the urge to eliminate while in the hospital. Constipation, incontinence, and discomfort can result and lead to an increased risk of urinary tract infection. Sensitivity, proper technique, and client education by the nurse support the client on bed rest.

▶ ASSESSMENT

1. Assess your equipment. Do you have the necessary items within reach? **Prevents having to stop the procedure and leave the client's bedside.**
2. Assess how much the client can assist in positioning and removing the bedpan. **Determines how the procedure will be done and whether assistance will be required.**
3. Check whether the client is confused, combative, in traction, or immobile. **Determines how the procedure will be done and whether assistance will be required.**

4. Check for casts, braces, or dressings, which need to be protected from accidental contamination with waste products. **Determines how much preparation will need to be done prior to toileting.**
5. Check for privacy and unexpected interruptions. **Determines whether extra steps need to be taken to ensure privacy prior to toileting.**
6. Assess whether the client has orders to record intake and output. **Determines need to take steps for measurement and may require containers with measurement markings.**

▶ DIAGNOSIS

Constipation

Bowel Incontinence

Stress Urinary Incontinence

Urinary Retention

Toileting Self-Care Deficit

Situational Low Self-Esteem

Powerlessness

Diarrhea

Total Urinary Incontinence

Urge Urinary Incontinence

Risk for Impaired Skin Integrity

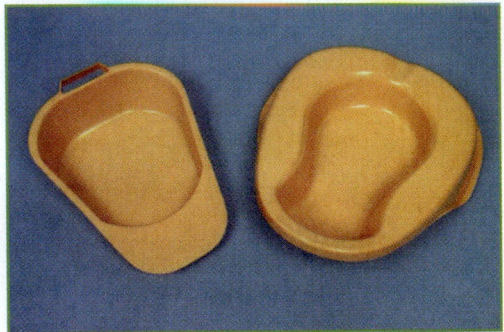

Figure 4-5-1 A fracture pan or bedpan are used for elimination when a client is confined to bed.

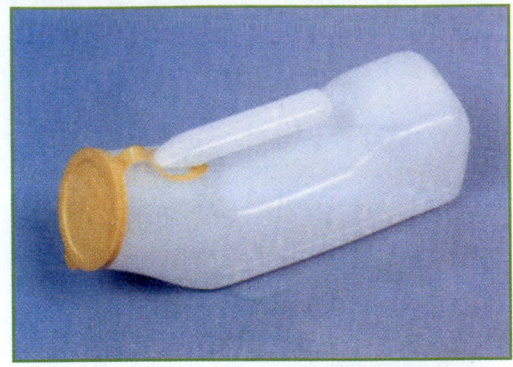

Figure 4-5-2 A urinal can be used by a male client for elimination when the client is confined to bed.

▶ PLANNING

Expected Outcomes:

1. Clients will be able to void and defecate when necessary.
2. Clients will have as much privacy and comfort as allowable, given their physical condition.
3. Intake and output will be accurately measured as needed.
4. The urinal or bedpan will be placed without skin damage.
5. The bedpan will be removed and emptied without spillage.

Equipment Needed (see Figures 4-5-1 and 4-5-2):

- Bedpan (regular or fracture) or urinal
- Disposable gloves
- Bedpan cover
- Toilet paper
- Washcloth and towel

▶ CLIENT EDUCATION NEEDED:

1. Educate the client about the need for using a bedpan instead of a bedside commode or bathroom.
2. Discuss privacy concerns.

Estimated time to complete the skill:
10–15 minutes

▶ DELEGATION TIPS

This skill is routinely delegated to ancillary personnel who have been trained in Standard Precautions and proper body positioning and to report color, odor, and amount of output to the nurse.

IMPLEMENTATION—Action/Rationale

Action	Rationale
Positioning a Bedpan	
1. Close curtain or door.	1. Provides privacy for the client.
2. Wash hands; apply gloves.	2. Reduces the transmission of microorganisms.
3. Lower head of bed so client is in supine position.	3. The supine position will increase ability of client to move to side-lying position.
4. Elevate bed.	4. Ensures proper body mechanics.

continues

Action	Rationale
5. Assist client to side-lying position using side rail for support.	5. Provides for best position for proper placement of bedpan.
6. Place bedpan under buttocks. Place a fracture pan with the lower end near the client's lower back region. Place large bedpans with the opening near the client's thighs.	6. Ensures proper placement of the bedpan before client rolls on top of bedpan.
7. While holding the bedpan with one hand, help the client roll onto his or her back while pushing against the bedpan (toward the center of the bed) to hold it in place.	7. Prevents dislocation or alignment of bedpan.
8. Alternate: Help the client raise the hips by using the overbed trapeze and slide the pan in place. Alternate: If the client is unable to turn or raise hips, use a fracture pan instead of a bedpan. With a fracture pan, the flat side is placed toward the client's head (see Figure 4-5-1).	8. Provides an alternate way to position the pan. Fracture pan reduces the amount of movement and lift required to place the pan.
9. Check placement of bedpan by looking between client's legs.	9. May prevent spillage from misalignment of bedpan.
10. If indicated, elevate head of bed to 45-degree angle or higher for comfort.	10. Check order of physician or qualified practitioner; bed remains flat if client has a spinal cord injury or spinal surgery. Elevating the head of bed creates a more normal elimination position.
11. Place call light within reach of client; place side rails in upright position, lower bed, and provide privacy.	11. Privacy allows for a more comfortable elimination environment; elevated side rails provide for safety.
12 Remove gloves; wash hands.	12. Reduces the transmission of microorganisms.

Positioning a Urinal

Action	Rationale
13. Repeat Actions 1 and 2.	13. See Rationales 1 and 2.
14. Lift the covers and place the urinal so the client may grasp the handle and position it. If the client cannot do this, you must position the urinal and place the penis into the opening (see Figures 4-5-3 and 4-5-4).	14. Ensures proper placement of the urinal and reduces the risk of spillage.
15. Remove gloves; wash hands.	15. Reduces the transmission of microorganisms.

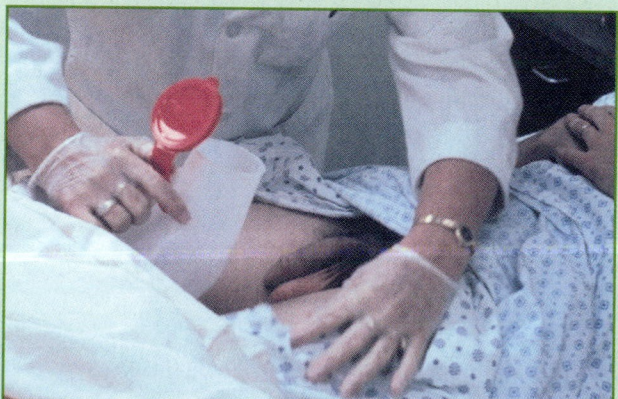

Figure 4-5-3   Lift the covers and place the urinal. Allow the client to adjust the position.

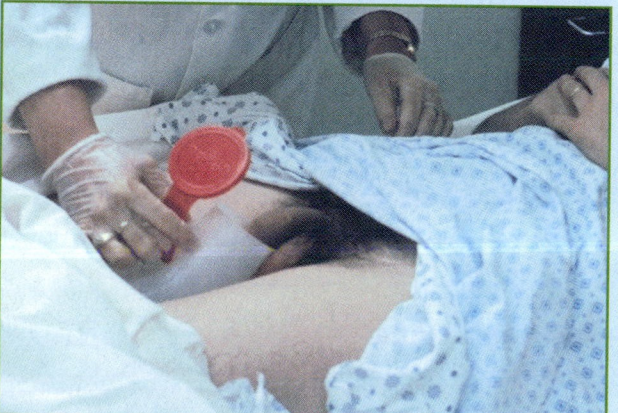

Figure 4-5-4   If the client is unable to assist, place the penis into the opening of the urinal.

continues

Action	Rationale
Removing a Bedpan	
16. Wash hands; apply gloves.	**16.** Reduces the transmission of microorganisms.
17. Gather toilet paper and washing supplies.	**17.** Having supplies at the bedside allows smooth and safe completion of the procedure.
18. Lower head of bed to supine position.	**18.** Increases client's ability to move to side-lying position.
19. While holding bedpan with one hand, roll client to side and remove the pan. Be careful not to pull or shear skin sticking to the pan and being careful not to spill contents (see Figure 4-5-5).	**19.** Prevents possible spillage of bedpan contents.

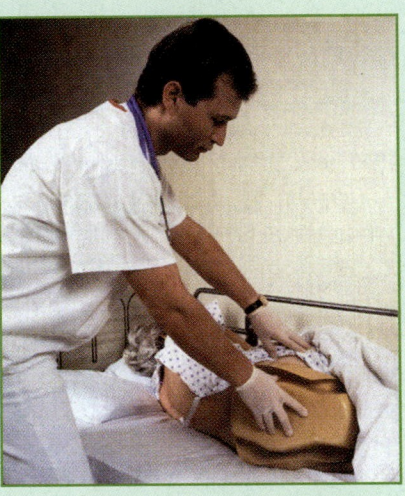

Figure 4-5-5   Place the bedpan against the client's buttocks while turning the client to the side.

Action	Rationale
20. Assist with cleaning or wiping; always wipe with a front to back motion.	**20.** Client may not be able to clean self; wiping from front to back decreases chances of cross-contamination from anus to urethra.
21. Empty bedpan (observe and measure urine output and check for occult blood if ordered), clean bedpan, and store it in proper place; if bedpan is to be emptied outside client's room, cover it during transport.	**21.** Promotes privacy and decreases the chance of spilling contents. Assessment of types of stool evaluates for constipation and diarrhea.
22. Remove soiled gloves. Wash hands.	**22.** Reduces the transmission of microorganisms.
23. Allow client to wash hands.	**23.** Provides for physical hygiene and comfort.
24. Place call light within reach; recheck that side rails are in the upright position.	**24.** Ensures client safety and comfort.
25. Wash hands.	**25.** Reduces the transmission of microorganisms.
Removing a Urinal	
26. Wash hands and apply gloves.	**26.** Reduces the transmission of microorganisms.
27. Empty the urinal, measuring urine output if ordered, rinse the urinal and replace it within the client's reach. Observe odor and color of urine before discarding.	**27.** Provides a way to measure the client's output. Keeping the urinal within reach promotes client autonomy. Helps evaluate for concentrated urine, infection, and renal problems.

continues

Action	Rationale
28. Remove soiled gloves. Wash hands.	28. Reduces the transmission of microorganisms.
29. Allow client to wash hands.	29. Provides for physical hygiene and comfort.
30. Place call light within reach; recheck that side rails are in the upright position.	30. Ensures client safety and comfort.
31. Wash hands.	31. Reduces the transmission of microorganisms.

▶ REAL WORLD ANECDOTES

Scenario 1

A 69-year-old woman was brought to the emergency room at approximately 3 a.m. with a fractured left hip. She had fallen in her home on her way to the bathroom. An IV inserted by paramedics at the scene has been running at a rapid rate for approximately 45 minutes. While waiting for the X-ray technician, the client appeared to be in distress but did not voice any complaints in the presence of the physician and the assistant. Alone with the nurse, the client explained that she had never made it to the bathroom and had to "go." She was certain she could not void without a bedpan under her, but attempting to place the fracture pan was too painful. The nurse solved the problem by moving the fracture pan as close as possible so the client could feel it under her, then placing absorbent padding and blue pads to catch the voided urine.

Scenario 2

A nursing student was working in a busy unit where one bathroom served two rooms, with a door to each. The student very efficiently flung open the bathroom door and in one smooth motion emptied the bedpan directly onto the lap of the other client, who was sitting on the toilet and had forgotten to lock the doors. The student quickly learned to always look first.

▶ EVALUATION

- The client was able to void or defecate as needed.
- The client's request for assistance was answered promptly.
- The bedpan or urinal was removed and emptied without spillage.
- Ordered tests were performed and samples were collected.
- The client's skin integrity was maintained without skin shear or tearing.
- The client was provided with as much privacy and comfort as possible.

▶ DOCUMENTATION

Nurses' Notes

- Document elimination and voiding. Include color, odor, consistency, and any unusual findings such as blood or mucus.

- Note any client complaints such as constipation or burning with urination.
- Document the condition of the client's skin.

Document on appropriate flow sheet or electronic medical record (EMR).

Intake and Output Record

- Record the time the client voided and the amount of urine voided.

▶ CRITICAL THINKING SKILL

Introduction

Toileting is a very private personal activity that has some unpleasant aspects. Some clients will be acutely embarrassed when they need assistance. The nurse must be as supportive as possible to lessen the discomfort of the client.

Possible Scenario

Mrs. Mun is an orthopedic client, confined to bed. In the evening, she needs to use the bedpan. Her anxiety over hospitalization has increased her peristalsis, causing her to have a very loose, gassy stool. Without thinking, the nurse reacts to removing the bedpan with a grimace and a loud "Phew!!"

Possible Outcome

The client is mortified by the nurse's reaction. Her anxiety over toileting increases, and she avoids further urges to defecate, especially during the evening shift. She experiences distress and discomfort and eventually requires treatment for constipation.

Prevention

The nurse's facial expressions, verbalizations, and actions need to convey support and avoid indications of disgust or displeasure when assisting the client with toileting. Providing privacy, odor-eliminating spray, and talking with the client about embarrassment will help decrease the trauma of using a bedpan.

► VARIATIONS

Geriatric Variations:

- *Geriatric clients often have thin, tender skin. Be careful not to shear or tear the skin when placing or removing the bedpan.*
- *Geriatric clients may have more difficulty with incontinence of urine or stool because of reduced muscle tone.*
- *The use of diuretics may increase the risk of incontinence.*
- *Reduced mobility in an elderly client may both increase the risk of constipation and increase the risk of incontinence because the client may not be able to "make it to the bathroom" in time. Clients may benefit by having a bedpan placed within reach.*

Pediatric Variations:

- *Children may be more comfortable with assistance from a parent.*
- *Adolescents may need extra privacy and control over their toileting time.*

Home Care Variations:

- *In the home care setting, the client does not have a call button. Make sure the client can summon you when needed.*
- *A pillowcase can be used as a bedpan cover in the home setting.*
- *A client who would be able to use a bedside commode in the hospital, but does not have one at home, can use a bedpan while sitting on the edge of the bed or on a bedside chair. Make sure there is adequate support and handholds. Assess for the potential risk of falling.*

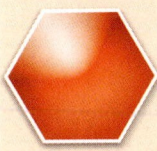

Long-Term Care Variation:

- *If the client is very thin, a folded towel placed on the bedpan to pad the bony sacrum area will increase comfort.*
- *If the bedpan will be used for an extended period of time, take extra care to keep the skin from sticking to the pan, which can increase the risk of pressure sores.*
- *The bedpan can contribute to breakdown over pressure points if the client is left on it too long.*
- *Try to promote independence in toileting when possible. Encourage the client to assist in positioning the pan and with perineal care as much as able.*

▶ COMMON ERRORS

Possible Error:

The nurse does not assist a male client to be as upright as possible to void.

Prevention:

Men usually void standing up. Assist the client into the most normal position possible to ease elimination.

Possible Error:

Not cleaning the bedpan completely.

Prevention:

Rinse the bedpan or urinal well. Be sure the outside is clean also. This eliminates odors and increases client comfort.

▶ NURSING TIPS

- To prevent the bedpan from sticking to the client, apply a small amount of powder to the outer edges of the bedpan.
- Place the towel or bedpan cover next to the side of the bed where you will be removing the pan. You may want to slip it between the mattress and springs so it is close and easy to reach after removing the pan.
- Never place a full bedpan on the bedside or bed table. Place it on a blue pad on a chair or take it away immediately.
- Men voiding large amounts of urine may be more comfortable with a second urinal within reach.
- It may help to remind the client that elimination and defecation are normal parts of everybody's functioning, and that assisting with these tasks does not make you uncomfortable or embarrassed.
- Leave deodorant spray within reach of clients so they can use the spray after defecating to help reduce embarrassment.
- Be aware that clients may have a regular schedule for bowel elimination, such as immediately after a meal or at a certain hour of the day. Note any such pattern and offer the bedpan or urinal at the appropriate times.
- The need to void or defecate can be sudden and intense, and delays in providing a bedpan or urinal may lead to incontinence and client embarrassment. Plan to offer privacy and the bedpan or urinal when the client requests it, and be responsive to urgent requests.

▶ SPECIAL CONSIDERATIONS

- *Clients are often required to share a room with a stranger. This further inhibits elimination because it is socially uncomfortable for many to void or move their bowels in such close proximity to another. If possible, ambulate one client while the other client is using the bedpan. This may provide the privacy that the client needs to complete the normal elimination pattern.*
- *The client with a urinary catheter in place may need the bedpan for a bowel movement. The catheter should be placed toward the front opening of the bedpan. Care should be taken to prevent pulling on the catheter. It is also important to cleanse the perineal area thoroughly from front to back when the bedpan is removed.*
- *Clients may find the use of urinals uncomfortable and drink less to reduce output. Monitor intake and output (I&Os) to encourage appropriate intake.*
- *Monitor color and odor of urine before discarding. Measure as appropriate.*
- *If clients have a hard stool, ascertain fluid intake and bowel program protocol. If the client has diarrhea, assess possible causes, such as diet and medications (especially certain antibiotics). Be aware of loss of electrolytes and the need to monitor for signs and symptoms of electrolyte imbalance. Seek to find the cause of diarrhea and treat with antidiarrheal medications as ordered. Clients may need skin protection to prevent excoriation of the perineal area.*
- *Use disposable bedpans in acute care facilities to avoid need for sterilizing equipment.*

Assisting with Feeding

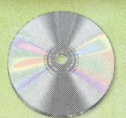

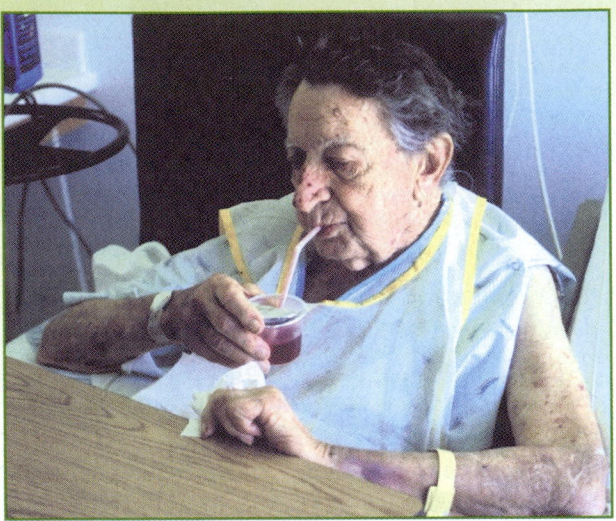

▶ OVERVIEW OF THE SKILL

Many clients, because of illness, weakness, paralysis, shortness of breath, or disorientation, are unable to take in the amount of nutrition required to sustain their bodies. If the client is able to swallow, oral feeding is preferred over tube feedings. Being fed involves complex cultural and esteem issues for clients and their family and patience in taking time to feed. Food preferences are often very specific and highly personal. As much as possible, a client's food preferences should be respected to promote increased nutritional intake.

▶ ASSESSMENT

1. Assess the appropriateness of the ordered diet for the client's needs. **The diet should take food preferences into consideration as well as abilities to swallow, chew, and digest foods.**
2. Assess the client's needs for specialized utensils, a specialized feeding area, or even a certain layout of food on the tray. **Mealtime should be as pleasant as possible, and the client should be provided with as many opportunities as possible to successfully enjoy the meal.**
3. Assess the client's immediate nutritional needs. If clients are diabetic, their nutritional needs may vary from day to day and meal to meal. **If clients are scheduled for lab tests or procedures, they**

may be NPO (nothing by mouth) until after the tests have been performed.
4. Assess the client's ability to chew and swallow. **The food should be served in a manner that is appropriate to the client's ability to chew and swallow while still being as palatable in taste and appearance as possible. Be aware of the possible need for thick liquids or foods with special textures.**
5. Assess the client's level of understanding. **Clients' level of understanding influences their ability to participate in eating the meal.**

▶ DIAGNOSIS

Imbalanced Nutrition: More Than Body Requirements

Imbalanced Nutrition: Less Than Body Requirements

Feeding Self-Care Deficit

Impaired Swallowing

Risk for Aspiration

Impaired Dentition

Nutrition: Readiness for Enhanced

▶ PLANNING

Expected Outcomes:

1. Clients will ingest calories adequate for their body requirements.

2. Clients will report their appetite being satiated and that they are comfortable.

Equipment Needed:

- Food appropriate to the client's condition
- Any specialized utensils the client may require
- Protective covering for the client's gown or bed linen

▶ CLIENT EDUCATION NEEDED:

1. If clients have trouble swallowing, encourage them not to talk while eating. Talking and eating at the same time may encourage choking.
2. Encourage clients to take small bites of food. This will make swallowing easier.
3. Educate the client or caregiver regarding the best foods for the client's needs. Thick food and thick fluids are easier to swallow than thin food and thin fluids. The client may need pureed food rather than food that is cut up into small pieces.
4. Teach the client to swallow twice after each bite. This promotes all the food being swallowed and decreases the chance of choking or aspiration.
5. Teach the client to sit up for at least 15 minutes after eating to encourage digestion and help prevent reflux.

Estimated time to complete the skill: **20–30 minutes**

▶ DELEGATION TIPS

This skill is routinely delegated to ancillary personnel who are properly trained in the use of Standard Precautions, proper positioning of the client, and reporting the amount of intake to the nurse.

IMPLEMENTATION—Action/Rationale

Action	Rationale
1. Wash hands.	1. Reduces the transmission of microorganisms.
2. Help the client wash hands and face in preparation for eating. Clean the client's dentures if needed and give the client his or her glasses, if appropriate.	2. This promotes client comfort and helps clients prepare mentally for a pleasant experience.
3. Remove or move any unpleasant visual stimuli such as commodes, bedpans, and urinals. Be sure there are no unpleasant smells noticeable.	3. Unpleasant sights and smells can decrease a client's appetite.
4. If possible, raise the head of the client's bed or have the client sit on the side of the bed or in a chair.	4. The upright position reduces the risk of aspiration and reflux.
5. Check to be sure that the food presented is in fact this client's food and corresponds to what the client ordered. Be sure the food is in a form the client can eat. Check for the presence of any specialized utensils the client may require. Check for tubes, braces, or dressings that may make eating more difficult.	5. The correct diet and the correct utensils promote increased intake.
6. Place a napkin or protective cover over the client, if needed.	6. Promotes cleanliness and improves client esteem.

continues

Action	Rationale

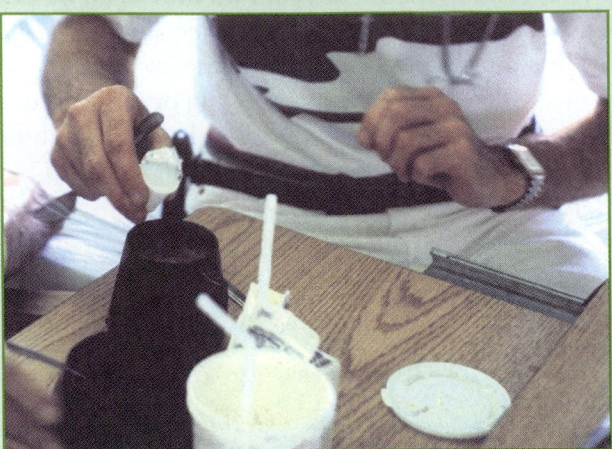

Figure 4-6-1   Prepare the food. Open cartons and cut up food, if needed.

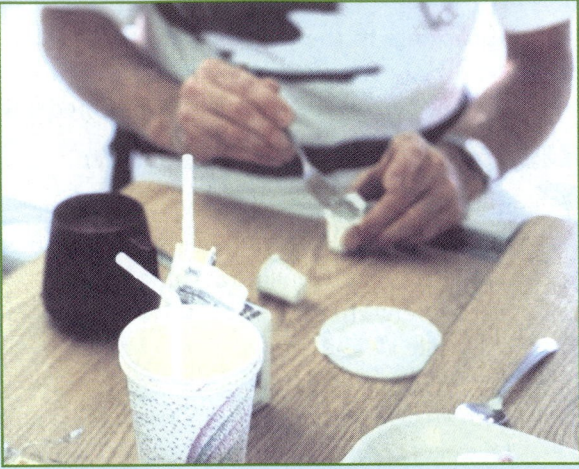

Figure 4-6-2   Place straws in cups and glasses to help the client drink.

7. Prepare the food on the tray in a manner that will help the client eat it. Cut up large pieces of food, open cartons and pour fluids (see Figure 4-6-1), open straws and place them in glasses (see Figure 4-6-2).

7. Doing some of the steps for the client encourages increased independence in the rest of the meal.

8. If you will be feeding the client, try to sit at the client's eye level. Try to sit on the client's unaffected side if the client has one-sided weakness.

8. This promotes a feeling of well-being and connection to the caregiver.

9. Allow the client to do as much as possible for him- or herself during the meal (see Figures 4-6-3 and 4-6-4). Allow client to make choices regarding the order food is eaten, the speed at which client eats, and the amount client will eat. Do not hurry the client through the meal.

9. This promotes client independence and self-esteem. If hurried, a client may aspirate in the rush to finish the meal.

10. Use this time as an opportunity to connect with the client. Discuss everyday subjects with the client, attempting to orient client, if needed. Do not discuss stressful events with the client.

10. Clients often view mealtime as a conversational time; feeling as though someone cares about them can help promote good nutrition via increased intake. Stressful topics at mealtime can delay digestion and decrease appetite, however.

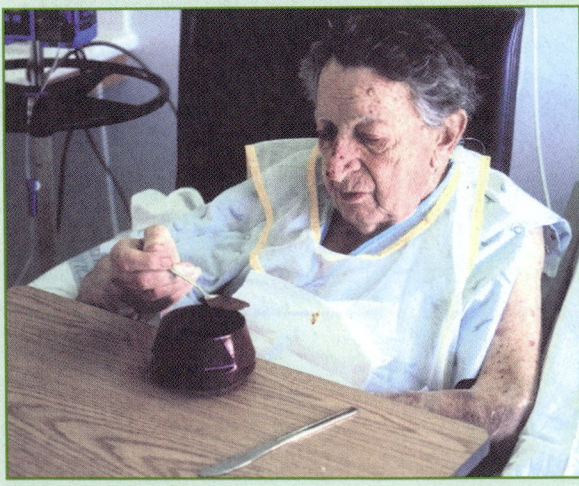

Figure 4-6-3   Promote client independence during the meal as much as possible.

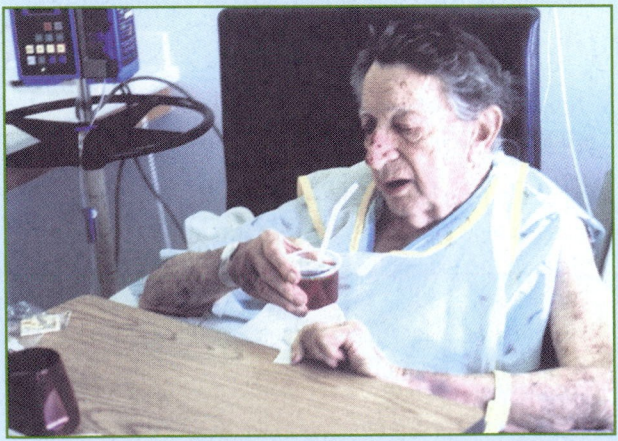

Figure 4-6-4   Encourage the client to feed him- or herself as much as possible, and do not hurry the client through the meal.

continues

Action	Rationale
11. When the client decides she or he is finished with the meal, remove the tray. Encourage the client to keep the head up or to continue to sit up for at least 15 minutes after the meal. Make sure the client is positioned properly and the call light is within reach (see Figure 4-6-5).	**11.** This decreases the risk of reflux and aspiration.
12. Help the client to clean up after the meal. Allow client to wash hands and face and clean dentures, if needed.	**12.** Helps promote client comfort.
13. Wash hands.	**13.** Reduces the transmission of microorganisms.

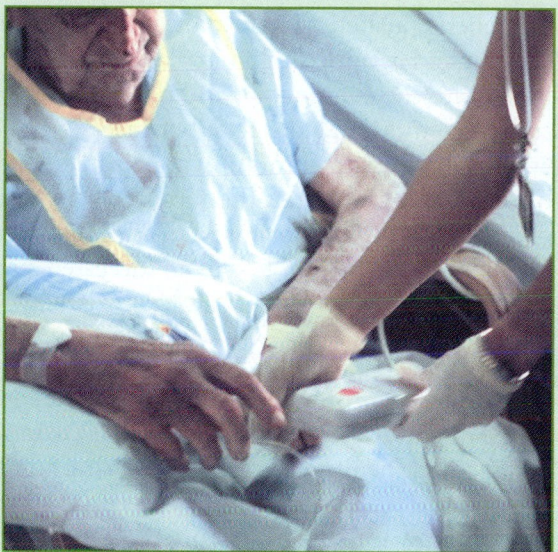

Figure 4-6-5   Place the call light within the client's reach.

▶ REAL WORLD ANECDOTES

Scenario 1

Penny was a client with advanced Huntington's disease. She had dementia and exaggerated choreiform movements, including thrashing and jerking, especially of her upper extremities. Penny was expending large amounts of energy and was often ravenously hungry but could not take in enough nutrition because of the high risk of aspiration. One day Penny was so hungry, she was gulping her food and choked. There was no portable suction available on the floor at the time. By the time a suction machine was brought to the bedside and her breathing was restored, she had suffered brain damage. Nurses and nursing assistants caring for Penny needed to make sure suction was available and ready for immediate use when feeding her. Her risk of aspiration during feeding should have been noted in the chart and at the bedside.

Scenario 2

Mrs. Scotts was an 87-year-old home care client. Once vibrant and active in community and charity events, she had experienced several strokes in the past year, which had left her almost completely disabled and very depressed. She slept most of the day and rarely spoke to friends or family. Mealtimes were often a dance of struggle and refusal. One day, her 93-year-old husband woke up early to make her a "special" breakfast—scrambled eggs, extra runny on toast, with a little nest of grape jelly buried inside the middle. That recipe was a secret they shared from many years ago, when they were newlyweds. The meal brought back vivid memories. They sat at her bedside, he fed her very slowly, and he talked to her about their lifetime and reminiscences together. She was more alert than she had been in weeks and was listening closely as she ate every bite. Later that day, she wanted to get up and go outside in her wheelchair for the first time in several months.

► EVALUATION

- Evaluate whether the client had an appetite for the meal.
- Evaluate whether there were certain foods that the client enjoyed more or less than others.
- Document any foods the client had trouble chewing or swallowing.
- Determine whether the meal was as relaxed and enjoyable as possible, given the limitations of the setting.
- Evaluate whether the client consumed adequate liquids with the meal.
- Evaluate whether the client's independence, intake, or enjoyment of the meal could be improved with alterations in the setting, time, or type of foods brought to the client.

► DOCUMENTATION

Nurses' Notes

- Document how much the client ate and how well the client tolerated the meal.
- Note any eating difficulties or food preferences the client exhibited.

Document on appropriate flow sheet or electronic medical record (EMR).

Intake and Output Record

- Record the time and amount of fluid intake.

► CRITICAL THINKING SKILL

Introduction

A nurse was feeding an elderly man of the Jewish orthodox faith who could not assist himself. As she carried the meal to the bedside, she noted that the meal slip indicated that the tray contained a kosher meal. She began to feed the client. After a few bites, she noticed there was no beverage on the tray, and the soup was clam chowder. She went to the floor refrigerator and obtained a carton of 2% milk.

Possible Scenario

The client resisted any attempts to be fed the meal. Impatient, the nurse tried to force the liquids—the chowder and the milk—on the client, who became increasingly agitated.

Possible Outcome

The client pushed the tray onto the floor and onto the nurse. He appeared angry and upset for several hours into the evening. He did not get his dinner and suffered emotional distress because of the mix-up and his inability to communicate his needs or control his environment. Later, the family paid a visit to the charge nurse and the hospital administrator, complaining that the client had been force-fed a meal that contained foods forbidden under Jewish law.

Prevention

As a nursing professional, this nurse needed to be aware of cultural, ethnic, and religious variations that might affect health care delivery. Orthodox Jews are not allowed to eat shellfish, and there are strict guidelines on how milk and meat are to be consumed. The nurse needed to check the chart for any cultural or religious food guidelines and to seek assistance if further clarification was needed. When this previously cooperative client became agitated, the nurse needed to stop and assess the situation and remember the special dietary needs of this client.

► VARIATIONS

Geriatric Variation:

- *Elderly clients may have teeth in poor condition or dentures. Check to make sure dentures are in place before feeding. Pay attention to complaints of inability to chew, or dental pain.*
- *The elderly client may have a less responsive thirst mechanism. Pay special attention to fluid intake.*

Pediatric Variation:

- *Adolescents are influenced by peer groups and peer pressure regarding what, where, and when to eat. Provide choice and independence where possible, and encourage the adolescent to participate in dietary choices.*

continues

▶ VARIATIONS *(continued)*

- Adolescents may be sensitive to needing assistance eating in front of others. Plan with the adolescent to set mealtimes and companionship.
- Children may do better if a parent helps them to eat.

Home Care Variations:

- Educate the primary caregiver who will be feeding the client. Educational needs include how to respond to choking, how to assist clients to eat while supporting their independence, and shopping for foods for clients on special diets. Monitor intake and output, and watch for signs of malnutrition.
- Allow the client to assist in food preparation when possible. Remember, the home setting is where the individual is generally used to being more independent. Placing a spoonful of jam on toast, or other simple tasks, helps reduce the feeling of dependence on a caregiver and may help lessen feelings of helplessness or depression that arise from losing independence over basic care.

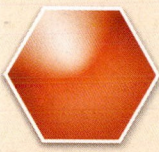

Long-Term Care Variations:

- For a client who has had a stroke, direct the food toward the unaffected side of the mouth.
- Long-term inactivity will decrease kilocaloric requirements because the individual is expending less energy in daily activities.
- Encouraging the intake of high-fiber foods and plenty of liquids will help the inactive client avoid constipation.
- Work with caregivers, friends, and family to have a familiar friend present at mealtimes to assist with meals when possible. Family and friends can create a more relaxed atmosphere and can make mealtime a social time as well.

▶ COMMON ERRORS

Possible Error:

Something on the bedside table along with the meal tray is mistaken for food and consumed by the client.

Prevention:

Assess with a critical eye. Remove any items that might be accidentally ingested. If a poisonous substance is ingested, review the emergency policy manual for accidental poisonings. Determine what was ingested, contact the physician, and follow the procedure manual for contacting the Poison Control Center and initiating poisoning responses.

Possible Error:

The client receives the wrong tray or the wrong diet.

Prevention:

Check the client's identification band. Check the chart to make sure the client's diet orders have not changed in the past several hours. Even if this is the right tray, check that it is the right meal.

Possible Error:

The meal is delayed and has become unappetizing.

Prevention:

Make every effort to schedule procedures so they do not overlap with mealtimes. If the meal is delayed, check that foods are hot enough and/or cold enough to still be enjoyable.

▶ **NURSING TIPS**

- Carry extra straws and prewrapped forks and spoons during mealtimes to save steps if items are dropped or missing from the trays.
- Test hot foods by placing a small portion on the inside of your wrist before feeding.
- If it is hard to get clients to open their mouth or accept the food, try using an extra-small spoon to begin. Then move to a regular spoon as the client becomes more comfortable.
- Start the meal with extra-small bites until the client gets used to food in the mouth, and starts to taste the food.
- Start the meal with a sip of cool beverage to lubricate the inside of the mouth.

- Many clients are used to water with their meals. Water is usually not delivered on the food tray. Placing a cold glass of water on the tray will encourage oral intake of fluids and may improve clients' enjoyment of the meal.
- Allow the client to pick what foods to eat in what order and to pick unusual combinations of foods. Some clients will eat dessert first and should have that freedom of choice, even when being fed.
- Although the client may appear to be chewing, check the oral cavity to make sure food is not being pocketed between the teeth and cheek.

▶ **SPECIAL CONSIDERATIONS**

- *Mealtime can provide a forum for social interaction. Eating a meal with others may improve the client's appetite.*
- *Carefully monitor clients with eating disorders during and just after meals. Observe the amount of food eaten at the meal and watch for signs of self-induced vomiting. Documentation should note any incidents.*
- *Using drinking straws increases the consumption of air into gastric pathway, causing stomach distension. Assist the client if necessary with drinking from a cup rather than using a straw.*
- *Feeding clients may take an extended period of time and present staffing problems. As it is important that clients receive adequate nutrition and not be rushed, plan time accordingly or seek volunteers or family assistance. Be sure to include adequate fluid with meals.*
- *Clients with dysphagia, or difficulty in swallowing, may tend to have food remain in the oral cavity. Assess that client is swallowing.*
- *Aspiration can occur during eating. Always have client sitting or in a high Fowler's position to prevent aspiration. Be aware if client is at risk for aspiration and take appropriate action. Report aspiration as this can lead to pneumonia. Monitor temperature.*

Bathing a Client in Bed

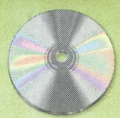

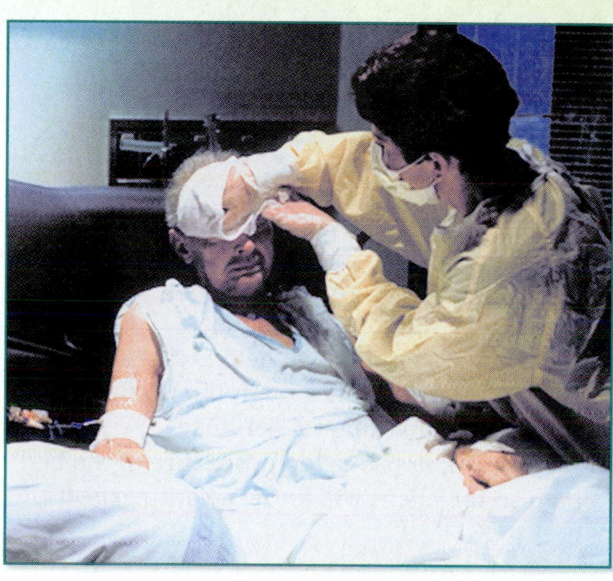

► OVERVIEW OF THE SKILL

Bathing clients is an essential component of nursing care and a critical time to assess the client. Whether the nurse performs the bath or delegates the activity to another health care provider, the nurse retains the responsibility for ensuring that the hygienic needs of the client are met. The type of bath provided will depend on the purpose of the bath and the client's self-care ability. The two categories of baths are cleaning and therapeutic. Cleaning baths are provided as routine client care. The purpose of a cleaning bath is personal hygiene. Following are the five types of cleaning baths:

• Shower
• Tub
• Self-help, or assisted bed bath
• Complete bed bath
• Partial bath

For clients who are confined to bed, the bed bath is used to provide hygienic care. There are several variations of bed bath depending on the client's ability to assist with care. The complete bed bath is provided to dependent clients confined to bed. The nurse washes the client's entire body during a complete bed bath. A partial bed bath and a self-help bed bath are variations of the complete bed bath.

► ASSESSMENT

1. Assess the client's level of ability to assist with the bath. **Determine whether the client is able to follow directions. Check the client's ability to assist with cleaning any portion of the body.**
2. Assess the client's level of comfort with the procedure. Check into potential cultural, sexual, or generational issues. **Determine whether the client is uncomfortable, tense, or nervous about being bathed by someone else.**
3. Assess the environment. Verify that the equipment needed is available. Assess if the client has skin intact or dressings, IV lines, or drainage tubes in place. Check whether clean, warm water is available. **Determine whether the need for modesty and privacy can be met. The environment should be conducive to a clean, safe, and comfortable procedure.**

► DIAGNOSIS

Risk for Compromised Human Dignity

Risk for Impaired Skin Integrity

Bathing/Hygiene Self-Care Deficit

► **PLANNING**

Expected Outcomes:

1. Clients will be cleaned without damage to their skin.
2. Clients' privacy will be maintained throughout the procedure.
3. Clients will participate in their own hygiene as much as possible.
4. Clients will not become overly tired or experience increased pain, cold, or discomfort as a result of the bath.

Equipment Needed (see Figures 4-7-1):

- Bath towels
- Washcloths
- Bath blanket
- Washbasin
- Soap
- Soap dish
- Lotion
- Deodorant
- Clean gown
- Clean linen
- Disposable, latex-free gloves

► **CLIENT EDUCATION NEEDED:**

1. Explain to the client the need for routine cleanliness, especially if you note that the

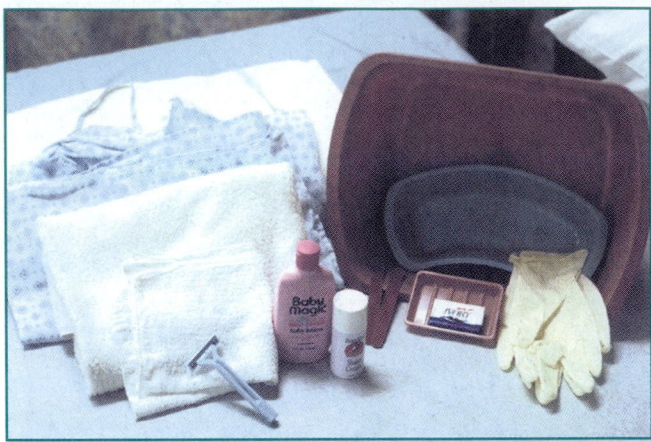

Figure 4-7-1 Emesis and bath basins, soap, towels, and lotion are used to bathe the client. A razor and shaving cream are used to groom the male client.

client does not seem to maintain a regular bathing routine.
2. Explain that bathing will help increase the client's comfort even though the client has not been doing anything to "get dirty."
3. Explain the step-by-step procedure of the bed bath so the client will know what to expect.

Estimated time to complete the skill:
30 minutes

► **DELEGATION TIPS**

This skill is routinely delegated to ancillary personnel who should allow the client to perform as much of the bath as possible or permitted. The caregiver employs Standard Precautions, properly positions the client, and observes and reports the client's skin condition and color to the nurse. The nurse retains the responsibility to assess the client.

IMPLEMENTATION—Action/Rationale

Action	Rationale
1. Assess the client's preferences about bathing.	1. Provides client opportunity to participate in care.
2. Explain procedure to client.	2. Enhances cooperation.
3. Prepare environment. Close doors and windows, adjust temperature, provide time for elimination needs, and provide privacy (see Figure 4-7-2).	3. Protects from chills during bath and increases sense of privacy.
4. Wash hands. Apply gloves. Gloves should be changed when emptying water basin.	4. Reduces the transmission of microorganisms.

continues

Action	Rationale

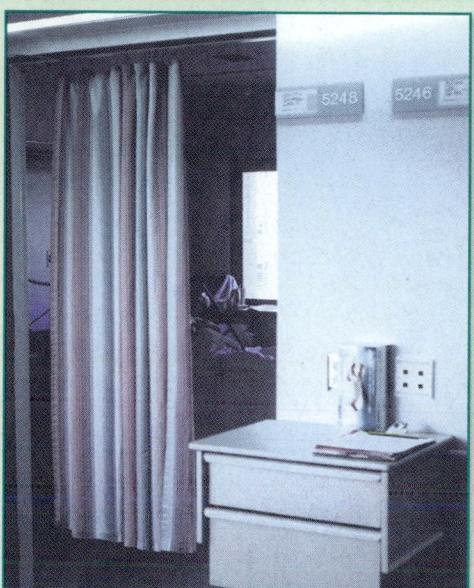

Figure 4-7-2   Close doors and/or curtains and provide privacy before beginning the bath.

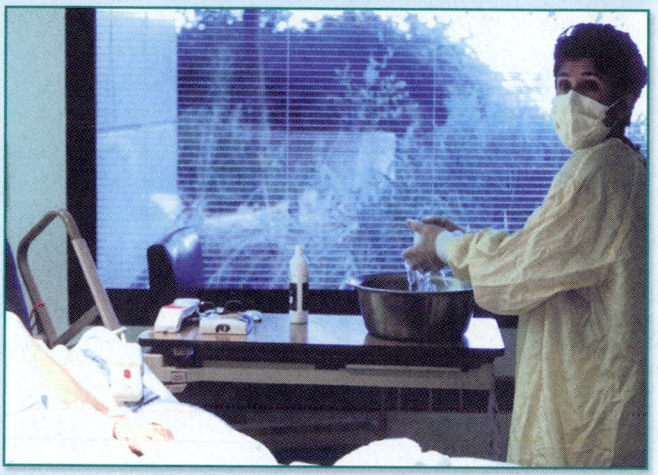

Figure 4-7-3   Wet the washcloth and wring out the excess water. The nurse is wearing a mask and gown because the client is in isolation.

5. Lower side rail on the side close to you. Position client in a comfortable position close to the side near you.

5. Prevents unnecessary reaching. Facilitates use of good body mechanics.

6. If bath blankets are available, place bath blanket over top sheet. Remove top sheet from under bath blanket. Remove client's gown. Bath blanket should be folded to expose only the area being cleaned at that time. (Top sheets or towels may also be used for bath blankets.)

6. Prevents exposure of client. Promotes privacy. Protects from chills.

7. Fill washbasin two-thirds of the way full. Permit client to test temperature of water with hand. Water should be changed when a soap film develops or water becomes soiled.

7. Prevents accidental burns or chills.

8. Wet the washcloth and wring it out (see Figure 4-7-3).

8. Prevents unnecessarily wetting of client.

9. Make a bath mitten with the washcloth. To make a mitten, grasp the edge of the washcloth with the thumb; fold a third over the palm of the hand; wrap remainder of cloth around hand and across palm, and grasp the second edge under the thumb; fold the extended end of the washcloth onto the palm and tuck under the palmar surface of the cloth.

9. Prevents ends of washcloth from dragging across skin. Promotes friction during bath.

10. Wash the face (see Figure 4-7-4). Ask the client about preference for using soap on the face. Use a separate corner of the washcloth for each eye, wiping from inner to outer canthus. Wash neck and ears. Rinse and pat dry. Male clients may want to shave at this time. Provide assistance with shaving as needed.

10. Some clients may not use soap on the face. Using separate corners of washcloth reduces risk of transmitting microorganisms. Patting dry reduces skin irritation and drying.

continues

Action	Rationale

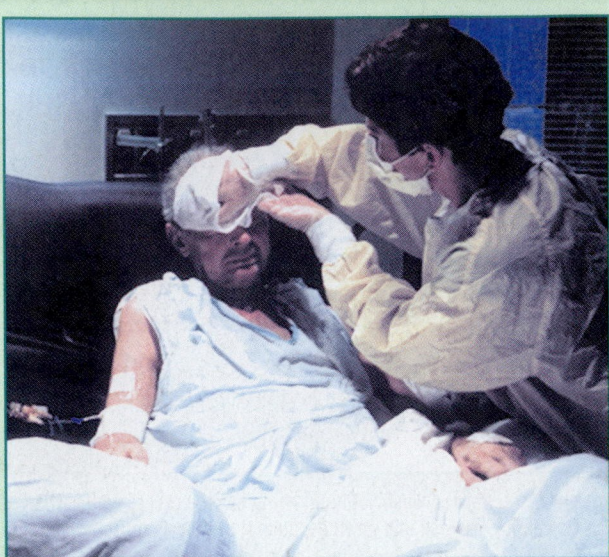

Figure 4-7-4   Wash the client's face first.

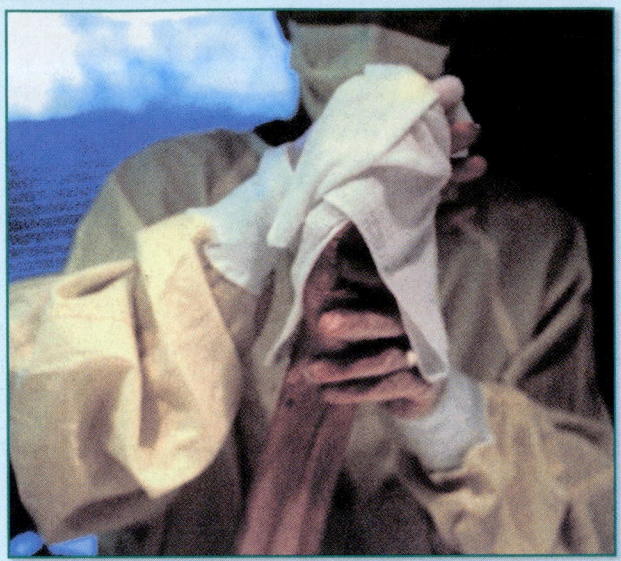

Figure 4-7-5   Wash the hands and arms next.

11. Wash arms, forearms, and hands (see Figure 4-7-5). Wash forearms and arms using long, firm strokes in the direction of distal to proximal (see Figure 4-7-6). Arm may need to be supported while being washed. Wash axilla. Rinse and pat dry. Apply deodorant or powder if desired. Immerse client's hand into basin of water. Allow hand to soak about 3 to 5 minutes. Wash hands, interdigit area, fingers, and fingernails. Rinse and pat dry.

12. Wash chest and abdomen. Fold bath blanket down to umbilicus. Wash chest using long, firm strokes. Wash skin fold under the female client's breast by lifting each breast. Rinse and pat dry. Fold bath blanket down to suprapubic area. Use another towel to cover chest area. Wash abdomen using long, firm strokes. Rinse and pat dry. Replace bath blanket over chest and abdomen. Cover chest or abdomen area in between washing, rinsing, and drying to prevent chilling.

13. Wash legs and feet. Expose leg farthest from you by folding bath blanket to midline. Bend the leg at the knee. Grasp the heel, elevate the leg from the bed, and cover bed with bath towel. Place washbasin on towel. Place client's foot into washbasin (see Figure 4-7-7). Allow foot to soak while washing the leg with long, firm strokes in the direction of distal to proximal. Rinse and pat dry. Clean soles, interdigits, and toes. Rinse and pat dry. Perform same procedure with the other leg and foot.

14. Wash back. Assist client into prone or side-lying position facing away from you. Wash the back and buttocks using long, firm strokes. Rinse and pat dry. Give back rub and apply lotion.

11. Long strokes promote circulation. Soaking hands softens nails and loosens soil from skin and nails. Strokes directed distal to proximal promote venous return.

12. Promotes privacy and prevents chills. Long strokes promote circulation. Perspiration and soil collect within skin folds.

13. Supports joints to prevent strain and fatigue. Soaking foot loosens dirt, softens nails, and promotes comfort.

14. Exposes back and buttocks for washing. Back rub promotes relaxation and circulation.

continues

Action	Rationale

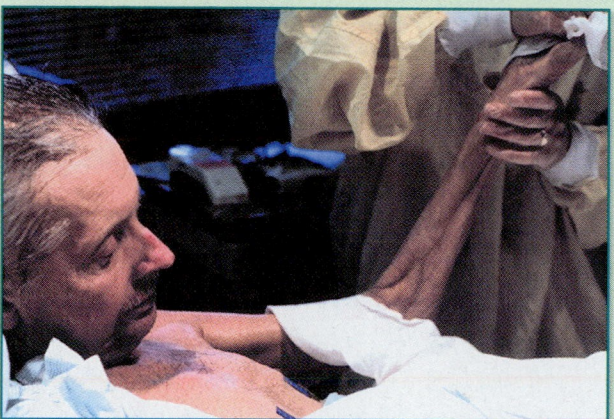

Figure 4-7-6 Wash from distal to proximal—from hands to forearms to upper arms.

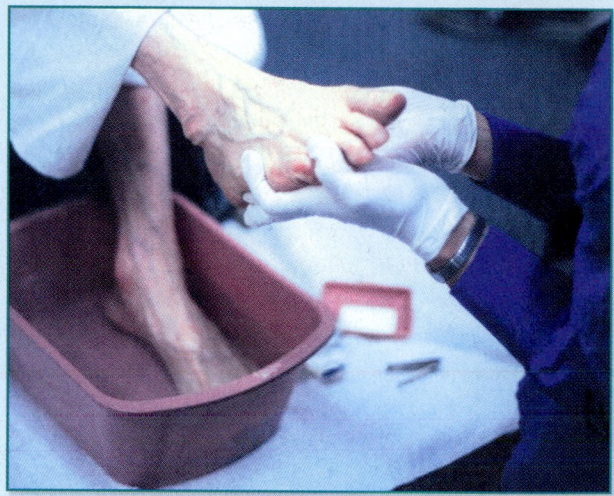

Figure 4-7-7 Place feet in basin. Clean interdigits and soles of feet.

15. Perineal care: Assist client to supine position. Perform perineal care (see Figures 4-7-8 and 4-7-9).

15. Removes genital secretions and soil.

16. Apply lotion as desired or needed. Apply clean gown.

16. Lotion lubricates skin. Powder absorbs excess perspiration.

17. Document skin assessment, type of bath given, and client outcomes and responses.

17. Provides evidence of nursing care.

18. Wash hands.

18. Reduces the transmission of microorganisms.

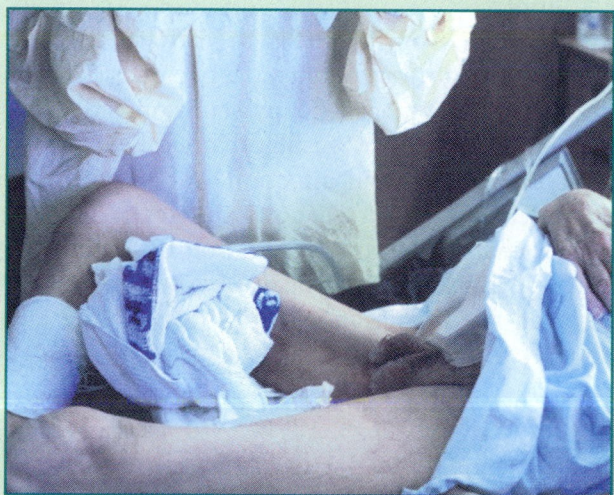

Figure 4-7-8 Wash perineal area.

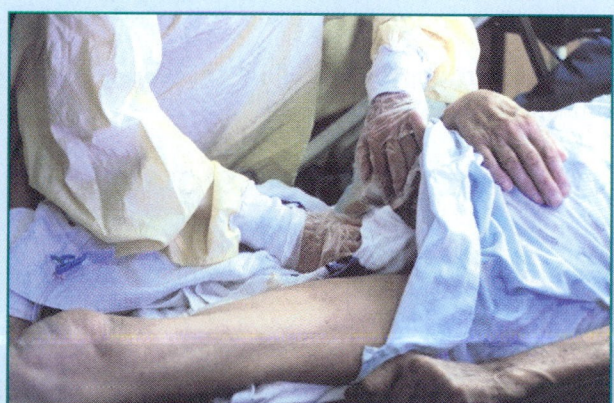

Figure 4-7-9 Dry perineal area carefully to prevent moisture from contributing to skin irritation or skin breakdown.

▶ REAL WORLD ANECDOTES

Nurse Duncan was assigned the newly admitted client from the emergency department, Mrs. White. She was an elderly woman admitted with a diagnosis of malnutrition. While doing the initial admission examination, the nurse noted that Mrs. White's hair was matted and her clothes and skin were quite dirty. After finishing the admission exam, Nurse Duncan set up Mrs. White for a bed bath. Mrs. White was weak and unable to assist much with the bath. During the bed bath, Nurse Duncan noticed small white spots, resembling dandruff, adhering to Mrs. White's pubic hair. Nurse Duncan finished Mrs. White's bath and proceeded to the nurse's station to chart the findings. While seated at the nurse's station, Nurse Duncan mentioned the white spots seen while bathing Mrs. White. The charge nurse asked Nurse Duncan to show her the spots. Upon examination the charge nurse noted that the white spots were, in fact, nits, or the white ovoid eggs deposited by lice. The charge nurse then checked for, and found, pubic lice. Nurse Duncan notified Mrs. White's doctor, who prescribed medicated shampoo for both Mrs. White and Nurse Duncan.

▶ EVALUATION

- The client was cleaned adequately without skin damage.
- The client's modesty was maintained throughout the procedure.
- The client participated in the procedure as much as possible.
- The client remained comfortable during the procedure.

▶ DOCUMENTATION

Nurses' Notes

- Note that the client was bathed. Indicate how much of the bath the client assisted with and how well the client tolerated the activity.
- Note any unusual findings including rashes, open sores, poor turgor, and so on.

Document on appropriate flow sheet or electronic medical record (EMR).

▶ CRITICAL THINKING SKILL

Introduction

Wash from the cleanest area to the dirtiest.

Possible Scenario

You are bathing Mr. Marshall. His biggest complaint at this time is that his wound site is draining and causing itching and discomfort. He is insistent that you wash around his dressing before doing anything else. You wash the skin around his dressing and note that the site is draining and the dressing is wet with drainage. You had already planned to change his dressing after the bath, and this decision is reinforced as you wash the skin around the dressing. Once Mr. Marshall is more comfortable at the dressing site, you rinse the washcloth in the basin and proceed to complete Mr. Marshall's bath.

Possible Outcome

If Mr. Marshall's wound is infected, you are potentially infecting other sites on Mr. Marshall's body while finishing his bath.

Prevention

Always wash from cleanest to dirtiest areas and change the bathwater when it becomes contaminated or soiled or has a soapy scum on the surface. Warm water and a wet washcloth are excellent media for contamination and infection. When performing routine care, ask yourself how you would feel about this procedure. If you would not be comfortable using the same washcloth and bathwater that had just been used to clean wound drainage, the client probably will not like it either.

► VARIATIONS

Geriatric Variations:

- *Elderly clients often have very thin skin. Handle the skin carefully to avoid tearing or shearing the delicate tissue.*
- *The bath is an excellent opportunity to scan the skin for possible skin cancers. Review photos of the basic appearance of skin cancers in a dermatology test or web site so they are recognizable to you.*
- *Make sure to check for hearing aids, and remove them before bathing the client's head and neck area. Water can damage many hearing aids.*
- *Be sure to replace necessary items such as eyeglasses, call light, bedside lighting, and hearing aids after the bath to help the elderly client remain independent.*
- *Note any inappropriate bruising that may be indicative of abuse.*

Pediatric Variations:

- *Children are easily embarrassed about strangers seeing and touching their bodies. Be sure to explain everything you are doing and why. Be sure to preserve the child's modesty as much as possible.*
- *With the heightened awareness regarding inappropriate touching, be aware of how you touch children while caring for them. If possible, have an appropriate family member present when you bathe a child.*
- *Make bath time play therapy if possible. A smaller child may enjoy playing with the slippery soap or hearing a nursery rhyme or song that changes with each part of the bath.*
- *Observe for signs of abuse, such as bruising, burns, or tender areas.*
- *Adolescents may be especially concerned over body image. The focus on the body during the bath draws attention to changes in body image caused by illness or surgery. Be sensitive and practice active listening to help adolescents communicate their concerns.*

Home Care Variations:

- *Take extra care not to spill bathwater or soak the mattress in the home care setting. It may not be protected with a waterproof cover like those in the hospital. Bring along protective linens to protect the bed against accidental spills.*
- *In the more relaxed home care setting, the bath can be a perfect opportunity to do range of motion and gentle stretching exercises.*

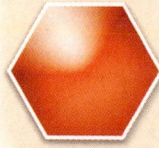

Long-Term Care Variations:

- *Focus on independence and autonomy in the bathing process as much as possible to help clients avoid developing unnecessary dependence on caretakers. A feeling of being overly dependent on others for basic care can lead to lowered self-esteem and possibly depression.*

► COMMON ERRORS

Possible Error:

The nurse does not change the bathwater and washcloth often enough.

Prevention:

Frequently assess the condition of the water, washcloth, and towels you are using. Are they clean and uncontaminated? Are the towels dry enough to dry the client's skin or so wet they are just pushing water around? How soapy is this washcloth? How soapy is the water? Is the soap floating in the water, keeping it from being clear enough to rinse with? When did you change the water last? How would you feel about bathing in the water now in the washbasin? Take the time to change the bathwater frequently and be sure to use enough linen to do the job right.

▶ **NURSING TIPS**

- Be sure to rinse the soap off the client well. Soap can cause drying and chafing.
- Be sure to dry the client well, especially in skin folds and areas that rub together often. Leaving water in these areas can cause cracking and irritation.

- Use this time to assess the client's skin integrity. Do you see any rashes, open areas, or reddened areas?
- Encourage clients to assist in the bath as much as they are able. Self-care of basic needs is a way to maintain a sense of control and self-esteem during illness.

▶ **SPECIAL CONSIDERATIONS**

- *Be aware of cultural variations in that some cultures do not allow the opposite sex to see the client unclothed or touch the client. Invite client's wishes on how he or she would prefer to have a bed bath done. Possibly involve family members if so desired. If family members bathe the client be sure to assess skin response to activity.*
- *A bed bath is a good opportunity to assess a client's skin integrity and peripheral circulation.*
- *Evaluate client's skin integrity for electrolyte imbalance, bruising, or skin breakdown.*

Oral Care

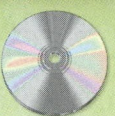

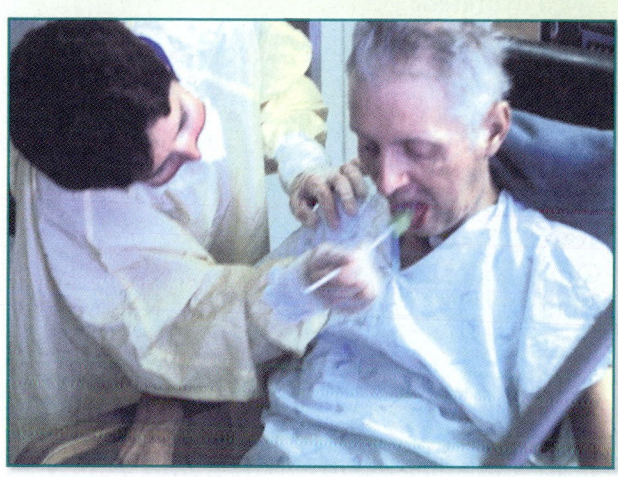

▶ OVERVIEW OF THE SKILL

The oral cavity functions in mastication, secretion of mucus to moisten and lubricate the digestive system, secretion of digestive enzymes, and absorption of essential nutrients. Common problems occurring in the oral cavity include the following:

- Bad breath (halitosis)
- Dental cavities (caries)
- Plaque
- Periodontal disease
- Inflammation of the gums (gingivitis)
- Inflammation of the oral mucosa (stomatitis)

Poor oral hygiene and loss of teeth may affect a client's social interaction and body image as well as nutritional intake. Daily oral care is essential to maintain the integrity of the mucous membranes, teeth, gums, and lips. Through preventive measures, the oral cavity and teeth can be preserved. Preventive oral care consists of fluoride rinsing, flossing, and brushing.

Fluoride

Researchers have determined that fluoride can prevent dental caries. This finding has led to the fluoridation of water supplies in many communities. Fluoride is a common component of many mouthwashes and toothpastes. However, people with excessive dryness or irritated mucous membranes should avoid commercial mouthwashes because of the alcohol content, which causes drying of mucous membranes.

Fluoride supplements are available without a prescription. Infants as young as 2 weeks of age can be given fluoride drops to prevent dental caries. Nurses should educate clients about fluoride being an excellent preventive measure against dental caries. However, excessive fluoride exposure can affect the color of tooth enamel.

Flossing

Flossing should be performed daily in conjunction with the brushing of the teeth. Flossing prevents the formation of plaque, removes plaque from between the teeth, and removes food debris. Dental caries and periodontal disease can be prevented by regular flossing. There are several methods of flossing. The nurse should instruct the client to use the technique that is most comfortable. Some clients find holding the floss difficult. There are many floss holders available to facilitate flossing.

Brushing

Teeth should be brushed after each meal. Brushing should be performed using a dentifrice (toothpaste) that contains fluoride to aid in preventing dental caries. An effective homemade dentifrice is the combination of two parts salt with one part baking soda. Brushing removes plaque and food debris and promotes blood circulation of the gums. Dentures should be brushed using the same brushing motion as that used for brushing teeth.

► ASSESSMENT

1. Assess whether the client is able to assist with oral care and to what extent. **Promotes independence where possible.**
2. Evaluate whether the client has an understanding of proper oral hygiene. **Promotes self-care and teaching.**
3. Check whether the client has dentures. **Determines how oral care will be performed.**
4. Assess the condition of the client's mouth. **Determines how oral care will be performed.**
5. Assess whether inflammation, bleeding, infection, or ulceration is present. **Determines how oral care will be performed. Determines the need for additional assessment and intervention.**
6. Assess what cultural practices must be taken into consideration. **Determines how oral care will be performed.**
7. Assess whether there are any appliances or devices present in the client's mouth such as braces, endotracheal tube, or bridgework. **Determines how oral care will be performed.**
8. Check that the proper equipment is available to perform oral care. **Ensures a smooth procedure.**

► DIAGNOSIS

Risk for Infection

Impaired Dentition

Impaired Oral Mucous Membrane

Bathing/Hygiene Self-Care Deficit

Deficient Knowledge of Oral Hygiene

► PLANNING

Expected Outcomes:

1. Client's mouth, teeth, gums, and lips will be clean and free of food particles.
2. Any inflammation, bleeding, infection, or ulceration present will be noted and treated.
3. The oral mucosa will be clean, intact, and well hydrated.

Equipment Needed (see Figure 4-8-1):
Brushing and Flossing

- Toothbrush
- Toothpaste with fluoride
- Emesis basin
- Towel
- Cup of water
- Nonsterile gloves
- Dental floss
- Mirror
- Lip moisturizer

Denture Care (see Figures 4-8-2 and 4-8-3)

- Denture brush
- Denture cleaner
- Emesis basin
- Towel
- Cup of water
- Nonsterile gloves
- Tissue
- Denture cup

Special Care Items for Clients with Impaired Physical Mobility or Who Are Unconscious (Comatose)

- Soft toothbrush or toothette
- Tongue blade

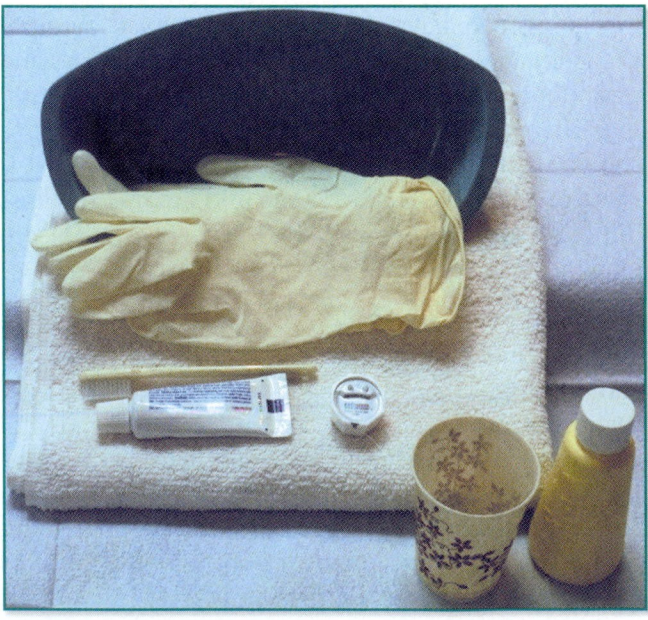

Figure 4-8-1 Toothbrush, dental floss, mouthwash, and emesis basin are still used in providing oral care.

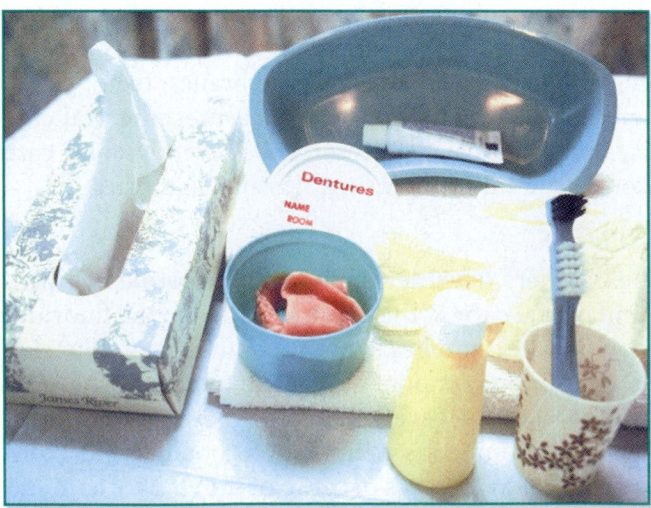

Figure 4-8-2 Denture brush and denture cup are added to oral care equipment when the client has full or partial dentures.

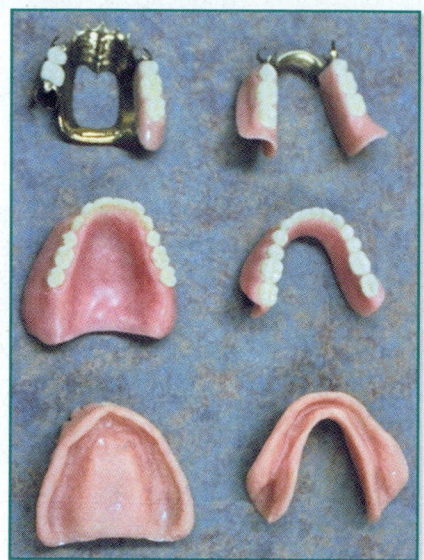

Figure 4-8-3   Dentures may include full upper or lower plates, or partial plates.

- 3 × 3 gauze sponges
- Cotton-tip applicators

- Prescribed solution
- Plastic Asepto syringe
- Suction machine and catheter

▶ CLIENT EDUCATION NEEDED:

1. Teach the client the importance of daily oral care, including flossing, fluoride, and brushing.
2. Instruct the client regarding brushing all surfaces of the teeth.
3. Instruct the client regarding the importance of flossing between all teeth.
4. Infants may benefit from fluoride drops as a supplement. Educate the child's family regarding the benefits of fluoride, even for very young children.

Estimated time to complete the skill: **20 minutes**

▶ DELEGATION TIPS

Oral care is routinely delegated to ancillary personnel who should allow the client to perform as much of the oral care as possible or permitted. The caregiver should be trained to employ Standard Precautions, to properly position the client, and to observe and report the client's mucous membrane condition and color to the nurse.

IMPLEMENTATION—Action/Rationale

Action	Rationale
Self-Care Client: Flossing and Brushing	
1. Assemble articles for flossing and brushing.	1. Promotes efficiency.
2. Provide privacy.	2. Relaxes the client.
3. Place client in a high Fowler's position (see Figure 4-8-4).	3. Decreases risk of aspiration.
4. Wash hands and apply gloves.	4. Reduces the transmission of microorganisms.
5. Arrange articles within client's reach.	5. Facilitates self-care.
6. Assist client with flossing and brushing as necessary. Position mirror, emesis basin, water with straw near the client, and a towel across the chest (see Figure 4-8-5).	6. Flossing and brushing decrease microorganism growth in the mouth. Use of a mirror permits cleaning back and sides of teeth.

continues

Action	Rationale

Self-Care Client: Flossing and Brushing
continued

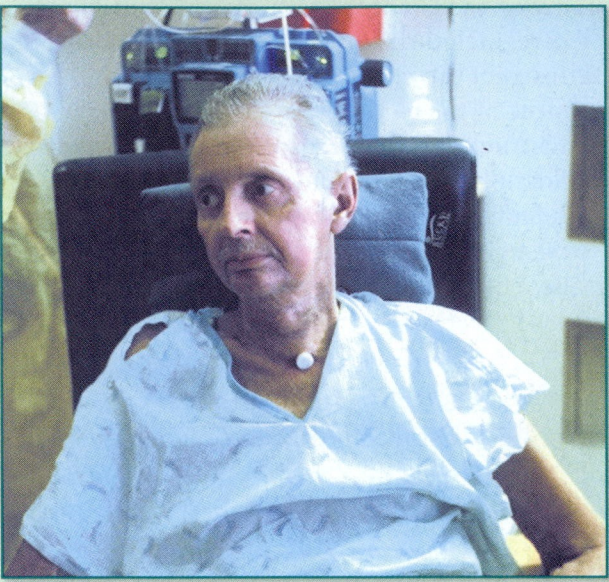

Figure 4-8-4 Place client in sitting position in a chair or in bed, if possible.

7. Assist client with rinsing mouth.

8. Reposition client, raise side rails, and place call button within reach.

9. Rinse, dry, and return articles to proper place.

10. Remove gloves, wash hands, and document care.

Self-Care Client: Denture Care

11. Assemble articles for denture cleaning.

12. Provide privacy.

13. Assist client to a high Fowler's position.

14. Wash hands and apply gloves.

15. Assist client with denture removal:
    a. Top denture:
       • With tissue, grasp the denture with thumb and forefinger and pull downward.
       • Place in denture cup.
    b. Bottom denture:
       • Place thumbs on the gums and release the denture. Grasp denture with thumb and forefinger and pull upward.
       • Place in denture cup.

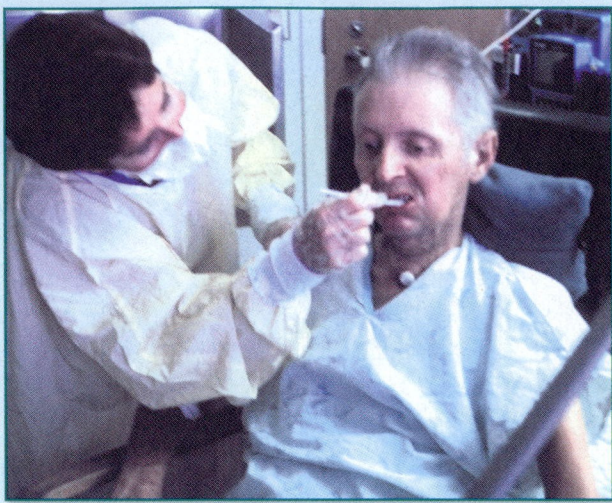

Figure 4-8-5 Promote independence, but assist with flossing or brushing as necessary.

7. Removes toothpaste and oral secretions.

8. Promotes comfort, safety, and communication.

9. Promotes a clean environment.

10. Reduces the transmission of microorganisms and documents nursing care.

11. Promotes efficiency.

12. Relaxes the client.

13. Facilitates removal of dentures.

14. Reduces the transmission of microorganisms and exposure to body fluids.

15. Breaks seal created with dentures without causing pressure and injury to oral membranes. Prevents breaking of dentures.

continues

Action	Rationale
16. Apply toothpaste to brush, and brush dentures either with cool water in the emesis basin or under running water in the sink. Pad sink with towel to protect dentures in case they are dropped.	16. Facilitates removal of microorganisms.
17. Rinse thoroughly.	17. Removes toothpaste.
18. Assist client with rinsing mouth and replacing dentures.	18. Freshens mouth and facilitates intake of solid food.
19. Reposition client, with side rails up and call button within reach.	19. Promotes comfort, safety, and communication.
20. Rinse, dry, and return articles to proper place.	20. Maintains a clean environment.
21. Remove gloves, wash hands, and document care.	21. Reduces the transmission of microorganisms and documents nursing care.
Full-Care Client: Brushing and Flossing	
22. Assemble articles for flossing and brushing.	22. Promotes efficiency.
23. Provide privacy.	23. Relaxes client.
24. Wash hands and apply gloves.	24. Reduces the transmission of microorganisms and exposure to body fluids.
25. Position client as condition allows: high Fowler's; semi-Fowler's; or lateral position, head turned toward side (see Figure 4-8-6).	25. Decreases risk of aspiration.
26. Place towel across client's chest or under face and mouth if head is turned to one side.	26. Catches secretions.
27. Moisten toothbrush or toothette, apply small amount of toothpaste, and brush teeth and gums.	27. Moistens mouth and facilitates plaque removal.
28. Grasp the dental floss in both hands or use a floss holder and floss between all teeth; hold floss against tooth while moving floss up and down sides of teeth.	28. Removes plaque and prevents gum disease.
29. Assist the client in rinsing mouth.	29. Removes toothpaste and oral secretions.
30. Reapply toothpaste and brush the teeth and gums using friction in a vertical or circular motion. On inner and outer surfaces of teeth, hold brush at 45-degree angle against teeth and brush from sulcus to crowns of teeth. On biting surfaces, move brush back and forth in short strokes. All surfaces of teeth should be brushed from every angle.	30. Permits cleaning of back and sides of teeth and decreases microorganism growth in mouth.
31. Assist the client in rinsing and drying mouth (see Figure 4-8-7).	31. Removes toothpaste and oral secretions.
32. Apply lip moisturizer, if appropriate.	32. Maintains skin integrity of lips.

continues

Action	Rationale

Full-Care Client: Brushing and Flossing *continued*

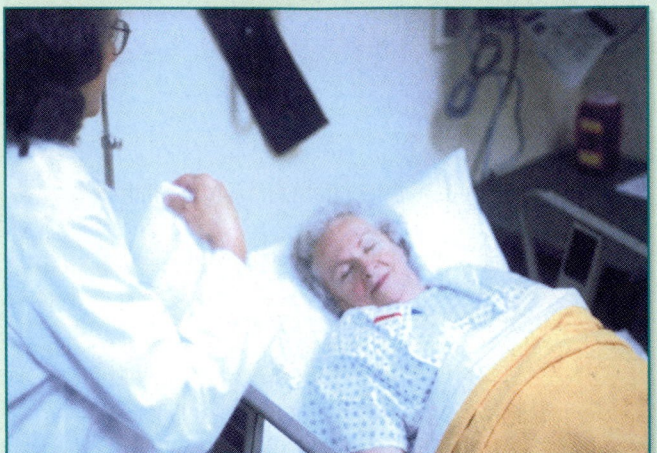

Figure 4-8-6   If client is unable to sit up, turn head to the side.

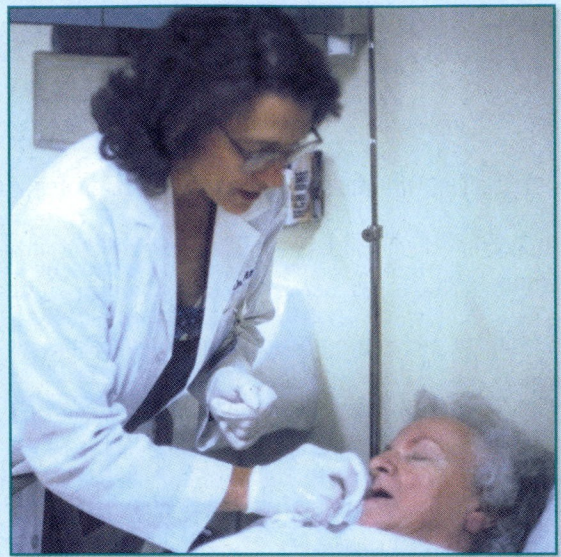

Figure 4-8-7   After completing oral care, dry the lips and face gently and carefully.

33. Reposition client, raise side rails, and place call button within reach.

34. Rinse, dry, and return articles to proper place.

35. Remove gloves, wash hands, and document care.

Clients at Risk for or with an Alteration of the Oral Cavity

36. Assemble articles for flossing and brushing.

37. Provide privacy.

38. Wash hands and apply gloves.

39. Bleeding:
    a. Assess oral cavity with a padded tongue blade and flashlight for signs of bleeding.
    b. Proceed with the actions for oral care for a full-care client except:
       • Do not floss.
       • Use a soft toothbrush, toothette, or a tongue blade padded with 3 × 3 gauze sponges to gently swab teeth and gums.

33. Promotes comfort, safety, and communication.

34. Provides an orderly environment.

35. Reduces the transmission of microorganisms and documents nursing care.

36. Promotes efficiency.

37. Relaxes client.

38. Reduces the transmission of microorganisms and exposure to body fluids.

39.
    a. Determines whether bleeding is present, amount, and specific areas.
    b.

       • Decreases risk of bleeding and trauma to gums.
       • Decreases risk of bleeding and trauma to gums.

continues

Action	Rationale
• Dispose of padded tongue blade into a biohazard bag according to institutional policy. • Rinse with tepid water.	• Promotes proper disposal of contaminated waste. • Cleanses mouth.
40. Infection: **a.** Assess oral cavity with a tongue blade and flashlight for signs of infection. **b.** Culture lesions as ordered. **c.** Proceed with the actions for oral care for a full-care client except: • Do not floss. • Use prescribed antiseptic solution. • Use a tongue blade padded with 3 × 3 gauze sponges to gently swab the teeth and gums. • Dispose of padded tongue blade into a biohazard bag according to institutional policy. • Rinse mouth with tepid water. • Apply additional solution as prescribed.	**40.** **a.** Determines appearance, integrity, and general condition. **b.** Identifies growth of specific microorganisms. **c.** • Prevents irritation, pain, and bleeding. • Antiseptic solutions decrease growth of microorganisms. • Promotes proper disposal of contaminated materials. • Cleanses mouth. • Provides a coating that promotes healing of the tissue.
41. Ulceration: **a.** Assess oral cavity with a tongue blade and flashlight for signs of ulceration. **b.** Culture lesions as ordered. **c.** Proceed with actions for oral care for a full-care client except: • Do not floss. • Use prescribed antiseptic solution. • Use a tongue blade padded with 3 × 3 gauze sponges to gently swab the teeth and gums. • Dispose of padded tongue blade into a biohazard bag according to institutional policy. • Rinse mouth with tepid water. • Apply additional solution as prescribed.	**41.** **a.** Determines appearance, integrity, and general condition. **b.** Identifies growth of specific microorganisms. **c.** • Prevents irritation, pain, and bleeding. • Antiseptic solutions decrease growth of microorganisms. • Promotes proper disposal of contaminated materials. • Cleanses mouth. • Provides a coating that promotes healing of the tissue.

Unconscious (Comatose) Client

Action	Rationale
42. Assemble articles for flossing and brushing.	**42.** Promotes efficiency.
43. Provide privacy.	**43.** Relaxes client.
44. Wash hands and apply gloves.	**44.** Reduces the transmission of microorganisms and exposure to body fluids.
45. Explain the procedure to the client.	**45.** Demonstrates respect for the client.
46. Place the client in a lateral position, with the head turned toward the side.	**46.** Prevents aspiration.
47. Use a floss holder and floss between all teeth.	**47.** Prevents transfer of microorganisms from a client bite.

continues

Action	Rationale
Unconscious (Comatose) Client *continued*	
48. Moisten toothbrush or toothette, and brush the teeth and gums using friction in a vertical or circular motion. Do not use toothpaste. On inner and outer surfaces of teeth, hold brush at 45-degree angle against teeth and brush from sulcus to crowns of teeth. On biting surfaces, move brush back and forth in short strokes. All surfaces of teeth should be brushed from every angle.	48. Permits cleaning of back and sides of teeth and decreases microorganism growth in mouth. Toothpaste may foam and cause aspiration.
49. After flossing and brushing, rinse mouth with an Asepto syringe (do not force water into the mouth) and perform oral suction.	49. Promotes cleansing and removal of secretions and prevents aspiration.
50. Dry the client's mouth.	50. Prevents skin irritation.
51. Apply lip moisturizer.	51. Maintains skin integrity of lips.
52. Leave the client in a lateral position with head turned toward side for 30 to 60 minutes after oral hygiene care. Suction one more time. Remove the towel from under the client's mouth and face.	52. Prevents pooling of secretions and aspiration.
53. Dispose of any contaminated items in a biohazard bag and clean, dry, and return all articles to the appropriate place.	53. Promotes proper disposal of contaminated materials.
54. Remove gloves, wash hands, and document care.	54. Reduces the transmission of microorganisms and documents nursing care.

▶ REAL WORLD ANECDOTES

Scenario 1
Nurse Rodriguez was assigned to care for Mr. Cunningham, a comatose, intubated client. Previous caregivers had charted that oral care had been performed and nothing unusual had been noted. When Nurse Rodriguez started Mr. Cunningham's oral care, she noticed that the interior of his mouth looked unusual. After repositioning the endotracheal tube, she found maggots thriving in Mr. Cunningham's mouth. Oral care and charting took longer than Nurse Rodriguez had expected that day.

Scenario 2
Mr. Chang, a client in the V.A. hospital for treatment of lung cancer, was experiencing a lot of nausea, dry mouth, cracked lips, and general discomfort. He was also experiencing a sense of loss of control and helplessness because he spent most of his day in bed waiting for tests and treatments. The nurse recognized his need for increased control over his care. She set him up with a pitcher and basin, soft toothettes, toothpaste, mouthwash, and lip balm. Mr. Chang was able to perform his own oral care as frequently as he desired. His comfort level improved, and his sense of control improved as well.

▶ EVALUATION

- The client's mouth, teeth, gums, and lips are clean and free of food particles.
- Inflammation, bleeding, infection, or ulceration are noted and addressed.
- The oral mucosa is clean, intact, and well hydrated.
- The oral care was performed with a minimum of trauma to the client.

▶ DOCUMENTATION

Nurses' Notes

- Note any unusual findings.

Document on appropriate flow sheet or electronic medical record (EMR).

▶ CRITICAL THINKING SKILL

Introduction

Simple oral care can be a life-threatening procedure if not performed correctly.

Possible Scenario

You have been assigned to perform oral care on Mr. Foster, a confused and very debilitated client. You have positioned Mr. Foster on his side with an emesis basin under his mouth. While rinsing his mouth, Mr. Foster begins to choke.

Possible Outcome

If the choking is not dealt with immediately, Mr. Foster could aspirate the fluid, leading to pneumonia or apnea, which could result in death.

Prevention

If a client chokes on the fluids used for oral care, position the head and mouth downward farther to allow gravity to drain the fluid. If this is not effective, hyperextend the neck and perform oral-pharyngeal suctioning to remove the fluid. Always have suction readily available when there is any possibility of aspiration during oral care.

▶ VARIATIONS

Geriatric Variations:

- *Elderly clients often wear dentures. Wet dentures are slippery; take care not to drop them in the sink and possibly break them. Broken dentures cause undue stress, extra expenses, lack of nutrition, and possibly mouth sores from adjusting to new dentures. Fill the sink halfway with water or pad the bottom of the sink with a towel to break the fall of the dentures if dropped.*
- *Assess an elderly denture wearer's mouth carefully for ulceration or inflammation caused by poorly fitting dentures.*

Pediatric Variations:

- *Children who do not have teeth yet should have their gums massaged and cleaned with a soft gauze.*
- *Be aware that children might bite. Keep your fingers out of harm's way.*
- *Use a pea-sized amount of toothpaste on a child's toothbrush as children often swallow toothpaste. Ingesting too much toothpaste causes excess fluoride consumption, which can affect tooth coloration.*
- *Braces or orthodontic appliances may require special handling. A child with appliances may need more thorough oral care to clean all surfaces of the appliance as well as the teeth. Ask the client or the client's parents about any special oral care needs the child may have and how to remove orthodontic devices, if applicable.*
- *Infants may benefit from fluoride drops given as a supplement.*
- *Children might be more comfortable using their own toothbrush or toothbrush brand. Parents can bring these items.*

Home Care Variations:

- *Oral care is especially important for clients who are receiving oxygen. Oxygen is drying to the mucous membranes. Teach home care clients the importance of diligent oral care.*
- *If clients have dentures, teach the clients or their caregivers to remove the upper dentures first and then the lower dentures.*
- *When replacing dentures in the mouth, the upper dentures should be placed first.*
- *When storing dentures in water, a few drops of white vinegar or mouthwash in the water can help prevent odor from clinging to the dentures.*

continues

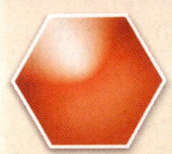

▶ VARIATIONS *(continued)*

Long-Term Care Variations:

- *Clients with nasogastric tubes or feeding tubes require diligent oral care. Their mouths are at a greater risk of dehydration, leading to cracking, bleeding, and infections.*
- *Do not use oral care products that contain lemon juice, which can etch the teeth, or glycerin, which actually absorbs moisture from the tissues.*
- *In unconscious clients, an oral cleansing solution of hydrogen peroxide and water (half and half; or one part peroxide to three parts water; or one-third water, one-third peroxide, and one-third mouthwash) may be used. If the stronger solution causes discomfort, use a weaker solution by increasing the percentage of water.*
- *In some facilities, milk of magnesia or buttermilk has been used in the oral care of unconscious clients. Both of these products can cause caries, so a noncarious solution, such as peroxide and water, is now preferred.*

▶ COMMON ERRORS

Possible Error:

Oral care is not done frequently enough.

Prevention:

Think about how often you brush your teeth and clean your mouth. Be aware of your client's comfort, especially if the client is unable to ask for self. In the conscious client, offer oral care opportunities frequently, especially if the client is to receive nothing by mouth (NPO). In the unconscious client, perform oral care at least as often as you would do it for yourself. Remember that unconscious clients often mouth breathe and require oral care more frequently than a conscious person.

▶ NURSING TIPS

- Never place your fingers in a client's mouth. A bite block or padded tongue blade can be used to hold the client's mouth open.
- The unconscious client's head should be turned to one side with a basin placed under the mouth. Oral suction should be available. Only small amounts of water should be used.
- Be careful when handling and cleaning dentures or other oral appliances. They can be slippery when wet and may break if dropped into the sink or on the floor.

- Clients with orthodontic appliances may have special oral care needs. Ask the client or the client's parents about any special cleaning needs or special appliance care.
- Avoid using oil-based products around oxygen and oxygen equipment because oil and grease are flammable. Petroleum jelly may be used on clients receiving oxygen, but it should not be used on oxygen equipment.
- Avoid breathing directly on client to avoid transmission of microorganisms.
- Wear a mask and goggles if within distance of splashes or sprays from the client's coughing.

► **SPECIAL CONSIDERATIONS**

- Clients with oral lesions may be sensitive to fluoride. Use mild or nonfluoride mouth-cleaning products to decrease irritation during oral care.
- Toothpaste with a greater concentration of fluoride may be prescribed to prevent dental caries. Because oral pH values differ among individuals, staining may occur with some clients. If this occurs, withhold the toothpaste and notify the health care practitioner.
- Report any signs of fungal infections, leukoplakia (white spots or patches on the mucous membranes), bleeding of gums, or reddened throat.
- Clients on anticoagulants may bleed and need soft toothbrushes or toothettes.

Perineal and Genital Care

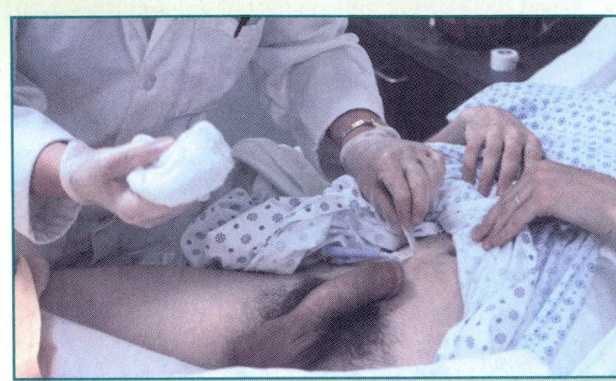

▶ OVERVIEW OF THE SKILL

The perineum is the external structure of the pelvic floor. It is composed of the skin and muscle surrounding the genitalia; it is the area between the scrotum and anus in the male and between the vulva and anus in the female. Care of the perineum and genitalia is directed toward maintaining a hygienic perineal environment. Perineal and genital care is usually self-care; however, alterations in the client's ability to perform self-care or alterations in the perineum and genitalia are reasons for nurses or other care providers to perform this skill. Perineal and genital care is an emotionally and culturally difficult subject. Many cultures have specific beliefs and taboos regarding the perineal/genital area. Many people are embarrassed by the idea of anyone else seeing or touching their genitals, particularly a stranger. The nurse must be aware of these possibilities when approaching genital/perineal care. In general, a professional, nonjudgmental approach will put the client more at ease with the procedure. Ask the client or the client's caregiver, if possible, about any preferences the client may have in this area. During labor, amniotic fluid, urine, and feces may be expelled. While the client is ambulatory, encourage frequent peri-care with urination. If the client is anesthetized, perform frequent peri-care to prevent infection and before any invasive procedure such as vaginal examination, internal monitoring, or rupture of membranes.

Obstetrics presents special perineal care needs. In the postpartum period for vaginal birth: If the client is ambulatory, perform peri-care at the toilet. Use a peri-bottle with water at a temperature comfortable to the mother. Teach her to use the entire contents of the bottle and spray from the front to the back, across the perineum (not into the vagina) to remove urine and fecal material. If there is an episiotomy or laceration, she will want to blot with tissue or a washcloth until the perineum is no longer sore. Also, if perineal medications are to be used (witch hazel, topical anesthetics, and so on), teach the client to do this with each urination and to use a clean sanitary pad. Ice should be considered to help alleviate pain and edema.

In the postpartum period for Cesarean birth: Until the mother is ambulatory, peri-care must be performed in the bed. Assist the mother to a bedpan, which has been padded underneath with waterproof pads. Use the water bottle to spray vaginal secretions from the perineum from the front to the back, across the perineum (not into the vagina). If an episiotomy is present, apply perineal medications as required and consider ice compresses for the first 12 hours to alleviate pain and edema. Once the mother is ambulatory, this care may be performed at the toilet and the client instructed in the technique.

▶ ASSESSMENT

1. Evaluate client status: level of consciousness, ability to ambulate, ability to perform self-care, frequency of urination and defecation, skin condition. **This allows the nurse to decide who, where, how, and when to perform perineal care.**
2. Identify cultural preferences for perineal care. **Perineal care is strongly associated with**

cultural practices for example, who may touch the perineal area and how, and the proper way to "wipe." To the extent possible, these preferences should be identified and incorporated into the client's care.

3. Assess the client's perineal health. Ask the male client if he has any perineal/genital itching or discomfort. Ask the female client if she has any urethral, vaginal, or anal discharge. **Determines the presence of signs and symptoms that may need additional assessment and intervention.**

4. Determine if the client is incontinent of urine or stool. **Affects how the procedure will be done and what additional procedures may be necessary.**

5. Assess whether the client has recently had perineal/genital surgery. **Affects how the procedure will be done and what additional procedures may be necessary.**

▶ DIAGNOSIS

Risk for Impaired Skin Integrity

Bathing/Hygiene Self-Care Deficit

Risk for Compromised Human Dignity

▶ PLANNING

Expected Outcomes:

1. Perineum and genitalia will be dry, clean, and free of secretions and unpleasant odors.
2. The client will report feeling comfortable and clean in the perineal area.
3. The client will not experience discomfort or undue embarrassment during the procedure.
4. The perineum will be free of skin breakdown or irritation.

Equipment Needed (see Figure 4-9-1):

- Personal protective equipment (gloves, gown)
- Toilet paper/washcloths
- Waterproof pads
- Cleansing solution, if needed
- Perineal wash bottle (fill with plain, warm water).
- Water receptacle (bedpan or toilet if client is ambulatory)

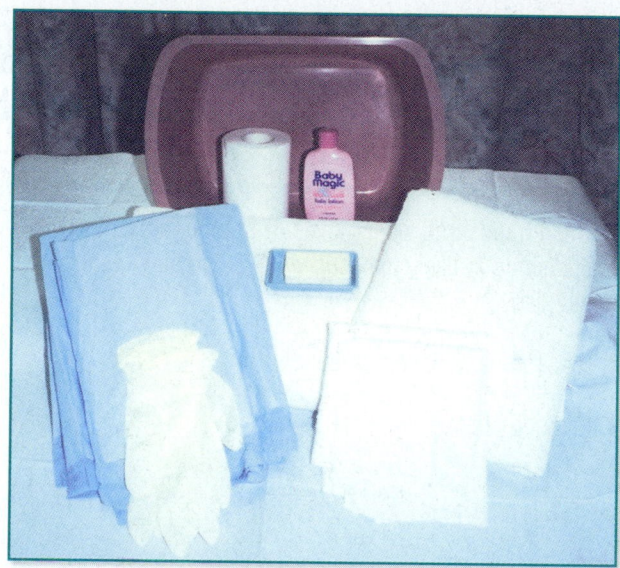

Figure 4-9-1 Toilet paper, soap, lotion, towels, gloves, and a basin are all used to provide perineal care.

- Dry towels
- Perineal treatment (i.e., ointment or lotions), if necessary
- Linen receptacle
- Room deodorizer

▶ CLIENT EDUCATION NEEDED:

1. Ask the client or the client's caregiver about preferences the client may have. Discuss the procedure with the client if this is the first time it is being done.
2. Teach clients to wash their hands after performing peri-care.
3. Warm water washes may provide comfort to the skin and reduce the need to repeatedly wipe the perineum if the area is tender.

Estimated time to complete the skill: **10 minutes**

▶ DELEGATION TIPS

This skill is routinely delegated to ancillary personnel who should be trained in Standard Precautions and proper client positioning and who are trained to report color, odor, and amount of any discharge, if present, to the nurse.

IMPLEMENTATION—Action/Rationale

Action	Rationale
1. Wash hands and wear gloves. If appropriate and splashing is likely to occur, wear gown, mask, and goggles.	1. Reduces the transmission of microorganisms.
2. Close privacy curtain or door.	2. Provides privacy.
3. Position client.	3. If client is ambulatory, perineal care may be done either with client on or standing at the toilet. If perineal care is to be performed in the bed, place the client on the side or over a deep bedpan.
4. Place waterproof pads under the client in the bed or under bedpan if used (see Figure 4-9-2).	4. Protects bed linen.
5. Remove fecal debris with disposable paper and dispose in toilet.	5. May require several attempts. If performing at the bedside, may collect paper in disposable pad or linens until end of procedure.
6. Spray perineum with washing solution if indicated. Alternatively, plain water may be used.	6. Several perineal solutions are available, which may or may not require rinsing. Carefully evaluate this requirement. Solutions that require rinsing may cause skin breakdown if left on the skin.
7. Cleanse perineum with wet washcloths (front to back on females), changing to clean area on washcloth with each wipe. Cleanse the penis if the client is a man (see Figure 4-9-3).	7. Maximizes cleaning; prevents spread of rectal flora to vagina.
8. Carefully examine gluteal folds and scrotal folds for debris. Gently visualize vulva for debris.	8. Fecal material causes irritation and skin breakdown rapidly when left in contact with skin.
9. If soap is used, spray area with clean water from the peri-bottle.	9. Rinses soap, which can irritate the skin, from the area.
10. Change gloves.	10. Reduces the transmission of microorganisms.
11. Dry perineum carefully with towel.	11. Residual moisture provides an ideal environment for the growth of microorganisms.
12. If indicated, apply barrier lotion or ointment.	12. Barrier ointments may be used if client is incontinent or skin folds tend to harbor moisture.
13. Reposition or dress client as appropriate.	13. Promotes client comfort.
14. Dispose of linens and garbage according to hospital policy.	14. Prevents spread of disease or bacteria.

continues

Action	Rationale

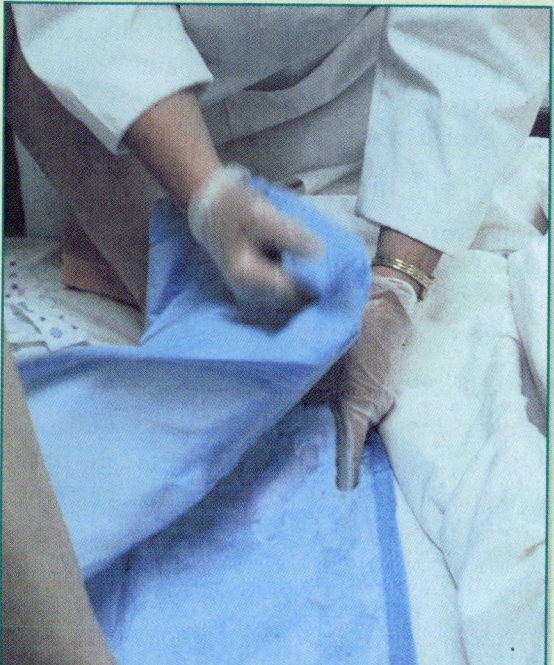

Figure 4-9-2 Use waterproof pads to protect mattress and linen from getting wet.

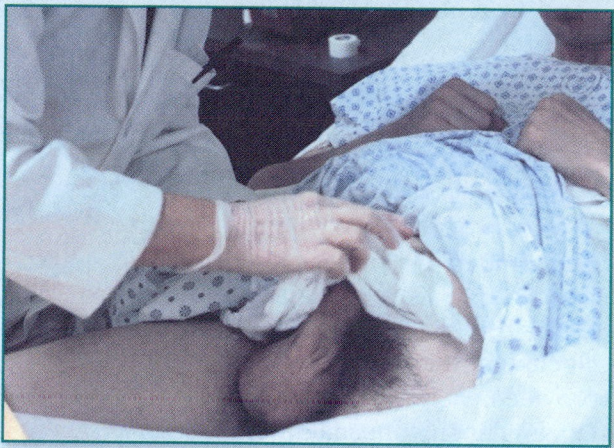

Figure 4-9-3 Cleanse the penis with a warm, wet washcloth.

15. Wash hands.

16. Deodorize room if appropriate.

15. Reduces the transmission of microorganisms.

16. Promotes client comfort. This may also be done at the beginning of the procedure.

▶ REAL WORLD ANECDOTES

Scenario 1

Arnold Green, age 72, was being treated for end-stage liver cancer and was receiving parenteral nutrition. He had severe diarrhea and was continent most of the time. However, the frequency of diarrhea stools caused irritation and pain. His compromised immune status and occasional incontinence predisposed him to infection. Arnold was embarrassed about his occasional incontinence and did not want to have the nursing staff help him clean himself. He was weak and often could not maintain his efforts to perform his own peri-care.

Scenario 2

Recognizing Arnold's high risk for skin breakdown and infection, Nurse Mark instituted a routine perineal care regime for Arnold. Perineal wash was provided for each defecation, and Arnold managed this himself. In cooperation with the primary care provider, a barrier skin cream was prescribed and Arnold administered this to himself per his request. Using therapeutic technique, Nurse Mark problem solved with Arnold about allowing staff to assist him when he was incontinent.

► EVALUATION

1. The perineum and genitalia are dry, clean, and free of secretions and unpleasant odors.
2. The client reports feeling comfortable and clean in the perineal area.
3. The client did not experience discomfort or undue embarrassment during the procedure.

► DOCUMENTATION

Nurses' Notes

- Document the time and type of perineal care provided.
- Document any unusual findings such as skin breakdown, infection, or unusual drainage.
- If the client has special preferences or cultural considerations, be sure to document that these were respected.

Document on appropriate flow sheet or electronic medical record (EMR).

► CRITICAL THINKING SKILL

Introduction

Sherry Jacobs just returned from surgery after her first baby by uncomplicated Cesarean birth. She had epidural anesthesia and is not having any pain. On admission from the recovery area, you note that she has moderate lochia and you assess that she needs peri-care.

Possible Scenario

Sherry wants to get up to go to the bathroom to wash up. She states she can feel her legs and would like to try. You, however, recognize that Sherry is 4 hours post-op and even though she can feel her legs, she may not be stable.

Possible Outcome

You discuss this situation with Sherry and together decide that you will provide her peri-care until she is ambulatory. You teach her the basic principles of peri-care as you perform them.

Prevention

Until Sherry is ambulatory, alternatives for perineal care must be provided for her safety.

► VARIATIONS

Geriatric Variations:

- *Incontinence in the elderly is a major influence in decisions to seek long-term care.*
- *Loss of ability to perform perineal self-care may be a source of embarrassment and a serious threat to ego integrity. Be sensitive to the emotional and self-image needs of the elderly client in need of perineal care.*
- *Some elderly clients, whether because of disease or as a way to compensate for poor self-image, may behave inappropriately during perineal care. Gently but firmly discourage the client from inappropriate touching or comments. If the behavior continues, a same-sex caregiver might be appropriate.*

Pediatric Variations:

- *Encourage parents to change the child's diapers frequently to minimize skin contact with urine and feces.*
- *Be sensitive to cultural concerns, particularly in regard to genital care for female children. Some societies have strict cultural taboos. Some societies have deep concerns regarding inappropriate touching. A same-sex caregiver is more appropriate in this situation. If there are concerns regarding touch, it may be appropriate to have two caregivers provide peri-care or perhaps have a same-sex family member present during care.*
- *Be aware that the child might revert to bedwetting because of the stress of hospitalization.*
- *Teach children to wipe from front to back when cleaning themselves.*

Home Care Variations:

- *Consideration should be given to using supplies that do not increase the caregiver burden. For example, linens should be minimized and soft disposable cloths may be a solution. Also, there are some products that can modify the toilet and provide a bidet-type cleansing alternative.*

continues

► **VARIATIONS** *(continued)*

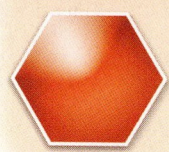

Long-Term Care Variation:
- *Incontinence may be a major factor in long-term care settings. Institutional practices must provide for sanitary and timely attention to perineal care needs.*

► **COMMON ERRORS**

Possible Error:
The nurse fails to clean the glans penis under the foreskin.

Prevention:
Cleaning under the foreskin of an uncircumcised male reduces the risk of urinary tract infections and infections under the foreskin.

► **NURSING TIPS**

- When performing perineal care on a client in bed, make sure the bed height is adjusted to permit proper body mechanics.
- Perineal care and bed linen changes may be performed at the same time. Begin by performing peri-care, then wrap soiled linens under the client and place clean linens to the edge of soiled linens. Roll the client to the other side and proceed with the linen change.
- Always wash your hands after performing perineal care. Gloves do not provide a flawless barrier.
- When performing peri-care for an adult or child, it is important to be sensitive to developmental considerations. Peri-care is usually learned early, and inability or difficulty performing this basic task for oneself can evoke feelings of embarrassment, worthlessness, and incompetence. It is critical that the nurse convey respect in an age-appropriate and culturally sensitive manner.

  Perineal care should be performed as often as necessary. Some procedures will necessitate a schedule. If peri-care is necessary after elimination, do not delay. Even short delays can result in unnecessary suffering.

- Ask the client about soap/iodine allergies. Often, clients will not disclose this on admission. Some perineal procedures will require use of iodine preparations.
- In uncircumcised males, gently retract the foreskin to clean smegma and other debris from the area around the glans. This procedure is not universal, however, and it is appropriate to ask the client whether this is acceptable. Care should be taken to replace the foreskin as soon as possible to prevent edema of the glans.
- Many cultures prescribe cleansing from the "front to the back" of the female perineum to prevent rectal debris and germs from coming in contact with the vulva. Be aware that this is also a cultural preference and if necessary may be followed for medical reasons (for example, interruptions in vaginal or perineal integrity).
- If possible, have a same-sex health care provider perform peri-care.
- Some clients may prefer to perform their own peri-care; however, they may not be able to complete adequate care and may require assistance.

▶ **SPECIAL CONSIDERATIONS**

- *Using a peri-bottle may facilitate cleansing of the perineum after toileting for the female client.*
- *Draw back the foreskin of the uncircumcised male client for thorough cleaning. The foreskin must be returned over the head of the penis after cleansing is completed.*
- *Incontinence can lead to skin breakdown and require protective barriers. If perineal skin breakdown is present, take actions such as additional treatment, drying lights, sitz baths, or topical ointments as ordered. Assess for urinary tract infections.*

Eye Care

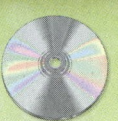

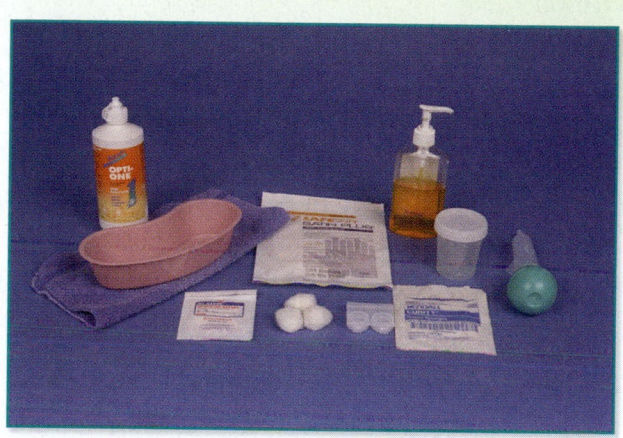

▶ OVERVIEW OF THE SKILL

Generally, the eye needs little daily care. Normally, eyes are continually cleansed by the production of tears and the movement of eyelids over the eyes. Some clients, however, do have special eye care needs.

Contact Lenses

Self-care is the best method of care for a client with contact lenses. However, accidents or illness may render a client unable to remove or care for the lenses. There are several kinds of contact lenses. Some may be left on the cornea for up to a week without damage. Most must be removed daily for cleaning and to prevent hypoxia of the cornea. It is the nurse's responsibility to determine whether the client is wearing contact lenses and to properly care for the lenses and the client's eyes. In acute care situations, the nurse should encourage the client to wear glasses if possible and send the contact lenses home with a family member.

Prosthetic Eyes

Some clients have an artificial eye (ocular prosthesis) in place. Artificial eyes are created to look identical to the client's biologic eye. They are generally made from glass or plastic. Some artificial eyes are permanently implanted in the eye socket, but others must be removed daily for cleaning. They should be removed daily and cleaned carefully. The eye socket should also be gently cleansed to remove crusts and mucus, and the prosthesis should be replaced in the eye socket.

▶ ASSESSMENT

1. Determine whether the client is wearing contact lenses or has an ocular prosthesis. If the client is unable to answer questions, you will need to find out another way. Does it indicate in the client's chart if the client wears contact lenses or has a prosthesis? Are there family members present to ask? **This will affect how eye care is given.**
2. Are the needed eye care supplies available? If the client can tell you what kind of eye care products he or she normally uses, ask or have a family member bring these products from home. **This will affect how eye care is given.**
3. Assess whether the client can do his or her own eye care. If not, evaluate what kind of assistance the client will need. **This promotes maximum independence in the client.**

▶ DIAGNOSIS

Ineffective Health Maintenance

Bathing/Hygiene Self-Care Deficit

Disturbed Sensory Perception (Visual)

▶ PLANNING

Expected Outcomes:

1. The client's contact lenses will be safely removed and stored.
2. The client's ocular prosthesis will be safely removed, cleaned, and either stored or returned to the client's eye socket.

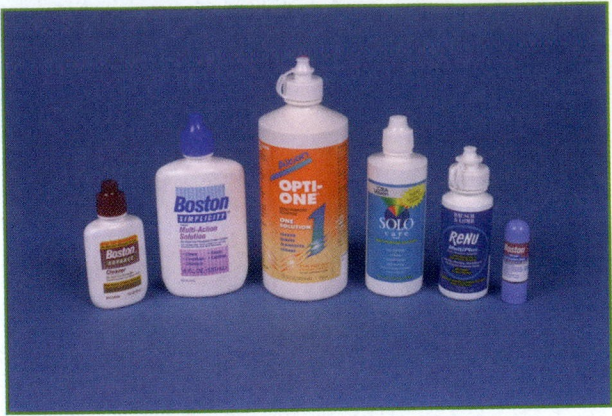

Figure 4-10-1 Commercial soaking and eye care solutions. There are many types of soaking solutions available. Select the type normally used by the client when possible.

3. The client's contacts or prosthesis will be cared for with a minimum of trauma to the client's eyes.
4. The client's eyes will be free of crusts and exudate.

Equipment Needed (see Figure 4-10-1):
Artificial Eye
- Storage container
- Mild soap
- 3 × 3 gauze sponges
- Cotton balls
- Towel
- Emesis basins
- Eye irrigation syringe (optional)

- Running water
- Sterile gloves
- Biohazard bag
- Saline solution

Contact Lenses
- Lens container
- Soaking solution—type used by client
- Towel
- Suction cup (optional)
- Scotch tape (optional)
- Nonsterile gloves

▶ CLIENT EDUCATION NEEDED:

1. Instruct the client to wash his or her hands before handling contact lenses or an ocular prosthesis.
2. Explain to the client that using saliva to wet lenses is hazardous to the cornea because of digestive enzymes in the saliva.
3. Instruct the client that daily wear lenses need to be removed at night to prevent hypoxia and possibly ulcers of the cornea
4. Ocular prostheses should be stored in saline or clean tap water, and not left on the bedside stand.

Estimated time to complete the skill:
15 minutes

▶ DELEGATION TIPS

Eye care requires the assessment and intervention of the nurse; delegation to ancillary personnel is inappropriate.

IMPLEMENTATION—Action/Rationale

Action	Rationale
Artificial Eye Removal	
1. Inquire about client's care regimen and gather equipment accordingly.	1. Promotes continuity of care.
2. Provide privacy.	2. Relaxes the client.
3. Wash hands; apply gloves.	3. Reduces the transmission of microorganisms.
4. Place client in a semi-Fowler's position.	4. Facilitates procedure and client participation.

continues

Action	Rationale
5. Place the cotton balls in an emesis basin filled halfway with warm tap water.	**5.** Dry cotton balls could cause irritation.
6. Place 3 × 3 gauze sponges in bottom of second emesis basin and fill halfway with mild soap and tepid water.	**6.** Gauze serves as padding to prevent breakage of the prosthesis.
7. Grasp and squeeze excess water from a cotton ball. Cleanse the eyelid with the moistened cotton ball, starting at the inner canthus and moving outward toward the outer canthus. After each use, dispose of cotton ball in biohazard bag. Repeat procedure until eyelid is clean (without dried secretions).	**7.** Eliminating the excess water prevents water from running down the client's face. Cleansing the eyelid prevents contamination of the lacrimal system (inner canthus area). Disposal of cotton balls reduces transmission of microorganisms to other health care workers.

8. Remove the artificial eye:
   a. Using dominant hand, raise the client's upper eyelid with index finger and depress the lower eyelid with thumb.
   b. Cup nondominant hand under the client's lower eyelid.
   c. Apply slight pressure with index finger between the brow and the artificial eye and remove it. Place it in an emesis basin filled with warm, soapy water.
	8. Cleanses the artificial eye.
	   a. Promotes removal of artificial eye.
	
	   b. Cupping reduces dropping and possible breaking of the eye.
	
	   c. Applying pressure will help the prosthesis to slip out.

9. Grasp a moistened cotton ball and cleanse around the edge of the eye socket. Dispose of the soiled cotton ball into biohazard bag.	**9.** Cleanses the eye socket. Disposal of cotton ball reduces transmission of microorganisms to other health care workers.
10. Inspect the eye socket for any signs of irritation, drainage, or crusting. *Note:* If the client's usual care regimen or physician order requires irrigation of the socket, proceed with Action 11; otherwise, go to Action 12.	**10.** Indicates an infection.

11. Eye socket irrigation:
   a. Lower the head of the bed and place the client in a supine position. Place protector pad on bed; turn head toward socket side and slightly extend neck.
   b. Fill the irrigation syringe with the prescribed amount and type of irrigating solution (warm tap water or normal saline).
   c. With nondominant hand, separate the eyelids with your forefinger and thumb while resting fingers on the brow and cheekbone.
   d. Hold the irrigating syringe in dominant hand several inches above the inner canthus; with thumb, gently apply pressure on the plunger, directing the flow of solution from the inner canthus along the conjunctival sac.
   e. Irrigate until the prescribed amount of solution has been used.
   f. Wipe the eyelids with a moistened cotton ball after irrigating. Dispose of soiled cotton ball in biohazard bag.
	11. Cleanses the eye socket and removes secretions.
	   a. Positioning of client facilitates ease in performing the procedure and client comfort.
	
	   b. Ensures compliance with client's regimen or prescribed orders.
	
	   c. Keeps the eyelid open and the socket visible.
	
	   d. Prevents injury to the client.
	
	   e. Ensures compliance with client's regimen of prescribed orders.
	   f. Reduces the transmission of microorganisms to prosthesis.

continues

Action	Rationale
Artificial Eye Removal *continued*	
g. Pat the skin dry with the towel.	g. Prevents maceration of the skin.
h. Return the client to a semi-Fowler's position.	h. Promotes client comfort.
i. Remove gloves, wash hands, and apply clean gloves.	i. Reduces the transmission of microorganisms.
12. Rub the artificial eye between index finger and thumb in the basin of warm, soapy water.	12. Creates cleaning with friction and prevents breakage of the prosthesis.
13. Rinse the prosthesis under running water or place in the clean basin of tepid water. Do not dry the prosthesis. *Note:* Either reinsert the prosthesis (Action 14) or store in a container (Action 15).	13. Removes soap and secretions. Keeping the artificial eye wet prevents irritation from lint or other particles that might adhere to it and facilitates reinsertion.

14. Reinsert the prosthesis:
  a. With the thumb of the nondominant hand, raise and hold the upper eyelid open.
  b. With the dominant hand, grasp the artificial eye so that the indented part is facing toward the client's nose and slide it under the upper eyelid as far as possible.
  c. Depress the lower lid.
  d. Pull the lower lid forward to cover the edge of the prosthesis.
	14. Allows for client comfort.
	  a. Facilitates reinsertion of the prosthesis without discomfort to the client.
	  b. Positions the prosthesis for insertion.
	  c. Allows the prosthesis to slide into place.
	  d. Holds the prosthesis in place.

15. Place the cleaned artificial eye in a labeled container with saline or tap water solution.	15. Protects the prosthesis from scratches and keeps it clean.
16. Grasp a moistened cotton ball and squeeze out excessive moisture. Wipe the eyelid from the inner to the outer canthus. Dispose of the soiled cotton ball in a biohazard bag.	16. Squeezing the cotton ball removes moisture. Cleansing the eyelid prevents contamination of lacrimal system. Disposal of cotton ball reduces the transmission of microorganisms to other health care workers.
17. Clean, dry, and replace equipment.	17. Promotes a clean environment.
18. Reposition the client, raise side rails, and place call light in reach.	18. Promotes client's comfort, safety, and communication.
19. Dispose of biohazard bag according to institutional policy.	19. Reduces the transmission of microorganisms to other health care workers.
20. Remove gloves and wash hands.	20. Same as Rationale 19.
21. Document procedure, client's response and participation, and client teaching and level of understanding.	21. Demonstrates that the procedure was done and the level of client participation and learning.
Contact Lens Removal	
22. Assemble equipment for lens removal.	22. Promotes efficiency.
23. Assess level of assistance needed, provide privacy, and explain the procedure to the client.	23. Level of assistance determines level of intervention. Privacy reduces anxiety. Explanation of procedure promotes cooperation.
24. Wash hands (see Figure 4-10-2).	24. Reduces the transmission of microorganisms.

continues

Action	Rationale

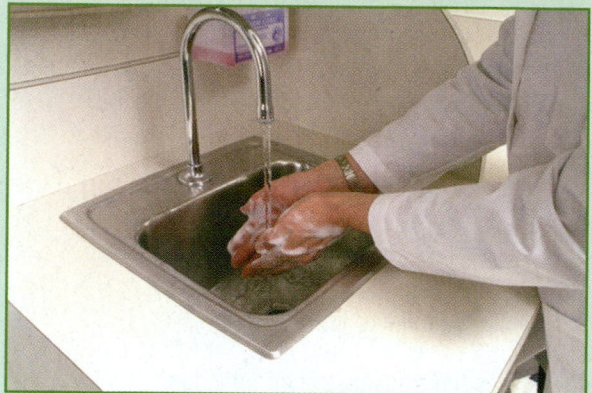

Figure 4-10-2 Wash hands before performing eye care. Have client wash hands if he or she will be performing own eye care.

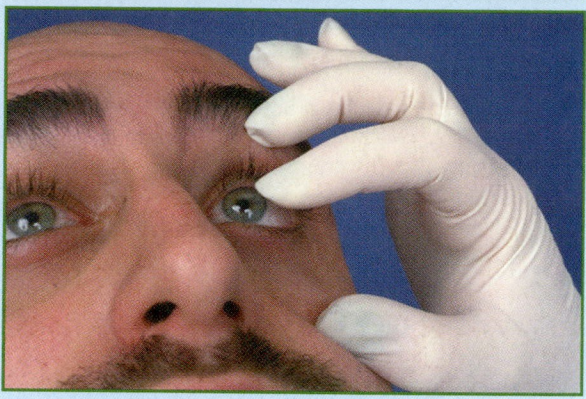

Figure 4-10-3 If the lens is not on the cornea, gently move it toward the cornea with the pad of the index finger.

25. Assist the client to a semi-Fowler's position if needed.

26. Drape a clean towel over the client's chest.

27. Prepare the lens storage case with the prescribed solution.

28. Instruct the client to look straight ahead. Assess the location of the lens. If it is not on the cornea, either you or the client should gently move the lens toward the cornea with the pad of the index finger (see Figure 4-10-3).

29. Remove the lens.
   a. Hard lens:
   - Cup nondominant hand under the eye.
   - Gently place index finger on the outside corner of the eye and pull toward the temple and ask client to blink. Catch the lens in your nondominant hand.

   b. Soft lens:
   - With nondominant hand, separate the eyelid with your thumb and middle finger.
   - With the index finger of the dominant hand gently placed on the lower edge of the lens, slide the lens downward onto the sclera and gently squeeze the lens.
   - Release the top eyelid (continue holding the lower lid down) and remove the lens with your index finger and thumb.
     Note: If Action 29 is unsuccessful, secure a suction cup to remove the contact lens. If you are unable to remove the lens, notify the physician or qualified practitioner.

25. Facilitates removal of lens.

26. Provides a clean surface and facilitates locating a lens if it falls during removal.

27. Hard lenses can be stored dry or in a special soaking solution. Soft lenses are stored in sterile normal saline without a preservative.

28. Client's position promotes easy removal of lens. Positioning lens on the cornea aids removal. Use of the finger pad of the index finger prevents damage to cornea and lens.

29. Provides for cleaning and storage of the lens.
   a.
   - Cupping the hand under the eye helps to catch the lens and prevent breakage.
   - Pulling the corner of the eye tightens the eyelid against the eyeball. Pressure on the upper edge of the lens causes the lens to tip forward.

   b.
   - Separating the eyelid exposes the lower edge of lens.
   - Positions lens for easy grasping with the pad of the index finger, which prevents injury to the cornea and lens. Squeezing the lens allows air to enter and release the suction.
   - Ensures control of the lens.
   - Suction cup is used to remove a lens from an unconscious or dependent client.

continues

Action	Rationale
Contact Lens Removal *continued*	
30. Store the lens in the correct compartment of the case ("right" or "left"). Label with the client's name.	30. Storage prevents damage to the lenses and ensures that each lens will be reinserted into the correct eye.
31. Remove and store the other lens by repeating Actions 29 and 30.	31. Refer to Rationales 29 and 30.
32. Assess the client's eyes for irritation or redness.	32. Signs of corneal irritation.
33. Store the lens case in a safe place.	33. Prevents damage or loss.
34. Dispose of soiled articles and clean and return reusable articles to proper location.	34. Reduces the transmission of infection.
35. Reposition the client, raise side rails, and place call light in reach.	35. Promotes client comfort, safety, and communication.
36. Remove gloves and wash hands.	36. Reduces the transmission of infection.
37. Document procedure, client's response and assessment findings, and the storage place of the lenses.	37. Documents the removal of lenses, condition of the cornea, and where the lenses are stored.

► REAL WORLD ANECDOTES

Student nurse Anderson was removing Mr. Molloy's artificial eye to clean it. Although she cupped her hand under his eye while removing the prosthesis, it was slippery and it slid out of her hand and onto the client's bed. While she searched through the blankets to find the prosthesis, the eye fell to the floor and rolled under the chair occupied by Mrs. Molloy. To retrieve the prosthesis, the student had to get down on her hands and knees and reach under the chair. Fortunately, the only damage was to the student's dignity; the eye survived intact.

► EVALUATION

- The client's contact lenses were safely removed and stored.
- The client's ocular prosthesis was safely removed, cleaned, and either stored or returned to the client's eye socket.
- The client's contacts or prosthesis were cared for with a minimum of trauma to the client's eyes.
- The client's eyes are free of crusts and exudate.
- The client is comfortable.

► DOCUMENTATION

Nurses' Notes
- Document that the client wears contact lenses.
- Note the location and condition of the lenses.

- Document whether the client requires assistance to place and remove the contact lenses.
- Document whether the client has an ocular prosthesis. Note which eye is prosthetic.
- Note the condition of the prosthesis and the condition of the eye socket.
- Indicate the care performed on the prosthesis and the socket and how the client tolerated the activity.
- Note any client teaching.

Document on appropriate flow sheet or electronic medical record (EMR).

► CRITICAL THINKING SKILL

Possible Scenario
While working in the emergency department, you are called upon to remove an unconscious client's contact

lenses. You remove the client's right lens only to realize that you have no container or solution ready.

Possible Outcome

The client's contact could get contaminated as you wander around with it in your hand searching for a container and sterile saline solution. It could become airborne, dropped, and lost, or it could dry out and become ruined. Any of these scenarios would be costly and inconvenient for the client (see Figure 4-10-4).

Prevention

Be sure you have the equipment ready and prepared before you start this or any procedure.

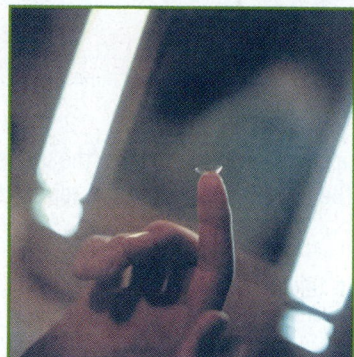

Figure 4-10-4   Be careful with the lens when it is out of the client's eye or out of the case. It may be easily dropped or lost.

▶ VARIATIONS

Geriatric Variations:

- *Elderly people often have very thin, delicate skin. When replacing or removing contacts or a prosthesis, be careful not to tear or bruise the skin surrounding the eye.*
- *Make sure eyewear is within reach. Clients can become more confused and less able to communicate if they cannot see clearly.*
- *If your client is an elderly person with limited income or restricted social contact, verify that the client's eyeglass prescription is up-to-date.*
- *If the elderly person is wearing or caring for contacts, mark the containers clearly with a large L and R for left and right eye. This will help keep the lenses in the correct place.*

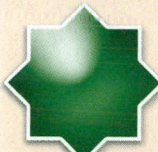

Pediatric Variations:

- *Children grow quickly and can outgrow an ocular prosthesis. When caring for a child with an ocular prosthesis, be sure to note the fit.*
- *If a child needs glasses to see, make sure they are within reach. A colorful cord or cloth may be attached to the glasses to help keep them around the neck and to help locate them in the bed. Do not fasten any cord too tightly to avoid the risk of strangulation.*
- *Young children may not be able to tell you if they have injured or scratched their eye. Carefully examine the eye for signs of infection or injury if a discharge, redness, or irritation is present.*
- *To remove contacts in a child, an additional staff member or parent may be needed to help hold and support the child.*

Home Care Variations:

- *Home care clients can become careless about the proper cleaning and storage of their contacts or prosthesis. Reinforce the proper techniques for cleaning and storage and the reasons proper technique is important.*
- *Bring a magnifying mirror on your home care visit to help clients do their own eye care when bedridden.*

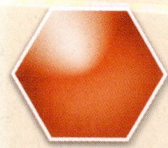

Long-Term Care Variations:

- *Long-term care clients may keep contacts or a prosthesis beyond the point of effectiveness. Examine the prosthesis or contacts to be sure they are not worn or ragged.*
- *Make sure eyewear prescriptions are kept up-to-date.*
- *Keep contacts in carefully labeled containers at the bedside to prevent damage or loss.*

► **COMMON ERRORS**

Possible Error:

When removing a client's contact lenses, the nurse becomes confused regarding her right and the client's left. As a result she placed the left lens in the container for the right lens.

Prevention:

The nurse should take her time to be careful and note which side is which.

► **NURSING TIPS**

- Be aware of right and left. Take care not to mix up a client's contacts.
- Prostheses are slippery. Be careful not to drop them while you are handling them.
- Place a towel or washcloth over the bottom of the sink when cleaning contacts or a prosthesis to prevent breakage if dropped and to prevent loss down the drain.

- If the client has glasses as well as contacts, encourage the client to send the contacts home with family and wear glasses while in the hospital.
- Place a towel in front of the client when an eye prosthesis is removed to catch it if it slips out of your hand.

► **SPECIAL CONSIDERATIONS**

- *Saline is often used to clean lenses but is also a medium for bacterial growth. Always check the date on the solution bottle and store it in the sealed container it was purchased in. Never allow clients to share solutions as accidental contamination may occur.*
- *Encourage clients to remove contact lenses at night. It is important to allow the vessels in the eye to have proper oxygen exchange at night.*
- *If a foreign body gets in the eye, it is important that the client does not rub the area. This will only further irritate the eye as well as introduce bacteria.*
- *If the client has eye pain, scratches, or possible corneal abrasions, seek appropriate medical attention.*

Hair and Scalp Care

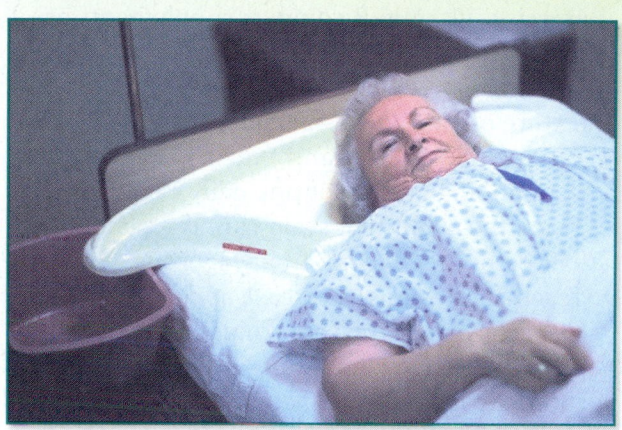

▶ OVERVIEW OF THE SKILL

Healthy hair is dependent on maintaining a healthy scalp. Combing, brushing, and shampooing stimulate circulation; remove dead cells, dirt, and debris; and distribute hair oils, thereby preventing skin irritation and producing a healthy sheen. These procedures, and styling the hair, relax clients and improve their appearance and self-esteem.

▶ ASSESSMENT

1. Assess client need for hair and scalp **care to determine what procedures need to be done.**
2. Assess structure and functional integrity of the hair and scalp **to identify possible need for medicated shampoo, conditioners, or treatments.**
3. Assess client preferences for frequency of care and care products **to determine possible allergies to products and client preferences for personal hygiene.**
4. Confirm client is not allergic to latex or any ingredients/products to be used during the procedure **to prevent adverse reactions to the procedures.**
5. Assess client's medical condition and health status such as contraindications to head manipulation and ability to tolerate sitting, prone, or side-lying positions **to prevent adverse reactions to the procedures.**
6. Assess client's knowledge of the procedure **to determine possible teaching needed.**

7. Assess client's ability to perform/assist with the procedure **to determine and plan how the procedure will be performed.**

▶ DIAGNOSIS

Risk for Impaired Skin Integrity

Dressing/Grooming Self-Care Deficit

Bathing/Hygiene Self-Care Deficit

Low Self-Esteem

▶ PLANNING

Expected Outcomes:

1. The client will have healthy hair and scalp free from infestation, infection, irritation, or alterations in hydration and oils.
2. The client will experience improved circulation to the scalp.
3. The client's comfort, self-esteem, and sense of well-being will be improved.

Equipment Needed (see Figure 4-11-1):

- Bedside/chairside table
- Clean comb (with dull teeth) and hairbrush (soft but firm bristles)
- Washcloth
- Two or three bath towels
- Shampoo tray
- Washbasin, plastic trash can, or pail
- Water pitchers/container: 1 or 2 large (1–2 gal.) and 1 small (2–3 cup)

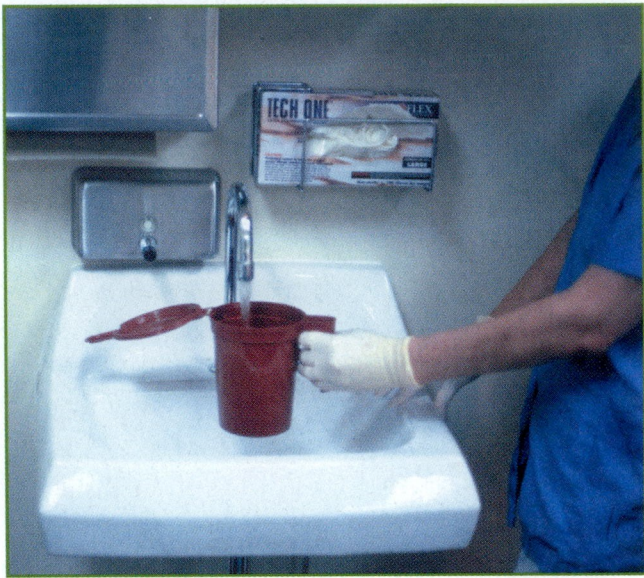

Figure 4-11-1 Warm water and a pitcher are used to provide hair care for the client confined to bed.

- Linen saver or plastic trash bag
- Nonsterile gloves
- Liquid shampoo
- Other: bath thermometer, conditioner, detangler (spray is convenient)
- Hair dryer (safety approved)

▶ **CLIENT EDUCATION NEEDED:**

1. Before the procedure, inform clients that you will be assisting them with care of their hair.

2. Explain each step of the procedure and help identify what assistance is needed.
3. During the procedure, educate the client about what potential problems to observe for and points to remember in self-care.
4. Jointly evaluate needs for the next time the procedure is to be performed.
5. Six glasses of water a day are essential, as is daily exercise. Vitamin B complex supplements are helpful.
6. Teach clients to use shampoo designed for their texture of hair and scalp condition.
7. Teach clients to recognize their hair's need for shampooing versus routine daily care.
8. Teach the client that scalp care is essential to hair care. Teach "gentle-but-vigorous care."
9. Teach about signs of disease and infection (persistent dandruff, breaking, falling out, sudden loss or growth, lesions, anything crawling, spontaneous color changes other than gray, and changes in texture).

Estimated time to complete the skill:
30 minutes

▶ **DELEGATION TIPS**

Hair and scalp care are routinely delegated to ancillary personnel who should be instructed to report any unusual findings, such as scaling or infections, to the nurse. Staff may also need training for cultural variations.

IMPLEMENTATION—Action/Rationale

Action	Rationale
1. Inform client you will be assisting with hair care.	1. Shows respect for client; maximizes cooperation and comfort.
2. Prepare room environment: provide privacy, adjust temperature, and eliminate drafts.	2. Maximizes client comfort and prevents chilling.
3. Review client history for allergies and confirm/obtain provider's orders for medicated shampoo or scalp treatment as needed.	3. Need prescription for medicated supplies.
4. Organize equipment at side of bed or chair.	4. Promotes efficiency.

continues

Action	Rationale
5. Adjust bed to comfortable height or position chair.	**5.** Prevents back strain.
6. Wash hands and apply gloves.	**6.** Reduces the transmission of microorganisms.
7. Remove pillow from under client's head or assist client to chair.	**7.** Positions for comfort and efficiency.
8. Place linen saver (or plastic bag) covered by a towel under client's shoulders and head.	**8.** Catches loose hair and dirt and prevents wetting of linens.
9. Fanfold a second bath towel and place around client's neck; pull the edge over the shoulders toward the midline of the chest to drape the shoulders.	**9.** Protects client's clothing, catches loose hair and dirt, and supports client's neck.
10. Gently comb/brush client's hair, observing scalp and hair for color, texture, distribution, scaling, infestation, or infection. • Comb fingers through hair with slight fingertip massage of scalp. • Turning the client's head away from you, hold the hair with one hand and comb/brush gently with the other on the hair side facing you. Work from the ends toward the scalp. • Part the hair into small sections and comb one section at a time, working from the ends toward the scalp. • Turn the client's head and repeat on the other side. • Facing back of client's head, brush entire head.	**10.** Removes tangles, loosens dead cells and debris, distributes oils, stimulates scalp circulation, and identifies abnormalities early. • Assesses degree of tangling and status of scalp and increases circulation to scalp. • Anchors each section above the area being brushed to avoid discomfort to the client. • Provides for easier handling. • Provides care to remainder of hair and scalp. • Stimulates circulation, loosens debris, distributes oils, and relaxes client.
11. Fill the large pitcher/s with warm water (105°–110° F), checking temperature with thermometer or volar surface of your arm. Place on bedside table.	**11.** Warm water promotes scalp circulation and prevents chilling and skin injury. Water at bedside promotes efficiency.
12. Place the shampoo tray under the client's neck and head with neck in the U-shaped opening. Adjust the fanfolded neck towel to cushion the tray.	**12.** Positions to facilitate drainage of water, maintain client comfort, and avoid pressure to neck.
13. Position pail/washbasin/trash can in direct line with the spout of the shampoo tray. Position as close to the spout as possible. You may need to set it on a chair, a stool, or a low table (see Figure 4-11-2).	**13.** Provides reservoir for water and minimizes splashing as water runs into the pail.
14. Offer washcloth for client to hold over or above eyes and cotton balls to place in ears during shampooing.	**14.** Prevents shampoo or water from irritating eyes/ears and moisture from collecting in ear canals.
15. Fill small pitcher with water by dipping it into the larger ptitcher. Double-check water temperature. Carefully pour the warm water over the hair, moistening thoroughly. Take care not to overfill the shampoo tray (see Figure 4-11-3).	**15.** Smaller container is easier to manipulate and prevents splashing. Water temperature can change while sitting. Moistened hair facilitates the cleansing action of the shampoo.
16. Place a small amount of shampoo into your palms and massage it into the hair, working the shampoo into a lather (see Figure 4-11-4). Using your fingertips, gently massage the shampoo into the scalp.	**16.** Shampoo lather facilitates removal of dirt, debris, and excess oils from scalp and hair. Massage promotes lather, stimulates scalp circulation, and relaxes client.

continues

Action	Rationale

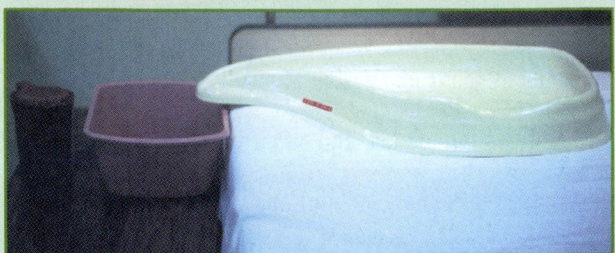

Figure 4-11-2   Position a basin to catch waste water from the shampoo tray.

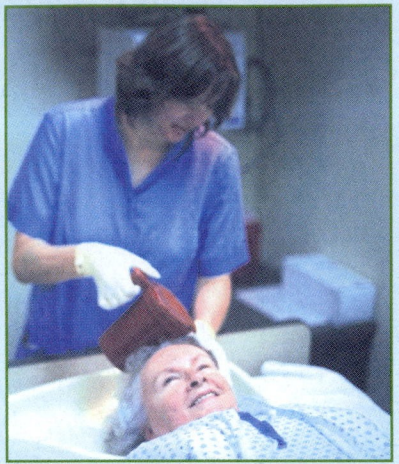

Figure 4-11-3   Pour the warm water over the hair and moisten thoroughly.

17. Rinse the hair by using the small pitcher to pour warm water over the hair and scalp (see Figure 4-11-5).

18. Repeat application of shampoo and massage scalp and hair gently but vigorously for a longer period of time. Observe hair and scalp for lesions, scaling, infection, and so on. Observe client for signs of relaxation and comfort.

19. Rinse again using several pitchers of water until hair and scalp are free of shampoo.

20. Apply conditioner or rinse as per product directions.

21. Support client's head while you remove the shampoo tray. Set to one side (see Figure 4-11-6).

17. Removes shampoo and debris.

18. Promotes thorough cleansing of hair and scalp, provides opportunity to observe hair and scalp abnormalities as fingers move through hair and across scalp, and massage relaxes scalp and shoulder muscles.

19. Removes remaining residue of shampoo.

20. Conditions hair and maintains client preferences.

21. Clears area for completion of procedure. Prevents inadvertent injury.

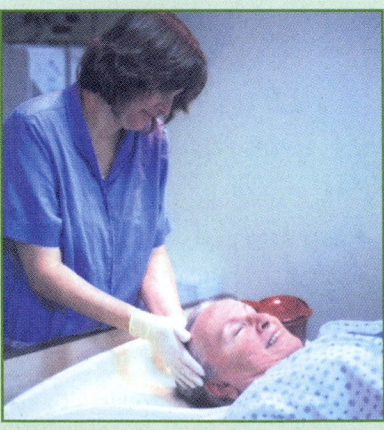

Figure 4-11-4   Massage the shampoo into a lather.

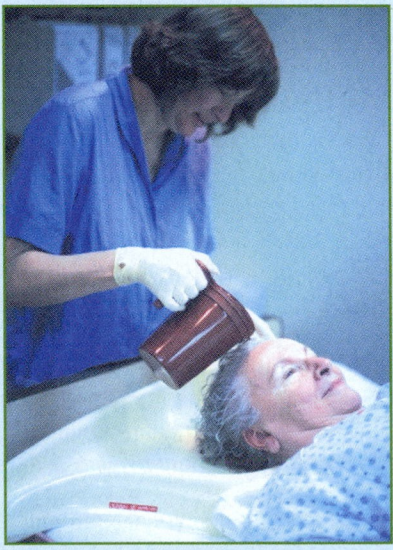

Figure 4-11-5   Rinse the hair using the pitcher to pour warm water over the scalp.

continues

Action	Rationale

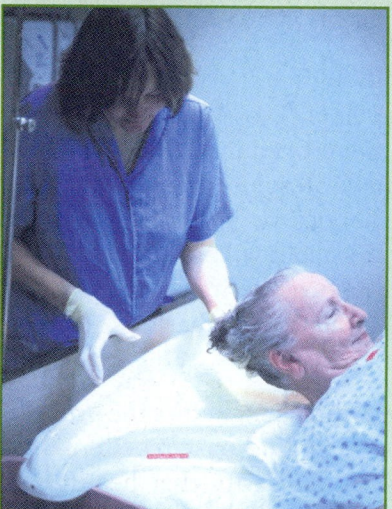

Figure 4-11-6   Support the client's head while removing the shampoo tray.

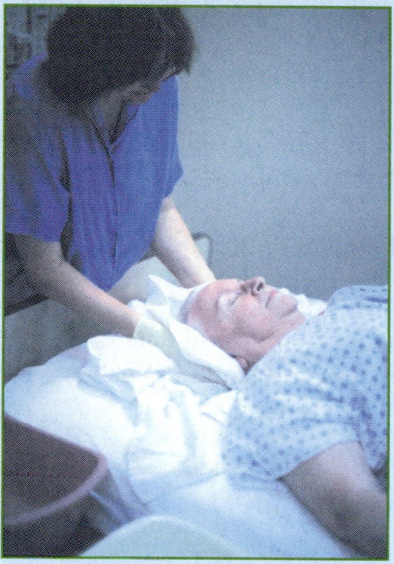

Figure 4-11-7   Dry the hair and scalp with a towel.

22. Wrap client's hair/head by gently pulling fanfolded bath towel from shoulders up and over scalp. Gently and briskly massage the scalp and hair with the towel (see Figure 4-11-7). Repeat with a dry towel as needed. Leave hair covered with the towel until ready to use the dryer.

22. Absorbs water from the hair and scalp while stimulating scalp circulation. Prevents chilling while waiting to dry the hair.

23. Remove the linen saver and towel from the bed by carefully folding inward.

23. Prevents debris from falling onto the bed or floor.

24. Elevate the head of bed to desired angle within prescribed and/or client-tolerated limits.

24. Promotes access to hair and client comfort.

25. Thoroughly dry your hands and/or change gloves.

25. Promotes safety in next steps.

26. Turn on hair dryer to warm setting and check the temperature on your inner arm.

26. Prevents injury from dryer heat.

27. Dry hair; concentrate on one section at a time, while moving your fingers, comb, or brush gently through the hair as it dries.

27. Facilitates drying and removes tangles.

28. Gently comb/brush the hair.

28. Removes all tangles and stimulates the scalp.

29. Style hair per client preference.

29. Maintaining personal appearance increases sense of well-being.

30. Reposition the client comfortably; adjust bed as requested within medical orders, safety measures, and communication needs (call light).

30. Maintains client comfort, rest, and safety.

31. Empty the water. Remove, clean, and return equipment.

31. Provides clean environment.

32. Remove gloves and wash your hands.

32. Reduces the transmission of microorganisms.

► EVALUATION

- The client has healthy hair and scalp free from infestation, infection, irritation, or alterations in hydration and oils.
- The client experienced improved circulation to the scalp.
- The client's comfort, self-esteem, and sense of well-being are improved.

► DOCUMENTATION

Nurses' Notes

- Document the time and date of the hair care.
- Note any unusual findings such as scaling, infestation, or infection.

Document on appropriate flow sheet or electronic medical record (EMR).

Medication Administration Record

- Record any prescription shampoo used or medications applied to the scalp.

► CRITICAL THINKING SKILL

Introduction

Client's hair is being washed and the client complains of itching and burning.

Possible Scenario

The client is sensitive or allergic to the shampoo or the health care provider inadvertently used an inappropriate solution.

Possible Outcome

The client develops hives, itching, and burning. Immediately stop the procedure, wash hair with lukewarm water to remove all solution, check the solution used, and verify allergies or past reactions to shampoos. Ascertain if the client will need medications for hives and itching. Report the incidence to the supervisor. Update allergy history in chart.

Prevention

Always check with client before the procedure regarding allergies, including past reactions to skin products or shampoos. Verify that health care provider used only labeled solutions and did not inadvertently use an iodine product or an irritating solution. Test solution on the client's skin before using.

► VARIATIONS

NOTE: The major variations are caused by the hair texture. Fine hair is typical in the elderly, those with fair skin (e.g., Scandinavians), and African Americans (whose hair is often mistaken as coarse). This is very important in their hair care. Fine hair usually does not need shampooing as frequently as other types. Twice a week is often appropriate.

Hair of medium texture is typical of Hispanics.

Coarse hair is typical in gray-haired individuals, Native Americans, and Asian clients. Blonde hair actually has fewer strands than brunette, and red hair generally has the greatest number of strands. Be sure to use a shampoo and conditioner designated for the texture of the hair.

Geriatric Variations:
- *Elderly clients may need adjustments in positioning because of loss of joint function or health restrictions.*
- *Gray hair needs routine (at least weekly) conditioning.*

Pediatric Variations:
- *Children may cooperate better if sitting, leaning forward, prone, or side-lying rather than lying supine.*
- *Encourage children to hold a washcloth over their eyes and use cotton in their ears to reduce the child's fear of getting soap and water in their eyes and ears.*
- *Infants and small children can be positioned on your lap for hair and scalp care.*

continues

▶ VARIATIONS *(continued)*

Home Care Variations:
- *Explore possible sites in the home. Be creative.*
- *A sprayer on the kitchen sink works well for rinsing. Inexpensive attachments are available for the tub as well.*
- *Plastic baby bathtubs can be used as a shampoo tray.*
- *Plastic shower liners are inexpensive protectors for under the towel. A liner can also be made into a shampoo tray by using rolled towels under it to shape a shallow U-reservoir that drains into a plastic pail on the floor.*

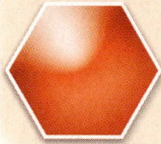

Long-Term Care Variations:
- *Long-term care clients often need adjustments in positioning as with geriatric clients.*
- *Hair should be combed two to three times a day. In addition to the traditional combing when the client is getting up or having company, combing the hair before the client rests may assist in relaxation.*

▶ COMMON ERRORS

Possible Error:

The nurse does not ask about the client's preferences and uses the wrong shampoo.

Prevention:

Determine whether the shampoo is appropriate for the client's hair. Assess the texture, client's activity level, medical condition, and medications. Ask clients what type of shampoo they normally use. Have a family member bring in shampoo.

Possible Error:

The nurse assumes that because clients are in bed all day they do not need shampooing as frequently.

Prevention:

The client needs hair care when the hair becomes oily, matted, or soiled with dandruff, perspiration, food, medications, or bodily fluids. This can be daily or every few days.

Possible Error:

The nurse does not assess the hair for possible problems that need treatment.

Prevention:

Do not assume hair loss results from "old age." Evaluate the client for poor circulation to the scalp; infection of hair follicles; overuse of conditioners, dyes, lubricants, straighteners, or braiding; poor nutrition; or medications. Dandruff may actually be dry skin. Real dandruff flakes are often greasy and may increase with stress, weather changes, poor hygiene, poor diet, or fungus.

▶ NURSING TIPS

- A folded bath blanket under the client's shoulders helps position the head in a slight hyperextension to facilitate water drainage during rinsing. A folded towel under the nondraining end of the shampoo tray helps drainage as well.

- If you detect flaking early, use a conditioner on the hair and avoid oils on the hair and scalp. Garlic shampoos or those with sulfur-containing compounds may help, too. Changing shampoo brands every 2 to 3 months seems to help as well.

- Broken hair strands indicate weakened hair usually secondary to dyes, tints, bleach, perms, medications, or poor nutrition. Hair preparations (other than shampoo and conditioning) must be stopped for 6 to 24 months (until hair has grown out naturally—about one-half inch per month) to restore hair.
- Perms can be imitated by braiding wet hair overnight and styling the next morning.
- Taking vitamin B complex two to three times a day promotes healthy hair.
- Hair that is naturally tightly curled is often configurated in whorls, which cause burrowing and trapped hairs. You must comb out carefully but thoroughly. Be gentle and take your time.
- Braiding is nice to prevent tangling in long or curly hair, but be sure braids and hair ties are loose at the scalp and positioned so they do not press against the scalp during the position assumed for the majority of the day or night.
- The less expensive hair care products often create a "waxy" buildup on the hair.
- Medications, especially for the thyroid and kidneys, often make hair oily and dirty faster.
- Braids (including cornrows) still need to be shampooed regularly. Dilute the shampoo by half and gently work it into the braids and over any exposed scalp. Rinse well as the lather can get trapped in the braids.
- Vitamin E oil, petrolatum, and mineral oil are often used to control and moisten what is perceived as dry hair. These occlude the pores and are not healthy for the scalp. The hair needs to be properly and consistently conditioned instead.
- Artificially colored hair requires more frequent conditioning—at every shampoo in addition to a deeper weekly conditioning.
- Oily hair is usually hereditary and can be helped by daily shampooing with warm water followed by rinsing with lemon juice or dilute vinegar then by a clear rinse.
- Styling can be facilitated by mousse to the roots, blow-drying small sections at a time with gentle guiding using a brush, and recurling the ends by wrapping them around a small round brush, hot rollers, or a medium curling iron (take care to avoid burns by keeping away from the scalp).
- A minimum of six glasses (8 oz. each) of water a day will significantly contribute to healthy skin and hair (and is inexpensive).
- Be sure to use a shampoo and conditioner designated for the texture of the hair.

▶ SPECIAL CONSIDERATIONS

- *Be aware of any cultural variations. For example, some cultures believe that hair washing immediately postpartum results in the client losing chi (energy) and is therefore prohibited. Involve client in the decision-making process for hair and scalp care.*
- *Client may choose to use over-the-counter products for hair loss. Client education should be provided regarding some of the possible overdose side effects such as hypertrichosis.*

Hand and Foot Care

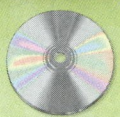

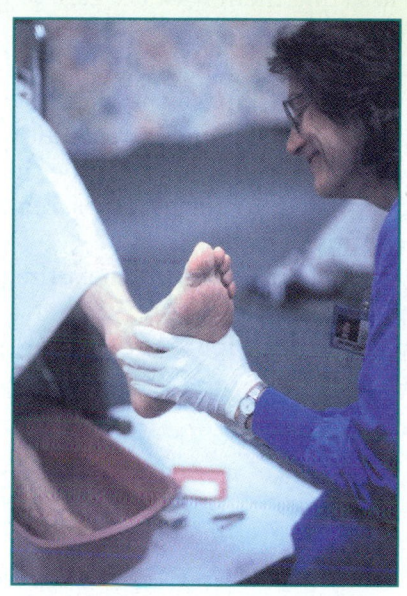

▶ OVERVIEW OF THE SKILL

Daily hand and foot care maintains the structure and function of two major body areas vital to mobility and the ability to carry out activities of daily living. It promotes cleanliness, controls odor, prevents infection, and stimulates circulation.

▶ ASSESSMENT

1. Assess skin integrity **to identify early intervention for abnormalities.**
2. Assess nail integrity **to identify present or potential disease or harm to skin.**
3. Assess structural integrity of hands and feet **to identify special needs of hands or feet.**
4. Assess functional status of hands and feet **to identify special needs of hands or feet.**
5. Identify allergies prior to the procedure **to avoid inadvertent client exposure.**
6. Assess client's knowledge and performance ability of basic hand and foot care **to identify baselines for client education.**
7. Assess client's preferences for cleansing agents, moisturizing agents, protective devices (socks, shoes, slippers), and equipment to be used in the procedure, and evaluate **them in light of function and safety.**

▶ DIAGNOSIS

Risk for Impaired Skin Integrity

Risk for Peripheral Neurovascular Dysfunction

Bathing/Hygiene Self-Care Deficit

▶ PLANNING

Expected Outcomes:

1. The client's hands and feet will be clean and odor-free, with soft, hydrated skin.
2. The client will experience maximized functional ability of hands and feet.
3. The client will be comfortable and relaxed.

Equipment Needed (see Figure 4-12-1):

- Gloves
- Bath/washbasin (plastic dishpan, bucket, or wastebasket will work as well)
- Warm water
- Towels (1–2)

425

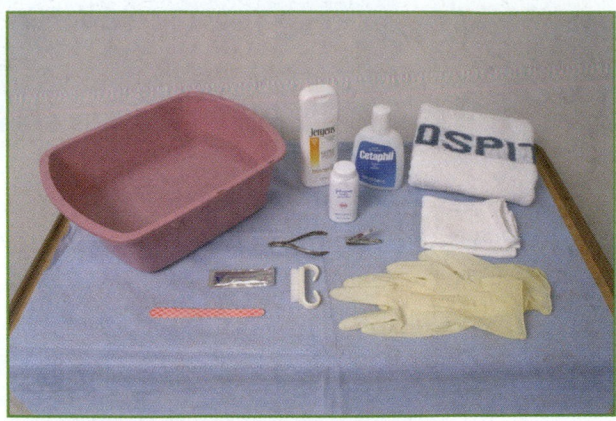

Figure 4-12-1 Equipment needed in providing hand and foot care.

- Washcloth (soft but textured)
- Soap (liquid preferable) or Cetaphil
- Nail brush (soft)
- Cotton-tip applicators
- Nail clippers: one for fingernails, plier-type for toenails
- Nail scissors (for cutting hangnails)
- Emery board
- Talcum powder (water absorbent without cornstarch)
- Body cream, petrolatum, or oil
- Optional/bath blanket
- Optional/linen-saver pad

- Optional/pillow
- Optional/cotton or lamb's wool pieces
- Optional/2 × 2 gauze pads
- Optional/bath thermometer

▶ **CLIENT EDUCATION NEEDED:**

1. Before the procedure, inform clients that you will be assisting them with the care of their hands and/or feet.
2. Explain each step of the procedure and help identify what assistance is needed.
3. During the procedure, educate about what to observe for and points to remember in self-care.
4. After the procedure, review steps, reminders, and recommendations.
5. Jointly evaluate needs for the next time the procedure is to be performed.
6. Offer the client tips for foot care (see Table 4-12-1).

Estimated time to complete the skill:
10–20 minutes

Table 4-12-1	Client Teaching Tips for Foot Care

1. The majority of foot problems are caused by tight-fitting shoes.

2. Report signs or symptoms of abnormalities in hands or feet:
   a. Pain, numbness, tingling
   b. Decreased sensation to touch or temperature
   c. Swelling, shiny appearance to skin
   d. Coldness (when previous sensation has been normal)
   e. Decreased hair growth or pulses
   f. Skin discoloration, bruising, cuts, cracks, scaling, itching
   g. Thickening or layering of skin or nails

3. Examine hands and feet daily. Report any changes. Use a mirror to see the bottoms of your feet.

4. Feel the inside of the shoes for foreign objects or rough spots before putting them on.

5. Check the water temperature before putting your hand or foot in. If using a thermometer, do not use glass; if no thermometer is available, test the temperature on the volar surface of the arm or place a few drops of water on your abdomen.

6. Avoid temperature extremes.

7. Put on extra socks if your feet are cold

8. Be sure shoes are wide enough and that there is room for a double pair of socks.

continues

Table 4-12-1   Client Teaching Tips for Foot Care (continued)

9. Shoes should provide good, gentle support and soft arch support (running shoes are usually good). Sandals, leather, and canvas also are good choice; they allow your feet to air.

10. Wear nonslip shower shoes in locker rooms, at camp, and so forth to protect your feet from injury and infection.

11. Break in new shoes slowly, that is, 30 minutes a day. Check your feet often for pressure points.

12. Shake shoes and slippers out as you take them off and before you put them on.

13. Change shoes two to three times a day to help prevent pressure areas. Change to a different style or brand so arch, sole, and heel supports vary. If this is not possible, change shoe inserts (soft ones) to vary the pressure.

14. Let your shoes "rest" every other day, if possible (don't wear the same shoes 2 days in a row).

15. Drink more water and juice if your skin is dry.

16. Exercise for 5 to 10 minutes every day to maintain good circulation.

17. Rest feet for brief periods throughout the day.

18. Maintain ideal body weight by eating a balanced diet filled with vegetables.

19. Avoid using a heating pad. Double your socks or gloves instead; put on a thin cotton sock and then a thicker wool sock (if not allergic).

20. Avoid hot water immersion. Use warm or cool water instead.

21. Avoid wearing high-heeled, narrow-heeled, or pointed-toe shoes.

22. Avoid knee-high stockings that leave a mark or indentation in your skin.

23. Avoid crossing legs at the knees.

24. Avoid smoking. It decreases the circulation to hands and feet.

▶ DELEGATION TIPS

Hand and foot care may be delegated to ancillary personnel in the nondiabetic client or client with peripheral vascular disease or peripheral neuropathy. Assessment of bilateral color, temperature, movement, and sensation should be a routine part of foot care. Any unusual appearance or condition of the skin and nails should be reported to the nurse.

IMPLEMENTATION—Action/Rationale

Action	Rationale
1. Explain to client planned procedure and confirm that client has no allergies (especially ask about latex, soaps, fragrances, creams, talc).	1. Enlist client compliance. Confirm that the client is not allergic to the materials to be used.
2. Assemble equipment.	2. Organization saves time, increases efficiency.

continues

Action	Rationale
3. Seat client in stable, comfortable chair. For feet: • Remind client not to sit on side of bathtub. • If bedridden, pull bedding out at the foot of the bed and fold upward to expose feet/lower legs. • If bedridden and bathing concurrently, cover client with bath blanket.	3. Ensures safety and maximizes client ability to assist. • Bathtub side becomes slippery and dangerous. • Keeps client warm while washing extremities.
4. Place linen saver (or towel) under client's hands/feet.	4. Protects the floor/bed from moisture.
5. Wash your hands; apply gloves.	5. Reduces the transmission of microorganisms.
6. Fill basin halfway with warm (not hot) water. Test temperature and place basin on the linen saver (see Figure 4-12-2).	6. Allows room for water to rise with immersion. Water temperature should not exceed 105° F (40.6° C).
7. Assist (place) client's hand/foot into the basin. Immerse. • If bedridden, have client bend knees to immerse foot in the water, place a pillow under the knees prn, and cushion the basin rim with the edge of the towel.	7. Provides support. • Prevents pressure on legs.
8. Soak hand/foot 2–10 minutes, depending on client's health and tolerance.	8. Softens skin, nails, and debris. Relaxes muscles and promotes client comfort. Limit time if systemic disease present: minimizes possible skin injury/infection.
9. Wash hand/foot with scant amount of a mild antibacterial soap; Cetaphil lotion may be used in place of soap (see Figure 4-12-3).	9. Soap is drying but a helpful surfactant. Cetaphil is a soapless, mild, antibacterial cleanser.
10. Rinse well to be sure all soap is removed.	10. Soap can irritate skin, so remove all residual.
11. Remove hand/foot from the basin and place directly onto clean towel.	11. Absorbs moisture.
12. Pat and then gently rub dry, paying close attention to between and under the fingers/toes.	12. Dries without harsh rubbing to prevent skin damage.

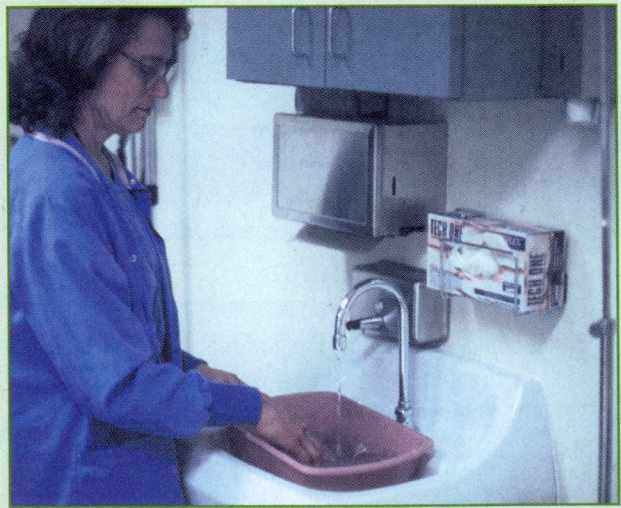

Figure 4-12-2 Fill basin halfway with warm water.

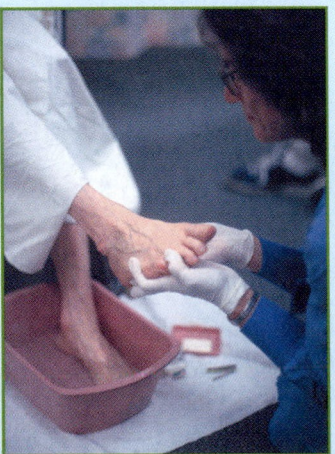

Figure 4-12-3 Wash with a small amount of antibacterial soap.

continues

Action	Rationale

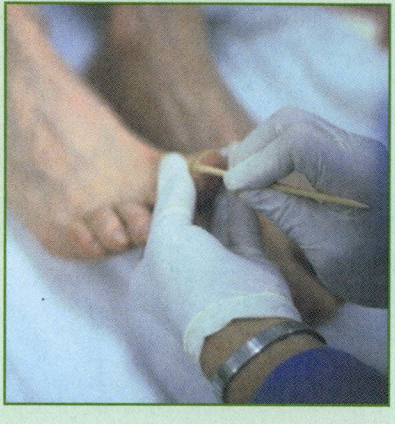

Figure 4-12-4   Using a cuticle stick, gently push the cuticle and subungual skin back.

13. Using the towel, or cuticle stick, gently push the cuticle and subungual skin back, checking nail edges. Do not "disturb" cuticles (see Figure 4-12-4).

13. Cuticle functions to prevent infection. Discourages ingrown nails and hangnails.

14. Use a towel or stone pumice on any thickened, dry skin areas (usually heels and medial side of large toe).

14. Discourages formation of corns and calluses.

15. Lightly powder between and under fingers/toes. (Do not shake directly onto client. Put in your hand or on a towel to apply.)

15. Maintains dryness between fingers and toes to discourage infection and skin breakdown. Talc absorbs moisture, but too much is counterproductive.

16. Concurrently assess skin and function. Observe color, shape, and texture. Note dryness, redness, cracks, blisters, discoloration, trauma, pain, numbness, tingling, swelling, muscle wasting, decreased sensation, hair growth, or pulses.

16. Observation for early prevention. Extremities are vulnerable to infections and need prompt treatment.

17. Check pulses, turgor, and capillary refill.

17. Assesses circulation and hydration to extremity.

18. Empty basin and refill. Repeat procedure with other hand/foot.

18. Provides warm water for opposite extremity.

19. While other hand/foot soaks, perform nail care on the first hand/foot.
    • Ask client's permission before cutting nails, especially the fingernails.
    • Note any areas where toenails may be injuring adjacent toes. Trim to prevent further damage.
    • Cut toenails straight across.
    • Trim fingernails according to client taste. If the client is confused or comatose, trim to prevent the client from injuring self or others.

19. Maximizes use of time.
    • Keep nails trimmed to avoid injury to skin on opposite limb as well as to the digit.
    • To prevent ingrown nails.

20. Lightly apply cream (not lotion), massaging into the hand/foot. Pay special attention to dry areas. Avoid between and under fingers/toes.

20. Maintains hydration, rehydrates skin.

21. "Towel" off any excess cream.

21. Avoids buildup and skin maceration.

continues

Action	Rationale
22. Perform range of motion exercises (repeat each movement 3–10 times): flex-extend, rotate clockwise, rotate counterclockwise, abduct-adduct fingers/toes.	22. Maintains function.
23. Place lamb's wool or cotton to protect areas that are rubbing or irritated. Put on clean, dry, absorbent (cotton) socks after foot care.	23. Protects skin.
24. Run your hand around the interior of shoes and slippers to be sure there are no foreign objects or scratchy edges prior to putting them on.	24. Protects skin.
25. Remove, clean, and/or replace equipment/supplies.	25. Avoids accidents and maintains cleanliness.
26. Dispose of gloves and wash hands.	26. Reduces the transmission of microorganisms.

▶ REAL WORLD ANECDOTES

Mr. Facundo was a middle-aged, grossly obese male with type II diabetes. Mr. Facundo lived independently and worked full time. Because of his size, he was unable to reach his feet to wash them or to perform foot care. When he went to see his endocrinologist, he complained of pain in his feet. The endocrinologist referred Mr. Facundo to a podiatrist. The podiatrist noted that Mr. Facundo's feet were heavily callused and covered in dead skin. While trimming the calluses from Mr. Facundo's feet with a razor blade, the podiatrist's hand slipped and cut Mr. Facundo's foot. Because of Mr. Facundo's diabetic peripheral vascular disease, the cut failed to heal properly and became infected, and required extensive treatment to prevent necrosis and the need for amputation.

▶ EVALUATION

- The client's hands and feet are clean and odor free, with soft, hydrated skin.
- The client experiences maximized functional ability of hands and feet.
- The client is comfortable and relaxed.

▶ DOCUMENTATION

Nurses' Notes

- Record the time and date care was performed.
- Note any unusual findings, open areas, or significant changes.
- Document on appropriate flow sheet or electronic medical record (EMR)

▶ CRITICAL THINKING SKILL

Introduction (see Figure 4-12-5)

Mr. Espinosa is a 75-year-old obese man with Alzheimer's, hypertension, and a family history of diabetes. Although he has not been diagnosed with diabetes, he does have symptoms of peripheral vascular disease. He kidded about his "wooden" ankle and feet, noting some pain but little feeling in them. His provider had not instructed him in foot care, usually addressing the more global, multiple concerns instead. His nurse neighbor was chatting one day midwinter in the

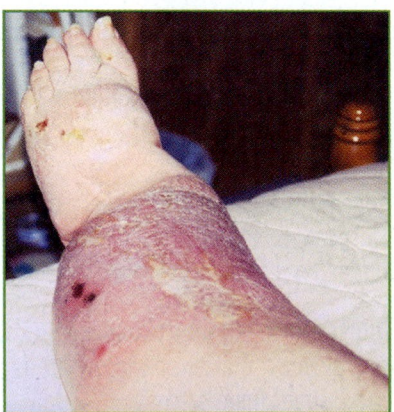

Figure 4-12-5   Clients may have feet in poor condition with skin breakdown, decreased sensation, or poor circulation.

yard with him when Mr. Espinosa mentioned that he thought he probably needed to go inside and change his socks. The nurse noticed him feeling his socks with his fingers to check for moisture. When she asked whether he could feel the cold and moisture, he admitted he could not feel it on his feet. She asked if his doctor had instructed him in foot care and how to take care of his feet if he could not feel them. Because he did not have a home health nurse, she offered to stop over later, when it would be convenient for him, to be sure his feet were all right and review some points of foot care that might help him.

Possible Scenario

As a result of his neighbor's visit, Mr. Espinosa remembered to soak his feet in warm water. However, because of his advanced peripheral vascular disease, he is unable to accurately assess the temperature of the water.

Possible Outcome

Mr. Espinosa's feet were numb secondary to his diabetic peripheral neurovascular disease. However, he was not aware of that and thought that his feet were numb from the winter cold. Despite soaking his feet, they did not seem to warm up. Mr. Espinosa continued to add more and more hot water to his footbath.

He was not aware that the water was too hot and scalding his feet. When his neighbor returned later in the week to check on Mr. Espinosa, she noticed that his feet were badly scalded and took him to see his doctor. The burns on his feet required months of daily dressing changes to heal.

Mr. Espinosa's neighbor was careful to explain about the need for temperature control. She was aware that he would not be able to accurately judge the water temperature without a thermometer. Before stopping over to show Mr. Espinosa some foot care techniques, his neighbor stopped by a drug store and purchased a bath thermometer as a gift for Mr. Espinosa.

Prevention

Instruct him to always test the temperature of the water before inserting his feet by using a thermometer (not glass) or by dropping a few drops onto the volar surface of his arm or onto his abdomen (check to be sure sensation there is normal). Instruct him to time how long his feet are in the water, recommending no more than 2 minutes at a time. Suggest that he put on a thin pair of cotton socks followed by a thicker pair of wool socks to warm up rather than keeping his feet in the water longer. Reinforce his self-discovered habit of checking his foot environment.

▶ VARIATIONS

Geriatric Variations:
- Elderly skin is very similar to that of premature infants: lacking subcutaneous tissue, frail, easily injured, and slow to repair. Use Cetaphil rather than soap, avoid tape on the skin, and exercise extra caution in preventive measures.

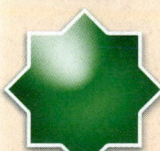

Pediatric Variations:
- Give the child a toy to play with in the water.
- Children's fingernails and toenails are much smaller. Be sure to use implements of the proper size.

Home Care Variations:
- Use whatever the client prefers for supplies and equipment as long as they are safe.
- Be sure to teach caregivers how to perform this care as well as teaching the client.

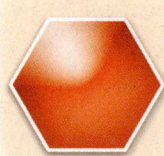

Long-Term Care Variations:
- If client is bedridden and foot care is part of bathing, soak the foot while you wash the leg.
- Place a pillow under the client's knees to increase comfort.

► **COMMON ERRORS**

Possible Error:

The nurse does not get the area between and under fingers and toes dry.

Prevention:

Skin between and under fingers and toes macerates easily if left moist. Warm, moist areas also promote the growth of fungal infections. Dry this area thoroughly.

► **NURSING TIPS**

- Observe hand posturing and, if necessary to maintain neutral position, position a hand roll in the client's hands after care.
- Insert 2 × 2 gauze pads or pieces of lamb's wool (if not allergic to wool) between overlapping toes to protect the adjacent skin.
- Check shoe size by drawing around the client's foot (standing if possible) and placing the shoe on the drawing. Be sure the forefoot has plenty of room. Teach the client to do likewise when shoe shopping.
- If the client is ticklish, use the heel of your hand and press firmly when massaging the bottom of the foot.
- Oil (olive, mineral, Vitamin E) or petroleum jelly may be used in place of cream if the skin is extremely dry or the client prefers it.
- If edema has been present, massage the foot 2 to 3 minutes in an elevated position and then leave it in a supported elevated position for 20 minutes if possible.
- Rub excess cream or oil on knees, elbow, or hands to use it up. Combine with exercise by rubbing the bottom of the foot down the opposite shin.
- An emery board may be used as a pumice stone if used very gently and the callus is large.

- Do not use a pumice stone or emery board on the skin of clients with peripheral vascular disease or systemic disease.
- If clients are "bored" with exercising, or need more variety, have them use their toes to pick up marbles and put them in a container. Also exercise and observe cerebellar function by touching thumb tip to each fingertip, counting them forward and backward: 1-2-3-4-4-3-2-1. Then rotate the wrist with rapid alternating hand movements by tapping the finger pads then backs of hand on the palm of the opposite hand in a "flipping the pancake" motion. Change hands.
- Shoes are not necessary for infants until they start walking. Infant shoes should be flexible (able to be flexed with one hand). A flat-footed appearance is normal. Large arch supports and rigid shoes are unnecessary and unhealthy (and usually the most expensive).
- Barefoot is healthy only if feet are safe from injury.
- Educate parents that it is normal for children to outgrow two to four pairs of shoes a year.
- A bilateral comparison of color, temperature, movement, and sensation should be a routine aspect of hand and foot care.

► **SPECIAL CONSIDERATIONS**

- *Special client precautions to prevent burns and cuts should be implemented when providing hand and foot care to diabetic, postoperative-anesthetic, or pain-medicated clients, or in cases of impaired peripheral sensory function.*
- *Clients with a decrease in circulation, such as those with peripheral vascular disease, are at a high risk for injury to extremities. As sensation may decrease with injury to nerves, clients may not be aware of sores. Alert clients to the need for daily inspection of feet and especially heels, tips of toes, and between toes. Once injury has occurred, the healing process is slowed; therefore, prevention is of utmost importance.*

Shaving a Client

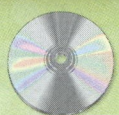

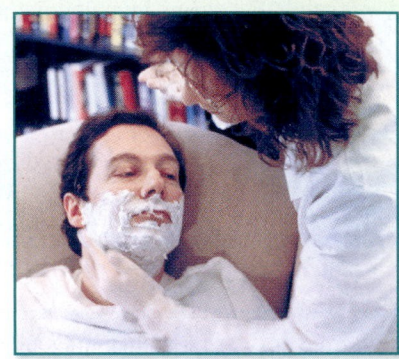

▶ OVERVIEW OF THE SKILL

Shaving the male client is done to remove facial hair if the client is unable to complete this self-care. It is usually done after a bath or shower and as often as required to remove unwanted facial hair. Most men shave every day, although the facial hair of older clients does not grow as rapidly. If a beard or mustache is present, it should be groomed daily and trimmed as appropriate. Do not shave off beards or mustaches without the client's permission.

▶ ASSESSMENT

1. Assess whether the client is able to perform self-care. **Promote independence when possible.**
2. Assess the client's skin for areas of redness, skin breakdown, moles, or skin lesions. **Shaving could irritate the skin further.**
3. Assess whether the client has a bleeding tendency or is on anticoagulants. **If there is an increased risk of bleeding, an electric razor should be used.**
4. If the client prefers to shave himself, assess the client's ability to manipulate the razor. **The client must be able to shave safely.**
5. Assess the client's preference for the type of shaving, type of equipment, and type of lotion (if there are options). **This promotes independence.**

▶ DIAGNOSIS

Dressing/Grooming Self-Care Deficit

Risk for Injury

Low Self-Esteem

▶ PLANNING

Expected Outcomes:

1. The client will be neat and well-groomed.
2. The client's skin integrity will remain intact.
3. If the client is able to shave or able to assist, the client will attain a sense of independence.
4. The client will be comfortable following the procedure.

Equipment Needed

- Electric razor or disposable razor
- Shaving cream or soap
- Warm water
- Washcloth and bath towel
- Washbasin
- After-shave lotion (if the client has no skin irritation and if the client prefers lotion)
- Mirror
- Sharp scissors and comb if mustache care is required
- Gloves

▶ CLIENT EDUCATION NEEDED:

1. Most male clients are usually experienced at shaving themselves and can share preferences and techniques with staff.

2. In clients who require facial surgery, all hair should be shaved to avoid microorganisms in the wound site.
3. If the client has unsteady hands, an electric razor should be used.

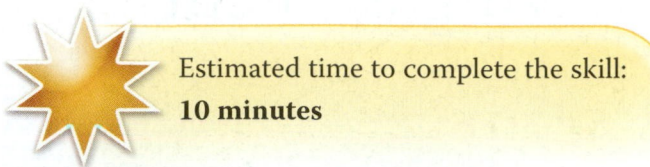

Estimated time to complete the skill:
10 minutes

▶ DELEGATION TIPS

Shaving the adult male client is routinely delegated. Caution must be exercised with intubated clients to maintain the integrity of their tubes.

IMPLEMENTATION—Action/Rationale

Action	Rationale
1. Wash hands and apply gloves (see Figure 4-13-1).	1. Reduces the transmission of microorganisms.
2. Assist the client to a comfortable position. If the client can shave himself, set up the equipment and supplies, including warm water, and watch the client for safety. Adjust lighting as needed.	2. Facilitates comfort and ease of shaving. Encourages sense of self-control and independence.
3. Place a towel over the client's chest and shoulder.	3. Protects the client and gown from soil.
4. Position the client. Raise the bed to a comfortable height, move the client to the sink, or have the client sit in a comfortable position.	4. Facilitates comfort of staff and prevents injury to client.
5. Fill a washbasin with water at approximately 44° C (110° F). Check temperature for comfort.	5. Warm water helps to soften the skin and beard. Warmth can be relaxing.
6. Place the washcloth in the basin and wring out thoroughly. Apply the cloth over the client's entire face.	6. Warm water helps to soften the skin and beard. Warmth can be relaxing.
7. Apply shaving cream.	7. Helps soften the whiskers.
8. Take the razor in the dominant hand and hold it at a 45-degree angle to the client's skin. Start shaving across one side of the client's face. Use the nondominant hand to gently pull the skin taut while shaving. Use short, firm strokes in the direction hair grows. Use short, downward strokes over the upper lip area (see Figure 4-13-2).	8. Holding the skin taut prevents razor cuts and discomfort during shaving.

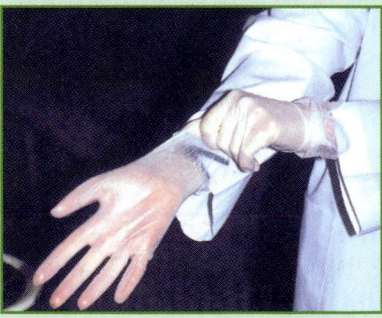

Figure 4-13-1 Wash hands and apply gloves.

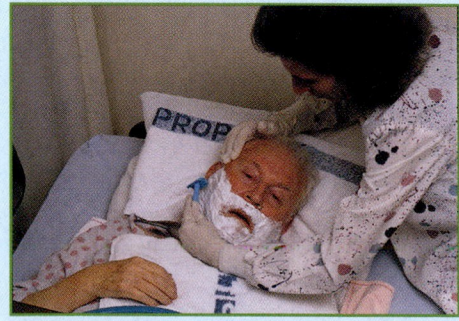

Figure 4-13-2 Shave with short, firm strokes in the direction the hair grows.

continues

Action	Rationale
9. Dip the razor in water as cream accumulates.	9. Keeps the cutting edge of the razor clean.
10. Check the face to see whether all the facial hair is removed.	10. Ensures a neat appearance.
11. After all the facial hair is removed, rinse the face thoroughly with a moistened washcloth.	11. Promotes comfort and cleanliness.
12. Dry the face thoroughly and apply after-shave lotion if desired.	12. Stimulates and lubricates the skin.
13. Assist the client to a comfortable position and allow him to inspect the results of your shave.	13. Facilitates comfort and a sense of control.
14. Dispose of equipment in proper receptacle.	14. Equipment should not be shared between clients in accordance with Standard Precautions as disruption of skin and bleeding may occur. The client may, however, keep his own razor. Clean and store it at the bedside.
15. Remove gloves. Wash hands.	15. Reduces the transmission of microorganisms.

► REAL WORLD ANECDOTES

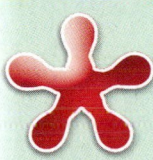

While performing Mr. Alfred's daily care, the nurse decided to trim his mustache, which had grown long enough to cover his upper lip. Mr. Alfred agreed that his mustache could use a trim and the nurse proceeded to snip away. As she was finishing the trim she noticed that Mr. Alfred's mustache was now lopsided. As she tried to even his mustache out, trimming first one side and then the other, Mr. Alfred watched in horror as his mustache slowly disappeared. Finally, in a desperate effort to save at least a little of his mustache, he stopped the nurse, explaining that he was very happy with its current look.

► EVALUATION

- The client is neat and well-groomed.
- The client's skin integrity remained intact.
- If the client was able to shave or assist, the client attained a sense of independence.
- The client is comfortable following the procedure.

► DOCUMENTATION

Nurses' Notes

- Document the procedure, if the client was able to assist, and how the client tolerated the activity.
- Note any unusual findings or injury that may have occurred.

Document on appropriate flow sheet or electronic medical record (EMR).

► CRITICAL THINKING SKILL

Introduction

You are caring for a client with a decreased platelet count. You grab a disposable razor and hand it to the client, who is quizzical but proceeds to shave. He mentions to his wife that he has brought his own electric razor from home.

Possible Scenario

Client cuts himself deeply. He starts bleeding.

Possible Outcome

He has prolonged bleeding, then continues to ooze the rest of the morning. He mentions that he has used an electric razor for 20 years and had lost the "knack" of shaving with foam and a blade.

Prevention

Remember to be aware when shaving any male client with bleeding problems. Use an electric razor that the family has brought from home. Listen to the client and assess skill level before allowing the client to perform any procedure.

▶ VARIATIONS

Geriatric Variations:
- *Older clients have thin, wrinkled skin and may be more easily cut.*
- *Older clients may have unsteady hands and require some assistance and patience.*
- *Some older clients have not used an electric razor or may prefer their own equipment.*
- *Older clients may need a warm towel in place for a longer time to soften the skin.*
- *Facial hair grows slower in elderly clients, and they may not require daily shaving.*

Pediatric Variations:
- *Adolescents may be embarrassed to have staff shave them and may feel a lack of independence.*
- *Provide privacy if needed.*
- *Adolescents may have unusual tastes in grooming and toiletries. Support choice, and enlist the aid of a parent if you are uncertain.*
- *Children need careful explanations if they must have their hair shaved that the hair will grow back and other reassurance to minimize bodily image disturbance.*

Home Care Variations:
- *If clients are unsteady, they may require an electric razor. Make sure the home razor has fresh, sharp blades.*
- *Listen to the routines of the client when you are in his or her home. Routines convey a sense of control and normalcy for the client. The client may be able to perform self-care tasks much more independently in the home setting than in the unfamiliar hospital setting. Facilitate independence as much as possible.*

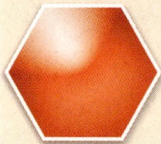

Long-Term Care Variation:
- *Do not overlook the psychosocial benefits of hands-on care. Shaving and grooming can be a special time for social contact and caring between the client and friends and family. Family members often feel a sense of helplessness watching a loved one struggle. These frustrations may be lessened if they can become involved in feeding and caring for someone they love. The client may enjoy the time and special attention and improved self-esteem as he is well-groomed for friends, family, and staff.*

▶ COMMON ERRORS

Possible Error:

The nurse is too rushed and does not involve the client.

Prevention:

Plan ahead so you are not rushed. A family member might wish to come in and assist with shaving.

continues

▶ **COMMON ERRORS** *(continued)*

Possible Error:

The nurse is too rushed and cuts the client.

Prevention:

Plan ahead so you are not rushed. Ask the client how best to shave him. He is the expert.

Possible Error:

Warm towels not kept in place long enough to soften skin.

Prevention:

Plan ahead so you are not rushed. Have the client or family member hold the towel in place long enough to soften the skin.

Possible Error:

Hair not shaved daily and allowed to grow longer will be more difficult to shave.

Prevention:

Set aside time to shave your client. If you do not have time, enlist the aid of a family member or other caregiver.

▪ **NURSING TIPS**

- Shave daily or as needed.
- Be careful to use a 45-degree angle to avoid cuts.
- Use new and disposable razors.
- Sometimes a client may be shaking and slow. This requires patience on the part of the staff.

▶ **SPECIAL CONSIDERATIONS**

- *Teach clients to never share the shaving blade or razor, even with partners, to prevent blood-borne transmitted diseases.*
- *Extra care should be taken to avoid cutting clients on anticoagulants. An electric razor should be used.*
- *Protect endotracheal or tracheostomy tubes with a towel. If client has a tracheostomy tube and is not intubated, do not completely cover tracheostomy to avoid blockage of air.*

Giving a Back Rub

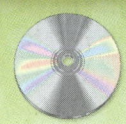

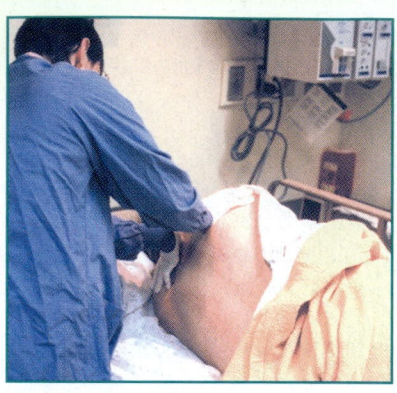

▶ OVERVIEW OF THE SKILL

Giving a back rub is a basic nursing skill. Back massage can be an effective means of building a sense of trust and increased rapport between the nurse and client. Clients are often touch-deprived in the busy health care industry of today. The small amount of time that it takes to do a simple back massage can often soothe and relax a "difficult" client and increase the effectiveness of the nurse–client relationship.

Massage can be performed in many different ways, from light strokes to heavy kneading. Various forms include effleurage, deep or gentle stroking, and pétrissage, a kneading performed with the tips of the fingers and thumbs or palm of the hand. Massage can stimulate circulation and promote lymphatic drainage, thereby helping to rid the body of metabolic wastes, speed healing, and provide gentle relaxation. Massage can open lines of communication and improve the therapeutic relationship between a nurse and client. A simple back massage is easily learned by nurses and caregivers and can be done in as little as 5 to 10 minutes.

▶ ASSESSMENT

1. Assess the client's willingness to have a massage. **The client may not want a massage or may not enjoy the tactile experience of a massage.**
2. Assess the client for contraindications of a back rub **to prevent injuring the client.** Conditions include open sores or lesions, vertebral fractures, burns, and signs of decubitus ulcers.

3. Assess any limitations the client has in positioning **to determine whether the client has any conditions that prohibit a side-lying or prone position.**
4. Assess the client for fatigue, stiffness, or soreness in the back and shoulders. **Knowing areas of particular concern allows you to focus your energies toward "trouble areas."**
5. Assess the client for anxiety or emotional disturbances. **Massage can help to reduce anxiety and calm people in distress.**
6. If possible, have the client quantify the degree of discomfort using a 1 to 10 rating scale. **Quantifying the results can provide more validity to the intervention.**

▶ DIAGNOSIS

Anxiety

Pain

Impaired Physical Mobility

Readiness for Enhanced Comfort

▶ PLANNING

Expected Outcomes:

1. The client will experience a reduction in tension, anxiety, pain, and fatigue.
2. The nurse will establish a better rapport with the client.

Equipment Needed:

- Quiet environment, free of interruptions, with a comfortable room temperature
- Comfortable bed or massage table that allows a client to lie in a side-lying or prone position
- Bath blanket
- Bath towel, to absorb excess moisture, oils
- Lotion, baby powder, or massage oil
- Gloves, if necessary

▶ **CLIENT EDUCATION NEEDED:**

1. Explain the procedure and potential benefits to the client.

2. Arrive at a mutually agreed upon time that you will massage.
3. Assure clients that they may discontinue the massage at any time.
4. Encourage clients to give you feedback regarding the amount of pressure you are giving them.

Estimated time to complete the skill:
5–10 minutes, as tolerated by client

▶ **DELEGATION TIPS**

Giving a back rub to a client is routinely delegated to properly trained ancillary personnel, who should communicate the client's response to the back rub to the nurse.

IMPLEMENTATION—Action/Rationale

Action	Rationale
1. Wash your hands and apply gloves, if necessary.	1. Reduces the transmission of microorganisms.
2. Help client to a prone or side-lying position (see Figure 4-14-1).	2. Exposes back and shoulder area.
3. Drape the bath blanket, and undo the client's gown, exposing the back, shoulder, and sacral area, but keeping the remainder of the body covered (see Figure 4-14-2).	3. Prevents chilling and excess exposure.

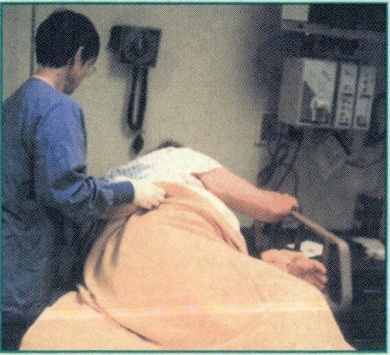

Figure 4-14-1   Position client in a prone or side-lying position.

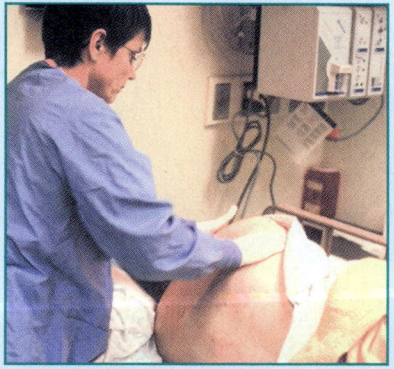

Figure 4-14-2   Expose the back, shoulder, and sacral area.

continues

Action	Rationale

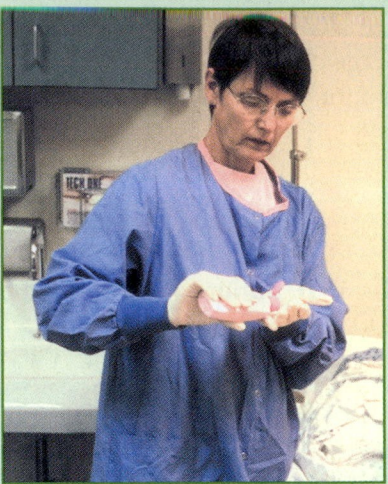

Figure 4-14-3 Pour lotion on your hand and warm between your palms.

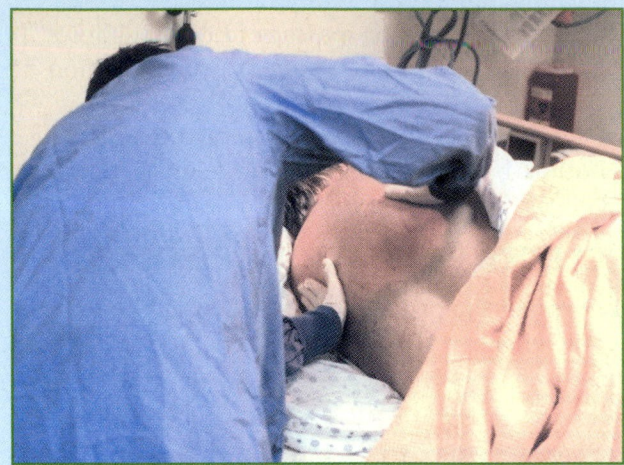

Figure 4-14-4 Apply firm continuous pressure without breaking contact between your hands and the client's skin.

4. Pour a small amount of lotion in your hand and warm between your palms for a few moments. The lotion bottle can also be submerged in a bowl of warm water for a few minutes to warm the lotion. Baby powder may be substituted for oils or lotions (see Figure 4-14-3).

4. Prevents the shock of cold lotion being applied to the body. Some clients may be sensitive to oils or lotions.

5. Begin in the sacral area with smooth, circular strokes, moving upward toward the shoulders. Gradually lengthen the strokes (effleurage) to the upper back, scapulae, and upper arms. Apply firm, continuous pressure without breaking contact with the client (see Figures 4-14-4 and 4-14-5).

5. Applying firm, continuous pressure increases circulation and relaxation.

6. Assess the client's back as you are massaging for areas of redness and signs of decreased circulation.

6. Monitors for signs of early skin breakdown.

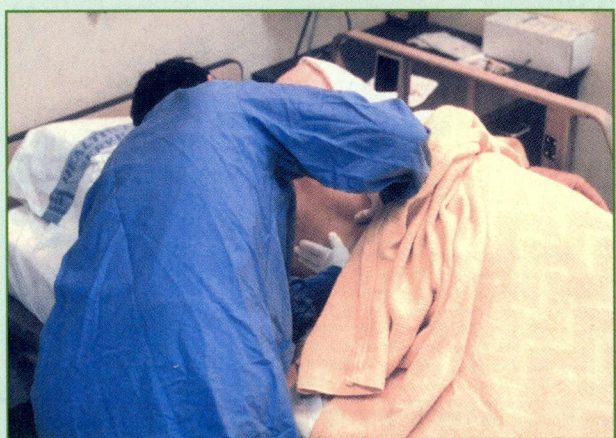

Figure 4-14-5 Use long circular strokes from the sacral area upward toward the shoulders.

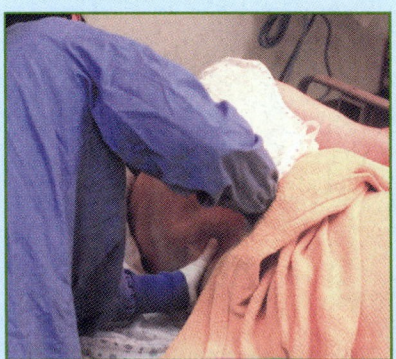

Figure 4-14-6 Use firm kneading massage on areas of increased muscle tension.

continues

Action	Rationale

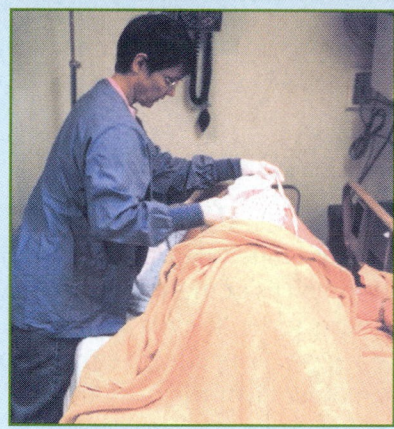

Figure 4-14-7 Finish the massage with light brush strokes, using the fingertips.

Figure 4-14-8 Cover the client after the massage for warmth and modesty.

7. Provide a firm, kneading massage (pétrissage) to areas of increased tension, if desired, in areas such as the shoulders and gluteal muscles (see Figure 4-14-6).

7. Firm, kneading strokes can decrease muscle tension, reducing pain and increasing relaxation.

8. Complete the massage with long, very light brush strokes, using the tips of the fingers (see Figure 4-14-7).

8. This is a very relaxing stroke and signals an end to the massage.

9. Gently pat or wipe excess lubricant off the client and cover the client (see Figure 4-14-8).

9. Prevents soiling of the bed with excess lotions and keeps the client warm.

10. Remove gloves. Wash hands.

10. Reduces the transmission of microorganisms.

▶ REAL WORLD ANECDOTES

Mrs. Mai was a client admitted to the hospital for failure to thrive. She was admitted to the oncology floor because it was the only floor with an available bed. Mrs. Mai was cold to the nurses, withdrawn, and obviously depressed. She told the nurses on many occasions that nobody really cared about her. During her morning bed bath, a nurse noticed that she was developing some redness over the bony areas of her shoulders and buttocks. The nurse informed Mrs. Mai that she was going to massage some lotion on her back. Mrs. Mai reluctantly agreed to the massage. After about 10 minutes of massage, Mrs. Mai stated that her back "felt a little better." The next morning, during her bed bath, Mrs. Mai asked the nurse if she would do another one of those "back rubs." This became an every-morning activity with Mrs. Mai with each nurse. She became more animated with the nurses and less withdrawn, looking forward to her morning massage.

▶ EVALUATION

- The client experienced a reduction in tension, anxiety, pain, and fatigue.
- The nurse established a better rapport with the client.

▶ DOCUMENTATION

Nurses' Notes

- Record the time and date the back rub was performed.
- Note the client's response to the back rub.

- Record any complaints of pain or tension the client reported.
- Document any unusual findings.

Document on appropriate flow sheet or electronic medical record (EMR).

► CRITICAL THINKING SKILL

Introduction

The aged are often touch-deprived, even though they need touch as much as or more than other age groups. Often, they have fewer friends or family members, and touch can serve as an effective means of communication when other channels of communication have been reduced.

Possible Scenario

Mrs. Zaricor, an 84-year-old woman, has been in a nursing home for a month. She is hard-of-hearing and has extremely poor eyesight despite glasses. She has had no visitors and has been reluctant to interact with any other clients in the home. She has been withdrawn from staff, and voices few complaints other than nagging aches and pains in her shoulders and back. The nurses doing her morning care have been giving her a 5- to 10-minute back massage this past week.

Possible Outcome

Mrs. Zaricor has reported fewer problems with her back and shoulders. She has been warming up to the nurses and has been talking about her past. She still is not taking part in group activities; however, she has been going to the group room to be around others.

Prevention

Taking the time for a simple back massage has opened up a channel of communication with Mrs. Zaricor that was otherwise inaccessible. Massage has built a level of trust and assurance that the nurses care about her as a person and are willing to take time to be with her.

► VARIATIONS

Geriatric Variations:
- *Assess for and avoid areas of chronic pain related to arthritis or injury.*
- *Assess for contraindications such as cancer within the past 5 years, blood-clotting disorders, or hypertension.*
- *Be sure to assess the client's cognitive and sensory abilities. You may need to speak louder or vary the pressure/intensity of the massage.*
- *Be sure to assess the client's willingness for massage. Some people are uncomfortable with touch.*

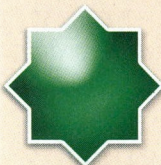

Pediatric Variations:
- *Children generally enjoy massage.*
- *Some are uncomfortable with touch, especially those with histories of physical or sexual abuse.*
- *Children may be more comfortable with their parent or guardian with them.*
- *Be sure to use very light pressure with children.*

Home Care Variations:
- *Encourage caretakers to take part in the session so that they can give massage in the future.*
- *Assess for ongoing changes in skin condition or complaints of pain.*

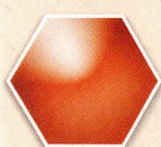

Long-Term Care Variations:
- *Be sure to assess cognitive and sensory abilities.*
- *Assess for ongoing changes in skin condition or complaints of pain.*
- *Make sure that massage is offered by all appropriate staff.*

▶ COMMON ERRORS

Possible Error:

The nurse gives a stressful massage.

Prevention:

Be sure that you are comfortable giving a massage. Do not do the massage hastily; "be with" the client. If you are in a hurry or are uncomfortable, the client will sense those feelings. Encourage frequent feedback regarding pressure or pain from the massage.

Possible Error:

The nurse experiences back strain from giving a massage.

Prevention:

Use good body mechanics. Adjust the level of the bed. Brace your feet to balance your weight and bend your knees rather than lean over the client.

▶ NURSING TIPS

- Be sure to use good body mechanics while doing massage. Elevate the bed and keep your center of balance. Try to let the movements come from your legs, not just your hands and arms. Try to keep shoulders in alignment with your hips (do not twist your spine) as you perform the procedure.
- Encourage clients to ask for a massage.
- If time allows, massage of the feet or hands can be very therapeutic.
- Pass on the client's response to massage at report.

- Be sure to chart the client's responses to massage in the nurses' notes.
- Be aware of your own feelings regarding massage. If you have difficulty with touch, these feelings will be transmitted to the recipient.
- Sometimes those who are uncomfortable with massage can feel better with simple handholding.
- Be aware that some clients' comfort levels are affected by the sex of the nurse and the area of the body being touched. Studies have shown that female clients are not as comfortable being touched by older male nurses, though handholding did not evoke such a response.

▶ SPECIAL CONSIDERATIONS

- *Therapeutic Touch (Skill 3-4), developed by nurses, incorporates the hand-heart maneuver as one of its therapies. This involves taking the client's left hand in yours and placing your other hand on the client's heart. It is important that the nurse is "present" with the client and sends a message of calm and healing. This can be taught to family members as well. Remember to withdraw the hand gradually by bringing it up to the shoulder and then down the left arm before release. This is a great way to end a massage with your client or to sit with a client when massage is not possible.*
- *Know cultural variations associated with touch. Some cultures do not accept touch as relaxing, but rather as an invasion of personal space.*

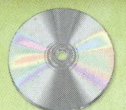

Changing the Gown in Clients with IVs

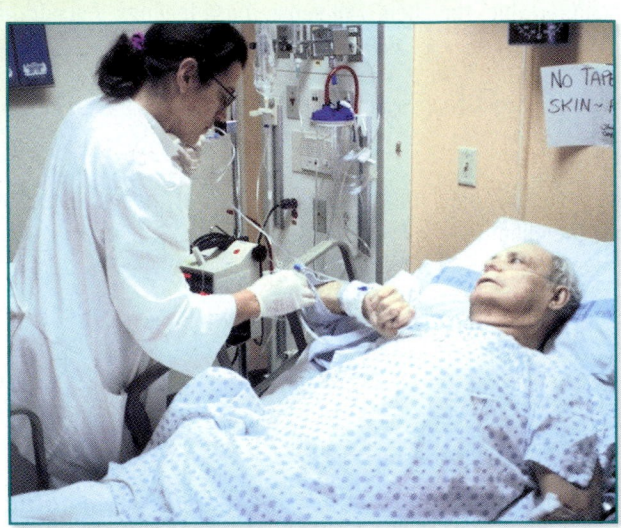

▶ OVERVIEW OF THE SKILL

All clients require clean gowns at regular intervals. Clients receiving IV therapy are no exception to this rule. However, clients with IV access in one or both arms require a different technique to change their gown without disrupting their IV access. Some institutions have special gowns with snaps at the shoulders, which provide an easy method of applying a client's gown over arms, with IV access. In this case, the snaps can be undone and the gown easily removed and changed. If the client's gown has no snaps, it can be changed by passing the IV bag through the sleeve of the gown, or briefly disconnecting the IV tubing, so the client can benefit from clean and comfortable linen. In some cases, it may be necessary to cut the gown sleeve to safely remove the gown; however, this step should only be taken if no other option is available. Care must be taken not to compromise the IV access. Also, some IV medication rates cannot be stopped or slowed without endangering the client.

▶ ASSESSMENT

1. Assess the client for the presence of an IV line or lines **so the necessary supplies can be gathered.**
2. Assess the client's current gown **to determine how the old gown will be removed.**
3. Assess the contents of the IV infusion to determine whether the infusion can be turned off

briefly **so the adjustment can be made using a special gown or procedure to change the gown.**
4. Assess availability of gowns made for clients with IVs.

▶ DIAGNOSIS

Dressing/Grooming Self-Care Deficit

Risk for Injury

Risk for Impaired Skin Integrity

▶ PLANNING

Expected Outcomes:

1. The IV line will remain intact while the gown is being changed.
2. The privacy of the client will be preserved.
3. The IV gown will be changed without becoming twisted or tangled in the IV line.
4. The client's gown will be changed without compromising the client's health.

Equipment Needed:

- Client gown
- Betadine or alcohol
- Tubing clamps
- Sterile gloves

▶ CLIENT EDUCATION NEEDED:

1. Instruct clients on the rationale for changing the gown.

444

2. Tell clients they will need to move their arms to change the gown.
3. Reassure clients that all precautions will be taken to guard the current IV access.
4. Tell clients not to remove their gowns by themselves because there may be an increased risk of dislodging their IV.

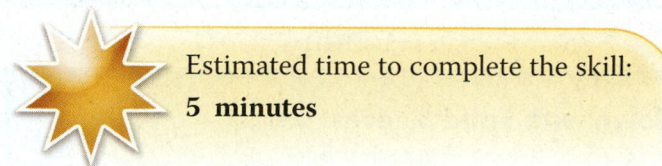

Estimated time to complete the skill:
5 minutes

► **DELEGATION TIPS**

Changing an IV gown may be delegated to properly trained ancillary personnel. However, they must be supervised and cautioned not to disrupt the integrity of the solution connections or the flow of the infusion. If this is required, the licensed nurse must not delegate the procedure.

IMPLEMENTATION—Action/Rationale

Action	Rationale
1. Wash hands.	1. Reduces the transmission of microorganisms.
2. Untie or unsnap the back fasteners on the old gown.	2. Facilitates removal of the old gown.
Gown with Shoulder Snaps	
3. Unsnap the gown sleeves.	3. Facilitates removal of the gown without disrupting the IV access.
4. Cover the client with the clean gown.	4. Provides privacy.
5. Keeping the client covered, pull the old gown out from underneath the clean gown. Be sure the IV lines are not tangled in the old gown.	5. Provides privacy.
6. Snap the sleeves of the clean gown around the client's arms.	6. Secures the gown, providing client privacy without disrupting the IV access.
Gown with Solid Sleeves	
7. Place the clean gown over the client with the sleeves in the proper orientation. Keep the client covered with the clean gown throughout the procedure (see Figure 4-15-1).	7. Provides privacy. Eases the transition from old gown to clean gown.
8. Remove the old gown from the arm without IV access. Slide the old gown to the IV access side.	8. Allows the old gown to be removed without pulling on the client's other arm.
9. Determine if the client can tolerate a brief interruption in the IV infusion.	9. Some infusions cannot be interrupted, even briefly, without endangering the client.

continues

Action	Rationale

Gown with Solid Sleeves *continued*

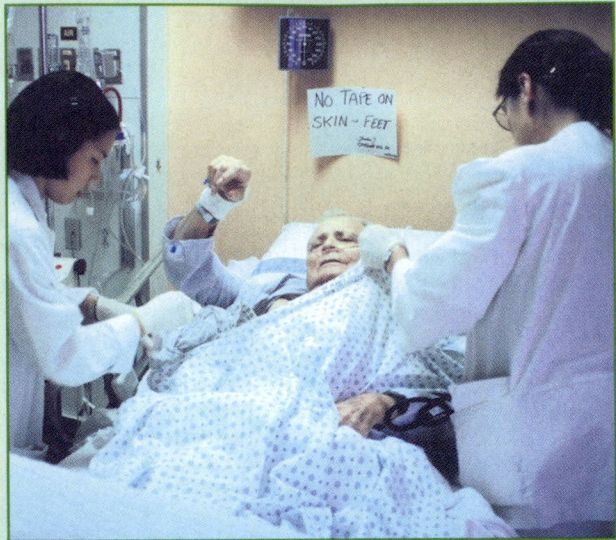

Figure 4-15-1   Place the clean gown over the client with the sleeves in the proper orientation.

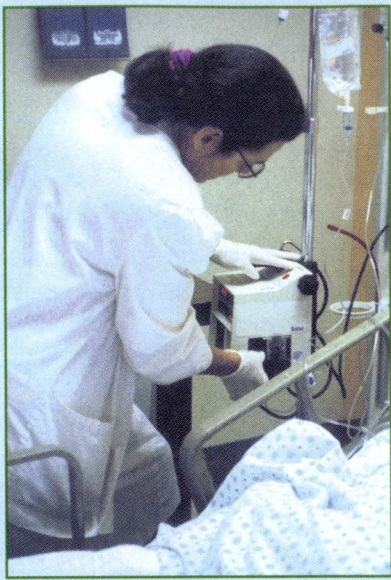

Figure 4-15-2   If the client can tolerate a brief interruption in the IV, clamp the tubing and shut off the IV pump.

10. If the IV can be shut off briefly or slowed, clamp the IV tubing. If the IV is regulated by a pump, shut off the IV pump and remove the tubing from the pump (see Figure 4-15-2). If the IV cannot be slowed or clamped, proceed to Action 11.

10. Frees the IV line and bag to be passed through the sleeve of the gown. Clamping the tubing prevents free flow of the IV fluids into the client.

11. Remove the IV bag from the IV stand.

11. Facilitates changing the gown. Do not hold the IV bag below the IV access site to prevent blood backflow into the IV tubing.

12. While holding the IV bag in the nondominant hand, use the other hand to slide the old gown off the arm with IV access, over the IV tubing, over the IV bag, and onto the nondominant hand (see Figure 4-15-3).

12. Allows removal of the old gown without disrupting IV access.

13. Take the IV bag in the dominant hand and remove the client's gown from the nondominant hand. Dispose of the old gown appropriately.

13. Promotes a clean environment.

14. With the IV bag in the dominant hand, place the nondominant hand through the sleeve of the clean gown, from the distal end of the sleeve toward the proximal end of the sleeve.

14. Prepares for placing the clean gown.

15. Place the IV bag in the nondominant hand, with the clean gown on it. Use the dominant hand to slide the sleeve of the clean gown over the IV bag, down the IV tubing, and over the client's arm.

15. Allows placement of the clean gown without disrupting IV access.

continues

Action	Rationale
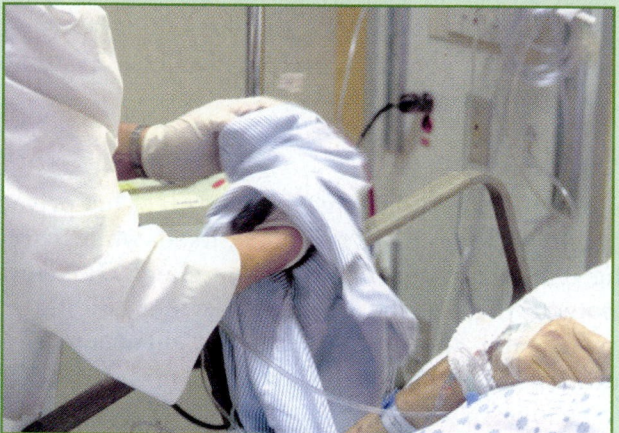 **Figure 4-15-3** Slide the IV bag through the arm of the gown.	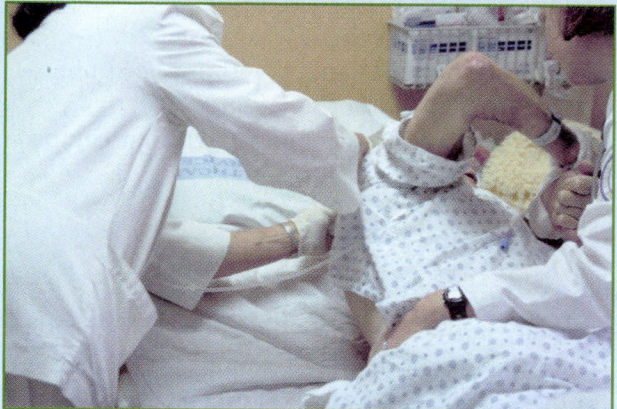 **Figure 4-15-4** Fasten the clean gown in back.

Action	Rationale
16. Replace the IV bag on the IV stand. Reinsert the IV tubing into the IV pump and open the clamp on the IV tubing.	**16.** Resumes the IV infusion.
17. Check the IV flow rate to ensure that it is still at the ordered rate. Check the IV access site to ensure the IV is still intact and patent.	**17.** Ensures proper infusion of the IV fluids without injury to the client.
18. Slide the gown sleeve over the client's other arm.	**18.** Provides client privacy.
19. Check the IV flow rate to ensure that it is still at the ordered rate and adjust appropriately (done by nurse). Check the IV access site to ensure the IV is still intact and patent.	**19.** Ensures proper infusion of the IV fluids without injury to the client.
20. Fasten the client's gown in back. Straighten the bedclothes and provide for the client's comfort (see Figure 4-15-4).	**20.** Provides privacy and client comfort.
21. Wash hands.	**21.** Reduces the transmission of microorganisms.

▶ REAL WORLD ANECDOTES

Randy was a 7-year-old boy who had an appendectomy. The day after his surgery, he got up to bathe at his bedside. The IV bag was too large to thread through the sleeve of his client gown, but the IV tubing had an extension set on it with a connector about 6 inches from the IV site. The nurse turned off the IV and clamped the extension tubing leading to the client. The nurse removed the gown from Randy's arm. Using sterile technique, she protected the IV tubing connection while slipping the tubing through the sleeve. She had already obtained a special gown with snaps at the shoulder to put on Randy until his IV was discontinued. The nurse was thankful that Randy's IV fluids could be interrupted briefly. If she could not have clamped and disconnected the IV, she may have had to cut the gown sleeve to safely remove the gown.

▶ EVALUATION

- The IV line remained intact while the gown was being changed.
- The privacy of the client was preserved.
- The IV gown was changed without becoming twisted or tangled in the IV line.
- The client's gown was changed without compromising the client's health.

▶ DOCUMENTATION

Nurses' Notes

- Document the date and time of the gown change when documenting the reason for the change such as daily care, client was incontinent, and so on.
- Note the condition of the IV access site.
- Note any unusual findings or client concerns.

Document on appropriate flow sheet or electronic medical record (EMR).

▶ CRITICAL THINKING SKILL

Introduction

Clients with IV lines need help changing their gowns because the risk of dislodging the IV is high.

Possible Scenario

A confused client has soiled his gown and tried to take it off by himself. The gown has become entangled in the IV tubing. The client says, "I have to go to the bathroom *now*." The client pulls at the IV tubing as he tries to remove it.

Possible Outcome

The nurse grabs a new gown to protect his privacy and folds the soiled gown on itself while carrying it to the bathroom with the client. The nurse protects the IV site and tubing while holding the gown. Later, the nurse settles the client and carefully removes the soiled gown and replaces it with a new one.

Prevention

Tell the client the nurse will help him change his gown to protect the IV needle, tubing, and bag. If the client is confused, reassure the client that the nurse will help him. Ask family members to reinforce this instruction to the client.

▶ VARIATIONS

Geriatric Variations:
- *Elderly clients may need more help changing their gowns with an IV in place.*
- *Careful handling of the IV site is especially crucial in elderly clients because they may have fragile veins.*

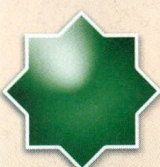

Pediatric Variations:
- *Children's gowns may be too small to slip the IV bag through the sleeve of the gown.*
- *Children may be more active and get their gown tangled more easily.*

Home Care Variations:
- *Clients receiving IV therapy at home will probably wear their own clothing, which can be altered to accommodate an IV.*
- *Caregivers should be taught how to change the clothing of a client with an IV in place.*

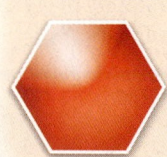

Long-Term Care Variations:
- *Special gowns may be necessary for clients receiving IV therapy in a long-term care facility.*
- *Staff should be taught how to manage a clothing change in clients receiving IV therapy.*

► COMMON ERRORS

Possible Error:

You remove the gown from the client's arm and forget to thread the IV bag through the sleeve. The tape at the IV site is pulled and the needle is slightly dislodged.

Prevention:

Remember to check that the gown is completely free of the tubing before pulling it away from the client. If this error does occur, assess the IV for patency. If it is intact, retape the needle in place. Then remove the gown and replace it with a fresh one.

► NURSING TIPS

- It may be easier in some situations to simply leave the gown off the arm where an IV is in place. Be sure to secure the gown as well as possible and use a second gown to cover the exposed arm.

- Position the gown over the client so it will be placed on the client correctly.
- Disconnect the IV only if other methods of removing the gown cannot be used. Disconnecting the IV increases the risk of infection.

► SPECIAL CONSIDERATIONS

- *IV therapy gowns with snaps may be available at some facilities. Check for the availability of the gown to promote the best quality of care.*
- *Avoid clamping the IV line when changing the gown. If clamping the IV line cannot be prevented during the procedure, make sure to unclamp the IV line and reassess the patency of the IV flow rate.*
- *If the client is receiving intermittent IV therapy and can be changed to a saline lock (Skill 8-8), wait to change the gown until the lock is in place.*
- *Needleless systems allow for a safe temporary disconnection of system to change the gown.*

Assisting from Bed to Stretcher

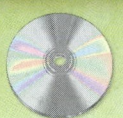

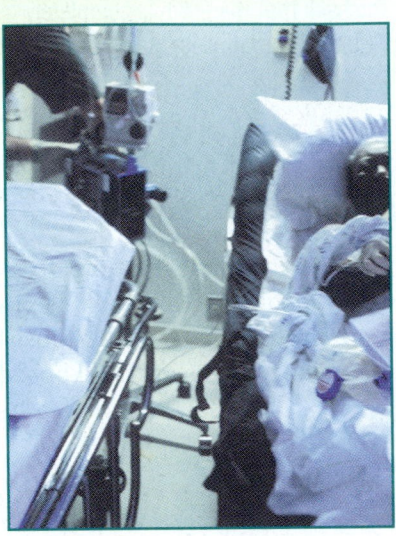

▶ OVERVIEW OF THE SKILL

Some clients must remain horizontal when they are moved. If they are not strong enough to sit erect in a wheelchair or there is some injury that prevents them from sitting, clients must be moved while lying flat. The most commonly used equipment for transferring a client is a stretcher or gurney. A stretcher is a narrow, cart-like bed that rolls on wheels. For client safety, stretchers are equipped with side rails or safety straps to prevent accidental falls during transport. The wheels on a stretcher lock to prevent accidental movement during client transfers.

▶ ASSESSMENT

1. Assess the client's current level of mobility. Knowing whether a client is able to assist with the transfer will affect how the transfer is performed.
2. Assess for injury. **Caregivers may need to keep the client in the same alignment as much as possible.**
3. Assess for any impediments to mobility such as a cast, drainage tubes, IVs, or intubation. **This will affect how the transfer is performed.**
4. Assess the client's level of understanding of the procedure. **This will affect client comfort, anxiety, and cooperation.**

5. Assess the client's environment. Assess how close the stretcher will move to the bed. Assess the height of the bed. **This allows for a safe transfer. Plan for good body mechanics.**
6. Make sure the stretcher is safe to use. Check for working brakes, side rails, safety straps that are intact and usable, and an IV pole attachment if needed. **This allows for a safe transfer. Plan for good body mechanics.**

▶ DIAGNOSIS

Impaired Physical Mobility

Activity Intolerance

Risk for Falls

▶ PLANNING

Expected Outcomes:

1. The client will be transferred from the bed to the stretcher without pain or injury.
2. Drainage tubes, IVs, or other devices will remain intact.
3. The client's skin will be intact and undamaged.

Equipment Needed:

Transferring a Client with Minimum Assistance

- Bed
- Stretcher

Transferring a Client with Maximum Assistance
(see Figure 4-16-1)

- Bed
- Stretcher

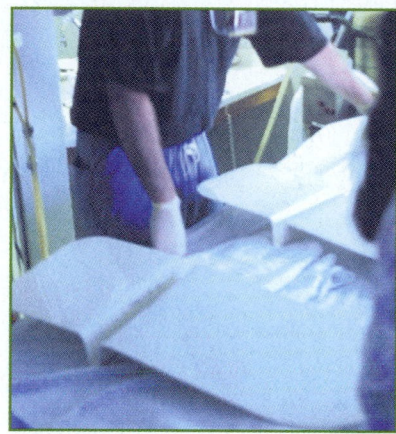

Figure 4-16-1 Transfer or slider boards reduce the friction when sliding the client on or off the stretcher.

- Pillows
- Transfer/slider boards
- Lift sheet
- Other qualified personnel to assist

▶ **CLIENT EDUCATION NEEDED:**

1. If the client has an injury or condition that requires immobility, explain the need and rationale for immobility to the client.
2. Be sure to remind the client that the gurney is narrow and to move carefully while on it. Remember that if the client is confused, and explanation will not help, safety straps and side rails are needed.

Estimated time to complete the skill:
5–10 minutes

▶ **DELEGATION TIPS**

Assisting a client from a bed to a stretcher is a skill routinely delegated to properly trained ancillary personnel.

IMPLEMENTATION—Action/Rationale

Action	Rationale
Transferring a Client with Minimum Assistance	
1. Wash hands and apply gloves.	1. Reduces the transmission of microorganisms.
2. Inform client about desired purpose and destination.	2. Reduces client anxiety and increases cooperation.
3. Raise the height of bed to 1 inch higher than the stretcher and lock brakes of bed.	3. Reduces distance nurse must bend, thus preventing back strain; prevents bed from moving.
4. Instruct client to move to side of bed close to stretcher. Lower side rails of bed and stretcher. Leave side rails on opposite side up (see Figure 4-16-2).	4. Decreases risk of client falling.

continues

Action	Rationale

Transferring a Client with Minimum Assistance *continued*

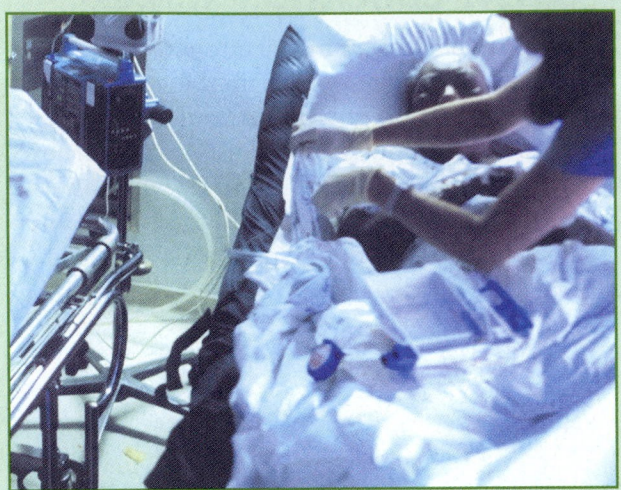

Figure 4-16-2   Lower side rails of bed and stretcher.

5. Stand at outer side of stretcher and push it toward bed.

5. Diminishes the gap between bed and stretcher; secures the stretcher position.

6. Instruct client to move onto stretcher with assistance as needed.

6. Promotes client independence.

7. Cover client with sheet or bath blanket.

7. Promotes comfort; protects privacy.

8. Elevate side rails on stretcher and secure safety belts about client. Release brakes of stretcher.

8. Prevents falls.

9. Stand at head of stretcher to guide it when pushing.

9. Pushing, not pulling, ensures proper body mechanics.

10. Wash hands.

10. Reduces the transmission of microorganisms.

Transferring a Client with Maximum Assistance

11. Repeat Actions 1 and 2.

11. See Rationales 1 and 2.

12. Assess amount of assistance required for transfer. Usually, two to four staff members are required for the maximum-assisted transfer.

12. Promotes client independence; ensures that enough staff are present before beginning transfer.

13. Lock wheels of bed and stretcher.

13. Prevents falls.

14. Have one nurse stand close to the client's head.

14. Supports the client's head during the move.

15. Logroll the client (keep in straight alignment) and place a lift sheet under the client's back, trunk, and upper legs. The lift sheet can extend under the head if client lacks head control abilities.

15. Prevents flexion and rotation of client's hips and spine; maintains correct body alignment.

continues

Action	Rationale

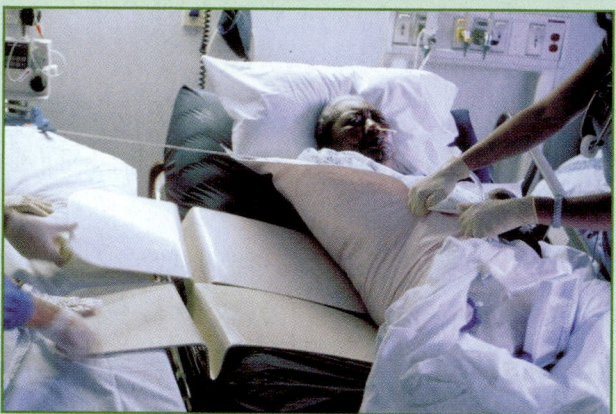

Figure 4-16-3   Place pillow or slider board overlapping the bed and stretcher.

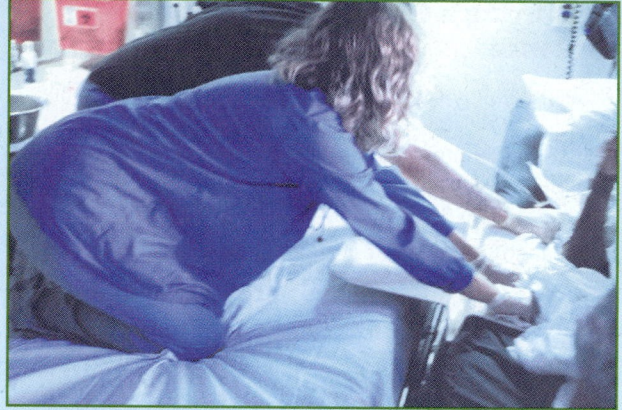

Figure 4-16-4   Firmly grasp edges of lift sheet.

16. Empty all drainage bags (e.g., T-tube, Hemo Vac, Jackson-Pratt). Record amounts. Secure drainage system to client's gown before transfer.

17. Move client to edge of bed near stretcher. Lift up and over to avoid dragging.

18. Because the client is now on the side of the bed, without the side rail up, the nurse on nonstretcher side of bed holds the stretcher side of the lift sheet up (by reaching across the client's chest) to prevent the client from falling onto the stretcher or off the bed.

19. Place pillow or slider board overlapping the bed and stretcher (see Figure 4-16-3).

20. Have staff members grasp edges of lift sheet. Be sure to use good body mechanics (see Figure 4-16-4).

21. On the count of three, have staff members pull lift sheet and the client onto the stretcher.

22. Position client on stretcher, place pillow under head, and cover client with a sheet or bath blanket (see Figure 4-16-5).

16. Decreases possibility of spills; prevents dislodging of tubes.

17. Prevents dragging, which causes shearing force.

18. Protects the client from falling.

19. Protects head from injury. Slider board eases movement of the client.

20. Provides surface for client to slide on. Prevents dragging and shearing.

21. Working in unison makes the overall job easier and prevents staff injury.

22. Promotes comfort and provides for privacy.

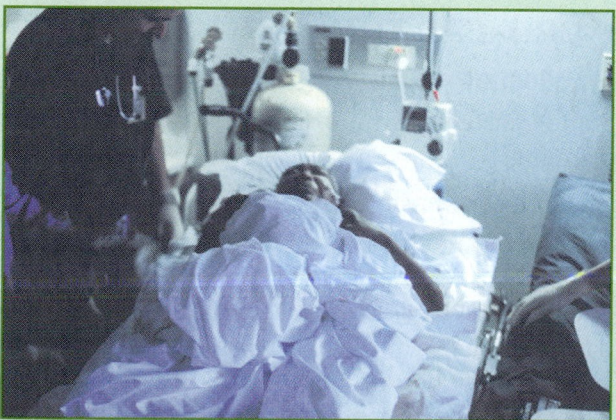

Figure 4-16-5   Place pillow under head and cover client with blanket.

continues

Action	Rationale
Transferring a Client with Maximum Assistance *continued*	
23. Secure safety belts and elevate side rails of stretcher.	23. Prevents falls.
24. If IV pole is present, move it from bed IV pole to stretcher IV pole after client transfer.	24. Prevents tubing from being pulled and IV from being dislodged.
25. Wash hands.	25. Reduces the transmission of microorganisms.

▶ REAL WORLD ANECDOTES

Scenario 1

Mr. Cao arrived in the emergency department (ED) on a backboard with a hard cervical collar on. He had been involved in an automobile accident. The ED doctor ordered a computed tomography (CT) scan to check for spinal damage. The client denied any numbness or tingling in any of his extremities. The client complained of pain from the discomfort of the backboard, and the restraining straps were loosened while the client waited for the scan. While he was being transferred from the stretcher back to the emergency room bed, the nurses performing the transfer did not keep Mr. Cao's lower back in alignment. Shortly after the CT scan had been read, showing a fractured lumbar vertebra but no nerve damage, Mr. Cao began to complain of tingling in his feet and legs. A second spinal CT showed new damage that had not been present in the first CT. Mr. Cao was taken to emergency surgery, but the damage had been done and Mr. Cao was paralyzed from the waist down. The nurse needed to take precautions to protect the spinal cord from movement until the possibility of a fracture had been ruled out.

Scenario 2

A small hospital ED was in a separate building from the main hospital. To admit a client on a gurney from the ED to the hospital, the gurney had to be pushed out the door, immediately swung hard left to avoid the sloping driveway, then pushed hard across the pavement to the main hospital elevator. Most of the regular ED nurses knew the tricks and often transferred clients alone. One night a 125-lb. nurse tried to transfer a 270-lb. client. She got him out the door but could not turn the stretcher left in time. The stretcher, the client, and the nurse started a slow descent down the sloping driveway. Fortunately, help was at hand, but the nurse strained her back, and the client was stressed. The nurse needed to assess the task and get help for this extra-heavy client.

▶ EVALUATION

- The client was transferred from the bed to the stretcher without pain or injury.
- All drainage tubes, IVs, or other devices remain intact.
- Assess whether the client's skin is intact and undamaged.

▶ DOCUMENTATION

Nurses' Notes

- Document how much assistance the transfer required and how much the client was able to assist.
- Document the time, date, reason for transfer, type of transfer, and how the client tolerated the activity.

Document on appropriate flow sheet or electronic medical record (EMR).

▶ CRITICAL THINKING SKILL

Introduction

Some transfers are more difficult and need a little extra planning.

Possible Scenario

Mr. Khalif is a client in the intensive care unit. He is comatose and intubated. His doctor has ordered a CT scan of Mr. Khalif's head to determine the extent of any damage. While Mr. Khalif is being transferred from the bed to a stretcher, you note that he has a multitude of lines, wires, and tubes that must be carefully coordinated during the move.

Possible Outcome

Some of the tubes, lines, or wires could become dislodged or pulled out entirely. With some of these devices, this could be a life-threatening situation. If Mr. Khalif's ET tube becomes dislodged or pulled out, he could die of respiratory failure. If a pacemaker wire becomes dislodged, he could die of cardiac failure.

Prevention

Carefully assess which devices can be safely removed before transferring a client and which ones must be carefully guarded to prevent accidental removal. Be sure to get enough help to move complex clients. It may take one or two nurses just to watch the lines and tubes to move a client safely.

▶ VARIATIONS

Geriatric Variations:

- *Geriatric clients may have contractures or other disabilities that impair their ability to lie flat. Be aware that your transfer technique may need to be altered to accommodate this.*
- *Elderly clients may have thin, fragile skin. Care should be taken during the transfer not to tear or damage their skin.*

Pediatric Variations:

- *A child may be small enough to lift onto a stretcher. If the parent is lifting, make sure the parent can hold the weight of the child. Give brief instructions on proper body mechanics prior to the lifting of the child.*
- *Children may be small enough to slip through the side rails on a gurney. Be sure to fasten any safety straps or restrain the child some other way.*

Home Care Variation:

- *Stretchers are rarely used in the home care situation.*

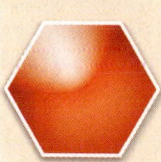

Long-Term Care Variation:

- *Long-term care clients may have contractures or other disabilities that impair their ability to lie flat. Be aware that your transfer technique may need to be altered to accommodate this.*

▶ COMMON ERRORS

Possible Error:

The nurse does not have enough help to move the client safely.

Prevention:

Think about what will happen if you try to move this client without enough help: You could be seriously injured. If you try to move this client with too much help, you may get in each other's way, but the client and the staff are more likely to be safe from harm. Be sure to ask for help when transferring a client. Unless the client is very capable, a bed-to-stretcher transfer usually requires at least two nurses. Do not be embarrassed to ask for help.

▶ NURSING TIPS

- Count to three and have everyone move the client on the count of three. Designate a "team leader" to coordinate the move and call the count.
- If possible, fold the client's arms across the chest to prevent them from being caught underneath the body during the transfer.
- Be careful to support the client's head and neck during the transfer.

- Do not allow the urinary catheter drain bag to be held above the level of the client's bladder. Holding it up encourages backflow of urine and can lead to bladder infections.
- Even though both the stretcher and bed wheels are locked, leaning your body into the stretcher will help prevent gaps between the stretcher and bed.

▶ SPECIAL CONSIDERATIONS

- *Some facilities may use a roller to transfer the client from bed to stretcher or gurney. A roller is a vinyl cover over several steel rollers that functions much like a conveyor belt. The client in bed is turned on his or her side and the roller is placed under him or her with a towel or draw sheet over it. Then the client is placed onto the roller and the sheet is used to pull the client towards the stretcher.*
- *When transferring a client from stretcher to operating room (OR) table, the client is moving from one narrow place to another. Before surgery, when the client is alert and able to assist in the move, the client is asked to stay on his or her back and lift his or her hips to move onto the OR bed. The surgical tech or scrub nurse (nurse who will "scrub in" during the operation) is asked to put the client's back to the opposite side of the OR bed to serve as a guide or reminder for the client. The circulating nurse (not "scrubbed in" during operation) stands on the locked stretcher side and gives the client instructions while ensuring that the stretcher stays in the locked position.*
- *When in the OR and moving an anesthetized client, the anesthesiologist or nurse anesthetist gives the signal to move. It is essential that the airway is maintained throughout the move.*
- *If the client has a chest tube in place, know institution protocol for transfer. Be alert to emergency procedure if the chest tube becomes displaced or accidentally pulled out.*

Assisting from Bed to Wheelchair, Commode, or Chair

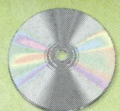

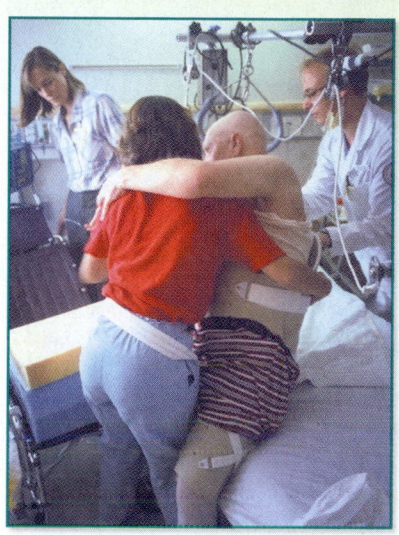

▶ OVERVIEW OF THE SKILL

Client activity is an important part of the healing process. Activity improves muscle tone, increases venous return to the heart, and stimulates peristalsis. Moving a client from the bed to a chair is an important part of client activity.

Moving a client from the bed to a chair, wheelchair, commode, or stretcher is called a transfer. Transferring a client requires good planning to avoid injury to the client and the nurse. When transferring a client, the nurse needs to consider the client's ability to assist with the transfer. If the client is unable to provide any assistance or is large, the nurse may need one or more staff members to help perform the transfer safely.

The most frequent complication in transferring a client is falling during the transfer. If a client does start to fall while being transferred, lower him or her gently to the floor, making sure the head does not strike anything. If a client does fall, obtain assistance and perform a thorough assessment of the client before moving him or her.

Another possible hazard in client transfers is pulling on or dislodging indwelling tubes or catheters. Think ahead about ways tubes will move with the transfer and try to avoid snagging them. Care should be taken to appropriately anchor all tubes and catheters prior to transferring a client.

Clients are also at risk of damage to their skin during a transfer. Sliding across the sheets, side rails, and wheelchair armrests can bruise or injure the client. Using a transfer board or padding any sharp exposed areas can help prevent injury to the client.

Be sure the client is wearing shoes or slippers with firm, nonslip soles when transferring a client. Even if the client will be standing only briefly, the feet need to be protected from potential injury and contamination from the floor. The client needs to be protected from slipping.

When transferring a client with weakness on one side of the body, use the "Good to go" maxim. This means that the client needs to lead off with the "good" or strong side of the body. Perform the transfer in the direction of the good side so the client pivots and supports the weight on the good side. This will allow for maximum strength and stability on the client's part.

▶ ASSESSMENT

1. Assess the client's current level of mobility. Determine how much the client is able to assist with the transfer. Assess for pain or confusion, which might impair ability to assist. Check for a "weak" side. **Affects how the procedure will be carried out.**

2. Assess for any impediments to mobility, including casts, drainage tubes, catheters, IVs, or intubation. **Affects how the procedure will be carried out. Prepares caregivers to keep tubes and equipment from becoming dislodged, tipping, or pulling.**

3. Assess the client's level of understanding and anxiety regarding the procedure. **Affects how the procedure will be carried out. Affects client teaching.**

4. Assess the client's environment. Assess the available space for maneuvering the wheelchair to the bed. **Affects how the procedure will be carried out. Affects safety and good body mechanics for caregivers.**

5. Assess the equipment. Check the bed and chair height. See whether they are adjustable. Check for chair footings and wheelchair brakes. **Affects safety for client and caregivers.**

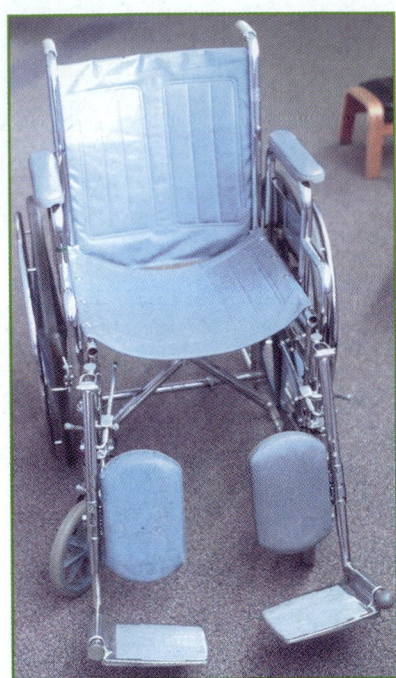

Figure 4-17-1   Wheelchair

▶ DIAGNOSIS

Impaired Physical Mobility

Activity Intolerance

Risk for Injury

Risk for Fall

▶ PLANNING

Expected Outcomes:

1. The client will be transferred from the bed to the wheelchair, commode, or chair without pain or injury.
2. Drainage tubes, IVs, or other devices will be intact.
3. The client's skin will be intact and undamaged.

Equipment Needed:

- Bed
- Wheelchair, chair, or commode (see Figure 4-17-1)
- Any splints, braces, or supportive equipment specific to the client
- Shoes or slippers with nonskid soles
- Gait belt
- Transfer board (if necessary)

■ CLIENT EDUCATION NEEDED:

1. Explain to the client the need for activity and its importance in the recovery process.
2. Teach the client about "Good to go" if one side of the client's body is weaker than the other. "Good to go" reminds the client to lead off with the stronger limb when walking or transferring.
3. Advise the client of the need for sturdy shoes or slippers with nonslip soles.

Estimated time to complete the skill:
20 minutes

▶ DELEGATION TIPS

Assisting a client from a bed to a wheelchair, commode, or chair is a skill routinely delegated to properly trained ancillary personnel.

IMPLEMENTATION—Action/Rationale

Action	Rationale
1. Wash hands.	1. Reduces the transmission of microorganisms.
2. Inform client about desired purpose and destination.	2. Reduces client anxiety and increases cooperation.
3. Assess client for ability to assist with the transfer and for presence of cognitive or sensory deficits.	3. Allows planning regarding the amount of assistance and cooperation to expect from the client.
4. Lock the bed in position.	4. Prevents the bed from rolling during the procedure.
5. Place any splints, braces, or other devices on the client.	5. Provides support and prevents injury to the client.
6. Place the client's shoes or slippers on the client's feet.	6. Provides a nonslip surface for stability.
7. Lower the height of the bed to lowest possible position.	7. Reduces distance client has to step down, thus decreasing risk of injury.
8. Slowly raise the head of the bed if this is not contraindicated by the client's condition.	8. Minimizes lifting.
9. Place one arm under the client's legs and one arm behind the client's back. Slowly pivot the client so the client's legs are dangling over the edge of the bed and the client is in a sitting position on the edge of the bed (see Figure 4-17-2).	9. Supports the client while sitting him or her upright.
10. Allow client to dangle for 2 to 5 minutes. Help support client if necessary (see Figure 4-17-3).	10. Allows time for assessing client's response to sitting; reduces possibility of orthostatic hypotension.
11. Bring the chair or wheelchair close to the side of the bed. Place it at a 45° angle to the bed. If the client has a weaker side, place the chair or wheelchair on the client's strong side.	11. Minimizes transfer distance. Allows the client to pivot on the stronger leg.

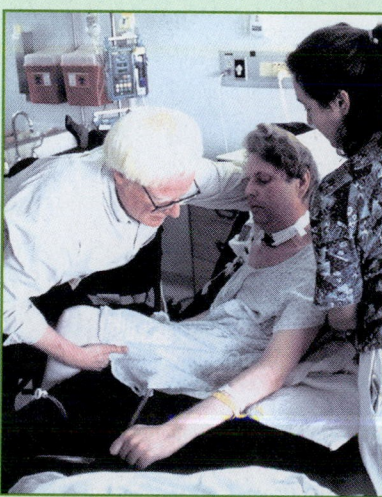

Figure 4-17-2 Pivot the client to a sitting position on the edge of the bed.

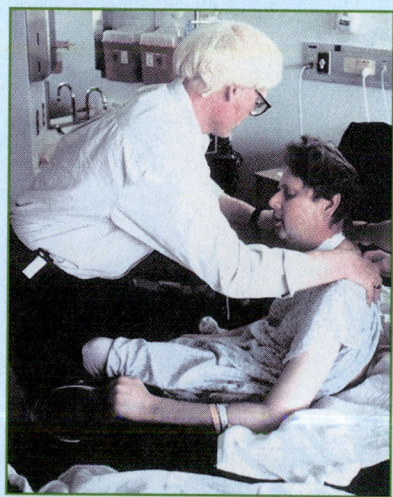

Figure 4-17-3 Support the client, if needed, while the client adjusts to the sitting position.

continues

Action	Rationale
12. Lock wheelchair brakes and elevate the foot pedals. For chairs, lock brakes if available.	12. Provides stability.
13. If you will be using a gait belt to assist the client, place it around the client's waist.	13. Provides a secure handhold for the nurse during the transfer.
14. Assist client to side of bed until feet are firmly on the floor and slightly apart.	14. Moves client into proper position for transfer. Provides stable footing for client.
15. Grasp the sides of the gait belt or place your hands just below the client's axilla. Using a wide stance, bend your knees and assist the client to a standing position (see Figure 4-17-4).	15. Wide stance increases nurse stability and minimizes strain on the back. Avoids putting pressure directly on the axilla, and risking nerve damage or shoulder subluxation.
16. Standing close to the client, pivot until the client's back is toward the chair.	16. Moves client into proper position to be seated.
17. Instruct the client to place hands on the arm supports, or place the client's hands on the arm supports of the chair.	17. Allows client to gain balance and judge distance to seat.
18. Bend at the knees and ease the client into a sitting position.	18. Increases stability and minimizes strain on back.
19. Assist client to maintain proper posture (see Figure 4-17-5). Support weak side with pillow if needed.	19. Increases client comfort.
20. Secure the safety belt, place client's feet on feet pedals, and release brakes if you will be moving the client immediately. Make sure tubes and lines, arms, and hands are not pinched or caught between the client and the chair (see Figure 4-17-6). If the client is sitting in a chair, offer a footstool if available (see Figure 4-17-7).	20. Ensures client safety; prepares client for movement.
21. Wash hands.	21. Reduces the transmission of microorganisms.

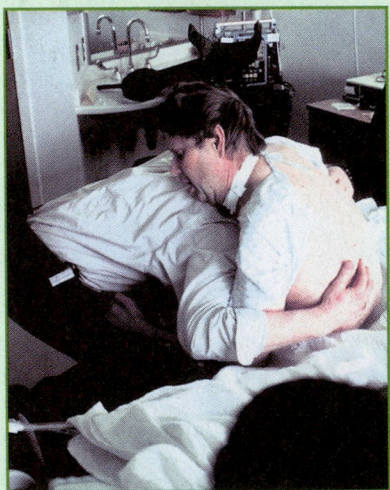

Figure 4-17-4   Bend your knees, grasp the client firmly, and help the client into a standing position.

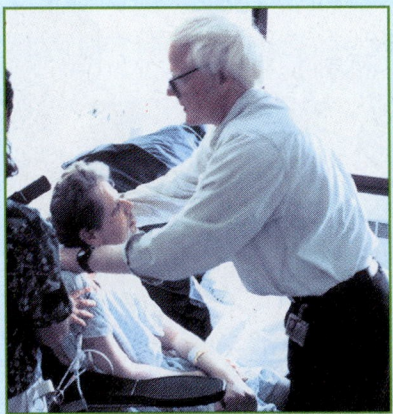

Figure 4-17-5   Assist client to maintain proper position.

continues

Action	Rationale
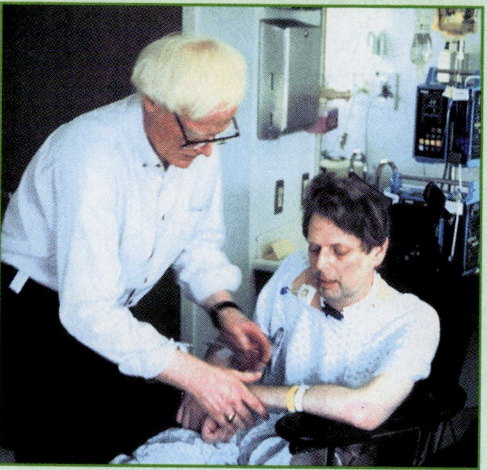	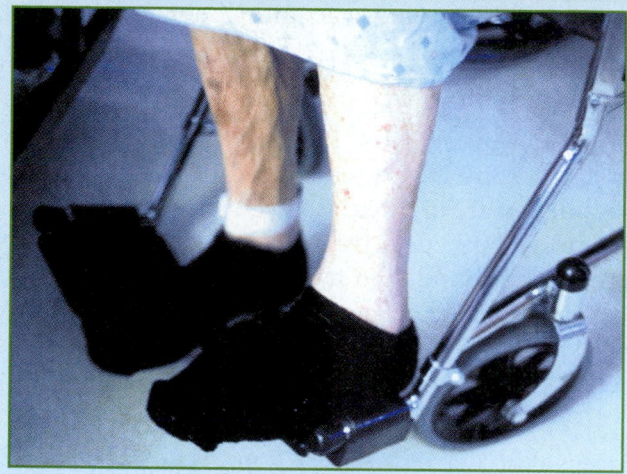
Figure 4-17-6 Once the client is moved, make sure skin, tubing, or equipment is not pinched between the client and the chair.	**Figure 4-17-7** Position the wheelchair footrests or use a footstool if the client is sitting in a chair.

▶ REAL WORLD ANECDOTES

Scenario 1

Mr. Bridges is an insulin-dependent diabetic. Because of his diabetes, he is now blind and his left leg was amputated above the knee. He is requesting an enema and the commode because of perceived constipation. After administering a tap water enema, the nurse prepared to transfer Mr. Bridges to the commode. As the nurse was pivoting from the bed to the commode, the commode slid out from under Mr. Bridges. Mr. Bridges fell to the floor and fractured his right leg. In the ensuing lawsuit, Mr. Bridge's nurse was found negligent for not securing the commode's wheel locks before attempting the transfer.

Scenario 2

A nurse is transferring a frail, anxious elderly person from a bed to a bedside chair. He reaches his arms behind him and grabs the armrests of the chair. He locks his elbows in place because he is so frightened. The nurse cannot sit him down, and his arms push the chair back. They both "walk" the chair across the room. Finally, the nurse literally lifts and carries the client and sets him back on the bed. The nurse needed to explain the procedure carefully to the client before attempting a transfer and to make sure he was comfortable and able to follow instructions prior to attempting a transfer with no one else in the room to assist.

▶ EVALUATION

- Determine whether the client was transferred from the bed to the wheelchair without pain or injury.
- Check that drainage tubes, IVs, or other devices remain intact.
- Assess whether the client's skin is intact and undamaged.

▶ DOCUMENTATION

Nurses' Notes

- Record the client's tolerance of the activity, any aids that were required, how much assistance was required, and the client's ability to assist.
- Note any unusual events during the transfer.

Document on appropriate flow sheet or electronic medical record (EMR).

► CRITICAL THINKING SKILL

Introduction

It takes only 1 second to acquire 2 months of pain.

Possible Scenario

You are preparing Mrs. Richards to go to radiology for X-rays. She is very sleepy and not very cooperative, but you are in a hurry. As you transfer Mrs. Richards from the bed to the wheelchair, Mrs. Richards sags to the ground. You try to hold her up and make it to the wheelchair, but she is too heavy. You lock your knees and bend at the waist as her weight pulls you down. As you gently lower her to the ground, you feel a sharp pain in your lower back.

Possible Outcome

You get help for the rest of your transfers and lifts, but it is too late. By the end of your shift, you are in agony. You visit the doctor for a series of muscle relaxants, exercises, and pain medications.

Prevention

You remembered reading about good body mechanics. Now you will practice them religiously. You also decide to always have enough assistance before starting any transfer, even if it is a "hassle" to find someone.

► VARIATIONS

Geriatric Variations:

- *Elderly clients are more likely to be weak or to get dizzy easily. Assess their abilities throughout the transfer. If dangling at the bedside does not ease the dizziness or if the client seems less stable than previously thought, lie the client back down and get assistance.*

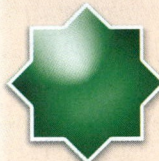

Pediatric Variations:

- *Children may be small enough to simply lift into the wheelchair. Be sure to use good body mechanics while lifting.*
- *Children need wheelchairs fitted to their size. Adult-size wheelchairs are uncomfortable and can be dangerous for a child.*

Home Care Variations:

- *The bed of a home care client may be at a poor height for safe transfer from bed to wheelchair. If the bed is too low, the nurse may be required to lift the client farther than is safe. If the bed is too high, the risk of a client fall is increased. Advise the client or caregiver of the proper height for bed-to-wheelchair transfers and the reason it is important. Problem-solve with the caregiver to outline ways to use proper body mechanics, adjust the height of the bed, or acquire an adjustable bed.*
- *Assess the wheelchair of home care clients. Home care clients may have modified their equipment or failed to maintain it for safe use. Check for sharp, exposed edges; frayed or damaged material; and other damage or modification that might be unsafe for the client.*

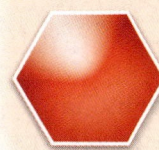

Long-Term Care Variation:

- *Long-term care clients may have contractures or pressure ulcers that will affect their ability to transfer safely and their ability to sit in a wheelchair comfortably. Be sure to assess for these possibilities prior to transferring a client.*

► COMMON ERRORS

Possible Error:

The nurse transfers a client with his weaker side first.

Prevention:

If the client has one-sided weakness, be sure to lead the transfer with strong leg and arm. This increases the client's stability and decreases the risk of injury to the client and the nurse.

► NURSING TIPS

- Be sure to place any splints, braces, or other appliances on the client prior to transfer.
- When transferring a client with weakness on one side of the body, use the "Good to go" maxim. Perform the transfer on the client's strong, or good, side for maximum strength and stability on the client's part.
- Sliding across the sheets, side rails, and wheelchair armrest can bruise or injure the client. A transfer board or placing padding on any sharp, exposed areas can help prevent injury to the client.

► SPECIAL CONSIDERATIONS

- *If the client loses his or her footing when transferring from bed to chair, and appears to be slipping, the nurse must gently lower the client to the floor. It is imperative to use good body mechanics and avoid injury to the back.*
- *The client may develop orthostatic hypotension (light-headedness) when getting up after being supine for a long period of time. Always let the client sit and dangle at the side of the bed before standing. This is a good time to explain how you will be moving the client and what is expected of him or her.*
- *If the client is planning to sit in the wheelchair for long periods of time, the nurse should provide a foam, gel, or egg-crate cushion for the seat of the chair.*
- *If the client is obese you may need to use a hydraulic lift (see Skill 4-19).*

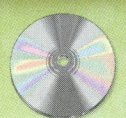

Assisting from Bed to Walking

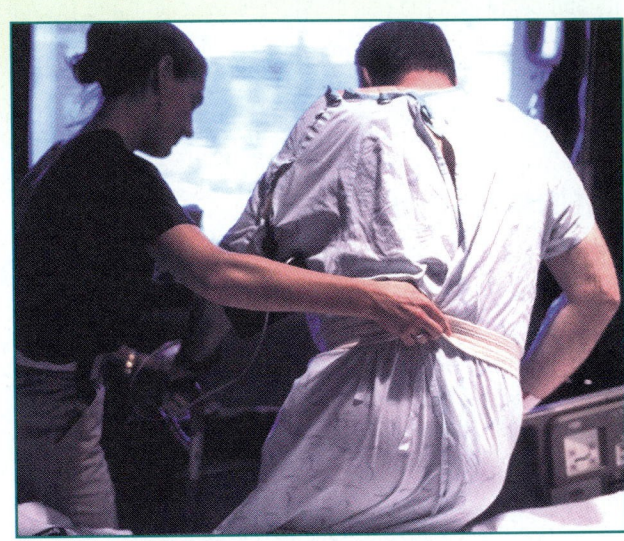

▶ OVERVIEW OF THE SKILL

Clients are often unable to get out of bed and ambulate independently while in the hospital. Because of the multisystem effects of prolonged bed rest, it is medically advantageous for clients to resume ambulating as quickly as possible and emotionally and mentally advantageous to resume purposeful activity within their environment. The adverse effects of bed rest include muscle weakness, decreased range of motion, decreased endurance, orthostatic hypotension, deconditioning, depression, as well as clots, constipation, decreased elimination leading to ulcer and abrasion responses, and possible consequences to skin integrity.

Depending upon how deconditioned the client is and the effects of orthostatic hypotension, the client may need to progress to ambulation slowly. After the client is comfortably able to tolerate sitting on the side of the bed and then standing at the side of the bed, progressive ambulation activities can be initiated. If a client is unable to bear full weight on either leg or has difficulty with balance and ambulation, aid is often necessary. It is often helpful to have the client set ambulation goals and to monitor progress either with ambulating distance, speed of ambulating, or by the amount of assistance necessary to ambulate.

For both client and caregiver safety, a gait belt should always be used during ambulation activities. The gait belt should be secured about the waist of the client. Because the gait belt is close to the client's center of gravity, the caregiver's ability to assist the client to maintain balance is enhanced. For foot protection, the client should also always wear a stable shoe while ambulating. Disturbances in balance, coordination, proprioception, as well as weakness, low endurance, and deconditioning often occur as a result of the consequences of medical/surgical procedures. This can cause clients to need assistance with ambulation. Therefore, the client's blood pressure, respiration rate, pulse rate, color and moisture of skin, and subjective comments should be monitored closely, as well as neurologic responses such as orientation, tremors, tetany change in consciousness state, or other neurologic, compromised states.

▶ ASSESSMENT

1. Assess the client's ambulating potential. This includes the client's age, medical diagnosis, cognitive status, and altered sensation, as well as assessment of the client's neuromuscular, musculoskeletal, and cardiovascular systems. Also, check the physician's

or qualified practitioner's orders for specific restrictions to client ambulation. **To determine the client's potential tolerance for the procedure as well as any limitations the client may experience.**

2. Assess client's limitations to functional mobility and ability to perform safe and effective activities of daily living (ADL). **To determine the safest way to perform the procedure.**

▶ DIAGNOSIS

Impaired Physical Mobility

Risk for Impaired Skin Integrity

Risk for Activity Intolerance

Risk for Falls

▶ PLANNING

Expected Outcomes:

1. The client's functional abilities will improve.
2. The client's strength and endurance will improve.
3. The effects of immobility on the client will be minimized or avoided.

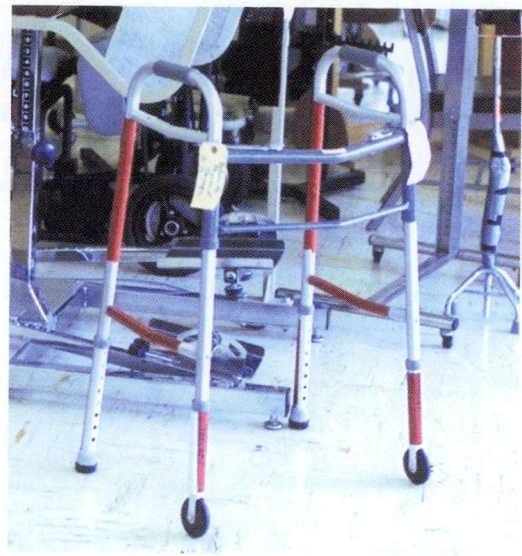

Figure 4-18-2 Walker

Equipment Needed (see Figures 4-18-1 and 4-18-2):

- Ambulation device, as required
- Proper-fitting shoes

▶ CLIENT EDUCATION NEEDED:

1. Inform the client of the adverse effects of prolonged immobility.
2. Inform the client of the advantages of progressive mobility. Help the client set reasonable and obtainable ambulation goals.
3. Encourage the client during progressive mobility activities.
4. Inform the client of the signs and symptoms of fatigue, orthostatic hypotension, disequilibrium, or other untoward responses to activity.
5. If necessary, problem-solve with the client to make necessary changes to the home environment to allow for safe and effective ambulation.

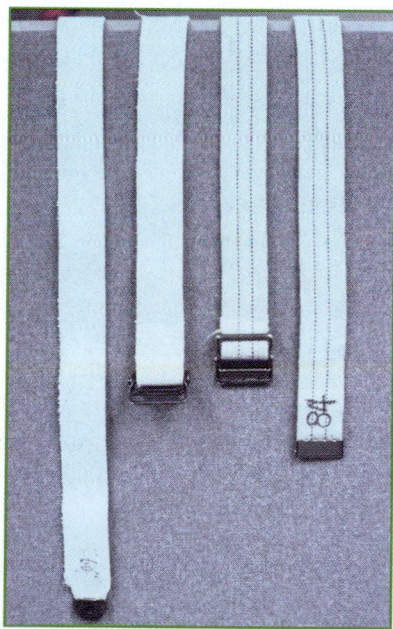

Figure 4-18-1 Gait belts

Estimated time to complete the skill:
10–20 minutes

▶ DELEGATION TIPS

This skill is routinely delegated to properly trained ancillary personnel.

IMPLEMENTATION—Action/Rationale

Action	Rationale
1. Wash hands.	1. Reduces the transmission of microorganisms.
2. Explain procedure to the client to elicit client cooperation and participation.	2. Decreases anxiety, improves client compliance and cooperation.
3. Provide for client privacy.	3. Practices respect and ensures client dignity.
4. Adjust bed to a comfortable working height. Lower side rail on side of bed from which you are assisting client.	4. Prevents caregiver back and muscle strain.
5. Gather all necessary equipment. Position drains, tubes, and IVs to accommodate for the new client position.	5. Prevents accidental dislodgment and/or discomfort from movement by reduced mechanical tension.
6. Flatten bed and assist client in rolling toward you in balanced, orthopedically sound movements. Encourage client to actively move legs, or this may be done passively.	6. Provides for client and caregiver safety. Client movement stimulates flow of blood, especially elevation of systolic blood pressure to prevent possible orthostatic hypotension.
7. While client is in the side-lying position, assist as necessary to bring the legs off the bed. Assist client into the sitting position. Client's feet should be resting on the floor for support. If this is not possible, a footstool can be used.	7. Provides for client and caregiver safety.
8. As necessary, assist client to maintain the sitting position and monitor vital signs, as appropriate.	8. Provides for client safety and prevents possible baroreceptor/orthostatic hypotension response.
9. Secure gait belt around client's waist. Place ambulation device such as a walker within reach of the client, if necessary (see Figure 4-18-3). Assist client into standing position. Make sure bed is locked and floor is not slippery. It is helpful if client has shoes with nonslip soles. If footstool is used, have client step down to the floor, then remove footstool.	9. Provides for client and caregiver safety.
10. As necessary, assist client to maintain the standing position and monitor vital signs, as appropriate (see Figure 4-18-4).	10. Provides for client safety and secures equilibrium prior to walking experience.
11. If client is able to proceed with ambulating, assume a position beside the client and assist the client as necessary using the gait belt. Place yourself in a guarding position so as to assist client quickly and safely, if necessary. Use additional assistance, as necessary (see Figure 4-18-5).	11. Provides for client and caregiver safety.

continues

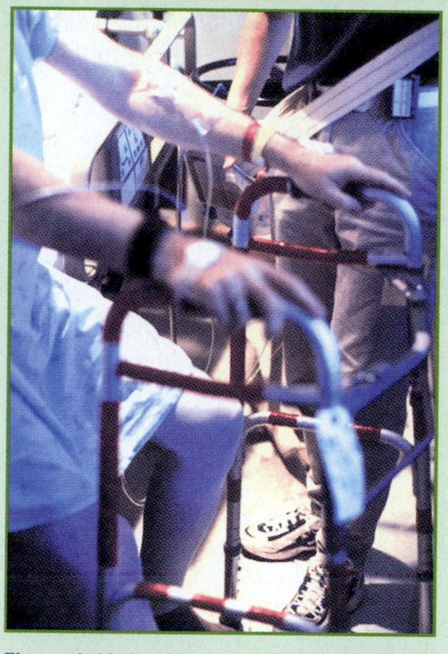

Action	Rationale

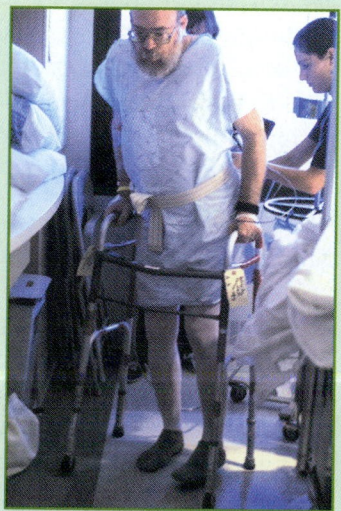

Figure 4-18-3   Place the walker in front of the client.

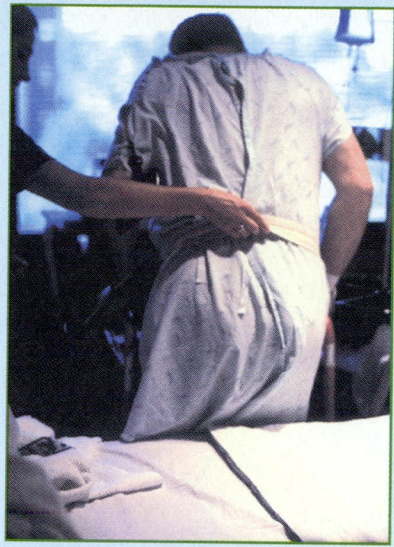

Figure 4-18-4   Assist the client into a standing position.

12. During ambulation, monitor client's vital signs, as necessary, including neurologic assessment.

13. After ambulation, return client to bed, remove gait belt, and monitor vital signs, as necessary. Note cardiovascular and neurologic "rest" responses in monitoring.

14. Replace side rails to upright position.

15. Place the call light within reach of the client.

16. Move the bedside table close to the bed and place items of frequent use within reach of the client.

17. Wash hands.

12. Provides for client safety.

13. Provides for client safety and comfort.

14. Provides for client safety.

15. Provides for client safety.

16. Provides for client safety.

17. Reduces the transmission of microorganisms.

Figure 4-18-5   Assist the client to maintain the standing position, if needed.

► **EVALUATION**

- Client's functional abilities improved.
- Client's strength and endurance improved.
- The effects of immobility were minimized or avoided.

► **DOCUMENTATION**

Nurses' Notes

- Distance walked
- Amount of assistance required
- Ambulation device used, if any
- Client response to ambulating (including vital sign assessment)
- Client/family education
- Client's response to activity, biophysical as well as psychosocial

Document on appropriate flow sheet or electronic medical record (EMR).

► **CRITICAL THINKING SKILL**

Introduction

Clients have a basic need for physical homeostasis and safety. Assisting, facilitating, strengthening, and maintaining this movement toward increased freedom and esteem is crucial.

Possible Scenario

A client has an orthopedic surgical procedure in which walking initially is not ordered or permitted.

The nurse recognizes that this loss of control is perceived to decrease self-control. During this period, the nurse actively promotes moving, turning, coughing, passive range of motion, and isotonic exercises. The goal is to help the client maintain muscular functioning and realize the effects of exercise, including better peripheral and central circulation, prevention of clots and subsequent possible embolism, decreased constipation, improved urinary elimination, and less depression.

Possible Outcome

The client keeps his muscle strength and suffers no complications from his period of immobility. His gradual return to walking strengthens his muscles, improves his neurologic responses, and equilibrium, as well as enhancing his ego strength and esteem. Throughout his recovery, the nurse is supportive of his continued ambulation, knowing that walking is vital to maintaining central and peripheral body perfusion, skin, and neurologic functioning.

Prevention

Movement, from changes in bed position to walking, prevents the effects of immobility. Walking is also important in the prevention of social isolation, improving orientation to time, place, or person by increasing contact with the external environment. Often during walking, memories, thoughts, and wishes are revisited, thus improving morale, temperament, and esteem.

► VARIATIONS

Geriatric Variations:

- *Compromised cardiovascular or neurologic systems may signal a need for slower, careful movements to lessen occurrence of faintness, change in pulse from baseline, disequilibrium, or other untoward sensory/motor responses to physical stress.*
- *Some cardiovascular, psychotropic, and sedative medications may lessen or compromise stability and equilibrium.*
- *The walking experience may also be a motivator for enhanced attention to self-care/hygiene and respect.*

Pediatric Variations:

- *Attention to age-appropriate movement, to improve balance and posture, facilitates the experience of walking.*
- *Specific, fun, age-appropriate goals, such as a trip to a social/creative/recreational activity, increases motivation for the walking experience.*

Home Care Variations:

- *Evaluate the home environment for obstacles to safe ambulation such as slippery floors, throw rugs, and narrow stairs.*
- *Remember to plan for the extra exertion that sloping walkways or driveways require.*
- *Lighting and visibility should be evaluated for safety.*
- *Evaluate the presence or lack of assistive devices, bearing in mind that this may be related to socio-economic/access issues.*

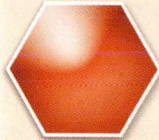

Long-Term Care Variations:

- *Environmental safety, including lighting, noise level, stair rails, and the condition of the floors, are essential in the long-term care setting.*
- *Combine the ambulation experience with a pleasurable motivation such as social, recreational, or creative activities.*

► COMMON ERRORS

Possible Error:

The nurse does not use a gait belt when assisting the client with ambulation.

Prevention:

Be sure to have the proper equipment available before starting any procedure. Be sure the equipment is in good working order.

Possible Error:

The client is not wearing nonslip supportive shoes.

Prevention:

Be aware of the footwear available to the client. Know how to obtain nonslip footwear if it is available. Have a family member or caregiver bring the footwear the client will be wearing most of the time, if possible.

► **NURSING TIPS**

- Have all equipment necessary for ambulating readily available in the client's room.
- If the client becomes dizzy after standing, check blood pressure in lying, sitting, and standing positions to assess for orthostatic hypotension.
- Progressively advance the client toward independent ambulation, as possible.
- Encourage the client with positive reinforcement during mobility activities.
- Attend to environmental or potential obstacles before the walking experience.

► **SPECIAL CONSIDERATIONS**

- *A postoperative client recovering from surgery may experience pain with ambulation. Offer the client pain medication 20 to 30 minutes before ambulation.*
- *If the client has had vascular surgery, such as a femoral-popliteal bypass, then it is necessary to carefully observe the wound for seepage when ambulating.*
- *If the client loses her or his footing or weakens to the point where she or he cannot stand, gently lower the client to the floor. Call for assistance and with two people assist the client to the standing position or get a wheelchair to return the client to her or his room.*
- *Set realistic goals for ambulation. Each day increase the distance by small increments until the client regains his or her strength.*

Using a Hydraulic Lift

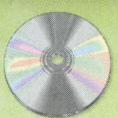

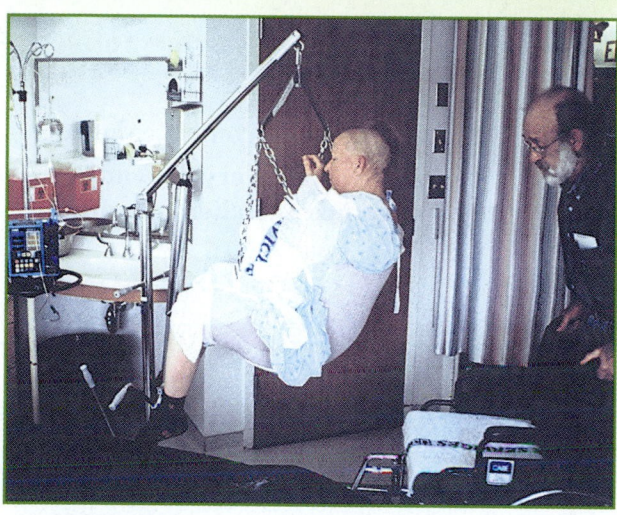

▶ OVERVIEW OF THE SKILL

The hydraulic or Hoyer lift may be used to transfer or weigh a client who is immobile or obese. The nurse may transfer a client to a stretcher, chair, bedside commode, or scale by using a hydraulic lift. Generally, the manufacturer's directions accompany equipment and should be followed. Weight limits should not exceed manufacturer's specifications. Two personnel are needed to use equipment safely. Do not use on spinal cord injury clients.

▶ ASSESSMENT

1. Identify clients with any injuries of the vertebrae. **The use of the lift may be contraindicated**.
2. Identify any equipment that is connected to the client, such as intravenous tubing or a catheter. **Determines how the procedures will be performed. Allows planning to avoid stretching, tipping, or dislodging tubes and equipment.**
3. Assess client's need for transfer and physical and mental condition, including assessment of vital signs before transfer. **Allows for safe transfer.**
4. Assess client's ability to assist and understand transfer. **Affects safety and good body mechanics for caregivers.**

5. Assess number of staff needed for transfer. Generally at least two staff members are needed for a safe transfer with a hydraulic lift. **Affects safety and good body mechanics for caregivers.**
6. Determine whether client is in appropriate clothes and ready for transfer. **Ensures the smoothness of the procedure.**

▶ DIAGNOSIS

Impaired Physical Mobility

Risk for Falls

▶ PLANNING

Expected Outcomes:

1. Client will be transferred safely.
2. Client will not experience anxiety during the transfer.
3. Client will incur no injuries.
4. Privacy will be maintained.

Equipment Needed (see Figure 4-19-1):

- Mechanical lift, such as hydraulic or Hoyer lift
- Equipment should include lift, plus canvas or mesh sheet and bars to slide into sheet
- Protective disposable cover or disinfectant to clean canvas
- Gloves (when applicable)

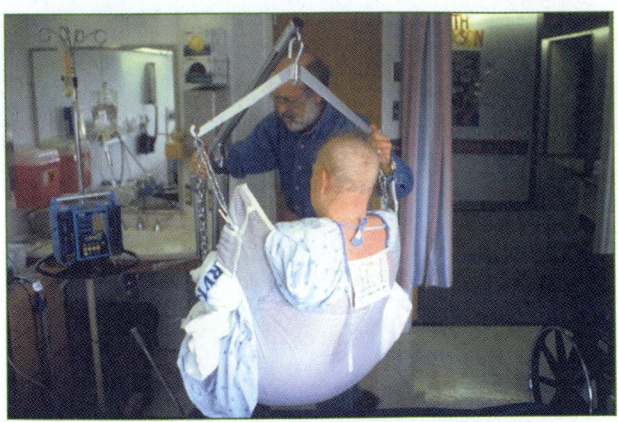

Figure 4-19-1   Raise the client from the bed and steer the lift away from the bed.

▶ **CLIENT EDUCATION NEEDED:**

1. The client understands the purpose of the procedure such as to obtain weight or to transfer.

2. The client understands that she or he will be suspended temporarily above the bed and moved to a chair or stretcher.
3. The client understands that she or he should lie still during the procedure.
4. The client understands the purpose of keeping hands crossed over the chest as the client is moved.

Estimated time to complete the skill: **15 minutes; may vary depending on assistance and client condition**

▶ **DELEGATION TIPS**

This skill is routinely delegated to properly trained ancillary personnel. Supervision by a licensed nurse may be required for the client with multiple invasive lines.

IMPLEMENTATION—Action/Rationale

Action	Rationale
1. Wash hands.	1. Reduces the transmission of microorganisms.
2. Check the physician's or qualified practitioner's order to determine the length of time the client may sit.	2. The physician or qualified practitioner may want the client to sit only for a specified length of time or for as long as possible.
3. Check the client's medical diagnosis and any other medical problems.	3. Assists you in determining any problems that sitting may cause or any restrictions needed.
4. Ask the client how long ago he or she last sat.	4. If the client has been in the bed several days, he or she may complain of dizziness or faintness.
5. Lock the wheels of the bed.	5. Prevents the bed from rolling when the client is moved.
6. Position the chair close to the bed.	6. Always transfer the client the shortest possible distance.
7. Position urine drainage, nasogastric, and IV tubing on the side of the bed where the chair will be placed. Ensure slack in the tubing.	7. Prevents the tubing from being dislodged when the client is moved.

continues

Action	Rationale
8. Clamp and disconnect any tubing, if permitted.	8. Nasogastric suction tubing and tube-feeding tubing are often allowed to be clamped. This makes moving the client easier.
9. Roll the client on his or her side and position the sling on the bed behind the client (see Figure 4-19-2).	9. The sling is positioned behind the client so the client can be turned in the opposite direction and the sling can be pulled through.
10. Roll the client on his or her opposite side, pull the sling through, and position the sling smoothly on the bed.	10. Prevents skin breakdown.
11. Roll the client back onto the sling and fold the arms over the chest (see Figure 4-19-3).	11. Prevents injury to the client's arms during the transfer.
12. Make sure the sling is centered.	12. Evenly distributes the client's weight.
13. Lower the side rail and position the lift on the side of the bed with the chair. Be sure to spread the base of the hydraulic lift as indicated in the manufacturer's instructions to provide stability (see Figure 4-19-4). Protect the client from falls while the side rail is down.	13. The side rail must be down to use the lift. Always transfer the client the shortest possible distance. The wheels and base of the lift should be spread to provide a wide, stable base to prevent the lift from tipping.
14. Lift the frame and pass it over the client. Carefully lower the frame and attach the hooks to the sling (see Figures 4-19-5 and 4-19-6).	14. Safely attaches the sling to the frame.
15. Raise the client from the bed by pumping the handle.	15. Read the manufacturer's directions to determine the mechanism for raising the particular lift you are using. The various models do not operate in the same manner.
16. Secure the client with a safety belt and cover the client with a blanket.	16. Provides safety and comfort.
17. Steer the client away from the bed and slide a chair through the base of the lift.	17. It is safer to slide the chair through the base than to slide the base around the chair.

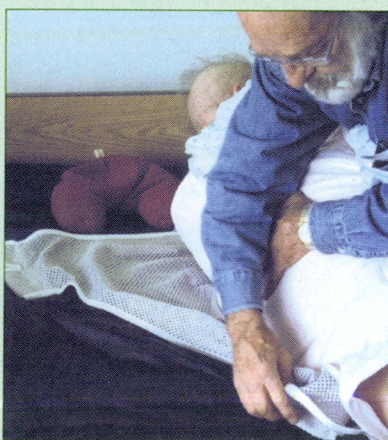

Figure 4-19-2   Adjust the sling so it is smooth and flat under the client.

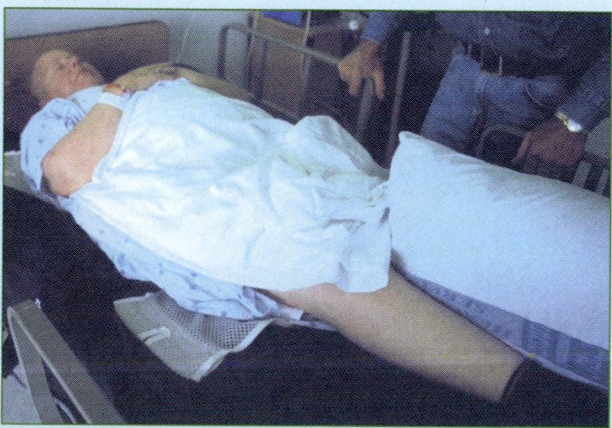

Figure 4-19-3   Roll the client back onto the sling. Position the client's arms across his or her chest.

continues

Action	Rationale

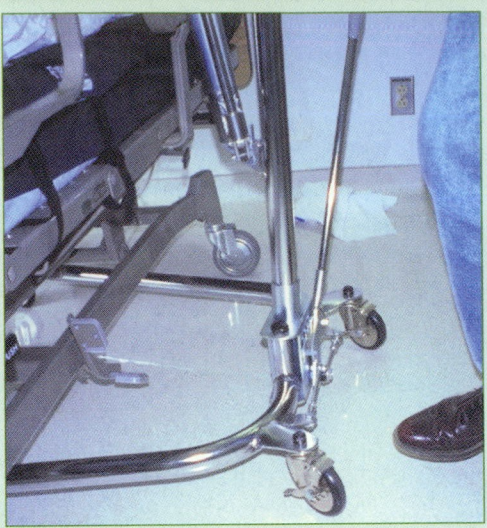

Figure 4-19-4 Spread the base of the hydraulic lift to provide stability.

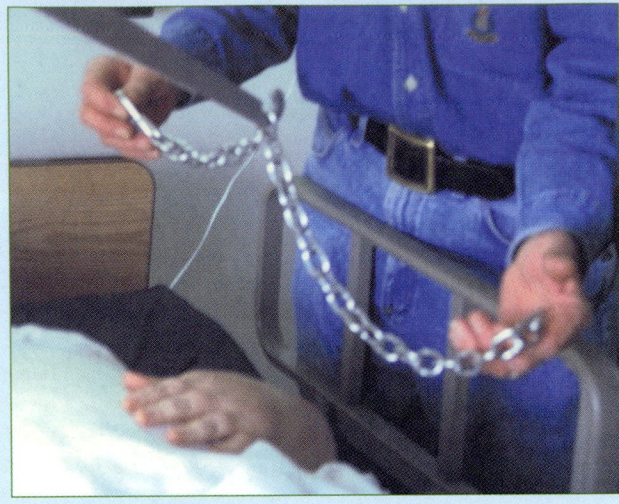

Figure 4-19-5 Locate the correct hook for each corner of the sling.

18. The sling can be disconnected and the lift can be moved out of the way while the client is sitting in the chair. If the lift will be used to return the client to bed, the sling may be left in place beneath the client.

18. The sling can be disconnected and the lift can be moved out of the way while the client is sitting in the chair.

19. Reposition and reconnect any tubing necessary.

19. Tubing should not be left disconnected. The client may sit for a while and will need all the equipment to function properly.

20. Assess how well the client tolerated the move and whether any dizziness was experienced.

20. The data are necessary for charting whether the client experienced any problems.

21. Place call light, appropriate covers, and padding as needed after transfer. Place protective restraints as needed. Cover feet with slippers if in sitting position.

21. Ensures privacy and protection.

22. Reverse the procedure to return the client to the bed.

22. Transfers client safely and comfortably.

23. Wash hands.

23. Reduces the transmission of microorganisms.

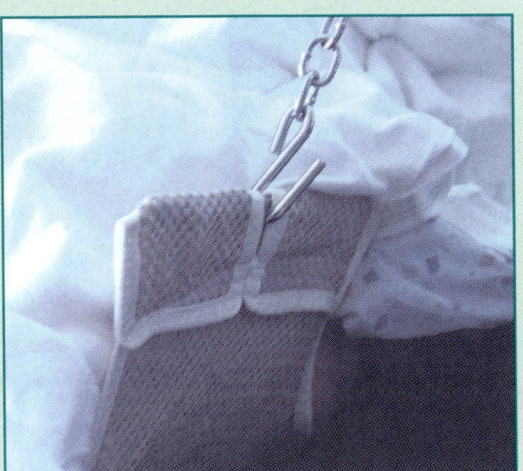

Figure 4-19-6 Attach the hooks to the sling.

▶ REAL WORLD ANECDOTES

Nurse Andrews was using the hydraulic lift to move Mrs. Gunderson from her wheelchair into the hydrotherapy tub. Mrs. Gunderson's primary care nurse had used a hydraulic lift and sling to move her into the wheelchair and had left the sling underneath Mrs. Gunderson to facilitate the move into the hydrotherapy tub. Because she had not been involved in the original transfer from bed to wheelchair, Nurse Andrews was not aware that the sling was badly worn and fraying. Nurse Andrews successfully lifted Mrs. Gunderson from the wheelchair and was maneuvering her over the water-filled hydrotherapy tub when she heard a tearing sound. As she heard the sound, Mrs. Gunderson cried out that she was falling. Nurse Andrews realized that the sling was tearing and that Mrs. Gunderson was in danger of falling and being injured. She quickly maneuvered the sling into position over the tub and lowered Mrs. Gunderson into the water. The sling gave way, just as Mrs. Gunderson was almost in place in the tub. Fortunately, the water cushioned Mrs. Gunderson as she fell the last few inches into the tub and she was unharmed. However, as a result of this incident, Mrs. Gunderson refused further hydrotherapy treatments and any other use of the hydraulic lift. This delayed her healing and prolonged her hospital stay.

▶ EVALUATION

- Client was transferred safely.
- Client did not experience anxiety during the transfer.
- Client incurred no injuries.
- Privacy was maintained.

▶ DOCUMENTATION

Nurses' Notes

- Document the date and time of the procedure.
- If the client was transferred to a chair, document how the client tolerated sitting and if he or she experienced any dizziness.
- Note how the client tolerated the transfer and any unusual findings.

Document on appropriate flow sheet or electronic medical record (EMR).

▶ CRITICAL THINKING SKILL

Introduction

A 400-lb man is to be moved to a cardiac chair in a room with limited space. He states that he is very frightened because the previous nurses had a hard time and the sling was swinging back and forth. It was also difficult to position him in this type of chair. He was sure he was going to fall.

Possible Scenario

If the client is moved too fast and the center of gravity changes abruptly, it can be frightening to the client as well as cause swinging back and forth and the lift might tip.

Also, cardiac chairs have high backs, and it can be difficult to position clients in them.

Possible Outcome

If the lift is moved too quickly, the center of gravity could change enough to cause the lift to tip, dropping the client. Because of the lack of space to maneuver the lift it may be difficult to adequately position the client in the cardiac chair.

Prevention

It is not always possible to have ideal circumstances when moving clients. If the room is too crowded to maneuver in, it may be necessary to move some of the furniture into the hallway temporarily. Be sure the bed and chair are positioned as close together as possible to avoid undue manipulation of the lift. Move them if necessary. Be sure to have adequate staff available to ensure client safety and client confidence.

▶ VARIATIONS

Geriatric Variations:

- *Older clients may have difficulty with sudden moves; therefore, take time to explain procedures and move slowly.*
- *Make sure the client can see and hear what you are doing.*
- *Make sure eyeglasses and hearing aids are in place.*

Pediatric Variations:

- *Children may be fearful of the suspension above the bed and being moved to the chair.*
- *Explain the procedure and first demonstrate how the lift is locked in place and then released to allow the sling to lower. Smaller children can often just be picked up. The weight of a child who must be moved with a hydraulic lift may be determined by hospital policy.*

Home Care Variations:

- *Check hydraulic fluid and functioning of the lift to ascertain that the equipment works.*
- *Have appropriate maintenance performed.*
- *Make sure any caregiver who is using the lift is trained in the procedure. The client can often instruct the caregiver and control the procedure in the home setting.*
- *Make sure there is enough space to maneuver the lift.*
- *Launder the sling periodically to keep it clean.*

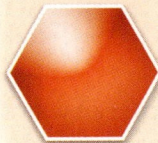

Long-Term Care Variation:

- *These are the same as home care variations. In the long-term setting, increase the independence and control the client has over the procedure as much as possible.*

▶ COMMON ERRORS

Possible Error:

The lift is lowered too rapidly.

Prevention:

Take your time; lower the handle slowly.

Possible Error:

Base is not widened to provide stability.

Prevention:

Be sure to know and understand the manufacturer's instructions regarding use of the equipment. Remember to widen the base of the lift to provide stability.

Possible Error:

The client is moved too fast and swinging occurs.

Prevention:

Take your time.

continues

► **COMMON ERRORS** *(continued)*

Possible Error:

Body parts, tubes, linens get pinched or pulled.

Prevention:

Plan ahead to move tubes and lines. Make sure the client's and caregiver's hands and fingers are away from the moving parts of the lift.

► **NURSING TIPS**

- Read directions before entering the room.
- Note open and closed position of hydraulic lift.
- Check that the handle is in the proper position.
- Ask clients to keep their hands crossed over the chest to provide stability and prevent hands changing the center of gravity.

► **SPECIAL CONSIDERATIONS**

- *Your hospital may use the "Arjo" style lift for your clients. This lift accommodates clients up to 190 kg and can work by battery when not plugged in. The special feature of this lift is that the client may be toileted while in the lift; it does not act like a sling because it comes around the shoulder and under the legs. This device allows the client to be lifted from the floor.*
- *Check manufacturer's directions and weight limits for equipment. Routinely test equipment for proper functioning.*
- *Remember that using a lift may be very frightening for the client, especially the first time it is used. Assure the client that you are there to support him or her and that you will not let the client fall.*

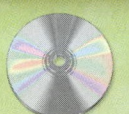

SKILL 4-20

Administering Preoperative Care

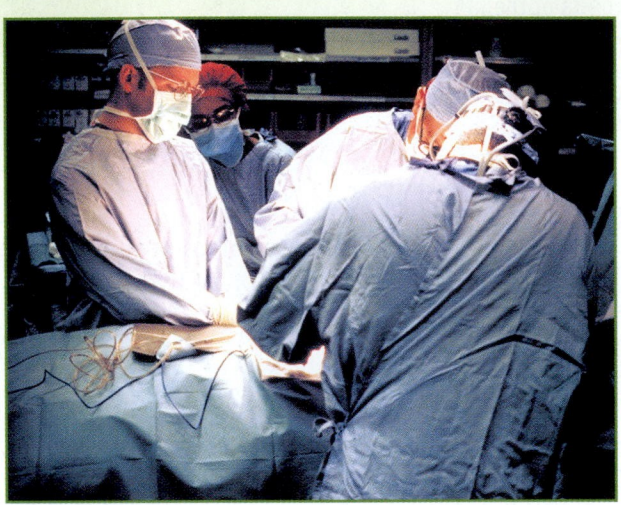

▶ OVERVIEW OF THE SKILL

For most people, surgery is a frightening prospect. Multiple fears, ranging from loss of control to death, are aroused in a client when confronted with the need for surgery. The preoperative period is the time to allay the client's fears by preparing the client mentally and physically for surgery. The preoperative phase starts when the client first considers surgery and ends when the client enters the operating room.

During the preoperative period, the nurse performs a baseline assessment of the client's mental, emotional, and physical condition. This baseline will be essential for evaluating the client's postoperative condition. The nurse determines the client's level of understanding regarding the surgery and what to expect postoperatively. Teaching during the preoperative phase is essential. The client is generally open to learning as much as possible at this time. Preoperative teaching includes teaching postoperative exercises; what to expect regarding pain, physical changes, and length of recovery; and the reason for the surgery and the various preoperative procedures. The nurse also determines the client's physical condition and prepares the client physically for surgery. This may include assisting with a preoperative shower, shaving the surgical site, administering cleansing enemas, or keeping the client from eating.

Most institutions have forms that outline the assessment and preparation required during the preoperative period. It is the nurse's responsibility to be sure that the client has been properly prepared for the next stage of surgery, the intraoperative period.

▶ ASSESSMENT

1. Assess the client's diagnosis and the planned surgery **to determine what care will be needed and what complications might be expected.**
2. Assess the client's surgical history. Determine if the client has had any previous surgical experiences that may affect the current surgery, such as a poor reaction to anesthesia or a particularly traumatic surgical history, **to reduce unnecessary frustration or discomfort and provide care that is optimal for the particular client.**
3. Assess for complicating factors, including diabetes, either treated or borderline; overweight; underweight; advanced age; malnourishment; addictions; or psychiatric disorders **to establish a baseline for intraoperative and postoperative care.**
4. Assess for any allergies, such as drugs, food, tape, latex, and iodine. Place an appropriate armband on the client and clearly note the allergy in the appropriate places in the chart **to reduce the risk of the client receiving a drug he or she is allergic to.**
5. Assess the client for false teeth, contact lenses, artificial eyes, rings, jewelry, or mementos that

cannot accompany the client to the operating room **to prevent possible loss or physical trauma resulting from wearing these items during surgery.**

6. Determine when nothing per mouth (NPO) status was initiated. In emergency situations, establish when the client last ate and what was eaten **to help the surgeon determine appropriate care and precautions.**

7. Assess the client's level of understanding regarding the plan of care during the recovery period **to determine what education and support will be needed.**

8. Make sure signed informed consents have been obtained **to provide legal coverage for the planned surgery and type of anesthesia.**

▶ DIAGNOSIS

Deficient Knowledge

Anxiety

Fear

Decisional Conflict

▶ PLANNING

Expected Outcomes:

1. The client will experience decreased anxiety subsequent to appropriate instruction.
2. The client will not experience any adverse reactions caused by inadequate physical preparation.
3. The client will not experience any loss of belongings or possessions during the surgery or recovery period.
4. The client will not experience any disruption or delay of the surgery caused by poor preoperative care or planning.

Equipment Needed (see Figure 4-20-1):

- Blood pressure cuff
- Stethoscope
- Flashlight
- Preoperative checklist
- Container for dentures, glasses
- Appropriate storage for valuables and clothes
- Information packets regarding surgery

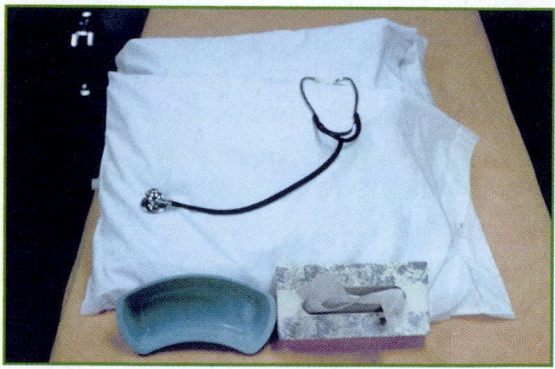

Figure 4-20-1   A stethoscope is used for preoperative assessment.

- Surgical consent forms indicating risks
- Intravenous fluids, needles, and equipment as needed
- Preoperative medications
- Transfer cart

▶ CLIENT EDUCATION NEEDED:

1. Ascertain what information has been provided to the client by the physician or qualified practitioner.
2. If the client has further questions, answer as appropriate.
3. Remind the client that there are no "dumb" questions.
4. Explain the need for removal of rings, dentures, prostheses, contacts, glasses, or studs from a pierced tongue.
5. Explain the reason for not eating before the surgery.
6. Inform the client of what to expect preoperatively and postoperatively. Long waits in the operating suite can be frightening if this is not anticipated, especially if clients do not know what to expect.
7. Transfer the client directly to another staff member. Do not move the client to the operating room waiting area and leave unattended.

Estimated time to complete the skill: **20–30 minutes**

▶ DELEGATION TIPS

Assessment of the physical condition and the learning needs of the preoperative client requires the skill of a nurse. Collection of clinical data such as vital signs, weights, and laboratory specimens may be delegated.

IMPLEMENTATION—Action/Rationale

Action	Rationale
1. Wash hands.	1. Reduces the transmission of microorganisms.
2. Verify admission orders regarding the type of surgery, any risks (including recent changes in vital signs), and client preparation.	2. Provides accurate information and baseline information.
3. Verify the client by checking name tag and asking name.	3. Provides safety and protects legally.
4. Check whether the client has any questions regarding the surgery and understands the procedure and explain accordingly.	4. Decreases anxiety. Clients who are uninformed may be more vulnerable and at higher risk for complications.
5. Complete the preoperative checklist, including history, physical assessment, and check of valuables.	5. Provides baseline data.
6. Perform neurologic assessment, including checks for orientation, eye coordination, handgrips, knee bends, and plantar and dorsiflexion of the feet (see Figure 4-20-2).	6. Provides baseline data for postoperative assessment and changes.
7. Perform vascular assessment (see Figure 4-20-3), including checks of pulse, blood pressure, and apical pulse rhythm, peripheral pulses, and temperature. Compare with previous information. Clients older than 50 years of age may require baseline electrocardiogram.	7. Provides baseline data. If any irregularities, notify physician to avoid complications.
8. Auscultate the lungs bilaterally front and back (see Figure 4-20-4). If any wheezes, rhonchi, coughs, upper respiratory infections, or increased temperature are noted, notify physician or qualified practitioner.	8. Provides baseline data and avoids potential complications such as postoperative pneumonia. Surgery may need to be rescheduled if there is an upper respiratory infection.

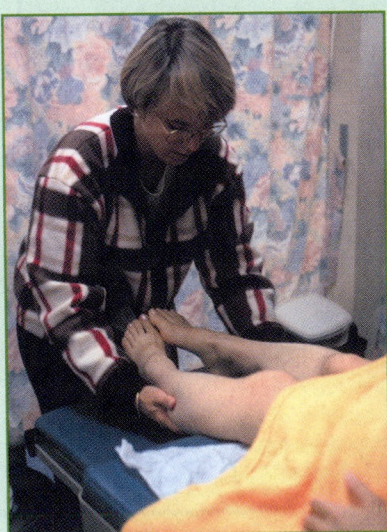

Figure 4-20-2   Perform a neurologic assessment.

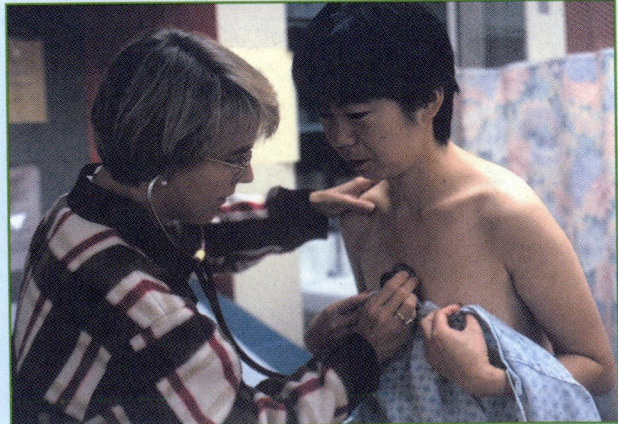

Figure 4-20-3   Perform a vascular assessment, including peripheral pulses.

continues

Action	Rationale
9. Assess the gastrointestinal system (time of last meal, food allergies, bowel sounds, last bowel movement, time of last fluids).	9. Provides baseline data and prevents postoperative nausea, vomiting, and aspiration pneumonia. If the client has eaten recently, surgery may need to be rescheduled. Usual instructions are NPO after midnight on the day of scheduled surgery.
10. Assess the genital/urinary system (last menstrual period, last void, state of pregnancy, estrogen replacement therapy).	10. Provides baseline data.
11. Assess skin and muscle tone for any skin breakdown, redness, bruises, or decreased skin integrity (see Figure 4-20-5).	11. Provides baseline data.
12. Ascertain any allergies, including any adverse reactions during previous surgeries or use of anesthesia.	12. Provides baseline data. Of special importance are allergies to iodine because povidone-iodine is a common antiseptic used in surgical site preparation.
13. Obtain medication history, including the time and date of the last dose of medication.	13. Provides baseline data and avoids drug interaction. Provides for daily medications that need to be administered. Ascertain that surgeon is cognizant of daily medications. Especially important is insulin use. Orders must be written regarding insulin use preoperatively and postoperatively. Other medications that can affect surgical outcome are aspirin, anticoagulants (increase bleeding); steroids (suppress immunity); nonsteroidal anti-inflammatories (increase risk of stress ulcers and displace other drugs from blood proteins); bromide medications (signs and symptoms of dementia); and drugs with anticholinergic effects (increase confusion).

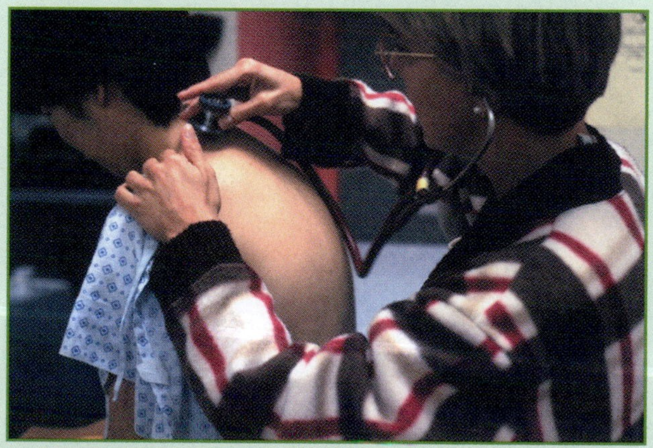

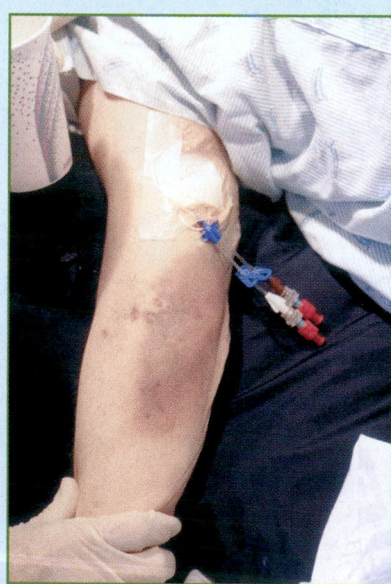

Figure 4-20-4 Auscultate the lungs.

Figure 4-20-5 Assess skin condition and look for signs of breakdown, redness, or bruises.

continues

Action	Rationale
14. Ascertain any history of drugs/alcohol use and when they were last used.	**14.** Prevents alcohol/drug withdrawal during or after surgery. Withdrawal from alcohol can occur 8 hours after the last drink and may require treatment. Withdrawal can cause major complications in combination with surgery. The use of drugs/alcohol could alter the way pain medications are used and their effect.
15. Obtain weight.	**15.** Provides a baseline for postsurgical assessment.
16. Check whether family is available and who is present.	**16.** Presence of family or significant others may decrease anxiety and provide support.
17. Ascertain whether client has signed the surgical consent. Determine whether the client has a living will or has designated resuscitation status.	**17.** Surgical consents must be signed by client, legal guardian, or next of kin to provide legal basis for surgery. A living will or resuscitation status provides legal guidelines for client requests.
18. Remove all valuables with the exception of wedding rings, if requested. Tape rings in place. Check and document whether valuables are placed in a locked area, safe storage area, or given to family.	**18.** Provides security for items.
19. Check if eyeglasses and dentures are removed; place in a labeled container.	**19.** Provides security and safety. Dentures can interfere with intubation and become dislodged, broken, or misplaced during surgery.
20. Administer intravenous fluids according to orders (see Figure 4-20-6).	**20.** Follows orders and protocol.
21. Administer medications according to orders.	**21.** Follows orders.
22. Ascertain that preoperative checklist is complete.	**22.** Appropriate protocol.

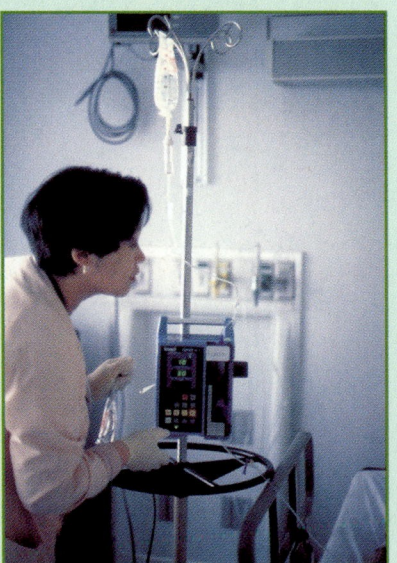

Figure 4-20-6 Administer intravenous fluids according to orders.

continues

Action	Rationale
23. Transport the client to appropriate area.	**23.** Appropriate protocol.
24. Inform family members where the surgical waiting area is and establish a way to contact them when the surgery is completed.	**24.** Provides assurance to the client and family.

▶ REAL WORLD ANECDOTES

Mrs. Avdic was admitted for an exploratory laparoscopy. When the nurse asked her to sign the informed consent, she wanted to wait until her husband was present. As the nurse prepared Mrs. Avdic for surgery, the unsigned informed consent was pushed to the bottom of the stack of paperwork to be filled out. By the time Mr. Avdic arrived to be with his wife, the CNA/PCA was waiting with a gurney to transport Mrs. Avdic to the operating room. Hurriedly, the nurse placed the entire stack of paperwork in the front of Mrs. Avdic's chart and sent it with the client to the operating room.

As Mrs. Avdic was being prepped in the operating room, the anesthesiologist asked her whether she had signed the informed consent. She told him that she had signed a bunch of papers and she was sure that was one of them. In a hurry, the anesthesiologist did not pursue the matter.

During surgery, Mrs. Avdic was found to have endometriosis. The surgeon decided to perform a hysterectomy because he felt that the endometriosis had spread too far. After surgery, when Mrs. Avdic was awake, the surgeon explained his findings and what he had done. Mrs. Avdic burst into tears and was inconsolable. She and her husband had been trying to have children for several years, and as a result of this surgery, they would never have a chance to have children of their own.

About a year later the surgeon received notice that the Avdics were suing him, the nurse who cared for Mrs. Avdic preoperatively, and the hospital. Without a signed consent in the chart, Mrs. Avdic was able to prove her case for malpractice. All signed consent forms must be in the chart before surgery and may have prevented the malpractice action.

▶ EVALUATION

1. The client experienced decreased anxiety subsequent to appropriate instruction.
2. The client did not experience any adverse reactions caused by inadequate physical preparation.
3. The client did not experience any loss of belongings or possessions during the surgery or recovery period.
4. The client did not experience any disruption or delay of the surgery caused by poor preoperative care or planning.

▶ DOCUMENTATION

Preoperative Checklist (see Table 4-20-1)

- Fill out and initial the preoperative checklist.
- Note any unusual findings.

Nurses' Notes

- Document on appropriate flow sheet or electronic medical record (EMR).
- Document any unusual findings from the preoperative checklist.
- Note any preoperative teaching.
- Document the disposition of client valuables, noting whether they were left at the client bedside, given to a family member, or placed in a locked area.

Medication Administration Record (MAR)

- Note any preoperative medications given and the IV insertion site if an IV was ordered.

Table 4-20-1   Preoperative Checklist

	(√)	CK Comments	Nurse CK (√)
COMPLETE NIGHT BEFORE SURGERY			
List allergies			
Procedure scheduled			
Surgical permit signed/witnessed			
History/physical on chart and/or dictated			
Preanesthetic evaluation done			
Able to state type and purpose of surgery			
Demonstrates ability to perform: Deep breathing, turning, and coughing exercises			
Leg exercises			
p.m. care with shower or bath given			
Nail polish removed and makeup removed			
Old chart requested and obtained			
Type and cross-match for _____ units of blood			
Blood consent signed and witnessed			
Labor work a. CBC _____ b. UA _____			
Tonsillectomy and Adenoidectomy clients: a. __PTT b. __PT c. __Platelets			
If ordered by MD: a. ECG ___ b. Chest X-ray _____			
Add other lab work ordered (specify)			
Notify surgeon of abnormal lab work			
New progress note and physician order sheet on chart			
Weight			
NPO after midnight (if applicable)			
Signature of Nurse _____		Date _____	
COMPLETE DAY OF SURGERY			
Jewelry removed and secured with responsible party			
Dental prosthesis, contact lenses, and tongue stud removed			
Hospital gown/cap on and undergarments removed			
Voided on call to surgery			
Indwelling catheter ordered and inserted			
Tampon removed			
Identiband and/or bloodband on/checked for accuracy			
Time _____ Pulse _____ Resp _____ BP _____ Temp. _____			
Pre-op medicine given Medication _____ Time _____ a.m. p.m.			
Side rails up and bed to lowest level			
Client instructed not to get out of bed without nursing assistance			
Addressograph plate/MARs on chart			
VS 30 minutes after pre-op (if remains on unit)			
BP _____ P _____ R _____ T _____			
Old chart sent to surgery per request			
Surgical prep done and checked			
To surgery Time _____ Via _____			

Signature of Nurse _____   Date _____
Holding Room Nurse Signature _____   Date _____

► **CRITICAL THINKING SKILL**

Introduction

A complete client history can turn up unexpected information.

Possible Scenario

A 62-year-old woman is being readied for surgery when the nurse discovers there is a history of diabetes in the family. Further questioning reveals that the client was diagnosed 4 years prior to admission with noninsulin-dependent diabetes. The nurse asks about her current diabetic treatment and monitoring. She states that she does not monitor her condition and that her surgeon is not aware of her diabetes.

Possible Outcome

The surgeon is informed and delays the surgery until a medical consult can be arranged. The client will have a longer hospital stay. However, the risk of serious complications will be lessened.

Prevention

Any client scheduled for surgery should have a complete medical and nursing history, a physical exam, and appropriate blood and diagnostic work before surgery.

► **VARIATIONS**

Geriatric Variations:
- *Elderly clients are at much greater risk for complications postoperatively, such as pneumonia and deep venous thrombosis.*
- *Elderly clients may be poor historians; therefore, the family may need to be consulted for history and medication use.*
- *Sensitivity to medications may be more pronounced in older adults; therefore, any potential sensitivity should be elicited.*
- *Skin integrity is decreased in elderly clients and tape sensitivity should be noted. Shear injuries can be caused by moving or transferring the client incorrectly.*
- *Previous fractures or the presence of osteoporosis should be noted because injuries can occur when transferring elderly clients.*
- *Because short-term memory or depth of understanding may be a problem, repeated explanations of surgery and purpose may be necessary.*
- *Hearing deficit may be present; therefore, ascertain whether the client can hear explanations.*

Pediatric Variations:
- *Because children usually are very frightened by the hospital and especially surgical experiences, explanations that are age-appropriate should be done. Parents should be present to assure the child while explanations are made and to answer questions.*
- *Drawings and the use of toys with explanations may help. Involving the child in explanations through play may be helpful.*
- *Allowing the child to take a favorite toy into surgery may allay some anxiety.*
- *Having the same nurse care for the child as much as possible may help decrease fear. Adequate time with the child may help gain trust.*
- *Medication doses are adjusted to weight, and both weight and dosage of the medications should be carefully checked.*
- *Allowing the parents to stay with the child as long as possible may be helpful unless the parent is overly anxious.*

Home Care Variation:

- *If the client is having outpatient surgery, be sure the client understands the surgical preparation she or he is being asked to perform at home, such as remaining NPO, taking laxatives or other medication prior to admission, or showering with antibacterial soap prior to admission.*

▶ COMMON ERRORS

Possible Error:

There is no name band or an inadequate name band on the client, thus making the surgical team unable to identify the sedated client or whether the client has allergies or sensitivities, especially if the chart is not with the client at all times.

Prevention:

Be sure the client has a legible name band in a place that will not interfere with IV placement or the surgical site. Be sure the name band or a second allergy band correctly identifies the client's allergies and sensitivities, even if this is "no known allergies" (NKA). This will indicate that the client has been asked about allergies.

▶ NURSING TIPS

- Recheck surgery consent forms for signature and type of surgery.
- If a client questions the type of surgery, follow up and obtain correct information and inform the surgeon.
- Recheck that presurgery forms are completely filled with assessment, valuables, and so on.
- Recheck the name band with the chart so that the appropriate chart is sent.
- Be careful not to provide inappropriate information because all laboratory and diagnostic tests may not be available to the nurse and certain questions should be referred to the physician or qualified practitioner. Inappropriate misinformation may increase unnecessary anxiety.

- If the client does not speak English as the native tongue, it may be necessary to involve an interpreter to obtain informed consent.
- If the client has a wedding ring that he or she does not remove, it should be taped to the finger and a note placed in the chart. If the surgery is going to be lengthy and the client could receive a large amount of IV fluids, every attempt should be taken to remove the ring prior to surgery.
- When listing valuables in the chart, do not specify the type of metals or stones present. Rather than list a "diamond ring with a gold band," it should be noted as a "ring with a clear stone and gold-colored band."

▶ SPECIAL CONSIDERATIONS

- *If the client is having vascular surgery (femoral-popliteal bypass) it is helpful to mark an X on the pedal pulses at dorsalis pedis and posterior tibial sites. This will help the circulating nurse (nurse not "scrubbed in") when she or he needs to locate these pulses during surgery.*
- *Inform the client that he or she may awaken to find a rectangular shape shaved on the upper leg. This site is often used for placement of the electrocautery pad and may need to be shaved to ensure proper placement.*

Preparing a Surgical Site

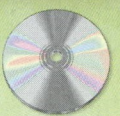

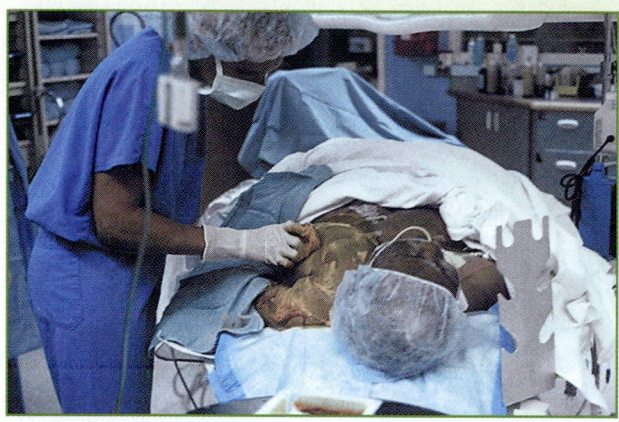

▶ OVERVIEW OF THE SKILL

Once the client arrives in the operating room, there are more preparations that are necessary to undertake before surgery can begin. The client must be positioned on the operating table in a way that will optimize the surgeon's access to the surgical site without compromising the client's neurovascular status. Once the client is in position the surgical site may need to be shaved and a final cleansing performed.

The client's position on the operating table will vary according to the type of surgery to be performed. There are several kinds of positions: the supine position, Trendelenburg position, reverse Trendelenburg position, lithotomy position, modified Fowler's position, prone position, jackknife (Kraske) position, lateral position for a chest operation, and lateral position for a kidney operation, to name just a few. The client must be positioned to allow optimal access to the needed body part. The nurse must also consider the client's inability to move during surgery when positioning a client. Because the client cannot move or tell anyone if the position is painful or impairing circulation, the nurse must position the client in a way that will not impair the client's neurovascular status during a lengthy procedure.

Once the client is positioned, the surgical site must be cleansed and prepared in a way that will reduce the possibility of infection. Site preparation is important to reduce infections, promote visualization

of the area, and to provide a clean surface for sutures and dressings. In general, surgical sites can be categorized as head and neck, lateral neck, chest, hand and forearm, thorax and abdominal, abdomen, abdominal and pubic, abdominal and perineal, perineal, thigh, lower extremity, lower leg, sacral and perineal, upper back, lower back, and flank. The prepared area should be larger than the anticipated incision site because of the possibility of an unexpected extension of the incision and to reduce possible accidental contamination of the surgical field.

Hair should be removed from the surgical site only as necessary. The three common methods of hair removal are clipping, depilatory, and wet shaving. To reduce the risk of infection, shaving should be performed as close to the time of surgery as possible. Shaving is the most common method of hair removal. It has the advantage of being easily performed with commonly available instruments. It has the disadvantage of causing microscopic cuts and skin irritation, damaging the skin's integrity, and increasing the possibility of infection. In some cases, a depilatory (hair removing cream) may be ordered the night before surgery. Depilatories use a chemical agent that destroys the hair at the root and causes the hair shaft to break down. The advantage of a depilatory is that it has less potential for cutting the skin compared with shaving. The disadvantage is that the chemical used in depilatories may cause skin irritation and possibly allergic reactions. A patch test using a small area of skin must be performed before using a depilatory on a surgical site. Clipping the hair close to the skin without actual shaving is gaining popularity as a method of surgical site preparation. It has the advantage of not causing skin damage or irritation. The disadvantage of this method is reduced visibility of the site during surgery as well as the increased possibility of harboring microorganisms among the hair shafts.

After the site is shaved, it must be thoroughly cleansed to remove as many microorganisms as possible. This further reduces the risk of infection. The solutions used for skin cleansing and disinfection vary according to each hospital policy. The solution should not irritate the skin or in any way interfere with the skin's normal functioning. The commonly used solutions are soap, detergent, and antiseptic agents such as povidone-iodine, tincture of iodine, 70% alcohol, hexachlorophene, benzalkonium chloride, chlorhexidine, and iodophor.

▶ ASSESSMENT

1. Assess the client for sensitivity or allergies to the scrub solution. Iodine preparations are most often used **to reduce the risk of skin irritation or allergic reaction.**
2. Assess skin integrity because open areas **may increase the risk of infection.**
3. Assess the client's knowledge of the surgical preparation procedure **to determine what teaching needs to be provided.**
4. Assess for existing appliances, catheters, or other instrumentation **to determine whether the preparation requires any modification.**
5. Assess the client's level of mobility at the surgical site **to determine any perioperative positioning modifications.**

▶ DIAGNOSIS

Risk for Infection

Risk for Impaired Skin Integrity

Deficient Knowledge, related to surgical preparation procedures

Risk for Perioperative Positioning Injury

▶ PLANNING

Expected Outcomes:

1. The surgical preparation will be performed without injury or trauma to the client.

2. The client will understand the procedure and the reason for it.
3. The client will not experience any allergic reaction or skin sensitivity secondary to the surgical preparation.
4. The client will not experience any infections secondary to poor site preparation.
5. The client will not experience disruption to any existing appliances, catheters, or other instrumentation.
6. The client will not experience any injury secondary to perioperative positioning.

Equipment Needed (see Figure 4-21-1):

- Gloves (clean for shaving; sterile for cleaning surgical site)
- Razor and sharp blades
- Sterile gauze (to clean the razor)
- Warm water
- Antibacterial cleansing agent
- Sterile cotton swabs
- Sterile cotton sponges
- Transfer forceps in antiseptic solution
- Solution for surgical site cleaning, such as 70% alcohol
- Solution basins
- Mask and protective goggles

▶ CLIENT EDUCATION NEEDED:

1. Explain the reason for the surgical preparation and any shaving of the area. If the area to be prepped and shaved is cosmetically important, reinforce the need for a thorough preparation of the site.

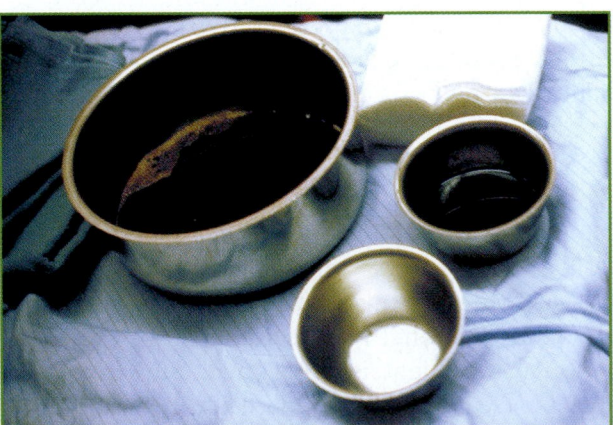

Figure 4-21-1 Basins, povidone-iodine, and sponges are used to prepare the surgical site.

2. Assure the client that the surgery may not involve the total area prepped.
3. Explain the need for proper positioning during surgery so the surgeon can easily access the site.

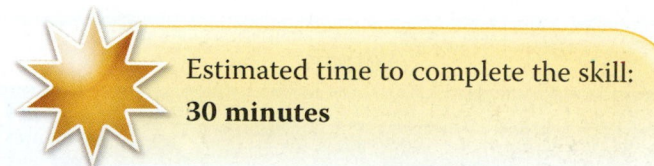

Estimated time to complete the skill:
30 minutes

▶ DELEGATION TIPS

The skill of preparing a surgical site is routinely delegated to properly trained surgical technicians. The nurse and ultimately the health care provider are responsible to ensure that the correct site is prepared.

Rectal surgery: Shave the buttocks from the iliac crest down to the upper third of the thighs, including the anal region. The area extends to the midline on each side.

Flank surgery: Extends anteriorly from the axilla, down to the upper thigh, including the external genital area. Posteriorly the area extends from the midscapular to the midgluteal regions (see Figure 4-21-6).

Hand and forearm surgery: The area includes the full circumference of the affected arm, from the axilla to the fingertips.

Lower-extremity surgery: The area includes the entire leg, toes, and foot of the affected leg from the umbilicus anteriorly and the top of the buttocks posteriorly.

Lower leg surgery: The area to be prepared includes the circumference of the entire region from midthigh to the distal toes of the affected leg.

IMPLEMENTATION—Action/Rationale

Action	Rationale
1. Review chart for surgery to be performed and determine the exact area to be prepped. Check the surgeon's preference card, which is a document that lists desired position, instruments, and suture required for the case.	1. Avoids errors regarding site to be prepped.
2. Wash hands. Don mask and protective goggles.	2. Reduces the transmission of microorganisms.
3. Assess client's level of consciousness and mobility.	3. Determines client's ability to cooperate with the skill.
4. Explain the procedure to client. Verify that the client has no allergies, especially to iodine or latex.	4. Provides comfort and support for the client. Protects client from exposure to allergenic materials.
5. Be sure that hairpins, jewelry, nail polish, contact lenses, prostheses, and dentures were removed during the preoperative preparation.	5. Removes artifacts that may interfere with the assessment and procedure.
6. Assist client with transfer from wheelchair or bed to the surgical table.	6. Ensures client safety.
7. Position the client for optimal access to the surgical site according to institutional protocol.	7. Allows the surgeon access to the body part requiring surgery.
8. Cover with blanket (see Figure 4-21-2).	8. Maintains body temperature and provides privacy. The temperature in the operation room is often lower than in the client's room.

continues

Action	Rationale

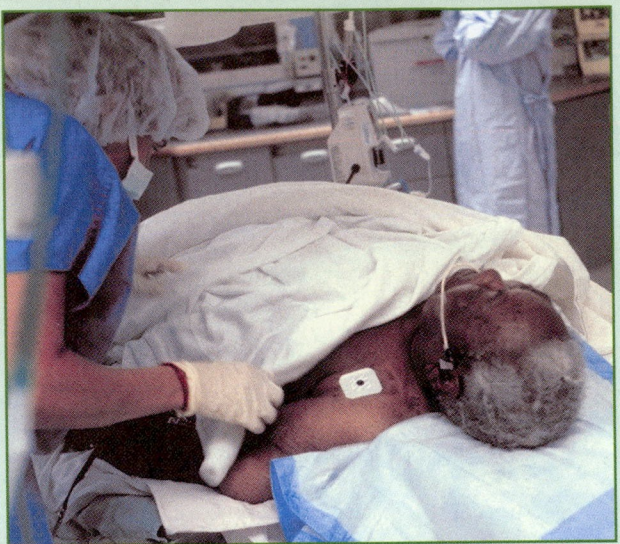

Figure 4-21-2   Covering the client with blankets helps maintain body temperature.

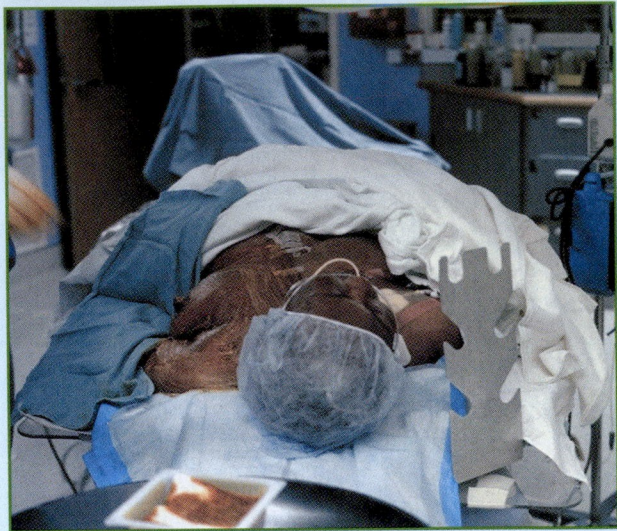

Figure 4-21-3   Covering the client's hair helps maintain a sterile field.

9. Cover hair if required (see Figure 4-21-3).

10. Assemble equipment needed (see Figure 4-21-4).

11. Remove ring(s) and watch. Wash hands and apply clean gloves.

12. The surgical prep sites follow, depending on the type of surgery to be performed.
    Head and neck: The site extends from above the eyebrows, over the top of the head, and includes the ears and both anterior and posterior areas of the neck. The face and eyebrows are not shaved (see Figure 4-21-5).

9. Keeps loose hairs from entering sterile field.

10. Ensures a smooth procedure.

11. Reduces the transmission of microorganisms. Provides infection control.

12. The area to be shaved and cleansed for surgery varies with the type of surgery to be performed. The prepared site should optimize the surgeon's access to the necessary body structures.

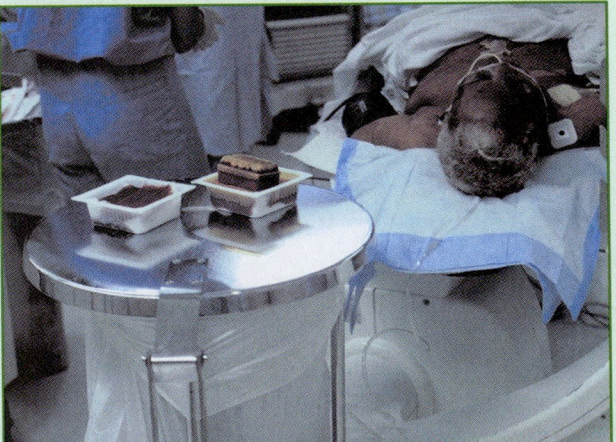

Figure 4-21-4   Assemble equipment next to the client.

continues

Action	Rationale
Lateral neck: Clean the external auditory canal with a cotton swab. Anteriorly, prepare the side of the face, from above the ear to the upper thorax to just below the clavicle. Posteriorly, prepare from the neck to the spine including the area above the scapula.	

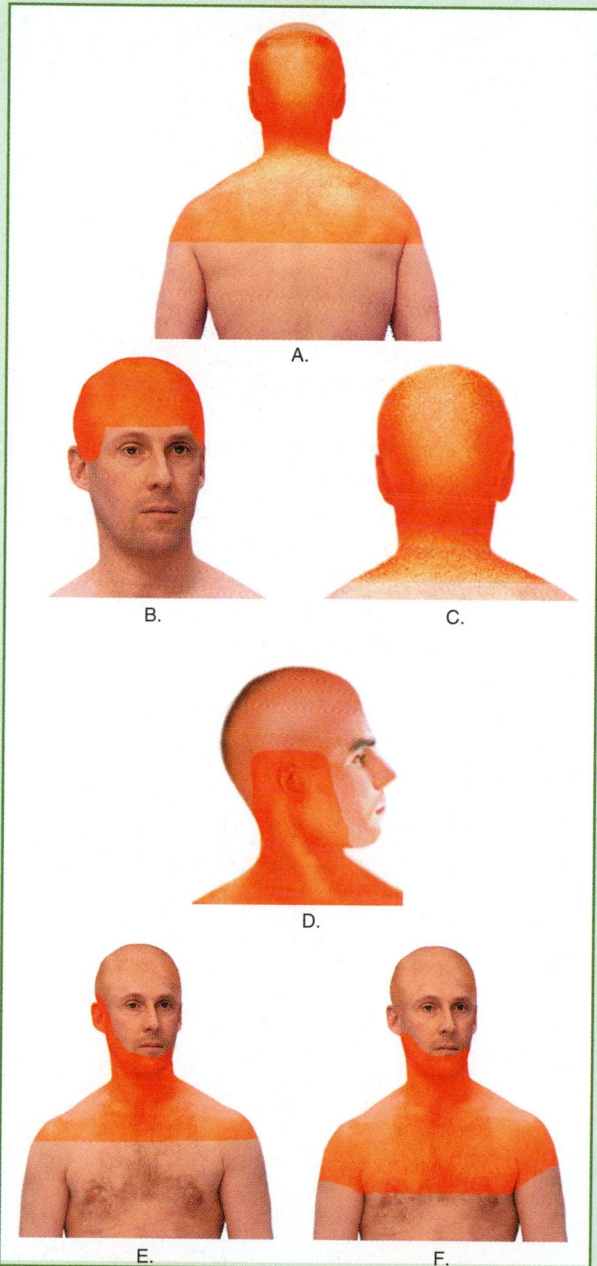

Figure 4-21-5 Preparation of the head for surgery: A–C. Head for craniotomy; D. Neck for otologic surgery; E, F. Upper thorax for thyroidectomy.

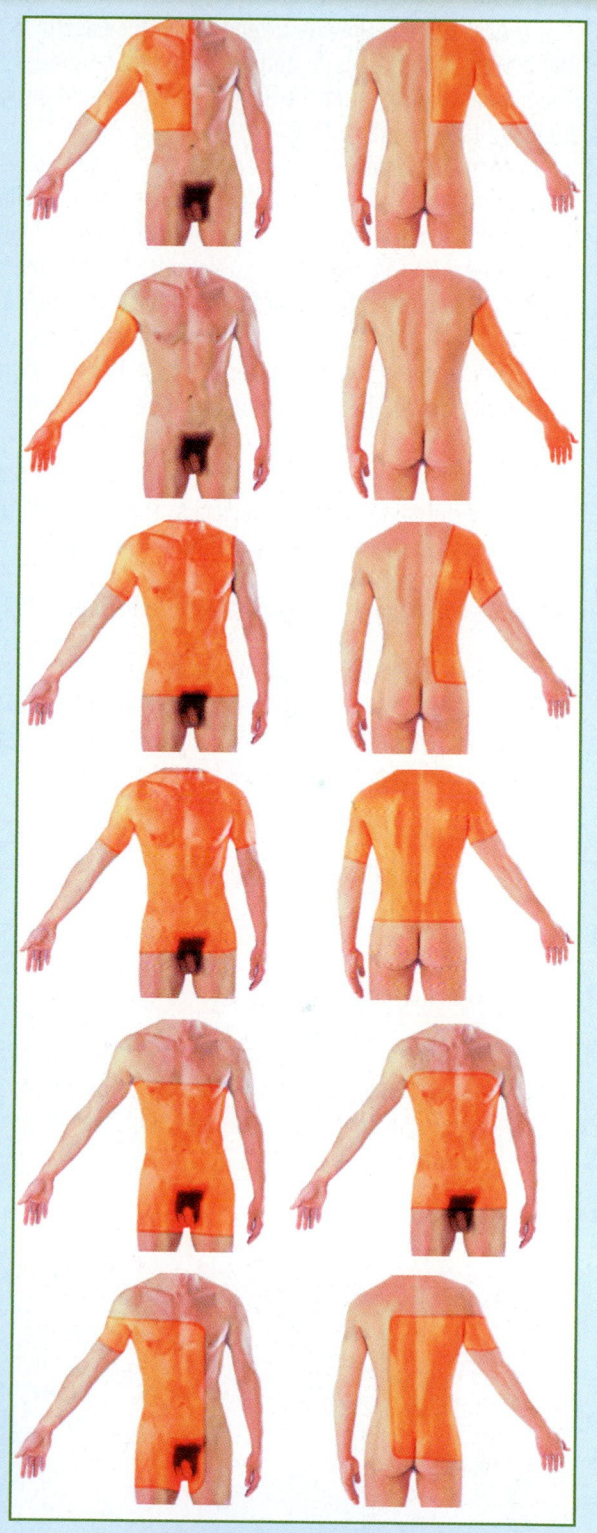

Figure 4-21-6 Preparation of the upper extremities and trunk for surgery.

continues

Action	Rationale
Chest surgery: The site extends from the neck to the bottom of the rib cage and to the lateral midline. The shoulder and arm of the operative side should be included (see Figure 4-21-6). *Abdominal surgery:* The preparation site extends from the axilla to the pubis extending bilaterally to the lateral midline. All visible pubic hair should be shaved (see Figure 4-21-6). *Perineal surgery:* Shave all pubic hair and the inner thighs to the midthigh. The area starts above the pubic bone anteriorly and extends beyond the anus posteriorly. *Cervical spine surgery:* Posteriorly from the top of the ears to the waist. The area extends on each side to the midaxillary line. *Lumbar spine surgery:* Posteriorly from the axilla down to the midgluteal level of the buttocks. The area extends on each side to the midaxillary line (see Figure 4-21-6).	
13. Arrange for adequate light on the area to be prepared.	13. Light provides for good visualization and safe shaving.
14. Using warm water, hold the skin taut and hold the razor at a 45-degree angle. Shave the area carefully by stroking in the direction of hair growth. Rinse the razor carefully to remove accumulated hair from the blade.	14. Holding skin taut will decrease chance of cutting the client. Stroking in the direction of hair growth will reduce ingrown hairs when the hair grows back. Rinsing the razor will improve performance of the blade, and decrease the amount of skin irritation.
15. Dry the client's skin with a sterile towel.	15. Prevents the spread of microorganisms.
16. Clear the shaving supplies from the preparation area.	16. Prevents contamination of the area with used supplies.
17. Apply sterile gloves.	17. Prevents the spread of microorganisms.
18. Scrub the surgical site with an antibacterial cleaner (see Figure 4-21-7). Using a rotary movement to clean the skin, begin in the center and gradually enlarge the area with each rotation.	18. Removes dirt and transient microbes from the skin. Reduces the resident microbial count as much as possible.

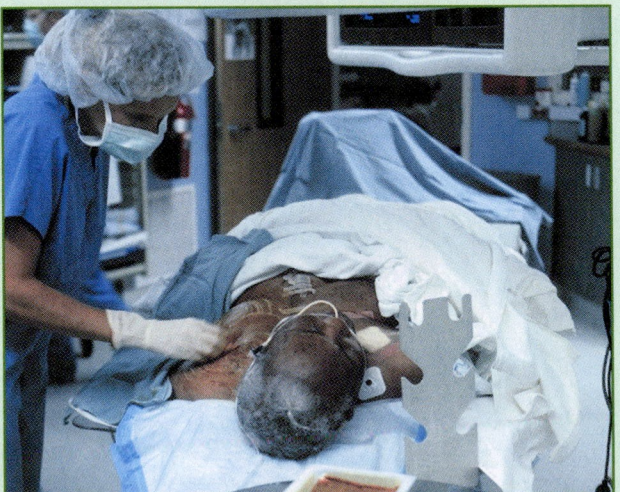

Figure 4-21-7 Scrub the surgical site using a rotary movement; start at the center and work outward.

continues

Action	Rationale
19. Continue this process for 3 to 10 minutes as prescribed by institutional policy.	**19.** Be sure to use a clean brush or swab whenever returning to the center of the surgical site to prevent recontamination of the site.
20. Clean any hidden areas in the surgical site (the ear canals, under the fingernails, the umbilicus) using cotton swabs.	**20.** Decreases transmission of microorganisms.
21. Rinse the area with sterile water. Wait for the site to dry or pat dry with a sterile towel.	**21.** Decreases transmission of microorganisms.
22. Cover the area with sterile drapes leaving the surgical site exposed (see Figures 4-21-8 to 4-21-11).	**22.** Provides a sterile field for the surgical procedure.

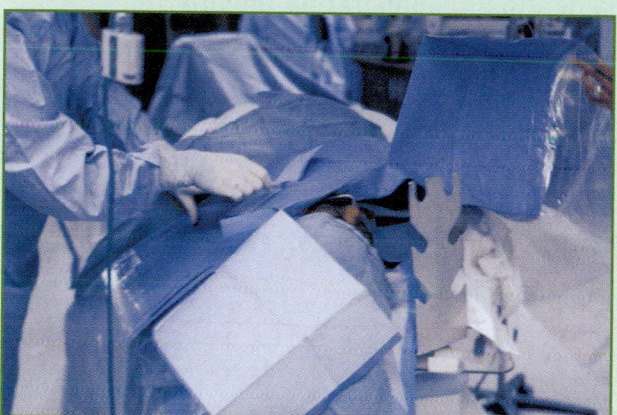

Figure 4-21-8   Cover the area with sterile drapes.

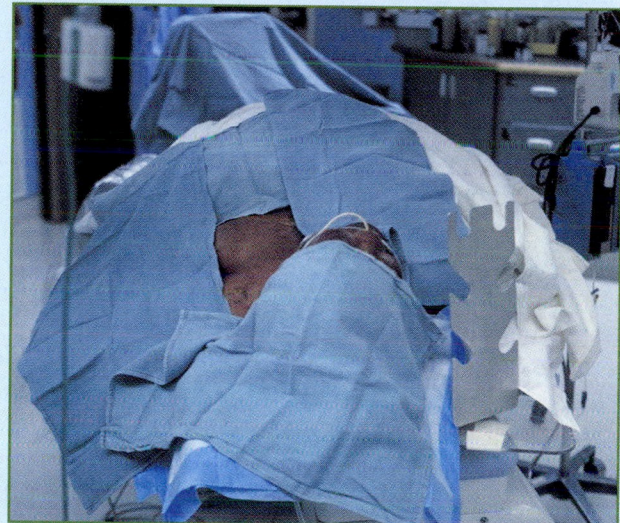

Figure 4-21-9   Follow institutional protocol for draping specific areas of the body.

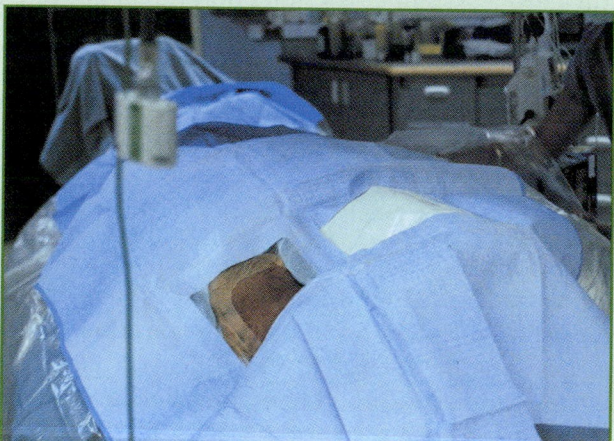

Figure 4-21-10   Use proper technique to avoid contaminating the drape or the client's skin.

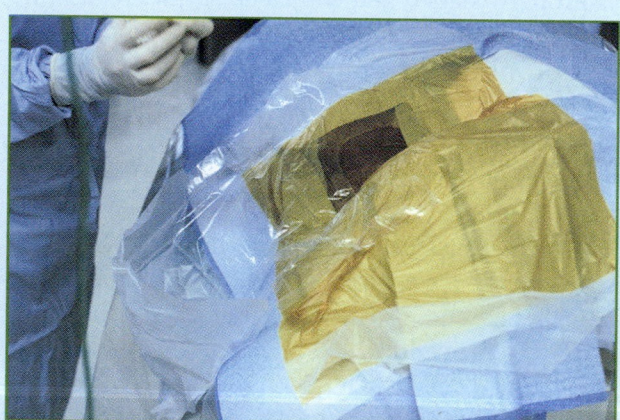

Figure 4-21-11   The scrubbed and draped surgical site.

▶ REAL WORLD ANECDOTES

Mrs. McKenzie, a 38-year-old woman, presented to the hospital for a vaginal hysterectomy. The surgery went well and she was to be released that evening. Before her discharge from the hospital, Mrs. McKenzie complained of numbness in her right leg. The nurse practitioner found that Mrs. McKenzie had movement, circulation, and some feeling in her leg. She reassured Mrs. McKenzie that the numbness would go away. When Mrs. McKenzie returned to see her physician for a postoperative follow-up, she complained that her leg was numb and weak. Her physician suggested that it might be secondary to nerve pressure from intraoperative positioning and reassured her that it would improve with time. Mrs. McKenzie's condition did not improve with time. Her leg continued to be numb and weak. She needed a cane to walk. After a year without improvement, Mrs. McKenzie sued the physician and the nurses for a perioperative positioning injury. Both the nurses and the physician needed to take Mrs. McKenzie's symptoms seriously from the onset. Documenting and reporting Mrs. McKenzie's symptoms early would have alerted the physician to the presence of a problem.

▶ EVALUATION

- The surgical preparation was performed without injury or trauma to the client.
- The client voices understanding of the procedure and the reason for it.
- The client did not experience any allergic reaction or skin sensitivity secondary to the surgical preparation.
- The client did not experience any infections secondary to poor site preparation.
- The client did not experience disruption to any existing appliances, catheters, or other instrumentation.
- The client did not experience any injury secondary to perioperative positioning.

▶ DOCUMENTATION

Preoperative Checklist

- Review checklist for completeness.
- Check the medical record to ensure the presence of a properly signed and witnessed surgical consent.
- Report client's response to surgical preparation.
- Report positioning of the client for surgery.

Nurses' Notes

- Document on appropriate flow sheet or electronic medical record (EMR).
- Record the method of shaving and site cleaning. Include the area, type of shaving, solution for sterilizing, client's responses before, during, and after the procedure.
- Note any discrepancies such as dentures still in or a lack of preoperative documentation in the chart.
- Report if the client requires any special preparation, such as medication or a new IV site.

Medication Administration Record

- If a new IV site was needed, record the date, time, location, and type of equipment used.
- Record any medications administered with date, time, route, and dosage.

▶ CRITICAL THINKING SKILL

Introduction

Client's skin is being prepped and the client complains of burning.

Possible Scenario

While prepping the surgical site for abdominal surgery, your client begins to complain of burning and itching at the preparation site.

Possible Outcome

The worst-case scenario is that the client could potentially have a systemic reaction and even anaphylactic shock. Lesser reactions may be hives, redness, itching, or burning sensation. Stop the procedure, evaluate the client's skin and overall condition, clean the solution off the surgical site and notify the client's physician or practitioner.

Prevention

Always check the client's chart for a history of allergies to iodine, other topical medications, or skin products. Note any earlier site preparation. Iodine preparations are often used for surgical site cleansing. Be sure to question the client specifically regarding any iodine or seafood allergies as well as any allergies to topical products. Using the cleaning solution, test for sensitivity on a small patch of the skin before the actual skin preparation.

▶ VARIATIONS

Geriatric Variations:
- *Elderly clients in general have very sensitive skin and even though no history of allergic reactions was reported, clients may react to cleaning solutions.*
- *Elderly clients have very thin skin that is difficult to hold taut during preparing and can easily tear or be cut during shaving or scrubbing.*

Pediatric Variations:
- *Children may be frightened by the skin preparation; therefore, this procedure may be performed after the child is sedated. Otherwise carefully explain the purpose, and have a parent or other trusted person in the room while the prep is being performed.*

Home Care Variation:
- *Not applicable.*

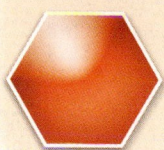

Long-Term Care Variation:
- *Not applicable.*

▶ COMMON ERRORS

Possible Error:

The nurse fails to remove the client's jewelry. After surgery, the client's hands may swell and rings may be difficult to remove. In a cold operating room, rings may fall off.

Prevention:

Explain to the client the reason for removing or taping jewelry. Remove as much jewelry as possible; ideally send it home with family members. Tape any jewelry that the client does not wish to remove or cannot remove. Ask the client about any piercings or other permanent body jewelry. If the client has permanent body jewelry in a critical area (mouth, nose, or at the surgical site) notify the physician prior to surgery. When in the surgical suite, double check the client's hands, neck, ears, nose, and mouth before draping the client.

▶ NURSING TIPS

- Double check the physician's orders regarding the type and location of the surgery.
- Check protocol regarding type of surgical prep required and positioning of client.
- If X-rays or other reports are available, ascertain that appropriate area is prepped.
- Check the most recent progress notes for any changes in preparation or positioning.
- Because operating rooms tend to be cold, drape the client and use warmed covers if available.

- Warm solutions if possible.
- Cleanse and shave an area greater than the anticipated surgical incision area to prevent accidental contamination of the surgical field.

- If a depilatory is used for hair removal, check the client's skin for sensitivity by applying a small amount to the skin of the forearm. Wait 10 minutes. If redness occurs, do not continue. Notify the physician or practitioner.

► **SPECIAL CONSIDERATIONS**

- *DuraPrep™ or prep solution containing iodine and alcohol is not to be removed immediately after surgery unless the client has a skin reaction and/or itching. The solution provides lasting antimicrobial effects and is not easily removed. After 24 hours, it may be removed with DuraPrep™ remover or you may use an alcohol solution for ease of removal.*
- *Abdominal cleansing begins at the site of incision and continues in a circular motion; overlap each circle as you widen the prepped area. Pay particular attention to cleansing the umbilicus; you may need to use a cotton-tipped applicator for this.*
- *If the client requires a vaginal and an abdominal prep then two separate prep trays should be used. The vagina is cleansed externally and then internally.*
- *When cleansing a traumatic or open wound, the open area is covered with sterile gauze and the surrounding area is cleansed first. It is important that solutions used to clean the surrounding area are not allowed to run into the open wound. Next, the sterile gauze is removed and the wound is flushed and irrigated extensively.*

Administering Immediate Postoperative Care

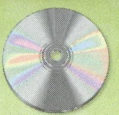

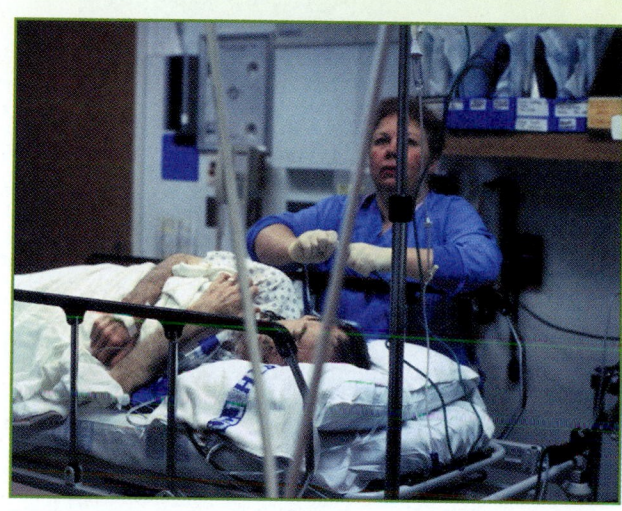

▶ OVERVIEW OF THE SKILL

The postoperative period extends from the completion of the surgical procedure through the time the client's condition is stabilized after surgery. During the immediate postoperative period, the client is usually sent to a special area called the recovery room, postoperative unit, or a postanesthesia care unit (PACU). During this time, the client is closely monitored while recuperating from the effects of the anesthesia and the surgical procedure. Both anesthesia and surgical procedures can have profound effects on the body, and this recovery period is critical. During the immediate postoperative period, the client is closely monitored to ensure that the body's systems are returning to normal.

As soon as the client is received from the operating room, the recovery room nurse assesses the client's baseline status and checks alertness, vital signs, cardiac rhythm, respiratory rate and efficiency, pain, blood oxygen saturation, IV patency, and the condition of the surgical site. Every 5 to 15 minutes for the next few hours, the nurse will reassess the client's status. Careful and frequent monitoring is essential during the immediate postoperative stage in order to detect and prevent potentially life-threatening complications. Once the client's condition is stabilized, as indicated by stable vital signs for at least 1 hour, an intact surgical site and an adequate respiratory status, the client is transferred to an area with less-intensive monitoring, generally a surgical intensive care unit or a surgical ward. After this transfer, the nurse assuming care will repeat the thorough baseline assessment and will continue to monitor the client's condition every 15 minutes for at least an hour.

▶ ASSESSMENT

1. Assess the client's sedation level and mental status **to evaluate the effects of anesthesia and any neurologic changes.**
2. Assess the client's cardiovascular status as indicated by heart rate, blood pressure, and electrocardiogram **to evaluate the stability of the client's condition after surgery.**
3. Assess the client's respiratory status as indicated by respiratory rate, oxygen saturation, and breath sounds **to evaluate the client's oxygenation after surgery.**
4. Assess the client's level of pain as indicated by appropriate pain scale **to determine the type and amount of medication and/or treatment needed to provide adequate pain control.**
5. Assess the surgical site and surgical appliances **to evaluate the client's needs and the client's response to the surgery.**
6. Assess the client's fluid status by reviewing the intake and output record **to determine the client's fluid status and respond appropriately.**

7. Assess the neurovascular status of the client's extremities **to evaluate for possible perioperative positioning injury.**

▶ DIAGNOSIS

Risk for Infection

Risk for Imbalanced Body Temperature

Ineffective Tissue Perfusion, cardiopulmonary, if general anesthesia was administered

Risk for Deficient Fluid Volume

Risk for Aspiration

Impaired Tissue Integrity

Risk for Perioperative Positioning Injury

Disturbed Sensory Perception, secondary to anesthesia

Pain

Fear

Impaired Gas Exchange

▶ PLANNING

Expected Outcomes:
1. The client's airway will be patent.
2. The client's vital signs will be stable for at least one hour.
3. The client will be alert and oriented when stimulated.
4. The client's respiratory status, including oxygen saturation, respiratory rate, and tidal volume will be adequate.
5. The client's pain control will be adequate.
6. In clients receiving regional anesthesia, motor and sensory function will be at an adequate level.
7. The client's surgical site will be intact with a dry or appropriately reinforced dressing present when the client is discharged from the recovery area.
8. The client's intravenous access will be intact and patent without signs or symptoms of infiltration or infection when the client is discharged from the recovery area.
9. The client's output will be within normal limits.
10. The client's temperature will be within normal limits.

Equipment Needed:
- Stethoscope
- Sphygmomanometer
- Oximeter
- Blankets
- Cardiac monitoring equipment
- Sterile dressings as needed
- Client's chart with postoperative orders

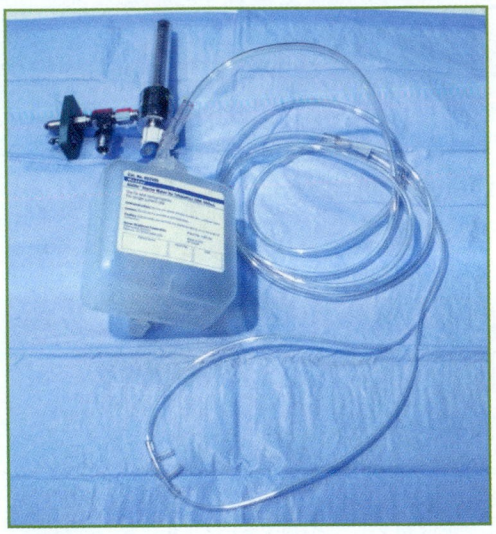

Figure 4-22-1 Supplemental oxygen equipment

- Incentive spirometer (may be optional)
- Supplemental oxygen, if needed (see Figure 4-22-1)
- Sequential stockings and/or antiembolic stockings (as ordered)
- Thermometer

▶ CLIENT EDUCATION NEEDED:

1. Inform client of purpose of various equipment to ease the fear of the unknown.
2. Inform the client of required position changes.
3. Inform the client to let nurse know when pain or shivering is noted.
4. Explain the reason deep breathing, turning, and coughing are encouraged right away despite the client's recent surgery and some discomfort.
5. Reinforce the client's preoperative teaching regarding postoperative expectations and exercises.
6. Explain the reason for frequent vital sign and neurovascular checks. Note that the frequent checks do not indicate anything is wrong. Assure client that regular checks are part of the routine to prevent problems.
7. Instruct the client to tell you if in pain, nauseated, or uncomfortable in other ways.
8. Encourage the client to ask questions regarding the surgical procedure, the postoperative routine, or any surgical changes that might have taken place.

Estimated time to complete the skill:
15 minutes for initial assessment; 1–2 hours for client to recover from anesthesia and stabilize, depending on surgery

IMPLEMENTATION—Action/Rationale

Action	Rationale
1. Wash hands and apply gloves.	1. Reduces the transmission of microorganisms.
2. Check the client's temperature, pulse, respiratory rate, and blood pressure upon the client's arrival in the unit.	2. Establishes a baseline and is indicative of the client's status.
3. Identify client via armband and verify the client's identity with the chart.	3. Protects the client from errors.
4. Inform the client that he or she is out of the operating room and in the recovery room.	4. Decreases anxiety. If the client has had general anesthesia, you may need to reorient the client several times.
5. If bedside electrocardiogram monitoring is available, attach the leads to the client (see Figure 4-22-2) and run a baseline electrocardiogram strip.	5. Establishes baseline rhythm and provides constant monitor of client's cardiac rate and rhythm.
6. Change oxygen from portable to wall-mounted unit, attach the oximeter to the client, and monitor the client's oxygen saturation (see Figure 4-22-3).	6. Establishes baseline data and ongoing monitor of client's need for supplemental oxygen.

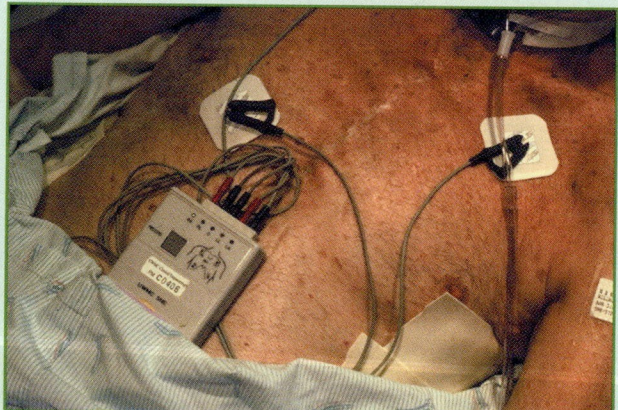

Figure 4-22-2   If bedside electrocardiogram monitoring is available, attach the leads to the client.

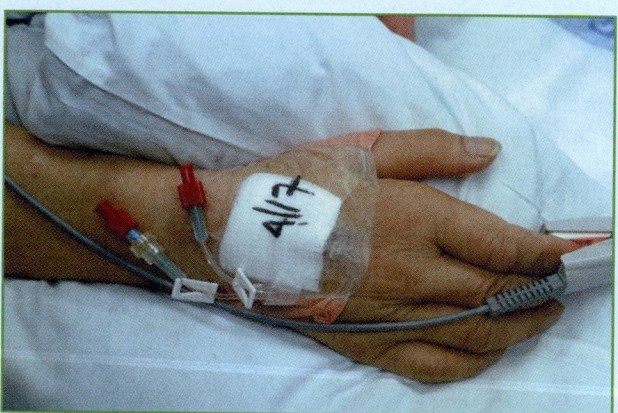

Figure 4-22-3   Attach the oximeter to the client.

continues

Action	Rationale

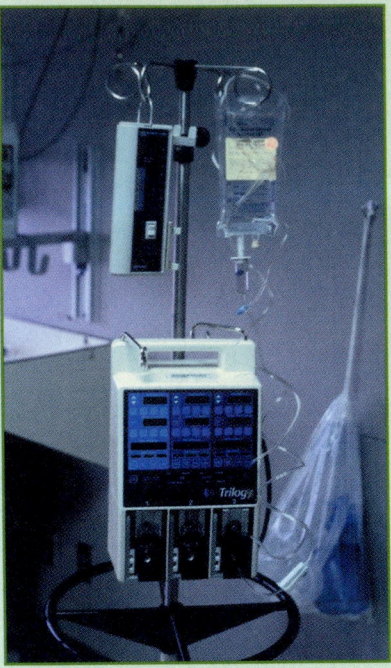

Figure 4-22-4 Check the intravenous (IV) site, pump, solution, and tubing.

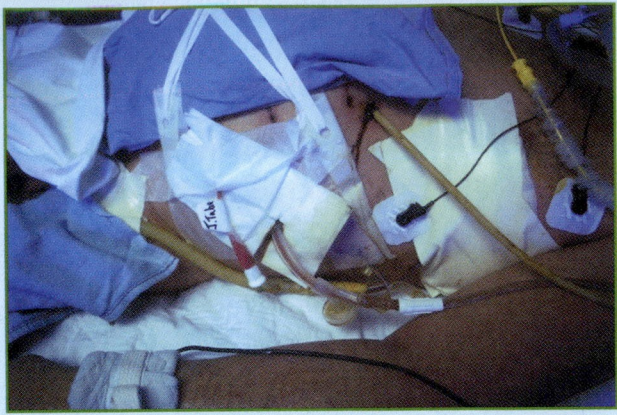

Figure 4-22-5 Check surgical dressing and site, if visible. Assess dressings for amount and type of drainage.

7. Check drainage tube placements. Check intravenous (IV) site using gloves. Check IV solution(s) (see Figure 4-22-4), flow rate, and that the IV line is taped as necessary.

8. Check surgical dressing and site, if visible (see Figure 4-22-5). Assess dressings for amount and type of drainage (see Figure 4-22-6). Reinforce the dressings as needed. Change the dressing only with the physician's approval.

9. Complete a total head to toe assessment. A complete assessment should include the following:

Airway

- Check the patency of the client's airway.
- Assess for the presence of breath sounds that are equal on both sides, especially if the client is intubated.
- Note the presence of rhonchi, rales, or wheezes while assessing breath sounds.

7. Tubes may become dislodged or disconnected during the transfer to PACU. Prevents complications from infiltration of IV, allows appropriate rehydration, verifies appropriate solution, prevents the line from disconnecting.

8. Establishes the condition of the surgical site, including the presence of any drains, bleeding, purulence, or other notable conditions.

9. Provides baseline data and prevents complications of surgery. Start with the ABCs of assessment: airway, breathing, circulation.

Oxygen is the primary need of all clients and without a patent airway all other measures are useless.

continues

Action	Rationale

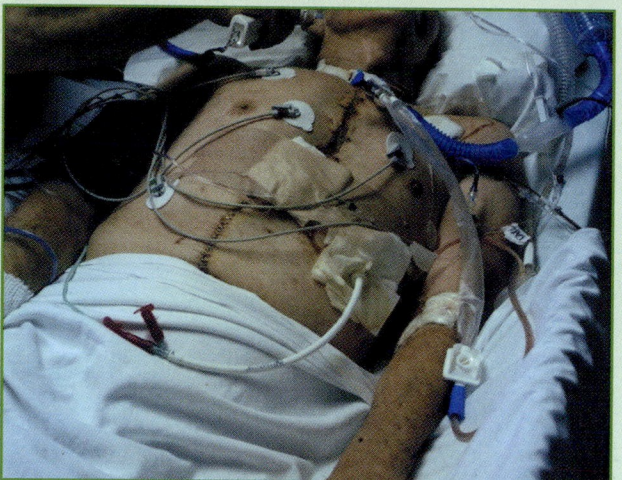

Figure 4-22-6 Check the surgical dressings and site(s). Assess dressings for amount and type of drainage.

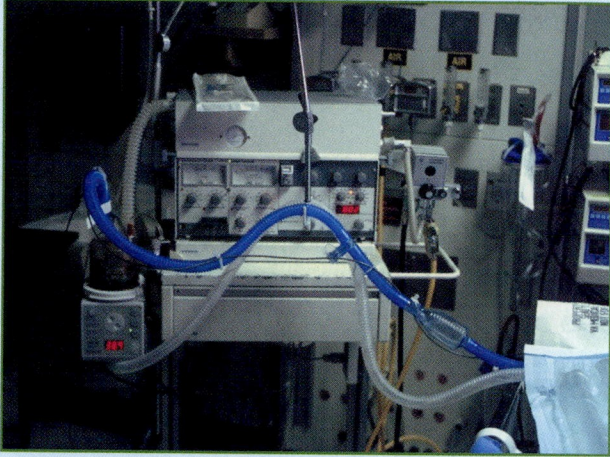

Figure 4-22-7 Oxygen is critical for all organs, especially the brain. Assess respiratory and oxygen supplemental or support systems.

Respiratory

- Note the presence of any supplemental oxygen and the type of oxygen delivery system (see Figure 4-22-7).
- Assess the client's blood oxygen saturation as well as the type, depth, and efficiency of the client's respirations.

Oxygen is critical for all organs, especially the brain. Lack of oxygen to the brain and other body organs can be life threatening. Poor oxygenation despite supplemental oxygen could indicate complications such as respiratory or cardiac failure, pulmonary embolus, atelectasis, inadequate lung expansion, mucus plugs, or lung consolidation.

Cardiovascular

- Check apical pulses, radial pulses, and peripheral pulses especially those distal to the surgical site.
- Note the color and temperature of extremities, and the capillary refill rate.
- Check the client's cardiac rate and rhythm, blood pressure, and any indications of bleeding.

- Changes in distal pulses could indicate blockage of circulation to the surgical site.
- Changes in blood pressure or cardiac rate or rhythm can indicate bleeding or life-threatening vascular failure.

Temperature

- Check the client's core temperature. Note any complaints of coldness or shivering.

Postoperative clients often have hypothermic body temperatures after surgery. A low core temperature can slow the metabolic rate and slow the client's recovery. Shivering, which often accompanies postoperative hypothermia, can increase the client's oxygen needs dramatically. Most institutions have standard postoperative treatments for warming postoperative clients.

Neurologic

- Assess the client's level of awareness, orientation, level of cooperation, equality of pupils, verbal response, equality of movement, and feeling in the extremities.

- Sedation level is one of the indicators of readiness to be transferred out of PACU. Any change in neurologic function could indicate brain damage, nerve damage, or circulatory changes.

continues

Action	Rationale
Gastrointestinal • Evaluate for the presence of nausea or vomiting. If a nasogastric (NG) tube is present, auscultate the placement of the tube. If the NG tube is hooked to suction, note whether the suction is intermittent or continuous and whether it is functioning properly. • Assess gastric secretions for color and amount. Record the amount of gastric output (check for bleeding and pH as indicated) and replace fluids if indicated. If the client is vomiting NG placement may be necessary.	• If the client is nauseated or vomiting, turn the client to the side, if indicated, to prevent aspiration. Treat nausea and vomiting with medication, NG tube insertion, or reevaluation of pain medications.
Genitourinary • Evaluate the amount and color of the client's urinary output. If indicated check for the presence of blood, evaluate the pH, specific gravity, presence of glucose, ketones, sediment, and so forth. • Assess that the catheter is draining appropriately.	• Urinary output can indicate the client's hydration state, pituitary dysfunction, or cardiac output status. Output should be at least 30 mL/hr.
Pain • Assess the client's level of pain on a 1- to 10-point pain scale and treat as appropriate. If a client-controlled analgesic (PCA) system is used, as the client recovers from sedation instruct the client on the use of the PCA. • Assess other means of controlling pain, such as repositioning. Sometimes anti-inflammatory agents are used alone or in conjunction with sedatives or narcotics. If the client experiences vomiting reevaluate pain medication employed.	• Clients who are in pain may not recover from surgery as fast and may experience complications. If clients are in pain, deep breathing and coughing may not be achieved and the client may get pneumonia. Increased pain may be indicative of complications. All complaints of pain should be taken seriously.
Fluid Balance • Evaluate the client's fluid status. Check the client's fluid intake and output status. • Check for peripheral edema or jugular venous distention. Note and report any extremes of intake or output.	• Peripheral edema or jugular venous distention might indicate fluid overload. Fluid loss or overload can further stress the client's cardiovascular status.
Vital Signs • Reevaluate the client's vital signs and status as needed, at least every 15 minutes. 10. Encourage the client to breathe deep, cough, and use the incentive spirometer (see Figure 4-22-8). For more information on the use of incentive spirometer, see Skill 7-3.	• Monitors any changes in the client's condition. 10. Improves lung expansion, prevents respiratory complications, and hastens clearance of anesthesia from the lungs.

continues

Action	Rationale
11. Check and implement postoperative orders.	**11.** Provides appropriate and safe postoperative care.
12. Inform the client's family or significant other that the client is in the recovery room.	**12.** Decreases anxiety for client and others.
13. Turn the client as needed for comfort (see Figure 4-22-9).	**13.** Prevents venous stasis and prevents decreased circulation and disruption of skin integrity. Turning increases lung expansion and reduces the chance of pneumonia.
14. Upon discharge by the postanesthesia caregiver, a full report of the postanesthesia phase and intraoperative course of events should be given to the nurse assuming care of the client.	**14.** Provides continuity of care after transfer.
15. Remove gloves and wash hands.	**15.** Reduces the transmission of microorganisms.

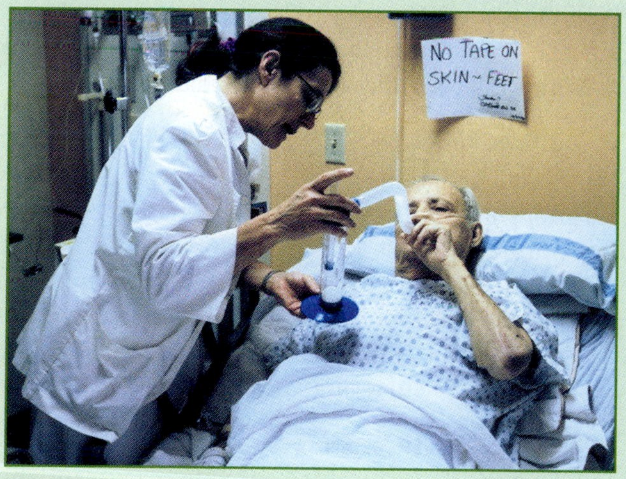

Figure 4-22-8 Encourage the client to use the incentive spirometer to reduce the risk of respiratory complications.

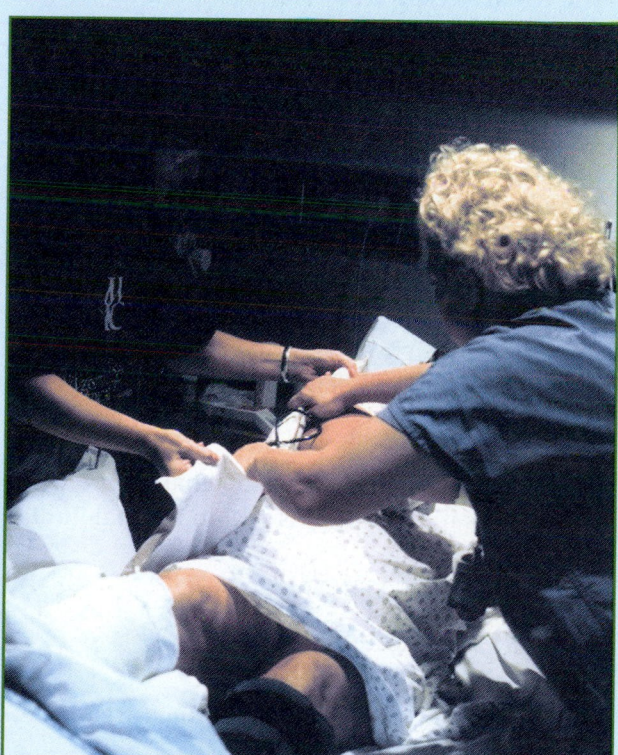

Figure 4-22-9 Turn the client every hour to reduce the risk of respiratory and circulatory complications, or skin breakdown.

> **REAL WORLD ANECDOTES**

Jason is an 8-year-old boy admitted for placement of Harrington rods to correct severe scoliosis. Before surgery, Jason had full movement and feeling in both feet and legs. After surgery, and 2 hours of recovery, Jason was moved to the pediatric surgery ward. When Jason arrived in the surgery ward, his nurse noted that he was sleepy, able to follow commands, and denied numbness or tingling in his feet and legs.

Following hospital protocol, Jason's nurse monitored his vital signs and neurovascular status every 15 minutes for the first hour and every 30 minutes for the next 2 hours. During the course of this 3-hour period, Jason began to complain of numbness in his toes, gradually spreading to his feet. Two and one-half hours after Jason returned to the surgical floor, he could no longer move or feel his feet. After patiently observing and recording the progress of Jason's paralysis for two and one-half hours, the nurse called the physician. Jason's doctor ordered emergency surgery to remove the Harrington rods. Unfortunately, the rods were not removed in time and Jason was rendered a spastic paraplegic. Conducting regular assessments did not help, because the nurse did not interpret the findings correctly, and did not recognize that the spreading numbness and paralysis was abnormal and should have been reported.

> **EVALUATION**

- The client's airway is patent.
- The client's vital signs are stable for at least 1 hour.
- The client is alert and oriented when stimulated.
- The client's respiratory status, including oxygen saturation, respiratory rate, and tidal volume is adequate.
- The client's pain control is adequate.
- In clients receiving regional anesthesia, motor and sensory functions are at an adequate level.
- The client's surgical site was intact with a dry or appropriately reinforced dressing present when the client was discharged from the recovery area.
- The client's intravenous access was intact and patent without signs or symptoms of infiltration or infection when the client was discharged from the recovery area.
- The client's output is within normal limits.
- The client's temperature is within normal limits.

> **DOCUMENTATION**

Vital Signs Flow Sheet

- Document the client's vital signs.
- Record neurologic checks, level of consciousness, and oxygen saturation.
- Note the condition of the surgical site and any drains or appliances.

Document on appropriate flow sheet or electronic medical record (EMR).

Intake and Output Record

- Record the client's IV and oral intake, urine output, and any drainage.

Medication Administration Record

- Record any medications administered, including date, time, route, and dosage.

Nurses' Notes

- Document the time the client was received.
- Record any unusual findings and note the findings of the total systems assessment.

> **CRITICAL THINKING SKILL**

Introduction

Operating rooms often are cooled to temperatures that are comfortable for the staff rather than for the client.

Possible Scenario

Mrs. Larkspur has just been moved to the recovery area after surgery. On initial assessment, her tympanic temperature is 96.2° F. You place warmed blankets over Mrs. Larkspur and send for a bed warmer to help raise her body temperature. Before the bed warmer arrives, Mrs. Larkspur begins to shiver violently. She complains of the shivering and of the cold.

Possible Outcome

Mrs. Larkspur's respiratory rate increases and her oxygen saturation level decreases because of the increased energy demands placed on her body. She requires an increase in supplemental oxygen and her body is unnecessarily stressed by the shivering.

Prevention

Shivering increases the body's oxygen use dramatically and places a stress on the cardiopulmonary system. In clients whose cardiopulmonary system is already compromised, this stress can be life-threatening. Be sure to have warm blankets and bed warming equipment ready when the client is admitted to the recovery area to prevent having to wait. IV Demerol is sometimes used postoperatively to control shivering, which can compromise the client's recovery.

► VARIATIONS

Geriatric Variations:
- *Elderly clients may become confused or agitated after the use of general anesthesia. Be prepared for possible confusion and the need for frequent reorientation to time and place.*
- *Elderly clients may be at risk for respiratory complications prior to surgery and may require a vigorous pulmonary toilet.*

Pediatric Variations:
- *Children recovering from anesthesia may not always understand directions. Physical restraint or client-repeated instructions may be necessary.*
- *If the child's parent is available and supportive, have the parent sit with the child as she or he comes out of anesthesia to provide emotional comfort.*
- *Children may suffer from postanesthesia excitement. They may be confused, delirious, uncooperative, or combative. Be sure to have enough help available. Restraints may be necessary.*

Home Care Variation:
- *Teach the client and caregiver about what will happen when the client returns home (e.g., follow-up care and appointments, caring for the wound, medication administration, returning to normal levels of activity, and assessing for short- and long-term complications of the surgery).*

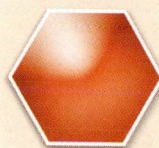

Long-Term Care Variation:
- *People with multiple surgeries may develop anticipatory fear. Assess the client for history and discuss the procedure.*

► COMMON ERRORS

Possible Error:

Not encouraging the client to cough and breathe deeply because of complaints of surgical site pain.

Prevention:

After general anesthesia, the lungs are not reexpanded properly, and some of the inhaled anesthesia lingers. Having the client breathe deeply and cough helps the anesthesia clear from the lungs faster and complications such as pneumonia and atelectasis can be prevented.

▶ **NURSING TIPS**

- Do not raise the client's head until you have determined the type of surgery and anesthesia used. Some procedures require the client to lie flat for several hours.
- Be sure to have emergency resuscitation equipment handy as well as functioning suction and oxygen.
- The motion of moving the client to a room may cause vomiting.
- Position the client to keep the airway clear and have suction available.
- Provide regular updates to family and friends to provide comfort during stressful times. What may be routine to the nurse can be a frightening experience for family members.
- A client may forget things she or he was told while recovering from anesthesia. Be prepared to explain more than once.

▶ **SPECIAL CONSIDERATIONS**

- *Adolescent clients tend to awaken fitfully from general anesthesia. You may need to have additional staff nearby to assist you when the client awakens.*
- *The postoperative client may not be aware of a catheterization that took place intraoperatively and may awaken with a sense that he or she needs to void. Carefully monitor the client and explain that there is a catheter in place that goes into the bladder to remove the urine.*
- *As clients awaken, they generally are quite frightened. Let clients know where they are and that the surgery is complete.*
- *Clients may pull at tubes as they awaken from anesthesia. Take precautions to monitor placement of tubes.*

Postoperative Exercise Instruction

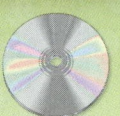

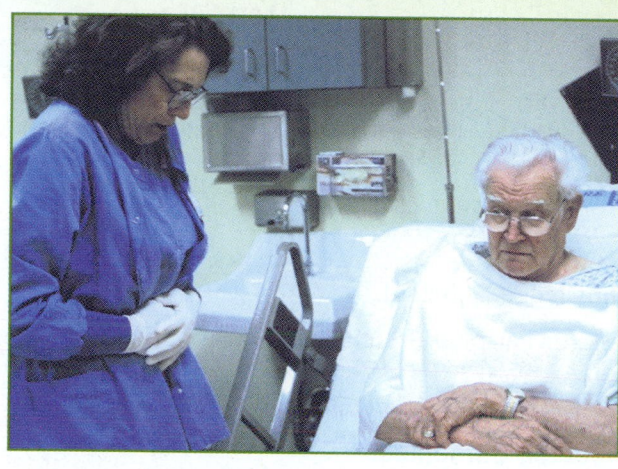

► OVERVIEW OF THE SKILL

Preoperative teaching of postoperative exercises prepares the client physically and emotionally for the impending surgery. The goal of instruction is to have the client demonstrate the performance of exercises while verbalizing why the exercises are used during the postoperative phase.

There are several postoperative exercises that help to speed recovery from surgery. Deep breathing and coughing facilitate removal of accumulated pulmonary secretions. Clients may experience their worst postoperative pain while coughing, deep breathing, and exercising. Clients with abdominal or chest surgery may avoid using muscles in the affected areas to take deep breaths or to cough effectively. Certain anesthetic agents depress the central nervous system and cause some clients to experience shallow respirations. Inhaled gases and oxygen have a direct drying effect on the respiratory mucosa, which increases the viscosity of mucus, and makes the secretions difficult to raise with coughing. These factors place the client at risk for respiratory complications.

To prevent respiratory complications, the nurse teaches clients to use a breathing technique in which the client turns, coughs, and breathes deeply to achieve sustained maximum inspiration (SMI). SMI promotes the reinflation of the alveoli and the removal of mucus secretions.

Several devices help encourage clients to perform SMI exercises. The breathing devices, called incentive spirometers, measure the client's ventilatory volume and provide the user with a tangible reward for generating an adequate respiratory flow. Devices range from simple types, a Ping-Pong ball in a plastic tube, to sophisticated models. When the client takes a deep breath, the ball moves upward and the amount of air is measured, thereby making the results visible to the client.

Turning, deep breathing, coughing, and using spirometry prevent respiratory complications by doing the following:

- Promoting pulmonary circulation
- Promoting the exchange of gases by increasing lung compliance
- Facilitating the removal of mucus secretions from the tracheobronchial tree

Postoperatively, the client is encouraged to move in bed and perform leg exercises. These exercises assist in preventing circulatory complications that can arise from anesthetic agents that depress the metabolic and heart rates. Early ambulation also increases respiratory function and the return of peristalsis.

Types of Surgical Incisions

Nurses need to be knowledgeable about common surgical incisions to reinforce the surgeon's teaching and to answer the client's questions. Two main

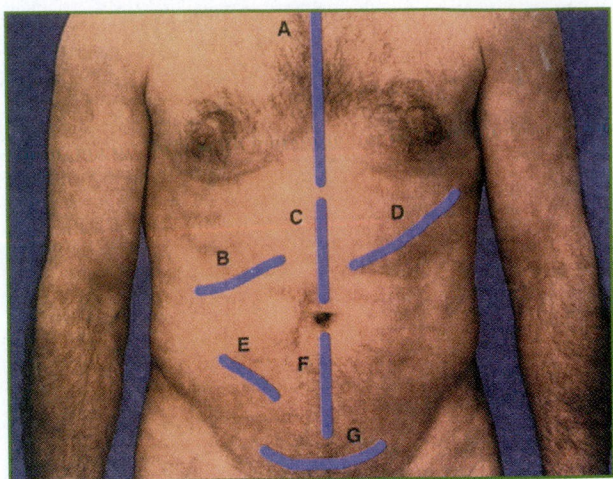

Figure 4-23-1   Location of common surgical incisions.

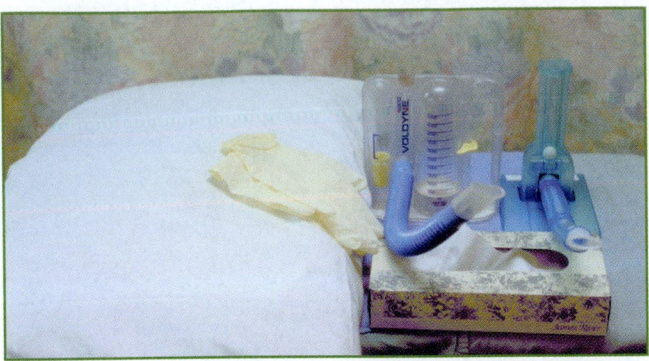

Figure 4-23-2   Incentive spirometers encourage deep breathing. A pillow may be used to splint the incision site. Tissues are used to cover the mouth when coughing.

factors govern incisions: direction and location. Incisions may be vertical, horizontal, transverse, or oblique. Figure 4-23-1 illustrates the location of common surgical incisions.

▶ ASSESSMENT

1. Assess the client's current understanding of postoperative procedures. **Establishes baseline for teaching.**
2. Assess the client's ability to understand the postoperative exercise instructions. **Establishes baseline for teaching. Affects how the teaching and the procedures will be performed.**
3. Assess any preoperative limitations the client may have that would prevent or impair the ability to perform the postoperative exercises accordingly. **Establishes baseline for teaching. Affects how the teaching and the procedures will be performed. Allows modification of the exercises.**

▶ DIAGNOSIS

Pain

Impaired Physical Mobility

Impaired Gas Exchange

Risk for Impaired Skin Integrity

Risk for Constipation

Knowledge Deficient

Risk for Peripheral/Neurovascular Dysfunction

▶ PLANNING

Expected Outcomes:

1. The client will be able to successfully demonstrate postoperative exercises, deep breathing, coughing, pillow splinting, turning and proper body alignment, leg and foot exercises, and out-of-bed transfers.
2. The client will be able to successfully demonstrate proper use of the incentive spirometer.

Equipment Needed (see Figure 4-23-2):

- Educational materials
- Pillow
- Tissue
- Nonsterile gloves
- Disposable, volume-oriented incentive spirometer

▶ CLIENT EDUCATION NEEDED:

1. Explain to the client the need for SMI.
2. Explain to the client the need for leg exercises.

Estimated time to complete the skill: **45 minutes**

▶ DELEGATION TIPS

Postoperative instruction requires the assessment and intervention of a nurse. Ancillary staff may reinforce the information and directions taught to the client.

IMPLEMENTATION—Action/Rationale

Action	Rationale
1. Wash hands and organize equipment.	1. Reduces the transmission of microorganisms and promotes efficiency.
2. Check the client's identification band.	2. Facilitates proper identification of client.
3. Apply gloves.	3. Reduces the transmission of microorganisms.
4. Place client in a sitting position.	4. Promotes full chest expansion.
5. Demonstrate deep breathing exercises. • Place one hand on abdomen (umbilical area) during inhalation. • Expand the abdomen and rib cage on inspiration. • Inhale slowly and evenly through your nose until you achieve maximum chest expansion. • Hold breath for 2 to 3 seconds. • Slowly exhale through your mouth until maximum chest contraction has been achieved. (For more information on deep breathing exercises, see Skill 7-2, "Assisting a Client with Controlled Coughing and Deep Breathing.")	5. Shows the client how to breathe deeply. • Exerts counterpressure during inhalation. • Promotes maximum chest expansion. • Maintains full expansion of the alveoli. • Increases the pressure, thereby preventing immediate collapse of the alveoli. • Promotes maximum chest contraction.
6. Have the client return-demonstrate deep breathing.	6. Fosters learning.
7. Have the client repeat the exercise 3 to 4 times.	7. Reinforces learning. Promotes increased air exchange.
8. Instruct the client on the use of an incentive spirometer (see Figure 4-23-3). • Hold the volume-oriented spirometer upright. • Take a normal breath and exhale, then seal lips tightly around the mouthpiece; take a slow deep breath to elevate the balls in the plastic tube, hold the inspiration for at least 3 seconds. • The client simultaneously measures the amount of inspired air volume on the calibrated plastic tube. • Remove the mouthpiece, exhale normally. • Take several normal breaths. (For more information on using the incentive spirometer see Skill 7-3, "Assisting a Client with an Incentive Spirometer.")	8. Reinflates the alveoli and removes mucus secretions. • Promotes proper functioning of the device. • Allows for greater lung expansion; holding the inspiration increases the pressure, preventing the immediate collapse of the alveoli. • Encourages the client to do respiratory exercises. • Allows normal expiration. • Provides the client the opportunity to relax.
9. Have the client repeat the procedure 4 to 5 times.	9. Encourages sustained maximal inspiration and loosens secretions.

continues

Action	Rationale

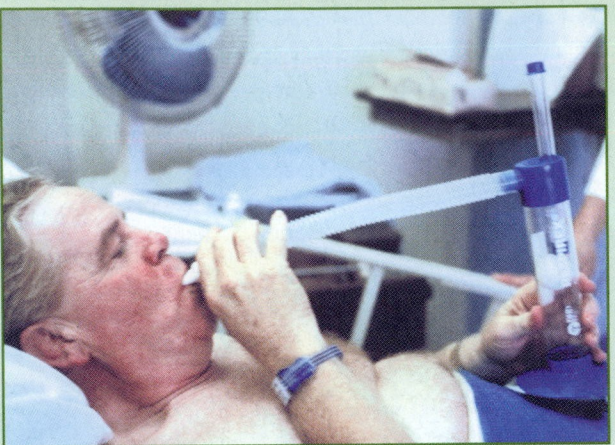

Figure 4-23-3   Instruct the client to take a slow deep breath to elevate the ball in the tube.

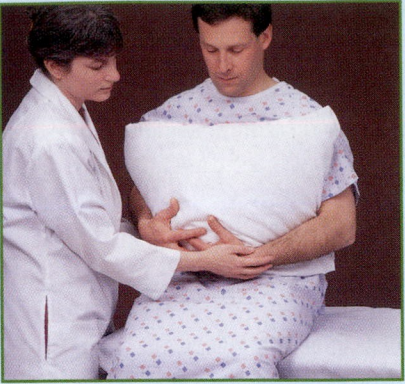

Figure 4-23-4   Use a pillow to support the abdominal muscles when coughing.

10. Have the client cough after the incentive effort. See the following section.

11. Demonstrate splinting and coughing.

   • Have the client slowly raise head and sniff the air.

   • Have the client slowly bend forward and exhale slowly through pursed lips.

   • Repeat breathing two to three times.

   • When the client is ready to cough, have client place a folded pillow against the abdomen with clasped hands.

   • Have client take a deep breath and begin coughing immediately after inspiration is completed by bending forward slightly and producing a series of soft, staccato coughs.
   • Have a tissue ready.
        (For more information on deep breathing exercises see Skill 7-2, "Assisting a Client with Controlled Coughing and Deep Breathing.")

12. Have the client return-demonstrate splinting and coughing (see Figure 4-23-4).

13. Wash the incentive spirometer mouthpiece under running water and store in a clean container. Disposable mouthpieces should be changed every 24 hours.

10. Facilitates the removal of secretions.

11. Shows the client how to raise mucus secretions from the tracheobronchial tree.
   • Increases the amount of air and helps to aerate the base of the lungs.
   • Dries the tracheal mucosa as air flows over it. There is a slight increase in carbon dioxide level, which stimulates deeper breathing.
   • Loosens mucus plugs and moves secretions to the main bronchus.
   • Elevates the diaphragm and expels air in a more forceful cough; supports the abdominal muscles and reduces pain while coughing, if the client has an abdominal incision.
   • Removes secretions from the main bronchus.

   • Preparation for sputum disposal.

12. Fosters learning.

13. Reduces the transmission of microorganisms.

continues

Action	Rationale

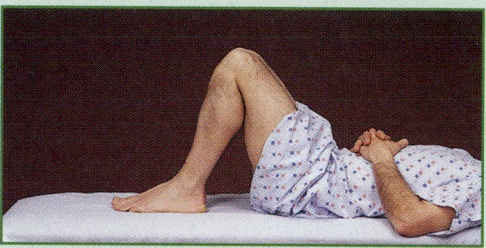

(A)

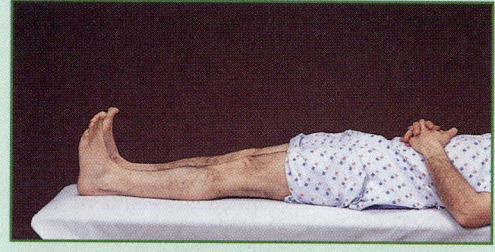

(B)

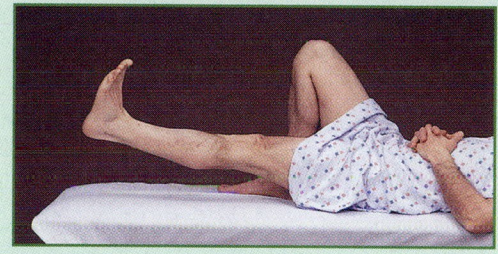

(C)

Figure 4-23-5 Leg exercises improve venous blood return. (A) Bend the knee. (B) Flex foot forward. (C) Lift leg up and flex foot forward.

14. Teach the client leg and foot exercises (see Figure 4-23-5).
- Have the client, with heels on bed, push the toes of both feet toward the foot of the bed until the calf muscles tighten, then relax feet. Pull the toes toward the chin, until calf muscles tighten; then relax feet (see Figure 4-23-5A and B).
- With heels on bed, lift and circle each ankle, first to the right and then to the left; repeat three times, relax.
- Flex and extend each knee alternately, sliding foot up along the bed; relax (see Figure 4-23-5C).

15. Have the client return-demonstrate the leg and foot exercises.

16. Explain how to turn in bed and get out of bed.

17. Instruct the client who has a left-sided abdominal or chest incision to turn to the right side of bed and sit up as follows:
- Flex the knees.
- With the right hand, splint the incision with hand or small pillow.

14. To improve venous blood return from the legs.
- Causes contraction and relaxation of the calf muscles.

- Causes contraction and relaxation of the quadriceps muscles.
- Causes contraction and relaxation of the quadriceps muscles.

15. Fosters learning of how to improve venous blood return.

16. Elicits client cooperation.

17. Fosters learning how to turn and get out of bed without putting pressure on the incision line.

continues

Action	Rationale
• Turn toward right side by pushing with the left foot and grasping the shoulder of the nurse or partial side rail of the bed with the left hand. • Raise up to a sitting position on the side of the bed by using the left arm and hand to push down against the mattress or side rail.	
18. Reverse instructions (use left side instead of right) for the client with a right-sided incision according to Action 17 (see Figure 4-23-6).	18. Same as Rationale 17.
19. Instruct clients with orthopedic surgery (e.g., hip surgery) how to use a trapeze bar.	19. Facilitates movement in bed without putting pressure on a leg or hip joint.
20. Wash hands.	20. Reduces the transmission of microorganisms.

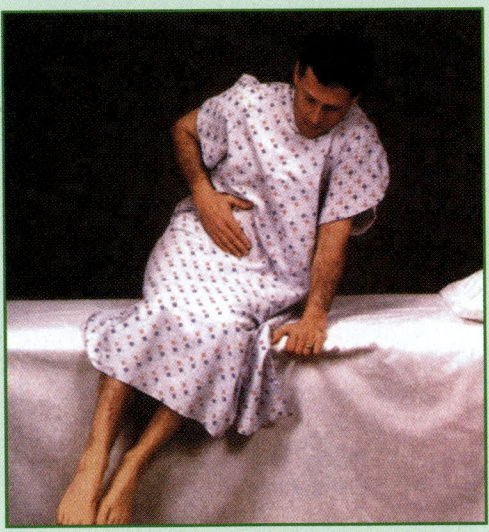

Figure 4-23-6 Using the hand to splint the incision site when sitting up in bed will reduce pain and pressure at the incision site.

► REAL WORLD ANECDOTES

Scenario 1

A student nurse is assigned to ambulate Mrs. Ross, who had abdominal surgery yesterday. The student enters the room and explains to Mrs. Ross that she needs to get up and walk today. Mrs. Ross is horrified. She explains that there must be some mistake because she just had major surgery and cannot possibly get out of bed yet. The student explains the need for exercise to prevent respiratory complications and to promote peristalsis. Mrs. Ross clearly did not expect to exercise postoperatively. She refuses to attempt even coughing and deep breathing until a "real" nurse has explained the reasons for early postoperative activity and reassured her that this was per doctor's orders. This is a good reminder to the nurse and the student nurse that preoperative teaching regarding postoperative exercises is an important element in a client's surgical recovery.

continues

▶ **REAL WORLD ANECDOTES** *(continued)*

Scenario 2
Margaret's postoperative recovery went well, partially because her children brought in several toys to help her do her postoperative exercises. Her favorite was a foam ball tied by a string to her bedside. She could squeeze the ball, or toss it at anyone or anything that annoyed her, then retrieve it unassisted.

▶ **EVALUATION**

- The client is able to successfully demonstrate post-operative exercises, deep breathing, coughing, pillow splinting, turning and proper body alignment, leg and foot exercises, and out-of-bed transfers.
- The client is able to successfully demonstrate proper use of the incentive spirometer.

▶ **DOCUMENTATION**

Nurses' Notes

- Document teaching the client postoperative exercises.
- Note the client's level of understanding and cooperation with the teaching.

Document on appropriate flow sheet or electronic medical record (EMR).

Preoperative Checklist

- Initial the check-off area for documentation of preoperative teaching.

▶ **CRITICAL THINKING SKILL**

Introduction
Understand the client's perspective when assessing for noncompliance.

Possible Scenario
Mr. Hays had gallbladder surgery yesterday. This morning the nurse is encouraging Mr. Hays to cough, take deep breaths, and use his incentive spirometer. Before surgery Mr. Hays had demonstrated an understanding of these skills and had been able to perform them well. However, this morning he is breathing shallowly and coughing poorly. The nurse encourages him to try harder, but he explains that it hurts too much.

Possible Outcome
The nurse knows that if Mr. Hays is not able to improve his respiratory volumes and move the mucus secretions out of his lungs, he is at risk of pneumonia and postoperative complications that could prolong his hospital stay and further endanger his health.

Prevention
The nurse gives Mr. Hays his pain medication before his exercises so he is able to perform the tasks with less pain. If Mr. Hays was on PCA, the nurse could either have manually bolused the medication or had Mr. Hays initiate a dose of medication in anticipation of the exercises.

▶ **VARIATIONS**

Geriatric Variation:
- *Geriatric clients are generally at higher risk of pulmonary complications, and their pulmonary treatment often must be more aggressive.*

Pediatric Variation:
- *Children are often very frightened of pain. They should be given pain medication before asking them to perform painful procedures. Other ways of encouraging deep breathing are with play activities such as blowing bubbles, mobiles, or paper windmills, or blowing a paper sailboat across a basin of water.*

continues

▶ VARIATIONS *(continued)*

Home Care Variation:
- *Teach the client's caregivers how to do and supervise these exercises so they can help and encourage the client.*

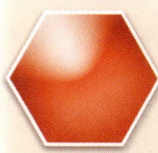

Long-Term Care Variation:
- *Long-term clients often have impaired mobility prior to surgery. The nurse should be more diligent about exercises to prevent circulatory stasis in these clients.*

▶ COMMON ERRORS

Possible Error:

The nurse is not being aggressive enough with postoperative exercises because of client pain.

Prevention:

Be prepared to be placed in the supportive "bad guy" role of gently but firmly helping clients to do therapies that hurt. When clients are in pain, it is difficult for them to evaluate the long-term complications of their behavior. The nurse must be able to insist that clients do what is healthy even if they complain. Allow clients as much control as possible over the timing and pace of the therapy.

▶ NURSING TIPS

- The best time to teach postoperative exercises is before surgery. Remember to assess the client's motivation to learn and ability to pay attention.

- Encourage the client to use a pillow or other splinting method to ease the discomfort of coughing, turning, and deep breathing.
- Keep the incentive spirometer close to the client to encourage its use.

▶ SPECIAL CONSIDERATIONS

- *The client may become dependent on the incentive spirometer to perform deep breathing exercises. The spirometer may be inadvertently moved across the room when the meal tray arrives; therefore, the client must be encouraged to continue hourly exercises with or without the spirometer. Teach the client to take a deep breath and hold it, then release it slowly. This is as effective as the incentive spirometer and does not delay recovery when the spirometer is misplaced.*
- *Encourage family members to remind the client to use the incentive spirometer and to exercise while on bed rest. When appropriate, encourage family members to participate in postoperative recovery by working with them and encouraging the client to breathe deeply and exercise. If a clock is in the room have the client and family member set up a schedule to take deep breaths and exercise hourly. When you involve the client and the family in the recovery process, the client learns self-care and may have decreased anxiety and a sense of control in the outcome. By scheduling hourly times, the activity occurs more frequently and is not solely dependent upon the nurse.*

Administering Passive Range of Motion (PROM) Exercises

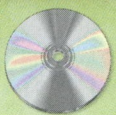

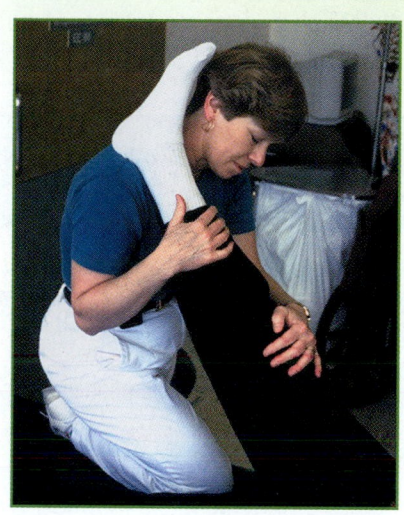

▶ OVERVIEW OF THE SKILL

Passive range of motion (PROM) exercises seek to maintain or improve the current level of functional mobility of a client's extremities. The nurse provides, assists with, and teaches the client functional movements in all available planes and directions of involved joints. PROM exercises prevent contractures and shortening of muscles and tendons, increase circulation to extremities, decrease vascular complications of immobility, and facilitate comfort for the client.

▶ ASSESSMENT

1. Be aware of the client's medical diagnosis. **Understand the expected functional limits of a client with this diagnosis.**
2. Familiarize yourself with the client's current range of motion. Note any joint pain, stiffness, or inflammation that might limit the client's motion. **Understanding the client's current PROM will help you assess the functional limits of movement of each joint.**
3. Assess client consciousness and cognitive function. **Client should be encouraged to participate in PROM as actively as possible.**

▶ DIAGNOSIS

Impaired Physical Mobility

Risk for Activity Intolerance

Pain

▶ PLANNING

Expected Outcomes:

1. Client will maintain or improve current functional mobility in all involved joints and extremities.
2. Client will regain or improve strength and/or voluntary movement in involved joints and extremities.
3. Client will avoid complications of immobility, including decubitus ulcers, contractures, decreased peristalsis, constipation, fecal impaction, orthostatic hypotension, pulmonary embolism, and thrombophlebitis.

Equipment Needed:

No special equipment is needed, except gloves when contact with body fluids is possible.

▶ CLIENT EDUCATION NEEDED:

1. Explain who you are and the purpose of PROM exercises.
2. Explain that PROM should not be painful and that any increase in pain or other symptoms should be reported immediately.
3. Discuss anticipated benefits of PROM exercises.

4. Use verbal cues to encourage the client to participate as actively as possible.
5. Verbally identify to the client each joint and movement to be exercised in turn.

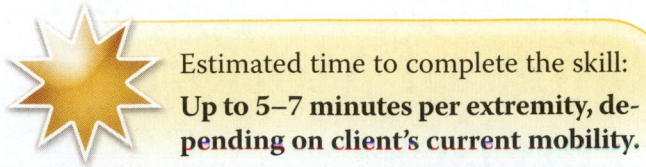

Estimated time to complete the skill:
Up to 5–7 minutes per extremity, depending on client's current mobility.

▶ **DELEGATION TIPS**

Administering PROM may be delegated to properly trained ancillary personnel. Outcomes must be reported to the nurse.

IMPLEMENTATION—Action/Rationale

Action	Rationale
1. Wash hands; wear gloves if contact with body fluids is possible.	1. Reduces the transmission of microorganisms.
2. Explain procedure to client, including estimated duration.	2. Decreases anxiety; encourages compliance and participation.
3. Provide for privacy, including exposing only the extremity to be exercised.	3. Decreases embarrassment.
4. Adjust bed to comfortable height for performing PROM.	4. Prevents muscle strain and discomfort for nurse.
5. Lower bed rail only on the side you are working.	5. Prevents falls.
6. Describe the PROM exercises you are performing, or verbally cue client to perform ROM exercises with your assistance. Include all applicable exercises (refer to Table 4-24-1).	6. Exercises all joint areas.
7. Start at the client's head and perform PROM exercises down each side of the body.	7. Provides a systematic method to ensure that all body parts are exercised.
8. Repeat each PROM exercise as the client tolerates, to a maximum of five times. Perform each motion in a slow, firm manner. Encourage full joint movement, but do not go beyond the point of pain, resistance, or fatigue.	8. Provides exercise to the client's tolerance or to a level that will maintain the joint function.

9. Head
    Perform these movements with the client in a sitting position, if possible.
    • *Rotation*: Turn the head from side to side.
    • *Flexion and extension*: Tilt the head toward the chest and then tilt slightly upward.
    • *Lateral flexion*: Tilt the head on each side so as to almost touch the ear to the shoulder.
	9. To optimize the performance of the movements.
	    • To preserve muscle tone and joint flexibility.

10. Neck
    Perform these movements with the client in a sitting position, if possible.
    • Rotation: Rotate the neck in a semicircle while supporting the head.
	10. To optimize the performance of the movements.
	    • To preserve muscle tone and joint flexibility.

continues

Action	Rationale
11. Trunk Perform these movements with the client in a sitting position, if possible. • *Flexion and extension*: Bend the trunk forward, straighten the trunk, and then extend slightly backward. • *Rotation*: Turn the shoulders forward and return to normal position. • *Lateral flexion*: Tip trunk to the left side, straighten trunk, tip to the right side.	**11.** To optimize the performance of the movements. • To preserve muscle tone and joint flexibility.
12. Arm • *Flexion and extension*: Extend the arm in a straight position upward toward the head, then downward along the side. • *Adduction and abduction*: Extend the arm in a straight position toward the midline (adduction) and away from the midline (abduction).	**12.** To optimize the performance of the movements. • To preserve muscle tone and joint flexibility.
13. Shoulder • *Internal and external rotation*: Bend the elbow at a 90-degree angle with the upper arm parallel to the shoulder; rotate the shoulder by moving the lower arm upward and downward.	**13.** To optimize the performance of the movements. • To preserve muscle tone and joint flexibility.
14. Elbow • *Flexion and extension*: Supporting the arm, flex and extend the elbow. • *Pronation and supination*: Flex elbow, move the hand in palm-up and palm-down position.	**14.** To optimize the performance of the movements. • To preserve muscle tone and joint flexibility.
15. Wrist • *Flexion and extension*: Supporting the wrist, flex and extend the wrist (see Figure 4-24-1). • *Adduction and abduction*: Supporting the lower arm, turn wrist right to left, left to right, then rotate the wrist in a circular motion.	**15.** To optimize the performance of the movements. • To preserve muscle tone and joint flexibility.
16. Hand • *Flexion and extension*: Supporting the wrist, flex and extend the fingers (see Figure 4-24-2). • *Adduction and abduction*: Supporting the wrist, spread fingers apart and then bring them close together. • *Opposition*: Supporting the wrist, touch each finger with the tip of the thumb. • *Thumb rotation*: Supporting the wrist, rotate the thumb in a circular manner.	**16.** To optimize the performance of the movements. • To preserve muscle tone and joint flexibility.

continues

Action	Rationale

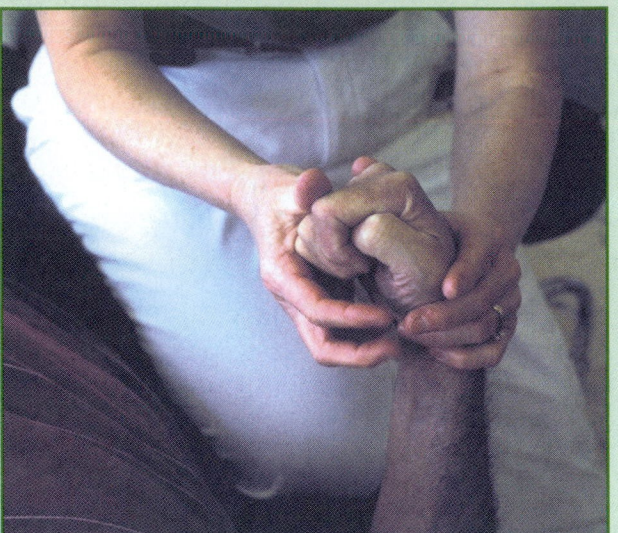

Figure 4-24-1   Flex and extend the wrist.

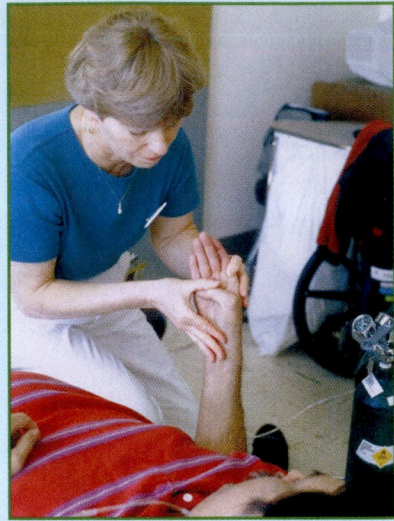

Figure 4-24-2   Flex and extend the fingers.

17. Hip and leg

   Perform these movements with the client in a supine position, if possible.

   • *Flexion and extension*: Supporting the lower leg, flex the leg toward the chest and then extend the leg.

   • *Internal and external rotation*: Supporting the lower leg, angle the foot inward and outward.

   • *Adduction and abduction*: Slide the leg away from the client's midline and then back to the midline (see Figure 4-24-3).

18. Knee

   • *Flexion and extension*: Supporting the lower leg, flex and extend the knee (see Figure 4-24-4).

19. Ankle

   • *Flexion and extension*: Supporting the lower leg, flex and extend the ankle.

20. Foot

   • *Adduction and abduction*: Supporting the ankle, spread the toes apart and then bring them close together.

   • *Flexion and extension*: Supporting the ankle, extend the toes upward and then flex the toes downward.

21. Observe client's joints and face for signs of exertion, pain, or fatigue during movement.

22. When finished, replace covers and position client in proper body alignment.

17. To optimize the performance of the movements.
   • To preserve muscle tone and joint flexibility.

18. To optimize the performance of the movements.
   • To preserve muscle tone and joint flexibility.

19. To optimize the performance of the movements.
   • To preserve muscle tone and joint flexibility.

20. To optimize the performance of the movements.
   • To preserve muscle tone and joint flexibility.

21. Alerts nurse to discontinue exercise.

22. Promotes comfort.

continues

Action	Rationale

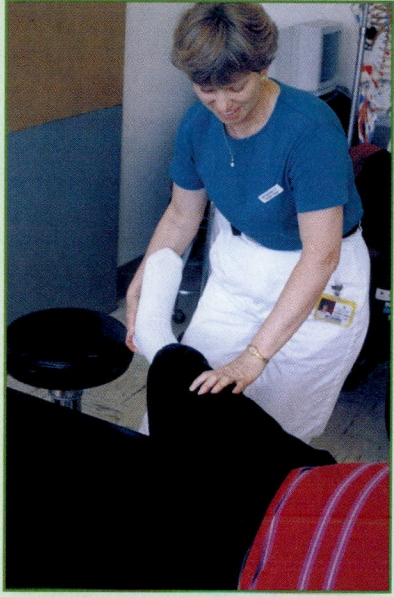

Figure 4-24-3   Slide the leg away from the client's midline, then return.

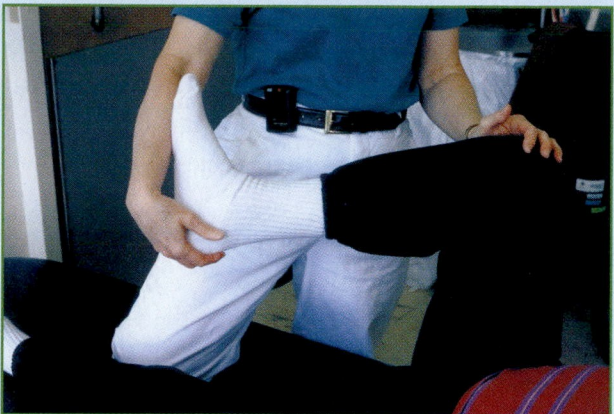

Figure 4-24-4   Flex and extend the knee.

Action	Rationale
23. Place side rails in original position.	23. Prevents falls.
24. Place call light within reach.	24. Facilitates communication.
25. Wash hands.	25. Reduces the transmission of microorganisms.

Table 4-24-1   Joint Range of Motion

JOINT MOVEMENT	RANGE	MUSCLE GROUP(s)	
1. Temporomandibular Joint (TMJ) (Synovial Joint)			
a. Open mouth.	1–2.5 in.		
b. Close mouth.	Complete closure	Masseter, temporalis	
c. *Protrusion*: Push out lower jaw.	0.5 in.	Pterygoideus lateralis	
d. *Retrusion*: Tuck in lower jaw.	0.5 in.		
e. *Lateral motion*: Slide jaw from side to side.	0.5 in.	Pterygoideus lateralis, pterygoideus medialis	

continues

Table 4-24-1   Joint Range of Motion (*continued*)

JOINT MOVEMENT	RANGE	MUSCLE GROUP(s)	
2. Cervical Spine (Pivot Joint)			
a. *Flexion*: Rest chin on chest.	45° each side	Sternocleidomastoid	
b. *Extension*: Return head to midline.	45°	Trapezius	
c. *Hyperextension*: Tilt head back.	10°	Trapezius	
d. *Lateral flexion*: Move head to touch ear to shoulder.	40° each side	Sternocleidomastoid	
e. *Rotation*: Turn head to look to side.	90° each side	Sternocleidomastoid, trapezius	
3. Shoulder (Ball-and-Socket Joint)			
a. *Flexion*: Raise straight arm forward to a position above the head.	180°	Pectoralis major, coracobrachialis, deltoid, biceps brachii	
b. *Extension*: Return straight arm forward and down to side of body.	180°	Latissimus dorsi, deltoid, triceps brachii, teres major	
c. *Hyperextension*: Move straight arm behind body.	50°	Latissimus dorsi, deltoid, teres major	
d. *Abduction*: Move straight arm laterally from side to a position above the head, palm facing away from head.	180°	Deltoid, supraspinatus	
e. *Adduction*: Move straight arm downward laterally and across front of body as far as possible.	230°	Pectoralis major, teres major	

continues

Table 4-24-1   Joint Range of Motion (continued)

JOINT MOVEMENT	RANGE	MUSCLE GROUP(s)	
f. *Circumduction*: Move straight arm in a full circle.	360°	Deltoid, coracobrachialis, latissimus dorsi, teres major	
g. *External rotation*: Bent arm lateral, parallel to floor, palm down, rotate shoulder so fingers point up.	90°	Infraspinatus, teres minor, deltoid	
h. *Internal rotation*: Bent arm lateral, parallel to floor, rotate shoulder so fingers point down.	90°	Subscapularis, pectoralis major, latissimus dorsi, teres major	
4. Elbow (Hinge Joint)			
a. *Flexion*: Bend elbow, move lower arm toward shoulder, palm facing shoulder.	150°	Biceps brachii, brachialis, brachioradialis	
b. *Extension*: Straighten lower arm forward and downward.	150°	Triceps brachii	
c. *Rotation for supination*: Elbow bent, turn hand and forearm so palm is facing upward.	70°–90°	Biceps brachii, supinator	
d. *Rotation for pronation*: Elbow bent, turn hand and forearm so palm is facing downward.	70°–90°	Pronator teres, pronator quadratus	
5. Wrist (Condyloid Joint)			
a. *Flexion*: Bend wrist so fingers move toward inner aspect of forearm.	80°–90°	Flexor carpi radialis, flexor carpi ulnaris	
b. *Extension*: Straighten hand to same plane as arm.	80°–90°	Extensor carpi radialis longus, extensor carpi radialis brevis, extensor carpi ulnaris	
c. *Hyperextension*: Bend wrist so fingers move back as far as possible.	80°–90°	Extensor carpi radialis longus, extensor carpi radialis brevis, extensor carpi ulnaris	

continues

Table 4-24-1   Joint Range of Motion *(continued)*

JOINT MOVEMENT	RANGE	MUSCLE GROUP(s)	
d. *Radial flexion*: Abduction—Bend wrist laterally toward thumb.	Up to 20°	Extensor carpi radialis longus, extensor carpi radialis brevis, flexor carpi radialis	
e. *Ulnar flexion*: Adduction—Bend wrist laterally away from thumb.	30°–50°	Extensor carpi ulnaris, flexor carpi ulnaris	
6. Hand and Fingers (Condyloid and Hinge Joints)			
a. *Flexion*: Make a fist.	90°	Interosseus dorsales manus, flexor digitorum superficialis	
b. *Extension*: Straighten fingers.	90°	Extensor indicis, extensor digiti minimi	
c. *Hyperextension*: Bend fingers back as far as possible.	30°–50°	Extensor indicis, extensor digiti minimi	
d. *Abduction*: Spread fingers apart.	25°	Interosseus dorsales manus	
e. *Adduction*: Bring fingers together.	25°	Interosseus palmares	
7. Thumb (Saddle Joint)			
a. *Flexion*: Move thumb across palmar surface of hand.	90°	Flexor pollicis brevis, opponens pollicis	
b. *Extension*: Move thumb away from hand.	90°	Extensor pollicis brevis, extensor pollicis longus	
c. *Abduction*: Move thumb laterally.	30°	Abductor pollicis brevis, abductor pollicis longus	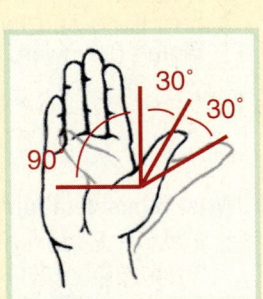
d. *Adduction*: Move thumb back to hand.	30°	Adductor pollicis transversus, adductor pollicis obliquus	
e. *Opposition:* Touch thumb to tip of each finger of same hand.	Touching	Opponens pollicis, flexor pollicis brevis	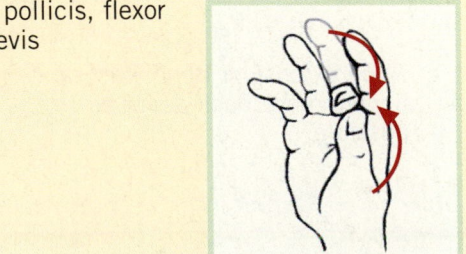

continues

Table 4-24-1   Joint Range of Motion (continued)

JOINT MOVEMENT	RANGE	MUSCLE GROUP(s)	
8. Hip (Ball-and-Socket Joint)			
a. *Flexion*: Move straight leg forward and upward.	90°–120°	Psoas major, iliacus, iliopsoas	
b. *Extension*: Move leg back beside the other leg.	90°–120°	Gluteus maximus, adductor magnus, semitendinosus, semimembranosus	
c. *Hyperextension*: Move leg behind body.	30°–50°	Gluteus maximus, semitendinosus, semimembranosus	
d. *Abduction:* Move leg laterally from midline.	40°–50°	Gluteus medius, gluteus minimus	
e. *Adduction:* Move leg back past midline.	20°–30° past midline	Adductor magnus, adductor brevis, adductor longus	
f. *Circumduction*: Move leg backward in a circle.	360°	Psoas major, gluteus maximus, gluteus medius, adductor magnus	
g. *Internal rotation*: Turn foot and leg inward, pointing toes toward other leg.	90°	Gluteus minimus, gluteus medius, tensor fasciae latae	
h. *External rotation*: Turn foot and leg outward, pointing toes away from other leg.	90°	Obturator externus, obturator internus, quadratus femoris	
9. Knee (Hinge Joint)			
a. *Flexion*: Bend knee to bring heel back toward thigh.	120°–130°	Biceps femoris, semitendinosus, semimembranosus	
b. *Extension*: Straighten each leg, place foot beside other foot.	120°–130°	Rectus femoris, vastus lateralis, vastus medialis, vastus intermedius	

continues

Table 4-24-1 Joint Range of Motion *(continued)*

JOINT MOVEMENT	RANGE	MUSCLE GROUP(s)	
10. Ankle (Hinge Joint)			
a. *Plantar flexion*: Point toes downward.	45°–50°	Gastrocnemius, soleus	
b. *Dorsiflexion*: Point toes upward.	20°	Peroneus, tertius, tibialis anterior	
11. Foot (Gliding Joint)			
a. *Eversion*: Turn sole of foot laterally.	5°	Peroneus longus, peroneus brevis	
b. *Inversion*: Turn sole of foot medially.	5°	Tibialis posterior, tibialis anterior	
12. Toes (Condyloid)			
a. *Flexion*: Curve toes downward.	35°–60°	Flexor hallucis brevis, lumbricales pedis, flexor digitorum brevis	
b. *Extension*: Straighten toes.	35°–60°	Extensor digitorum longus, extensor digitorum brevis, extensor hallucis longus	
c. *Abduction*: Spread toes apart.	Up to 15°	Interosseus dorsales pedis, abductor hallucis	
d. *Adduction*: Bring toes together.	Up to 15°	Adductor hallucis, interosseus plantares	

► REAL WORLD ANECDOTES

Scenario 1

Mrs. Takashima had fractured her right humerus near the shoulder when she fell from a ladder. Her physician had done an open reduction and internal fixation of the humerus and now Mrs. Takashima was being taught passive and active range of motion of the right arm. When Mrs. Takashima returned for her third appointment, the nurse noted that Mrs. Takashima's range of motion had decreased. Mrs. Takashima insisted that she had been performing the range of motion exercises regularly and she did not understand why she wasn't getting better. Upon closer examination the nurse noted an unusual lump at the fracture site. When the nurse performed passive range of motion on Mrs. Takashima's arm, the nurse noted that the lump changed in size and shape. Fearing that the fracture was no longer reduced, the nurse immobilized Mrs. Takashima's arm and notified the physician. X-rays revealed that the fracture had indeed dislocated and a second surgery was required for fixation of the fracture.

continues

> ► **REAL WORLD ANECDOTES** (continued)

Scenario 2

Mr. Rewolinski, a postpolio syndrome client, was ventilator dependent and received active/assisted PROM 6 days a week. Functional shoulder rotation movement was normal and strong, but all other upper extremity movements were weak, especially shoulder flexion. The nurse could have easily accepted Mr. Rewolinski's inability to raise his arms and simply perform PROM. This would have maintained the client's shoulder mobility. For Mr. Rewolinski to have any reasonable hope of performing self-care, however, the nurse needed to continually encourage Mr. Rewolinski to participate in his exercises, assisting in the full range of motion but encouraging the client to expand his functional PROM. At the time of this printing, Mr. Rewolinski continues to slowly regain his strength and mobility.

Scenario 3

Mrs. Evangelista suffered subarachnoid trauma around her brain stem. PROM was ordered to minimize the complications of the resulting paralysis and extended bedrest. Though Mrs. Evangelista was largely unresponsive when PROM began, it later became obvious that she was awake and conscious of her surroundings at that time. Therefore, it is extremely important to communicate verbally with all clients, especially those who are unresponsive. Since suffering her trauma, Mrs. Evangelista has made substantial improvements. She is able to track and participate in conversations; assist in transfers into and out of a wheelchair; and perform limited self-care, including eating by herself. Mrs. Evangelista has communicated with the staff how appreciative she is to those who talked to her when she could not respond.

► **EVALUATION**

- Client has maintained or improved current functional mobility in all involved joints and extremities.
- Client has regained or improved strength and/or voluntary movement in involved joints and extremities.
- Client has avoided complications of immobility, including decubitus ulcers, contractures, decreased peristalsis, constipation, fecal impaction, orthostatic hypotension, pulmonary embolism, and thrombophlebitis.

► **DOCUMENTATION**

Nurses' Notes

- Document the performance of PROM exercises. Include the joints and extremities on which ROM was performed, the types and degrees of limitation observed, the extent of the client's active involvement in exercises, any reports of pain or discomfort, and any observations of intolerance to exercise.
- Record any unusual findings.

Document on appropriate flow sheet or electronic medical record (EMR).

► **CRITICAL THINKING SKILL**

Introduction

Nurses must be able to evaluate the true functional limit of a client's PROM.

Possible Scenario

A client with a closed head injury or another type of upper motor neuron damage often exhibits spastic paralysis. ROM is indicated to reduce muscle spasticity and lengthen contractures. Because the client's muscles are working against the nurse, it is much more difficult to assess true functional limits as compared to a client with flaccid paralysis.

Possible Outcome

If ROM is attempted quickly with a client exhibiting spastic paralysis, the nurse could easily conclude that the client's functional limits were narrow and discontinue movement as soon as any resistance was felt. Very little motion would be accomplished and comparatively little therapeutic benefit would be achieved.

Prevention

Care must be taken to exercise slowly through all repetitions and encourage movement to functional limits as muscles relax. As long as one repetition accomplishes a longer arc of movement than the previous, even by a few degrees, the nurse may conclude that functional limits have not been reached. The nurse must take care, however, to monitor not only the joint being exercised but also the face of the client for signs of pain or fatigue.

► VARIATIONS

Geriatric Variations:
- *The ultimate goal of PROM exercise is client independence, so encourage as much participation as possible.*
- *Arrange for PROM to be performed at the same time each day, at the client's convenience.*
- *Various chronic conditions (chronic obstructive pulmonary disease, hypertension, and so on) require extra caution and careful observation for fatigue, pain, and respiratory difficulty.*

Pediatric Variation:
- *For a child of appropriate age, demonstrate each movement to be performed either on yourself, a doll, or some other nonthreatening surrogate.*

Home Care Variation:
- *Instruct family members and caregivers to perform PROM between scheduled visits. Lower extremity ROM is best performed on a flat, raised surface, whereas upper-extremity PROM can be executed in a seated position.*

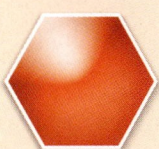

Long-Term Care Variations:
- *Various chronic conditions (chronic obstructive pulmonary disease, hypertension, and so on) require extra caution and careful observation of the client for fatigue, pain, and respiratory difficulty.*
- *The ultimate goal of PROM exercise is client independence, so encourage as much participation as possible.*
- *Arrange for PROM to be performed at the same time each day, at the client's convenience.*

► COMMON ERRORS

Possible Error:

Exercises place the client in pain or discomfort.

Prevention:

Watch the client's face as well as the joint being moved. Observe changes in expression when nearing the limits of movement. If the client does indicate feeling pain or discomfort, discontinue exercise immediately and assess client for pain management.

Possible Error:

PROM exercises were administered incorrectly because orders were written for only specific joints or planes.

Prevention:

Do not assume PROM exercises will be ordered for both upper and lower extremities. Be sure to read orders each shift. If PROM exercises are administered incorrectly, admit the error to the client and perform any omitted PROM exercises correctly.

Possible Error:

The nurse ignores a nonresponsive client.

Prevention:

Do not assume that nonresponsive means unaware. Talk each client through every exercise.

► **NURSING TIPS**

• Perform all needed ROM exercises on one extremity, then move to the other side of the client, and perform ROM on the other extremity.

• If a joint or plane of motion is especially tight, hold the joint close to the end range for up to 30 seconds to stretch the area, then move the joint again through the PROM.

► **SPECIAL CONSIDERATIONS**

• *Many clients will need continued range of motion exercises when they return home from the hospital. Encourage them to learn the exercises that they can participate in and include family members. You may want to introduce music along with the exercises to encourage the client to work on a skill for a certain length of time. For example, when doing hip and leg exercises you can encourage the client to hold the leg adducted for this many beats, then abduct the leg, and so on. Set up a schedule of exercises that the client can independently perform. For example, if a client has hip surgery, he or she may be able to perform arm PROM exercises independently instead of depending solely on the therapist. Reinforce the need for exercise to prevent complications.*

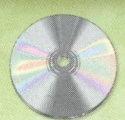

Postmortem Care

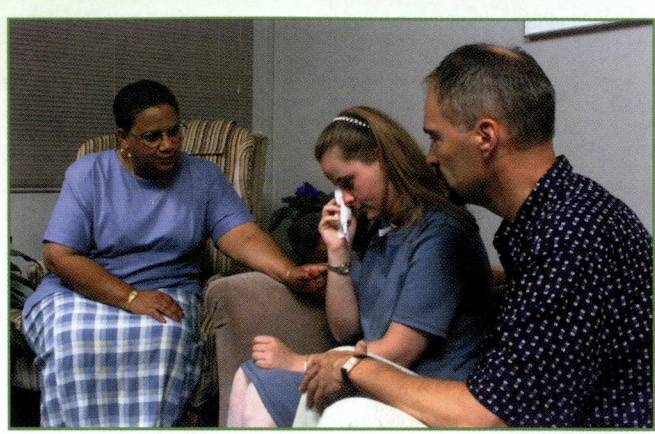

▶ OVERVIEW OF THE SKILL

Postmortem care involves the physical caring for the body after death, while respecting the wishes of the deceased and family as much as possible. In some institutions, the physician or qualified practitioner is responsible for notifying the next of kin and obtaining permission for an autopsy and organ donation. In others, nurses notify the family.

▶ ASSESSMENT

1. Verify that respiration and heart activity have ceased before initiating postmortem care. Verify that the physician has pronounced the death. **As a client nears death, respiratory and cardiac systems become more difficult to assess. A client may develop stridor from pooled secretions or exhibit Cheyne-Stokes breathing with long periods of apnea. The heart rate eventually slows and usually becomes quite irregular. Peripheral pulses will become weaker, thready, and difficult to palpate. Documentation of the death will include when the heartbeat and respiration ceased.**

2. Assess the family's response to the news of the client's death. **Providing emotional support to the family during the acute grieving stage is essential.**

3. If not already known or required, ask the family's preference for an autopsy. **Usually asking the family's permission for an autopsy is the physician's or qualified practitioner's responsibility, but that can vary at institutions.**

4. Follow hospital policy regarding seeking permission from the family for organ donation if not already known. **Some organs must be harvested within hours of the death in order to be transplanted.**

▶ DIAGNOSIS

Grieving

Deficient Knowledge

Death Anxiety

▶ PLANNING

Expected Outcomes:

1. Next of kin will be informed of the client's death in a timely manner and offered the option to visit the deceased, if desired, before postmortem care.

2. The client will be bathed and prepared for the morgue according to hospital policies.

3. The client's body alignment will be maintained during family visitation.

4. The family will experience no undue emotional shock or trauma from resuscitation debris left

around the bedside, blood or secretions staining the sheets, or needles or tubes protruding from the body.

Equipment Needed:

- Clean client gown and bed linens
- Basin, soap, and other bathing supplies
- Morgue pack, which may include shroud, tags for labeling the body
- Equipment to remove tubes if indicated (i.e., a syringe to remove the Foley catheter, a suture removal kit, and so on)
- Morgue cart, or stretcher

▶ **CLIENT EDUCATION NEEDED:**

1. The family should be informed when the body will be sent to the mortuary.
2. The family needs to be aware of hospital or institution resources such as a chaplain or priest, or facilities such as chapels.

Estimated time to complete the skill: **Depends on the length of the family visit. Preparing the body for the morgue will take approximately 20–30 minutes.**

▶ **DELEGATION TIPS**

Postmortem care is a skill that can be routinely delegated to properly trained ancillary personnel.

IMPLEMENTATION—Action/Rationale

Action	Rationale
1. Close the drapes and/or door. Allow the family to stay in the room, if desired (see Figure 4-25-1).	1. Privacy is maintained.
2. Notify the physician in charge when death has occurred. Have physician and/or other qualified person pronounce the client's death.	2. The physician is responsible for pronouncing the client's death, completing the death certificate, notifying the next of kin, and obtaining permission for an autopsy and/or organ donation. The physician may assign some of these duties to another person.

Figure 4-25-1   The morgue cart and morgue pack are used to prepare the body and transport it to the morgue.

continues

Action	Rationale
3. Notify the nursing supervisor, admitting department, and any other departments that need to know of the client's death.	3. Informing the proper personnel is essential to be sure that policy is followed.
4. Wash hands and apply gloves and other protective equipment (see Figure 4-25-2).	4. Handwashing reduces the transmission of microorganisms. Wearing gloves and other protective equipment protects the nurse from exposure to body fluids.
5. Bathe the body and remove all tubes (or leave tubes in place for autopsy according to the institution's policy). Put a gown on the client if the family will view the body. Also, clean the immediate environment as indicated.	5. Showing consideration for the family and friends of the deceased includes cleaning of the body and environment before viewing.
6. Follow the institution's policy about removing or inserting dentures, dental plates, artificial eyes, limbs, and hair, and removing contact lenses.	6. Institutional policy will determine the appropriate disposition of these items.
7. Gently close the client's eyes, if open. Do not use tape.	7. Tape may mark the face.
8. Allow family and friends of the deceased time to view the deceased, if desired. Be available to answer questions and provide support. Be sensitive to different cultural beliefs surrounding the deceased immediately after death (see Figure 4-25-3).	8. Family and friends of the deceased may want to view the body alone for varying lengths of time. If the family was not present at the time of death, they may have questions about the immediate steps leading up to the death. If at all possible, allow for cultural variations.
9. Inventory the client's belongings if this has not already been done.	9. Inventory of the client's belongings is preliminary to their disposition.
10. Send all the client's belongings, jewelry, and personal effects home with the family, if possible. Document the name of the person who received the items. If the family is not available, follow the institution's policy regarding disposition of belongings.	10. Sending belongings home with the family prevents their loss during transport or in the morgue.

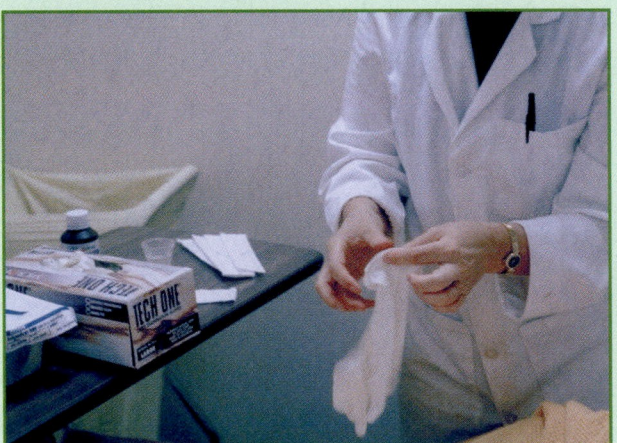

Figure 4-25-2 Apply gloves before preparing the body.

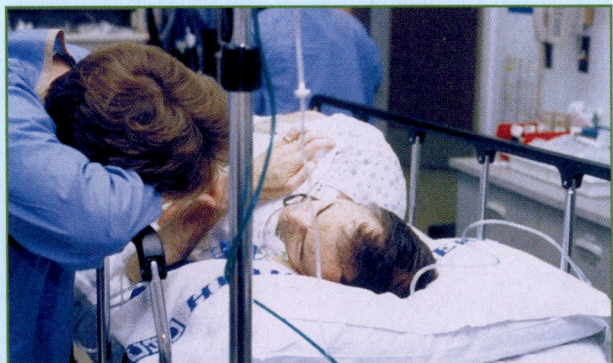

Figure 4-25-3 Allow family and friends time to view the deceased.

continues

Action	Rationale

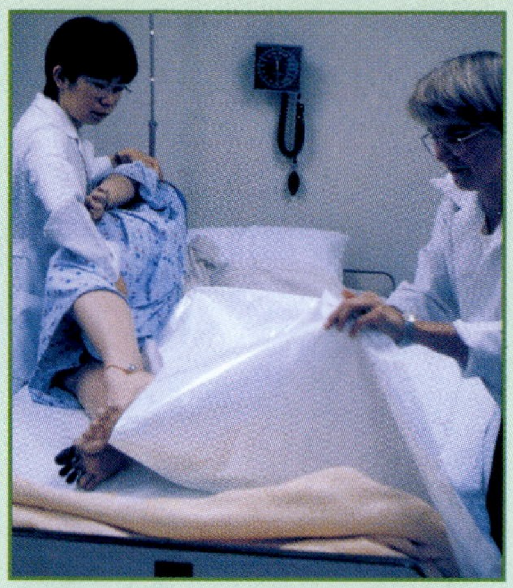

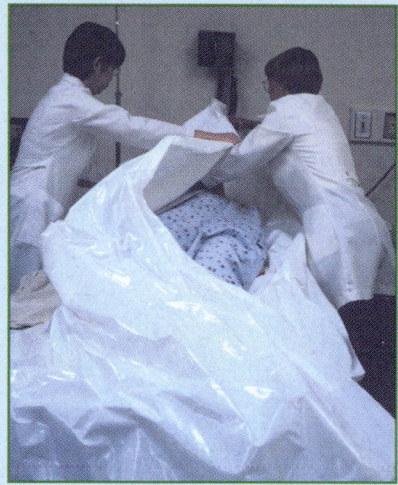

Figure 4-25-4 Roll the body to one side and open the shroud. Roll the body back on top of the open shroud.

Figure 4-25-5 Wrap the body in the shroud.

11. Obtain postmortem kit, if available. Place identifying tags on the deceased according to the institution's policy.

11. The policy will determine how the body should be identified.

12. Wrap the body in a sheet or shroud (see Figures 4-25-4, 4-25-5, and 4-25-6).

12. Follow policy to ensure that the body is properly prepared for the morgue.

13. Transfer the body to the stretcher or morgue cart (see Figures 4-25-7 and 4-25-8).

13. Ensures safe transport of client.

14. Arrange for transportation to the morgue.

14. Ensures proper disposition of the body.

15. Leave the morgue cart in the room until ready to transport.

15. Ensures client privacy.

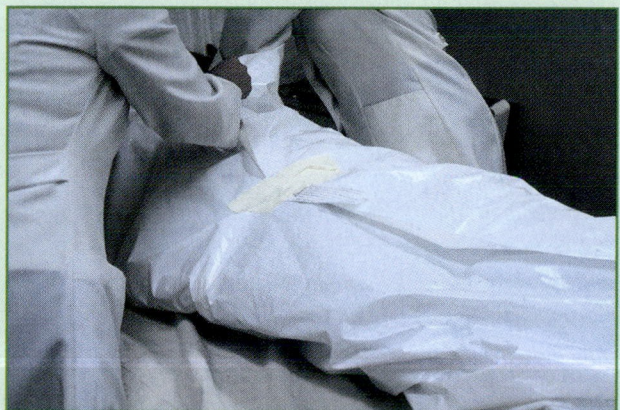

Figure 4-25-6 Secure the shroud around the body.

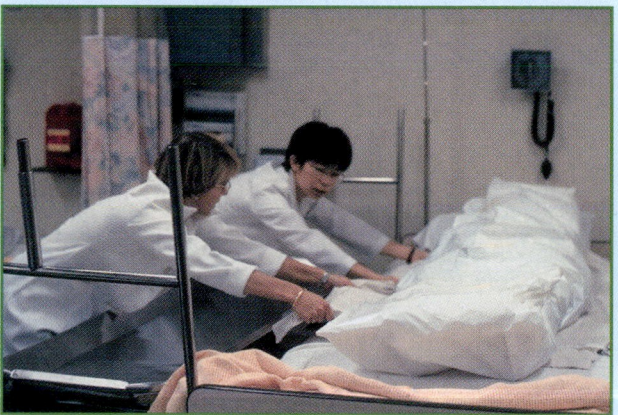

Figure 4-25-7 Transfer the body to the morgue cart. Obtain assistance with heavy lifting.

continues

Action	Rationale

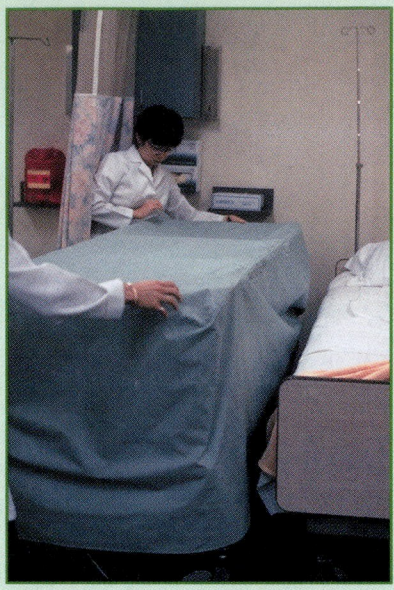

Figure 4-25-8   Replace the cover on the morgue cart before moving it.

16. Document in the progress notes the time the pulse and respiration ceased; the time the physician was notified; the time the family was notified; absence or presence of the family; and disposition of jewelry, personal effects, and the body.

16. Accurate documentation of disposition is essential if there are questions asked regarding the whereabouts of belongings and so on.

17. Wash hands.

17. Reduces the transmission of microorganisms

► REAL WORLD ANECDOTES

Clarissa Stubb's death was expected and she had been receiving terminal care for several days. Her family, who had recently decided on a "no code" status because of the irreversibility of her illness, had been visiting Mrs. Stubb every day. Usually, one or more members were with the client at all times, even at night. The family decided to meet together for dinner one evening because there were a number of personal issues to discuss as a group, on the assumption that the client was stable enough to be left alone for a few hours.

Shortly after the family left the unit, Mrs. Stubb died. Unfortunately, the family had not left the telephone number or name of the restaurant, so the physician was unable to notify them of the death. When the family returned to the ward several hours later, they were informed that Mrs. Stubb had died. Several members of the family began blaming themselves for leaving the client alone during her last moments of life. Other members of the family blamed the nursing staff for not properly informing them of the imminent death so that they could have decided to stay.

The nurse allowed the family to talk about their concerns before gently stating that the point of death is not predictable. The family had many questions about the immediate events leading up to the death, including whether their absence had hastened the death. By not taking the family's comments personally, the nurse was able to calmly and sensitively listen to their questions before focusing the discussion on whether the family wanted to spend some time with Mrs. Stubb and say good-bye. The family did want to visit with the deceased. The nurse allowed them privacy with the body but made himself available to answer any questions. By the time the family left the unit, they were visibly less angry and thanked the nurse for caring for their family member.

► EVALUATION

- Ensure that the client's body is prepared for the morgue appropriately by following the institution's policy.
- Check the inventory of the client's belongings against the disposition of belongings prior to transporting the client to the morgue to be sure that all personal effects are accounted for.

► DOCUMENTATION

Nurses' Notes

- Document the client's condition immediately before and at the time of death. Include the time of and situation surrounding client's death, and the cessation of pulse and respirations.
- Note the date and time the physician or qualified provider was notified.
- Document if and when the family was notified. Record which family members were notified of the client's demise.
- Record whether the family visited. Include the family's reaction and any special requests the family may have.
- Note the disposition of the client's belongings, including jewelry, personal effects, and so on.
- Indicate that postmortem care was completed. Include which tubes were discontinued or left in place. Note any special postmortem preparations or instructions.
- Document notification of the mortuary or transport to the morgue.

Document on appropriate flow sheet or electronic medical record (EMR).

► CRITICAL THINKING SKILL

Introduction

An elderly Chinese-American client died after a long illness at the hospital. Many of his family were present during the death and requested that the body be wrapped in a special cloth brought from home.

Possible Scenario

After the death of the client, the family approached the nurse and requested that they be allowed to bathe the body. The nurse agreed and granted privacy to the family. Upon the nurse's return to the room, she discovered the body had been wrapped in a special cloth, which the family requested be transported with the client to the morgue. The nurse checked with the nursing supervisor and the morgue to be sure that the family wishes would be honored. After careful documentation of her actions, including the family's request and approval from the morgue, the nurse sent the body shrouded in the special cloth to the morgue.

Possible Outcome

By honoring the family's request, the nurse was sensitive to the client's desires even during postmortem care. If the nurse had refused to allow the family to bathe and prepare the body in accordance with their beliefs, she would have negatively interfered with the grieving process.

Prevention

Exercising culturally sensitive nursing care allowed the nurse to facilitate a grieving process rather than create an obstacle.

► VARIATIONS

Geriatric Variation:
- *If the death has been expected and/or the client is old or debilitated, family and friends may feel a mixture of sadness, happiness, and relief upon learning of the death. Such feelings may be distressing to them. They may be remorseful that they are not feeling overwhelming grief.*

Pediatric Variation:
- *Parents may feel tremendous guilt if the death was accidental or unexpected. If applicable, remind the parents of the good care and love they gave to the child.*

continues

> ## ► VARIATIONS *(continued)*

Home Care Variations:
- *Assist the family in making funeral arrangements and contacting relatives.*
- *Plan before the death whom to call and how the body will be removed from the house. Discuss with the family if they wish to be present when the body is being removed.*

Long-Term Care Variation:
- *Consider the needs of other residents of a long-term care facility. Often friends and family are deceased, live far away, and do not visit often. Fellow residents become "family" to each other. When a fellow resident dies, consider the needs of other residents to grieve and to view the body. Remember that the death may remind them of their own mortality, especially if they are in a similar situation.*

> ## ► COMMON ERRORS

Possible Error:
The client's family reports a missing ring. The nurse remembers that a family member took the valuable ring home, but it was not documented.

Prevention:
Document disposal of all client property, the client's chart, and the personal property records used at the institution, including property taken by the family.

► NURSING TIPS

- Allow uninterrupted time to talk with the family about the client's death.
- If death is imminent, check to see whether the client is an organ donor before the death occurs. Refer to institutional policies regarding how families are to be approached.
- Careful documentation of the client's belongings, including disposition, will provide answers if there are questions about belongings.

- If appropriate, the nurse may want to call the family after the death to address any unanswered questions and provide some closure.
- Be sure the nursing unit has current contact information for the next of kin of clients admitted.
- If the family desires to be with the body immediately, and you do not have time to clean the body and the environment, you can wash the client's hands, and cover the client with a clean sheet, leaving the hands on the outside. Remove debris in the room or cover with clean sheets.

> ## ► SPECIAL CONSIDERATIONS

- *Sometimes clients are in semiprivate rooms when one client expires. If the client in bed A expires, you may want to move the client in bed B to another room. This will facilitate room for the postmortem care and allow the family some time and space to grieve.*
- *Some institutions do not allow removal of tubes when the case is a trauma. Check with your institution's policy regarding removal of tubes from trauma clients.*

Medication Administration

Administering Oral, Sublingual, and Buccal Medications

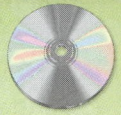

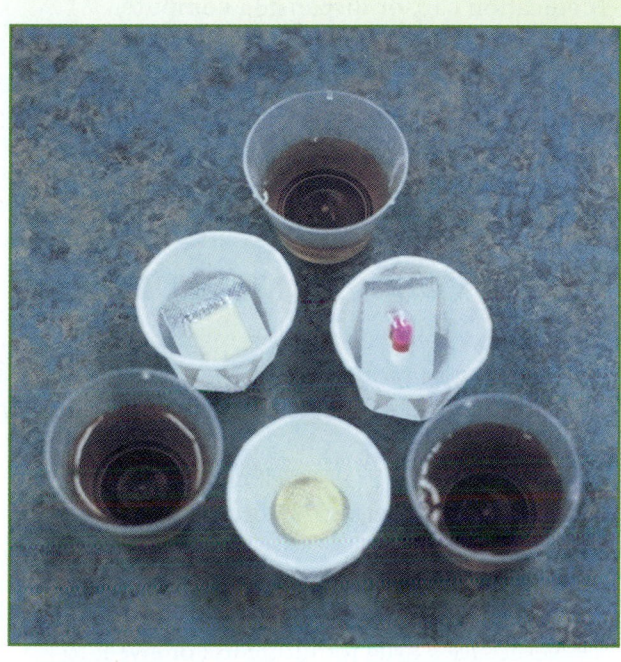

▶ OVERVIEW OF THE SKILL

The easiest and most common method of administering a medication is usually by mouth. Clients may be taught to administer the medication by themselves at home or a nurse can prepare the medications and dispense to clients. Oral medications are contraindicated for clients who have gastrointestinal alterations, who are using a nasogastric tube or a gastrostomy tube, or who have a poor gag reflex. Clients with an inability to swallow because of neuromuscular disorder, esophageal stricture, or lesion of the mouth or those who are unresponsive or comatose are also ineligible to receive oral administration of medication.

Nurses need to know the action, normal dosage, side effects, and nursing implications for each drug they administer. In some settings, medications for several clients may be prepared at one time in the medication room or medication cart by carefully identifying each client's doses (see Figure 5-1-1). Most hospitals use a computerized limited access medication system.

▶ ASSESSMENT

1. Assess the five rights: right client, right medication, right route, right dose, and right time. **Prevents errors in medication administration.**

2. Review the action, purpose, normal dosage and route, common side effects, time of onset and peak action, and nursing implications of each

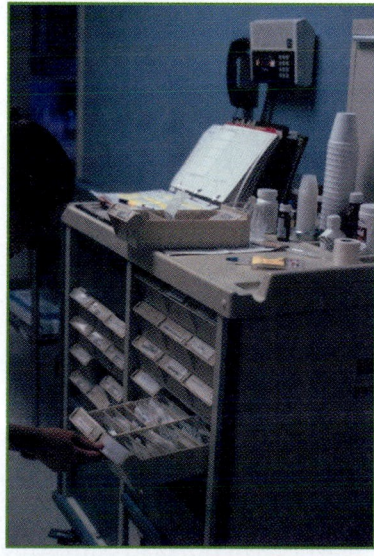

Figure 5-1-1 In some settings, medications for several clients are prepared at the medication cart at one time.

drug **so the client's response to the medication may be monitored.**

3. Assess the client's condition to be sure the order of the health care provider is appropriate **as the client's condition may have changed since the order was written.**

4. Assess the client's ability to swallow food and fluid **as he or she may be unable to swallow a pill and an alternate route for medication may be needed.**

5. Assess for any contraindications for administering an oral medication such as nausea and vomiting, gastric suction, or gastric surgery resulting in decreased peristalsis **as alterations in gastrointestinal function may interfere with drug absorption and excretion.**

6. Assess the client's medical record for a history of allergies to food or medications **so these medications can be avoided.**

7. Assess the client's knowledge about the use of medications **so client teaching can be tailored to his or her needs. This may also assess compliance for taking the drugs at home or reveal drug dependence or abuse.**

8. Assess the client's age **as pediatric or geriatric clients may have special needs according to their ability to swallow a pill.**

9. Assess the client's need for fluids **as swallowing a pill is usually easier with fluid and promotes fluid intake. However, fluid restrictions may be necessary to observe.**

10. Assess the client's ability to sit or turn to the side. **The client must be able to swallow the pill without aspiration.**

11. Assess the client for allergies. **The client may be allergic to the medicine.**

▶ DIAGNOSIS

Noncompliance

Impaired Swallowing

Deficient Knowledge

Risk for Allergic Response

▶ PLANNING

Expected Outcomes:

1. The client will swallow the prescribed medication.
2. The client will be able to explain the purpose and schedule for taking the medication.
3. The client will have no gastrointestinal discomfort or alterations in function.

4. The client will show the desired response to the medication such as pain relief, regular heart rate, or stable blood pressure.

5. The client will have no allergic reaction.

Equipment Needed (see Figure 5-1-1):

- Health care provider's order for the medication
- Medication administration record (MAR)
- Medication cart or dispensing computer
- Medication tray
- Disposable medication cups
- Glass of water, juice, or other liquid
- Drinking straw
- Mortar and pestle, if needed
- Paper towels

▶ CLIENT EDUCATION NEEDED:

1. Provide written information regarding each medication as requested.

2. Clients should be taught the basic guidelines for drug safety:
   - Keep each drug in its original, labeled container.
   - Discard any outdated medication through approved methods.
   - Always finish a prescribed drug unless instructed otherwise.
   - Never save a drug for future use or give it to another person.
   - Keep drugs out of reach of children.
   - Refrigerate medications that require it.
   - Read labels carefully and follow all instructions.

3. Instruct clients on which foods, medications, or other elements, such as alcohol or sunlight, are to be avoided while taking this medication.

4. Teach client how to store the medication at home, such as in the refrigerator or in a clean, dry place.

5. Clients need to be cautioned on which drugs can cause gastric irritation and need to be taken with food.

6. Remind the client that medications taken sublingually should not be swallowed or they will have little effect as gastric juices will destroy them.

7. Caution clients taking medications intended for buccal administration to allow them to dissolve against the mucous membrane of the cheek and swallow the saliva.

8. Instruct clients to allow lozenges to dissolve and not to chew or swallow them whole as the drug acts slowly through oral absorption and not through gastric mucosa.

9. Clients with drug allergies should wear an identification bracelet listing the drugs to which they have an allergy.

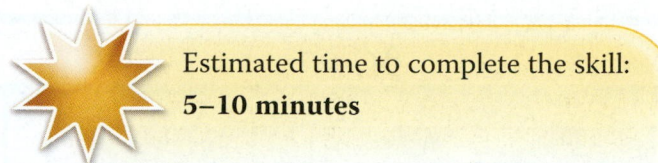

Estimated time to complete the skill:
5–10 minutes

IMPLEMENTATION—Action/Rationale

Action	Rationale
1. Wash hands and put on clean gloves.	1. Reduces the number of microorganisms.
2. Arrange the medication tray and cups in the medication room or on the medication cart outside the client's room. Most hospitals use a computerized limited access medication cart. Follow institutional protocol.	2. Organizing medications and equipment saves time and reduces the possibility of error.
3. Unlock the medication cart or log on to the computer.	3. Medications need to be safeguarded.
4. Prepare the medication for one client at a time following the five rights. Select the correct drug from the medication drawer according to the MAR (see Figure 5-1-2). Calculate the drug dosage, if needed.	4. The five rights are right client, right time, right medication, right dose, and right route. Comparing the MAR with the label reduces error. Double checking reduces error in calculation.
5. To prepare a tablet or capsule: Pour the required number of tablets or capsules into the bottle cap and transfer the medication to a medication cup without touching them.	5. Avoids wasting expensive medications and avoids contamination of medication.
• Scored tablets may be broken, if necessary, using gloved hands or with a pill cutting device (see Figure 5-1-3).	• Tablets that are not scored are not meant to be broken. The medication's effectiveness would be diminished if the tablet were broken or crushed.
• A unit-dose tablet should be placed directly into the medicine cup without opening it until it is administered to the client.	• The wrapper maintains cleanliness and identification until it is administered.
• For clients with difficulty in swallowing, some tablets may be crushed into a powder using a mortar and pestle or by being placed between two paper medication cups and ground with a blunt object, then mixed in a small amount of applesauce or custard. Be aware that time-released or specially coated medications must not be crushed. Check with the pharmacy if you are uncertain (see Figure 5-1-4).	• A large tablet is usually easier to swallow if it is ground and mixed with soft food.

continues

Action	Rationale

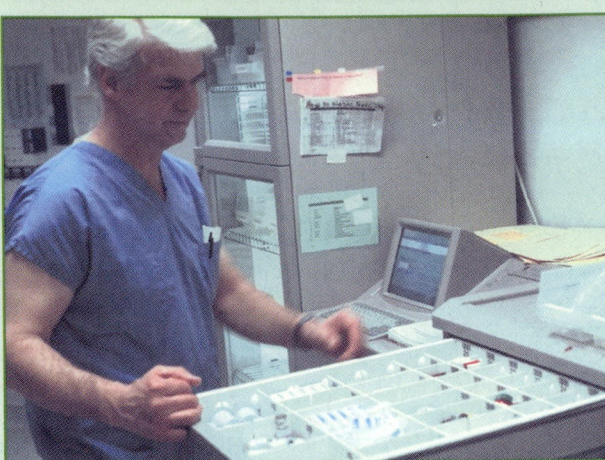

Figure 5-1-2 Prepare oral medications following the five rights—right client, time, medication, dose, and route.

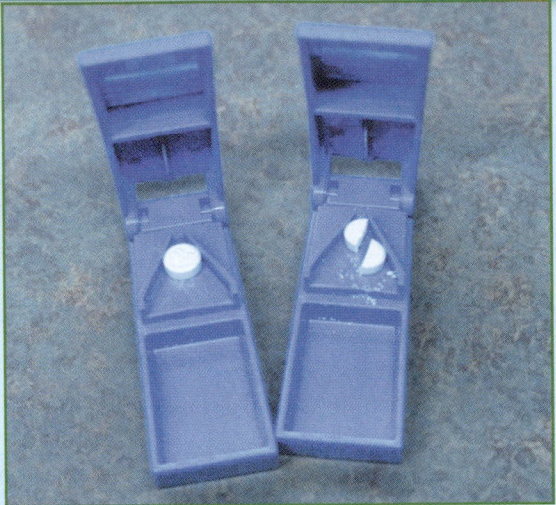

Figure 5-1-3 Scored tablets may be broken, if necessary.

6. To prepare a liquid medication: Remove the bottle cap from the container and place cap upside down on the cart. Hold the bottle with the label up and the medication cup at eye level while pouring (see Figure 5-1-5). Fill the cup to the desired level using the surface or base of the meniscus as the scale, not the edge of the liquid on the cup. Wipe lip of bottle with paper towel.

6. Placing the bottle cap upside down on the cart prevents contamination of the inside of the container. Holding the bottle with the label up keeps spilled liquid from obliterating the label. Holding the medication cup at eye level ensures an accurate dose. Wiping the lip of the bottle prevents the bottle cap from sticking.

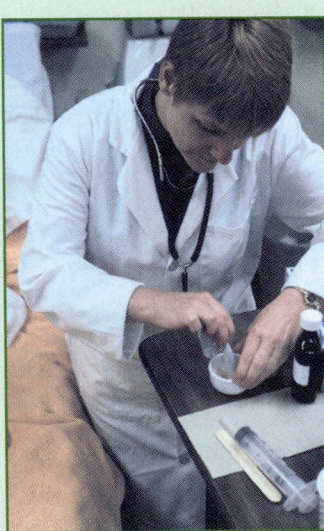

Figure 5-1-4 Some medications may be crushed and mixed with a soft food, such as applesauce, for clients who have difficulty swallowing.

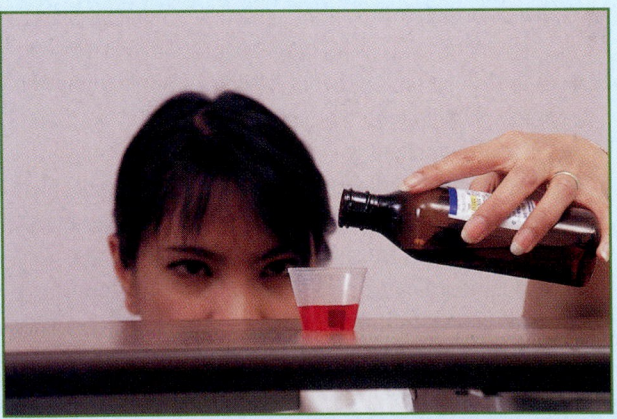

Figure 5-1-5 Measure oral medications at eye level.

continues

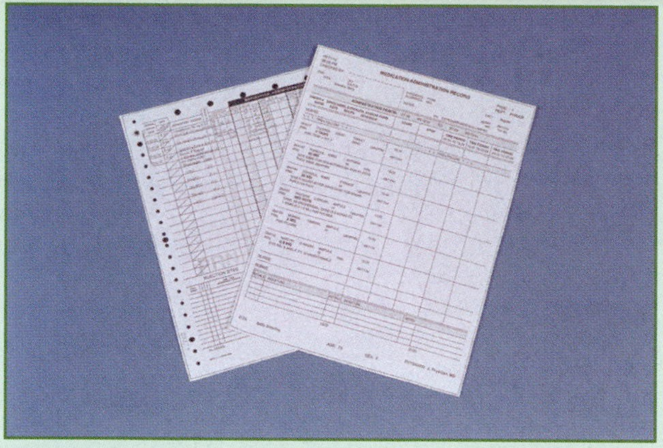

Action	Rationale

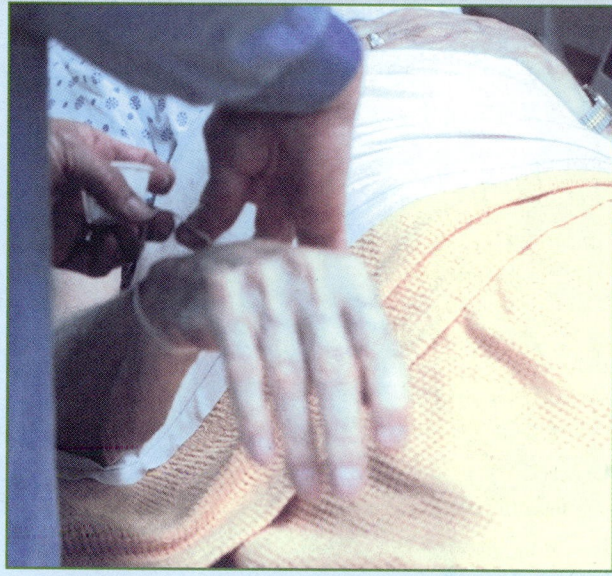

Figure 5-1-6   Controlled substance laws require records of each narcotic dose dispensed.

Figure 5-1-7   Identify the client by reading the client's name bracelet and asking his or her name before administering medication.

7. To prepare a narcotic, obtain the key to the narcotic drawer and check the narcotic record for the drug count when signing out the dose (see Figure 5-1-6). If the drug count does not agree with the records, report to the charge nurse immediately. The institution may require an incident report be filed.

7. Controlled substance laws require records of each dose dispensed. Early identification of errors assists in corrective action.

8. Check expiration date on all medications.
- Double-check the MAR with the prepared drugs.
- Return stock medications to their shelf or drawer.
- Place MARs with the client's medications.
- Do not leave drugs unattended.

8. Expired medications may lose their effectiveness.
- Reduces risk of error.
- Ensures safety of stock medications.
- Ensures identification of medications.
- Drugs are safeguarded by nurse.

9. Administer medications to client: Observe the correct time to give the medication.
- Identify the client by reading the client's name bracelet, repeating the name, and/or asking the client to state his or her name (see Figure 5-1-7). Additionally, check the hospital number if name alert or client is not reliable.
- Check the drug packaging, if it is present, to ensure the medication type and dosage.
- Assess the client's condition and the form of the medication.
- Perform any assessment required for specific medications, such as a pulse or blood pressure.
- Explain the purpose of the drug and ask if the client has any questions.
- Assist the client to a sitting or lateral position.

9. Ensures the therapeutic effect of the drug when given within 30 minutes of the prescribed time. (Right time.)
- Identification bracelets made at the time of admission are the most reliable source of identification even if the client is unable to state his or her name. (Right client.)

- Prevents giving the wrong medication or wrong dose. (Right medication, right dose.)
- Allows you to assess the route of the medication and if this route is appropriate. (Right route.)
- Determines whether the medication should be given at that time or not.
- Improves compliance with drug therapy.

- Prevents aspiration during swallowing.

continues

Action	Rationale

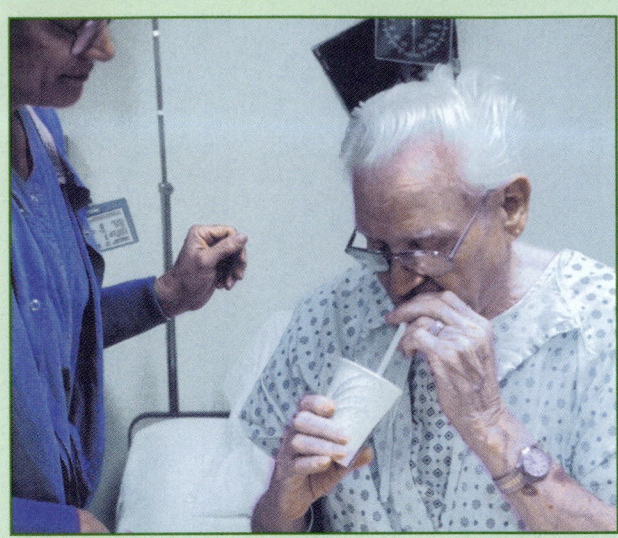

Figure 5-1-8   Allow the client to hold the tablet, and give water or juice to help him or her swallow the medication.

Action	Rationale
• Allow client to hold the tablet or medication cup.	• Client becomes familiar with medications.
• Supply a glass of water or other liquid, and straw if needed, to help the client swallow the medication (see Figure 5-1-8).	• Promotes client comfort in swallowing and can improve fluid intake.
• For sublingual medications, instruct client to place medication under the tongue and allow it to dissolve completely.	• Drug is absorbed through the mucous membranes into the blood vessels. If swallowed, the drug may be destroyed by gastric juices or detoxified in the liver too quickly so that its intended effects will not occur.
• For buccal administration of drugs, instruct the client to place the medication in the mouth against the cheek until it dissolves completely.	• Promotes local activity on mucous membranes.
• For oral medications given through a nasogastric tube, crush tablets or open capsules and dissolve powder with 20 to 30 mL of warm water in a cup. Be sure medication will still be properly absorbed if crushed and dissolved. Check placement of the feeding tube or nasogastric tube before instilling anything but air into the tube.	• Allows medication administration via nasogastric or feeding tube. Ensures that the medication is absorbed and utilized correctly.
• Remain with the client until each medication has been swallowed or dissolved.	• Nurse is responsible for ensuring that the client receives the dose and does not save it or discard it.
• Assist the client into a comfortable position.	• Maintains client's comfort.
10. Dispose of soiled supplies and wash hands.	10. Reduces transmission of organisms.
11. Record the time and route of administration on the MAR and return it to the client's file.	11. Prevents administration error.
12. Return the cart to the medicine room; restock the supplies as needed. Clean the work area.	12. Assists other staff in completing duties efficiently.

> ## ▶ REAL WORLD ANECDOTES
>
> *Fred was a 91-year-old resident of a long-term care facility who was having increasing difficulty swallowing after a series of small strokes. His favorite breakfast consisted of a bowl of bran buds with milk and two glasses of prune juice. The tablets his physician ordered for him were large, so the nurse crushed them by putting them between two paper medication cups and crushing them with a pestle. This made it easy to remove the top cup and add a teaspoon of applesauce to the powder just before she approached Fred to give him his medications. She gave him the cup and he spooned the medication-containing applesauce into his mouth and washed it down with his prune juice.*

▶ EVALUATION

- Evaluate the client's response to the drug within 30 minutes of administration or sooner if an allergic reaction is anticipated.
- Ask client or caregiver to discuss the purpose, action, dosage schedule, and side effects of the drug.

▶ DOCUMENTATION

Medication Administration Record

- Date and time each drug was administered including initials and signature.
- If drug is withheld, circle the time the drug was scheduled on the MAR.

Document on appropriate flow sheet or electronic medical record (EMR).

Nurses' Notes

Document:
- Date, time, and reason a drug was withheld
- Response to drug administered

▶ CRITICAL THINKING SKILL

Introduction

Oral medications are manufactured under aseptic conditions. They should be administered under the same conditions. The nurse does not touch the medications with fingers during the preparation of the medications.

Possible Scenario

The nurse prepares the medications for a client. When handing the medication cup containing two tablets and one capsule to the client, one of the tablets falls to the floor.

Possible Outcome

The nurse administers the tablet and capsule to the client, then picks up and discards the contaminated tablet and goes back to the medication cart to obtain another tablet, following the same procedure as before. After returning to the client, the nurse administers the remaining tablet.

Prevention

The client's ability to handle the medication cup needs to be assessed. The nurse may assist the client to a comfortable position in order to take the prescribed dose.

> ## ▶ VARIATIONS
>
> ### Geriatric Variations:
> - *Elderly clients may be more at risk for fluid overload; if so, any fluid intake restrictions should be considered when giving oral medications.*
> - *Older clients may have increased difficulty swallowing and therefore be at greater risk of aspiration.*
> - *Older clients should be encouraged to take one tablet at a time and not rush.*
> - *Elderly clients may have dry mouth caused by loss of elasticity in oral mucosa or reduction in parotid gland secretion.*

continues

► VARIATIONS *(continued)*

- *Difficulty swallowing may be caused by delayed esophageal clearance.*
- *Physiologic changes with aging may include reduction in gastric acidity and stomach peristalsis and reduced colon motility, which may slow drug absorption and excretion.*

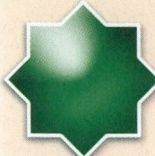

Pediatric Variations:

- *Liquid oral medications are the preferred route of administration for children.*
- *Solid preparations such as tablets and capsules are not recommended for children less than 5 years old.*
- *An oral syringe (without needle), plastic cup, and teaspoon for dispensing liquid medication are helpful in administering medications to pediatric clients.*
- *Offering carbonated beverages poured over finely crushed ice after giving medications to a client may reduce nausea in both children and adults.*
- *Use small amounts of flavorings when mixing with medications.*

Home Care Variations:

- *Clients need to be compliant in order to successfully self-administer their medications.*
- *Clients may benefit from a special medication container with compartments for times of the day and days of the week to assist them in remembering and complying with the medication schedule.*

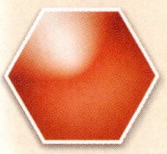

Long-Term Care Variations:

- *Maintain medication cart with a mortar and pestle, spoons, and a supply of applesauce.*
- *Keep a record on each client's MAR of how they need their medications given.*

► COMMON ERRORS

Possible Error:

The teenager with pain after arthroscopic knee surgery holds on to his pain pill so he can take several doses at one time.

Prevention:

Careful assessment of the client may reveal a drug abuse problem. When a client requests a repeat dose of pain medication sooner than the medication is ordered, the nurse may question the client's level of pain. The nurse may also ask the client about previous use of pain medication. If a pain tablet is found in the client's possession, the nurse should remain with the client until sure the client has taken it. The nurse can then record that it was taken so that the next dose can be administered according to the orders.

Possible Error:

The client takes a tablet but becomes nauseated and vomits it 10 minutes later.

Prevention:

The client should be assessed for nausea before administering the medication. If the client complains of nausea, give an antiemetic first, wait for a positive response, and then administer the medication ordered. If the nausea is mild, giving the medication with a saltine cracker may help reduce the nausea so the medication can be taken.

► NURSING TIPS

- Remember that checking a medication five times reduces the risk of a medication error by:

  –Checking the medication name with the order

  –Calculating or verifying the dose

  –Determining the ordered route of the medication

  –Checking the name of the client the medication is ordered for with the client's identification bracelet

  –Checking the frequency and times the medication is ordered

- Obtain the key to the narcotics drawer if you are anticipating the client's need for a controlled medication.

- Keep a calculator on the medication cart for use in dosage calculations. If in doubt about a medication calculation, have a second nurse perform the calculations as well.

- Maintain a pill cutting device, a mortar and pestle, and a supply of gloves on the medication cart for use in breaking scored tablets.

- Powdered medications such as Metamucil should be mixed with liquid immediately before administration or it will become thick or even solid, making swallowing impossible.

- Effervescent powders and tablets should be given immediately after dissolving as this improves its taste and is therapeutic.

- If the client is alert, call the client by name or ask his or her name prior to giving the medication to ensure the right client gets the medication.

- Enteric-coated pills should not be crushed as the purpose of the coating is to delay absorption, thus preventing gastric irritation.

- Tablets for buccal or sublingual administration should not be crushed.

- Offering a nonfat snack with medications that can be taken with food will reduce gastric distress.

► SPECIAL CONSIDERATIONS

- To facilitate the client swallowing medication tablets, fluid such as carbonated water may be used to assist passing the tablet through the esophagus. However, be aware of the medication specifications as some medications can only be taken with plain water.
- Be aware of the cultural variation; some clients may prefer ice water, whereas others may favor warm water. Ask client's preference before administering the oral medication.
- Always obtain information and perform a thorough assessment about the medication or vitamin supplements that clients are taking other than those prescribed. Clients may consume over-the-counter medications or vitamins on a regular basis and not realize that interactions or countereffects among medications may occur.

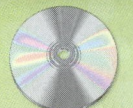

SKILL 5-2

Administering Eye and Ear Medications

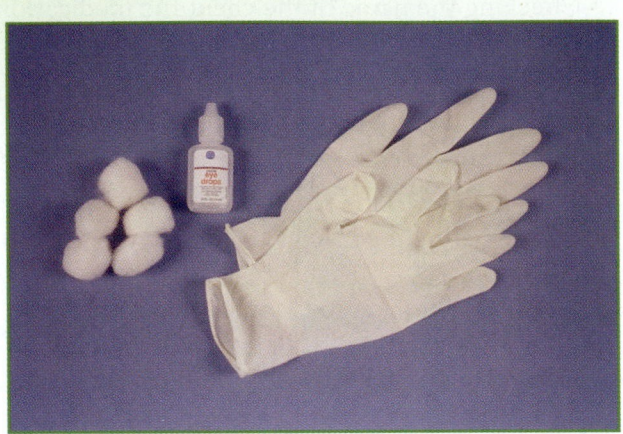

▶ OVERVIEW OF THE SKILL

Medications can be administered by various routes. The route of administration depends on many factors: client condition, type of medication, area to be medicated, and desired effect of the medication. An accurate understanding of the anatomy and physiology of the area being medicated is essential to the safe and effective administration of the medications.

Eye Medications

Eye medications refer to drops, ointment, and disks. These drugs are used for diagnostic and therapeutic purposes—to lubricate the eye or socket for a prosthetic eye and to prevent or treat eye conditions such as glaucoma (elevated pressure within the eye) and infection. Diagnostically, eye drops can be used to anesthetize the eye, dilate the pupil, and stain the cornea to identify abrasions and scars.

The nurse should review the abbreviations used in medication orders to ensure that the medication is instilled in the correct eye. Cross-contamination is a potential problem with eye drops. The nurse should adhere to the following safety measures to prevent cross-contamination:

- Each client should have his or her own bottle of eye drops.
- Discard any solution remaining in the dropper after instillation.

- Discard the dropper if the tip is accidentally contaminated, as by touching the bottle or any part of the client's eye.

Ear Medications

Solutions ordered to treat the ear are often referred to as otic (pertaining to the ear) drops or irrigation. Eardrops may be instilled to soften ear wax, to produce anesthesia, to treat infection or inflammation, or to facilitate removal of a foreign body, such as an insect. External auditory canal irrigations are usually performed for cleaning purposes and less frequently for applying heat and antiseptic solutions.

Before instilling a solution into the ear, the nurse should inspect the ear for signs of drainage, which is an indication of a perforated tympanic membrane. Eardrops are usually contraindicated when the tympanic membrane is perforated. If the tympanic membrane is damaged, all procedures must be performed using sterile aseptic technique; otherwise, medical asepsis is used when instilling medication into the ear.

Certain conditions have contraindications for specific drugs; for example, hydrocortisone eardrops are contraindicated in clients with a fungal infection or a viral infection such as herpes.

▶ ASSESSMENT

1. Assess the five rights: right client, right medication, right route, right dose, and right time. **Prevents errors in medication administration.**

546

2. Assess the condition of the client's eyes and/or ears. Are there any contraindications present to administering this medication present? Is there drainage from the ear indicating a possible tympanic rupture? If so, the medication administration must be done using sterile technique. **Reassessing the client before every medication dose prevents possibly injuring the client.**

3. Assess the medication order. Is the medication for only one eye/ear or both? With eye medications be sure to understand the abbreviations used for right eye (OD), left eye (OS), and both eyes (OU). **Prevents errors in medication administration.**

▶ DIAGNOSIS

Risk for Injury

Deficient Knowledge

Disturbed Sensory Perception

▶ PLANNING

Expected Outcomes:

1. The right client will receive the right dose of the right medication via the right route at the right time.

2. The client will encounter minimum discomfort during the medication administration procedure.

3. The client will receive maximum benefit from the medication.

Equipment Needed (see Figure 5-2-1):
Eye Medication

- Medication administration record (MAR)
- Eye medication
- Tissue or cotton ball
- Nonsterile latex-free gloves (if needed)

Ear Medication

- Medication administration record (MAR)
- Medication

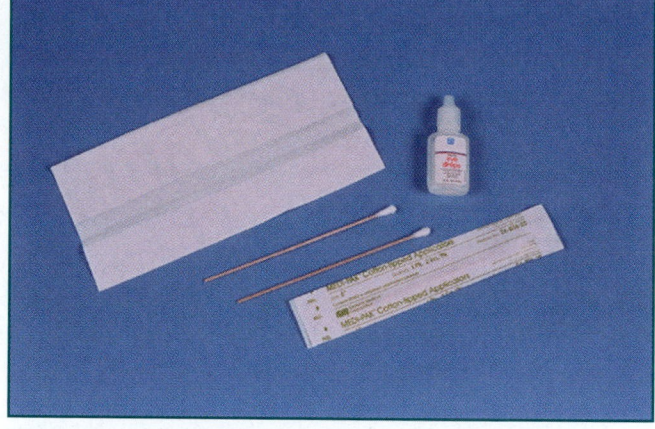

Figure 5-2-1   Many over-the-counter and prescription drops and ointments are dispensed directly into the eye.

- Nonsterile latex-free gloves
- Cotton-tipped applicator
- Tissue

▶ CLIENT EDUCATION NEEDED:

1. Educate the client regarding the reason for this medication, including the importance of taking the right dose at the right time.

2. Instruct the client in ways to prevent contamination and cross-contamination, especially when using eye drops.

3. Teach the client to gently press the tear duct closed while administering eye drops to prevent loss of the medication and possible systemic complications.

Estimated time to complete the skill: **5 minutes**

▶ DELEGATION TIPS

The skill of medication administration is not delegated to ancillary personnel in acute care settings. This may vary in state or federal institutions. Ancillary personnel are generally informed about the medications the client is receiving if adverse effects are anticipated or are being monitored.

IMPLEMENTATION—Action/Rationale

Action	Rationale

Eye Medication

1. Check with the client and the chart for any known allergies or medical conditions that would contraindicate use of the drug.

2. Gather the necessary equipment.

3. Follow the five rights of drug administration.

4. Take the medication to the client's room and place on a clean surface.

5. Check client's identification armband.

6. Explain the procedure to the client; inquire if the client wants to instill medication. If so, assess the client's ability to do so.

7. Wash hands, don nonsterile latex-free gloves, if needed.

8. Place client in a supine position with the head slightly hyperextended.

Instilling Eye Drops

9. Remove cap from eye bottle and place cap on its side.

10. Squeeze the prescribed amount of medication into the eyedropper.

11. Place a tissue below the lower lid.

12. With dominant hand, hold eyedropper one-half to one-third inch above the eyeball; rest hand on client's forehead to stabilize.

13. Place hand on cheekbone and expose lower conjunctival sac by pulling down on cheek.

14. Instruct the client to look up and drop prescribed number of drops into center of conjunctival sac (see Figure 5-2-2).

15. Instruct client to gently close eyes and move eyes. Briefly place fingers on either side of the client's nose to close the tear ducts and prevent the medication from draining out of the eye (see Figure 5-2-3).

---

1. Prevents occurrence of adverse reactions.

2. Promotes efficiency.

3. Promotes safety.

4. Decreases risk of contamination of bottle cap.

5. Accurately identifies client.

6. Reduces client's anxiety and enhances collaboration; some clients are used to instilling their own medication.

7. Decreases contact with bodily fluids.

8. Minimizes drainage of medication through the tear duct.

9. Prevents contamination of the bottle cap.

10. Ensures correct dose.

11. Absorbs the medication that flows from the eye.

12. Reduces risk of dropper touching eye structure, and prevents injury to the eye.

13. Stabilizes hand and prevents systemic absorption of eye medication.

14. Reduces stimulation of the blink reflex; prevents injury to the cornea.

15. Distributes solution over conjunctival surface and anterior eyeball.

continues

Action	Rationale

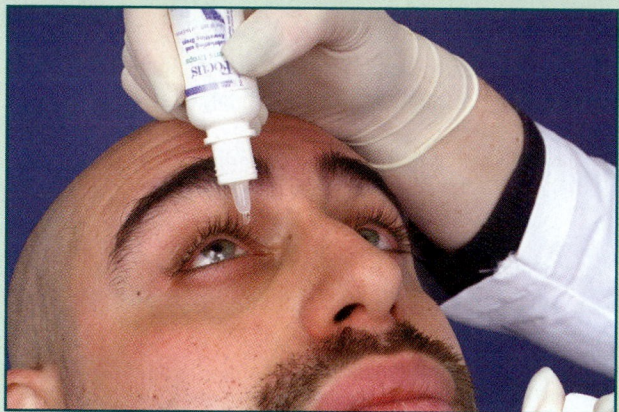

Figure 5-2-2 Instruct the client to look up. Administer prescribed number of drops into the center of the conjunctival sac.

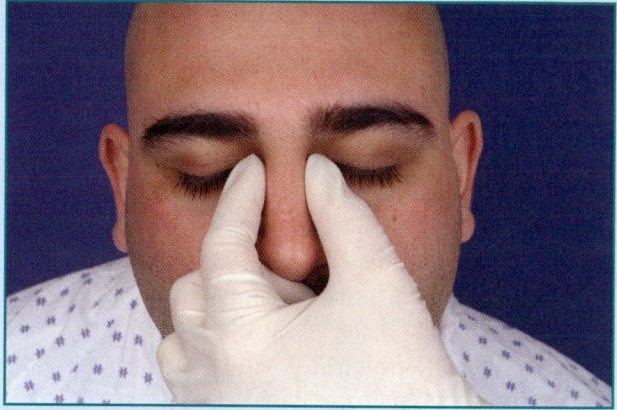

Figure 5-2-3 Placing the fingers on the sides of the client's nose closes the tear ducts and prevents the medication from draining out of the eye.

16. Remove gloves; wash hands.

17. Record on the MAR the route, site (which eye), and time administered.

Eye Ointment Application

18. Repeat Actions 1 to 8.

19. Lower lid:
   - With nondominant hand, gently separate client's eyelids with thumb and finger and grasp lower lid near margin immediately below the lashes; exert pressure downward over the bony prominence of the cheek.
   - Instruct the client to look up.

   - Apply eye ointment along inside edge of the entire lower eyelid, from inner to outer canthus.

20. Upper lid:
   - Instruct client to look down.
   - With nondominant hand, gently grasp client's lashes near center of upper lid with thumb and index finger, and draw lid up and away from eyeball.
   - Squeeze ointment along upper lid starting at inner canthus.

21. Repeat Actions 16 and 17.

Medication Disk

22. Repeat Actions 1 to 8.

23. Open sterile package and press dominant, sterile gloved finger against the oval disk so that it lies lengthwise across fingertip.

16. Reduces the transmission of microorganisms.

17. Provides documentation that the medication was given.

18. See Rationales 1 to 8.

19.
   - Provides access to the lower lid.

   - Reduces stimulation of the blink reflex and keeps cornea out of the way of the medication.
   - Ensures drug is applied to entire lid.

20.
   - Keeps cornea out of the way of the medication.
   - Ensures medication is applied to entire length of lid.

21. See Rationales 16 and 17.

22. See Rationales 1 to 8.

23. Promotes sticking of disk to fingertip.

continues

Action	Rationale
Medication Disk *continued*	
24. Instruct the client to look up.	**24.** Reduces stimulation of the blink reflex and keeps cornea out of the way of the medication.
25. With nondominant hand, gently pull the client's lower eyelid down and place the disk horizontally in the conjunctival sac. • Then pull the lower eyelid out, up, and over the disk. • Instruct the client to blink several times. • If disk is still visible, repeat steps. • Once the disk is in place, instruct the client to gently press the fingers against the closed lids; do not rub eyes or move the disk across the cornea. • If the disk falls out, pick it up, rinse under cool water, and reinsert.	**25.** Allows the disk to automatically adhere to the eye. • Secures the disk in the conjunctival sac. • Allows the disk to settle into place. • Ensures correct placement of the disk. • Secures disk placement. Prevents corneal scratches. • Preserves medication. This is not a sterile procedure. Health care provider must wear gloves to pick up disk.
26. If the disk is prescribed for both eyes (OU), repeat Actions 23 to 25.	**26.** Ensures both eyes are treated at the same time.
27. Repeat Actions 15 to 17.	**27.** See Rationales 15 to 17.
Removing an Eye Medication Disk	
28. Repeat Actions 3 and 5 to 8.	**28.** See Rationales 3 and 5 to 8.
29. Remove the disk: • With nondominant hand, invert the lower eyelid and identify the disk. • If the disk is located in the upper eye, instruct the client to close the eye, and place your finger on the closed eyelid. Apply gentle, long, circular strokes; instruct client to open the eye. Disk should be located in corner of eye. With your fingertip, slide the disk to the lower lid, then proceed. • With dominant hand, use the forefinger to slide the disk onto the lid and out of the client's eye.	**29.** • Exposes the disk for removal. • Safely moves the disk to the lower conjunctival sac. • Safely removes the disk without scratching the cornea.
30. Remove gloves; wash hands.	**30.** Reduces transmission of microorganisms.
31. Record the removal of the disk on the MAR.	**31.** Provides documentation that the disk was removed.
Ear Medication	
1. Check with client and chart for any known allergies.	**1.** Prevents the occurrence of hypersensitivity reactions.
2. Check the MAR against the health care provider's written orders.	**2.** Ensures accuracy in identification of the medication.

continues

Action	Rationale
3. Wash your hands.	3. Reduces the transfer of microorganisms.
4. Calculate the dose (see Figure 5-2-4).	4. Ensures the administration of the correct dose.
5. Use the identification armband to properly identify the client (see Figure 5-2-5).	5. Ensures correct client.
6. Explain the procedure to the client.	6. Enhances cooperation.
7. Place the client in a side-lying position with the affected ear facing up.	7. Facilitates the administration of the medication.
8. Straighten the ear canal by pulling the pinna down and back for children less than 3 years of age or upward and outward in adults and older children.	8. Opens the canal and facilitates introduction of the medication.
9. Instill the drops into the ear canal by holding the dropper at least 1/2 inch above the ear canal (see Figure 5-2-6).	9. Prevents injury to the ear canal.
10. Ask the client to maintain the position for 2 to 3 minutes.	10. Allows for distribution of the medication.
11. Place a cotton ball on the outermost part of the canal.	11. Prevents the medication from escaping when the client changes to a sitting or standing position.

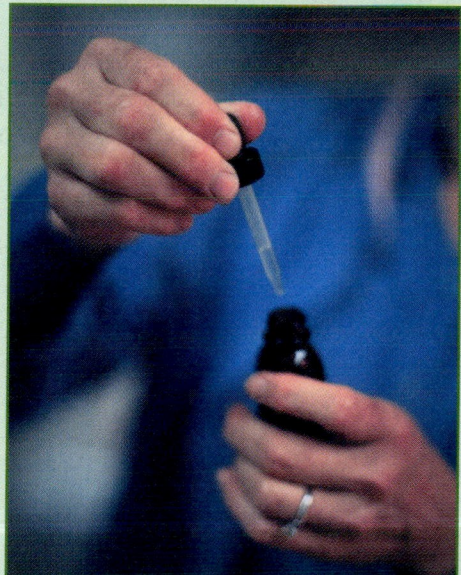

Figure 5-2-4 Calculate the correct dose and draw medication into the ear dropper.

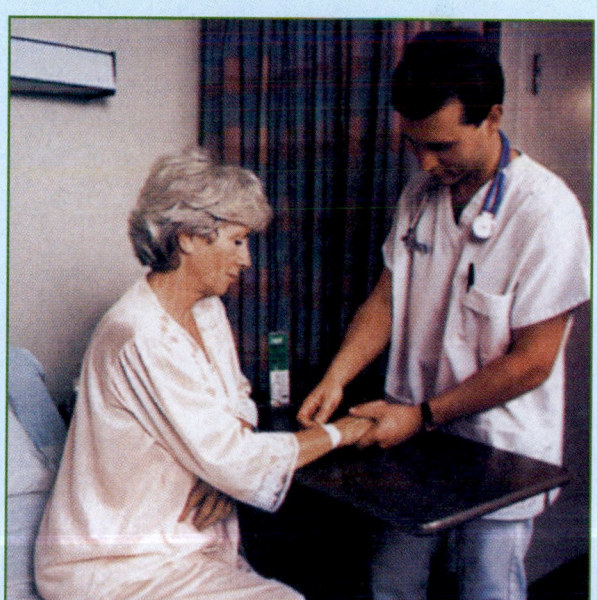

Figure 5-2-5 Check the client's identification band before administering medication.

continues

Action	Rationale
Ear Medication *continued*	
12. Wash hands.	12. Reduces the transmission of microorganisms.
13. Document the drug, number of drops, time administered, and ear medicated.	13. Documenting the actions of the nurse will reduce the number of medication errors.

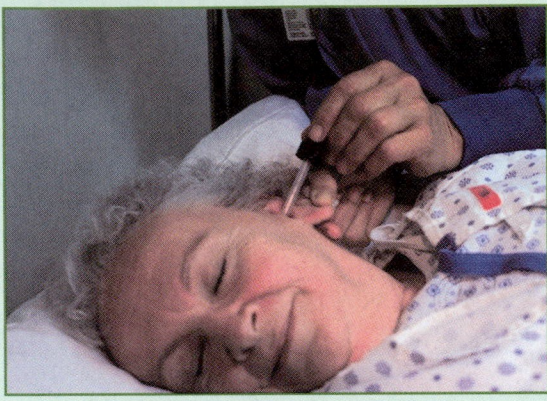

Figure 5-2-6 Slowly instill the drops, holding the dropper at least one-half inch above the ear canal.

▶ REAL WORLD ANECDOTES

Nurse Woodard has volunteered to work as a summer camp nurse for a week. Shortly after the arrival of this week's campers, Darla, a 9-year-old girl, presents to the infirmary complaining of an earache in her left ear. On examination the nurse finds no inflammation or drainage in the outer ear or the ear canal. During the exam Darla talks to the nurse about her mother being away on her honeymoon this week. The nurse notes that when she is discussing her feelings Darla's ear pain seems to disappear. After examining Darla's eardrum with the otoscope to be sure it is intact, the nurse gently instills some warm sterile saline into Darla's ear and inserts a cotton ball to hold the saline in. She tells Darla to be sure and come back later in the day for another check of her ear. Nurse Woodard continues to check Darla's ear and ear canal twice a day for the remainder of the week. There is no evidence of inflammation or drainage and Darla reports pain relief after the instillation of the warm saline. During Darla's visits Nurse Woodard encourages Darla to discuss her feelings about her mother's marriage and the changes that will be occurring after she returns home.

▶ EVALUATION

- The right client received the right dose of the right medication via the right route at the right time.
- The procedure was performed with minimum trauma and/or discomfort to the client.
- The client received maximum benefit from the medication.
- All the prescribed medication went into the eye or ear and none was spilled.

▶ DOCUMENTATION

Medication Administration Record (MAR)

- Record the date, time, location, and dosage of medication administered.
- If an ordered medication was not given, note this, usually by circling the time of the missed medication.

Nurses' Notes

- If an ordered medication was not given, record the reason.

• If an as-needed medication was given, note the reason for giving the medication and the client's response.

Document on appropriate flow sheet or electronic medical record (EMR).

▶ CRITICAL THINKING SKILL

Introduction

Always assess for potential interactions between a medication and a client.

Possible Scenario

Mrs. Wagner has been receiving cortisone eye drops for several weeks to treat an inflammation of her eyes. She presents to her physician's office today complaining of irritability, weight gain, and facial puffiness. While taking her initial vital signs, you recognize that these symptoms are characteristic of systemic cortisone usage.

Possible Outcome

If Mrs. Wagner has other medical problems, systemic cortisone may be seriously contraindicated. If the cortisone is affecting Mrs. Wagner systemically, she may need to be weaned off the eye drops carefully, rather than simply stopping them, to prevent systemic withdrawal.

Prevention

To prevent systemic contamination by a local eye drop, be sure to gently compress the tear duct at the inner corner of the eye. This helps to keep the medication in the eye rather than running through the tear duct and down the back of the throat.

▶ VARIATIONS

Geriatric Variations:

• *Elderly clients may be treated with eye drops for glaucoma or cataracts. These conditions make it difficult to read the small print on eye drop bottles. Be sure to mark the bottles in an easily identifiable manner so the client will be sure to get the right medication at the right time in the correct eye.*

• *Small bottles may be hard to hold if the elderly client has reduced fine motor skills, trembling, or reduced sensation in his or her hands. The nurse can help the client devise ways of stabilizing the bottle by bracing the other fingers of the hand on the face (for eye drops) or the side of the head (for eardrops). The nurse can demonstrate how to make an eye drop or ear drop bottle easier to hold by wrapping it with a cloth to increase its diameter.*

Pediatric Variation:

• *Children tend to rub their eyes and noses when tired. A child with an eye infection, such as pink-eye, can easily cross-contaminate from one eye to another. Parents need to be taught the importance of keeping the child's hands away from the eyes as well as keeping the child's hands and eyes clean.*

Home Care Variations:

• *Clients who use eye drops routinely at home can become careless about identifying the right medication for the right time and the right use. Help the client mark the eye drop bottles so they are clearly identifiable.*

• *Contact wearers have been known to confuse eye drop bottles with liquid glue or nail adhesive bottles. Be sure the client is aware of the similarity and teach the client to carefully identify anything before he or she puts it in the eyes.*

• *Make sure there is adequate lighting in the home care setting. A client who is having trouble with vision may have difficulty seeing medication in the dropper or reading the medication labels. Good lighting makes it easier to read and see without eyestrain.*

continues

▶ **VARIATIONS** *(continued)*

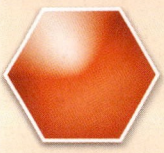

Long-Term Care Variations:
- *Long-term care clients who are self-medicating may be reluctant to dispose of outdated or contaminated eye drops/ear drops. Explain the importance of not using contaminated or outdated medications.*
- *The risk of contamination of an eye drop or eardrop bottle rises if that bottle is used repeatedly, especially if proper technique is not followed. Make sure that proper technique is taught and reinforced for caregivers and clients in the long-term care setting.*

▶ **COMMON ERRORS**

Possible Error:

Mr. Adams is scheduled to receive antibiotic ointment in both eyes. At this time he only has an infection in his right eye, but his physician is concerned that treating only one eye will lead to a back-and-forth cross-contamination. As you instill the antibiotic ointment, you have difficulty in separating the ointment ribbon from the tube nozzle. In order to end the ribbon, you gently nudge the nozzle against the inside of Mr. Adams's lower eyelid. The tip of the antibiotic ointment tube is now contaminated.

Prevention:

In this case the nurse should medicate the noninfected eye first if using the same tube of ointment for both eyes. The safer and cleaner method would be to use two tubes of the same ointment and designate one for the clean left eye and one for the contaminated right eye. Cross-contamination when only one eye or ear is infected is a common error that can be prevented with careful attention to aseptic technique. If the tip of the medication dropper touches the client or anything else, it is contaminated and must be cleaned or discarded immediately. Gently pull, twist, or rotate the tube away from the eye to end the ribbon, rather than touch the tip of the tube to the eyelid.

▶ **NURSING TIPS**

- Insert medication disks at bedtime because they usually cause blurring of the eyes on insertion.
- Apply pressure to the inner canthus when instilling eye drops that have potential systemic effects such as atropine, Timoptic, or hydrocortisone to prevent the drug from flowing into the tear duct and being absorbed systemically.
- Remember that the client always has the right to refuse any and all treatment, including medications.
- Unused medication in the medication dropper should be discarded rather than returned to the medication bottle. This avoids contaminating the medication remaining in the bottle.
- Clean any drainage or old medication from the eye or ear prior to administering the medication.

- Warm eardrops to room temperature unless this is specifically contraindicated. Cold medication against the eardrum can cause pain and dizziness.
- Have the client gently close the eye and move the eyeball back and forth under the lid to disperse the medication. If the client squeezes the eye shut, the medication will be squeezed out.
- If an ointment was instilled, have the client hold the eye gently closed for 1 minute to allow the ointment to melt. If the client squeezes the eye shut, the ointment may be squeezed out.
- When instilling eardrops, the client should remain on his or her side for 2 to 3 minutes to allow the medication maximal contact with the ear canal.

▶ **SPECIAL CONSIDERATIONS**

- When administering eye medication, make sure the client is not wearing contact lenses. In addition, wearing contact lenses may be prohibited within 30 minutes after the eye medication has been administered as medication may damage the contact lenses.
- Some eye medications cause pupil dilation and make the client's eyes sensitive to light and, therefore, require protective measures such as sunglasses. Most often after the pupils are dilated, it is difficult for the client to read for several hours. Proper client education should be addressed to promote client comfort and safety.

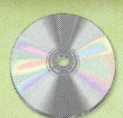

Administering Skin/Topical Medications

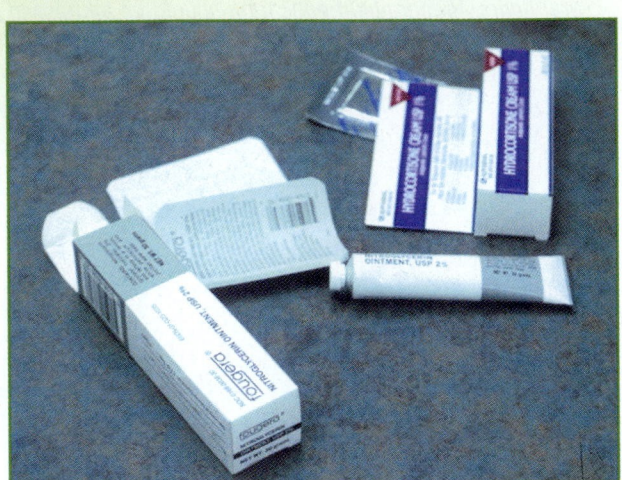

▶ OVERVIEW OF THE SKILL

Topical medications are applied directly to the skin or mucous membranes. These types of medications are used for their local effect or to produce systemic effects by absorption from percutaneous routes. Topical medications include creams, ointments, and lotions. Topical medications applied to the skin are commonly used to relieve itching, prevent local infections, moisten the skin, or for vasodilatation. Most topical medications are used for local effects; however, certain medications can be absorbed percutaneously to provide systemic effects, such as topical nitroglycerin, nicotine patches, or certain estrogen products.

▶ ASSESSMENT

1. Assess the five rights: right client, right medication, right route, right dose, and right time. **Prevents errors in medication administration.**
2. Assess the area where treatment will be applied **to establish a baseline condition of the skin for future comparison.**
3. If the drug is being used for systemic effect, assess for an area free of scars, moles, or other skin aberrations **to facilitate selection of a site with no barriers to absorption.**
4. Assess for allergies to **determine previous response to medications.**

▶ DIAGNOSIS

Risk for Impaired Skin Integrity

Risk for Allergy Response

▶ PLANNING

Expected Outcomes:
1. Good skin integrity
2. Relief of itching, irritation, or pain
3. Improved circulation

Equipment Needed (see Figure 5-3-1):
- Correct medication
- Correct applicator (cotton balls, sterile gauze pad, tongue blades, or cotton applicator)
- Gloves (sterile if broken skin integrity)
- Basin with warm water

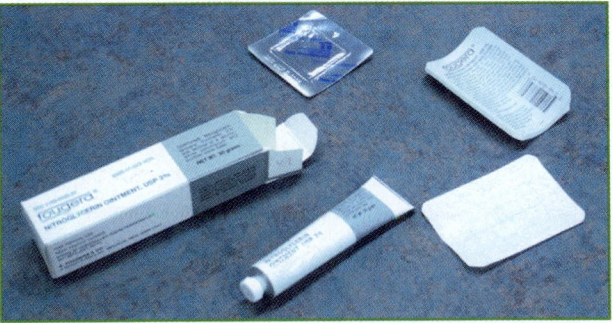

Figure 5-3-1 Creams, lotions, ointments, and patches are all used to dispense topical medications.

- Mild soap (if appropriate and not contraindicated by skin condition or interaction with medication)
- Wash cloth and towel
- Gauze dressing, tape as indicated
- Disposable waterproof pad
- Chart or medication sheet for medication verification
- Latex-free gloves

▶ CLIENT EDUCATION NEEDED:

1. Instruct the client regarding the reason for the topical medication.
2. Explain the need to allow for absorption without disturbing the area of application.

3. Teach the client what possible adverse effects can occur and to report any symptoms.
4. Explain to the client the need to wear gloves if self-administering systemically absorbed topical medications to avoid overmedicating.
5. Note the danger of inhaling topical aerosolized medications or powders.
6. Instruct the client to apply only the ordered amount of medication to avoid over or undermedication.

Estimated time to complete the skill:
5–15 minutes, depending on if a dressing change is needed

▶ DELEGATION TIPS

The application of some creams, lotions, and ointments may be delegated to properly trained ancillary personnel, but these medications are generally over-the-counter preparations and not prescription medications.

IMPLEMENTATION—Action/Rationale

Action	Rationale
1. Wash hands.	1. Reduces the transmission of microorganisms.
2. Obtain order for medication from health care provider.	2. Prevents inappropriate medication administration. An order is needed for any medication.
3. Ascertain client's allergic status.	3. Avoids allergic reactions. Nurses are responsible for medication errors, including reactions. Charts may not always be current regarding allergies or an oversight might have occurred.
4. If unfamiliar with medication, read label and paper insert or seek appropriate information.	4. Prevents inappropriate medication administration and errors. Medications should never be administered without knowledge about the medication.
5. Select medication and verify medication with orders (first medication verification).	5. Prevents medication errors.
6. Check expiration date.	6. Outdated medications may not be effective.
7. Read medication label again before leaving medication room or cart as available in facilities (second medication verification).	7. Avoids medication errors.
8. Take medication to client's room and introduce self. In some facilities, topical medication used for skin irritations are kept in the client's room and therefore verification may be done at the bedside.	8. Helps establish rapport with the client and identifies credentials of person administering the medications. If the medications are kept in the client's room, the nurse must still verify appropriate medication with right client.

continues

Action	Rationale
9. Ask the client if he or she has had the medication before and to describe its effect; ascertain whether the client has any drug allergies or untoward reactions.	**9.** Provides another verification for the medication. If the client has had adverse effects to medication, revalidate.
10. Explain the purpose of the medication.	**10.** Helps to inform the client and assists him or her in taking some responsibility for his or her care. Provides the client with involvement in learning more about the condition.
11. Read the label for the third time (third medication verification) and check the client's identification band.	**11.** Avoids medication errors.
12. Position the client appropriately for administration of medication. Keep client draped for privacy.	**12.** Keeps the client in a comfortable position for medication administration. Protects privacy.
13. Put on gloves. If a dressing is over the area to be treated, remove, discard, and change gloves (see Skill 9-6, Changing Dressings Around Therapeutic Puncture Sites).	**13.** Decreases contact with microorganisms.
14. If an open wound, clean area to be treated with mild soap (if no allergies or reactions to soap) and water. If skin is irritated, use only warm water. If administering a systemically absorbed topical medication, clean the skin surface thoroughly and pat skin dry, leaving no residues of soap. Do not rub vigorously as absorption can be altered (see Figure 5-3-2).	**14.** Soap can irritate an open wound. If skin is already irritated, soap may cause more irritation. Systemically absorbed medication can be effected by residue on the skin or rubbing, which causes vasodilatation.
15. Assess the client's skin condition, making notation of circulation, drainage, color, temperature, or any altered skin integrity.	**15.** Information can be compared with future assessment and effect of medication.
16. Change gloves.	**16.** Prevents spread of microorganisms and avoids absorption of medication by caregivers. (This is especially important with systemically absorbed medication.)
17. Apply medication according to label. If lotion or ointment, apply a thin layer and smooth into skin as indicated.	**17.** Medication dosages have been studied and are recommended according to certain standards.
18. If an aerosol spray is used, shake the container and administer according to direction. Spray evenly over affected area and avoid spraying close to client's or caregiver's face.	**18.** Aerosol may need to be mixed to be effective. Avoid inhalation as doing so may have adverse effects on the mucous membranes and lungs.

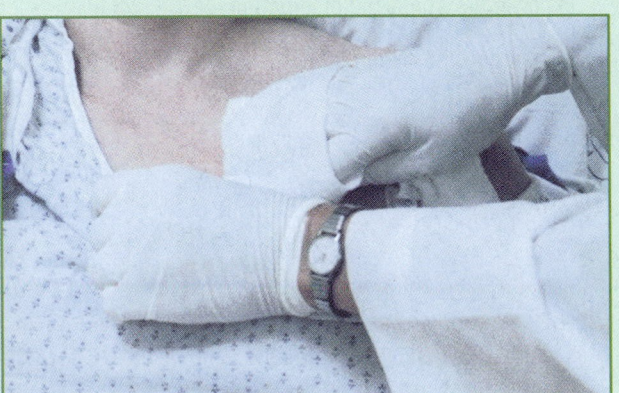

Figure 5-3-2 Cleanse the skin before applying topical medication.

continues

Action	Rationale
19. If gels or pastes are used, applicators may be needed. Apply evenly. If applying over an area with hair growth, follow direction of hair.	**19.** Apply evenly to affected areas. Excess gel or paste will be wasted because absorption can only occur at skin level. The client will experience less discomfort if hair growth pattern is followed.
20. If powders are used, dust lightly and avoid inhalation by client and caregiver.	**20.** Excess powder will be wasted because absorption can only occur at skin level. Inhalation can cause untoward effects on the lungs and mucous membranes.
21. If nitroglycerin ointment or paste is used, follow instructions and orders carefully to administer correct dosage.	**21.** Nitroglycerin is systemically absorbed and accurate dosing is essential. If thick lines of ointment are applied, the dose will be different; therefore, the manufacturer's suggestions must be followed carefully for safe use of this drug.
• Remove the old ointment strip and clean the old site thoroughly. New ointment will be applied in a different area.	• If areas of ointment from previous doses are not removed, the client will be receiving more than one dose at a time.
• Cleanse the new site with the appropriate cleaner.	• Ensures proper absorption of the medication.
• Squeeze the dose out onto the enclosed medication measuring strip (see Figure 5-3-3). Nitroglycerin paste dosages are measured in inches and applied to the paper measuring strip before being applied to the client.	• Use care not to over- or undermedicate by squeezing out a line of ointment that is too thick or too thin.
• Flatten the roll of nitroglycerin so the ointment will be spread over a wider area when applied to the client.	• The wider area of contact and thinner coating of ointment increases absorption.
• Apply the measuring paper, ointment side down, to a portion of the client's body without hair.	• Using a nonhairy area increases the absorption of the medication.
• Tape the paper in place.	• Keeps the medication in place.
22. If a transdermal patch is used, follow the manufacturer's directions and apply the patch to a smooth, cleaned skin surface.	**22.** Patches offer a more reliable means of controlling dosage; however, patches are generally more expensive than ointments.
• Remove the old patch and wash the site of the old patch.	• Prevents overdose.
• Wash and prepare the skin at a new site.	• Allows for maximal medication absorption.

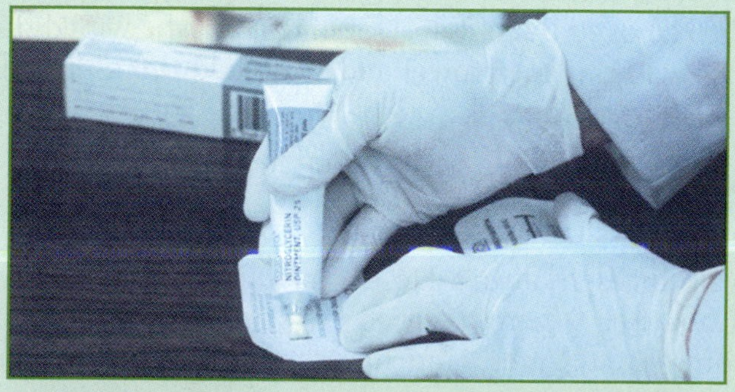

Figure 5-3-3 Squeeze the correct dose out onto the enclosed medication measuring strip.

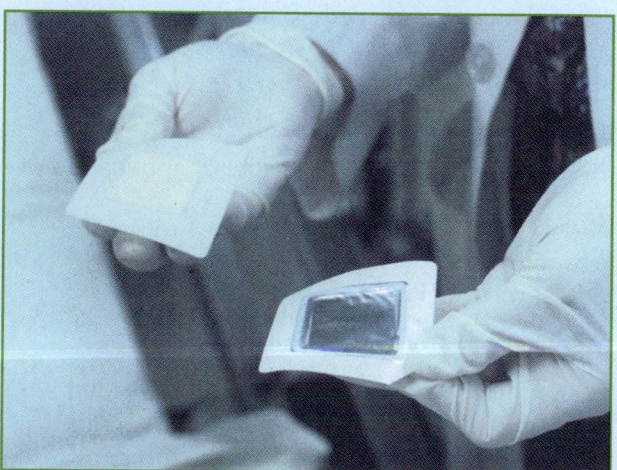

Figure 5-3-4 When applying a transdermal patch, remove the protective covering and apply the patch.

continues

Action	Rationale
• Remove the protective covering over the transdermal portion of the patch and apply the new patch (see Figure 5-3-4). • Write the date and time on the patch.	• Removing the protective covering allows the medication to be absorbed. • Alerts caregivers when the patch was applied.
23. Remove gloves; wash hands.	23. Reduces the transmission of microorganisms.
24. Document the medication given, the site it was applied to, and the client's response to the medication.	24. Proper documentation is essential for client care.

▶ REAL WORLD ANECDOTES

Mrs. Hayes brought her 7-month-old son, Darren, to the walk-in clinic. While the nurse did her intake evaluation, Mrs. Hayes noted that Darren had been in a week earlier because of diaper rash. Mrs. Hayes had brought Darren back because his rash was worse despite regular use of the cream ordered a week earlier. Upon examination, the nurse noted that Darren's diaper area was quite red and seemed to be painful for Darren. While examining the redness, the nurse noticed that it seemed to have abrupt edges right at the edge of Darren's diaper. When asked about it, Mrs. Hayes noted that it had not been that way 1 week earlier. Upon closer questioning, the nurse realized that the abrupt edges of the redness represented the limit of Mrs. Hayes's application of the cream. The nurse suspected that the worsening diaper rash actually represented an allergic reaction to the prescription cream. The nurse explained what symptoms to look for with topical allergies and Mrs. Hayes was advised to stop using the cream and to leave Darren's buttocks open to air as much as possible. Within a week both Darren's diaper rash and his topical redness were gone.

▶ EVALUATION

• The client's skin integrity was maintained.
• The client experienced relief of itching, irritation, or pain if this was the intent of the medication.
• The client experienced maximum effect from the topical medication.
• The client experienced no allergic reaction

▶ DOCUMENTATION

Medication Administration Record

• Record the date, time, and site of application of the topical medication.

Document on appropriate flow sheet or electronic medical record (EMR).

Nurses' Notes

• Document any changes in the client's skin integrity, coloration, or sensation.
• If medication was for irritation, itching, or rash, document any improvement or change.
• Note any unusual findings or client complaints.

▶ CRITICAL THINKING SKILL

Introduction
A little medication can go a long way.

Possible Scenario
Mr. Carr, a 62-year-old man, was receiving 1 inch of nitroglycerin ointment every 4 hours. The nurse caring for Mr. Carr was distracted while measuring his ointment. She inadvertently applied 2 inches of ointment to the measuring paper instead of one. When she removed the old dose of ointment, she wiped the area with a paper towel and reapplied the ointment to the same spot.

Possible Outcome
An hour later the nurse returned to help Mr. Carr walk in the hallway. He complained of a pounding headache. When he tried to stand, he was overcome by dizziness and had to sit back down right away. When the nurse took his vital signs, his blood pressure was low. The nurse realized that these were

all signs of a high dose of nitroglycerin ointment. She removed the nitroglycerin ointment and washed the site with soap and water. She had Mr. Carr remain sitting and monitored his condition until his blood pressure had improved and Mr. Carr felt able to return to bed.

Prevention

Topical preparations can have serious systemic effects. Be sure to use the right amount of medication. It is even more important to pay attention when dispensing a medication that is difficult to measure, such as nitroglycerin paste. Carefully follow the manufacturer's recommendations for applying any ointment. Measure carefully.

▶ VARIATIONS

Geriatric Variations:
- *As skin changes with age, elderly clients may be more sensitive to topical medications.*
- *When using systemically absorbed topical medications, locate an area of skin with minimal wrinkles for administration.*

Pediatric Variation:
- *Children may move about causing topical medication to be wiped off.*

Home Care Variations:
- *Continuous use of systemically absorbed topical ointments may require a systematic tracking system to ensure the medication is administered at different sites.*
- *Teaching proper use of topical medications is essential.*

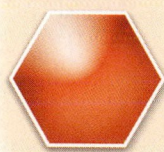

Long-Term Care Variation:
- *Caregivers should be aware of the adverse signs and symptoms associated with the topical medication the client is receiving and how to respond to them.*

▶ COMMON ERRORS

Possible Error:

Overapplication of ointments is both costly and wasteful.

Prevention:

Apply medications carefully and according to directions.

Possible Error:

When topical medications are kept in the client's room, they may overtreat self.

continues

▶ **COMMON ERRORS** *(continued)*

Prevention:

Keep medications in secure or designated areas only.

Possible Error:

Overapplication of systemically absorbed topical medication can lead to adverse effects.

Prevention:

Apply medications carefully and according to directions. Keep appropriate records of medications administered.

▶ **NURSING TIPS**

• Latex-free gloves should be worn to avoid absorption of medications by the health care worker. If soothing lotions are used, gloves should be worn if the skin is not intact.

▶ **SPECIAL CONSIDERATIONS**

• *Shaved areas should be avoided as the skin site could be sensitive or irritated. Shaving cream (hair remover) should be avoided as well, as the chemical in the hair remover could have interaction with the applied topical medication.*
• *To avoid contact dermatitis or allergic reaction, non-latex gloves should be used when administering topical medications.*

Administering Nasal Medications

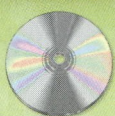

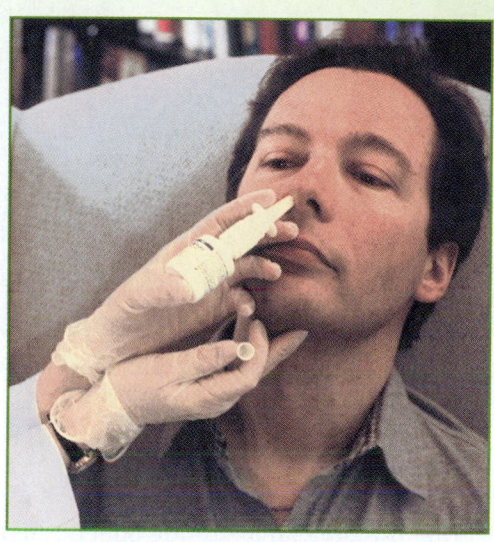

▶ OVERVIEW OF THE SKILL

Nasal medications may be administered by drops or sprays. Sprays may be packaged as pump sprays, sprays in aerosolized containers (pressurized containers, sometimes called nasal nebulizers), or powdered turbo inhalers. Prescribed medications are generally available in pump sprays or aerosolized sprays, whereas sprays and nasal drops are available in over-the-counter medications. Since the advent of environmental controls on fluorocarbons, some aerosolized medications (which use fluorocarbons in pressurized dispensers) are being replaced by pump sprays. Nasal medications may be used to achieve local effects on the nasal mucosa, indirect effects on the sinuses, or a systemic effect. Examples of medications that have systemic effects and are available in nasal sprays are insulin, agents for suppression of nicotine use, and agents for the treatment of migraine headaches. The four groups of sinuses (frontal, ethmoid, sphenoid, and maxillary) communicate with the nasal fossae and are lined with mucous membranes similar to those that line the nose. Although it is unlikely that nasal medications penetrate the sinuses, positioning may aid in decreasing inflammation and congestion in the mucous membranes adjacent to the sinuses, thereby indirectly decreasing pressure in the sinuses. To medicate the mucous membranes adjacent to the frontal sinuses, the client will assume a supine position with the head turned to the affected side to be treated (Parkinson position). To medicate the mucous membranes adjacent to the ethmoid sinuses, the client will lie supine with his or her head leaning back over the side of the bed with the client's head supported by the nurse's hand to avoid muscle strain on the client's neck (Proetz position). Although the nose is not considered a clean or sterile cavity, because of its connection with the sinuses, the nurse should employ medical asepsis when performing nasal instillation.

▶ ASSESSMENT

1. Assess the five rights: right client, right medication, right route, right dose, and right time. **Prevents errors in medication administration.**
2. Assess the client's nasal congestion and nasal obstruction **to determine whether the medicine can be inhaled to reach the nasal mucosa and to determine the effectiveness of the medication.**
3. Assess the color, quantity, and odor of the client's discharge and the color and moistness of the nasal mucosa **to check for signs and symptoms of infection, to discern tissue damage, and to establish a baseline for future assessments.**
4. Assess the client's pain and/or discomfort level in the areas of the sinuses **as this is another**

563

symptom of infection. May determine whether the client can use the inhaler or drops.

5. Assess the client for systemic conditions that may be adversely affected by nasal medications (see manufacturer's information). **Clients with cardiovascular conditions and hypertension may need to use caution with medications containing sympathomimetic ingredients.**

▶ DIAGNOSIS

Impaired Oral Mucous Membrane

Ineffective Therapeutic Regimen Management

▶ PLANNING

Expected Outcomes:

1. The client will be free of nasal congestion.
2. The client will be free of nasal discharge and odor.
3. The client will breathe freely through the nasal passages.
4. The client will be free of sinus pain and nasal pain.
5. The client's nasal passages will be moist and pink.

Equipment Needed (see Figure 5-4-1):

- Medication in spray, drops, or aerosolized form
- Latex-free gloves
- Tissue as needed
- Dropper as needed

▶ CLIENT EDUCATION NEEDED:

1. Teach client the purpose of the medication.
2. Explain the need for certain positioning with administration of medication and the need to retain positioning for a few minutes.
3. Help client understand the need for compliance with the prescribed regimen.
4. Explain the purpose of closing one nostril while administering the medication to the other nostril.
5. Discuss the effects of the overuse of nasal decongestants.
6. Teach the client to clear the nostril before treatment and to administer the medication during inhalation.

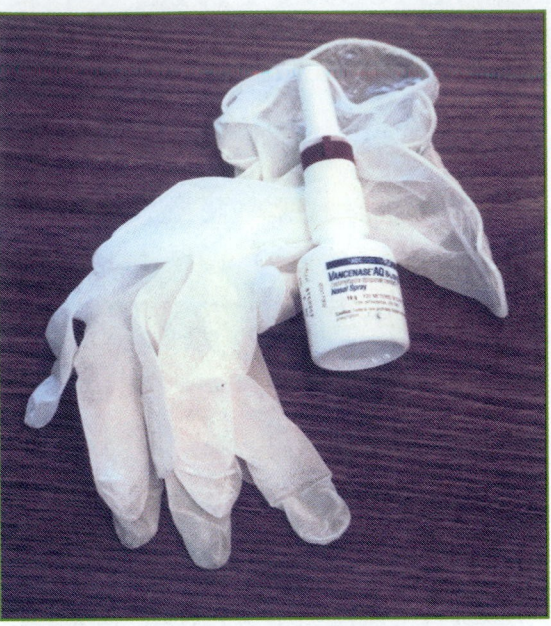

Figure 5-4-1   Nasal medication spray. Wear latex-free gloves when administering nasal medication to a client.

7. Describe possible adverse side effects, such as increased temperature, increased sinus headache, nasal mucosa that remain inflamed and tender, increased nasal discharge, or a change in color of nasal discharge, and teach the client to report these to health care provider.
8. Some clients may feel nauseated or even vomit after unpleasant side effects of nasal medication, such as with nose drops or sprays that drip into the oral pharynx.
9. Teach the client the purpose of closing one nostril while administering the medication to the other nostril.

Estimated time to complete the skill:

5 minutes to administer medication. Assess the client 15–30 minutes after treatment.

▶ DELEGATION TIPS

The skill of medication administration is not delegated to ancillary personnel in acute care settings. This may vary in state or federal institutions. Ancillary personnel are generally informed about the medications the client is receiving if adverse effects are anticipated or are being monitored.

IMPLEMENTATION—Action/Rationale

Action	Rationale
1. Wash hands. Wear a mask if the client is coughing or sneezing. Don latex-free gloves.	1. Reduces transmission of microorganisms. Respiratory-related microorganisms are easily transferred by the hands and air droplets. Gloves prevent absorption of medication through the skin of health care worker.
2. Explain the purpose of the medication and the position desired for the client (see Figure 5-4-2).	2. The client will be more compliant with medication if he or she understands the purpose and proper use of medication. Proper positioning is necessary with nose drops so the drops will reach the area of treatment by gravity with the client assuming a dependent position.
3. Explain to the client the sensation of the local effects of the medications, such as burning, tingling, and the effect on taste buds. If drops are used, explain to the client that a sensation of medications may be felt in the posterior oral pharynx.	3. Some nasal medications cause undesirable tastes. If this occurs, the health care provider may order other medications or encourage mouthwashes after treatment. Warning of postnasal sensations of the medication will prepare the client. Some clients may feel a quick sensation of choking. This can be frightening if the client has not been alerted to this consequence.
4. If a nasal inhaler is prescribed, explain the manufacturer's directions and how inhalers work. Follow the five rights of drug administration (check identification and orders at five different stages of administration).	4. Clients will be more compliant if they understand the use of the inhalers and that a fine cold mist will be released into the nasal passage via a pressurized container. Nasal medications that are prescribed must be considered to have the same safety precautions of administration as any medication.
5. Have the client assume a comfortable position. If inhalers are to be used, this will generally be an upright position. If drops are to be instilled, the client should assume the appropriate position as mentioned above to medicate specific sinuses that need treatment. Before the instillation of drops or the use of an inhaler, ask the client to blow his or her nose and clear the nostrils of discharge as much as possible. Squeeze nose drops into dropper.	5. Nose drops are effective only if they reach the areas to be medicated. The client should be as comfortable as possible, otherwise he or she may not stay in desired position an adequate time. If the client is in a position with the neck hyperextended, a pillow or support by the nurse's hand under the neck may be necessary. Medications can only be effective if they are in contact with the mucous membranes. If large amounts of discharge are present, medications cannot be effective.
6. Have the client exhale and close one nostril.	6. As the client will be asked to inhale with the use of nasal medications, exhalation will first be necessary.
7. Ask the client to inhale while the spray is pumped or sprayed into the first nostril (see Figure 5-4-3). If nose drops are used, insert nasal dropper only about three-eighths of an inch into the nostril, keeping the tip of the dropper away from the sides of the nostril. Insert the prescribed dosage of medication into the nostril. Discard any unused medication in dropper.	7. Nasal medications are more effective if instilled during inhalation as they will be carried and distributed farther into the nasal passages. Droppers should be kept away from the nostril to avoid inserting bacteria into the medication bottle. Excess medication is discarded for the same reason.

continues

Action	Rationale

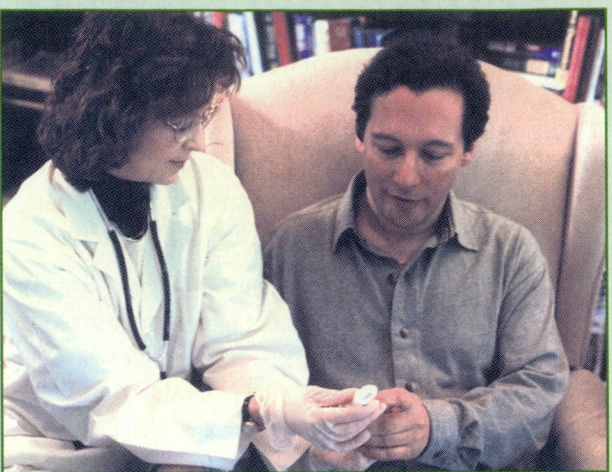

Figure 5-4-2   Explain the purpose of the medication to the client.

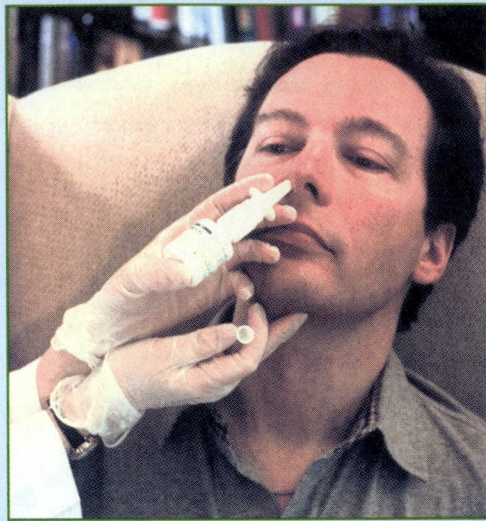

Figure 5-4-3   Ask the client to inhale while the spray is administered into the nostril.

8. Ask the client to blot excess drainage from the nostril; however, do not have the client blow his or her nose.

8. Blowing the nose will remove medication and therefore should not be done. However, excess medication should be removed from dripping out of the nostrils onto the facial areas in order to avoid discomfort.

9. Repeat the procedure on the other nostril.

9. Most often, both nostrils contain congestion and therefore need to be treated.

10. Help the client resume a comfortable position. If nose drops are used, the client should stay in the appropriate position as indicated by manufacturer's suggestions, generally 5 minutes. Ask the client to breathe through the nose after the decongestion administration. It may be necessary to occlude one nostril at a time and breathe deeply.

10. Nose drops need positions that by gravity will allow medications to reach areas of desired treatment.

11. Remove all soiled supplies and dispose according to Standard Precautions. Remove gloves. Wash hands carefully.

11. Use of gloves and proper disposal decreases the chance of transmission of microorganisms. Respiratory diseases are especially easily transmitted.

12. Evaluate the effect of the medication in 15 to 20 minutes.

12. It is necessary to note if the medication is effective without adverse side effects; otherwise, other medications may be considered. If the client experiences bothersome or unpleasant symptoms, such as a bad taste, other medications may be considered. Clients generally will not comply with medications that have too many unpleasant side effects.

► REAL WORLD ANECDOTES

Sharon was taking aerosolized medication for her migraine headaches. She complained that it did not work as well as the injections she had been using previously; it dripped out of her nose and it left a bad taste in her mouth. The nurse reviewing the medication administration procedure with Sharon realized that Sharon was not taking the time to allow the medication to be absorbed through the mucous membranes near her sinuses. The nurse suggested to Sharon that she position her head to allow the medication to contact the mucous membranes for better systemic absorption. The nurse recommended mouthwash or crackers for the bad taste left by the medication.

► EVALUATION

- The client is free of nasal congestion.
- The client is free of nasal discharge and odor.
- The client breathes freely through the nasal passages.
- The client is free of sinus pain and nasal pain.
- The client's nasal passages are moist and pink.
- The client is free of adverse side effects secondary to the nasal medication.

► DOCUMENTATION

Medication Administration Record

- Indicate the time and date the medication was given, the amount (number of drops may be necessary), and the nostril medicated.

Document on appropriate flow sheet or electronic medical record (EMR).

Nurses' Notes

- Document the results of the treatment.
- Document any adverse or unpleasant side effects.

► CRITICAL THINKING SKILL

Introduction

Nose drops can enter the oral pharynx and cause coughing, choking, and possibly vomiting.

Possible Scenario

Three-year-old Tommy is prescribed nose drops for a persistent nasal discharge. The nurse gives Tommy his first dose, showing his mother how the procedure is done. Tommy wiggles and cries during the procedure and then starts to cough and choke. The nose drops have dripped into his oral pharynx causing a choking sensation. Tommy continues to cough and choke, crying and becoming increasingly agitated. After much difficulty, Tommy's mother calms him, but the mere sight of the nose drop bottle starts him crying and struggling again.

Possible Outcome

Tommy will continue to fight whenever his mother attempts to give him the nose drops. If forced, Tommy may aspirate and develop pneumonia. Before long, Tommy's mother will give up trying to give him the nose drops and Tommy will not receive any medication for his nasal discharge.

Prevention

When instilling any nasal medications, be prepared to position clients so as to avoid aspiration. Alert clients that medication may enter the oral pharynx and give a sensation that may cause them to cough. Sometimes swallowing before taking the medication, using mouthwash after the medication, or at least preparing the client for this sensation may avert the client from choking or vomiting. Some forms of medication are not appropriate for some age groups. Children, who are less likely to be cooperative, need a medication that will be pleasant or at least nonthreatening to use.

► VARIATIONS

Geriatric Variations:
- *Elderly clients may not be able to tolerate positions with the head dependent for long periods of time; therefore, pump sprays may be more useful.*
- *Aerosolized containers may be too difficult for elderly clients to apply appropriate pressure to be effective.*

Pediatric Variations:
- *Small children may not be cooperative and may need to be restrained. Sometimes the use of a reward system may be beneficial.*
- *Position infants using a football hold and slightly hyperextend the neck.*

Home Care Variations:
- *If nasal congestion persists, clients may have chronic sinus infections that require the adjunct of humidifiers or different medications.*
- *Saline nose sprays or drops may be effective for simple nasal congestion or as adjunct therapy and can be made by dissolving 1 teaspoon of salt in 1 pint of warm water.*
- *Saline solutions should not be kept over 24 hours because bacterial growth will occur. Clients should assess temperature and report long-lasting sinus headaches.*

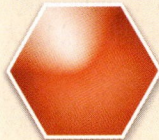

Long-Term Care Variations:
- *Tolerance can develop with some nasal decongestants and, therefore, cannot be used on a routine basis.*
- *Other categories of drugs may be needed.*
- *Clients with persistent nasal congestion should seek medical attention and be evaluated for allergies, chronic sinus problems, or other health problems.*

► COMMON ERRORS

Possible Error:
The client does not effectively blow the nose, and medication cannot penetrate the nasal mucosa.

Prevention:
Carefully explain to the client how to effectively clear the nasal passages by blowing the nose. Explain the importance of clearing the nasal passages before using the medication.

Possible Error:
The client does not use proper head positioning or allow enough time for the medication to be absorbed through the mucous membranes.

Prevention:
Teach the client the appropriate head position for the ordered medication. Explain the importance of positioning and of allowing time for the medication to be absorbed.

▶ **NURSING TIPS**

- Explain medication and needed positions before administering medication. Allow the client time to find a comfortable position if asked to assume a Proetz or Parkinson position.
- Ask the client to review risks of overuse of decongestants and methods of administration.
- Ask the client to demonstrate use of nasal medication (see Figure 5-4-4).
- Clients with a history of hypertension or cardiovascular disease should not instill nasal medications that contain vasoconstrictors. If sympathomimetic drugs are absorbed, elevated blood pressure may result.
- If the nasal route of administration is used for medications with systemic effects, evaluate the patency of nasal passage before administration of the medication.
- Certain nasal medications may cause an unpleasant taste. Using a mouthwash after administration of the medications may aid in compliance with the prescribed regimen.

- Some clients may feel nauseated or even vomit after use of nasal medication, such as with nose drops or sprays that drip into the oral pharynx.

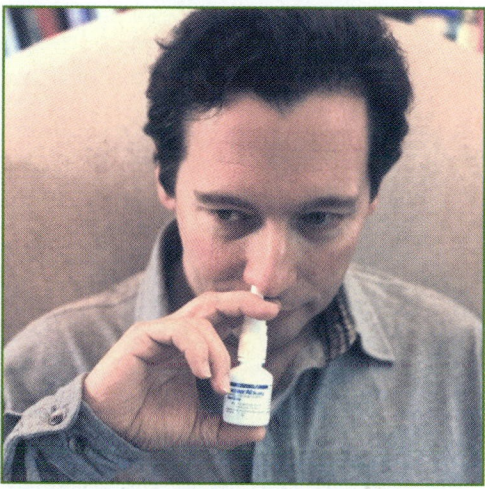

Figure 5-4-4 If the client will be self-administering the medication, have the client demonstrate how to administer the medication.

▶ **SPECIAL CONSIDERATIONS**

- *Client should not use over-the-counter nose sprays for more than 3 to 5 days, depending on the medication. Tolerance develops to nasal sprays and, therefore, it is generally recommended that the client stop using these for 1 to 2 days before resuming use. Follow medication instructions. If sprays contain sympathomimetic drugs, a rebound vasodilatation may occur or nasal congestion symptoms may worsen.*
- *Health care practitioners should take care not to be in close proximity and inhale medication that may be in the air close to the client.*

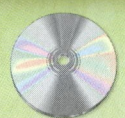

Administering Rectal Medications

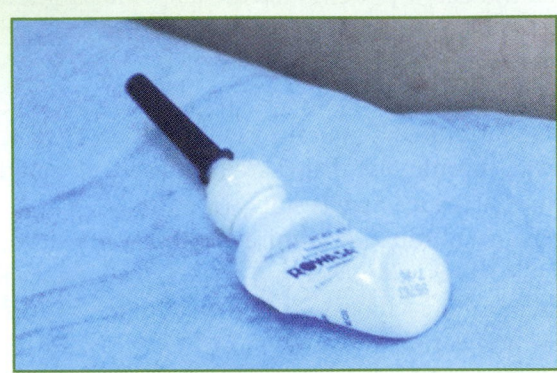

▶ OVERVIEW OF THE SKILL

The administration of rectal medications is an important responsibility for nurses in numerous health care settings. Rectal suppositories include medications that produce both local and systemic effects. Suppositories that produce a local effect include laxatives, which promote defecation. Medications to help relieve nausea, fever, or bladder spasms can also be administered via rectal suppository but produce a systemic effect.

As with all medications, nurses must understand the drug's action in order to assess the positive outcome or harmful side effects. To ensure safe and accurate medication administration, the nurse should always follow the five rights: the right client, the right medication, the right route, the right dose, and the right time.

▶ ASSESSMENT

1. Assess the five rights: right client, right medication, right route, right dose, and right time. **Prevents errors in medication administration.**
2. Review the health care provider's order and identify the medication to be delivered, verifying dosage, route, time, and correct client. **This ensures safe and correct administration of medications.**
3. Assess the client's need and appropriateness for rectal medication administration and review the client's history for contraindications. **A history of rectal surgery or bleeding may contraindicate use of a suppository.**
4. Consider any adjustments that may need to be taken in delivery of medications resulting from the age of the client. **This allows the nurse to deliver the medication in a correct manner if the client is an infant, child, or adult.**
5. Observe the client for the desired therapeutic effects or any adverse reactions, and document this response appropriately **to determine the effectiveness of the treatment.**
6. Assess the client's knowledge and understanding of the procedure. **Explaining the procedure not only will allay fear and anxiety but will also promote understanding and cooperation. If physically able, the client may wish to self-administer the medication.**
7. Assess the client's rectal area to determine condition of skin, mucosa, and presence of hemorrhoids or other rectal conditions. **Preventive action can be taken to protect injured skin and ensure client comfort.**

▶ DIAGNOSIS

Constipation

Risk for Caregiver Role Strain

Risk for Compromised Human Dignity

▶ PLANNING

Expected Outcomes:

1. The medication will be delivered appropriately and safely following the five rights of medication administration.
2. The desired outcome will be verbalized by the client and documented appropriately by the nurse.

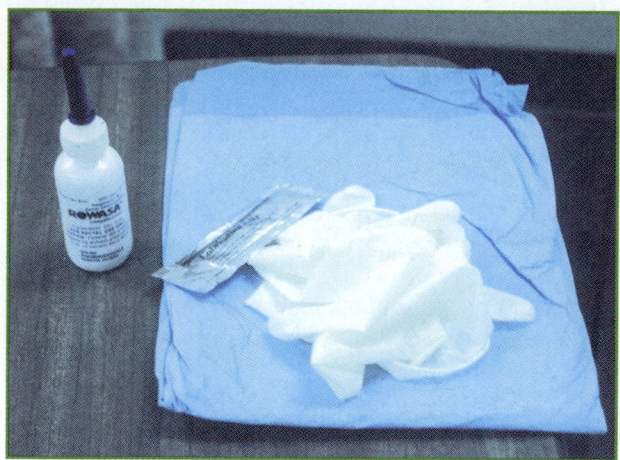

Figure 5-5-1 Protective pad, latex-free gloves, lubricant, and rectal medication.

3. The treatment will be completed as quickly and efficiently as possible to decrease discomfort and anxiety.
4. Client will state relief of complaint after medication administration.

Equipment Needed (see Figure 5-5-1):
- Medication (suppository or medicated enema)
- Water-soluble lubricant
- Latex-free gloves
- Tissue or washcloth
- Bedpan if client is physically immobile
- Medication administration record
- Towels or pads (such as disposable "Blue pads")

▶ CLIENT EDUCATION NEEDED:

1. Explain the type of medication, including purpose, onset of action, and any side effects.
2. Explain the procedure in detail, including client position, any sensations such as coolness from the lubricant, or any discomfort. A thorough explanation may empower the client to self-administer medications.
3. Teach the client to take slow, deep breaths not only to help allay anxiety but also to relax the anal sphincter.

Estimated time to complete the skill: **5–10 minutes**

▶ DELEGATION TIPS

The skill of medication administration is not delegated to ancillary personnel in acute care settings. This may vary in state or federal institutions. Ancillary personnel are generally informed about the medications the client is receiving if adverse effects are anticipated or are being monitored.

IMPLEMENTATION—Action/Rationale

Action	Rationale
1. Assess the client's need for the medication.	1. Allows nurse to determine effectiveness of the medication.
2. Check health care provider's written order.	2. Ensures safe and accurate administration of medication.
3. Check the medication administration record against the medication order, verifying correct client, medication, dose, route, and time.	3. Ensures accuracy and decreases chance of medication error.
4. Check for any drug allergies.	4. Decreases risk of allergic reaction.

continues

Action	Rationale
5. Review the client's history for any previous surgeries or bleeding.	**5.** Contraindications for rectal administration may be discovered.
6. Gather the equipment needed for the procedure before entering the client's room.	**6.** Prevents numerous trips to gather supplies and helps the procedure flow smoothly.
7. Assess the client's readiness to receive the medication. Encourage visitors to leave until the procedure is completed and close the door or curtain.	**7.** Promotes privacy and maintains self-image.
8. Wash hands.	**8.** Reduces transmission of microorganisms.
9. Ask the client's name and check the identification band.	**9.** Ensures correct client.
10. Apply disposable gloves (see Figure 5-5-2).	**10.** Prevents contact with fecal material.
11. Assist client into correct position; side-lying Sims' position, preferably the left side with upper leg drawn up toward chest. Provide protection under client such as towel or pad.	**11.** The descending colon is on the left side; this is a more anatomically correct position. This position exposes the anus to identify placement. Pads can provide comfort to client who may fear soiling linen.
12. Visually assess the client's external anus.	**12.** Determines presence of any active bleeding.
13. Remove suppository from wrapper and lubricate rounded end along with insertion finger. If a medicated enema is used, lubricate the enema tip if it is not lubricated beforehand (see Figure 5-5-3).	**13.** Lubrication decreases friction and decreases discomfort.

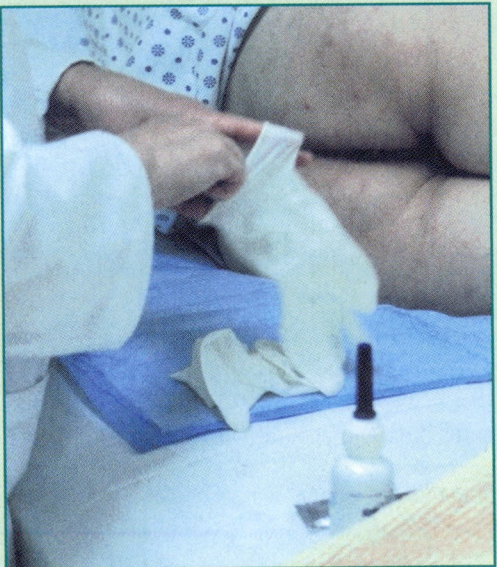

Figure 5-5-2   Apply latex-free gloves before administering rectal medications.

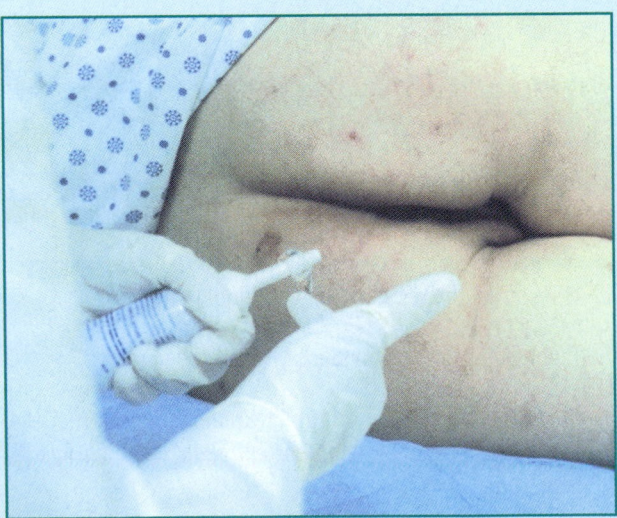

Figure 5-5-3   Lubricate the enema tip if it is not prelubricated.

continues

Action	Rationale
14. Tell client he or she will experience a cool sensation and pressure during administration. Encourage slow deep breaths.	**14.** Prepares the client for administration. Relaxes the rectal sphincter.
15. Retract buttocks with nondominant hand, visualizing the anus (see Figure 5-5-4). Using the dominant index finger, slowly and gently insert the suppository through the anus, past the internal sphincter, and against the rectal wall. Depth of insertion will differ if client is a child or infant. If instilling a medicated enema, gently insert the enema tip past the internal sphincter and instill the contents by slowly squeezing (see Figure 5-5-5).	**15.** Slow insertion minimizes pain. Correct placement ensures adequate absorption and less chance for expulsion of medication.
16. Remove finger or enema tip and wipe client's anal area with a washcloth or tissue.	**16.** Removes lubricant externally. Promotes cleanliness and comfort.
17. Discard gloves.	**17.** Reduces transfer of microorganisms.
18. Wash hands.	**18.** Reduces transfer of microorganisms.
19. Discuss with client a 10-minute time frame to remain in bed or on side.	**19.** Keeps suppository or medicated fluid in place for better absorption.
20. Place call light in client's reach if administering suppository containing laxative to assist once client has sensation to defecate.	**20.** Gives client control over situation and nurse response once sensation to defecate occurs.
21. Record administration of medication.	**21.** Provides documentation of administration of medication.
22. Document effectiveness or any side effects of treatment on nursing flow sheet or progress note, if applicable.	**22.** Communicates with other caregivers the effectiveness of treatment.

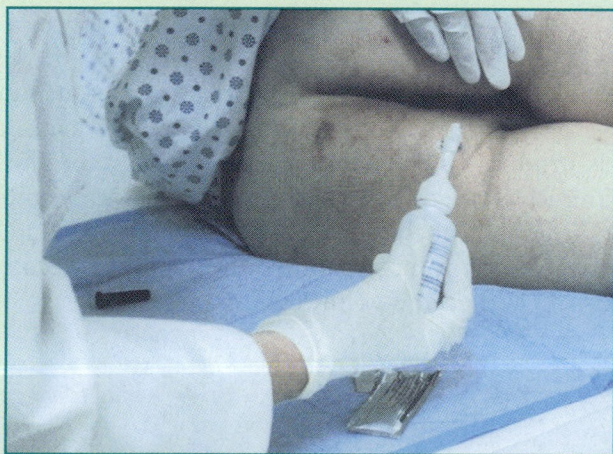

Figure 5-5-4   Retract the buttock and visualize the anus.

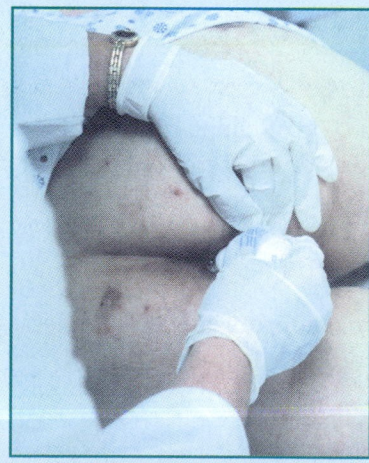

Figure 5-5-5   Gently insert the enema tip and instill the contents by slowly squeezing the bottle.

Mrs. Upton is a 57-year-old woman who had surgery 2 days previously. She has not been tolerating any oral intake and is requiring maintenance intravenous fluids to keep her hydrated. You are called to her room because her IV is infiltrated and other nurses have been unable to restart it. Mrs. Upton is also complaining of severe nausea. To provide immediate relief of the nausea until IV access is achieved, you administer a Compazine suppository. After about 15 minutes, Mrs. Upton feels less nauseated and is relaxed enough to cooperate with the IV restart.

▶ EVALUATION

- The medication was delivered appropriately and safely following the five rights of medication administration.
- The desired outcome was verbalized by the client and documented appropriately by the nurse.
- The treatment was completed as quickly and efficiently as possible to decrease discomfort and anxiety.
- Client stated relief of complaint after medication administration.

▶ DOCUMENTATION

Medication Administration Record
- Name of medication
- Dosage
- Route of administration
- Time administered
- Initials and signature of nurse administering medication

Nurses' Notes
- Time and type of client complaint
- Medication administered
- Outcome of treatment (client response)
- Health care provider notified, if needed
- Nurse's signature

Document on appropriate flow sheet or electronic medical record (EMR).

▶ CRITICAL THINKING SKILL

Introduction
Numerous systemic and local reacting medications can be given rectally when clients cannot take oral or IV medications.

Possible Scenario
Mr. Woodall is complaining of nausea and begins complaining of feeling hot and chilled. You take his temperature and note that it is 39.2° C. Blood cultures, a chest X-ray, and a urine sample are collected. Mr. Woodall's health care provider orders acetaminophen to reduce Mr. Woodall's fever. Mr. Woodall takes the acetaminophen but within minutes vomits. The intact acetaminophen tablets are noted to be in the emesis.

Possible Outcome
Without a method to retain and assimilate the acetaminophen, Mr. Woodall's fever will not be treated, and he will continue to be uncomfortable.

Prevention
Many oral medications are also available in suppository form. If a client is complaining of nausea, it is prudent to consider and request an alternative administration method as well as the oral route. An acetaminophen suppository would have treated Mr. Woodall's fever without the discomfort accompanying nausea and vomiting.

▶ VARIATIONS

Geriatric Variations:
- *Absorption may vary in older adults.*
- *Elderly people are more prone to constipation because of such factors as insufficient fluid intake, insufficient dietary fiber and bulk, decreased activity or sedentary lifestyle, or side effects of medications.*
- *Older clients may be physically unable to self-administer the medications and require assistance.*
- *Fecal impaction may occur more often, thereby interfering with suppository placement.*
- *If the suppository is a laxative, provide bedpan or bedside commode if client is immobile or at risk to not make it to the bathroom on time.*

Pediatric Variations:
- *Consider the age of the client when explaining the procedure. Provide simple and brief explanations and answer questions honestly to facilitate open communication.*
- *Never leave the medication unsupervised near the client.*
- *After the medication has been inserted into the rectum, press the buttocks together for several minutes to prevent expulsion.*
- *Provide extra assurance of privacy for adolescent clients during the procedure.*

Home Care Variations:
- *Teach client or family members the procedure of administration. If the rectal suppository is ordered on an as-needed basis, teach the caregivers how to determine whether the medication is needed.*
- *Make sure rectal suppositories are stored correctly in the home setting, refrigerated if needed, and discarded when they have expired.*

Long-Term Care Variations:
- *Review medications given over extended periods of time to determine any long-term side effects that might occur.*
- *Review with primary caregivers how to assess and document these side effects.*

▶ COMMON ERRORS

Possible Error:

The nurse is unable to visualize the external anus clearly enough to safely place the suppository.

Prevention:

Pressing the hard suppository into the wrong area can cause trauma to the anus and surrounding tissue. Be sure you can see where you are placing the suppository before inserting it. This may require extra help to position the client or you may need to clean the rectal area before inserting the suppository.

Possible Error:

The nurse inserts the suppository into stool in the rectum rather than placing it against the rectal wall.

Prevention:

Slide the suppository along the rectal wall as you are passing it through the anal sphincter. This will keep it in contact with the rectal mucosa, thereby increasing the absorption of the medication.

► **NURSING TIPS**

- Adjust the height of the bed to decrease back strain during insertion.
- Communication helps decrease anxiety and promotes cooperation.

- Observe the client's nonverbal and verbal cues during the procedure.
- Provide for privacy: Close the door, pull the curtains, and ask visitors to leave until the procedure is complete.

► **SPECIAL CONSIDERATIONS**

- The sphincter muscle around the rectum may start to contract as a normal response to the insertion of the medication bottle tip. Wait a few seconds until the muscle relaxes before instilling the medication.
- Special attention should be given to the client with a rectal fistula. Observe for signs of perforation such as leaking in the perineal area and abdominal cramping.
- If excoriation is present, protect the skin with topical creams or lubricants as allowed by institutional policy prior to administration of suppositories or enemas.

Administering Vaginal Medications

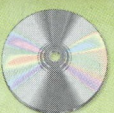

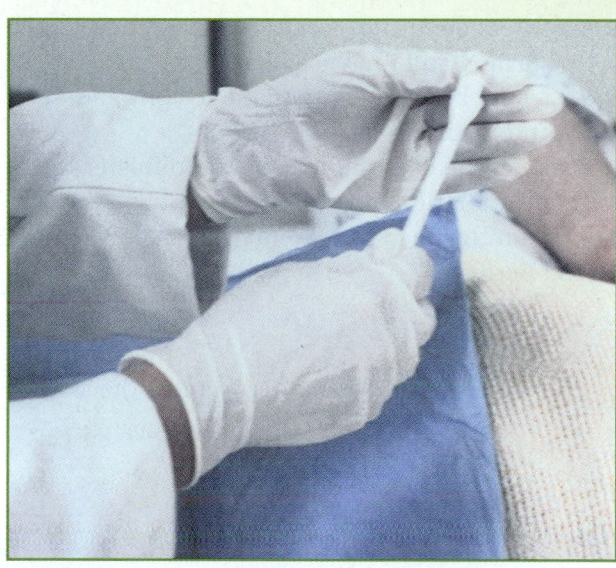

▶ OVERVIEW OF THE SKILL

Vaginal medications come in the form of creams, suppositories, foams, jellies, or irrigations (commonly known as douches). Vaginal medications are generally used to treat infections, irritations, or pruritus requiring topical treatment. These medications may be prescribed by a physician or nurse practitioner or many vaginal medications can be purchased over-the-counter (OTC). Irrigations or douches can be used to soothe, cleanse, change vaginal acidity/alkalinity, or disinfect the vagina; however, if used excessively, they can cause vaginal irritation. Most often, creams, foams, or jellies are administered with an applicator or inserter. Suppositories are individually foil-wrapped, oval-shaped solids that require refrigeration. Once the suppository is inserted by an applicator or directly with a finger (gloved hand), body temperature causes the suppository to melt and the medication to be distributed. Clients often prefer to administer their own vaginal medications. Once a vaginal medication is administered, a perineal pad may be placed to collect excess drainage and discharge. Pericare and personal hygiene (see Skill 4-9, Perineal and Genital Care) are essential as many vaginal infections cause foul-smelling discharge and irritation. Assess the client's level of pain, pruritus, burning, or general discomfort to establish a baseline for future assessment.

▶ ASSESSMENT

1. Assess the client's comfort level. Evaluate the level of burning, irritation, pruritus, pain, and odor **to establish a baseline for assessment of treatment.**
2. Assess the client's knowledge of the purpose of the medication and treatment. Enables client to understand and monitor effects of medication.
3. If the client prefers to self-administer the medication, assess the client's ability to do so, such as ability to manipulate the applicator or insert a suppository the appropriate distance. **Clients may prefer to self-administer vaginal medications for privacy, but if medication is not properly inserted it will not be effective.**

▶ DIAGNOSIS

Impaired Tissue Integrity

Ineffective Sexuality Patterns

Risk for Compromised Human Dignity

▶ PLANNING

Expected Outcomes:

1. Client will experience an absence of vaginal infection, pruritus, burning, or irritation.

2. Client will experience an absence of foul-smelling, curdlike, or blood-tinged discharge.
3. Client will understand the importance of continued treatment until infection is absent.
4. Client will understand the importance of personal hygiene in combination with medication.
5. Client will understand the need to properly clean and store equipment.

Equipment Needed (see Figure 5-6-1):

- Vaginal medication: cream, foam, jelly, or suppository
- Applicator (if needed)
- Water-soluble lubricating jelly (for suppository)
- Nonsterile latex-free gloves
- Perineal pad
- Paper towel, toilet tissue, or tissue paper
- Washcloth and warm water (optional)

▶ CLIENT EDUCATION NEEDED:

1. Instruct client of need to be in proper position and to stay in position.

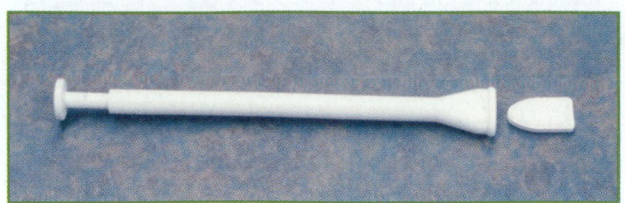

Figure 5-6-1 Vaginal medication and applicator

2. Instruct client to report adverse reactions, such as burning and increased irritation.
3. Instruct client to advise nurse if signs and symptoms improve.
4. Instruct the client how to self-administer the medication (if appropriate).
5. Explain the need for careful personal hygiene and pericare.

Estimated time to complete the skill:
15–10 minutes if vaginal irrigation

▶ DELEGATION TIPS

The skill of medication administration is not delegated to ancillary personnel in acute care settings. This may vary in state or federal institutions. Ancillary personnel are generally informed about the medications the client is receiving if adverse effects are anticipated or are being monitored.

IMPLEMENTATION—Action/Rationale

Action	Rationale
1. Verify orders.	1. Prevents medication errors.
2. Ascertain whether the client has ever received vaginal medications before and understands the procedure.	2. Enables understanding and compliance.
3. Ask the client to void.	3. Provides for client comfort during the procedure.
4. Wash hands.	4. Reduces transmission of microorganisms.
5. Arrange equipment at client's bedside.	5. Promotes organization.
6. Provide complete privacy by closing door and curtains.	6. This procedure can be embarrassing, and this protects the client's privacy.
7. Assist the client into a dorsal-recumbent or Sims' position (see Figure 5-6-2).	7. Allows positioning for administration and for medication to remain in vagina.

continues

Action	Rationale

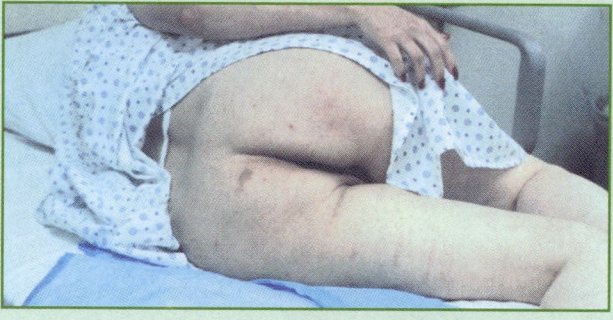

Figure 5-6-2   This client is placed in the Sims' position for administering vaginal medications.

8. Drape the client as appropriate, such as over the client's abdomen and lower extremities. Provide towel or protective pad on bed.

8. Provides privacy. Prevents linen from becoming soiled.

9. Position lighting to illuminate vaginal orifice.

9. Assists in visualization of vagina and proper administration of medication.

10. Don latex-free gloves and assess the perineal area for redness, inflammation, discharge, or foul odor.

10. Decreases risk of transmission of microorganisms. Provides baseline data. Decreases risk of reaction to latex.

11. If using an applicator, fill with medication. If using a suppository, remove the suppository from the foil and position in the applicator (applicator is optional) (see Figure 5-6-3). An applicator may be used for suppositories or a gloved finger may be used. The foil is discarded. Apply water-soluble lubricant to suppository or applicator (optional for applicator).

11. The medication is prepared for insertion. Lubricant provides comfort and ease of insertion.

12. For suppository, with nondominant hand, retract the labia (see Figure 5-6-4).

12. Allows visualization of the vaginal orifice and eases insertion of medication.

13. With dominant hand, insert the applicator 2 to 3 inches into the vagina, sliding the applicator posteriorly (see Figure 5-6-5). Push the plunger to administer the medication (see Figure 5-6-6). With a suppository, insert the tapered end first with the index finger or applicator along the posterior wall of the vagina (approximately 3 inches).

13. Medication must be inserted completely to provide coverage of the entire vagina. When medication is deposited at the posterior end of the vagina, gravity will allow medication to move toward the orifice.

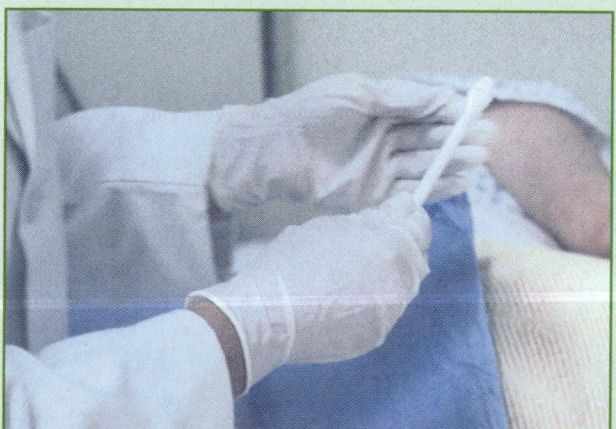

Figure 5-6-3   Place the suppository in the applicator.

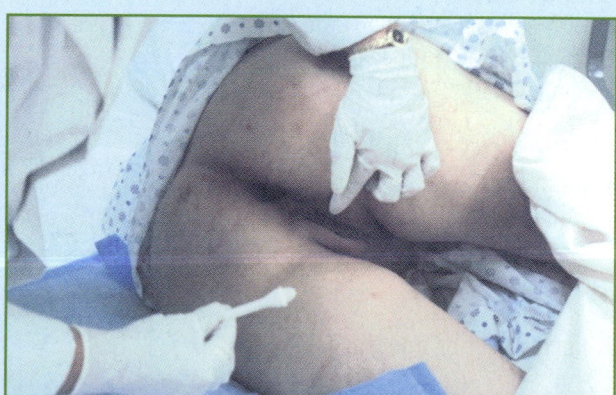

Figure 5-6-4   Retract the labia with the nondominant hand.

continues

Action	Rationale

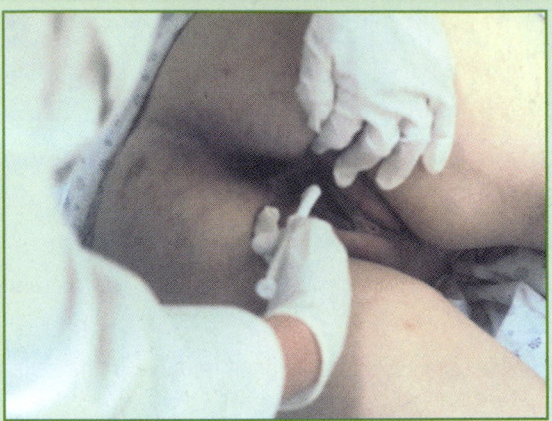

Figure 5-6-5   Slide the applicator 2 to 3 inches into the vagina.

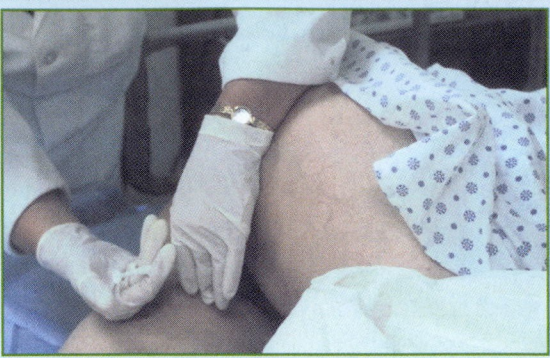

Figure 5-6-6   Push the plunger to administer the medication.

14. Withdraw the applicator and place on a towel.

15. If administering a douche or irrigation:
    - Warm solution to slightly above body temperature (105° to 110° F). Check using the back of the hand or the wrist.
    - Position the client in a semi-recumbent position on a bedpan, on a toilet seat, or in a tub.
    - Apply lubricant to the irrigation nozzle and insert approximately 3 inches into the vagina.
    - Hang the irrigant container approximately 2 feet above the client's vaginal area.
    - Open the clamp and allow a small amount of solution to flow into the vagina.
    - Move the nozzle and rotate around the entire vaginal area. If the labia are inflamed, allow the solution to flow over the labia as well. If the client is on the toilet seat, alternate between closing off the labia and allowing solution to be expelled.

16. Wipe and clean the client's perineal area, including the labia, from the front to the back with toilet tissue. Some clients may prefer that the perineal area is also cleaned with a washcloth and warm water.

17. Apply a perineal pad.

18. Wash the applicator (if reusable) with soap and warm water and store in appropriate container in client's room.

19. Remove gloves and wash hands.

14. Reduces the transmission of microorganisms.

15.
    - Avoids burning the client. The mucous membranes of the vagina are sensitive.
    - Provides comfort during procedure and allows for appropriate drainage of irrigation solution.
    - Provides comfort.

    - Height is necessary for drainage by gravity. If the container is too high, the flow will be too forceful and uncomfortable.
    - Allows the client to evaluate the temperature.

    - Rotation allows for irrigation throughout vagina. Closing off labia allows medication to stay in and flush total vagina.

16. Provides comfort for client and avoids spread of infective agents to perineal area.

17. Protects client from discomfort of drainage and spread of infection or irritation to perineal area.

18. Applicator can only be used for individual clients; however, some applicators and inducers are reusable and must be appropriately cleaned and stored to prevent reinsertion of infective agents.

19. Reduces the transmission of microorganisms.

continues

Action	Rationale
20. Instruct the client to remain flat for at least 30 minutes.	**20.** Allows maximum contact between the medication and the vaginal mucous membranes.
21. Raise side rails and place the call light in reach.	**21.** Provides for client comfort and safety.

▶ REAL WORLD ANECDOTES

Mrs. Lopez is an elderly woman who presented to the clinic with complaints of foul-smelling discharge and vaginal irritation 1 week earlier. She returns complaining that the medication the doctor prescribed has not helped at all. She speaks very little English and has brought her granddaughter along to translate. While questioning Mrs. Lopez about her medication, the nurse realizes that Mrs. Lopez had been unable to read the use directions and had been too embarrassed to ask anyone to translate them for her. Mrs. Lopez had been taking the suppositories orally, not realizing that they were intended for vaginal insertion. The nurse carefully explained where the medication was to be applied and how to use the applicator. Mrs. Lopez was initially embarrassed to be discussing this with her granddaughter present, but the nurse's matter-of-fact demeanor put her at ease. By the time Mrs. Lopez left the clinic, the nurse was confident that Mrs. Lopez would be able to correctly apply her medication and was on the way to recovery.

▶ EVALUATION

- Client experiences an absence of vaginal infection, pruritus, burning, or irritation.
- Client experiences an absence of foul-smelling, curd-like, or blood-tinged discharge.
- Client understands the importance of continued treatment until infection is absent.
- Client understands the importance of personal hygiene in combination with medication.
- Client understands the need to properly clean and store equipment.

▶ DOCUMENTATION

Nurses' Notes

- Document the procedure performed and the results.
- Note any unusual findings or client complaints.
- Document client's response to treatment.
- Document client's signs and symptoms associated with vaginal condition.

Document on appropriate flow sheet or electronic medical record (EMR).

Medication Administration Record

- Record the date and time the medication/treatment was administered.

▶ CRITICAL THINKING SKILL

Introduction

Client education is an important part of nursing care.

Possible Scenario

Mrs. Davies frequently presented to the clinic with complaints of vaginal irritation and tenderness. Despite a number of medication regimes, she continued to suffer with these problems. Mrs. Davies' complaints had become so common that her doctor had started simply calling in prescriptions when she notified the office of another episode of vaginal irritation and tenderness, hoping to save her the cost of an office visit.

Possible Outcome

Mrs. Davies continues to have vaginal irritation and tenderness. The constant mess of the medication as well as the vaginal tenderness she experiences has affected her relationship with her husband. The next time she calls the office complaining of vaginal irritation and tenderness, the office nurse takes the time to sit and talk to Mrs. Davies. One of the questions the office nurse asks regards douches. The office nurse had noticed in Mrs. Davies chart that she had previously reported using vinegar douches. When the nurse asks Mrs. Davies if she uses premixed douches from the store or if she mixes her own, Mrs. Davies notes that she mixes her own. The nurse then asks about the ratio of vinegar to water Mrs. Davies uses. Mrs. Davies seems surprised and replies that she uses plain white vinegar as a douche liquid. She had read that vinegar douches tighten the vagina and improve the sexual experience. She had not noted that the article called for a vinegar/water mix and advised not douching too frequently. In an effort to improve relations with her husband, Mrs. Davies had increased the frequency of the vinegar douches, increasing her irritation and tenderness. The mystery was solved with some insightful nursing communication.

Prevention

Do not assume that clients have the advantage of information that you have. Many clients do not understand the workings of the human body and many harbor ideas that seem odd to a nurse educated in anatomy and physiology. Do not ask yes/no questions when gathering client information. Ask questions that require the client to explain, and then listen carefully, without preconceived notions. If the nurse had assumed that "vinegar douche" meant the same thing to her and to Mrs. Davies, the client might have suffered until her relationship ended, only to then discover that her irritation improved. Especially in an area where many people are reluctant to discuss concerns or to ask questions, good communication and client teaching are essential.

► **VARIATIONS**

Geriatric Variations:
- *The labia may be more difficult to hold apart because of decreased turgor in elderly clients.*
- *Elderly clients may be more sensitive to temperature variations of irrigation fluids.*
- *Assess the client's previous use of vaginal irrigations as some elderly clients may use douches frequently.*

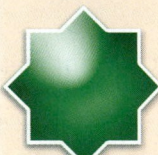

Pediatric Variations:
- *Vaginal medications can be very embarrassing for children. The staff need to be extremely sensitive to the child's privacy.*
- *Inappropriate touching can be an issue with children. Have a trusted female family member or a second staff member present when giving vaginal medications to children.*

Home Care Variations:
- *Assess the home environment to see if there is a place where equipment can be properly cleaned and stored.*
- *Instruct the client or the client's caregiver how to administer the medication, if necessary.*

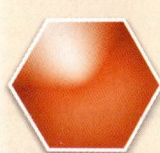

Long-Term Care Variations:
- *The client's ability to assume a Sims' or recumbent position may be limited. Alternative positioning or medication administration may be necessary.*
- *Most vaginal medications are not designed to be used over long periods. Regular reevaluation of the need for a vaginal medication should be performed.*

► **COMMON ERRORS**

Possible Error:

The nurse does not insert the medication deeply enough into the vagina.

Prevention:

Visualize the vaginal opening before trying to insert the applicator. Be sure to insert the medication 2 to 3 inches into the vagina.

Possible Error:

The client does not remain in the recumbent position long enough to allow the medication to effectively contact the vaginal mucosa.

Prevention:

Educate the client regarding the need to lie flat for 30 minutes to allow the medication time to work. Explain that this is as important a step as proper insertion of the medication

► **NURSING TIPS**

- Insert medication 2 to 3 inches.

- Clean client carefully after inserting medication to avoid perineal irritation.

► **SPECIAL CONSIDERATIONS**

- *The client can have allergic reactions to vaginal medications or to latex gloves. Assess for reactions. If redness persists, it may be an allergic reaction instead of a reaction to the infection process. A case has been reported of anaphylaxis to latex gloves used in a vaginal exam.*

Administering Nebulized Medications

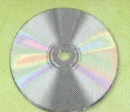

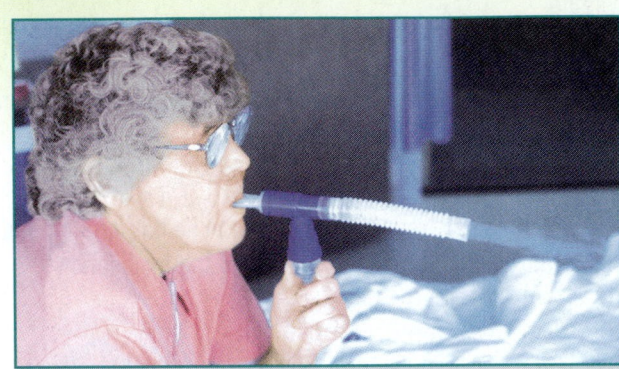

▶ OVERVIEW OF THE SKILL

A nebulizer is a device that is used to aerosolize medications into a mist for delivery directly into the lungs. Medication that is inhaled in the form of small droplets is absorbed immediately into the mucosa and bloodstream and is available to the body within minutes. This method of medication delivery is one of the fastest, noninvasive methods of medication delivery. A large number of medications can be delivered by inhalation, but currently this delivery method is used primarily for medications designed to ease respiratory distress symptoms such as those seen with asthma.

This skill deals with two types of nebulizers: the single-dose nebulizer, which is driven by an air compressor, wall air, or wall oxygen; and the portable metered-dose inhaler. Both nebulizers have advantages and disadvantages. The single-dose, compressor-driven nebulizer delivers smaller droplets, allowing faster, more complete assimilation of the medication. The single-dose nebulizer can be filled with any type of medication that is ordered and it can be used by clients who cannot coordinate the use of the metered dose inhaler. The primary drawback of the single-dose nebulizer is its lack of portability. The nebulizer itself is portable, but to function it must be connected to a compressor. The nebulizer must also be loaded with medication for each use, thus delaying the client's relief.

The metered-dose inhaler has the benefit of being small and portable. It can be carried in the client's pocket. Because the meter dispenses measured doses of the preloaded medication, no special training is needed to prime the inhaler. The primary drawback of a metered-dose inhaler is the need to coordinate dispensing the dose and inhalation. Very small children, clients with coordination impairment, and clients with cognitive difficulties may not be able to use the metered-dose inhaler.

▶ ASSESSMENT

1. Assess the five rights: right client, right medication, right route, right dose, and right time. **Prevents errors in medication administration.**

2. Assess the client's respiratory status. Note if the client is using accessory muscles for respiration or if there is flaring of the nares. Auscultate the client's chest for wheezes and crackles. **Respiratory distress is the primary reason to administer nebulized medications.**

3. Evaluate the history of this episode of the client's distress. Take a complete history from the client or a reliable informant about the symptoms and length of time the client has had them. Respiratory distress can have many causes. Asthma, bronchitis, a foreign object in the airways, and chronic obstructive pulmonary disease can all cause respiratory distress. **Assessing the client's current symptoms provides more accurate diagnosis and care. The client's history of asthma does not mean that this episode of distress is asthma.**

4. Assess the client's ability to use the nebulizer or metered-dose inhaler. Determine the client's ability to understand and follow the directions, the client's ability to hold and manipulate the equipment, and the client's ability to coordinate

the release of the medication with inhalation. **This will determine the type of equipment used for the client. Very young children may need a mask instead of a mouthpiece on the nebulizer. The elderly may need specialized dispensers for their metered-dose inhalers.**

5. Assess the medication(s) currently ordered by the health care provider: action, purpose, common side effects, time of onset, and peak of action. **This permits the nurse to anticipate what to observe from the client.**

6. Assess the medications the client is currently taking, including over-the-counter drugs. **Some medications can interact. Beta blockers (Propranolol, Atenolol, and Betalol) can antagonize the beta agonists and cause or increase asthma symptoms.**

7. Assess the client's knowledge regarding the medications and the use of the nebulizer or metered-dose inhaler. **This allows the nurse to determine the need for client education to promote compliance.**

8. Check the client's drug allergy history, as **an allergic reaction could occur.**

▶ DIAGNOSIS

Impaired Gas Exchange

Ineffective Breathing Pattern

Deficient Knowledge

Anxiety

Fear

▶ PLANNING

Expected Outcome:

1. The client will experience improved gas exchange.

2. The client's breathing pattern will become effective.

3. The client will demonstrate understanding of the need for the medication and the use of the nebulizer or metered-dose inhaler.

4. The client will not experience any adverse effects secondary to medication interactions.

5. The client's anxiety level will decrease following treatment.

Equipment Needed (see Figure 5-7-1 A and B):

Handheld Nebulizer

- Medication administration record
- Nebulizer set (cup, tubing, cap, T-shaped tube, mouthpiece, or mask) or prepackaged nebulizer and applicator
- Medication(s)
- Saline
- Air compressor, wall air, or wall oxygen

Metered-Dose Inhaler

- Metered-dose inhaler
- AeroChamber, if appropriate

▶ CLIENT EDUCATION NEEDED:

1. Explain the purpose of the procedure.

2. Teach the client how to use the nebulizer properly, holding it upright to prevent spillage of medication, sealing the mouth around the mouthpiece, and breathing in slowly and deeply through the mouth. Observe the client for about 1 minute during the nebulization treatment to ensure that proper technique is being followed.

3. Describe how long the treatment should take.

4. Teach the client the importance of measuring medication to be nebulized properly. Have the client demonstrate the instructions given.

5. Explain the medication(s) the client will be using for the nebulization. This includes the

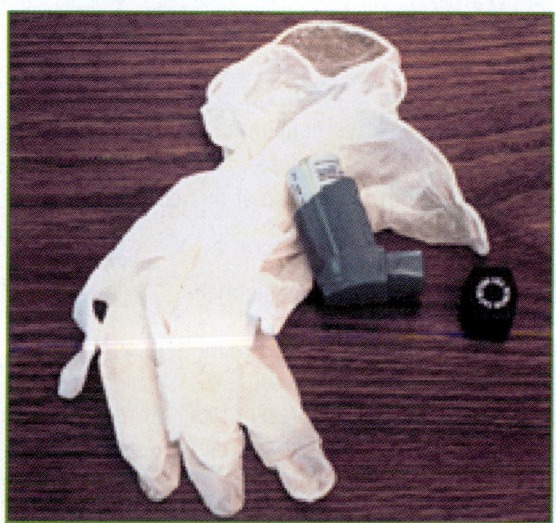

Figure 5-7-1A Handheld metered dose inhaler

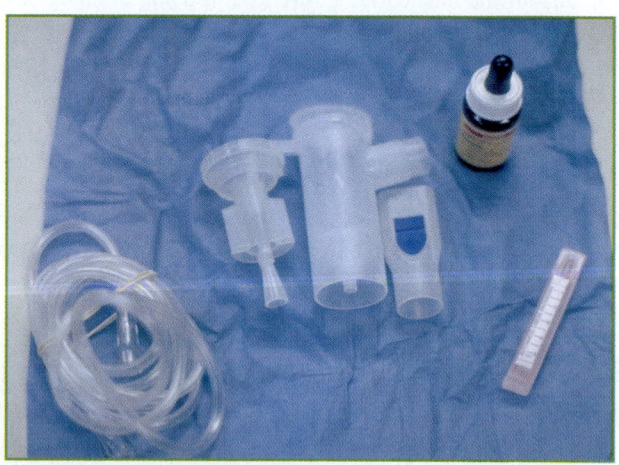

Figure 5-7-1B Nebulizer cup, tubing, cap, T-shaped tube, medication, and mouthpiece

purpose, time of onset, peak of action, and common side effects.

6. Teach the client how to use an AeroChamber if unable to coordinate the inhalation in a metered-dose inhaler.

7. Explain how long the task will last and the expected outcome.

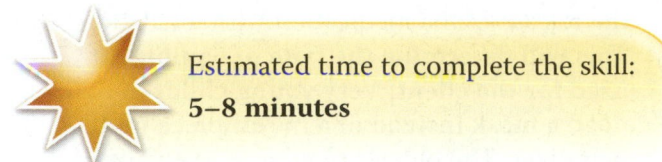

Estimated time to complete the skill:
5–8 minutes

▶ DELEGATION TIPS

The skill of medication administration is not delegated to ancillary personnel in acute care settings. This may vary in state or federal institutions. Ancillary personnel are generally informed about the medications the client is receiving if adverse effects are anticipated or are being monitored.

IMPLEMENTATION—Action/Rationale

Action	Rationale
Handheld Nebulizer	
1. Assess client's ability to use the nebulizer.	1. Ensures client compliance.
2. Check the medication administration record against the health care provider's orders.	2. Ensures accuracy in the administration of medication. (Right drug.)
3. Check for drug allergies and hypersensitivity.	3. Decreases the risk of allergic reaction such as hives, urticaria, or anaphylactic shock.
4. Wash your hands before setting up the nebulizer.	4. Reduces the transmission of microorganisms.
5. Set up the medication(s) for one client at a time.	5. Ensures that the client receives the right medication(s). (Right drug.)
6. Look at the medication at eye level if using droppers to dispense the solution into the nebulizer.	6. Increases accuracy. (Right dose.)
7. Pour the entire amount of the drug(s) into the nebulizer cup carefully. • Avoid touching the drug while pouring into the nebulizer cup.	7. Determines the correct amount of medicine and ensures accurate dosage. (Right dose.) • Reduces the transmission of microorganisms.
8. Cover the cup with the cap and fasten.	8. Prevents spillage of the medication.
9. Fasten the T-piece to the top of the cap.	9. Provides a connector for the mouthpiece.
10. Fasten a short length of tubing to one end of the T-piece.	10. Provides dead space to prevent room air from entering the system and medicated aerosol from escaping.

continues

Action	Rationale
11. Fasten the mouthpiece or mask to the other end of the T-piece. • Avoid touching the nebulizer mouthpiece or the interior part of the mask.	**11.** Provides a portal for the client to inhale the aerosolized medication. • Reduces the transmission of microorganisms.
12. Identify the client prior to administration of medication(s).	**12.** Ensures the right client gets the medication. (Right client).
13. Identify the medication(s) to the client and clearly explain the therapeutic purpose(s) of the medication.	**13.** Promotes client's cooperation and awareness of the medication's effects.
14. Advise the client to sit in an upright position.	**14.** Promotes better expansion of the lungs.
15. Attach tubing to the bottom of the nebulizer cup and attach the other end to the air compressor or wall air. • Before turning it on, adjust the wall oxygen valve to 6 liters/min. (or less per health care provider's orders). • Leave the air on for about 6 to 7 minutes until the medication gets used up.	**15.** Provides a conduit for the compressed air. • Drives the medication into a mist or wet aerosol form.
16. Instruct the client to breathe in and out slowly and deeply through the mouthpiece/mask. • The client's lips should be sealed tightly around the mouthpiece.	**16.** Promotes better deposition and efficacy of the medication in the airways.
17. Remain with the client long enough to observe the proper inhalation-exhalation technique.	**17.** Ensures the correct use of the nebulizer to get the full effects from the medications administered.
18. Wash your hands with soap and water.	**18.** Reduces the transmission of microorganisms.
19. Record the medications administered along with the date, time, and dosages on the chart.	**19.** Provides documentation of administration of drugs.
20. When the nebulizer cup is empty, turn off the compressor or wall air. • Detach the tubing from the compressor and the nebulizer cup. • If the nebulizer is disposable, dispose of the nebulizer in the appropriate container. • If the nebulizer is to be reused for this client, carefully wash, rinse, and dry the nebulizer components.	**20.** Stops the aerosolization. • Prepares components for cleaning or disposal. • Prevents the transmission of microorganisms. • Prevents the transmission of microorganisms.
21. Assess the client immediately following the treatment for results or adverse effects from the treatment.	**21.** Allows the nurse to determine the effectiveness of the treatment.
22. Reassess the client 5 to 10 minutes following the treatment.	**22.** Some effects may be delayed.
23. Wash your hands.	**23.** Reduces the transmission of microorganisms.

continues

Action	Rationale
Metered-Dose Nebulizer (see Figure 5-7-2)	
24. Assess the client for ability to use the metered-dose nebulizer.	24. Ensures client compliance.
25. Check the medication administration record against the health care provider's orders.	25. Ensures accuracy in the administration of medication.
26. Check for drug allergies and hypersensitivity.	26. Decreases the risk of allergic reaction, such as hives, urticaria, or anaphylactic shock.
27. Wash your hands before administering medication and don latex-free gloves.	27. Decreases risk of the transmission of microorganisms and prevents reaction to latex.
28. Shake the prepackaged nebulizer.	28. Thoroughly mixes the medication.
29. Place the nebulizer into the applicator.	29. Allows for proper administration of the medication.
30. Place the AeroChamber onto the nebulizer if needed (see Figure 5-7-3).	30. The AeroChamber provides dead space for the medicated mist while the client inhales.
31. Have the client place the mouthpiece in his or her mouth.	31. Delivers medication to the lungs through the proper route.
32. Have the client press down on the prepackaged dispenser as the client simultaneously inhales.	32. Allows delivery of the medication to the lungs.
33. If there is an AeroChamber attached to the nebulizer, have the client inhale slowly and deeply.	33. Allows proper delivery of the medication.
34. Observe the client for several minutes to assess for possible adverse effects from the medication.	34. Nebulized medication is delivered into the bloodstream almost immediately and reactions can occur right away.
35. Have the client rinse his or her mouth.	35. The medication may leave a metallic taste.

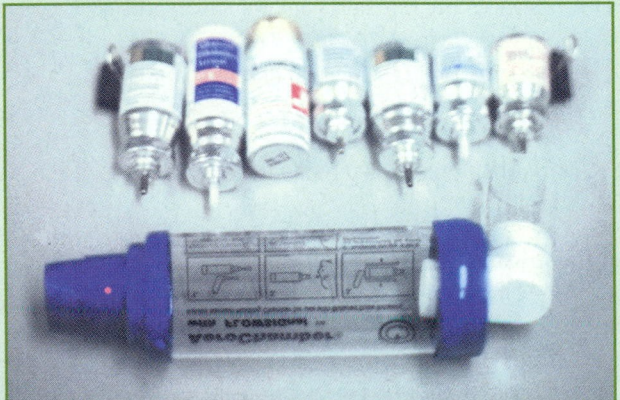

Figure 5-7-2   Metered-dose nebulizer and medications

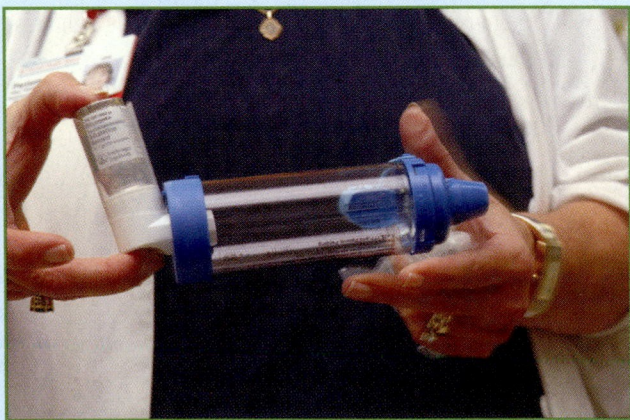

Figure 5-7-3   Preparation of a metered-dose inhaler and medication.

continues

Action	Rationale
36. Wash your hands.	**36.** Prevents the transmission of microorganisms.
37. Record the medication administration and your observations.	**37.** Provides a record of care and ensures continuity of care.

▶ REAL WORLD ANECDOTES

An ambulatory 15-year-old boy arrived at the clinic for his regular 4-month checkup. He does not remember the names of the two regular metered-dose inhalers prescribed for his asthma. He uses the medications irregularly. He can only recall the colors of the containers; one is teal green and the other is pink. He uses the "yellow one" as a rescue medication at least once a day. His pulmonary lung function test results showed mild-to-moderate obstruction in his airways. The physician decided to give him bronchotherapy via a nebulizer. The client did not want to listen to the instructions of the nurse because he apparently knew how to do it and had done it a couple of times before. The nurse left, assuming that the client knew the correct way of using the nebulizer. The client decided to lie on his side on the exam table while reading a sports magazine. Lung function tests were repeated 10 minutes after the treatment was over. Because the nebulizer was not used correctly, the client's results did not show significant improvement as expected. The nurse should have instructed or reviewed with the client how to inhale slowly and deeply through the mouthpiece even if he had "done it before." This ensures good client compliance.

▶ EVALUATION

- The client experienced improved gas exchange.
- The client's breathing pattern became effective.
- The client demonstrated understanding of the need for the medication and the use of the nebulizer or metered-dose inhaler.
- The client did not experience any adverse effects secondary to medication interactions.
- The client's anxiety level decreased following treatment.

▶ DOCUMENTATION

Medication Administration Record

- Name of medication(s)
- Dosage
- Route
- Site
- Time of administration
- Initials of the nurse who administered the medication(s)
- Signature of the nurse identifying the initials

Nurses' Notes

- Client's assessment parameters
- Name of medication, dosage, route, and time of administration
- Amount of oxygen delivered per minute from wall oxygen or air compressor machine
- Signature and initials of the nurse
- Client's response

Document on appropriate flow sheet or electronic medical record (EMR).

▶ CRITICAL THINKING SKILL

Introduction

Be aware of client limitations.

Possible Scenario

A 75-year-old woman was evaluated for asthma. Pulmonary function tests showed moderate-to-severe airway obstruction. The client was given two nebulization treatments of albuterol 0.5 mL and Atrovent 2.5 mL with 6 liters/min. of oxygen. The client became stabilized and was prescribed metered-dose inhalers to be used at home. The client was told to come back for a 2-week follow-up visit.

Possible Outcome

Two nights later, the client had to go to the emergency room. She told the physician that her asthma inhalers did not seem to help her. When questioned regarding her use of the inhalers, she seemed to understand how to dispense the dose while inhaling. When asked to demonstrate her use of the inhalers, however, it was clear that she was unable to coordinate dispensing the dose and inhalation.

▶ VARIATIONS

Geriatric Variations:

- Some older clients may have arthritis or some disabling condition that may make it difficult for them to set up a nebulizer or manipulate a metered-dose inhaler. There are aids designed for clients with manual dexterity difficulties that can make these tasks easier.
- Older clients have trouble seeing the lines on the medicine dropper. Use of unit-dose inhalers or premixed solutions will make it easier and ensures accuracy for the right amount of medicines to be given.
- Older clients may have hand tremors, so it may be hard for them to keep the nebulizer mouthpiece in place. Provide the client with a mask so the nebulizer does not have to be held during treatment.

Pediatric Variations:

- Infants and toddlers will not be able to hold the nebulizer mouthpiece properly. Use of appropriately sized mask can be used for this age group.
- Young children might get upset or cry when they see the mist coming out of the nebulizer cup. Continue giving the nebulizer treatment because crying can actually increase the chance of medication being deposited in the airways/lungs.
- Metered-dose inhalers are often prescribed for asthmatic children. Be sure to reinforce the correct usage and dosage frequently. Children may become dependent on their inhalers and use them more often than prescribed.

Home Care Variations:

- Clients who will be in nebulization treatment at home are advised to purchase or rent an air compressor machine. A multiuse nebulizer can be recommended, but it is exclusively for a single client's use only. The nebulizer set should be changed every 6 months depending on its use.
- Client should be advised to clean and disinfect the nebulizer. Dishwasher-safe nebulizers are available, and rinsing off with soap and water and letting all parts air dry on a clean cloth or paper towel are advised after each use. Store in a clean Ziploc bag if nebulizer is totally dry. Disinfecting with diluted bleach (1:100) is recommended at least once a day. Soaking the nebulizer with one part vinegar and three parts distilled or sterile water will remove the clog in the nebulizer cup after using it several times. The tubing does not need to be washed, but it can be cleaned from the outside with alcohol or a wet towel with bleach and then air dried.

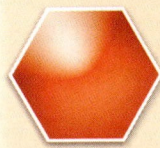

Long-Term Care Variations:

- Clients on long-term nebulizer treatment are advised to purchase two kinds of nebulizer machines. One is portable and the other is the regular air compressor machine. The portable nebulizer will allow the client to have nebulization treatments wherever he or she goes. Charged or regular batteries or a cigarette lighter adapter can power it.
- Some clients, especially the elderly, usually get a regular supply of unit or premixed dose medications from the pharmacy or health care agencies so that they will not fail to have nebulizer treatments. The respiratory therapist visits from the health care agencies can provide free monitoring of client compliance.

▶ **COMMON ERRORS**

Possible Error:

Nebulizer medication and saline solution is beyond the maximum 5-mL capacity of the cup.

Prevention:

Use caution in handling medications. Examine the medicine dropper at eye level and pour the entire amount into the cup carefully without spilling. Discard the medication, obtain the replacement, repeat the preparation, and administer the correct medication.

Possible Error:

The client exhales while using the metered-dose inhaler.

Prevention:

Have the client demonstrate the use of the metered-dose inhaler. If the client is unable to adequately coordinate inhaling while dispensing the metered dose, provide the client with an AeroChamber to provide a holding chamber for the medication while the client breathes in and out normally.

Prevention

Although the client understood the instructions, she lacked the physical dexterity to carry them out. The nurse should not only explain how to perform the skill but require a return demonstration. Clients may voice understanding without actually being able to perform the skill.

▶ **NURSING TIPS**

- Evaluate the client's need for medication delivery. Some clients, such as young clients (usually younger than 5 years of age), clients with coordination problems, and clients with severe or acute asthma, will benefit more from using a nebulizer. Some clients, such as school-aged children, active adults, and clients with exercise-induced asthma, will benefit more from the ease and portability of a metered-dose inhaler.
- Be aware of the client's ability to use the nebulizer device. Young children and clients with acute or severe exacerbation may not be able to use the mouthpiece for the nebulizer. A mask may provide better delivery of the medication(s).
- Measure the medication accurately by looking at the medicine dropper at eye level, and pour the exact amount of medication needed into the cup.
- Familiarize yourself with all the asthma medications in order to be aware of any outcomes the client may have from treatment. Some medications that the client might be taking can interact with each other. Beta blockers (Propranolol, Atenolol, and Betalol) can antagonize the beta agonists, increasing asthma symptoms. The nurse needs to be familiar with the medications in order to anticipate possible reactions.
- Be aware of the advantages and disadvantages of using the nebulizer or the metered-dose inhaler. The particle size of medication used via a nebulizer, which is in a mist form, is smaller compared to using metered-dose inhalers. Therefore, the medication gets deposited into the receptor sites quicker and the effects are faster. It takes about 6 to 7 minutes to finish up a nebulizer treatment of 2.5 to 3 mL of solution, whereas it only takes about a minute to use one to two puffs of a metered-dose inhaler.
- Health care practitioner should avoid close proximity and risk of inhaling medications.

► **SPECIAL CONSIDERATIONS**

- *Clients need good oral care after using a nebulizer. In some clients, rashes may form around the lips or the mucus of the mouth caused by concentrated particles in the medication. Closely monitor rashes; if symptoms persist or progress to a larger area, notify the health care provider.*
- *Observe for white patches or fungal infections and report observation to health care provider.*
- *As nebulized medications may leave an unpleasant taste in the mouth, rinsing after use may improve compliance.*

Administering an Intradermal Injection

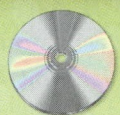

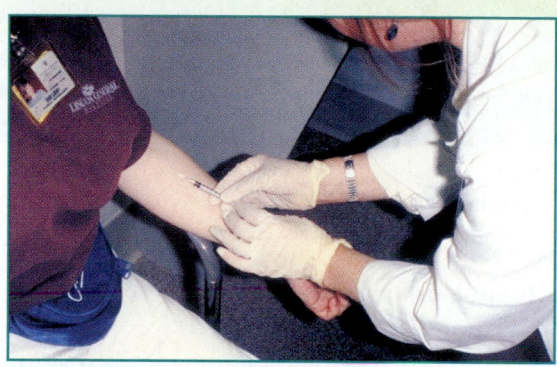

▶ OVERVIEW OF THE SKILL

An intradermal injection is a method used to administer medications just below the skin. Potent medications that should be absorbed slowly are given intradermally because of the less richly supplied blood vessels of this layer. However, the client may respond rapidly and should be monitored for allergic reactions.

The most common reason for an intradermal injection is skin testing such as tuberculin screening or allergy testing. Only small amounts (0.01–0.10 mL) of fluid are given intradermally.

The most common sites for injections are forearms, upper chest, and upper back. The site should be lightly pigmented, free of lesions, and hairless. As these areas are easily accessible, the nurse can monitor the reaction (see Figure 5-8-1).

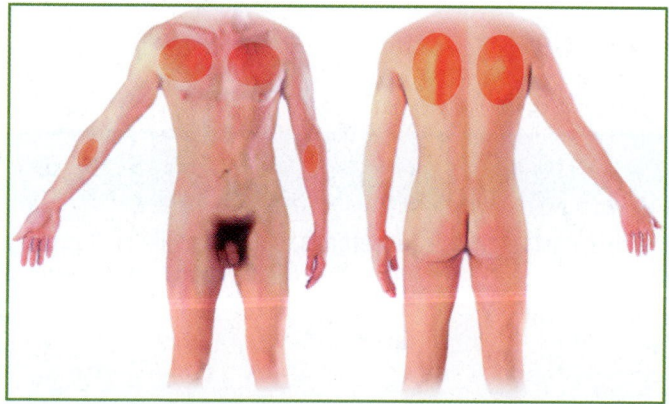

Figure 5-8-1   Common intradermal injection sites: A. Inner aspect of the forearm; B. Upper chest; C. Upper back.

A syringe, consisting of the barrel with plunger and tip of syringe where a needle can be attached, is used. The needle's hub screws into the tip of the syringe and its hollow shaft ends at a beveled point. A tuberculin or small hypodermic syringe is used with a short (one-quarter to one-half inch), fine (26 to 27) gauge needle.

As of April 2001 a Federal Needle Stick Safety and Prevention Law requires safe medical devices. The position of the Occupational and Safety Health Act (OSHA) provides that whenever exposure to blood-borne pathogens is anticipated, the use of controls to eliminate employee exposure should be used, hence, safe devices. Examples of such devices are needle-protected or needleless systems. In the case of intradermal injections, safety syringes or needles should be used. These can be safety-glide needles or safety-retraction or slide syringes. Instruction should be provided appropriate to the manufacturers' specifications.

▶ ASSESSMENT

1. Assess the five rights: right client, right medication, right route, right dose, and right time. **Prevents errors in medication administration.**
2. Review health care provider's order **so that the drug is administered safely and correctly.**
3. Review information regarding the expected reaction to the allergen **to anticipate the type of reaction a client may have.**
4. Assess for the indications for intradermal injection including the client's allergy history **so**

the nurse will not administer a substance to which the client is known to be sensitive.

5. Check the expiration date of the medication vial **as the drug loses its potency over time.**

6. Assess client's knowledge regarding the medication to be received **so that client education may be tailored according to need.**

7. Assess the client's response to discussion about an injection **as some clients may express anticipatory anxiety, which may increase pain.**

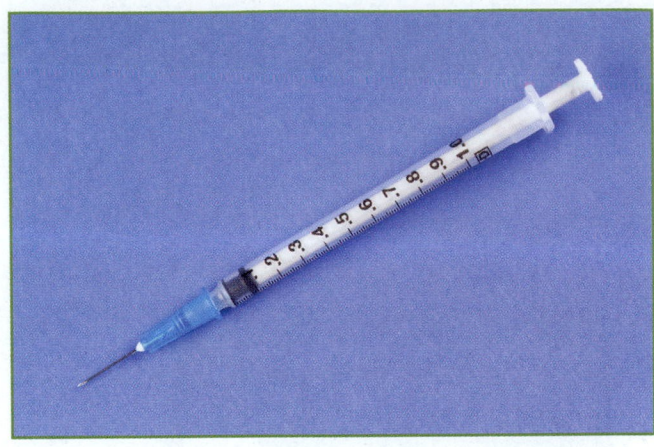

Figure 5-8-2 Syringes come in many sizes. Select a 1-mL tuberculin safety syringe for intradermal injections.

▶ DIAGNOSIS

Risk for Infection

Impaired Skin Integrity

Deficient Knowledge

Anxiety

Fear

▶ PLANNING

Expected Outcomes:

1. The client will experience only minimal pain or burning at the injection site.
2. The client will experience no allergic reaction or other side effects from the injection.
3. The client will be able to explain the significance of the presence or absence of a skin reaction.
4. The client will keep follow-up appointments within the recommended time frame to have responses to the medication evaluated.

Equipment Needed (see Figure 5-8-2):

- Tuberculin syringe, 1 mL
- Needle (25- to 27-gauge, 1/4- to 5/8-inch)

- Antiseptic or alcohol swabs
- Medication ampule or vial
- Medication card or medication administration record
- Disposable gloves

▶ CLIENT EDUCATION NEEDED:

1. Teach the client the rationale for administering the medication intradermally.
2. Reassure client that the injection will look and feel like a mosquito bite.
3. Teach the client to report any bleeding, itching, pain, or other skin reactions.

Estimated time to complete the skill:
5–10 minutes

▶ DELEGATION TIPS

The skill of medication administration is not delegated to ancillary personnel in acute care settings. This may vary in state or federal institutions. Ancillary personnel are generally informed about the medications the client is receiving if adverse effects are anticipated or are being monitored.

IMPLEMENTATION—Action/Rationale

Action	Rationale
1. Wash hands and put on clean gloves.	1. Reduces the transmission of microorganisms.
2. In the inpatient setting, close door or curtains around bed and keep gown or sheet draped over body. In the outpatient setting, close door to exam or treatment room. Identify client.	2. Provides privacy. Ensures medication is given to right client.
3. Select injection site (see Figure 5-8-1). • Inspect skin for bruises, inflammation, edema, masses, tenderness, and sites of previous injections. • Forearm site should be 3 to 4 finger widths below antecubital space and one hand width above wrists on inner aspect of forearm.	3. Injection site should be free of lesions. Repeated daily injections should be rotated. Ensures a clear site for interpreting results.
4. Select 1/4- to 5/8-inch 25- to 27-gauge needle (see Figure 5-8-3).	4. Ensures that the needle will be injected into the intradermis.
5. Assist client into a comfortable position. *Forearm site:* Relax the arm with elbow and forearm extended on a flat surface. Distract client by talking about an interesting subject.	5. Relaxation minimizes discomfort. Distraction reduces anxiety.
6. Use an antiseptic swab in a circular motion to clean the skin at the site.	6. Circular motion and mechanical action of swab remove secretions containing microorganisms.
7. While holding the swab between the fingers of the nondominant hand, pull cap from needle.	7. Swab remains accessible during procedure. Prevents contamination of needle.
8. Administer injection: • With nondominant hand, stretch skin over site with forefinger and thumb. • Insert needle slowly at a 5- to 15-degree angle, bevel up, until resistance is felt; then advance to no more than 1/8 inch below the skin. The needle tip should be seen through the skin. • Slowly inject the medication. Resistance will be felt. • Note a small bleb, like a mosquito bite, forming under the skin surface (see Figure 5-8-4).	8. • Needle penetrates tight skin easier than loose skin. • Ensures needle tip is in the dermis. • Dermal layer is tight and does not expand easily when fluid is injected. • Indicates the medication was deposited in the dermis.
9. Withdraw the needle while applying gentle pressure with the antiseptic swab.	9. Supporting tissue around injection site minimizes discomfort.
10. Do not massage the site.	10. Prevents medication from being dispersed into the tissue and altering test results.

continues

Action	Rationale

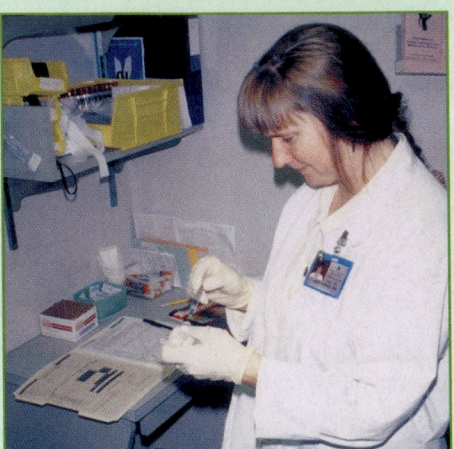

Figure 5-8-3   Select a 1/4- to 5/8-inch 25- to 27-gauge needle for the injection.

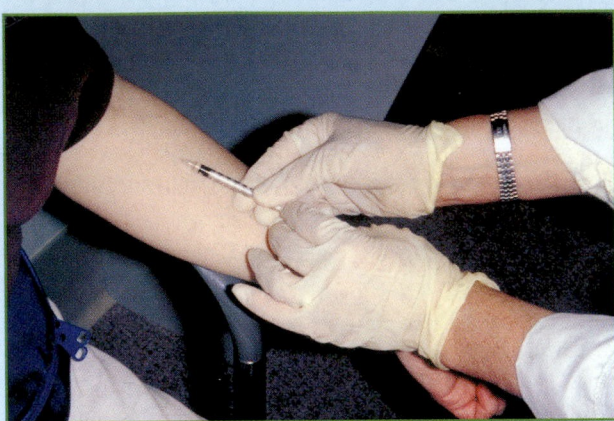

Figure 5-8-4   Note a small bleb, like a mosquito bite, forming under the skin surface as the medication is injected.

11. Assist the client to a comfortable position.	11. Promotes comfort.
12. Discard the uncapped needle and syringe in a safe receptacle.	12. Decreases risk of needle stick.
13. Remove gloves and wash hands.	13. Reduces transmission of organisms.

▶ REAL WORLD ANECDOTES

Sharon, a teenager, suddenly developed sneezing, watery eyes, and sinus congestion. Her mother thought it was allergies and took her to a doctor. Skin testing was ordered after a history and physical examination. The nurse talked with Sharon about the intradermal injections before bringing the vials and syringes into the room. It seemed that Sharon was concerned about the marks the injections might make on her skin as well as the pain. So the nurse explained that the injections would be on her forearms. She discussed ways to cover the sites, such as wearing a long-sleeved blouse, until the redness disappeared. When the nurse explained that the injection would be similar to a mosquito bite, Sharon relaxed and allowed the nurse to prepare the injection.

▶ EVALUATION

- The client experienced only minimal pain or burning at the injection site.
- The client experienced no allergic reaction or other side effects from the injection.
- The client was able to explain the significance of the presence or absence of a skin reaction.
- The client kept all follow-up appointments within the recommended time frame to have responses to the medication evaluated.

▶ DOCUMENTATION

Medication Administration Record

- Document date, time, dose, route, site of medication, and signature or initials.

Nurses' Notes

Document:
- Date and time of skin reaction
- Date and time of any systemic side effects of the medication. Report to health care provider.

Document on appropriate flow sheet or electronic medical record (EMR).

► CRITICAL THINKING SKILL

Introduction

Potent medications are used in skin testing so the dermis is used because the drug is absorbed slowly in this area of fewer blood vessels.

Possible Scenario

A bleb does not appear after an intradermal injection and a small amount of blood oozes from the site after the needle is removed.

Possible Outcome

The client test results are invalid because the drug has entered the circulation or the client experiences an anaphylactic reaction due to an IV dose of the potent drug.

Prevention

When inserting the needle into the dermis, be sure the needle meets resistance, an indication that the needle is in the dermis. When injecting, if no resistance is felt, pull the needle out, clean another site, and start again with a new syringe.

► VARIATIONS

Geriatric Variation:
- *Aging skin may be fragile. Use extra caution and guide the needle into position slowly. Apply gentle pressure when withdrawing the needle.*

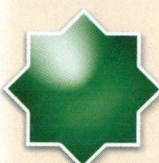

Pediatric Variations:
- *Distracting a child so he or she does not see the syringe and needle may help relieve anxiety.*
- *Lightly tap the skin before inserting the needle. This may decrease pain by focusing the child's attention on the touch rather than the needle. Be sure not to contaminate the clean site.*
- *Elicit the child's cooperation to sit still and enlist the parent's or caregiver's help to assist the child to remain still. Discuss a reward, such as a play opportunity after the injection, to elicit cooperation.*
- *Draw a rabbit, cat, or flower around the site instead of just a circle.*

Home Care Variation:
- *Clients may call the nurse to report skin reactions at various time points after the injection.*

► COMMON ERRORS

Possible Error:

The needle is inserted too deeply and no bleb forms during the injection.

Prevention:

Check placement of needle by visual inspection of the needle tip below the skin and observing the bleb formation. Remove the needle and perform the injection at another site.

continues

▶ **COMMON ERRORS** *(continued)*

Possible Error:

The needle is inserted too deeply and no bleb forms during the injection.

Prevention:

Check placement of needle by visual inspection of the needle tip below the skin and observing the bleb formation. Remove the needle and perform the injection at another site.

▶ **NURSING TIPS**

- A flat surface with a towel or cushion will provide a comfortable place for the client to rest his or her arm.
- Remember to inject the needle with the bevel up so the medication is not injected into the subcutaneous tissue.
- Remember when documenting the site of the injection to indicate left or right arm, as markings often wash off.
- Mark sites with skin marking pen, if appropriate. This avoids confusion when evaluating results.
- If a bleb or wheal does not appear after an intradermal injection, select another site and repeat injection.

▶ **SPECIAL CONSIDERATIONS**

- *The intradermal injection method is usually used in diagnostic tests such as allergy or tuberculin tests. To promote an accurate test result, choose a skin site that is not bruised or discolored.*
- *Aspiration is generally not recommended for intradermal injections; however, some health care providers may apply gentle backward pressure to plunger to verify absence of blood.*

Administering a Subcutaneous Injection

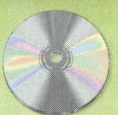

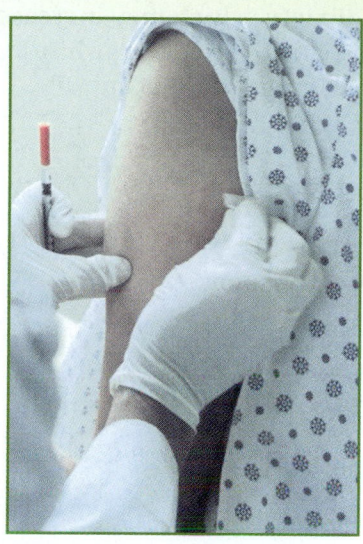

▶ OVERVIEW OF THE SKILL

A subcutaneous injection is a method used to administer medications into the loose connective tissues just below the dermis of the skin. Medications that do not need to be absorbed as quickly as those given intramuscularly are given subcutaneously because of the less richly supplied blood vessels in the subcutaneous tissue. However, the client may respond more rapidly to a subcutaneous injection than to oral medication and should be monitored for potential side effects, allergic reactions, the risk of infection, or bleeding.

Only small (0.5- to 1-mL) doses of isotonic, nonirritating, nonviscous, and water-soluble medications should be given subcutaneously, such as anticoagulants, insulin, tetanus toxoid, allergy medications, epinephrine, and vitamin B_{12}. If larger volumes of medications remain in these sensitive tissues, a sterile abscess could form, causing a hard, painful lump.

The most common sites for subcutaneous injections are the vascular areas around the outer aspect of the upper arms, the abdomen, and the anterior aspect of the thighs (see Figure 5-9-1). As these areas are easily accessible, the client may learn how to self-administer medications. Rotation of sites of injections should be observed so that no site is used more often than every 6 to 7 weeks.

For a subcutaneous injection, a 2- to 3-mL syringe or a 1-mL syringe is recommended. U-100 insulin syringes in 30-, 50-, and 100-unit sizes are used for subcutaneous insulin injections. The most commonly used needle for a subcutaneous injection is a 5/8-inch 25-gauge needle. Adjustments need to be made for pediatric, obese, or cachectic clients.

As of April 2001 a Federal Needle Stick Safety and Prevention Law requires safe medical devices. The position of the Occupational and Safety Health Act (OSHA) provides that whenever exposure to

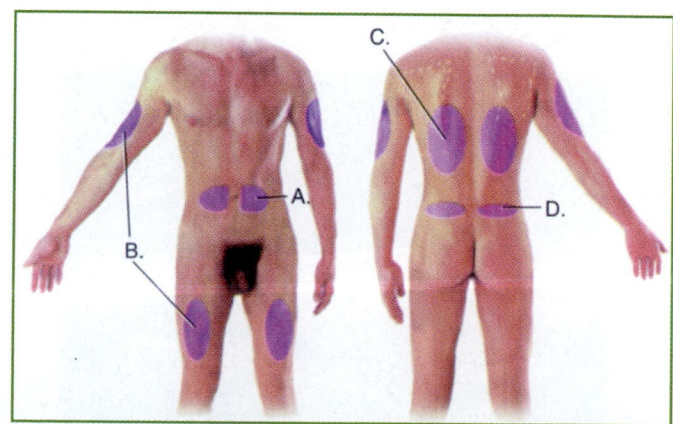

Figure 5-9-1 Subcutaneous injection sites: A. Abdomen; B. Lateral and anterior aspects of the upper arm and thigh; C. Scapular area of back; D. Upper ventrodorsal gluteal area.

blood-borne pathogens is anticipated, the use of controls to eliminate employee exposure should be used, hence, safe devices. Failure to comply with using safe devices and safe disposal can result in fines. Examples of safe devices are needle-protected or needleless systems with proper disposal in sharps containers clearly marked. In the case of subcutaneous injections, safety-syringes or needles should be used. These can be safety-glide or retraction needles or slide syringes. Instruction should be provided appropriate to the manufacturers' specifications.

▶ ASSESSMENT

1. Assess the five rights: right client, right medication, right route, right dose, and right time. **Prevents errors in medication administration.**
2. Review health care provider's order **so that the drug is administered safely and correctly.**
3. Review information regarding the drug ordered such as action, purpose, time of onset and peak action, normal dosage, common side effects, and nursing implications **to anticipate the drug's effects and anticipate a reaction.**
4. Assess client for factors that may influence an injection such as circulatory shock or reduced local tissue perfusion **as reduced tissue perfusion will interfere with the absorption and distribution of the drug.**
5. Assess for previous subcutaneous injections **in order to rotate sites and avoid repeating a dose in the same site.**
6. Assess for the indications for subcutaneous injection **as an injection is preferred for clients who are confused or unconscious, are unable to swallow a tablet, or have a gastrointestinal disturbance including the use of nasogastric suction.**

7. Assess the client's age **as older clients or pediatric clients have special needs based on their physiologic status.**
8. Assess client's knowledge regarding the medication to be received **so that client education may be tailored according to need.**
9. Assess the client's response to discussion about an injection **as some clients may express anticipatory anxiety, which may increase pain.**
10. Check the client's drug allergy history **as an allergic reaction could occur.**

▶ DIAGNOSIS

Risk for Infection

Impaired Skin Integrity

Risk for Allergic Response

Anxiety

Deficient Knowledge

Fear

▶ PLANNING

Expected Outcomes:

1. The client will experience only minimal pain or burning at the injection site.
2. The client will experience no allergic reaction or other side effects from the injection.
3. The client will be able to explain the action, side effects, dosage and schedule of the medication, and rationale for rotation of sites.

Equipment Needed (see Figures 5-9-2 and 5-9-3):

- Syringe appropriate for the medication being given
- Needle (25- to 27-gauge, 3/8 to 5/8 inch)
- Antiseptic or alcohol swabs
- Medication ampule or vial

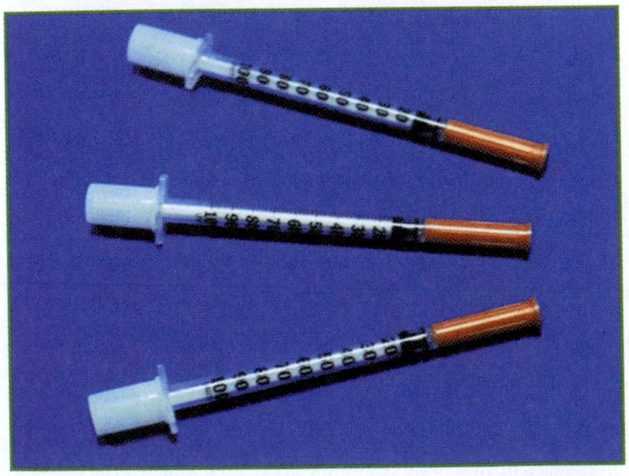

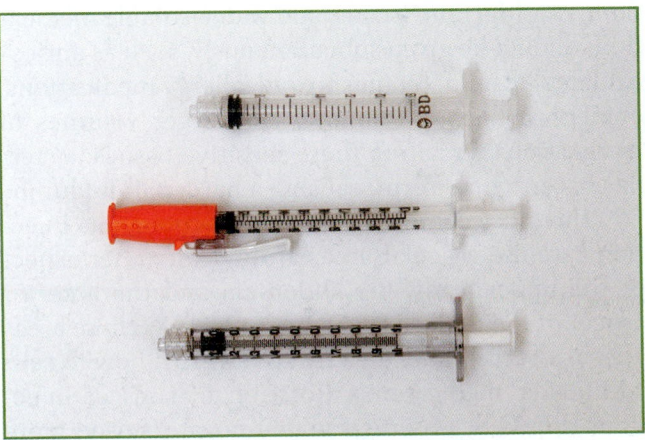

Figure 5-9-2   100-unit insulin syringes are used to administer insulin subcutaneously.

Figure 5-9-3   Syringes that may be used for a subcutaneous injection include a 3-mL syringe, an insulin syringe, and a tuberculin syringe.

- Medication record
- Disposable gloves

▶ **CLIENT EDUCATION NEEDED:**

1. Teach the client the rationale for administering the medication subcutaneously rather than orally.
2. Teach the client what to expect when receiving a subcutaneous injection.
3. Teach the client to report any bleeding, itching, pain, or other side effects as a result of the injection.
4. Instruct clients and caregivers to administer subcutaneous injections.
5. Provide the client with written, illustrated instructions on administration of a subcutaneous injection.

▶ **DELEGATION TIPS**

The skill of medication administration is not delegated to ancillary personnel in acute care settings. This may vary in state or federal institutions. Ancillary personnel are generally informed about the medications the client is receiving if adverse effects are anticipated or are being monitored.

IMPLEMENTATION—Action/Rationale

Action	Rationale
1. Wash hands and put on clean gloves.	1. Reduces the number of microorganisms.
2. Close door or curtains around bed and keep gown or sheet draped over client. Identify client.	2. Provides privacy. Ensures medication is given to the right client.
3. Select injection site (Figure 5-9-1). • Inspect skin for bruises, inflammation, edema, masses, tenderness, and sites of previous injections and avoid these areas (Figure 5-9-4). • Use subcutaneous tissue around the abdomen, lateral aspects of upper arm or thigh, or scapular area (Figure 5-9-1).	3. Injection site should be free of lesions. • Repeated daily injections should be rotated. • Avoids injury to underlying nerves, bone, or blood vessels.
4. Select needle size: • Measure the skinfold by grasping skin between thumb and forefinger. • Be sure needle is one-half the length of the skinfold from top to bottom (see Figure 5-9-5).	4. Ensures that the needle will be injected into subcutaneous tissue.
5. Assist client into a comfortable position: • Relax the arm, leg, or abdomen. • Distract client by talking about an interesting subject or explaining what you are doing step by step.	5. Relaxation minimizes discomfort. Distraction reduces anxiety.
6. Use an antiseptic swab to clean the skin at site.	6. Circular motion and mechanical action of swab remove microorganisms.
7. While holding swab between fingers of nondominant hand, pull cap from needle.	7. Swab remains accessible during procedure. Prevents contamination of needle.

continues

Action	Rationale

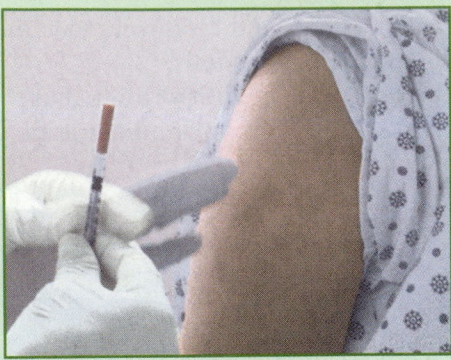

Figure 5-9-4   Select injection site. Inspect for bruises, tenderness, swelling, or other skin conditions prior to administering the injection.

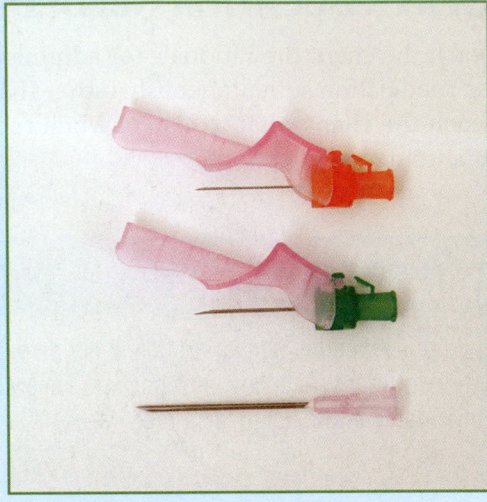

Figure 5-9-5   Different types of needles used for an injection. The needles shown have safety shields to protect against accidental needle sticks after the injection is given.

8. Administer injection:
   - Hold syringe between thumb and forefinger of dominant hand like a dart.
   - Pinch skin with nondominant hand (see Figures 5-9-6 and 5-9-7).
   - Inject needle quickly and firmly (like a dart) at a 45- to 90-degree angle (see Figure 5-9-8).

   - Release the skin.

   - Grasp the lower end of the syringe with nondominant hand and position dominant hand to the end of the plunger. Do not move the syringe.

8.
   - Quick, smooth injection is easier with proper position of syringe.
   - Needle penetrates tight skin easier than loose skin. Pinching skin elevates subcutaneous tissue.
   - Quick, firm injection minimizes discomfort. Angle depends on amount of subcutaneous tissue present and the site used.
   - Injection requires smooth manipulation of syringe parts. Movement of syringe may cause discomfort.
   - Aspiration of blood indicates intravenous placement of needle so procedure may have to be abandoned.

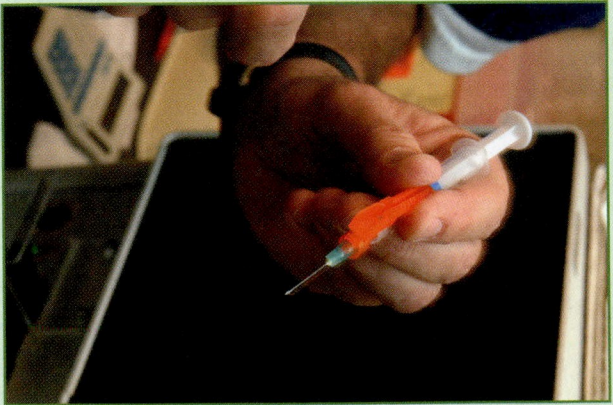

Figure 5-9-6   Hold the syringe between the thumb and forefinger of the dominant hand.

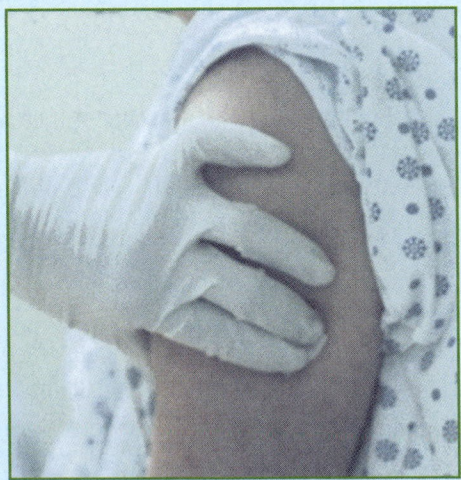

Figure 5-9-7   Pinch the skin with the nondominant hand.

continues

Action	Rationale
9. Remove hand from injection site and quickly withdraw the needle. Apply pressure with the antiseptic swab. Do not push down on the needle with the swab while withdrawing it, as this will cause more pain.	9. Supporting tissue around injection site minimizes discomfort. Removing hand before withdrawing needle reduces chance of needle stick.
10. Apply pressure. Some medications should not be massaged. Ask the pharmacy if you are unclear.	10. Stimulates circulation and improves drug distribution and absorption.
11. Discard the uncapped needle and syringe in a disposable needle receptacle (see Figure 5-9-9).	11. Promotes comfort and encourages client to remain still.
12. Assist the client to a comfortable position.	12. Decreases risk of needle stick.
13. Remove gloves and wash hands.	13. Reduces transmission of microorganisms.

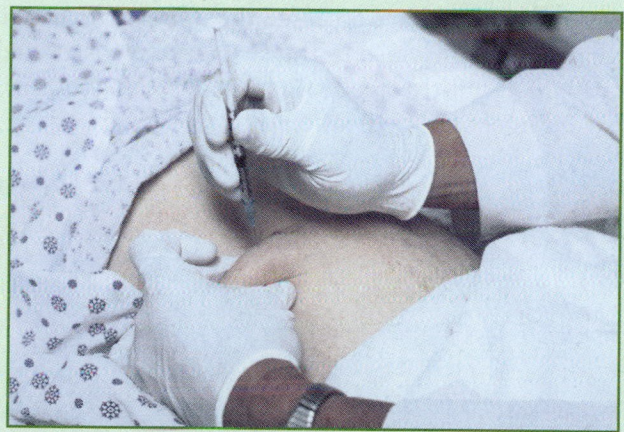

Figure 5-9-8 When injecting at a 90-degree angle, hold the syringe like a dart and pierce the skin quickly and firmly.

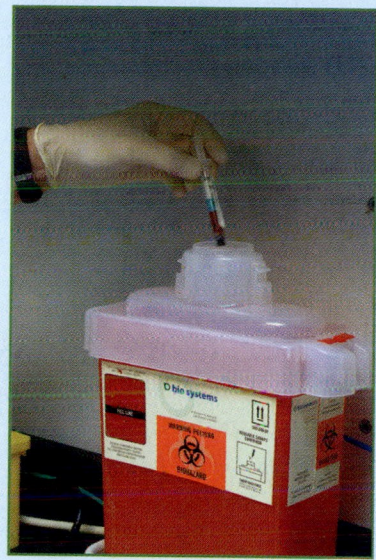

Figure 5-9-9 Dispose of the uncapped needle in the specified biohazard sharps container.

▶ REAL WORLD ANECDOTES

Dorothy was receiving chemotherapy for treatment of her breast cancer. After the first cycle of Adriamycin, cyclophosphamide, and 5-fluorouracil (5FU), her neutrophil count decreased to less than 500. She was admitted to the hospital for treatment of a presumed infection after she reported a fever of 38.5° C to her physician. In addition to IV antibiotics, Dorothy's doctor ordered subcutaneous injections of granulocyte colony-stimulating factor (G-CSF), a hematopoietic growth factor to stimulate her bone marrow to produce more neutrophils. Because she weighed over 90 kg, the daily dose was more than 2 mL, an amount of fluid too large to inject subcutaneously. Therefore, the nurse divided the dose into two syringes and gave the dose in two separate sites in Dorothy's abdomen one day and rotated the sites to each upper thigh the next day. This also enabled the nurse to teach Dorothy how to give herself the injections once she left the hospital or when she needed the medication after her next cycle of chemotherapy.

► EVALUATION

- Ask the client about pain, burning, numbness, or tingling at the injection site.
- Assess the client's response to the medication 30 minutes later.
- Ask the client to discuss the purpose, action, schedule, and side effects of the medication.

► DOCUMENTATION

Medication Administration Record

- Document the date, time, dose, route, site of injection, and signature or initials.

Nurses' Notes

- Document date and time of response to the medication.
- Document date and time of any side effects of the medication.

Document on appropriate flow sheet or electronic medical record (EMR).

► CRITICAL THINKING SKILL

Introduction

A subcutaneous injection is intended for the tissue below the skin, not a vein. It is important to check the needle position before injecting the medication.

Possible Scenario

A thin client with prominent superficial veins requires a subcutaneous injection so the nurse assesses the client for the best site. When the client states that she prefers the upper arm, the nurse honors her request and inserts the needle. When she aspirates to check for position of the needle, blood appears in the syringe.

Possible Outcome

The nurse removes the needle and syringe and applies pressure to the injection site. Then she discards the needle, medication, and syringe and prepares a new dose of the medication in another syringe. She assesses the abdomen and successfully injects the medication into subcutaneous tissue and not a vein.

Prevention

The nurse should have assessed the upper arm for the presence of veins close to the surface and instructed the client about the rationale for using the abdomen to avoid injecting medication into a vein.

► VARIATIONS

Geriatric Variations:
- *Older clients have less subcutaneous tissue and the skin is less elastic. Adjust site and angle as appropriate.*
- *Clients may have an increased need for daily subcutaneous injections such as insulin or heparin. Rotate sites.*

Pediatric Variations:
- *Distracting a child so he or she does not see the syringe and needle may help relieve anxiety.*
- *Lightly tapping the skin before inserting the needle may decrease pain by focusing the child's attention on the touch rather than the needle. Make sure not to tap the clean area, so it does not become contaminated.*
- *Demonstrate the injection procedure on a doll or teddy bear using a syringe without a needle.*
- *A parent or another caregiver may be needed to help hold the child for a safe procedure.*

Home Care Variation:
- *A safe method of disposing of needles and syringes should be maintained, especially if children or animals are present.*

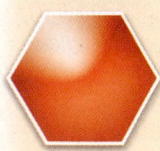

Long-Term Care Variations:
- *Clients who receive subcutaneous injections over long-term periods should be taught to rotate injection sites to prevent the buildup of scar tissue and poor absorption at any one site.*
- *Periodically reassess the client's injection technique. Over the long-term, clients can become careless with technique. Be sure the client continues to use the proper technique.*

► **COMMON ERRORS**

Possible Error:

The needle hits a bone when the nurse inserts it.

Prevention:

The client should be assessed for a suitable needle length and gauge according to weight and skinfold measurement. Remove the needle. Reassess the client and choose an appropriate needle. Change needles and reinsert.

Possible Error:

After inserting the needle, the client jerks and the syringe moves in the nurse's hand, causing pain to the client.

Prevention:

Tell the client when you are going to insert the needle and keep a hand on the syringe at all times. Reassure the client. Hold the syringe firmly. Support the tissue around the needle with the alcohol swab.

► **NURSING TIPS**

- A simple rule to follow: If 2 inches of tissue can be grasped, the needle should be inserted at a 90-degree angle. If 1 inch of tissue can be grasped, the needle should be inserted at a 45-degree angle.
- Do not push a needle through the skin; insert it quickly and smoothly.
- Divert the client's attention by engaging in conversation.
- Use an alcohol swab to stabilize the skin around the needle while removing it to reduce pulling of the tissue.
- Keep an anatomic chart with the medication record to document the sites used.

► **SPECIAL CONSIDERATIONS**

- *If a client receives a subcutaneous injection routinely, prevent repeated trauma to the tissue by alternating the site each time the injection is given. Create a chart or grid pattern to identify rotation sites.*
- *Aspirating for signs of blood prior to administering the injection may be adopted as part of the procedure to prevent the medication from accidentally entering the bloodstream and causing irritation, allergic reaction, or shock. Check the institutional policy for guidelines.*

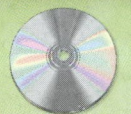

Administering an Intramuscular Injection

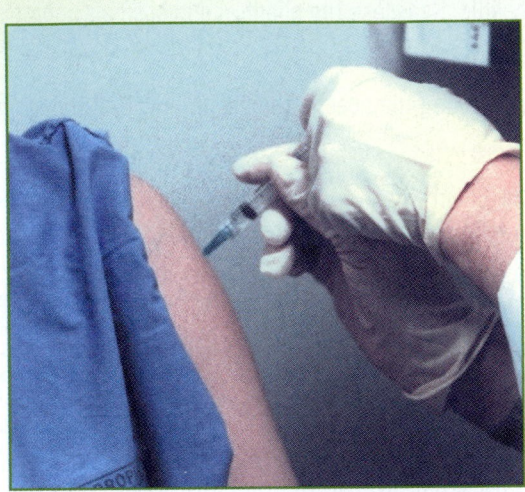

► OVERVIEW OF THE SKILL

An intramuscular injection is a method used to administer medications into the deep muscle tissue. Medications will be absorbed quickly because of the richly supplied blood vessels in the muscle. Most aqueous medications are absorbed in 10 to 30 minutes. Average-sized adults can tolerate up to 3 mL of medication injected into a large muscle because muscle is less sensitive to irritating and viscous drugs than subcutaneous tissue.

The most common sites for intramuscular injections are the vastus lateralis, the ventrogluteal, the dorsogluteal, and the deltoid muscles (see Figure 5-10-1). The vastus lateralis muscle is located on the anterior lateral aspect of the thigh. This easily accessible site is the preferred site for clients of all ages as it has no major blood vessels or nerves nearby. The ventrogluteal site is the preferred site in adults because it is located deep and away from major blood vessels and nerves. It is preferred over the dorsolateral for the following reasons: there is less risk of damage to the sciatic nerve and blood vessels and this site is less painful as the muscle is most often not tense even in an anxious client. The dorsogluteal muscle in the upper outer quadrant of the buttock poses greater risk of damage to the sciatic nerve, major blood vessels, and the greater trochanter bone. It should not be used in children younger than

5 years of age as this muscle is not developed. The deltoid muscle is found on the upper arm about 1 to 2 inches below the acromion process. Major nerves and blood vessels are beneath this site and only small volumes of medication should be injected.

There are many different types and sizes of syringes. For intramuscular injections, the basic syringe, consisting of a barrel with plunger and tip of syringe where a needle can be attached, can be used. The needle's hub screws into the tip of the syringe and the needle's hollow shaft ends at a beveled point. Prefilled syringes that consist of a prefilled barrel and needle assembly placed in a reusable plunger are often used (see Figure 5-10-2). For an intramuscular injection, a 2- to 3-mL syringe is recommended with a 1-1/4- to 1-1/2-inch, 19- to 23-gauge needle. Adjustments need to be made for pediatric, obese, or cachectic clients.

As of April 2001 a Federal Needle Stick Safety and Prevention Law requires safe medical devices. The position of the Occupational and Safety Health Act (OSHA) provides that whenever exposure to blood-borne pathogens is anticipated, the use of controls to eliminate employee exposure should be used, hence, safe devices. Failure to comply with using safe devices and safe disposal can result in fines. Examples of safe devices are needle-protected or needleless systems with proper disposal in sharps containers clearly marked. With intramuscular injections, safety-syringes or needles should be used. These can be safety-glide or retraction needles

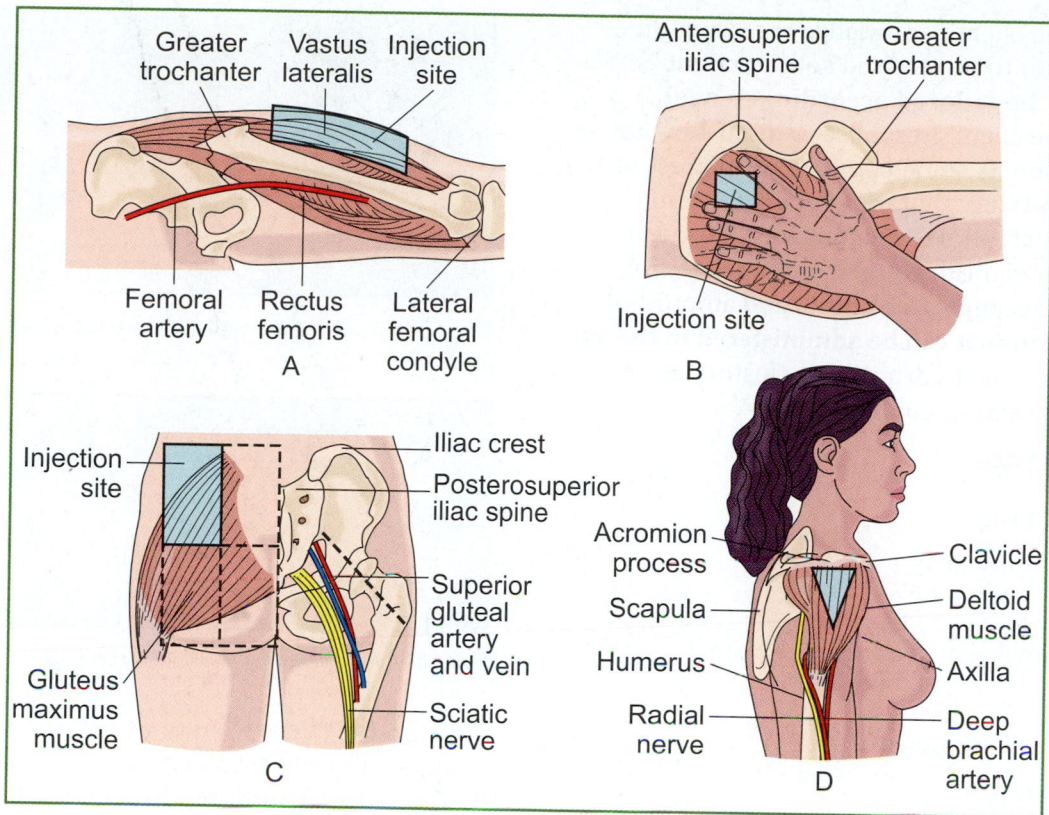

Figure 5-10-1 Intramuscular injection sites. A. Vastus lateralis: Identify greater trochanter; place hand at lateral femoral condyle; injection site is middle third of anterior lateral aspect. B. Ventrogluteal: Place palm of left hand on right greater trochanter so that index finger points toward anterosuperior iliac spine; spread first and middle fingers to form a V; injection site is the middle of the V angle. C. Dorsogluteal: Place hand on iliac crest and locate the posterosuperior iliac spine. Draw an imaginary line between the trochanter and the iliac spine; the injection site is the outer quadrant. D. Deltoid: Locate the lateral side of the humerus from two to three finger widths below the acromion process in adults or one finger width below the acromion process in children.

or slide syringes. Instruction should be provided appropriate to the manufacturers' specifications.

▶ ASSESSMENT

1. Assess the five rights: right client, right medication, right route, right dose, and right time. **Prevents errors in medication administration.**
2. Review health care provider's order **so that the drug is administered safely and correctly.**
3. Review information regarding the drug ordered such as action, purpose, time of onset and peak

action, normal dosage, common side effects, and nursing implications **to anticipate the drug's effects and to anticipate a reaction.**

4. Assess the client for factors that may influence an injection, such as circulatory shock, reduced local tissue perfusion, or muscle atrophy **as reduced tissue perfusion will interfere with the absorption and distribution of the drug.**
5. Assess for previous intramuscular injections **to rotate sites and avoid repeating a dose in the same site.**
6. Assess for the indications for intramuscular injection **as an injection is preferred for clients who require the fast action of the medication, are confused or unconscious, are unable to swallow a tablet, or have a gastrointestinal disturbance including the use of nasogastric suction.**
7. Assess the client's age **as older clients or pediatric clients have special needs based on their physiologic status.**

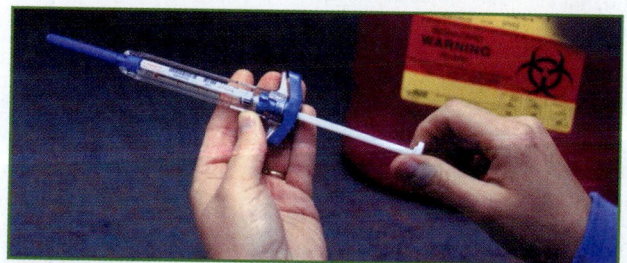

Figure 5-10-2 A prefilled syringe consists of a prefilled barrel and needle assembly placed in a reusable plunger.

8. Assess the client's knowledge regarding the medication to be received **so that client education may be tailored according to need.**

9. Assess the client's response to discussion about an injection **as some clients may express anticipatory anxiety that may increase pain.**

10. Assess the client's size and muscle development. **Assists in identification of appropriate site, needle size, angle to be used, and amount of medication that can be administered in the site.**

11. Check the client's drug allergy history **as an allergic reaction could occur.**

▶ DIAGNOSIS

Risk for Infection

Impaired Skin Integrity

Anxiety

Deficient Knowledge

Fear

Risk for Allergic Response

▶ PLANNING

Expected Outcomes:

1. The client will experience only minimal pain or burning at the injection site.
2. The client will experience no allergic reaction or other side effects from the injection.
3. The client will be able to explain the action, side effects, dosage, and schedule of the medication.

Equipment Needed (see Figures 5-10-3 and 5-10-4):

- Safety-syringe (1- to 3-mL)
- Safety-needle (19- to 23-gauge, 1-1/4- to 1-1/2-inches)
- Antiseptic or alcohol swabs
- Medication ampule or vial
- Medication record
- Disposable gloves

▶ CLIENT EDUCATION NEEDED:

1. Teach the client the rationale for administering the medication intramuscularly rather than orally.

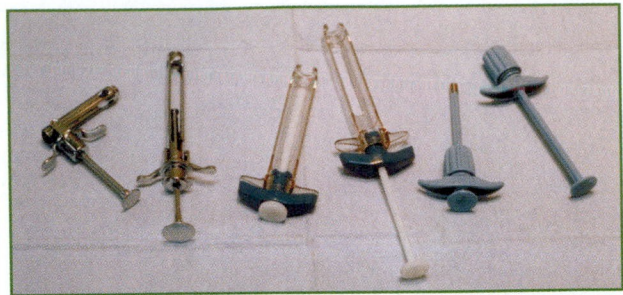
Figure 5-10-3   There are many types of prefilled syringe plungers in use today.

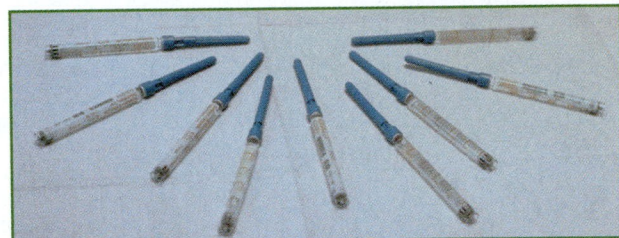
Figure 5-10-4   Prefilled barrel and needle cartridges.

2. Teach the client what to expect when receiving an intramuscular injection.
3. Teach the client to report any bleeding, itching, pain, or other side effects as a result of the injection.
4. Instruct the client who has allergies to be sure to wear a bracelet stating what he or she is allergic to.
5. Teach clients who require regular injections to record how they rotate the sites.
6. Instruct clients and caregivers to observe injection sites for complications and side effects of medications.
7. Teach clients and caregivers to administer intramuscular injections.
8. Provide written, illustrated instructions on administration of an intramuscular injection.

Estimated time to complete the skill:
5–10 minutes

▶ DELEGATION TIPS

The skill of medication administration is not delegated to ancillary personnel in acute care settings. This may vary in state or federal institutions. Ancillary personnel are generally informed about the medications the client is receiving if adverse affects are anticipated or are being monitored.

IMPLEMENTATION—Action/Rationale

Action	Rationale
1. Wash hands and put on clean gloves.	1. Reduces the number of microorganisms.
2. Close door or curtains around bed and keep gown or sheet draped over client. Identify client.	2. Provides privacy. Ensures medication is given to the right client.
3. Select injection site (Figure 5-10-1). • Inspect skin for bruises, inflammation, edema, masses, tenderness, and sites of previous injections. • Use anatomic landmarks.	3. Injection site should be free of lesions. • Repeated daily injections should be rotated. • Avoids injury to underlying nerves, bone, or blood vessels. Site should be selected based on muscle development, type and amount of medication, and comfortable access to site.
4. Select needle size: Assess size and weight of client and site to be used.	4. Ensures that needle will be injected into the muscle.
5. Assist client into a comfortable position: • For vastus lateralis, lying flat or supine with knee slightly flexed. • For ventrogluteal, lying on side or back with knee and hip slightly flexed. • For dorsogluteal, lying prone with feet turned inward or on side with upper knee and hip flexed and placed in front of lower leg. • For deltoid, standing with arm relaxed at side or sitting with lower arm relaxed on lap or lying flat with lower arm relaxed across abdomen (see Figure 5-10-5). • Distract client by talking about an interesting subject.	5. Relaxation minimizes discomfort. Distraction reduces anxiety.
6. Use antiseptic swab to clean skin at site.	6. Circular motion and mechanical action of swab remove secretions containing microorganisms.
7. While holding swab between fingers of nondominant hand, pull cap from needle.	7. Swab remains accessible during procedure. Prevents contamination of needle.
8. Administer injection: • Hold syringe between thumb and forefinger of dominant hand like a dart (see Figure 5-10-6). • Spread skin tightly or pinch a generous section of tissue firmly—for cachectic clients. • Inject needle quickly and firmly (like a dart) at a 90-degree angle (see Figure 5-10-7). • Release the skin. • Grasp the lower end of the syringe with nondominant hand and position dominant hand to the end of the plunger. Do not move the syringe.	8. • A quick, smooth injection is easier with proper positioning of the syringe. • Needle penetrates tight skin more easily than loose skin. • Quick, firm injection minimizes discomfort. • Injection requires smooth manipulation of syringe parts. Movement of syringe may cause discomfort.

continues

Action	Rationale

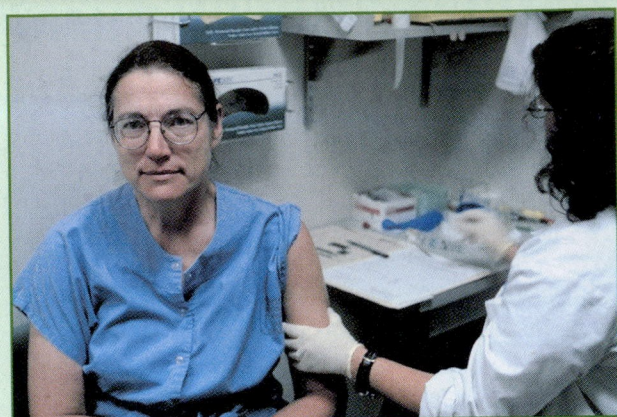

Figure 5-10-5 Have the client stand or sit with arm relaxed at side.

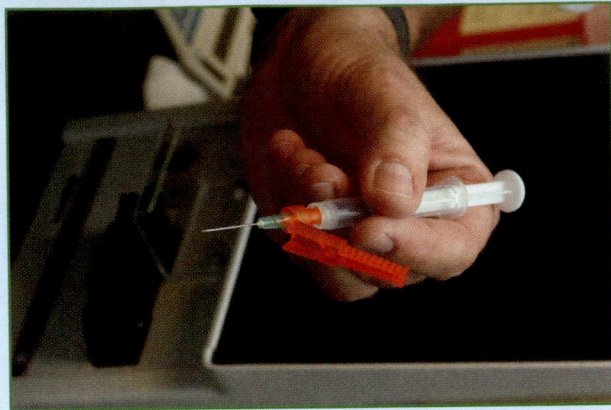

Figure 5-10-6 Hold the syringe between the thumb and forefinger of the dominant hand.

- Pull back on the plunger and aspirate to ascertain if needle is in a vein. If no blood appears, slowly inject the medication.

9. Remove nondominant hand and quickly withdraw the needle. Apply pressure with the antiseptic swab.

10. Apply pressure. Certain protocols suggest gentle massage action.

- Aspiration of blood indicates intravenous placement of needle so procedure may have to be abandoned.

9. Supporting tissue around injection site minimizes discomfort. Removing hand prior to withdrawing needle prevents needle stick.

10. Pressure prevents medication from leaking out of site. Gentle massage stimulates circulation and improves drug distribution and absorption.

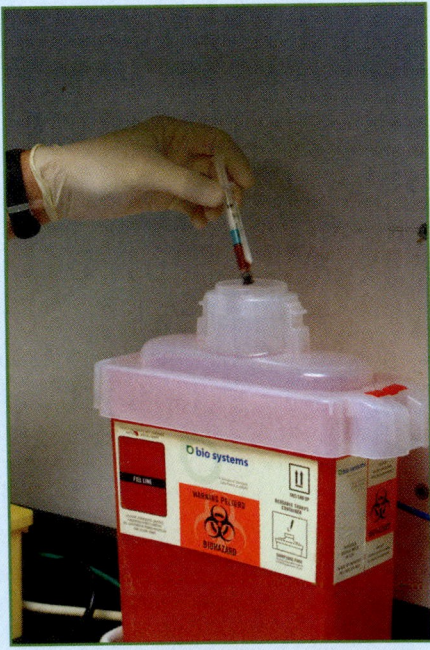

Figure 5-10-8 Dispose of the uncapped needle in the specified biohazard sharps container.

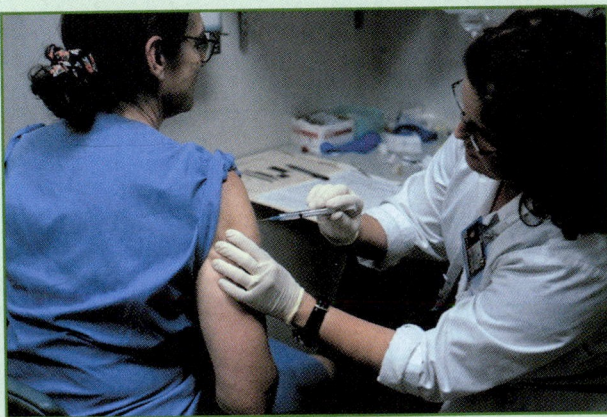

Figure 5-10-7 Inject needle quickly and firmly at a 90-degree angle.

Action	Rationale
11. Discard the uncapped needle and syringe in a specified biohazard sharps container (see Figure 5-10-8).	**11.** Decreases risk of needle stick.
12. Assist the client to a comfortable position.	**12.** Promotes comfort.
13. Remove gloves and wash hands.	**13.** Reduces transmission of microorganisms.

▶ REAL WORLD ANECDOTES

Mr. Germeau was to receive an IM injection of Demerol. The nurse carefully located the landmarks on Mr. Germeau's ventrogluteal site. She held her nondominant hand on Mr. Germeau's hip to mark the site as she inserted the needle, dart-like, into the muscle. Unfortunately, she darted the needle through the skin between her fingers as she darted the needle into Mr. Germeau's hip. While maintaining a straight face, the nurse injected the Demerol and withdrew the needle from his hip and her hand. Making sure Mr. Germeau was safe, the nurse proceeded to the sink to wash her hands and stem the bleeding from her nondominant hand. Once she had stopped the bleeding, she made sure Mr. Germeau was comfortable and proceeded to the nurses' station where she cleaned and dressed the injury and filled out an incident report.

▶ EVALUATION

- Ask the client about any pain, burning, numbness, or tingling at the injection site.
- Assess the client's response to the medication 10 to 30 minutes later.
- Ask the client to discuss the purpose, action, schedule, and side effects of the medication.

▶ DOCUMENTATION

Medication Administration Record

Document:
- Name of medication
- Dosage
- Route of administration
- Location of injection
- Time administered
- Initials and signature of nurse administering medication

Nurses' Notes

- Time and type of client complaint
- Medication administered
- Outcome of treatment (client response)
- Nurse's signature

Document on appropriate flow sheet or electronic medical record (EMR).

▶ CRITICAL THINKING SKILL

Introduction

The deltoid muscle is easily accessible, although not well developed in some adults and older clients. It may be difficult to avoid the nerves and blood vessels underlying the muscle.

Possible Scenario

A young woman injured in a car accident has a fractured pelvis and is in a knee-to-chest body cast. She has recovered from her acute injuries and no longer needs an IV, but she still requires IM injections of pain medication.

Possible Outcome

The only available muscle for an IM injection is the deltoid, so the nurse assesses her muscle and finds it is not well developed. She knows that pain medications are available in different concentrations. She draws up the dose of medication equal to 1.5 mL and injects it into the deltoid muscle.

Prevention

The only site for an IM injection was assessed and a suitable amount of medication was administered.

► VARIATIONS

Geriatric Variations:
- *Older clients who have had a cerebrovascular accident may have muscle atrophy.*
- *Elderly clients may require shorter and smaller gauged needles because of muscle atrophy.*
- *Older clients should receive no more than 2 mL of medication.*

Pediatric Variations:
- *No more than 1 mL of medication should be injected into the muscle of a small child. Small infants should not be given more than 0.5 mL IM.*
- *A tuberculin syringe and a 1/2- to 1-inch, 25- to 27-gauge needle are more appropriate for infants who require small doses of medications.*
- *Distracting a child so he or she does not see the syringe and needle may help relieve anxiety.*
- *Lightly tapping the skin before inserting the needle may decrease pain by focusing the child's attention on the touch rather than the needle.*
- *Parents can comfort their child after an injection.*
- *Band-Aids with cartoon pictures help soothe a child after an injection.*
- *Assistance may be required to help the child hold still.*

Home Care Variation:
- *Clients need an approved method of discarding needles and syringes when giving injections at home.*

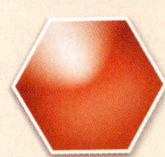

Long-Term Care Variation:
- *If the client requires routine doses of IM medication, be sure to rotate the sites to prevent tissue damage and poor absorption of the medication.*
- *Reassess the client's need for ongoing IM medications regularly. It may be more appropriate to deliver the medication via a different route.*

► COMMON ERRORS

Possible Error:

When the elderly, obese client turned on her side for an IM injection into her dorsogluteal muscle, the nurse could not identify the landmarks for the site.

Prevention:

Use the vastus lateralis muscle as it is accessible, safe, and easy to assess for correct injection site. Ask the client to turn onto her back and flex her knee slightly. Reassure her that an injection in her leg will be no more painful than in her buttock.

Possible Error:

The nurse felt the needle tip hit a bone when she gave an intramuscular injection in the dorsolateral muscle.

Prevention:

Assess the client for size and weight in order to select the most appropriate site. Be sure the needle length is also suitable for the client's weight. Pull back on the needle, then pull back on the plunger, to see if the needle is in a vein. If not, inject the medication.

► **NURSING TIPS**

- Avoid giving an injection into atrophied muscles as they absorb medication poorly.
- Do not push a needle through the skin; insert it quickly and smoothly.
- Divert the client's attention by engaging in conversation.

- Use an alcohol swab to stabilize the skin around the needle while removing it to reduce pulling of the tissue.
- Keep an anatomic chart with the medication record to document the sites used.

► **SPECIAL CONSIDERATIONS**

- Avoid administering the injection at sites that are close to a nerve. Be alert for signs such as shooting pain or numbness. Stop injection if client complains of shooting pain or numbness and report to the health care provider or supervisor.
- To avoid tissue irritation from the injected medication, gently rub the injection site. Massaging the injection site promotes local circulation and facilitates absorption of the medication.
- Air locks may be used with irritating medications. The air lock technique clears medication from the needle after injection and, therefore, prevents leaking into the subcutaneous muscle. Generally 0.2 mL of air ensures an air lock. Adjust medication accordingly.
- When a prefilled syringe contains a controlled substance, the wasting of the drug must be witnessed and documented according to institutional policy.
- When locating landmarks for intramuscular injections, inform clients of actions. When feeling for anatomic landmarks, such as in the ventrogluteal sites, clients may be alarmed that the injection site is close to the bones.
- The amount of medication that can be administered in a site is limited by the client's muscle development. If large amounts are to be given it is better to divide it into two different sites.

Administering Medication via Z-Track Injection

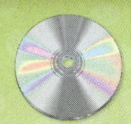

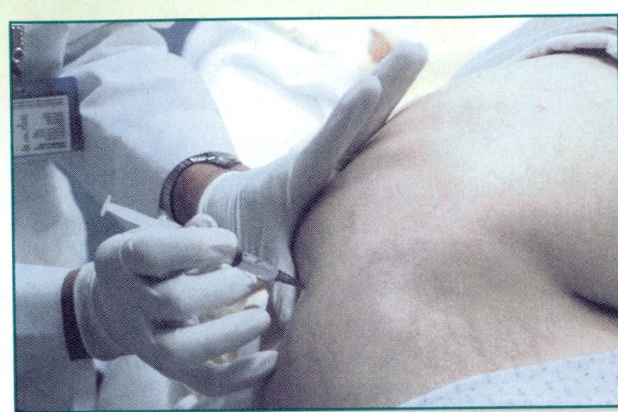

▶ OVERVIEW OF THE SKILL

Originally, the Z-track method of intramuscular injections was used as a special procedure for only certain medications. Medications such as iron dextran and hydralazine hydrochloride can be irritating to the tissues and stain the skin. Using the Z-track method prevents potentially irritating medications from being tracked up through the tissues by interrupting the injection tract. This method can also help reduce pain with nonstaining or irritating substances.

As of April 2001 a Federal Needle Stick Safety and Prevention Law requires safe medical devices. The position of the Occupational and Safety Health Act (OSHA) provides that whenever exposure to blood-borne pathogens is anticipated, the use of controls to eliminate employee exposure should be used, hence, safe devices. Failure to comply with using safe devices and safe disposal can result in fines. Examples of safe devices are needle-protected or needleless systems with proper disposal in sharps containers clearly marked. With intramuscular injections, safety-syringes or needles should be used. These can be safety-glide or retraction needles or slide syringes. Instruction should be provided appropriate to manufacturers' specifications.

▶ ASSESSMENT

1. Assess the five rights: right client, right medication, right route, right dose, and right time. **Prevents errors in medication administration.**

2. Assess the client's understanding of the proposed injection. **Allows the nurse to provide education and support as needs are identified.**

3. Verify the health care provider's order. **Ensures appropriate medication, route, dose, side effects, time of onset and peak action, and nursing implications. This allows the nurse to anticipate effects of the drug and to observe the client's response.**

4. Consider the appropriateness of the therapy. If the medication is a narcotic, how has the client responded to intramuscular narcotics in the past? **Knowing what dose and medication have been effective in the past for this client will enable the nurse to be a better client advocate.**

5. Replace any missing or faded identification bracelets. **Identification bracelets provide positive client information.**

6. Check the client's drug allergy history **as an allergic reaction could occur.**

▶ DIAGNOSIS

Risk for Allergic Response

Risk for Infection

Impaired Skin Integrity

Anxiety

Deficient Knowledge

Fear

▶ PLANNING

Expected Outcomes:

1. The correct client will receive the correct medication.
2. The client will not experience pain or skin staining secondary to the medication.
3. The client will obtain the expected benefit from the medication.
4. The client will not experience an allergic response.

Equipment Needed (see Figures 5-11-1 A, B, and C):

- Syringe with larger-bore needle for drawing up the medication
- Safety-needle to place on syringe for client injection
- Alcohol swab
- Medication
- Medication administration record (MAR)

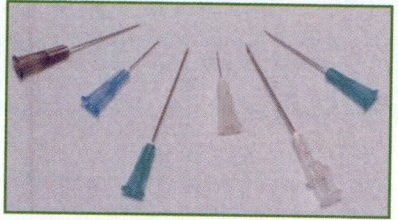

Figure 5-11-1B Select the correct gauge and length of needle for the size of the client and the type of medication being administered.

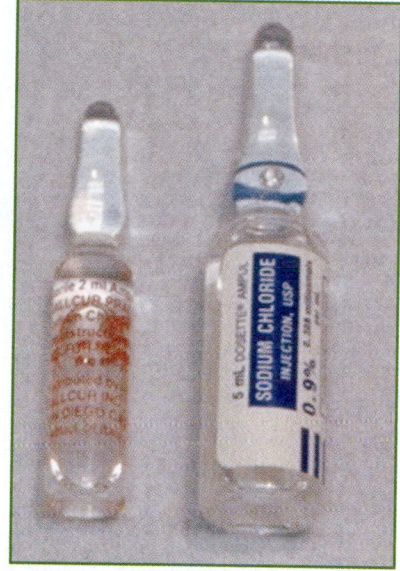

Figure 5-11-1C Medication ampules.

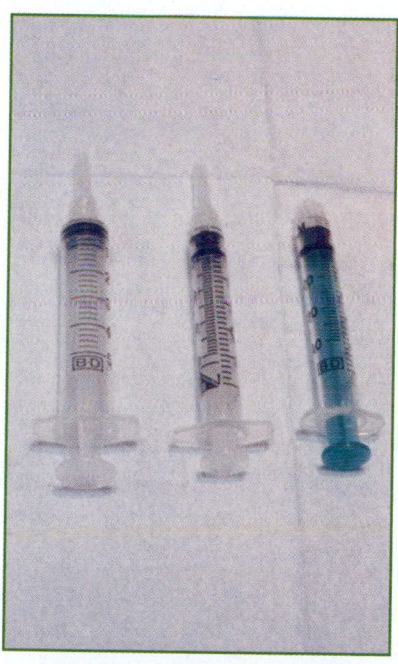

Figure 5-11-1A Various sizes of syringes. Select the appropriate syringe for the amount of medication being administered.

▶ CLIENT EDUCATION NEEDED:

1. Instruct client on appropriate positioning to maximize comfort during the procedure.
2. Explain the purpose of the injection and probable side effects and duration.

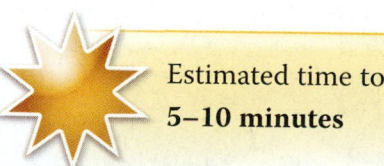

Estimated time to complete the skill: **5–10 minutes**

▶ DELEGATION TIPS

The skill of medication administration is not delegated to ancillary personnel in acute care settings. This may vary in state or federal institutions. Ancillary personnel are generally informed about the medications the client is receiving if adverse effects are anticipated or are being monitored.

IMPLEMENTATION—Action/Rationale

Action	Rationale
1. Wash hands.	1. Reduces the transmission of microorganisms.
2. Assess the client for knowledge of planned injection.	2. Decreases client anxiety.
3. Check the MAR against the health care provider's order.	3. Ensures accuracy in the administration of the medication.
4. Check for drug allergies.	4. Decreases risk of allergic reactions such as hives, urticaria, or anaphylactic shock.
5. Prepare the medication for only one client at a time.	5. Ensures that the right client receives the right medication.
6. Select the correct medication and double check against the MAR.	6. Increases accuracy and decreases potential errors.
7. Calculate the medication dose, if necessary.	7. Determines the correct amount of medication to be given.
8. With the syringe at eye level, draw up the medication with a large-bore needle. Remove the large-bore needle and replace it with a needle of the appropriate size and length for the client (see Figure 5-11-2).	8. Syringe at eye level increases precision. Changing the needle prevents introducing any potentially irritating medication into the client.
9. Create an air lock. Add 0.1 to 0.2 mL of air to the dose in the syringe. The air will push the medication out of the needle when the last of the medication has been injected (see Figure 5-11-3).	9. The injected medication is followed by air to clear the medication from the needle.
10. Identify client. Locate the appropriate injection site (see Figure 5-11-4). • *Quadriceps:* For children younger than 3 years of age • *Dorsogluteal:* For adults while lying prone with the feet internally rotated • *Ventrogluteal:* Desirable site for all ages • *Deltoid:* Use only for small volumes of fluid	10. Ensures medication is given to the right client. Selecting the most appropriate injection site for an IM shot is a critical factor. A large, healthy muscle should always be used. If client is receiving multiple injections, the injection site should be rotated. Rotating the injection site avoids overuse and muscle irritation.

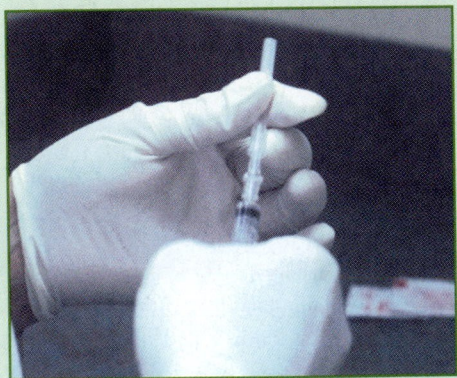

Figure 5-11-2   Replace the large-bore needle with a needle of appropriate size and length for the client.

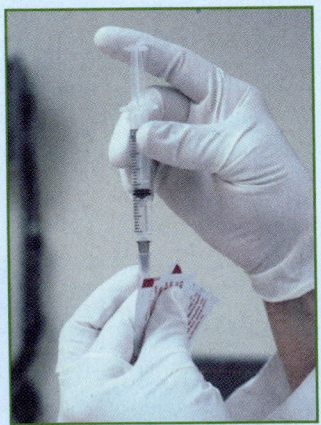

Figure 5-11-3   Add 0.1 to 0.2 mL of air to the medication in the syringe.

continues

Action	Rationale

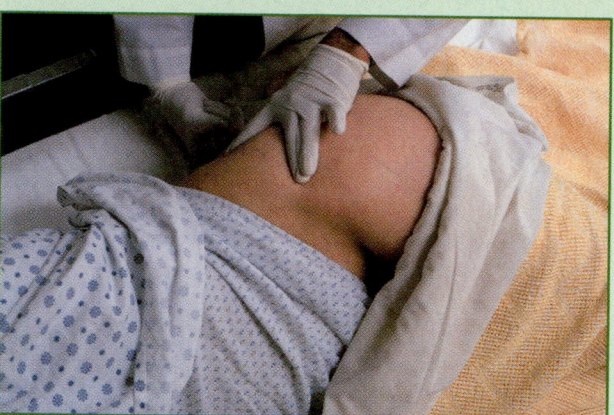

Figure 5-11-4 Locate the appropriate injection site for the Z-track injection.

11. Wash your hands using an antibacterial soap.

11. Decreases the potential of equipment and client contamination.

12. Clean the injection site thoroughly and allow it to dry.

12. The mechanical action of cleaning along with the alcohol at the injection site helps reduce microflora and decreases the potential of introducing pathogens into the client's tissue. Alcohol can cause skin irritation and burning if the skin is not allowed to dry before injection.

13. Using your nondominant hand, pull the skin and subcutaneous tissue to the side or downward about an inch.

13. Pulling the tissue to the side or downward prior to the injection will break the injection track after removing the needle and not allow the medication to track back up to the surface of the skin. Also, by pulling the tissue tight, the skin becomes firm and facilitates entry of the needle.

14. Using sterile technique, remove the needle guard using your nondominant hand.

14. Ensures the needle is not contaminated with microorganisms.

15. While maintaining traction on the skin, using your dominant hand, dart the needle into the skin at a 90° angle.

15. Darting the needle is more comfortable for the client. A 90° angle will ensure the needle reaches muscle tissue and is not trapped in the subcutaneous or adipose tissue.

16. Aspirate for a minimum of 5 seconds. Observe for a blood return.

16. Blood from small vessels can take up to 5 seconds to appear in the syringe.

17. If no blood return is present, slowly (at a rate of 1 mL/ 10 seconds) inject the medication.

17. Allows the medication to diffuse, causing less stretch on the muscle fibers and thus is better tolerated by the client.

18. If injecting iron dextran or other irritating substance, allow the needle to stay in place for 10 seconds after the medication is injected.

18. Allows the medication to diffuse before the needle is removed, which decreases the chance that any medication will be tracked back up through the skin.

19. While still maintaining traction on the skin with the nondominant hand, smoothly remove the needle and allow the skin to slide over the now-interrupted injection track.

19. Holding traction on the tissue prevents any irritation caused by the needle being removed. Allowing the tissue to slide over the track seals the track and does not allow any medication to penetrate the skin surface.

continues

Action	Rationale

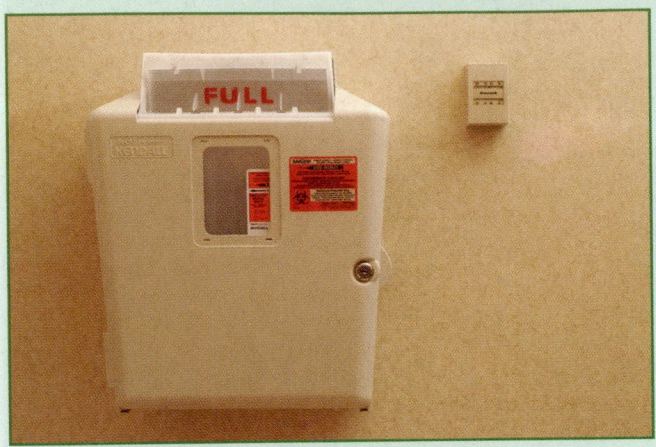

Figure 5-11-5   Dispose of the uncapped needle in the specified biohazard sharps container.

20. Do not rub or wipe the skin after removal of the needle.

20. This can cause seepage of the medication back to the surface and result in irritation.

21. Dispose of needle in an appropriate biohazard sharps container (see Figure 5-11-5).

21. Avoids needle sticks to self and colleagues.

22. Wash hands.

22. Reduces the transmission of microorganisms.

► REAL WORLD ANECDOTES

Mr. Arango had just returned postoperative from a lumbar laminectomy. He was supine in bed and complaining of severe back pain. Dr. Bowden ordered 100 mg of meperidine IM now. Nurse Kennedy knew that 100 mg of meperidine comes in a prefilled syringe of 2 mL. She also knew that she should not inject this large volume into the client's deltoid. The ventrogluteal site was ideal. This way Mr. Arango would not have to roll over, and the ventrogluteal was the ideal site for this large volume of meperidine. To increase client comfort, she gave the injection by Z-track.

► EVALUATION

- The correct client received the correct medication.
- The client did not experience pain or skin staining secondary to the medication.
- The client obtained the expected benefit from the medication.

► DOCUMENTATION

Medication Administration Record

- Document the date, time, medication, and dose.
- Record the injection site used.

Nurses' Notes

- Document the efficacy of the medication.
- Note any unusual findings.

Document on appropriate flow chart or electronic medical record (EMR).

► CRITICAL THINKING SKILL

Introduction

Dr. Smith orders a dose of an experimental medication for Mr. Kane. The medication comes with a package insert stating that the medication can be irritating to the skin; in addition it has been known to cause staining.

Possible Scenario

The nurse consults the pharmacist in regard to this medication to find out more information. The pharmacist says that this medication has been known to cause irritation and discoloration and to be very careful with its administration.

Possible Outcome

The nurse gives the medication in the ventrogluteal site with a 1-1/2-inch needle, via Z-track method. The client tolerates the procedure well and suffers no irritation or skin staining.

Prevention

Be familiar with any medication you are giving. The Z-track method is usually the preferred method for intramuscular administration.

▶ VARIATIONS

Geriatric Variation:
- *The ventrogluteal site is a preferred site for clients who are elderly and may have muscle wasting. It avoids the risk of injuring the sciatic nerve and is less painful.*

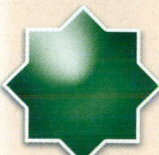

Pediatric Variations:
- *Adjust the needle size to the size of the child. Inspect and palpate the site prior to injection. The goal is to deliver the medication deep within a large muscle mass and to seal the medication into the muscle using the Z-track technique.*
- *The vastus lateralis site is usually used for children and infants.*
- *The dorsogluteal site should not be used for a child younger than 3 years of age.*

Home Care Variations:
- *Assess that the caregiver knows all the possible sites for Z-track administration and is comfortable rotating sites to decrease the impact of repeated injections at any one site.*
- *The vastus lateralis site is the most accessible for self-injections using the Z-track method.*

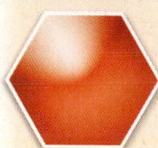

Long-Term Care Variations:
- *Set up a schedule for rotating sites to decrease the impact of repeated injections at any one site.*
- *Avoid injections into any site that shows bruising, swelling, or tenderness. Let it heal.*

▶ COMMON ERRORS

Possible Error:

Not using the correct length of needle.

Prevention:

Assess the site carefully, including the size and weight of the person. Visualize where the medication needs to go prior to selecting the needle.

Possible Error:

Letting go of the subcutaneous tissue before the needle is completely removed.

continues

> **COMMON ERRORS** (continued)

Prevention:

Watch carefully, and remember to hold the skin in the correct position until after the needle is out. Do not be in a hurry.

Possible Error:

Not palpating landmarks prior to injection.

Prevention:

Remember not to get overconfident, especially when repeating injections on the same client. Palpating landmarks prior to injection is a "must do" for every injection, every time.

Possible Error:

Attempting to give too large a volume in one shot.

Prevention:

If the volume to be administered is at or exceeds the recommended amount, either divide the amount into two injections or select a different dosage strength.

> **NURSING TIPS**

- Practice injecting the ventrogluteal site and become comfortable with it.
- Use the Z-track method routinely.

- Palpate your landmarks. Do not just visualize them.
- At times the medication itself causes pain for the client. Giving the medication slowly will decrease the client's discomfort.

> **SPECIAL CONSIDERATIONS**

- *The Z-track injection method can be used in most intramuscular injection sites, thereby decreasing the chance of bruising the site. Combining the methods of Z-track injection with air-lock injection technique is a good approach to decrease medication irritation at the injected site.*

Withdrawing Medication from a Vial

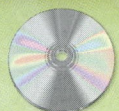

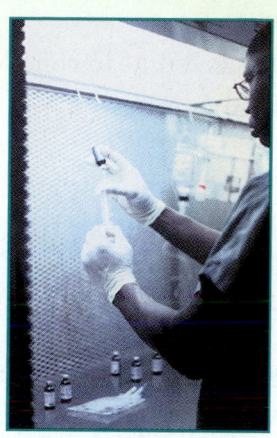

▶ OVERVIEW OF THE SKILL

Vials often are used to package multidose or single-dose parenteral medication. A vial is a small glass or plastic bottle with a rubber seal at the top. Vials come with a protective plastic or metal cap that prevents the rubber from being punctured before use. The rubber top must be cleaned with 70% alcohol with every usage of the medication. In order to aspirate the medication from the vial, an equal amount of air must be injected into the vial before attempting to withdraw any medication. In order to draw the medication out of the vial, the entire vial should be turned upside down. The syringe should be held at eye level to ensure an accurate amount of medication is drawn into the syringe.

▶ ASSESSMENT

1. Assess the expiration date on the vial to be sure it is current **to avoid administering outdated medications.**
2. Assess the contents of the medication vial you are about to use for the correct medication in the correct dosage strength **to avoid medication error.**
3. Assess the contents of the vial for color, consistency, and debris **to avoid administering contaminated medication.**
4. Assess the integrity of the vial and its stopper **to avoid using a vial that may be contaminated.**

5. Assess the integrity of the syringe and needle that will be used to withdraw the medication **to avoid using equipment that may be contaminated.**

▶ DIAGNOSIS

Risk for Infection

Risk for Injury

▶ PLANNING

Expected Outcomes:

1. The correct medication will be drawn from the vial using sterile technique.
2. The correct dose will be drawn from the vial.
3. The remaining contents of multiuse vials will not be contaminated.
4. The date will be marked on the vial after opening using an ink pen.

Equipment Needed (see Figure 5-12-1):

- Medication vial
- Syringe with needle
- Alcohol sponge pad
- Gloves (optional)
- Clean work space
- Medication administration record (MAR)

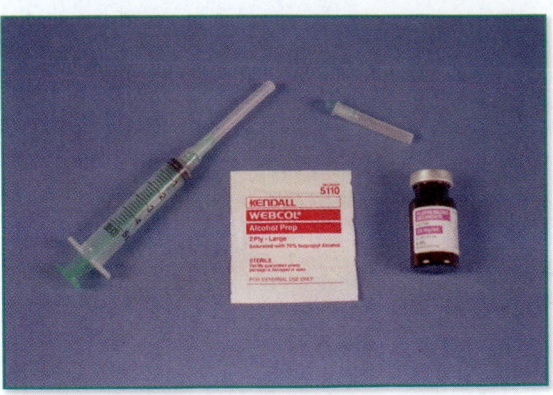

Figure 5-12-1 Syringe, needle, vial of medication, and alcohol wipe are used to withdraw medication from a vial.

▶ **CLIENT EDUCATION NEEDED:**

1. If the client or caregiver will be drawing up medications from a vial, educate the client regarding the correct technique.

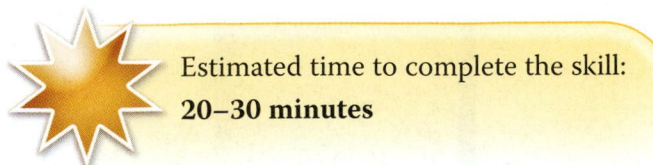

Estimated time to complete the skill:
20–30 minutes

▶ **DELEGATION TIPS**

The skill of medication administration is not delegated to ancillary personnel in acute-care settings, although this may vary in state or federal institutions. Ancillary personnel are generally informed about the medications the client is receiving if adverse effects are anticipated or are being monitored.

IMPLEMENTATION—Action/Rationale

Action	Rationale
1. Wash hands. Apply gloves (optional).	1. Decreases the transmission of microorganisms.
2. Select the appropriate vial (see Figure 5-12-2).	2. Prevents medication errors.
3. Verify health care provider's orders.	3. Prevents medication errors.
4. Check expiration date.	4. Avoids giving expired medication, which may have altered potency.
5. Determine the route of medication delivery and select the appropriate size syringe and needle.	5. The route of medication delivery is essential to knowing what size syringe and needle will be needed.
6. While holding the syringe at eye level, withdraw the plunger to the desired volume of medication.	6. Holding the syringe at eye level makes it easier to read the syringe calibrations and increases accuracy.
7. Clean the rubber top of the vial with a 70% alcohol pad. Use a circular motion starting at the center and working out (see Figure 5-12-3).	7. Ensures that the center of the rubber top is the cleanest area for needle entry. Reduces potential contamination with microorganisms.

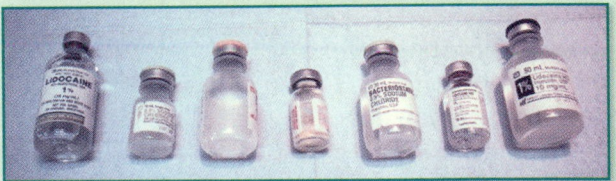

Figure 5-12-2 Carefully select the medication ordered.

continues

Action	Rationale

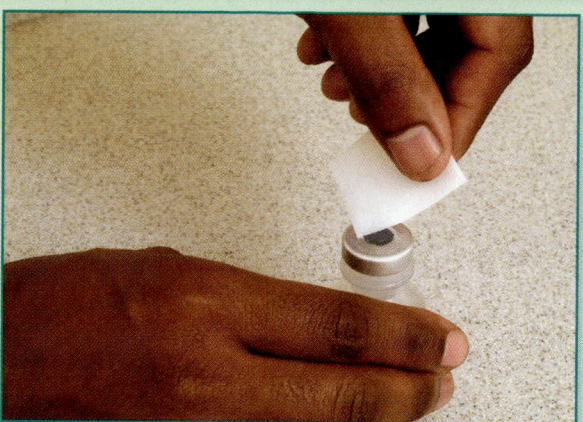

Figure 5-12-3 Wipe off the rubber top of the vial with a 70% alcohol pad.

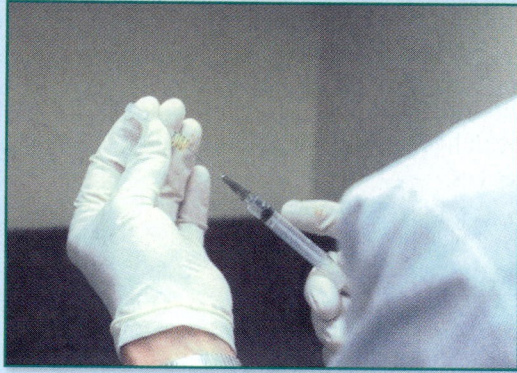

Figure 5-12-4 Using sterile technique, uncap the needle.

8. Using sterile technique, uncap the needle (see Figure 5-12-4).

8. Prevents spread of microorganisms.

9. Lay the needle cap on a clean surface.

9. Prevents spread of microorganisms.

10. Placing the needle in the center of the vial, inject the air slowly. Do not cause turbulence (see Figure 5-12-5).

10. Adding air prevents the buildup of negative pressure in the vial. Injecting quickly may cause turbulence, which can result in air bubbles forming within the vial, which could affect the accuracy of the volume of liquid being withdrawn.

11. Invert the vial and slowly, using gentle negative pressure, withdraw the medication. Keep the needle tip in the liquid (see Figure 5-12-6).

11. Decreases the number of air bubbles that tend to form with unsteady, fast, jerky motions. Keeping the needle tip in the liquid prevents drawing in air.

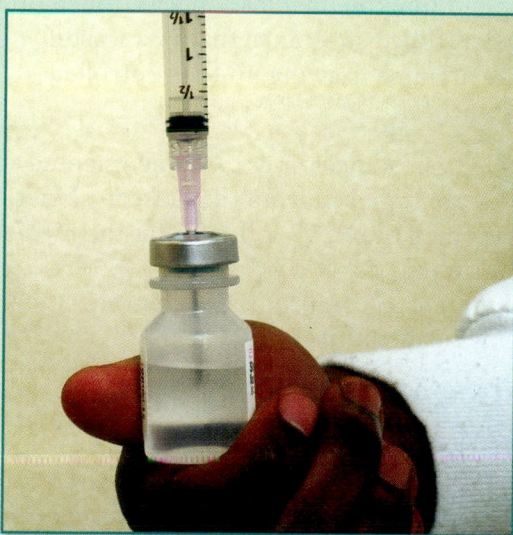

Figure 5-12-5 Place the needle into the vial through the center of the rubber top.

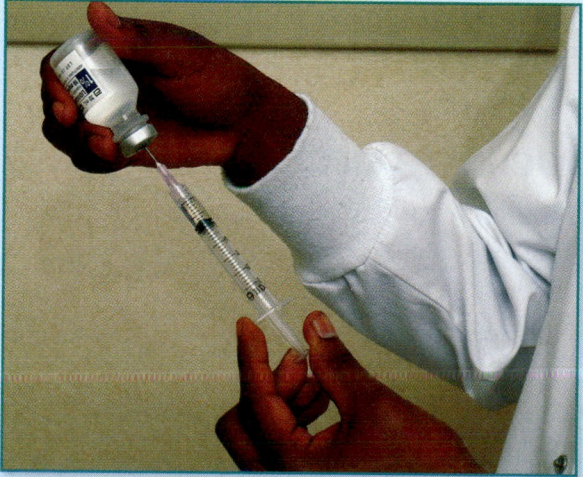

Figure 5-12-6 Invert the vial and slowly withdraw the medication until the appropriate dosage has been reached.

continues

Action	Rationale
12. With the syringe at eye level determine that the appropriate dose has been reached by volume.	12. Ensures client receives the ordered dose of medication.
13. Slowly withdraw the needle from the vial. Follow the institution's policy regarding recapping and changing needles.	13. Avoids splatter of medication and potential contamination of nearby supplies. Keeps the needle sterile.
14. Using ink, mark the current date and time and initials on the vial.	14. Prevents using a medication that has been opened too long per institutional protocol.
15. Label the syringe with drug, dose, date, and time.	15. Prevents medication errors.
16. Wash hands.	16. Decreases the transmission of microorganisms.

► REAL WORLD ANECDOTES

Dr. Saari ordered Mrs. Srsen's central line flushed every 12 hours with 10 mL of normal saline, followed by 3 mL of 100 U/mL heparin. Nurse Eubanks draws up the correct amount of normal saline in one syringe and heparin in another syringe and places them on her medication cart while she answers the phone. When she returns, one syringe is missing, and her notes have been moved. Concerned about the disappearance of the medication, Nurse Eubanks asks fellow staff members if they took the filled syringe. She discovers that a very busy float nurse had left two filled syringes on a different medication cart. In his hurry and disorientation on the unit, the float nurse had returned to the wrong cart and grabbed the wrong syringe. Luckily, the float nurse checked the "five rights" again before administering the medication. By double-checking he avoided delivering the wrong medication to the client.

► EVALUATION

- The vial was current and the rubber seal intact.
- The correct amount of medication was given.
- The needle did not become contaminated or damaged.

► DOCUMENTATION

Medication Administration Record

Document:
- Name of the medication
- Dosage drawn up
- Date and time the medication was drawn up

If the medication drawn up is a controlled substance, document in the Controlled Substances Record Book:
- Name of the medication
- Dosage drawn up

- Date and time the medication was drawn up
- Any controlled substance that was wasted
- Name of nurse drawing up the controlled substance

Controlled substances must be documented at the time they are removed from the locked cabinet. Documentation on the MAR is done after the medication is administered.

Document on appropriate flow sheet or electronic medical record (EMR).

► CRITICAL THINKING SKILL

Introduction

Carefully examine the label of your desired medication. Several drug manufacturers use very similar labels for very different medications. During a busy shift, errors can happen if the nurse does not pay particular attention to the medication label.

Possible Scenario

While drawing up normal saline to flush a heparin lock, the nurse reaches into the medication cupboard and into the box marked normal saline. She withdraws a vial. The vial is the same size and shape as the multidose normal saline vials and, distracted, she does not carefully check the label as she is drawing up the medication.

Possible Outcome

The multidose lidocaine is kept on the same shelf in the medication cupboard. The lidocaine vial is the same shape and size as the normal saline vial. The primary difference between the two vials is the color of the type on the label. If the label is not carefully checked, the client is at risk of receiving a potentially toxic dose of lidocaine rather than a therapeutic dose of saline.

Prevention

Be aware of the medication packaging. If two different types of medication are packaged very similarly, do not store them close to each other, as this invites confusion. Always check the label on the medication you are preparing to administer. Two different vials of insulin can look the same and yet have very different effects on the client.

► **VARIATIONS**

Geriatric Variations:

- If an older adult is drawing up medication from a vial, assess that his vision is adequate to read the syringe calibrations and the vial label.
- Assess that the client has sufficient flexibility in the hands to manipulate the syringe and hold the vial.

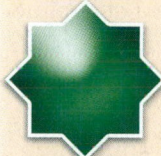

Pediatric Variations:

- Keep this and all medications out of the reach of children, especially on an unattended medication cart.
- If the setting requires drawing up the medication at the bedside, do not leave capped needles within reach of a child.
- Make sure all sharps go completely in the sharps container and that a small hand cannot reach into the opening.

Home Care Variations:

- Correct disposal of used vials and needles in the home health setting is extremely important to avoid needle-stick injury or cuts from broken glass. Sharps boxes are often not available in the home setting. An empty labeled bleach container can make a useful and safe sharp object container. Encourage clients to return their filled bleach containers to a medical facility instead of dispensing in the trash.
- Periodically reassess the client's or caregiver's technique when withdrawing medication from a vial to evaluate for any lapses in technique.
- Teach the client or caregiver to question any vial of medication that looks different from normal (color, amount, consistency, label).

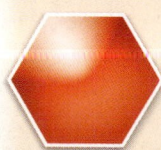

Long-Term Care Variations:

- Multiuse vials should be checked regularly for expiration, labeling with date they were opened, and any changes in appearance of the medication.
- Multiuse vials are more prone to contamination than single-use vials. Take care not to contaminate the contents of a vial. If there is any doubt, throw it out.

▶ COMMON ERRORS

Possible Error:

The medication in the vial is not good.

Prevention:

Question any medication that appears contaminated, discolored, or has a precipitate. Do not administer it.

Possible Error:

The vial has been opened too long.

Prevention:

Question any multidose vial where the prior-use information is smeared or unreadable. Do not administer it.

Possible Error:

Vials often look very similar. If similar vials are stored side by side and things get hectic or you are tired, you could possibly grab the wrong one.

Prevention:

Store similar vials apart. Label them clearly. Train yourself to always check and double-check, so checking becomes automatic.

▶ NURSING TIPS

- Double-check the vial for the appropriate medication. Be certain that a medication error does not happen.
- Verify that the generic name on the vial is the same trade medication that is desired. Many new medications are coming on the market, often with similar names. Always verify that the medication you are about to use is the medication desired. Take the extra time to look it up or call the pharmacy if you are unsure.
- If performing a drug calculation, have a colleague verify your calculation. Even nurses with years of experience have a colleague verify calculations to ensure client safety.
- If this is the first usage of the vial, use an ink pen to record the date the vial was opened.

▶ SPECIAL CONSIDERATIONS

- *A needle may become dull from penetrating the cap while withdrawing the medication from a vial. When this is a concern, the needle should be changed prior to giving the injection to a client. Account for medication in the needle when making adjustments.*
- *Rubber tops on vials usually contain latex. If a client has a history of latex allergy, contact the health care provider to ascertain risk.*

Withdrawing Medication from an Ampule

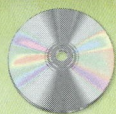

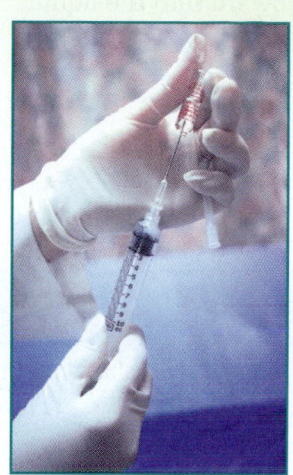

▶ OVERVIEW OF THE SKILL

Ampules are containers that hold a single dose of medication. The ampules are made of clear glass and have a distinctive shape with a constricted neck. The head of the ampule is broken off at the neck, and the medication is withdrawn with a needle and syringe.

The neck of the ampule is often colored and usually scored. This scoring allows the neck to be broken off easily from the body to obtain the medication. The nurse places a sterile piece of gauze around the neck of the ampule and breaks the neck in an outward motion. The gauze protects the nurse's fingers from the glass.

Medication can become trapped in the uppermost portion of the ampule. Before opening the ampule, nurses frequently need to flick the upper portion of the ampule with their fingernail to drop the medication from the upper segment down into the body of the ampule. This step may need to be repeated several times.

▶ ASSESSMENT

1. Identify the correct ampule, including medication, dosage strength, dosage volume, dosage route, and expiration date **to avoid medication errors.**
2. Assess the syringe, filter needle, and injection needle for expiration date and package intactness **to evaluate the suitability of the equipment.**
3. Assess the fluid in the ampule for cloudiness, particulate matter, or color changes **to evaluate for usability of the medication.**

4. Identify the medication's intended action, purpose, normal dosage range, time of action, common side effects, and nursing implications **to avoid medication errors.**

▶ DIAGNOSIS

Risk for Impaired Skin Integrity

Risk for Infection

▶ PLANNING

Expected Outcomes:

1. The correct medication ampule will be selected.
2. The medication will be drawn into an appropriate syringe.
3. Microorganisms will not be introduced into the sterile system.
4. Foreign objects will not be introduced into the sterile system.

Equipment Needed (see Figure 5-13-1):

- Medication ampule
- Sterile gauze pad or alcohol pad
- Syringe with filter needle
- Replacement needle
- Clean work space
- Medication administration record (MAR)

627

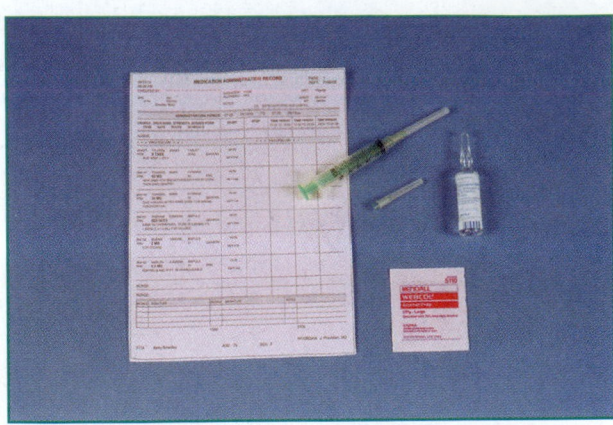

Figure 5-13-1 Syringes, needles, alcohol wipes, and medication ampules are used to withdraw medication from an ampule.

▶ **CLIENT EDUCATION NEEDED:**

1. When teaching a client to withdraw medication from an ampule, show how to hold the ampule away from the cut edges to prevent a hand laceration.
2. Clients or caregivers might find it easier to place the medication on a countertop and insert the needle downward into the liquid.

Estimated time to complete the skill: **2–5 minutes**

▶ **DELEGATION TIPS**

The skill of medication administration is not delegated to ancillary personnel in acute care settings, but this may vary in state or federal institutions. Ancillary personnel are generally informed about the medications the client is receiving if adverse effects are anticipated or are being monitored.

IMPLEMENTATION—Action/Rationale

Action	Rationale
1. Wash hands.	1. Decreases the transmission of microorganisms.
2. Select appropriate ampule (see Figure 5-13-2).	2. Ensures client receives correct medication.
3. Select syringe with filter needle (see Figure 5-13-3).	3. Filter needle entraps any glass fragments.

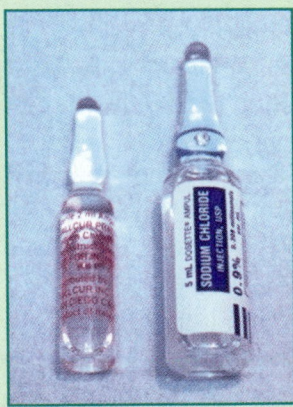

Figure 5-13-2 Medication ampules

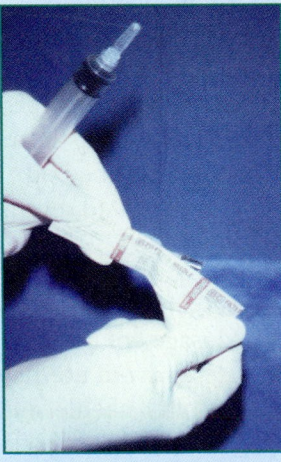

Figure 5-13-3 Select a syringe and filter needle.

continues

Action	Rationale

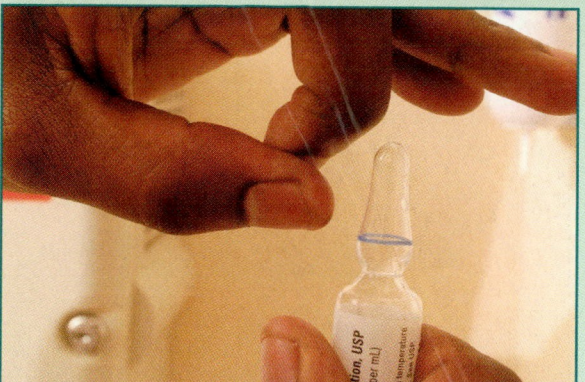

Figure 5-13-4 Flick the neck of the upright ampule to dislodge medication from the top of the vial.

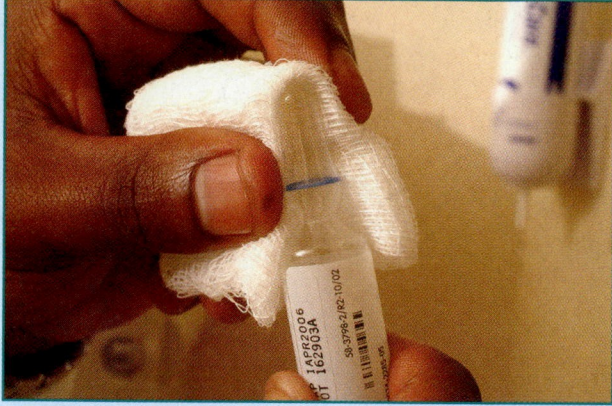

Figure 5-13-5 Wrap gauze or alcohol pad around the neck to protect fingers.

4. Obtain a sterile gauze pad.

4. Using a gauze pad prevents the nurse from being cut on the jagged edge of the broken ampule.

5. Select and set aside the appropriate length of safety-needle for planned injection.

5. Accurate needle length ensures the medication is administered where it is intended.

6. Clear a work space.

6. Prevents contamination of microdroplets that may spill when the ampule is broken.

7. Observe ampule for location of the medication.

7. The medication frequently becomes trapped in the top of the ampule.

8. If the medication is trapped in the top, flick the neck of the ampule repeatedly with your fingernail while holding the ampule upright (see Figure 5-13-4).

8. Flicking the neck and top of the ampule moves the medication into the body of the ampule.

9. Wrap the sterile gauze pad around the neck and snap off the top in an outward motion directed away from self (see Figures 5-13-5 and 5-13-6).

9. The gauze prevents the nurse from being cut by the jagged edge of the broken ampule. The outward motion provides added safety for the nurse.

10. Invert ampule and place the needle into the liquid. Gently withdraw medication into the syringe (see Figure 5-13-7).

10. Inverting the ampule allows all the medication to be withdrawn into the syringe. Surface tension will hold the medication in the ampule until the negative pressure of the syringe barrel draws it into the syringe.

11. Alternately, place the ampule on the counter, hold and tilt slightly with the nondominant hand. Insert the needle below the level of liquid and gently draw liquid into the syringe, tilting the ampule as needed to reach all the liquid.

11. Although it is more difficult to read the syringe calibrations, it is easier to hold the ampule steady. Choose the method most comfortable for you.

12. Remove the filter needle and replace with the safety injection needle (see Figure 5-13-8).

12. The filter needle is designed to trap glass particles and must not be used for client injections.

13. Dispose of the filter needle and glass ampule (including lid) in appropriate sharps container (see Figure 5-13-9).

13. Needles or sharp glass objects must always be disposed of in puncture- and leak-proof containers in order to provide safety for clients and health care workers.

continues

Action	Rationale

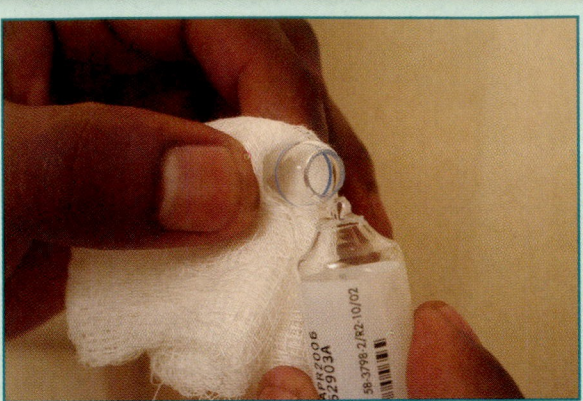

Figure 5-13-6 Snap the top of the ampule off in an outward motion away from self.

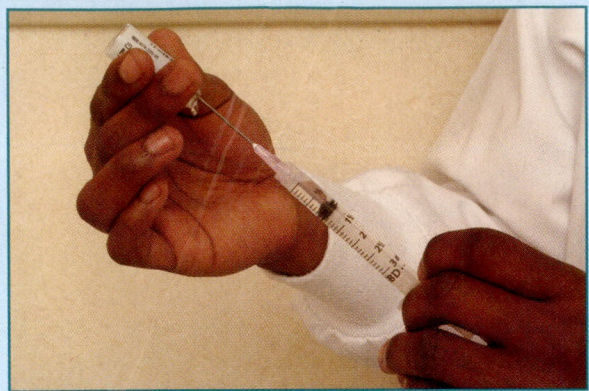

Figure 5-13-7 Invert ampule and gently draw the liquid into the syringe.

14. Label the syringe with drug, dose, date, and time.

15. Wash hands.

14. Prevents medication errors from taking place.

15. Decreases the transmission of microorganisms.

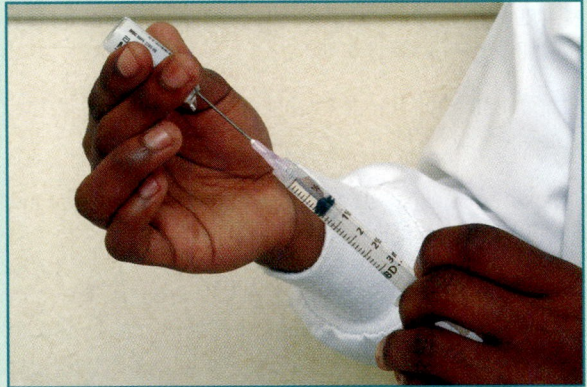

Figure 5-13-8 Remove the filter needle and replace with the injection needle.

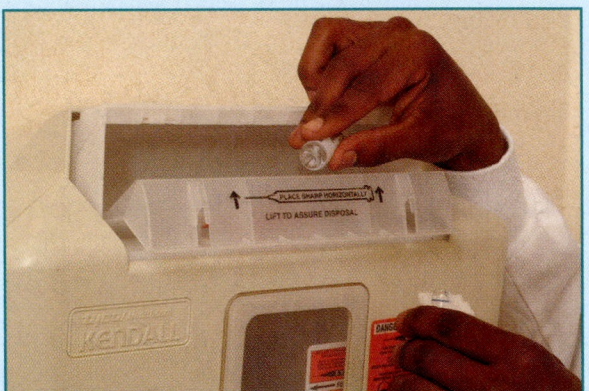

Figure 5-13-9 Dispose of the filter needle, ampule, and ampule top in an appropriate container.

▶ REAL WORLD ANECDOTES

Scenario 1

Kim followed the appropriate technique of wrapping the neck of an ampule with a sterile 2 × 2 gauze pad before breaking. Because of the force needed to break the ampule, she inadvertently allowed the broken neck of the ampule to jerk back and cut her finger. The necks of the ampules are not always of uniform thickness. In order to break them, a different amount of force is used for some rather than others. Kim did some experimentation after this injury and found that wrapping an unopened alcohol sponge around the gauze helped protect her fingers from injury.

Scenario 2

A client proudly showed his homemade sharps container (a converted olive-oil can) to the visiting nurse. It was puncture proof, leak proof, and well labeled. Unfortunately, the jagged edges of the opening he had cut had sharper edges than many of the sharps inside. The nurse helped with some redesign, and the sharps container worked well after that.

► EVALUATION

- The correct medication ampule was selected.
- The medication was drawn into an appropriate syringe.
- Microorganisms were not introduced into the sterile system.
- Foreign objects were not introduced into the sterile system.

► DOCUMENTATION

Medication Administration Record (MAR)

Document:
- Name of the medication
- Dosage drawn up
- Date and time the medication was drawn up

If the medication drawn up is a controlled substance, document in the Controlled Substances Record Book:
- Name of the medication
- Dosage drawn up
- Date and time the medication was drawn up
- Any controlled substance that was wasted
- Name of nurse drawing up the controlled substance

Document on appropriate workflow sheet or electronic medical record (EMR).

Controlled substances must be documented at the time they are removed from the locked cabinet. Documentation on the MAR is done after the medication is administered.

► CRITICAL THINKING SKILL

Introduction

Always double-check the amount of medication drawn up with the expected dosage. Do not assume that a single-dose ampule contains the exact amount needed for the dose.

Possible Scenario

Mrs. Ruden's pain medication order was for morphine sulfate 10 mg IM. Her nurse removed a 10-mg ampule of morphine from the controlled substances cupboard, opened it, and drew up the medication. The nurse was busy documenting the use of the controlled substance and did not pay attention to the amount of fluid she had drawn up in the syringe.

Possible Outcome

If the ampule was slightly overfilled, Mrs. Ruden would have received more morphine than had been ordered. Depending on her condition, this could have results ranging from negligible to serious. If some of the medication had been trapped in the top of the ampule and discarded, Mrs. Ruden would have received less pain medication than ordered. Potentially, Mrs. Ruden would not have received effective pain relief, thus causing unnecessary suffering for the client.

Prevention

Ampules usually contain one dose of medication. Manufacturers sometimes overfill ampules by a small amount to compensate for medication caught in the top of the ampule. If medication is caught in the top of the ampule, the dose drawn up may be too small. Do not assume that the amount of fluid in a single-dose ampule is the correct dose. Always double-check the amount of fluid against the label on the ampule.

Always double-check your math. There are three main ways to calculate dosages: ratio proportion, formula, and dimensional analysis. Study and use the method that feels most comfortable to you. Never feel embarrassed to have a second party verify your results. Ideally state the dosage calculation problem and do not tell the answer until you can compare it. This will be an added safety measure in calculating math problems.

► VARIATIONS

Geriatric Variation:
- *If an older adult is drawing up medication from an ampule, assess that the client's vision is adequate to see the contents of the ampule and to check for glass. Check that the client can clearly read the syringe calibrations and the medication label.*

continues

▶ VARIATIONS (continued)

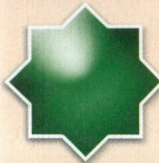

Pediatric Variations:
- *Keep this and all medications out of the reach of children.*
- *If the setting requires drawing up the medication at the bedside, do not leave the empty ampule within the reach of a child.*
- *Make sure all sharps go completely into the sharps container and that a small hand cannot reach into the opening.*

Home Care Variations:
- *Correct disposal of a used ampule in the home health setting is extremely important as it has sharp and jagged edges and may cut someone. A glass jar or metal container with a small mouth may be used. Make sure there is a lid that fits. Label the container clearly and place where it is accessible to the caregiver. Empty the container regularly.*
- *Change the needle before injection if you suspect any contamination has occurred or if there is irritating medication on the outside of the needle.*

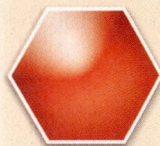

Long-Term Care Variations:
- *Change the needle prior to injection if you suspect any contamination has occurred or if there is irritating medication on the outside of the needle.*
- *Empty sharps containers regularly.*

▶ COMMON ERRORS

Possible Error:
The top of the ampule cannot be broken off its body.

Prevention:
Discard in the appropriate container and begin again with a new ampule.

Possible Error:
When the ampule is broken, some medication is spilled.

Prevention:
Make sure the medication left in the ampule has not been contaminated in any way. Lifting the syringe to eye level, determine if you still have the prescribed amount of medication. If not, you will need to open an additional ampule.

Possible Error:
The nurse uses a freshly opened alcohol swab to protect her fingers. Some of the alcohol runs into the ampule, contaminating the medication.

Prevention:
Use only unopened alcohol wipes or a gauze pad to protect fingers.

▶ **NURSING TIPS**

- An alcohol swab package wrapped around the sterile gauze adds extra protection for the nurse.
- Handle the top and bottom of the ampule when separated with extreme caution as one can be easily cut.

- Dispose of the parts in a sharps-proof container.
- Always move the ampule away from your face prior to breaking the neck to prevent glass from flying back at you.

▶ **SPECIAL CONSIDERATIONS**

- *Medication fluid can often be stuck in the neck of the ampule, making it difficult to flick down. Before breaking the neck, gently rotate the ampule in a circular motion. This will cause the fluid in the narrow space above the neck to easily come down.*
- *A filter needle should be used to draw medication from an ampule. If a filter needle is not available, use a regular needle to draw the medication and then change the needle prior to administering the medication to the client. If a filter needle was not used to draw up the medication, carefully assess for glass pieces in the medication solution throughout the process.*

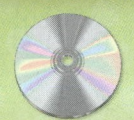

Mixing Medications from Two Vials into One Syringe

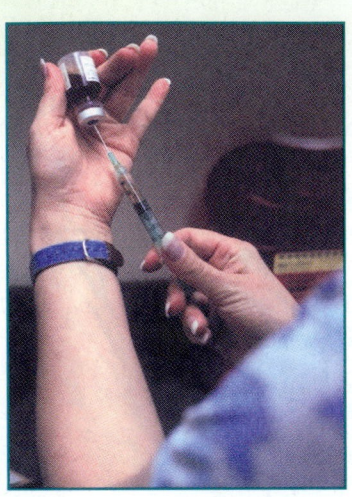

▶ OVERVIEW OF THE SKILL

When giving ordered subcutaneous or intramuscular medication to a client, it sometimes becomes necessary to mix medications in one syringe from two separate vials. In doing so, it is often important that the medications are removed from the vials in a specific order. Learning which medications must be mixed in a specific order is necessary to avoid contamination of the vials. It is also important for the nurse drawing up the medications to be familiar with this skill to ensure that the correct dose of medication is given to the client and that vials are not contaminated with other medications.

▶ ASSESSMENT

1. Identify the medications ordered. **Prevents medication errors.**
2. Consider whether the order of drawing up medications makes a difference. **This will vary based on the type of medications to be mixed.**
3. Assess client's knowledge regarding drawing medications up from two vials if the client will be performing this skill at home. **Determines need for drug education and assists in identifying client's compliance with drug therapy at home.**
4. Check the client's drug allergy history **as an allergic reaction could occur.**

▶ DIAGNOSIS

Risk for Injury, secondary to medication error

Risk for Infection

Risk for Allergic Response

▶ PLANNING

Expected Outcomes:

1. The ordered medications will be drawn up safely using sterile technique.
2. The correct dose of medications will be drawn from the vial.
3. The remaining contents of multiuse vials will not be contaminated.
4. The client will be instructed, if needed, on preparing an injection that requires mixing medications from two vials.

Equipment Needed (see Figure 5-14-1):

- Medication administration record (MAR)
- Medication vials
- Syringe
- Alcohol wipes

▶ CLIENT EDUCATION NEEDED:

1. If the client or caregiver will be performing this skill, explain the order of drawing up medications and the reason this order is important.

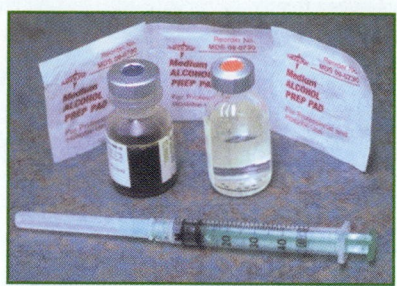

Figure 5-14-1   Syringe with needle, vials, and alcohol wipes are used to draw two medications into one syringe.

2. Have the client or caregiver perform a return demonstration after being shown how to draw up medication.

3. Make sure the client or caregiver knows whom to call with questions.
4. Reinforce verbal teaching with written instructions.

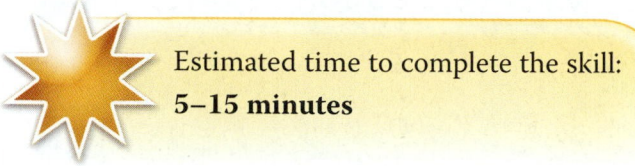

Estimated time to complete the skill: **5–15 minutes**

▶ DELEGATION TIPS

The skill of medication administration is not delegated to ancillary personnel in acute care settings. This may vary in state or federal institutions. Ancillary personnel are generally informed about the medications the client is receiving if adverse effects are anticipated or are being monitored.

IMPLEMENTATION—Action/Rationale

Action	Rationale
1. Check MAR against the health care provider's written orders.	1. Ensures accuracy in the administration of the medication.
2. Check for drug allergies.	2. Decreases risk of allergic reaction such as hives, urticaria, or anaphylactic shock.
3. Wash your hands.	3. Decreases transmission of microorganisms.
4. Gather the equipment needed. Prepare the medication for one client at a time.	4. Promotes organization. Ensures that the right client receives the right medications.
5. Check need for one medication to be drawn up before the other.	5. Determines the order in which medications will be drawn up.
6. Determine the total medication volume (in milliliters) you will have in the syringe when you have finished drawing both medications into the syringe.	6. Determines how much of the second medication will need to be drawn into the syringe.
7. Swab the top of each vial with alcohol (see Figure 5-14-2).	7. Decreases the transmission of microorganisms.

continues

Action	Rationale

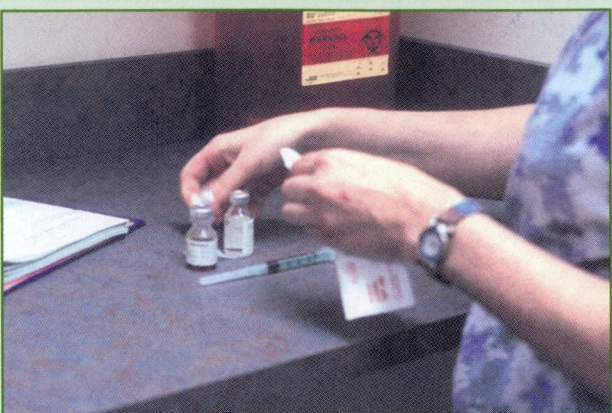

Figure 5-14-2 Swab the top of each vial with alcohol.

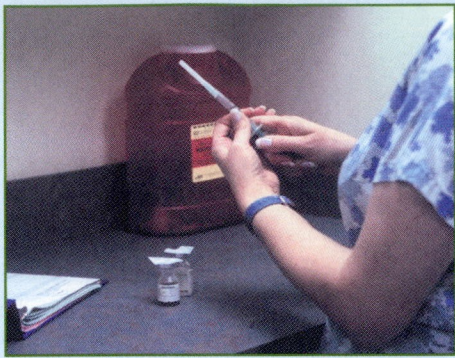

Figure 5-14-3 Draw air into the syringe equal to the amount of medication to be drawn up from the second vial.

8. Draw air into the syringe equal to the amount of medication to be drawn up from the second vial (see Figure 5-14-3). Inject air into the second vial and remove the syringe and needle from the vial (see Figure 5-14-4). Some protocols require changing needles.

8. Avoids creating a vacuum in the second vial. When you draw medication from the second vial, you will not be able to inject air at that time because your syringe will already contain medication from the first vial. If you inject air, you will also risk injecting medication and contaminating the second vial.

9. Draw air into the syringe equal to the amount of medication to be drawn up from the first vial. Inject air into the first vial. Keep the needle and syringe in the vial (see Figure 5-14-5).

9. Avoids creating a vacuum in the first vial.

10. Pulling back on the plunger, withdraw the correct amount (in milliliters) of medication from the first vial (see Figure 5-14-6).

10. Draws up the first medication.

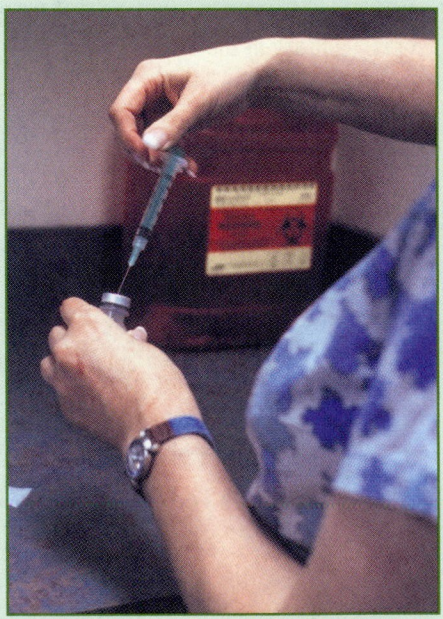

Figure 5-14-4 Inject air into the second vial.

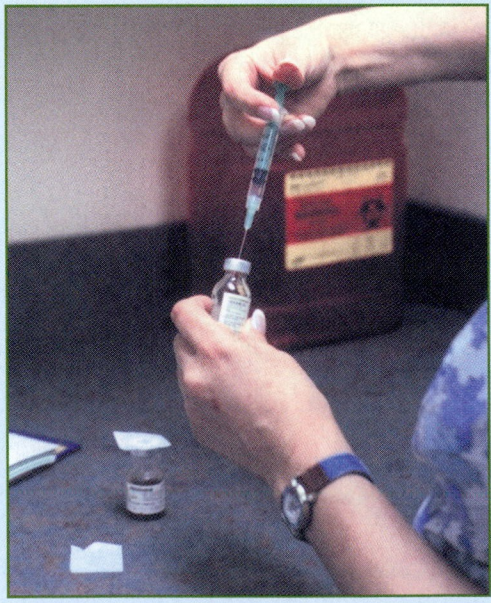

Figure 5-14-5 Inject air into the first vial.

continues

Action	Rationale

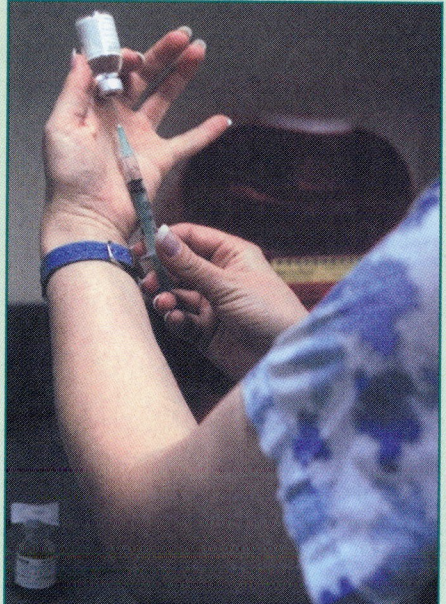

Figure 5-14-6 Withdraw the correct amount of medication from the first vial.

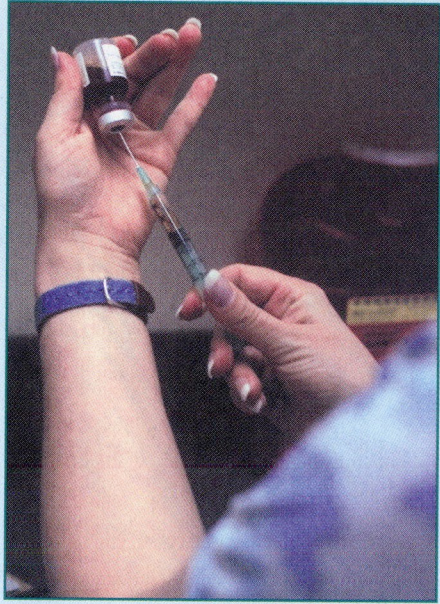

Figure 5-14-7 Withdraw medication from the second vial to the volume of both medications summed together.

11. Remove the syringe from the first vial and insert it into the second vial. Withdraw medication from the second vial to the volume (in milliliters) total of both medications summed together (see Figures 5-14-7 and 5-14-8).

11. Draws up the second medication. Drawing up medication equal to the total of both medications ensures the correct amount of second medication is withdrawn.

12. Either leave the needle in the second vial until just prior to injecting the medication or follow the institution's policy regarding recapping needles.

12. Prevents needle-stick injuries.

13. Wash hands.

13. Reduces the transmission of microorganisms.

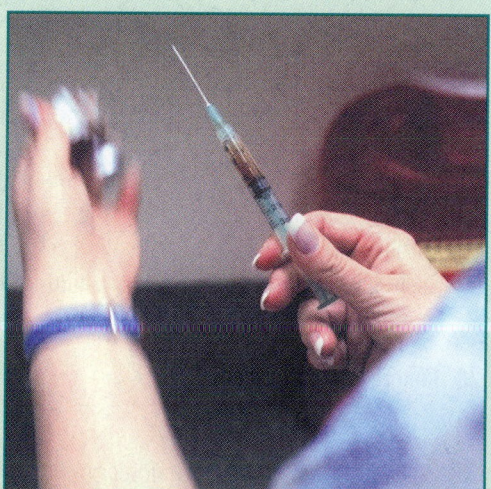

Figure 5-14-8 Double-check the syringe to make sure it contains medication equal to the total volume of both medications summed together.

continues

Action	Rationale

Mixing Insulin

Insulin solutions come premixed and in insulin pens; however, if these are not available, certain insulin solutions can be mixed. The clear insulin (regular, short-acting) is generally drawn up first then the cloudy solution (intermediate or long-acting). Mixing insulin can change time of action, absorption, and bioavailability; therefore, check the manufacturers' information regarding types of insulin and carefully assess response of client. Before administering insulin, dosage must be double-checked by two professionals. An inaccurate dose of insulin can be life-threatening.

14. Check client's most recent blood-glucose level, dietary intake, oral intake status (i.e., is it NPO), and signs and symptoms related to glucose level.

14. Prevents hypoglycemic episodes. May need to check with health care provider regarding insulin dosage. Prevents wasting of insulin if not to be given.

15. Repeat steps 1 to 4.

15. See Rationales 1 to 4.

16. Remove caps from insulin vials (if necessary). Gently rotate (never shake) the suspension insulin, such as NPH, intermediate, or long-acting insulin, until no sediment is at the bottom of the vial.

16. Long-acting insulin is a cloudy suspension and needs to be completely and gently mixed to ensure that all particles are distributed equally in suspension.

17. Wipe off tops on insulin vials with alcohol sponge.

17. Removes surface microorganisms.

18. Draw back the amount of air into the syringe that equals the total dose of both insulin solutions. Insert the needle and syringe into the vial with the cloudy, suspension (intermediate or long-acting insulin) and inject air equal to the amount to be given of that insulin. Do not touch solution with needle.

18. Prevents negative pressure from pulling solution into vial for next use; prevents contamination with different types of insulin.

19. Insert needle and syringe into vial of short-acting or regular insulin and inject air equal to the amount to be given.

19. Prevents negative pressure in vial.

20. Keep needle and syringe in solution. Invert vial and withdraw medication slowly and accurately.

20. Slow withdrawal can help prevent air trapping and ensure accuracy.

21. Withdraw needle and expel any air bubbles and check dose with another nurse.

21. Insulin must be double-checked for accuracy because of the dangers of administration of an inaccurate dose.

22. Invert the vial with longer-acting insulin, holding plunger carefully, and withdraw long-acting insulin, being careful not to inject any regular insulin into vial. Check dose with another nurse.

22. Prevents withdrawal of air and too much insulin. If too much insulin is withdrawn the solution must be discarded and the procedure repeated. If regular insulin is accidentally injected into vial of cloudy insulin the vial must be discarded.

23. Store insulin properly according to the manufacturer's specifications.

23. Ensures effective product.

24. Wash hands and prepare to administer injection.

24. Prevents transmission of microorganisms.

▶ REAL WORLD ANECDOTES

Jane is a diabetic woman who goes to the pharmacy to pick up her regular insulin and NPH as well as a new supply of syringes. Upon returning home, she gets out her medications to draw them both up in one syringe, as she is used to, to give herself her 12:00 dose. She realizes that the syringes look different, and is unable to read the numbers. She is confused about how to mix the two medications in the new syringes. She calls the pharmacy to tell them that she has the wrong syringes, and the pharmacist tells her that they have switched brands of syringes, and even though they look different, these are the syringes she is to use. She waits until her daughter gets home to help her draw up her medication. Her daughter helps her label the new syringes with tape to mark the numbers clearly.

▶ EVALUATION

- The ordered medications were drawn up safely using sterile technique.
- The correct doses of medications were drawn from the vials.
- The remaining contents of multiuse vials were not contaminated.
- The client was instructed, if needed, on preparing an injection that requires mixing medications from two vials.

▶ DOCUMENTATION

Medication Administration Record (MAR)

Document:

- Name of the medications
- Dosages drawn up
- Date and time the medications were drawn up

If either or both of the medications drawn up are controlled substances, document in the Controlled Substances Record Book:

- Name of the medication
- Dosage drawn up
- Date and time the medication was drawn up
- Any controlled substance that was wasted
- Name of nurse drawing up the controlled substance

Controlled substances must be documented at the time they are removed from the locked cabinet. Documentation on the MAR is done after the medication is administered.

▶ CRITICAL THINKING SKILL

Introduction

For diabetic clients who need insulin injections, it is important for that person to be comfortable drawing up and administering these medications. Careful teaching must occur to ensure that the diabetic client is comfortable with this skill.

Possible Scenario

Jim is a newly diagnosed diabetic client who must learn how to administer regular insulin and NPH when he goes home tomorrow. The nurse shows Jim how to draw up the medication out of the regular vial and then the NPH vial. She stresses the importance of doing this in the correct order so that the regular insulin is not contaminated with the cloudy NPH. She also shows him how to inject air into the vials before drawing up the medication and how to withdraw the units of regular insulin, then withdraw the units of both medications combined. For example, Jim needs to take 5 units of NPH and 7 units of regular insulin. After injecting air into each vial, Jim should first withdraw 7 units of regular insulin, and then, using the same syringe, he should withdraw NPH insulin to the 12-unit line.

Possible Outcome

Jim goes home the next morning. While trying to draw up his first dose of insulin at home, he realizes that he is unsure how to draw it up correctly. He calls the hospital asking if someone can give him directions. By the time he finally gets connected to the diabetic teaching nurse, he is angry and desperately in need of his insulin. After talking Jim through drawing up this dose of insulin, the diabetic teaching nurse arranges for a home care nurse to visit Jim and do some additional teaching.

Prevention

It is important to watch the client perform this skill one or two times to make sure the client understands the instructions. It is also important to give written information, if available, to reinforce the teaching that was done. Follow-up visits to the client's home may be in order as well. This is a skill that does not come easily, and clients who are already stressed regarding their disease may have a difficult time assimilating information they receive in the hospital.

▶ VARIATIONS

Geriatric Variations:
- *Client's vision must be clear enough to ensure that the correct dose of medication is drawn up.*
- *Manual dexterity must also be checked because of the difficulty in drawing up medications.*
- *Write down instructions in a step-by-step format in large print to help clients with vision or short-term memory difficulties self-administer the medication.*
- *Follow up teaching immediately to verify the client can perform the skill. Follow up in 1 to 2 weeks to verify client has retained the skill correctly.*

Pediatric Variations:
- *Determine with the health care provider, parent, and hospital policy at what age a child or adolescent may begin to participate in the preparation and administration of own medications.*
- *Check manual dexterity and motor skills.*
- *Determine areas where the child can participate, such as observation, play therapy, and hands-on activities, with supervision.*
- *Allow the child to participate in the process as much as possible.*

Home Care Variations:
- *Care must be taken in this setting to ensure the client is comfortable with the skill and that all needed supplies are available.*
- *Make sure medication vials are clearly labeled and the client or caregiver can read the labels.*
- *Check that the medication is being stored in a safe place at the proper temperature.*
- *Assess the client or caregiver to determine that he or she understands the basics of medication safety. Can he or she locate the expiration date on the vials, for example. Remind him or her to question, and not to administer, medications that have been improperly stored, look discolored, or do not look like his or her usual medication.*
- *In the home care setting, it is more difficult to replace medications if an error has contaminated a vial. The client, nurse, or caregiver needs to know the exact procedure for quickly replacing a medication during the day or after hours should the need arise. This will reduce the anxiety associated with mixing medications from two vials as well as reduce the temptation to overlook a possible contamination or mixing medication error.*
- *Make sure lighting is adequate to see the calibration numbers on the syringe.*

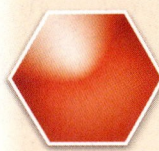

Long-Term Care Variations:
- *A client who self-administers the same medication over time may need a "refresher" course on how to correctly maintain his or her technique. This will reduce the temptation to adopt "short-cuts," such as not adequately cleaning the vial stopper. It may reduce the risk of damage to skin integrity, infection, or medication errors caused by poor technique.*

▶ COMMON ERRORS

Possible Error:

The medication vial becomes contaminated.

Prevention:

Always use an alcohol swab to clean the top of the vials before injecting the syringe. Assist any client with sensory or motor deficits when drawing up medications. Discard, obtain replacement, repeat preparation, and administer the medication.

Possible Error:

No air was injected into the vial before drawing up medication.

Prevention:

Follow the same set of steps listed in the Implementation section of this chapter. If previous users have not injected air and the negative pressure inside the vial is too high to withdraw medication, clean the top of the vial with an alcohol swab and insert a sterile needle into the stopper. The needle provides a sterile opening to allow the passage of air. This procedure should be done in a clean area to prevent the introduction of airborne bacteria into the vial.

▶ NURSING TIPS

- Become familiar with types of medications commonly ordered at your facility and which ones can be mixed together in one syringe.
- Find out the maximum number of milliliters that can be injected SQ and IM in one syringe at your facility.
- Think through the steps of drawing up two medications into one vial before you begin this procedure.
- Teach client this skill using the same equipment he or she will be using at home.

▶ SPECIAL CONSIDERATIONS

- *Insulin comes in both short- and long-acting medications and clients are often prescribed a combination of both. Compatible medications may be mixed in the same vial; however, care must be taken not to contaminate one medication with the other. The nurse must also carefully calculate the correct dose of the insulin for the client.*
- *Certain medications are cloudy in appearance. In the situation in which medications from two vials are mixed into one syringe, change the needle before drawing the medication from a different vial. If the needle cannot be changed, for example, an insulin syringe, first draw the medication from the clear vial and then the cloudy one. This will prevent the clear solution being contaminated by the cloudy one. The outcome could be fatal from the masking effect if the short-acting medication was contaminated by the long-acting one.*
- *To remember which insulin is withdrawn first, remember a clear day is preferable to a cloudy day.*
- *Insulin can be absorbed through the skin and should, therefore, be washed off immediately. Gloves can be worn prophylactically.*

Preparing an IV Solution

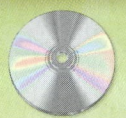

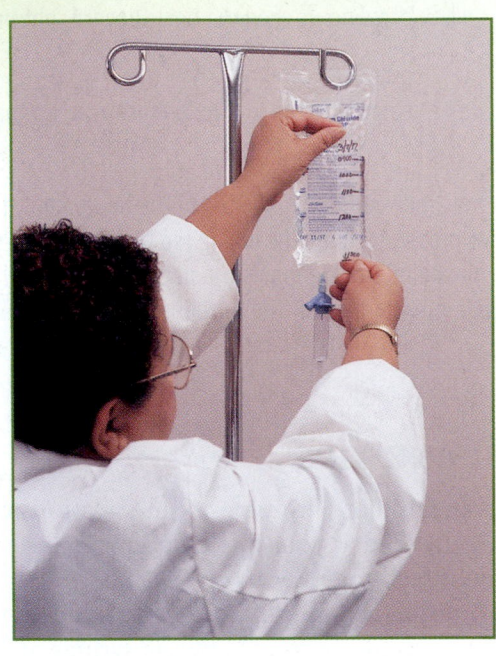

► OVERVIEW OF THE SKILL

An intravenous solution is a method of replacing fluid lost, or correcting an electrolyte imbalance. Clients who are acutely ill, are NPO after surgery, or have severe burns are examples of those who require IV therapy. The solution in an IV bag is ordered by the health care provider according to the client's needs and is changed at least every 24 hours, or per the institution's policy, to decrease the risk of infection. Tubing is used to connect the solution in the IV bag with the client's IV catheter or needle. Use needleless systems if available. OSHA requires safe devices.

► ASSESSMENT

1. Check the health care provider's order for the IV solution to be infused and rate of flow **to ensure accurate administration.**
2. Review information regarding the solution and nursing implications **to administer the solution safely.**
3. Check all additives in the solution and other medications **so that there will be no incompatibilities of additives with the solution.**

4. Assess whether the client understands the purpose of the IV infusion **so that client teaching can be tailored to his or her needs.**

► DIAGNOSIS

Risk for Infection

Risk for Impaired Skin Integrity

► PLANNING

Expected Outcomes:

1. The appropriate fluids at the ordered dosages will be available for IV infusion.
2. The IV infusion will be sterile, without precipitate or contamination.

Equipment Needed (see Figure 5-15-1):

- IV solution in a bag
- Medication administration record (MAR)
- IV flow sheet
- IV tubing, as needed

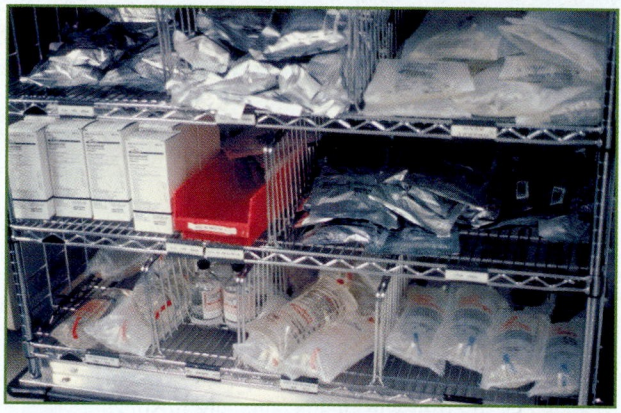

Figure 5-15-1 Many types of prepackaged IV solutions are available.

▶ **CLIENT EDUCATION NEEDED:**

1. If the client or caregiver will be administering IV fluids at home, provide clear, step-by-step instructions regarding the procedure.
2. Explain to the client or caregiver the need to store the solution in a clean, dry area.

Estimated time to complete the skill:
5–10 minutes

▶ **DELEGATION TIPS**

The skill of intravenous solution administration is not delegated to ancillary personnel in acute care settings. This may vary in state or federal institutions. Ancillary personnel are generally informed about the medications the client is receiving if adverse effects are anticipated or are being monitored.

IMPLEMENTATION—Action/Rationale

Action	Rationale
1. Check health care provider's order for the IV solution.	1. Ensures accurate administration of the solution.
2. Wash hands. Apply gloves if required by institutional policy.	2. Reduces the transmission of microorganisms.
3. Prepare new bag by removing protective cover from bag.	3. Allows for access to the solution container.
4. Inspect the bag for leaks, tears, or cracks. Inspect the fluid for clarity, particulate matter, and color. Check expiration date (see Figure 5-15-2).	4. Prevents infusing contaminated or outdated solution.

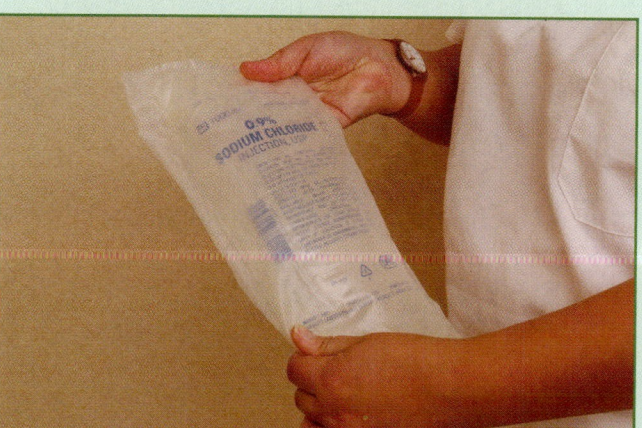

Figure 5-15-2 Inspect the bag for the proper solution, clarity of solution, and expiration date.

continues

Action	Rationale
5. Prepare a label for the IV bag: • On the label, note date, time, and your initials. • Attach the label to the bag. Keep in mind the bag will be inverted when it is hanging. Make sure the label can be read when the IV is hanging.	5. • Communicates when the bag was opened.
6. Store the prepared IV solution in the area assigned by the institution.	6. Keeps the prepared solution readily available for when it is needed.
7. Remove gloves and dispose of gloves with all used materials.	7. Reduces the transmission of microorganisms.
8. Wash hands.	8. Reduces the transmission of microorganisms.
9. Document the preparation of the IV solution.	9. Provides a record to ensure continuity of care.

Hanging the Prepared IV

Action	Rationale
10. Wash hands.	10. Reduces the transmission of microorganisms.
11. Obtain the IV solution for the client as ordered. Check the label on the IV bag to see that it matches the order.	11. Ensures the ordered medication is administered.
12. Inspect the bag for leaks, tears, or cracks and inspect the fluid for clarity, particulate matter, and color.	12. Prevents infusing contaminated solution.
13. Check client's identification bracelet.	13. Ensures IV solution is given to the correct client.
14. Make sure the clamp on the tubing is closed (see Figure 5-15-3). Grasp the port of the IV bag with your nondominant hand, remove the plastic tab covering the port (see Figure 5-15-4), and insert the full length of the spike into the bag's port (see Figure 5-15-5).	14. Promotes rapid flow of solution through new tubing without air bubbles.
15. Compress drip chamber to fill halfway (see Figure 5-15-6).	15. Filling chamber halfway allows the chamber to provide a clear measurement of drip rate when the IV is flowing.

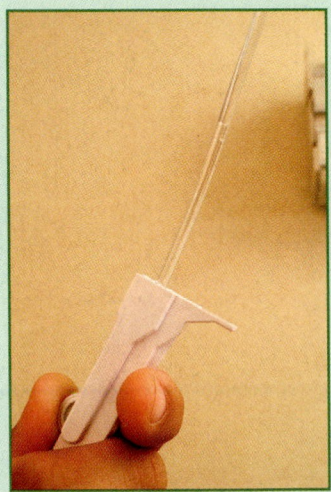

Figure 5-15-3   Roll the clamp down on the tubing.

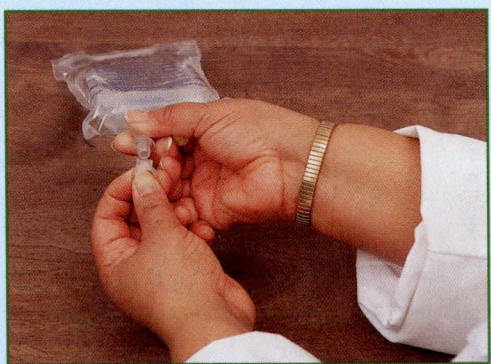

Figure 5-15-4   Open the IV plastic bag and pull down the plastic tab covering the port with one hand while pinching the port with the other hand.

continues

Action	Rationale

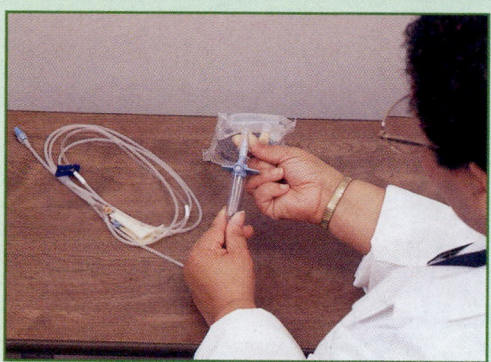

Figure 5-15-5 Remove the cap from the spike and spike the IV port.

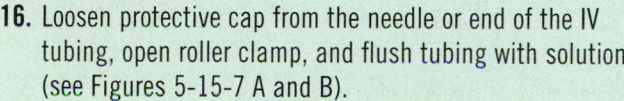

Figure 5-15-6 Make sure the drip chamber is filled halfway.

16. Loosen protective cap from the needle or end of the IV tubing, open roller clamp, and flush tubing with solution (see Figures 5-15-7 A and B).

17. Close roller clamp and replace cap protector.

16. Removes air from tubing.

17. Prevents fluid from leaking and maintains sterility of the needle.

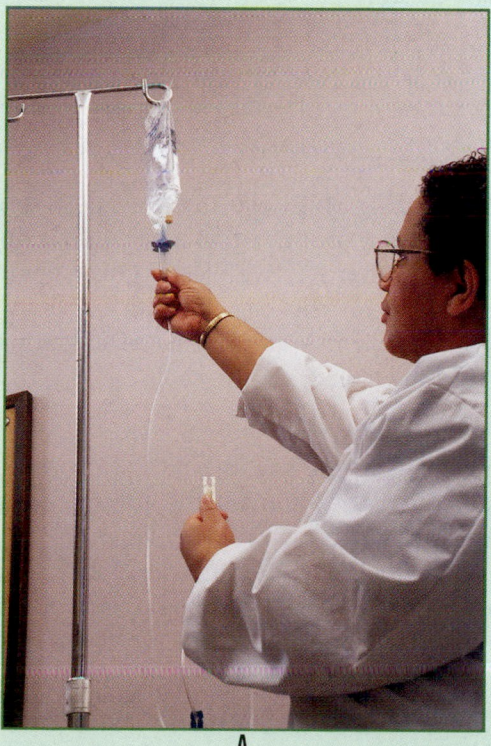

A

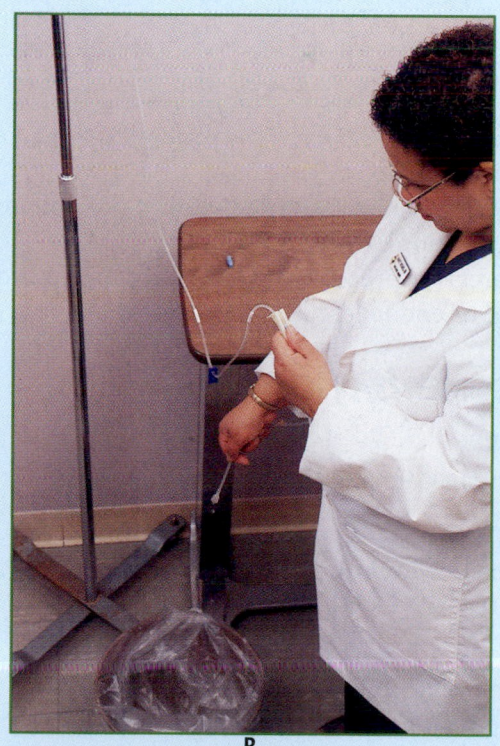

B

Figure 5-15-7 A, B Priming the IV tubing. Open the roller clamp on the tubing to allow the fluid to enter the tube and expel the air.

continues

Action	Rationale
Hanging the Prepared IV *continued*	
18. When ready to initiate infusion, remove the cap protector from the tubing. Attach the IV tubing to venipuncture catheter (see Skill 8-2, Starting an IV).	**18.** Initiates infusion.
19. Open clamp and regulate flow or, if applicable, attach tubing to infusion device or rate controller, if used. Turn on pump and set flow rate (see Skill 8-5, Setting the IV Flow Rate).	**19.** Allows flow rate to be regulated.
20. Wash hands.	**20.** Reduces the transmission of microorganisms.

> ▶ **REAL WORLD ANECDOTES**
>
> *While preparing an IV solution for her client, Tamekia grabbed a bottle of D_5W to mix the medication into. As she was drawing up the ordered additive, she glanced at the bottle of D_5W and noticed something unusual about it. On closer inspection, Tamekia noticed what appeared to be crystals in the bottom of the IV bottle. Tamekia disposed of the bottle and checked the rest of the stock of IV D_5W bottles. When she found several other bottles that were contaminated, she notified her supervisor and the old bottles were replaced with a new lot.*

▶ EVALUATION

- The appropriate fluids at the ordered dosages were available for IV infusion.
- The IV infusion was sterile, without precipitate or contamination.
- The caregiver preparing the IV solution was not injured or endangered.

▶ DOCUMENTATION

Flow Sheet

- Document date and time IV solution was prepared.

Document on appropriate flow sheet or electronic medical record (EMR).

▶ CRITICAL THINKING SKILL

Introduction

Some IV solutions are commercially made or prepared by the pharmacist, but others may require the nurse to prepare them. Reading the labels carefully will ensure that the correct solution is infused into the client.

Possible Scenario

On a busy evening shift, the nurse walked quickly into the medication room to grab a bag of IV solution for her client. The protective plastic cover obscured the label printed on the bag with its contents. He wanted 5% dextrose in water but he mistakenly took 10% dextrose in water from the shelf.

Possible Outcome

As the nurse spiked the bag and hung it from the IV pole, he watched the fluid fill the tubing. Then he noticed the 10% dextrose in water label on the bag. He had not connected the tubing with the IV solution to the client yet, so he took the bag down, discarded the bag and tubing, and went to obtain the correct IV solution and new tubing to start over again.

Prevention

The nurse should remember the five rights of drug administration: the right drug, the right dose, the right client, the right route, and the right time.

▶ VARIATIONS

Geriatric Variation:
- *Older clients may be at higher risk of fluid overload. IV solutions containing sodium may increase fluid retention in older clients.*

Pediatric Variations:
- *Small children require smaller volumes of fluid.*
- *Special effort needs to be taken to keep an IV site clean, dry, and intact in very young clients.*

Home Care Variation:
- *Be sure the client or caregiver has a clean, dry area to store IV solutions.*

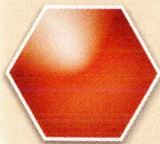

Long-Term Care Variation:
- *Regularly reassess the solution a client is receiving based on the client's current fluid and electrolyte status.*

▶ COMMON ERRORS

Possible Error:

The IV solution appears cloudy when the nurse takes it from the shelf.

Prevention:

The nurse should check the expiration date on the bag to make sure it is not out of date. The nurse should also check for any cracks or leaks in the bag. Do not use the cloudy IV solution. Return it to the pharmacy or stockroom with information about what the problem is. Obtain a fresh bag and proceed to prepare the IV solution.

▶ NURSING TIPS

- Anticipate the need for the next bag of IV solution to avoid the risk of an IV clotting caused by the solution running out.
- Keep in mind the client's laboratory results and need for fluid to be sure the correct solution is given.
- Hold the bag up against both a light and dark solid background to check for discoloration.

▶ SPECIAL CONSIDERATIONS

- *To help prevent medical errors, always consider the rationale and purpose for the designated therapy when preparing an IV solution. For example, a nurse should question a dextrose IV solution prescribed to a client who is going to receive a blood transfusion.*

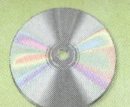

Adding Medications to an IV Solution

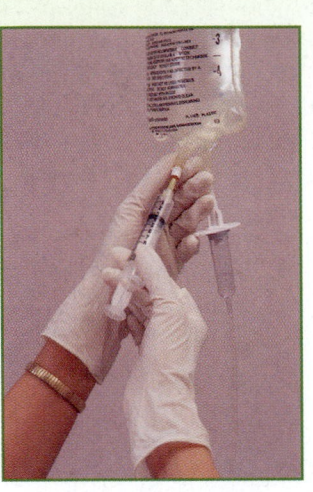

▶ OVERVIEW OF THE SKILL

The intravenous route carries the highest risk for a client as the response to the drug and solution are immediate. Great care and precise calculations are required when preparing a medication to add to an intravenous (IV) solution. The drug is diluted and mixed into a larger volume (50–1000 mL) of compatible solution and then infused into the primary or secondary IV line. Medications such as vitamins or potassium chloride are commonly added to IV solutions.

Mixing the drugs into large volumes of fluids is safe and easy. Although institutional policies vary, the nurse, pharmacist, or pharmacist technician can add the medication into a compatible solution of either normal saline, 5% dextrose in water, or lactated Ringer's solution. Use needleless systems if available. Safe devices, such as safety-needles or syringes, are required by OSHA.

It is important to note that some medications, such as potassium, can be irritating to the lining of blood vessels. Other medications injected into a traumatized vein can infiltrate tissue to such an extent that affected tissue could slough, become abscessed, or become necrotic.

▶ ASSESSMENT

1. Assess the five rights: right client, right medication, right route, right dose, and right time. **Prevents errors in medication administration.**

2. Check the health care provider's order for the client, medication, dosage, and time and route of administration **to ensure accurate administration.**

3. Review information regarding the drug, including action, purpose, side effects, normal dose, peak onset, and nursing implications, **in order to administer the drug safely.**

4. Determine the additives in the solution of an existing IV line **to determine whether the medication is compatible with the solution. If the medications are not compatible, a new IV site will be needed, unless the existing site is a double or triple-lumen catheter.**

5. Assess the patency of the IV **to ensure that the medication will enter the vein and not the surrounding tissue.**

6. Assess the skin at the IV site **so that the medication will not be administered into an inflamed or edematous site, which could cause injury to the tissue.**

7. Check the client's drug allergy history **as an allergic reaction could occur rapidly and be fatal.**

8. Assess the client's understanding of the purpose of the medication **so that client teaching can be tailored to client needs.**

▶ DIAGNOSIS

Risk for Infection

Risk for Impaired Skin Integrity

Risk for Allergic Response

► PLANNING

Expected Outcomes:

1. The appropriate fluids and medications at the ordered dosages will be mixed for IV infusion.
2. The IV infusion will not be contaminated during the procedure.
3. The caregiver mixing the IV will not be injured or endangered.
4. The medication will be infused without injury or trauma to the client.
5. The medication added will have the desired effect.

Equipment Needed (see Figure 5-16-1):

- Prescribed medication in vial or ampule
- Prescribed diluent for medication
- Sterile syringe of appropriate size (5–20 mL)
- Sterile needle (1- to 1.5-inch, 19- to 21-gauge)
- Sterile IV bag (500–100 mL)
- Antiseptic swab
- Label for IV bag
- Medication administration record

► CLIENT EDUCATION NEEDED:

1. Teach the client the rationale for the medication.
2. Teach the client the rationale for IV administration of the medication.

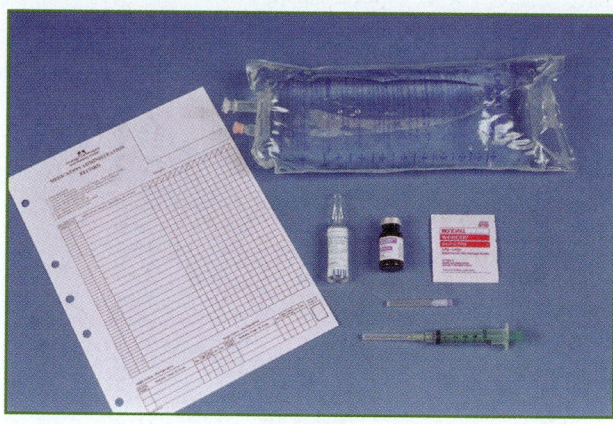

Figure 5-16-1 Medications may be ordered to be added to IV solutions for administration.

3. Teach the client to report any side effects he or she experiences immediately.
4. Instruct clients with an allergy history to wear a bracelet listing allergies.

 Estimated time to complete the skill: **5–10 minutes**

► DELEGATION TIPS

The skill of medication administration is not delegated to ancillary personnel in acute care settings but may vary in state or federal institutions. Ancillary personnel are generally informed about the medications the client is receiving if adverse effects are anticipated or are being monitored.

IMPLEMENTATION—Action/Rationale

Action	Rationale
1. Check health care provider's order for the IV solution and additives ordered.	1. Ensures accurate administration of the solution and additives.
2. Determine whether the ordered additives are compatible with the IV solution and with each other.	2. Multiple additives increase the possibility of incompatibility. Some medications can be mixed only in saline.
3. Wash hands. Apply gloves if required by institutional policy.	3. Reduces the transmission of microorganisms.

continues

Action	Rationale

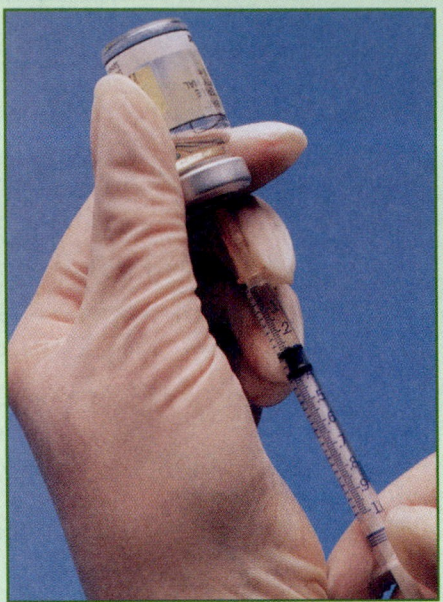

Figure 5-16-2   Draw the medication into the syringe.

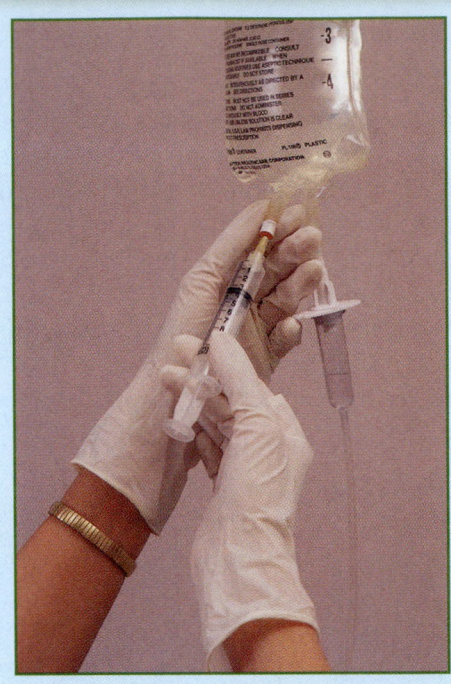

Figure 5-16-3   Inject the medication into the bag.

4. Using the appropriate technique, draw up any additives ordered by the health care provider (see Figure 5-16-2).

Adding Medication to a New Solution

5. Prepare new bag by removing protective cover from bag.

6. Inspect the bag for leaks, tears, or cracks. Inspect the fluid for clarity, particulate matter, and color. Check expiration date.

7. Add medication to IV solution:
- For plastic IV bag, locate port with rubber stopper.
- Wipe off port or site with antiseptic swab.
- Insert needle into center of port or site.
- Inject medication into bag (see Figure 5-16-3).
- Remove needle from bag.

8. Mix medication into IV solution by gently turning the bag from end to end.

9. Label the bag: See Figure 5-16-4
- Write the name and dose of medication. Write date, time, and nurse's initials.
- Apply to bag upside-down.

10. Store the prepared IV solution in the area assigned by the institution.

4. Ordered additives may come in vials, ampules, or bags.

5. Allows for access to the injection port.

6. Prevents infusing contaminated or outdated solution.

7.
- Avoids use of port of the IV tubing or the air vent.
- Reduces transmission of microorganisms.
- Facilitates adding medication to bag.
- Facilitates adding medication to bag.
- Injection ports are self-sealing.

8. Ensures even distribution of medication throughout the solution.

9.
- Informs nurses and doctors regarding medications added to the solution.
- Allows easy visualization when bag is hanging.

10. Keeps the prepared solution readily available for when it is needed.

continues

Action	Rationale

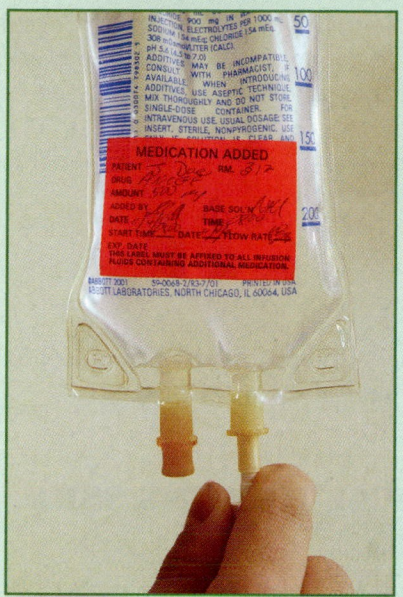

Figure 5-16-4 The medication label placed on the IV bag whenever a medication is added to the IV.

Adding Medication to an Existing Solution

11. Identify client using armband and calling name.

12. Explain the purpose of the medication and how it will be given.

13. Clamp the IV tubing and remove bag from IV pole.

14. Add medication to IV solution:
    - For plastic IV bag, locate port with rubber stopper.
    - Wipe off port or site with antiseptic swab.
    - Insert needle into center of port or site.
    - Inject medication into bag.
    - Remove needle from bag.

15. Mix medication into IV solution by gently turning the bag from end to end.

16. Apply a new label:
    - Write the name and dose of medication. Write date, time, and nurse's initials.

17. Unclamp the tubing and regulate the flow (see Skill 8-5, Setting the IV Flow Rate).

18. Remove gloves and dispose of all used materials appropriately.

19. Wash hands.

20. Document the preparation of the IV solution.

---

11. Ensures correct client received the medication.

12. Information reduces anxiety.

13. Prevents medication from being infused rapidly.

14.
    - Avoids use of port of the IV tubing or the air vent.
    - Reduces transmission of microorganisms.
    - Facilitates adding medication to bag.
    - Facilitates adding medication to bag.
    - Injection ports are self-sealing.

15. Ensures even distribution of medication throughout the solution.

16.
    - Informs nurses and doctors regarding medications added to the solution.

17. Prevents rapid infusion of the medication.

18. Reduces transmission of organisms.

19. Reduces transmission of organisms.

20. Provides a record to ensure continuity of care.

► **EVALUATION**

- The appropriate fluids and medications at the ordered dosages were mixed for IV infusion.
- The IV infusion was not contaminated during the procedure.
- The caregiver mixing the IV was not injured or endangered.
- The medication was infused without injury or trauma to the client.

► **DOCUMENTATION**

Medication Administration Record

- Document the name, dosage, time, and date of medication added to the IV solution.

Flow Sheet

- Note the date, time, solution, volume, and medications added.

Nurses' Notes

- Record the client's response to the medication and condition of the IV site.
- Document any serious side effects. These should also be reported to the health care provider immediately.

- Document on appropriate flow sheet or electronic medical record (EMR).

► **CRITICAL THINKING SKILL**

Introduction

A minimum amount of solution is necessary in which to dilute certain medications.

Possible Scenario

The physician ordered 40 mEq of KCl to be added to an existing IV solution of D_5NS already containing 40 mEq KCl. The nurse noted that there was only 120 mL of the solution left in the bag and that it was infusing at 100 mL per hour. Should she add the dose of potassium the physician prescribed?

Possible Outcome

The nurse realized that the amount of potassium that would infuse per hour at that concentration could be potentially dangerous. She notified the physician, who changed the IV order to a safe concentration.

Prevention

The nurse needs to know the action of medications that are added to IV solutions in order to give them safely.

continues

▶ VARIATIONS *(continued)*

Pediatric Variations:

- Giving a medication to a child through an established IV may be less traumatic than an IM or subcutaneous injection.
- Special effort needs to be taken to keep an IV site clean, dry, and intact in very young clients.
- Remember that there is even less room for fluid and electrolyte and fluid volume administration errors in infants and children. Double-check all orders to make sure the additives and the infusion amounts are appropriate for the age of the child.

Home Care Variations:

- Medications should be added to IV solutions by the pharmacist before dispensing them for home use.
- Make sure the caregiver can clearly read and understand the labels on the IV bag and any additive labels.
- Assess that the client or caregiver can determine if an additive has been added to an IV bag.

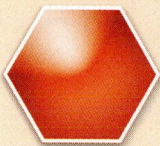

Long-Term Care Variation:

- Clients receiving IV additives over the long-term need to be assessed regularly for continued need of those additives. For example, if the client is receiving a potassium supplement, regular laboratory tests should be performed to track the client's blood potassium level.

▶ COMMON ERRORS

Possible Error:

The medication needle is inserted into the air vent and fluid leaks through the vent.

Prevention:

Be sure to visually assess the injection port or site before inserting the needle. Make sure you can tell the difference between the air vent and the injection port. Clamp the IV tubing to the client. Turn the bag upright to allow the fluid to return to the bag. Assess for contamination of the medication, the IV fluid, or the needle. Replace contaminated items, if needed.

▶ NURSING TIPS

- Prepare medication and label in the medication room before approaching the client.

- Some IV solutions should be prepared by the pharmacist under the laminar air flow hood to ensure a sterile solution.
- Check with the pharmacist or drug text regarding drug compatibility.

▶ SPECIAL CONSIDERATIONS

- Be aware of the minimum dilution requirements for medications. If there is a question regarding the adequacy of the amount of fluid in an existing IV bag, check with the pharmacist. A new IV solution may be used to replace the old one if the client does not have intake restriction.
- Nursing documentation should clearly state the medication information added to the IV solution. The amount and type of IV solution used for dilution should be recorded as well.
- Some medications have certain characteristics such as photosensitivity and should be protected from light.

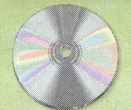

Administering Medications via Secondary Administration Sets (Piggyback)

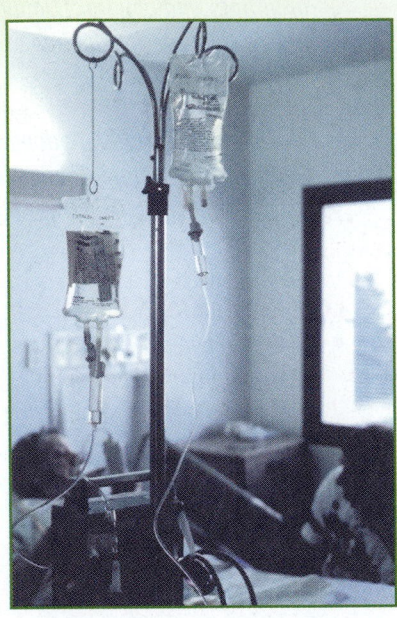

▶ OVERVIEW OF THE SKILL

A medication is given intravenously when a rapid response to a drug is required or when several medications need to be given intravenously (IV) on a regular schedule. This task is best accomplished by using an existing IV as the basic infusion and adding medications by "piggyback" when they are ordered. It also carries the highest risk of side effects because of the immediate response of the medication and the inability to correct a medication administration error.

The drug is diluted and mixed with a small volume (50–100 mL) of compatible solution and then joined to the primary IV line for infusion. The bag is connected to the upper Y-port of the primary infusion line and hung higher than the primary IV bag, thus the name "piggyback." The piggyback infusion works because of the backflow valve. When the piggyback infusion starts flowing, the valve stops the flow of the primary infusion. After the piggyback infusion is complete and the solution within the tubing falls below the level of the primary infusion drip chamber, the valve opens and the primary infusion flows.

It is important to note that some medications can be irritating to the lining of blood vessels. Other medications, when injected into a vein that is beginning to infiltrate, will injure the tissue to such an extent that tissue could slough, become abscessed, or become necrotic. No IV medication should be administered through IV sites that are suspected to be inflamed or infiltrated. Use needleless systems if available. Safety-needles and syringes are required by OSHA standards.

▶ ASSESSMENT

1. Check the health care provider's order or the medication administration record (MAR) for the medication, dosage, and time and route of administration **to ensure accurate administration.**
2. Review information regarding the drug, including action, purpose, side effects, normal dose, peak onset, and nursing implications, **in order to administer the drug safely.**
3. Determine additives in the solution of an existing IV line **so that the medication will be compatible with the solution.**
4. Assess the placement of the IV catheter in the vein **to ensure that the medication will enter the vein and not the surrounding tissue.**
5. Assess the skin at the IV site so that the medication will not be administered into an

654

inflamed or edematous site, which could cause injury to the tissue.

6. Check the client's drug allergy history as an allergic reaction could occur rapidly and be fatal.

7. Assess the client's understanding of the purpose of the medication so that client teaching can be tailored to needs.

8. Assess the compatibility of the piggyback IV medication with the primary IV solution to avoid an adverse reaction such as the formation of precipitate in the IV tubing.

▶ DIAGNOSIS

Risk for Infection

Risk for Injury

Impaired Skin Integrity

Deficient Knowledge

Risk for Allergic Reaction

▶ PLANNING

Expected Outcomes:

1. The drug is infused into the vein without complications.

2. The IV site remains free of swelling and inflammation.

3. The client will be able to discuss the purpose of the drug.

4. The client is free from allergic reaction.

Equipment Needed (see Figure 5-17-1):

- Disposable gloves
- Medication prepared in a labeled infusion bag
- Short microdrip or macrodrip tubing set for piggyback (needleless system preferred)
- Safety sterile needles, 21- or 23-gauge, if needleless system not available
- Antiseptic swab

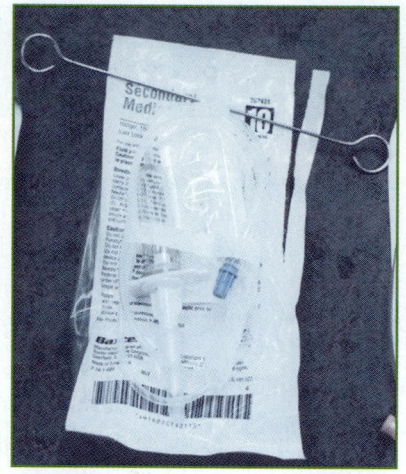

Figure 5-17-1   IV tubing set for piggyback administration.

- Adhesive tape
- IV pole
- Medication administration record

▶ CLIENT EDUCATION NEEDED:

1. Teach the client the rationale for the medication.

2. Teach the client the rationale for IV administration of the medication.

3. Teach the client to report any side effects he or she experiences immediately.

4. Reassure the client that the administration of an IV medication into an existing IV line may be uncomfortable but not painful.

5. Instruct the client with an allergy history to wear a bracelet listing allergies.

Estimated time to complete the skill: **5–10 minutes to set up the IV piggyback**

▶ DELEGATION TIPS

The skill of medication administration is not delegated to ancillary personnel in acute care settings. This may vary in state or federal institutions. Ancillary personnel are generally informed about the medications the client is receiving if adverse effects are anticipated or are being monitored.

IMPLEMENTATION—Action/Rationale

Action	Rationale
1. Check health care provider's order.	1. Ensures accurate administration of medication.
2. Wash hands. Gloves are not necessary if you are adding fluids to an existing infusion line.	2. Reduces the transmission of microorganisms.
3. Check client's identification bracelet.	3. Ensures medication is given to the correct client.
4. Explain procedure and reason the drug is being given.	4. Information decreases anxiety.
5. Prepare medication bag: • Close clamp on tubing of infusion set. • Spike medication bag with infusion tubing (see Figure 5-17-2). • Open clamp (see Figure 5-17-3). • Allow tubing to be filled with solution to evacuate air from tubing (see Figure 5-17-4).	5. • Prevents leakage of solution. • Provides a method of infusing the medication into the system. • Allows the solution to fill the tubing. • Prevents air embolus.
6. Hang piggyback medication bag above level of primary IV bag. One way to do this is to lower the primary bag using an extender (found in the piggyback tubing package) (see Figure 5-17-5).	6. Relationship between height of the bags affects the flow rate to the client.
7. Connect piggyback tubing to primary tubing at Y-port: • For needleless system, remove cap on port and connect tubing (see Figures 5-17-6 and 5-17-7) • If a needle is used, clean port with antiseptic swab and insert small-gauge needle into center of port. • Secure tubing with adhesive tape.	7. Ensures medication in piggyback bag is infused. • A needleless system is preferred to prevent accidental needle sticks. • A small-gauge needle does less damage to the rubber stopper on the port. • Prevents accidental removal of tubing.

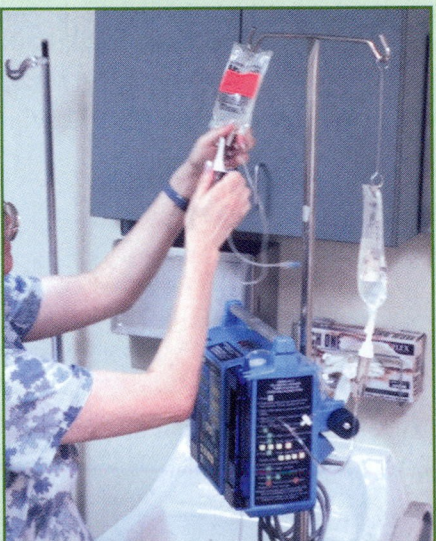

Figure 5-17-2   Spike the medication bag with the infusion tubing.

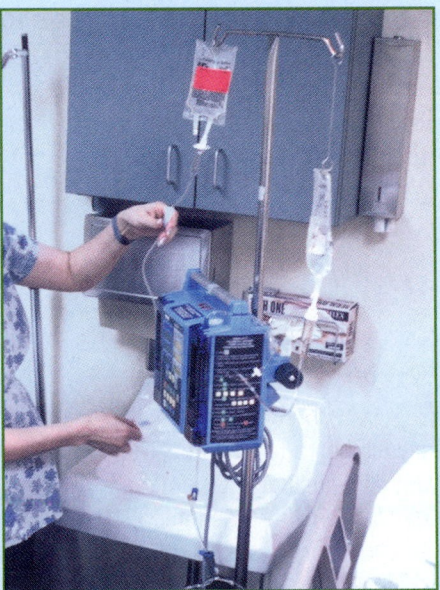

Figure 5-17-3   Open the clamp on the IV tubing.

continues

Action	Rationale

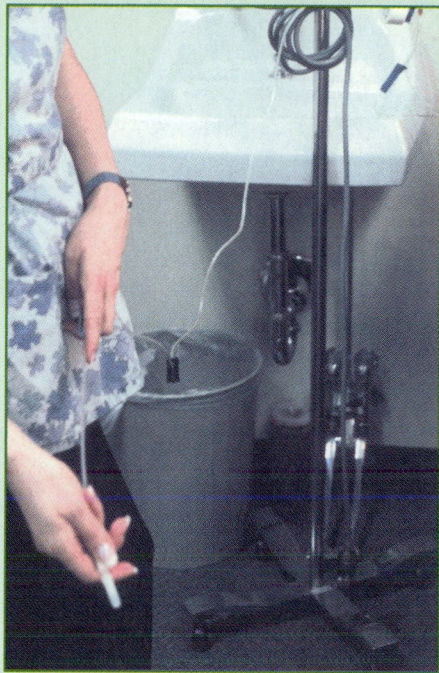

Figure 5-17-4   Allow the tubing to fill with solution.

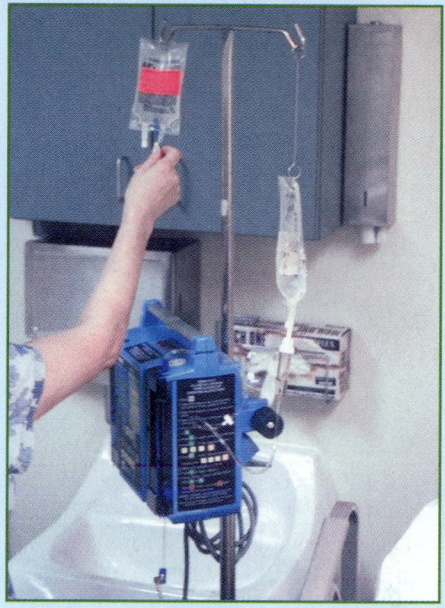

Figure 5-17-5   Hang the piggyback bag higher than the primary IV bag.

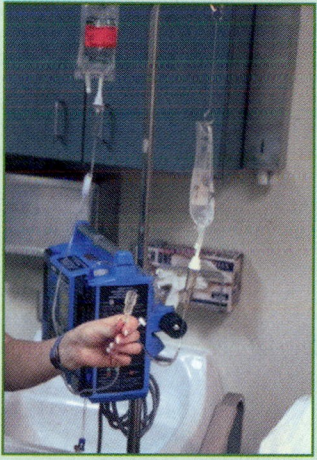

Figure 5-17-6   Remove the cap on the needleless system port.

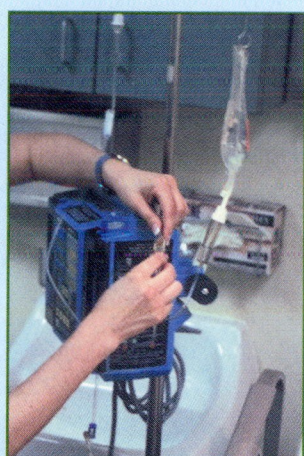

Figure 5-17-7   Connect the needleless system tubing.

8. Administer the medication:
   - Check the prescribed length of time for the infusion.

   - Regulate the flow rate of the piggyback by adjusting the regulator clamp (see Figure 5-17-8).
   - Observe whether backflow valve on piggyback has stopped flow of primary infusion during drug administration (see Figure 5-17-9).

8.

   - Each medication has a recommended rate for IV piggyback administration.
   - Medication infuses through primary line.

   - Prevents backup of medication into primary infusion line.

continues

Action	Rationale

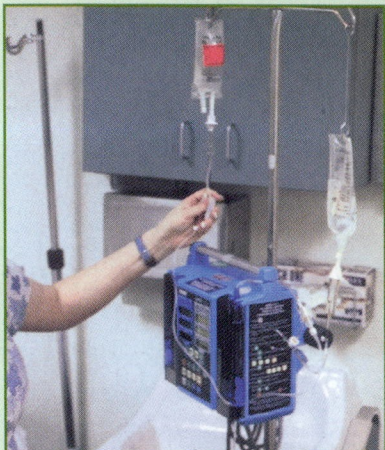

Figure 5-17-8   Regulate the flow rate of the piggyback by adjusting the regulator clamp.

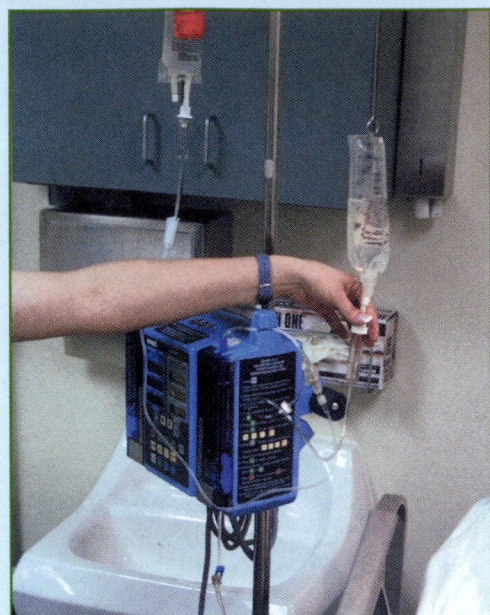

Figure 5-17-9   Double-check that the primary infusion has stopped flowing.

9. Check primary infusion line when medication is finished:
   - Regulate primary infusion rate.
   - Leave secondary bag and tubing in place for next drug administration.

10. Dispose of all used materials and place needles in needle biohazard sharps container.

11. Wash hands.

9.
   - Reestablishes primary infusion.
   - Reduces risk for entry of microorganisms by repeated changes of tubing.

10. Reduces transmission of microorganisms.

11. Reduces transmission of microorganisms.

▶ **REAL WORLD ANECDOTES**

Steven was hospitalized for meningitis. He received a continuous infusion of IV fluids to treat dehydration and fever as well as scheduled infusions of IV antibiotics. Steven was receiving ampicillin every 4 hours via IV piggy-back and amphotericin every 12 hours via IV piggyback. Steven's nurse was preparing to infuse his 4 p.m. dose of ampicillin. She checked the MAR and reached into the medication refrigerator for Steven's piggyback bag of ampicillin. Intent on getting to her meal break, she only glanced at the label long enough to verify that the bag was labeled for Steven. The medication name looked similar to ampicillin and she hurried to Steven's room to hang the medication. As she was preparing to spike the new piggyback she took a longer look at the label. Realizing that it said amphotericin, not ampicillin, she returned to the medication room with the piggyback and retrieved the bag of ampicillin, being careful this time to confirm that this was the correct medication for the correct client at the correct time.

▶ **EVALUATION**

- The drug was infused into the vein without complications.
- The IV site remained free of swelling and inflammation.
- The client was able to discuss the purpose of the drug.

▶ **DOCUMENTATION**

Medication Administration Record (MAR)

- Document the date, time, dose, and route of medication.

Flow Sheet

- Document the date, time, and volume of fluid infused IV piggyback.

Nurses' Notes

- Document the client's response to the medication.
- Record any serious side effects and report them to the health care provider immediately.

Document on appropriate flow sheet or electronic medical record (EMR).

Intake and Output Record

- Note the amount of fluid infused.

▶ **CRITICAL THINKING SKILL**

Introduction

The piggyback bag should be hung higher than the primary bag so the backflow valve will operate correctly.

Possible Scenario

A client has an IV of D_5W infusing at 75 mL per hour. The physician orders an antibiotic to be given via IV piggyback every 6 hours. The nurse connects the piggyback tubing into the primary IV line but does not hang it high enough, causing blood to back up 1 inch into the primary IV line.

Possible Outcome

If left in the tubing, the blood could clot and occlude the primary IV line, requiring a new IV start and unnecessary trauma for the client. In this case the nurse checked on the client within 5 minutes and noticed the blood in the primary tubing. The nurse raised the piggyback bag of medication, watched to be sure the piggyback fluid was infusing, and verified that the blood infused into the client's vein.

Prevention

The IV piggyback bag must be hung higher than the primary IV fluid. If it is not, the piggyback medication could flow into the primary IV fluid or the primary IV fluid could flow into the piggyback bag. In either scenario the client would not be receiving any IV fluid and the IV site would be in danger of occluding. Take the time to be sure the piggyback is infusing correctly before proceeding on to other duties.

▶ **VARIATIONS**

Geriatric Variation:

- *The veins of elderly clients may be more fragile and sensitive to irritating solutions.*

Pediatric Variations:

- *Giving a medication to a child through an established IV may be less traumatic than an IM or subcutaneous injection.*
- *Special precautions need to be taken to maintain an intact IV in very young clients.*
- *Adaptation to promote optimum mobility for a child while piggyback medication is infusing will increase the child's compliance with the procedure.*

continues

► VARIATIONS *(continued)*

Home Care Variation:

- *Medications can be given by IV piggyback at home after teaching caregiver and client how to perform the procedure.*

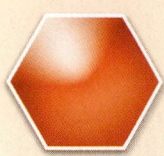

Long-Term Care Variation:

- *Clients who are receiving IV medication over the long-term generally have central lines in place to prevent repeated trauma to their peripheral veins. The procedure for administering a piggyback medication through a central line is the same.*

► COMMON ERRORS

Possible Error:

The IV piggyback tubing was not primed with fluid before it was connected to the primary IV line so air enters the primary tubing.

Prevention:

Be sure to visually assess the IV tubing for the presence of fluid before connecting it to the primary IV line. Stop the infusion. Assess the amount and location of the air. If it is close to the IV piggyback line, clamp the primary line, lower the piggyback bag, and allow gravity to fill the tubing up to the drip chamber. If the air is closer to the client, clean the port with the alcohol prep, use a new, empty syringe, insert it at the nearest port, and aspirate the air.

► NURSING TIPS

- The IV piggyback sets have specific instructions about the tubing and setup.
- An extra hanger may be used to lower the primary IV bag on the IV pole to ensure that the piggyback bag is higher than the primary IV bag.
- An alternative method of priming the IV tubing in the piggyback line is to connect it to the primary line, unclamp, then lower the piggyback bag and tubing below the level of the primary IV bag. This will allow solution from the main IV to backflow into the piggyback tubing. When the solution has flowed to fill half the drip chamber in the piggyback tubing, raise the piggyback and hang in place. Make sure to keep the piggyback bag upright during this process.
- Medication can never be piggybacked into a blood transfusion.

► SPECIAL CONSIDERATIONS

- *If an infusion pump is used with the primary and secondary IV lines, make sure to monitor the infusion rate and the solution residual. An infusion pump assists the nursing intervention and should not replace the autonomy of nursing assessment.*
- *In a situation when a secondary IV line is used to administer medication on a regular basis, maintain sterility of the IV line and ports between each intervention.*

Administering Medications via IV Bolus or IV Push

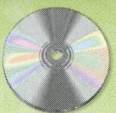

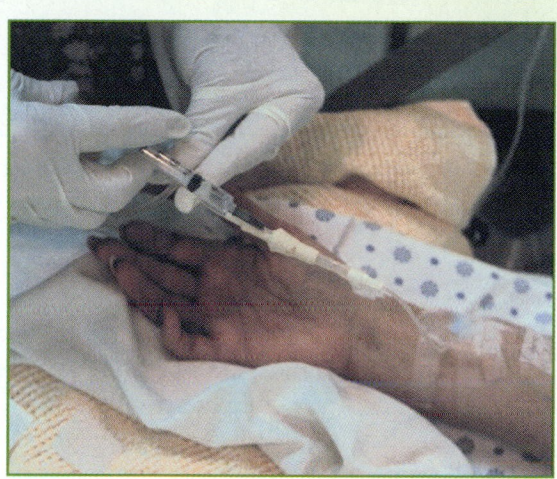

▶ OVERVIEW OF THE SKILL

An intravenous bolus is the administration of a medication directly into a vein through the injection port of an existing intravenous (IV) line or through a previously placed IV catheter with a saline lock. The method of administering the bolus dose of medication is called IV push. The nurse must follow institutional as well as pharmacologic guidelines regarding which medication may be given IV push.

An IV bolus is used when a rapid response to a drug is required such as a cardiac emergency. It also carries the highest risk of side effects because of the immediate response of the medication and the inability to correct a medication administration error.

Some medications can be irritating to the lining of blood vessels. Other medications, when injected into a vein that is beginning to infiltrate, will injure the tissue to such an extent that tissue could slough, become abscessed, or become necrotic. Some medications can be given directly while others require dilution.

▶ ASSESSMENT

1. Check the health care provider's order for the medication, dosage, time, and route of administration **to ensure accurate administration.**
2. Review information regarding the drug, including action, purpose, side effects, normal dose, peak onset, nursing implications, required dilution,

length of time for administration, and incompatibility with IV or other medications, **in order to administer the drug safely.**
3. Determine the additives in the solution of an existing IV line **so that the medication will be compatible with the solution.**
4. Assess the placement of the IV needle **to ensure that the medication will enter the vein and not the surrounding tissue.**
5. Assess the skin at the IV site **so that the medication will not be administered into an inflamed or edematous site, which could cause injury to the tissue.**
6. Check the client's drug allergy history **as an allergic reaction could occur rapidly and be fatal.**
7. Assess the client's understanding of the purpose of the medication **so that client teaching can be tailored to needs**.
8. Assess the medication to be given **to determine how much time is needed to administer the medication safely.**

▶ DIAGNOSIS

Risk for Infection

Risk for Injury

Impaired Skin Integrity

Deficient Knowledge

Risk for Allergic Response

▶ PLANNING

Expected Outcomes:

1. The drug will be infused into the vein without complications.
2. The IV site will remain free of swelling and inflammation.
3. The client will be able to discuss the purpose of the drug.
4. Any adverse reactions to the drug will be identified and treated.

Equipment Needed (see Figure 5-18-1):

- Disposable gloves
- Medication in vial or ampule
- Syringe, 3- to 5-mL
- Sterile needles, 21- and 25-gauge
- Antiseptic swabs (follow agency protocol)
- Two syringes with saline flush solution. Label syringe.
- Watch with second hand

▶ CLIENT EDUCATION NEEDED:

1. Teach the client the rationale for the medication.
2. Teach the client the rationale for IV administration of the medication.
3. Teach the client to report any side effects he or she experiences immediately.

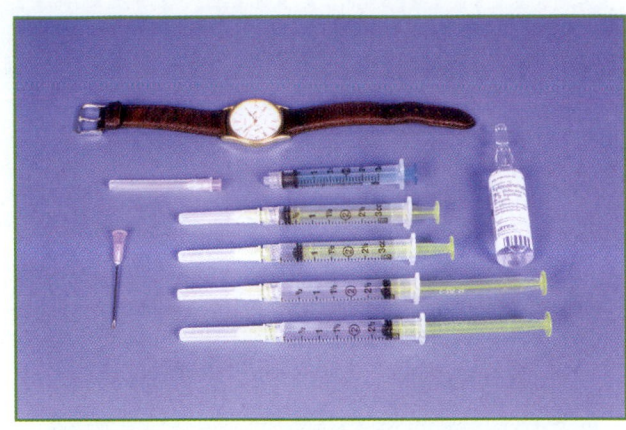

Figure 5-18-1 Povidone-iodine, chlorhexidine, or alcohol swabs are used to clean the injection site. Syringes are used to inject the medication. Saline is used to flush the injection port before and after medication is administered.

4. Reassure the client that the administration of an IV medication into an existing IV line or saline lock may be uncomfortable but not painful.
5. Provide clients with an allergy history a bracelet listing allergies.

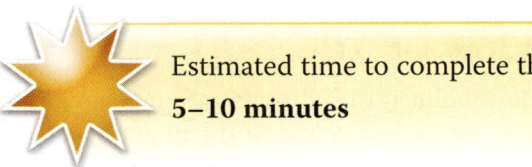

Estimated time to complete the skill: **5–10 minutes**

▶ DELEGATION TIPS

The skill of medication administration is not delegated to ancillary personnel in acute care settings. This may vary in state or federal institutions. Ancillary personnel are generally informed about the medications the client is receiving if adverse effects are anticipated or are being monitored.

IMPLEMENTATION—Action/Rationale

Action	Rationale
1. Check health care provider's order to give drug and ascertain if drug must be diluted or given over a certain time period. Check for IV and medication incompatibilities.	1. Ensures accurate administration of medication.
2. Wash hands and put on clean gloves.	2. Reduces the transmission of microorganisms.
3. Using the appropriate technique, draw the medication up into a syringe.	3. Prepares the medication bolus while preserving its sterility.

continues

Action	Rationale
4. Check client's identification bracelet.	4. Ensures medication is given to the correct client.
5. Explain procedure and reason the drug is being given.	5. Information decreases anxiety.
6. To inject medication using an injection port on an existing primary IV use a needleless system or safety-needle: • Select an injection port close to the IV insertion site. • Check for a blood return by pinching the tubing above the injection port and pulling back on the plunger of the syringe. • Clean the selected site with antiseptic solution. Administer the medication by continuing to pinch the tubing and slowly injecting the medication over the prescribed time period (see Figure 5-18-2). • After the medication bolus is infused, clear the tubing of medication by releasing the pinched tubing and allowing the infusion rate of the IV to resume. (If the medication is not compatible with the IV solution, a saline flush may be needed.) Check with the pharmacy if you are unclear.	6. • Selecting the closest insertion site decreases the amount of medication in the IV line if an immediate reaction occurs. • Ensures the IV is patent so that medication will enter the blood circulation and not the surrounding tissues. • Each medication has a recommended rate for IV push administration. Some medications can lead to death if given too rapidly. • Ensures that the entire dose of medication has been infused. Maintains the patency of the infusion catheter.
7. To inject medication using a saline lock: • Clean the saline lock with antiseptic solution and insert a saline syringe with a 25-gauge safety-needle into the center of the diaphragm. It is preferable to use a needleless system. • Check for blood return by pulling back gently on the plunger of the syringe then flush the lock with saline. • Remove the saline syringe. • Clean the injection port again with an antiseptic swab. • Insert the syringe with the medication into the injection port and slowly inject the medication over the prescribed time (see Figure 5-18-3). • Remove the medication syringe. • Clean the injection port with an antiseptic swab.	7. • Prevents the introduction of microorganisms into the client's circulatory system. Using a small-gauge needle causes less damage to the rubber diaphragm. • Ensures the IV is patent so that medication will enter the blood circulation and not the surrounding tissues. • Allows access for the medication syringe. • Prevents the introduction of microorganisms into the client's circulatory system. • Each medication has a recommended rate for IV push administration. Some medications can lead to death if given too rapidly. • Allows access for the saline syringe. • Prevents the introduction of microorganisms into the client's circulatory system.

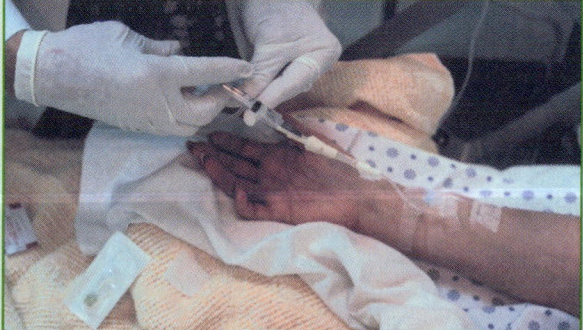

Figure 5-18-2 Pinch the tubing and slowly inject the medication over the prescribed time period.

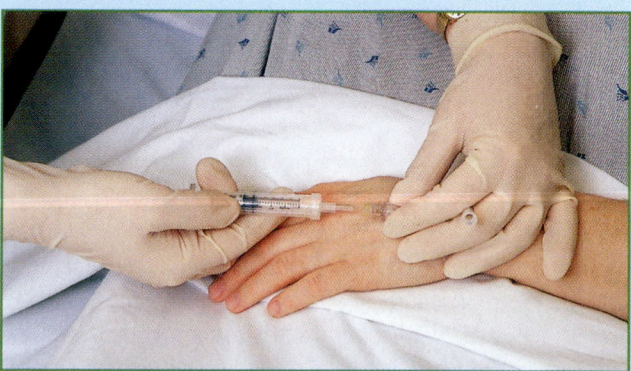

Figure 5-18-3 Injecting a bolus of medication into a peripheral saline lock.

continues

Action	Rationale
• Insert another syringe with saline into the injection port and slowly flush.	• Ensures that the entire dose of medication has been infused. Maintains the patency of the infusion catheter.
• Insert syringe of saline into the injection port and slowly flush. This step may vary depending on the policies at your institution.	• Saline prevents occlusion of the catheter.
8. To bolus medication using a three-way stopcock: • Turn off the stopcock to the port that will be used.	**8.** • Prevents the accidental infusion of air into the intravenous system. • Provides access to the infusion system.
• For a stopcock without an injection port, remove the stopcock cap and attach the needleless syringe to the uncapped port. • For a stopcock with an injection port, clean the port with an antiseptic swab and insert a small-gauge needle into the center of the port. • If the stopcock is attached to a catheter that is used intermittently, attach a syringe of saline rather than the syringe containing medication. • Open the stopcock so the fluid flow will progress from the syringe to the client. • Check for blood return by gently pulling back on the plunger of the syringe. • If flushing with saline, turn off the stopcock, remove the syringe, clean the cap, if present, insert the syringe filled with medication, and turn on the stopcock to the injection port. • Slowly inject the medication over the prescribed time period. • Turn off the stopcock to the injection port. • Reinitiate the flow of IV fluid, if applicable. • Flush the tubing or catheter with saline using the preceding technique, if there is no continuous IV flow.	• Prevents the introduction of microorganisms into the client's circulatory system. Using a small-gauge needle causes less damage to the rubber diaphragm. • Flushing with saline clears the existing fluid out of the catheter and tubing, decreasing the possibility of medication interactions. • Allows access to the client's circulatory system. • Ensures the IV is patent so that medication will enter the blood circulation and not the surrounding tissues. • Prevents the introduction of microorganisms and the accidental introduction of air into the client's circulatory system. • Each medication has a recommended rate for IV push administration. Some medications can be lethal if given too rapidly. • Prevents the accidental introduction of air into the system. • Maintains the patency of the infusion catheter. • Flushing with saline clears the medication out of the catheter.
9. Remove the needle from the port or diaphragm and swab the port with an antiseptic swab.	**9.** Prevents transmission of microorganisms.
10. Remove gloves and dispose in the appropriate container.	**10.** Reduces transmission of microorganisms.
11. Wash hands.	**11.** Reduces transmission of microorganisms.

▶ REAL WORLD ANECDOTES

Ralph was in the cardiac telemetry unit 4 days after experiencing a myocardial infarction. His IV infusion had been discontinued and a saline lock placed. That evening, the nurse noticed several premature ventricular beats on the cardiac monitor. When the arrhythmia persisted, she notified the physician, who ordered lidocaine to be given IV push immediately. The nurse prepared one syringe with saline and one with the lidocaine, flushed the lock with saline, then gave the lidocaine. An IV solution with tubing was prepared and attached to the saline lock for other emergency drugs to be given if needed.

► **EVALUATION**

- The drug was infused into the vein without complications.
- The IV site remained free of swelling and inflammation.
- The client was able to discuss the purpose of the drug.
- Any adverse reactions to the drug were identified and treated.

► **DOCUMENTATION**

Medication Administration Record

- Document the date, time, name, dose, and route of medication.

Nurses' Notes

- Record the client's response to the medication.
- Record any serious side effects and report them to the health care provider immediately.

Document on appropriate flow sheet or electronic medical record (EMR).

► **CRITICAL THINKING SKILL**

Introduction

Some medications are not compatible with a dextrose in water IV solution. They may form a precipitate that occludes the tubing or IV catheter.

Possible Scenario

A client has an IV of D_5W infusing at 75 mL per hour. The physician orders dilantin to be given IV as the client is unable to take oral medications. The nurse uses the port closest to the client to inject the dilantin, but after the first few seconds of starting the IV push notices a white precipitate forming in the tubing.

Possible Outcome

The nurse immediately stops pushing the dilantin and stops the IV infusion. As the precipitate did not reach the IV catheter, the nurse quickly obtains new tubing and replaces the contaminated tubing using sterile technique. After flushing the tubing with D_5W, the nurse attaches the new tubing to the IV catheter, draws up a new dose of dilantin, and starts the IV bolus dose again, this time flushing the line with normal saline before and after the dilantin.

Prevention

The nurse must always check the compatibility of a medication with the IV solution before giving it IV push.

► **VARIATIONS**

Geriatric Variations:
- *Elderly clients may react to an IV bolus more slowly because of circulatory deficits.*
- *The veins of elderly clients may be more fragile and sensitive to irritating solutions.*

Pediatric Variations:
- *Giving a medication to a child through an established IV may be less painful and traumatic than an IM or subcutaneous injection.*
- *Special precautions need to be taken to maintain an IV intact in very young clients.*
- *A child may react strongly to the feelings of pressure or coolness when IV medication is injected. Carefully observe the child and the site to determine if the reaction is related to anxiety or actual problems with the IV site.*
- *Explain the procedure carefully to children. Make sure that they do not think there is another "needle" going to be inserted into their skin.*

continues

▶ VARIATIONS *(continued)*

Home Care Variation:
- Clients may be taught how to flush an intravenous line to maintain patency, but IV push medications should be administered only by a nurse.

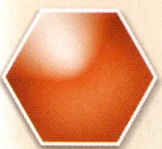

Long-Term Care Variations:
- Long-term IV push medications should be reevaluated periodically for effectiveness of the medication.
- Most clients receiving long-term IV push medications have a central line in place rather than a peripheral IV line.

▶ COMMON ERRORS

Possible Error:
Medication pushed slowly through a saline lock causes swelling around the needle.

Prevention:
Be sure to assess the IV for patency before administering the IV medication. Stop pushing the IV medication. Using another syringe, pull back to check for a blood return. If there is none, remove the needle and saline lock and start an IV in another site. When you are sure the needle is in the vein, administer a new dose of the medication.

▶ NURSING TIPS
- Sometimes no blood will return from a saline lock even though it is patent.
- Be sure the IV site is visible and free of tape or dressing while injecting the medication.
- A patent vein should allow a free flow of medication during an IV push.

▶ SPECIAL CONSIDERATIONS
- *Medications given through the IV push should be administered at a slow pace because the highly concentrated solution could irritate the surrounding vessel tissue. Watch for signs of infiltration and allergic reaction.*
- *Never attempt to force medication through an IV line or saline lock that may be clotted. This action may push the clot into the circulatory system.*

Administering Medications via Volume-Control Sets

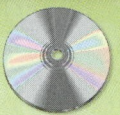

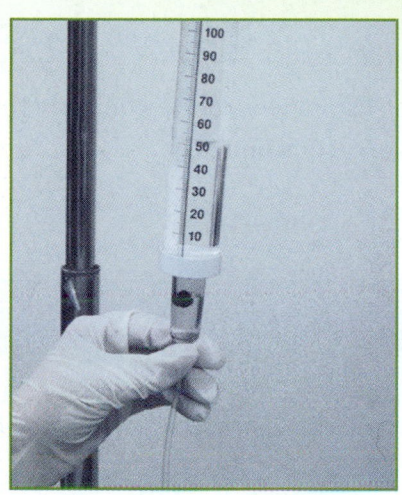

▶ OVERVIEW OF THE SKILL

Volume-control sets are often referred to by brand name such as Soluset, VoluTrol, or Buretrol. They allow the nurse or caregiver to dilute medication in a small to moderate quantity of intravenous (IV) fluid in a calibrated chamber. The drip rate is then adjusted using the roller clamp or a dial-a-flow to deliver a set volume over a set time. This makes it easier for the nurse to accurately regulate and manage the intermittent infusion of IV medications.

▶ ASSESSMENT

1. Identify the drug(s) ordered: action, purpose, normal dosage and route, common side effects, time of onset and peak action, possible interactions with IV solution, and nursing implications. **This allows the nurse to anticipate effects of the drug and to observe the client's response.**
2. Check allergies and replace any missing or faded identification bracelets. **Identification bracelets provide positive client identification.**
3. Assess client's knowledge regarding medications **to determine the need for drug education and to assist in identifying the client's compliance with drug therapy at home.**
4. Assess client's IV access **to determine the need for a new IV site or access to existing site.**

▶ DIAGNOSIS

Excess Fluid Volume

Risk for Infection

Risk for Injury

Risk for Allergic Response

▶ PLANNING

Expected Outcomes:

1. Correct dose of medication will be administered to client over correct time period.
2. Client will be instructed, if needed, on use of intermittent infusion or additive set.
3. The client will not suffer any adverse effects from the medication administration method.

Equipment Needed (see Figure 5-19-1):

- Primary IV set
- Volume-control infusion set
- Medication administration record (MAR)
- Medication
- Syringe (may be needed)
- Alcohol pads

▶ CLIENT EDUCATION NEEDED:

1. If client is going to be administering medication at home using volume-control sets, have client

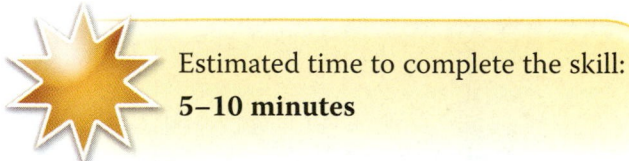

Figure 5-19-1 Volume-control infusion set.

do a return demonstration setting up the set independently.
2. Make sure client knows where to call with questions.
3. Reinforce verbal teaching with written instructions.

Estimated time to complete the skill:
5–10 minutes

▶ **DELEGATION TIPS**

The skill of medication administration is not delegated to ancillary personnel in acute care settings but this may vary in state or federal institutions. Ancillary personnel are generally informed about the medications the client is receiving if adverse effects are anticipated or are being monitored.

IMPLEMENTATION—Action/Rationale

Action	Rationale
1. Wash hands.	1. Reduces the transmission of microorganisms.
2. Check MAR against the health care provider's written orders.	2. Ensures accuracy in the administration of the medication.
3. Check for drug allergies.	3. Decreases risk of allergic reaction such as hives, urticaria, or anaphylactic shock.
4. Prepare the medication for one client at a time.	4. Ensures that the right client receives the right medication.
5. Decide what type of infusion set is needed. If a volume-control infusion set is your choice, assemble equipment.	5. Select the infusion device that will offer the best control and regulation for the type and delivery schedule of medication you are administering.
6. If you are unfamiliar with the brand of equipment where you are working, seek assistance before you need to use it to deliver medication to a client.	6. Reduces the chance of medication errors. Reduces the chance of anxiety or stress for the client.
7. Close clamps and open air vent on chamber (see Figure 5-19-2). Connect the primary IV bag to the volume-control set. Then connect the IV tubing to the volume-control set.	7. Opening the air vent prevents the buildup of negative pressure in the volume-control set, allowing the solution to flow out of the chamber.
8. Open the upper clamp and let the IV solution partially fill the chamber. Close the clamp (see Figure 5-19-3).	8. Fills the chamber so medication may be diluted.

continues

Action	Rationale

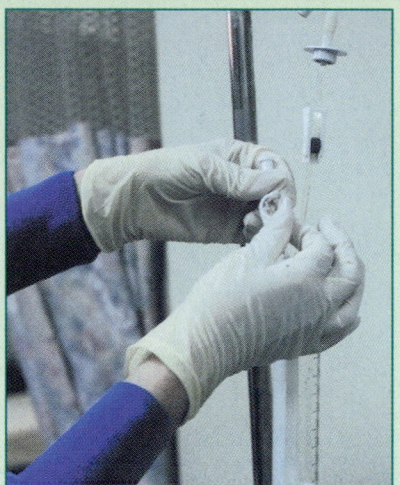

Figure 5-19-2 Close the clamps and open the air vent on the chamber.

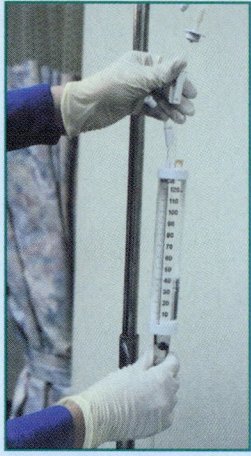

Figure 5-19-3 Open the upper clamp and let the IV solution partially fill the chamber.

9. Open the lower clamp. Squeeze the drip chamber and close the lower clamp at the same time. Allow the fluid to fill the drip chamber, and then open it and allow the solution to flow down to fill the tubing.

9. Primes the tubing to prevent air from entering the vein.

10. Prepare the medication for delivery. Draw up the medication into a syringe.

10. Allows for a smooth and accurate medication administration procedure.

11. Check the client's armband before administering the medications.

11. Ensures right client.

12. Identify the drug for the client and its therapeutic purpose.

12. Encourages client cooperation and increases client awareness of what to expect from the medication.

13. Clean the injection port with alcohol.

13. Reduces the transmission of microorganisms.

14. Inject the medication into the chamber and gently mix (see Figure 5-19-4).

14. Adds medication to chamber for dilution.

15. Open upper clamp and add additional IV solution to bring the volume of medication and diluent to the prescribed amount (see Figure 5-19-5). Close clamp.

15. Allows infusion of desired dosage strength in desired amount of diluent.

16. Adjust the flow rate, or set the dial-a-flow, to infuse the medication over the prescribed rate.

16. Allows infusion of desired medication in desired amount of time.

17. Label the chamber with medication information, date, time, and initials.

17. Reduces the chance of medication error.

18. Observe the client for side effects or adverse reactions.

18. Assesses for potential problems related to the medications administered.

19. When the volume in the chamber has infused, close the air vent and reset the flow rate to the prescribed IV infusion rate.

19. Allows resumption of IV therapy.

continues

Action	Rationale

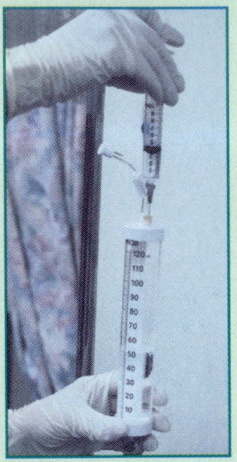

Figure 5-19-4 Inject the medication into the chamber.

20. Wash hands.

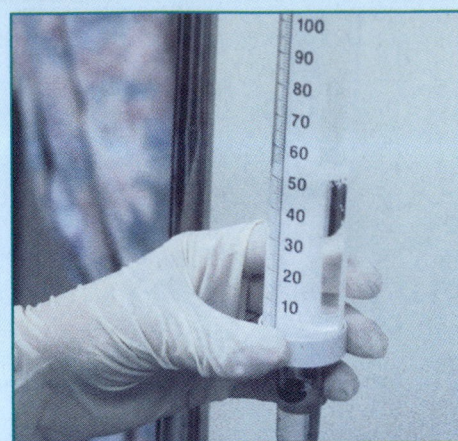

Figure 5-19-5 Open the upper clamp and add the additional IV solution to bring the volume of medication and diluent to the prescribed amount.

20. Decreases transmission of microorganisms.

► REAL WORLD ANECDOTES

The nurse brought the syringe filled with medication to be administered through the additive set into the client's room. He injected the medication into the Buretrol and left the room. When he returned to the room 20 minutes later, the Buretrol was still full. The nurse realized that he had forgotten to open the clamp on the Buretrol, which would allow it to empty and administer all the medication to the client. The nurse was reminded to always check the clamps.

► EVALUATION

- The correct dose of medication was administered to the client over the correct time period.
- The client was instructed, if needed, on the use of the intermittent infusion or additive set.
- The client did not suffer any adverse effects from the medication administration method.

► DOCUMENTATION

Medication Administration Record (MAR)

- Record the name and dosage of the medication.
- Record the date and time the medication was administered.

If the medication is a controlled substance, document in the Controlled Substances Record Book:

- The name and dosage of the medication.
- The date and time the medication was removed from the locked cabinet.

- Any controlled substance that was wasted.
- The name of the nurse administering the controlled substance.

Controlled substances must be documented at the time they are removed from the locked cabinet. Documentation on the MAR is done after the medication is administered.

Nurses' Notes

- Note the client's response to the medication.

Document on appropriate flow sheet or electronic medical record (EMR).

► CRITICAL THINKING SKILL

Introduction

Volume-control sets are helpful for administering IV medications over a period of time. The medication can be mixed with a certain volume of the primary IV fluid and then infused.

Possible Scenario

The nurse checks the MAR and notices that Bill is scheduled to receive potassium as well as a corticosteroid at noon today. She decides to put them both in the Buretrol at the same time and infuse them.

Possible Outcome

If the medications are incompatible, the effectiveness may be altered. A precipitate may also be formed causing the IV line to clog and become nonfunctioning. Precipitate could potentially be infused into the client.

Prevention

Always check the compatibility of drugs before mixing them together. When in doubt, infuse the two medications separately.

▶ VARIATIONS

Geriatric Variation:
- *The elderly may be susceptible to fluid overload. Be aware of the amount of diluent you are infusing.*

Pediatric Variations:
- *Only use microdrip IV tubing and an infusion pump for small children.*
- *Do not use too much diluent when infusing IV medications in small children. They are very susceptible to fluid overload.*

Home Care Variation:
- *Clients may try to reuse equipment more often than is safe. Teach the client the importance of regularly changing the infusion set.*

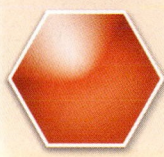

Long-Term Care Variation:
- *Periodically reassess the client's need for IV medication. Long-term IV access leaves the client susceptible to infection and thrombi.*

▶ COMMON ERRORS

Possible Error:

After the medication in an additive set is infused, not adjusting the rate of the primary infusion back to the original set rate.

Prevention:

Always check back within 20 to 30 minutes after setting up the medication infusion to see if the medication infusion is complete or on schedule and to adjust the rate as needed. Note the amount of fluid that was infused. Consider adjusting the rate of the primary infusion to make up for the incorrect amount of fluid that was infused. Follow institutional policy regarding adjusting an IV rate.

▶ NURSING TIPS

- Become familiar with types of volume-control sets used at the facility where you work.
- Think through the steps and review written instructions if unsure about how to assemble volume-control sets.
- If teaching the client this skill, use the same equipment he or she will be using at home.
- Learn the difference between the air vent and the injection port (see Figure 5-19-6).

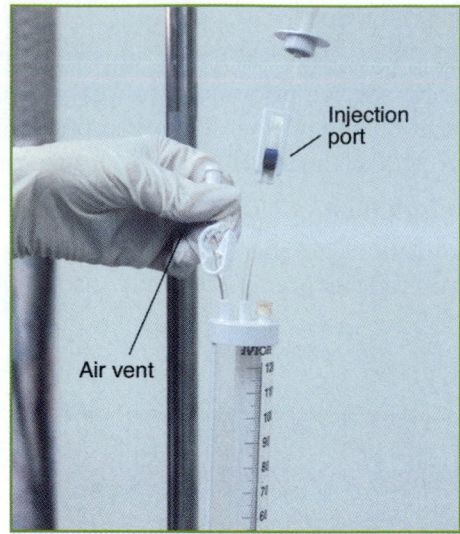

Figure 5-19-6 Learn the difference between the air vent and the injection port.

▶ SPECIAL CONSIDERATIONS

- *Volume-control sets are useful devices when smaller infusions are required. They can also be used for administering medications such as antibiotics. If the client has a continuous IV infusion order, and the volume-control is an add-on for medication purposes, always check at the end of each volume-controlled infusion to shift back and unclamp the primary tubing, readjusting the drip rate as ordered.*

Administering Medication via a Cartridge System

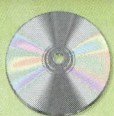

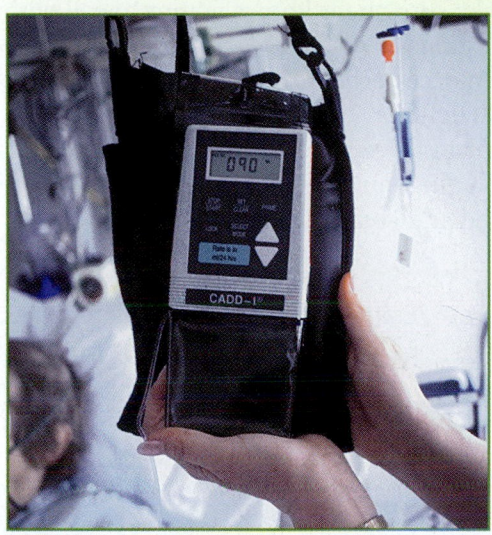

▶ OVERVIEW OF THE SKILL

Cartridge systems were designed to make IV or subcutaneous infusion of medications more portable for the client. Cartridge systems are widely used in various settings, including hospitals, outpatient infusion areas, clinics, long-term care settings, and home care. There are a number of different cartridge systems currently being used across the United States. They are compact. Many allow the client to put the entire cartridge system in a pocket or over the shoulder in order to move about freely. Cartridge systems can infuse a continuous rate of medication and can also be programmed to deliver a bolus of medication as needed. They are simple enough to program that the client or family member can often be instructed on how to operate them.

▶ ASSESSMENT

1. Assess the five rights: right client, right medication, right route, right dose, and right time. **Prevents errors in medication administration.**
2. Identify the drug ordered: action, purpose, normal dosage and route, common side effects, time of onset and peak action, and nursing implications. This allows the nurse **to anticipate effects of the drug and to observe client's response.**
3. Check allergies and replace any missing or faded identification bracelets. **Identification bracelets provide positive client identification.**

4. Assess client's knowledge regarding medications **to determine need for drug education and to assist in identifying client's compliance with drug therapy at home.**
5. Assess IV or SQ access **to determine whether a new site is needed.**
6. Assess rate of infusion to be run **to determine whether the volume to be infused and the infusion rate are feasible using a cartridge system.**

▶ DIAGNOSIS

Risk for Infection

Effective Therapeutic Regimen Management

Risk for Activity Intolerance

Deficient Knowledge

Risk for Allergic Response

▶ PLANNING

Expected Outcomes:

1. Correct dose of medication will be administered to the client in a set time period.
2. Client will demonstrate knowledge regarding the use of the cartridge system and, if appropriate, how to program system.

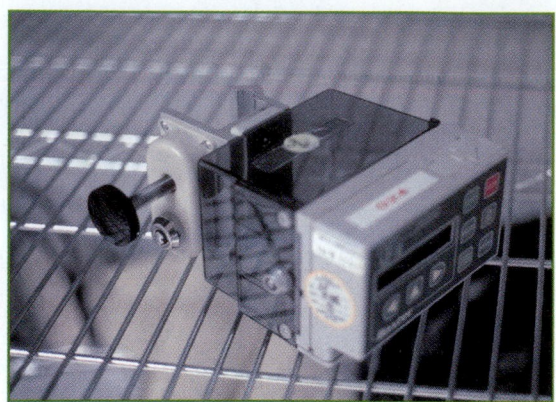

Figure 5-20-1 Cartridge system.

3. Client will not suffer any adverse effects secondary to the use of the cartridge system.

Equipment Needed (see Figure 5-20-1):

- Cartridge system
- Medication
- Tubing

- Alcohol pads
- Medication administration record (MAR)

▶ **CLIENT EDUCATION NEEDED:**

1. If client is going to be administering medication at home using an infusion set, have client do a return demonstration setting up the infusion set independently.
2. Make sure client knows whom to call with questions.
3. Reinforce verbal teaching with written instructions.
4. Explain the expected actions of the medication, including purpose for which it is being administered and common side effects.

Estimated time to complete the skill:
5–15 minutes

▶ **DELEGATION TIPS**

The skill of medication administration is not delegated to ancillary personnel in acute care settings. This may vary in state or federal institutions. Ancillary personnel are generally informed about the medications the client is receiving if adverse effects are anticipated or are being monitored.

IMPLEMENTATION—Action/Rationale

Action	Rationale
1. Wash hands.	1. Reduces the transmission of microorganisms.
2. Check MAR against the health care provider's written orders. Determine with the physician if a cartridge system is appropriate for this medication and this client. Check the five rights.	2. Ensures accuracy in the administration of the medication.
3. Check for drug allergies.	3. Decreases risk of allergic reaction such as hives, urticaria, or anaphylactic shock.
4. Prepare the medication for one client at a time. • Decide whether a cartridge infusion replacement set is needed. • Assemble needed equipment (check battery of cartridge system). • Ensure air is completely expelled from tubing.	4. Ensures that the right client receives the right medication.

continues

Action	Rationale
5. Check the client's identification bracelet before administering the medications (if appropriate).	5. Ensures right client.
6. Review the drug information with the client, including side effects, and therapeutic purpose.	6. Encourages client cooperation and increases client awareness of what to expect from the medication.
7. Administer the medication using the cartridge set through central, peripheral, epidural, or subcutaneous catheter site as ordered. Use a needleless system if available.	7. Cartridge sets can be used with many types of IV access. Needleless systems prevent needle sticks.
8. Observe the client for side effects or adverse reactions.	8. Assesses for potential problems related to the medications administered.
9. Wash hands.	9. Decreases transmission of microorganisms.

► REAL WORLD ANECDOTES

Scenario 1

Mary is an insulin-dependent diabetic. Recently her endocrinologist recommended that Mary start using an insulin pump. She received instructions from the diabetic teaching nurse and started to use the pump routinely. She had no problem with the pump until one day when she noticed that her blood-sugar level kept rising despite several boluses from the pump. Worried, Mary called the diabetic teaching nurse. The nurse recommended that Mary check the placement of the subcutaneous needle and the tubing to be sure they were intact. After careful inspection, Mary realized that the insulin syringe was not properly seated in the pump. After repositioning the syringe, Mary was able to successfully inject a bolus of insulin and control her blood-sugar level.

Scenario 2

Sally has been on pain medication using a cartridge system since surgery this morning. She is quite uncomfortable but has not used the bolus button to give herself a bolus of the pain medication because she is afraid she will give herself too much. Sally mentions this to the nurse and the nurse explains that the cartridge system is set up to give Sally a specific dose for a bolus, so she cannot get too much medication. The important thing is for her to have good pain control.

► EVALUATION

- Correct dose of medication was administered to the client in a set time period.
- Client demonstrates knowledge regarding the use of the cartridge system and, if appropriate, how to program the system.
- Client does not suffer any adverse effects secondary to the use of the cartridge system.

► DOCUMENTATION

Medication Administration Record (MAR)

- Document the name, dosage, and route of the medication.
- Note the site of medication administration, if appropriate.
- If the client is receiving a controlled substance, record the amount removed from the locked cabinet and any controlled substance wasted in the Controlled Substance Record.

Nurses' Notes

- Record client's response to medication and any adverse effects noted.
- Note client teaching performed.

Document on appropriate flow sheet or electronic medical record (EMR).

► CRITICAL THINKING SKILL

Introduction

Medications in cartridge systems can be mixed at different strengths. For instance, morphine can be mixed to infuse 5 mg/mL of morphine or 10 mg/mL of morphine. For this reason, when changing the cartridge, it is important to verify the strength of the medication being infused.

Possible Scenario

Jim has been receiving morphine through a cartridge set for the last week. His pain has been increasing, so his dose of morphine was increased over the last 2 days. The medication in the cartridge ran out so the nurse replaced it. Because of Jim's increased morphine use, the pharmacy decided to make the morphine cartridge a different strength. The nurse did not realize that the morphine cartridge that was sent up was a different concentration and was twice as strong as the previous medication cartridge. The nurse programmed the cartridge set at the same rate that was previously used.

Possible Outcome

Jim became very sleepy and somewhat disoriented. His respiratory rate decreased to seven breaths per minute. The nurse discovered the error, turned off the morphine infusion, and called Jim's doctor. In an hour, Jim was wide awake and once again oriented. The morphine infusion was restarted at the correct rate.

Prevention

Always check the concentration of new medication cartridges before setting up the infusion. Check the dose of the infusion against both the MAR and the doctor's original order. Have another nurse double-check the infusion rate, if needed. Sometimes the pharmacy will change the label of a medication to look different on cartridges of different concentrations.

► VARIATIONS

Geriatric Variation:
- *Elderly clients may be more sensitive to some medications. Carefully assess the client's reaction to the cartridge medication and report your findings to the client's health care provider.*

Pediatric Variation:
- *Be sure the cartridge system is either out of a small child's reach or locked to prevent the child from accidentally interfering with the cartridge system's function.*

Home Care Variations:
- *Arthritic clients or clients with impaired coordination may require a cartridge system that is easy to load and unload.*
- *Teach the client how to determine whether the battery is low in the cartridge system.*

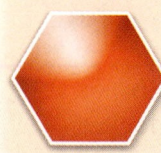

Long-Term Care Variations:
- *Periodically reassess the effectiveness of the medication being delivered by the cartridge system.*
- *Regularly monitor the condition of the cartridge system, including the battery strength.*

▶ COMMON ERRORS

Possible Error:

The cartridge set is programmed for the incorrect medication administration rate.

Prevention:

Always check the MAR and health care provider's orders for the correct dose of medication. Make sure that the concentration of medication in the cassette is the same as the concentration in the previous cassette. Turn medication cartridge set down or off. Assess client for medication side effects. Determine how the error occurred. Report the error.

Possible Error:

Medication is leaking from tubing connection between the cartridge set and client's IV access.

Prevention:

Always double-check that connections are secure. Secure connections. Assess amount of medication that was leaked and the need to replace medication. Document any leakage to explain any discrepancies between the amount in the cartridge and the amount the client used.

▶ NURSING TIPS

- Always check the connections in the tubing to make sure they are secure.
- Always check the concentration of the medication to ensure the right dose is being delivered to the client.
- Become familiar with types of infusion sets used at the facility where you work.
- Think through the steps and review written instructions if unsure about how to assemble an infusion set.

▶ SPECIAL CONSIDERATIONS

- *The cartridge system is designed to be portable and is often used in the outpatient or home setting where a medical professional is not immediately available. To avoid medical complications, client education on the operation and maintenance of the device should be emphasized. Emergency contacts should be established and the client should be well informed about the contact system.*

Administering Patient-Controlled Analgesia (PCA)

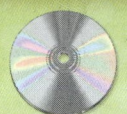

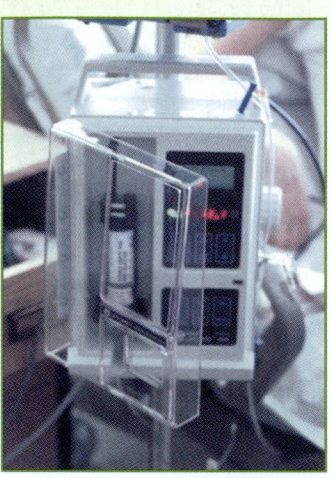

▶ OVERVIEW OF THE SKILL

Patient-controlled analgesia (PCA) is a method to relieve pain through self-administration of analgesics (usually opioids, e.g., morphine) by a client using a programmable pump connected to a subcutaneous, intravenous, or epidural catheter. It is commonly used for controlling postoperative pain or cancer pain in hospital and home. By pressing a button of the PCA pump, the client can bolus administer the prescribed analgesic as demanded. Clients need to operate the PCA as instructed. The use of PCA is contraindicated for sedated and confused clients.

Nurses should obtain an order with clear indication of the analgesic used, route of administration, bolus dose (amount of analgesic received when pressing the button), lock-out interval (the time period in which pressing the button more than once results in only one dose of analgesic received), and maximum dose limit (the maximum amount of analgesic that can be received within a certain period of time, e.g., 1 hour); loading dose (first bolus dose) and basal infusion rate (continuous infusion rate) should be prescribed if applicable. To administer PCA, nurses should maintain a patent catheter line as route, install the analgesic solution into the PCA chamber, and program the PCA pump according to the prescribed parameters.

▶ ASSESSMENT

1. Assess the five rights: right client, right medication, right route, right dose, and right time. **Prevents errors in medication administration.**
2. Assess client consciousness level and cognitive function **to determine whether the client has the ability to correctly operate the PCA pump.**
3. Identify the PCA ordered: the analgesic, action, purpose, common side effects, route, loading dose, bolus dose, lock-out interval, maximum dose, and basal rate. **Nurses should prepare the analgesics, program the PCA pump as prescribed, and observe client responses to the pain therapy.**
4. Assess client pain: Initial assessment should include the location, intensity, characteristics, and pattern of the pain as well as factors increasing and decreasing the pain; ongoing assessment includes the degree of pain intensity and pain relief, amount of analgesic administered, and times of button being pressed. **Evaluates the appropriateness of the pain therapy and titration of the pain medication.**
5. Measure client blood pressure and respiratory rate if opioid is prescribed. Low blood pressure or respiratory depression may occur if using opioid. **Reducing the dose, changing the drug,**

or administering naloxone (opioid antagonist) may be necessary.

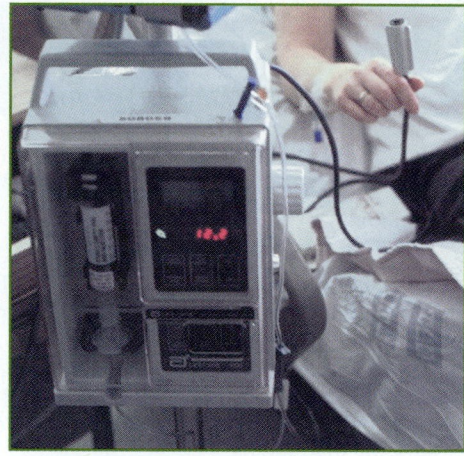

Figure 5-21-1 PCA pump.

▶ DIAGNOSIS

Pain

Deficient Knowledge

Anxiety

Risk for Allergic Response

▶ PLANNING

Expected Outcomes:

1. Client reports lessening or absence of pain.
2. Client can correctly press the PCA button to self-administer analgesic.
3. Client experiences no unwanted change in consciousness level, blood pressure, and breathing pattern.
4. Client experiences no uncontrollable side effects.

Equipment Needed (see Figure 5-21-1):

- A patent and indwelling subcutaneous, intravenous, or epidural line installed as the prescribed route of administration; see other skills about inserting an intravenous (IV) or subcutaneous (SC) catheter and assisting with epidural catheter placement.
- A PCA pump with manufacturer's instruction guide for operation: PCA pumps usually consist of a programmable infusion pump with syringe inside, a button linked to a timing unit that is activated by the client when demanded, and a tube that can be connected to an indwelling catheter (e.g., IV line).
- Properly prepared pain medication as ordered by the health care provider
- Label for drug identification and time tape
- Adhesive tape
- Disposable gloves
- Naloxone solution (0.4 mg in 10 mL of saline) if giving opioid agonists (e.g., morphine)

▶ CLIENT EDUCATION NEEDED:

1. Explain the purpose of PCA and the goal for pain therapy.
2. Teach client how to report pain (e.g., using a 0- to 10-point scale to indicate how much pain is experienced and how much pain relief is felt).
3. Coach when and how to press the PCA button to administer bolus dose of analgesic. Remind clients that they cannot overdose because of the lock-out interval.
4. Explain action and potential side effects of the pain medication.
5. Remind well-meaning family members or visitors not to push the PCA button for the client.
6. Explain the actions and side effects of the narcotic being used to both the client and family members.

Estimated time to complete the skill:
10–15 minutes

▶ DELEGATION TIPS

The skill of medication administration is not delegated to ancillary personnel in acute care settings. This may vary in state or federal institutions. Ancillary personnel are generally informed about the medications the client is receiving if adverse effects are anticipated or are being monitored.

IMPLEMENTATION—Action/Rationale

Action	Rationale
1. Wash your hands.	1. Reduces the transmission of microorganisms.
2. Assess the client's comfort level: pain location, intensity, characteristics, pattern, and factors that increase or decrease the pain.	2. Identifies pain problem, purpose of pain therapy, and other adjuvant therapies. Establishes baseline to measure improvement.
3. Assess the client's consciousness level and ability to understand the instruction.	3. PCA is contraindicated for sedated and confused clients.
4. Check the PCA order for drug, concentration, route, basal infusion rate, bolus dose, lock-out interval, maximum dose, and any loading dose.	4. Opioid administration requires a health care provider's order. Dosing parameters are necessary for programming a PCA pump.
5. Check the PCA medication label against health care provider's order and follow the five rights principle. PCA medication usually has been placed in the PCA syringe at the pharmacy.	5. Minimizes medication error and harm to client.
6. Read the manufacturer's instruction guide before assembling and programming the PCA pump.	6. Different manufacturers or models may require different operation. Follow the manufacturer's instruction to ensure proper operation of the pump.
7. Place the filled PCA syringe into the chamber in the PCA pump and detect any leaking or damage to the system (see Figures 5-21-2, 5-21-3, and 5-21-4).	7. Assemble PCA pump and inspect damage of the system to avoid medication error and harm to client.
8. Program the pump according to the prescribed parameters, usually including basal infusion rate (mg/hr), bolus dose (mg), lock-out interval (min), and maximum dose limit (mg/hr) (see Figure 5-21-5).	8. Avoids overmedication and ensures accuracy of the medication given.

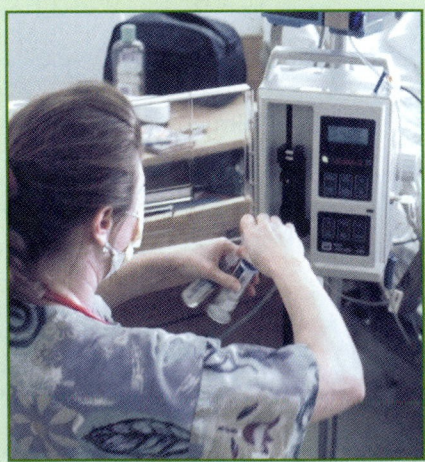

Figure 5-21-2 Remove the empty PCA syringe.

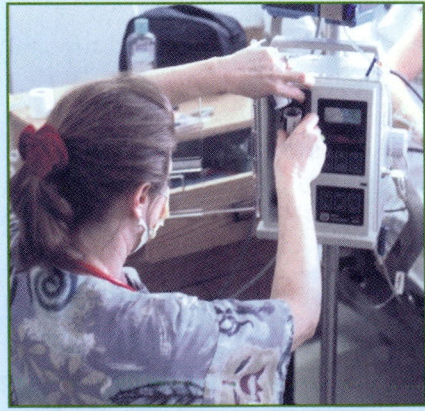

Figure 5-21-3 Place new PCA syringe into the chamber in the PCA pump.

continues

Action	Rationale
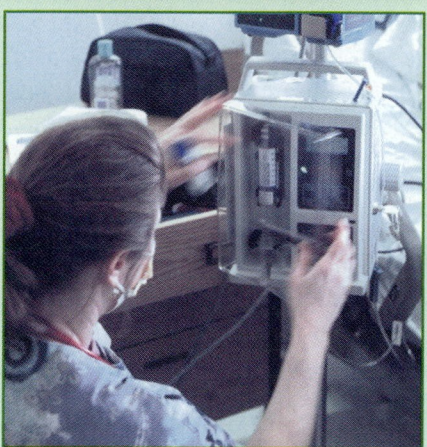 **Figure 5-21-4** Check for any leaking or damage to the system, and close the door to the chamber.	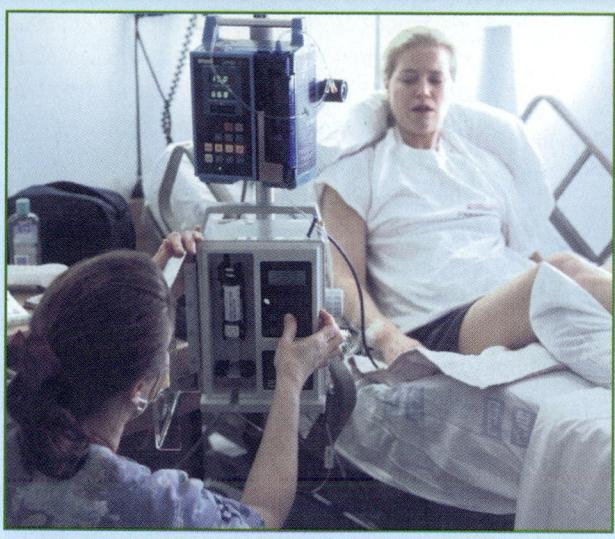 **Figure 5-21-5** Program the pump.
9. Wear gloves.	9. Sterile technique reduces transmission of microorganisms.
10. Inspect the existing infusion line and puncture site for any inflammatory sign and check any occlusion or leakage of the infusion line. Check IV catheterization or epidural catheter placement if client needs an infusion line.	10. Avoids skin breakdown and infection for safely administering medication. Infusion line must be patent to deliver medication to vessels.
11. Prime the PCA pump tubing. Connect the PCA pump tubing with the infusion line using aseptic technique and secure the connection with adhesive tape.	11. Reduces risk of infection and leakage. Prevents air embolism.
12. Give the client the control button and instruct how and when to press the button.	12. Client teaching ensures appropriate use of PCA.
13. Record the procedure, including starting time, type of medication used, route, dosage, lock-out interval, and maximum dose limit.	13. Prevents document errors by timely recording.
14. Wash your hands.	14. Reduces the transmission of microorganisms.

► REAL WORLD ANECDOTES

Mr. Franco, a 70-kg adult, received abdominal surgery. He complained of severe pain associated with position change. His wife was with him and asked the physician to give the client pain medication. The physician then prescribed PCA with IV infusion of morphine, starting with a loading dose of 10 mg, basal infusion rate of 0 mg, and bolus of 2 mg if demanded, lock-out interval of 15 minutes, with maximum dose of 20 mg in 3 hours. The nurse started the PCA and instructed the client how to use the PCA. Two hours after initiating the PCA, the nurse found Mr. Franco was quite drowsy and could not answer the nurse's questions. The nurse found Mrs. Franco was looking at a watch and then pressing the PCA button. Mrs. Franco admitted that she has pressed the button every 15 minutes to help relieve her husband's pain when she felt he might be in pain. The nurse immediately checked the vital signs of Mr. Franco and monitored any sign of overmedication. The nurse then communicated with Mrs. Franco about the purpose of PCA and the actions of morphine. The nurse was reminded to include family members in teaching and to emphasize the control of administration by the client to avoid overmedication. This incident served as a reminder to the nurse that even with the lock-out feature of the PCA, a client could be overmedicated for pain.

► EVALUATION

- Assess the degree of pain intensity and pain relief.
- Assess the consciousness level, blood pressure, and pattern of breathing.
- Check the presence and degree of nausea, vomiting, urinary retention, and constipation if opioid is administered.
- Assess the insertion site for inflammatory or infection sign.

► DOCUMENTATION

Medication Administration Record

- Record the route, drug name, concentration and volume prepared, dosage, loading dose, basal rate, lock-out interval, maximal hourly dose, and total dose of the PCA.

Nurses' Notes

- Record the pain location, intensity, characteristics, and pattern for initial assessment.
- Record the consciousness level, blood pressure, respiratory rate, and change in respiratory depth.
- Record any side effects associated with the drug use.

Document on appropriate flow sheet or electronic medical record (EMR).

► CRITICAL THINKING SKILL

Introduction

Nurses must be able to evaluate the effectiveness of PCA by assessment of the pain intensity and pain relief.

Possible Scenario

A client posthysterectomy was given PCA morphine for controlling pain. The client was lying stiff on her bed and breathing shallowly. The nurse asked how she was doing. She indicated that she was OK but could not rest. Assessing the client's pain intensity using a 0- to 10-point scale, the nurse found that her pain was 5 now and most of the time but could be 9 when she moved. The pain relief was about 2 to 3 when a 0- to 10-point scale was used. The nurse checked the PCA and discovered that she pressed the PCA button every 1 to 2 minutes. The nurse then reported to the physician. The physician changed the prescription to add continuous infusion of morphine and escalate the PCA bolus dose of morphine.

Possible Outcome

If the nurse did not assess the client's pain and detect insufficiency of morphine dose, the client would continuously suffer from pain. Restlessness and immobilization may occur from pain, and may impede recovery.

Prevention

The nurse prevented undermedication by assessing the client's pain intensity, pain relief, and medication used.

► VARIATIONS

Geriatric Variations:

- *The elderly may present with cognitive impairment or confusion, which is contraindicated with the use of PCA.*
- *In addition, the dosing should be carefully monitored and titrated in elderly with decreased kidney or liver function.*

Pediatric Variations:

- *Children need to be mature enough to understand the relationship between pain, pushing the button, and pain relief in order to operate the system.*
- *Most children older than the age of 7 understand this concept, and some younger children can learn to use PCA safely.*

Home Care Variations:

- *PCAs are commonly used in the home care setting.*
- *Family members need to be reminded not to press the button for the client if the client does not ask for it to avoid overmedication.*
- *Make sure the client will have access to the button at all times in the home setting and that a way to summon help is at hand if the button falls or is moved out of reach.*

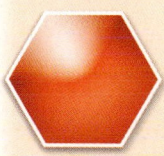

Long-Term Care Variations:

- *PCAs are usually used for a short period of time.*
- *Long-term use may be seen in clients with cancer or chronic pain, especially those who had break-through or incidence pain.*
- *Encourage the client to become an active participant in pain control.*
- *The client may be exploring other options to support for pain control, such as acupuncture, imagery, massage, or over-the-counter remedies.*

► COMMON ERRORS

Possible Error:

Opioid was not delivered because the infusion line was occluded or leaked.

Prevention:

Assess patency of the infusion line and detect any leakage. Secure the line to avoid kinking.

Possible Error:

Client was over- or undermedicated because of a mistake in PCA programming.

Prevention:

Check each parameter programmed against the health care provider's order. Have another nurse double-check the programming. Assess the client's condition such as pain, consciousness level, and vital signs. Intervene immediately if adverse effects occur. Correct or stop the infusion. Notify the health care provider for further intervention.

▶ NURSING TIPS

- Read manufacturer's instruction guide before assembling and programming the PCA pump.
- Identify the actions of the prescribed medication and necessary parameters to be programmed.
- Periodically assess pain intensity, pain relief, and side effects.

- Remember that if the medication is discontinued, any narcotic left in the pump must be wasted. Another nurse must witness the wasting procedure, and the amount, reason, time, and date of the wasting must be documented.

▶ SPECIAL CONSIDERATIONS

- *A patient-controlled analgesia (PCA) system can be fully used as a clinical tool for pain relief. PCA works best when the client's cognitive functioning is at an optimal level. A client's cognitive level may fluctuate during the pathologic process. Be aware of these changes as the client may experience pain if the system is not operated properly.*
- *Be aware of individual or cultural variations when instructing the client using a PCA system as some clients may not feel comfortable with self-administration of medication.*

Administering Epidural Analgesia

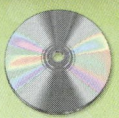

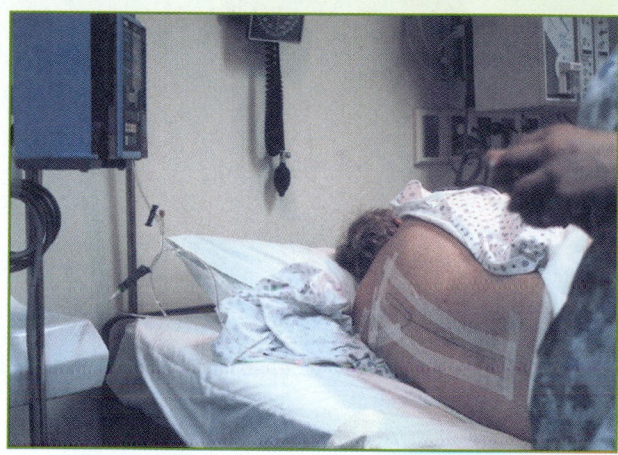

▶ OVERVIEW OF THE SKILL

Epidural catheters have long been used for administration of opioid analgesics for chronic intractable pain and for chemotherapy. They have become a popular and widely accepted vehicle for the management of acute postoperative pain. An epidural catheter frequently is used in clients during the childbirth process for the administration of opioids. Epidural opioid use is beneficial to the client because pain is controlled with lower dosages of drugs while producing fewer side effects.

The catheter is usually placed by the anesthesiologist into the epidural space. If the catheter is intended for long-term use, it is tunneled subcutaneously, exiting on the side of the body or on the abdomen. Epidural catheters intended for short-term use may not be sutured in place and will exit from the insertion site on the back.

▶ ASSESSMENT

1. Assess the five rights: right client, right medication, right route, right dose, and right time. **Prevents errors in medication administration.**
2. Although epidural analgesia is relatively safe, clients may experience headache, backache, shivering, and a drop in blood pressure. Care should be taken to carefully assess clients beforehand and to monitor afterwards. Clients may be frightened by the aspect of a line close to the spinal column. Clients should be assessed for relief from pain. The level of pain should be assessed, using a 0 to 10 scale, with 0 being pain free and 10 being excruciating pain. The type of pain and location of pain should also be assessed. **This will help establish a baseline to gauge the effectiveness of the pain medication.**
3. The catheter site should be assessed for erythema, purulent drainage, edema, and tenderness. **Denotes signs and symptoms of infection.**
4. Temporarily placed catheters should be assessed **to ensure that they are intact and have not been dislodged.**
5. Assess vital signs prior to infusing medication through the catheter **to establish a baseline for later assessment of the effects of the medication.**
6. Assess for a history of allergies **as an allergic response may occur from the analgesia.**

▶ DIAGNOSIS

Deficient Knowledge

Pain

Risk for Infection

Risk for Injury

Risk for Allergic Response

▶ PLANNING

Expected Outcomes:

1. Client's pain will be relieved.
2. Client's mobility will be improved by relief from pain.
3. Catheter and tubing will be taped securely in place.
4. There will be no signs or symptoms of infection.
5. The client will be able to void without difficulty.
6. The client will not experience an allergic reaction.

Equipment Needed (see Figure 5-22-1):

- Sterile gloves
- Prediluted, preservative-free medication
- Labels for the injection port and tubing
- Infusion pump for medication administered by continuous infusion
- IV tubing that does not have Y-ports if medication is administered by continuous infusion
- Tape
- Povidone-iodine swabs
- Syringe, 10- to 12-mL, if administering medication by bolus injection
- Filter needle
- Needle, 20-gauge, 1-inch, or needleless system

▶ CLIENT EDUCATION NEEDED:

1. Describe the epidural catheter to the client prior to placement. Showing the client a picture of the catheter or letting the client talk to another

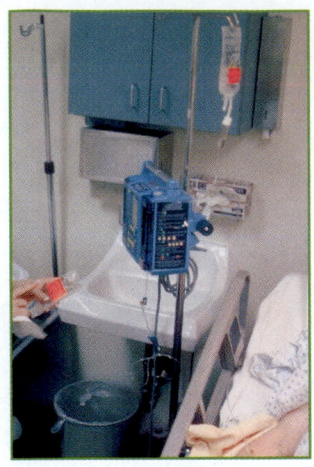

Figure 5-22-1 Infusion pump and infusion tubing are used to administer medication by continuous infusion.

client who has had an epidural catheter may relieve fears for the client.
2. Teach the client how to assess pain on a scale of 0 to 10.
3. Teach the client that pain relief will be obtained within 30 to 60 minutes after the injection.
4. Teach the client the side effects of the opiates and reassure the client that the side effects can be treated.

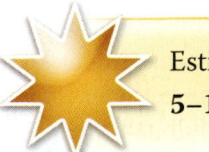

Estimated time to complete the skill: **5–10 minutes**

▶ DELEGATION TIPS

The skill of medication administration is not delegated to ancillary personnel in acute care settings. This may vary in state or federal institutions. Ancillary personnel are generally informed about the medications the client is receiving if adverse effects are anticipated or are being monitored.

IMPLEMENTATION—Action/Rationale

Action	Rationale
1. Wash hands.	1. Reduces the transmission of microorganisms.
2. Verify medication with order.	2. Decreases risk of medication error.
3. Gather equipment needed and verify client.	3. Ensures all equipment needed is available and saves time. Verifying correct client decreases risk of medication error.

continues

Action	Rationale
4. Set up sterile field.	4. Minimizes risk of infection by using sterile technique.
For Bolus Injection	
5. For bolus injection: draw up prediluted, preservative-free narcotic solution through filter needle in 10-mL syringe (see Figure 5-22-2).	5. Preservatives are toxic to neural tissue. Filter needles remove any microscopic glass particles.
6. Change from filter needle to regular 20-gauge needle or needleless system, if in use.	6. Prepares medication to be injected.
7. Clean injection cap with povidone-iodine.	7. Never use alcohol, as it is toxic to neural tissue. Povidone-iodine cleans injection cap and minimizes introduction of microorganisms during needle insertion. Allow povidone-iodine to dry for 2 to 3 minutes to maximize effectiveness.
8. Insert safety-needle into injection cap and aspirate.	8. Aspiration of clear fluid of 0.5 mL or less is indicative of epidural catheter placement. If more than 0.5 mL cerebrospinal fluid or blood is obtained, notify health care provider as catheter may be in subarachnoid space or in a blood vessel.
9. If clear fluid returns are 0.5 mL or less, inject drug slowly. Assess vital signs prior to and after administration.	9. Slowly injecting medication minimizes client discomfort by lowering the pressure exerted. Client's blood pressure may decrease and require treatment.
10. Remove needle from the injection cap and dispose of properly.	10. Prevents accidental needle sticks and complies with biosafety guidelines for disposal of contaminated material.
For Continuous Infusion	
11. For continuous infusion, attach preservative-free opioid to infusion pump tubing and prime tubing (see Figure 5-22-3).	11. Priming eliminates air bubbles to prevent air embolus.

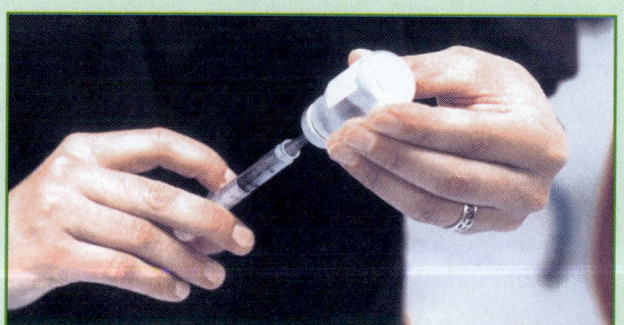

Figure 5-22-2 For bolus injection, draw up prediluted, preservative-free narcotic solution through filter needle in 10-mL syringe.

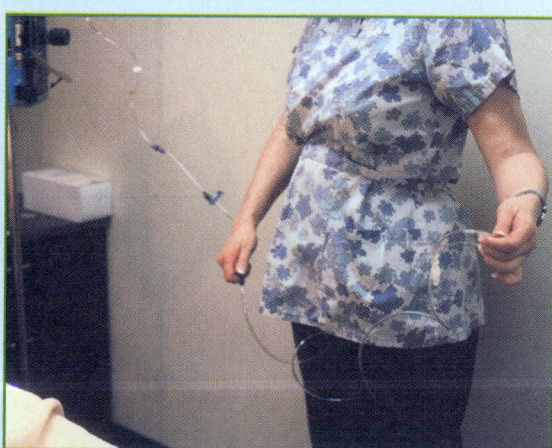

Figure 5-22-3 For continuous infusion, attach preservative-free opioid to the infusion pump tubing and prime tubing.

continues

Action	Rationale
For Continuous Infusion *continued*	
12. Attach the proximal end of the tubing to the pump and the distal end to the catheter (see Figure 5-22-4). Luer-lock all connections. Tape a tension loop of tubing to client's body. Start pump.	12. Luer-locking connections minimize the risk of accidental leakage from separation of catheter and tubing. This also minimizes risk of infection. Taping tension loop minimizes risk of dislodging catheter by pulling on tubing.
13. Ensure pump is infusing at desired rate.	13. Ensures client is receiving correct dose.
14. Label tubing as epidural catheter tubing and with name of drug, date, and time.	14. Protects against inadvertent use of line for other reasons.
15. Dispose of gloves and wash hands.	15. Reduces transmission of microorganisms.
16. Document in client's chart.	16. Records dose, route, and time drug was administered.

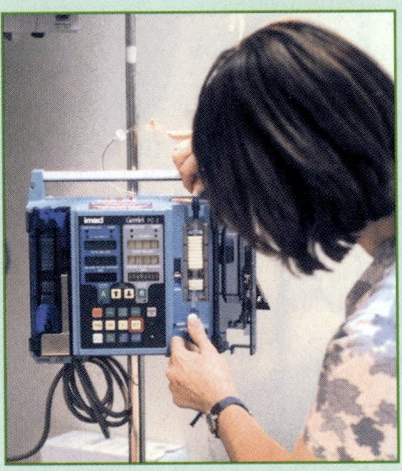

Figure 5-22-4 Attach the proximal end of the tubing to the pump.

▶ REAL WORLD ANECDOTES

Maria Rodriguez was status post an exploratory laparoscopy and total abdominal hysterectomy. Her anesthesiologist placed an epidural catheter with morphine infusing for control of the pain. The nurse caring for Ms. Rodriguez assessed her pain level, and according to the client, the pain score was 2 on a scale of 0 to 10. Upon assessment, the exit site of the epidural catheter was clean, with no tenderness noted. The catheter was securely taped in place. Ms. Rodriguez had a Foley catheter that was draining clear yellow urine. Her vital signs were stable, and her only complaint was of mild nausea. The nurse administered 10 mg of prochlorperazine as ordered, with relief of nausea obtained. Four hours later, Ms. Rodriguez was sitting in a chair at the bedside.

▶ EVALUATION

- Client's pain was relieved.
- Client's mobility was improved because of relief from pain.
- Catheter and tubing were taped securely in place.
- There are no signs or symptoms of infection.
- The client is able to void without difficulty.
- The client did not experience an allergic reaction.

▶ DOCUMENTATION

Medication Administration Record

- Record the type of drug, dose, time, and route (either by bolus injection or continuous infusion).

- In the Controlled Substance Record, record the type of drug, dose, and time. Note any controlled substance that is wasted.

Nurses' Notes

- Record the effectiveness of the medication in relieving the client's pain.
- Note the status of the epidural catheter site.
- Document any client teaching performed.
- Record the client's vital signs and neurologic status.

Document on appropriate flow sheet or electronic medical record (EMR).

Intake and Output Record

- Note the amount of fluid infused from the previous cassette or the current bolus.

▶ CRITICAL THINKING SKILL

Introduction

A client has a tunneled epidural catheter for continuous infusion morphine to treat intractable cancer pain. The client has had the catheter for a month and has not had any complications. She is being admitted to the hospital for a temperature of 102° F.

Possible Scenario

Upon initial assessment, the nurse caring for the client notes that the client flinches when the nurse lightly touches her back along the spinal cord. The nurse also notes some erythema and edema at the lower lumbar spine. She notifies the physician, who orders intravenous antibiotics, blood cultures, and a consult to the anesthesiologist who placed the epidural catheter.

Possible Outcome

Twenty-four hours after initiation of antibiotics, the client became afebrile. The site of the epidural catheter was still tender but less erythematous and the edema disappeared. The client was kept on intravenous antibiotics for an additional 24 hours, but when cultures were negative and the client remained afebrile, she was changed to oral antibiotics and discharged to home. However, a visiting nurse was ordered to follow up at home and reinforce teaching on how to care for the epidural catheter to the client and her husband.

Prevention

Maintaining good technique in caring for the epidural catheter as well as carefully monitoring for signs and symptoms of infection can decrease the risk of infection. However, when immunocompromised clients have any indwelling foreign object, they are automatically at an increased risk for infection.

▶ VARIATIONS

Geriatric Variations:

- *The elderly are more sensitive to side effects of medication and may need to be titrated carefully to relieve pain yet minimize side effects of the opiates.*
- *They may become easily confused, so it is important that the catheter is well secured and tubing Luerlocked to minimize displacement if the client becomes restless or confused.*
- *It is important to assess other medications the elderly client is taking to ensure that there is no synergism of side effects from the multiple medications the client may be taking.*

Pediatric Variations:

- *Children have the same needs for pain relief as adults do, yet research has shown that children are chronically undermedicated.*
- *Children can safely use epidural analgesia, but it is important that the catheter is well secured and tubing Luer-locked to minimize displacement if the child becomes restless.*
- *Check the catheter frequently in an active child to make sure tubing connections are secure.*

Home Care Variation:

- *Temporary epidural catheters should remain in place for only 7 days to decrease the risk of infection. If the client is to be discharged with an epidural catheter in place, a permanent catheter may be required to decrease risk of infection and dislodgement.*

continues

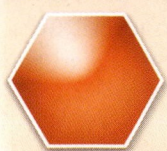

▶ VARIATIONS *(continued)*

Long-Term Care Variations:
- *Epidural catheters placed in clients in long-term care facilities should be permanent catheters.*
- *The employees at the long-term care facility need information on how to care for the client as well as what signs and symptoms to look for that will alert for catheter malfunction as well as infection.*

▶ COMMON ERRORS

Possible Error:

Injecting the wrong medication into the catheter.

Prevention:

Often clients coming out of surgery have a multitude of intravenous lines. It is imperative that intravenous tubing used for the epidural catheter be clearly marked so that medications other than the preservative-free opioids are not injected.

Possible Error:

Misinterpreting rest and undermedicating the client.

Prevention:

Many times health care professionals do not administer the necessary amount of opiates because of fear of overmedicating the client. A client who has been in chronic pain may sleep for an extended period of time when opioid analgesia is initiated, not because of oversedation, but because the client is pain-free and is able to rest.

▶ NURSING TIPS

- A client receiving intravenous opiates will need to have them titrated down once epidural opiates are initiated. The intravenous to epidural morphine equivalent is 10:1. However, each individual is different and must be closely observed to ensure that pain is controlled but the client is not oversedated.
- All medication should be clearly marked as preservative-free if it is to be used epidurally.
- It is advisable to keep a patent IV in place for 24 hours after the epidural catheter has been initiated for easy access of IV medications needed to treat side effects of the medication used in the epidural catheter.
- A client with an epidural catheter should not be using heparin.
- Observe for side effects of opioid, including nausea/vomiting, urinary retention, constipation, headache, increased sedation, and, in rare cases, respiratory depression.
- Observe for paresthesias and/or change of level of consciousness, suggesting displacement of epidural catheter.
- An in-line filter may be required depending on institutional policy.

▶ SPECIAL CONSIDERATIONS

- *The epidural catheter should be marked clearly and set apart so that it will not be mistakenly treated as a regular IV line. The results can be fatal if the wrong solution is injected into the epidural catheter.*
- *Aspirate to check the placement and patency of the epidural catheter prior to administering medication through the epidural route. If more than 1 mL of blood or fluid is returned, the intervention should be withheld and the health care provider notified.*
- *Clients may shiver with the administration of epidural medications and require warm blankets. Ascertain vital signs and report abnormal findings. Blood pressure may decrease with an epidural and require treatment or increased monitoring.*

Managing Controlled Substances

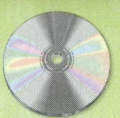

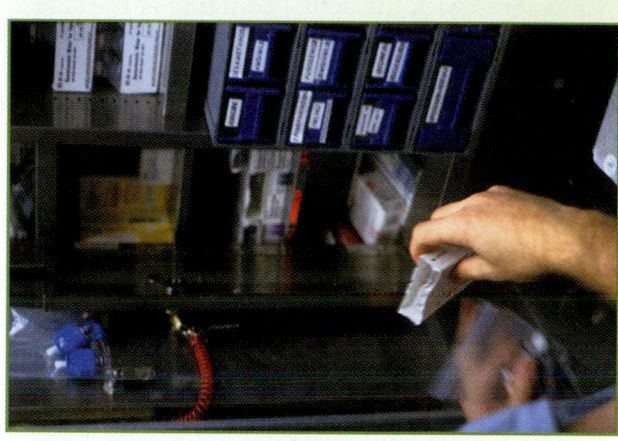

▶ OVERVIEW OF THE SKILL

A controlled substance is a chemical or drug designated by the Drug Enforcement Agency (DEA) as having a potential for abuse by humans. They are identified by a capital "C" and Roman numerals (IV) on the label. Potential for abuse is thought to exist if the chemical is being used in amounts sufficient to create a hazard to the individual or community, there is diversion of the chemical from legitimate uses, or the chemical is being used without licensed medical advice. Evidence of actual abuse of a substance is indicative that a drug has a potential for abuse.

Controlled substances are categorized according to their abuse potential. There are five categories known as schedules:

- Schedule I substances have no acceptable medical use in the United States. This category includes heroin, LSD, and mescaline.
- Schedule II substances have a high potential for psychological or physical dependency, but have legitimate medical uses. This category includes narcotic, stimulant, and depressant drugs.
- Schedule III substances have a lesser potential for abuse than Schedule II substances. This category includes some preparations containing narcotics and barbiturates. Because of the widespread abuse of anabolic steroids, many states now consider them to be a Schedule III substance.
- Schedule IV substances have a lesser potential for abuse than Schedule III substances. This category includes phenobarbital, chloral hydrate, and Valium.
- Schedule V substances have a lesser potential for abuse than Schedule IV substances. This category includes preparations containing small amounts of narcotics such as antitussive medication and antidiarrheal medication.

Controlled substances must be stored, accounted for, and distributed according to strict legal guidelines. All substances must be accounted for in the record and the record must match the actual substance on hand. Controlled substances must be kept in a double-locked safe that is either attached to a wall or weighs greater than 2,000 lbs. Nothing else can be locked in the same safe including paperwork and nonscheduled substances. The keys to the safe must be in the possession of a licensed person at all times and must remain in the facility at all times.

When controlled substances are routinely stored and administered by the registered nurse, it is the nurse's responsibility to safeguard the keys and record all controlled substances received, given, and wasted, as well as monitoring the current inventory. Because these medications have a high potential for abuse, the responsible nurse should monitor all personnel who come in contact with the narcotics safe. Nurses are not immune from substance abuse leading to workplace theft. Suspicions regarding potential theft of controlled substances or impaired staff members must be dealt with according to institutional policy. In most major facilities controlled substances are now dispensed using an automated medication and supply dispensing system, one example being PYXIS. Through these automated and secured access systems, inaccuracies in counts of controlled substances have decreased. A secured access code is required and keys are not needed. By using these streamlined computerized systems, the incorrect count of controlled substances can be identified immediately instead of waiting for a count at the end of the shift.

▶ ASSESSMENT

1. Assess the security of the controlled substance storage safe **to remain within legal guidelines and to ensure the safety of the substances.**
2. Assess the contents of the safe for any evidence of tampering with substance containers **to detect possible theft.**
3. Assess the controlled substance record for integrity regarding records of substances given to clients and substances wasted **to detect possible diversion of substances.**
4. Assess the method used for the storage and safeguarding of the safe keys **to remain within legal guidelines and ensure the safety of the substances.**
5. Assess the method used for signing out controlled substances that are to be administered to clients **to detect possible diversion of substances.**
6. Assess the method used for wasting unused controlled substances **to detect possible diversion of substances.**
7. Assess the method used to document controlled substances received from and returned to the pharmacy **to detect possible diversion of substances.**

▶ DIAGNOSIS

Risk for Caregiver Role Strain

Deficient Knowledge

Decisional Conflict

▶ PLANNING

Expected Outcomes:

1. The controlled substances will be stored in a legal, safe, and secure manner.
2. The controlled substance packaging will be intact without evidence of tampering.
3. The Controlled Substance Record will be accurate and agree with the actual contents of the safe.
4. The keys to the controlled substance safe will be maintained in a secure place and manner.
5. Controlled substances removed from the safe will be recorded and dispensed in a safe and legal manner.
6. Unused portions of controlled substances will be disposed of in a safe and legal manner.
7. Controlled substances will be received from and returned to the pharmacy using a secure and legal method.

Equipment Needed:

- Controlled substance safe
- Controlled substance count sheet
- Keys
- Client's medical administration record (MAR)
- Sharps box
- Sink
- Pen
- Automated medication-dispensing system

▶ CLIENT EDUCATION NEEDED:

1. Educate the client regarding the potential for abuse and addiction inherent in a controlled substance.
2. Reinforce the need to take the controlled substance as ordered. Educate the client that if the substance is not working effectively, to notify the caregiver rather than take an extra dose of medication.

 Estimated time to complete the skill: **10 minutes**

▶ DELEGATION TIPS

The skill of medication administration is not delegated to ancillary personnel in acute care settings. This may vary in state or federal institutions. Ancillary personnel are generally informed about the medications the client is receiving if adverse effects are anticipated or are being monitored.

IMPLEMENTATION—Action/Rationale

Action	Rationale
Dispensing a Controlled Substance to a Client	
1. Wash hands.	1. Reduces the transmission of microorganisms.
2. Obtain the client's MAR to determine the type and dosage of the controlled substance.	2. Verifies the order for the controlled substance.
3. Obtain the keys to the controlled substance safe.	3. Provides access to the controlled substance safe.
4. Making sure that the area is secure, open both locks on the controlled substance safe (see Figure 5-23-1).	4. Promotes a secure area to prevent pilferage while the safe is open.
5. Remove the ordered controlled substance and check the medication and dosage against the client's MAR (see Figure 5-23-2).	5. Ensures the right medication and dosage for the right client.

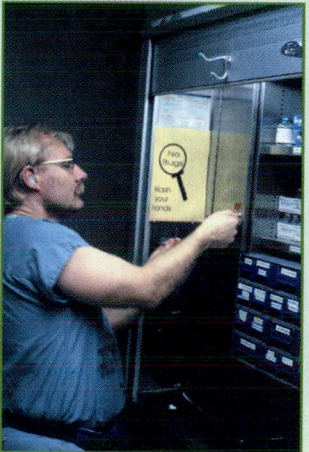

Figure 5-23-1 Make sure the area is secure, then open both locks.

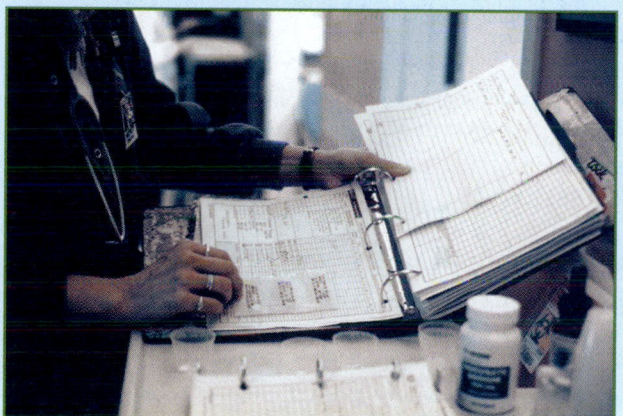

Figure 5-23-2 Check the medication and dosage against the client's MAR.

Action	Rationale
6. Remove the ordered dosage from the safe and relock the safe.	6. Secures the remaining controlled substances.
7. On the controlled substance sign-out record, note the date, time, client, drug, and dosage. Sign the record.	7. Provides a legal record of the disposition of the controlled substance.
8. Secure the controlled substance safe keys.	8. Prevents pilferage from the safe.
9. Dispense the controlled substance using the appropriate method according to the form of the substance.	9. Ensures the appropriate method of medication administration—IM, oral, SQ, and so forth.

continues

Action	Rationale
Disposing of Unused Portions of Controlled Substances	
10. Obtain the assistance of a second registered nurse.	10. Provides a legal witness to the disposal of the controlled substance.
11. Have the second registered nurse verify the medication to be disposed (see Figure 5-23-3).	11. By law, any controlled substance that is disposed must be witnessed by a second registered nurse.
12. With the second nurse as a witness, safely dispose of the unused controlled substance. If it is a liquid, pour it down the sink. Pills may be crushed and disposed of in the biohazard container or the powder may be flushed down the sink (see Figure 5-23-4).	12. Disposes of the controlled substance in an irretrievable manner.
13. On the Controlled Substance Record, note the amount of substance wasted, the method of disposal, the date, and the time. Sign the proper area and have the witnessing nurse also sign.	13. Provides a legal record of the disposition of the entire amount of the controlled substance.
14. If using an automated medication-dispensing system, the second nurse will log in and verify the amount of medication to be disposed (see Figure 5-23-5).	14. By law, any controlled substance that is disposed of must be witnessed by a second registered nurse.
15. Dispose of any needles or biohazardous substances in the appropriate containers.	15. Follows Standard Precautions.
16. Wash hands.	16. Reduces the transmission of microorganisms.
Inventorying Controlled Substances	
17. Obtain the assistance of a registered nurse from the next or previous shift.	17. Provides a legal witness for the procedure.

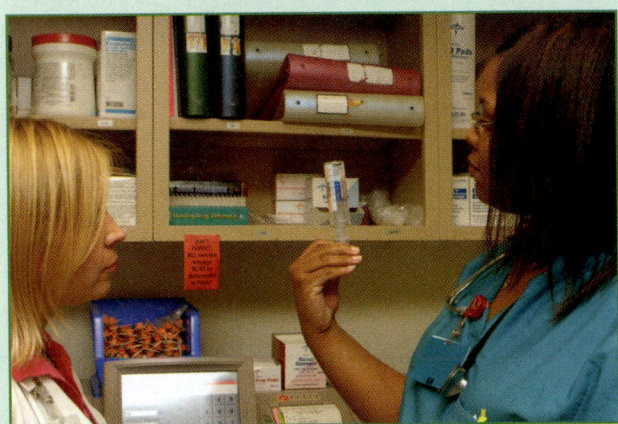

Figure 5-23-3   A second nurse verifies the medication to be disposed.

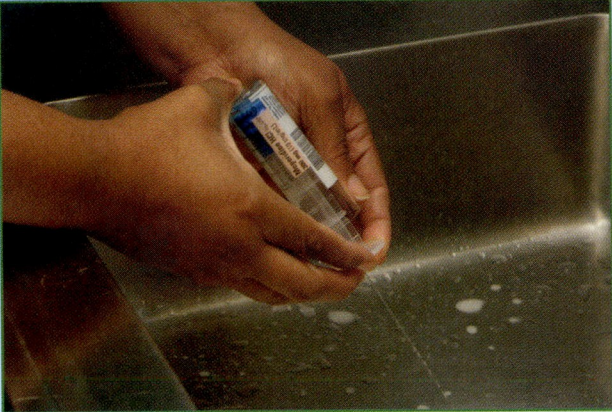

Figure 5-23-4   With the second nurse as a witness, dispose of the liquid by pouring it down the sink.

continues

Action	Rationale

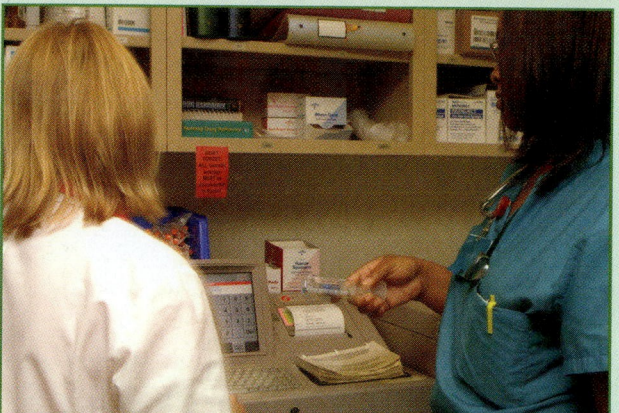

Figure 5-23-5   The second nurse will log into the automated medication dispensing system and verify the amount of the medication disposed.

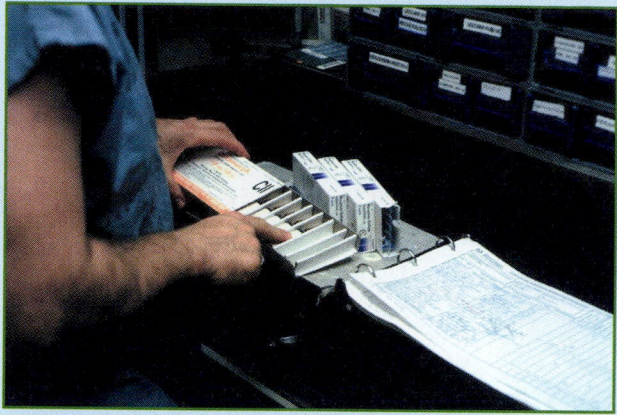

Figure 5-23-6   One nurse counts the amount of each type and dosage of controlled substance in the safe.

18. Obtain the keys to the controlled substance safe.

18. Provides access to the controlled substance safe. This is a good time to collect all sets of keys for the safe.

19. One nurse physically counts the amount of each type and dosage of controlled substance in the safe, informing the second nurse of each total (see Figure 5-23-6).

19. Physically verifies the presence of each medication. This is the time to examine the various medication containers to assess for possible tampering.

20. The second nurse records the counted totals in the appropriate space in the Controlled Substance Record (see Figure 5-23-7).

20. Checks the physical total against the written totals. These amounts must tally exactly. This is a good time to examine the Controlled Substance Record for excessive use of controlled substances, suspicious waste documentation, or other suspicious documentation.

21. Any discrepancies must be accounted for and accompanied by the signature of the responsible nurse before the administering nurses can be dismissed.

21. By law all controlled substances, dispensed or in the safe, must be accounted for before the dispensing nurse can leave.

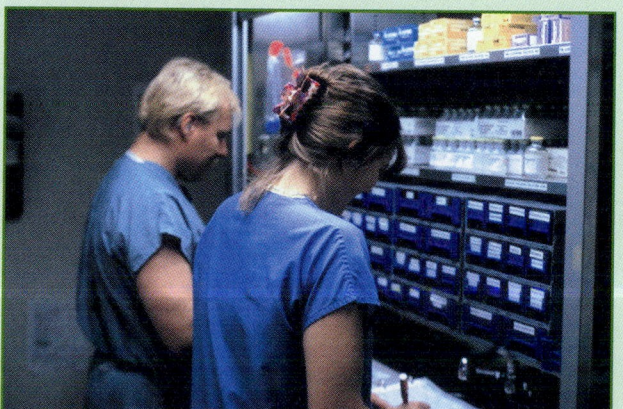

Figure 5-23-7   The second nurse records the counted totals in the Controlled Substance Record.

continues

Action	Rationale
Inventorying Controlled Substances *continued*	
22. All sets of keys must be accounted for and collected before the administering nurses can be dismissed.	22. By law all sets of keys to the controlled substance safe must remain on the institution premises to prevent tampering or copying.
23. Relock the controlled substance safe and secure the keys.	23. Secures the controlled substances and limits access to the controlled substances.

► REAL WORLD ANECDOTES

While working her shift in labor and delivery, Mary has a set of keys to the controlled substance safe. She uses the keys several times throughout the shift and appropriately signs out the substances she gives. As the time for change of shift approaches, Mary notes that there are no clients in the labor and delivery area. She has an appointment soon and asks Vera, the other RN in labor and delivery, to count the controlled substances while she changes out of her scrubs. Vera agrees and counts the controlled substances with the oncoming shift. As Vera hands over her set of keys, the oncoming nurse asks about the second set of keys. Realizing that Mary must still have the second set, Vera hurries to the changing room. Unfortunately, Mary is already gone and so is the dirty laundry. Vera and the oncoming nurses have to contact the laundry and everyone has to go through dirty scrubs in search of the keys to the controlled substance safe.

► EVALUATION

- The controlled substances are stored in a legal, safe, and secure manner.
- The controlled substance packaging is intact and shows no evidence of tampering.
- The controlled substance record is accurate and agrees with the actual contents of the safe.
- The keys to the controlled substance safe are maintained in a secure place and manner.
- Controlled substances removed from the safe have been recorded and dispensed in a safe and legal manner.
- Unused portions of controlled substances are disposed of in a safe and legal manner.
- Controlled substances are received from and returned to the pharmacy using a secure and legal method.

► DOCUMENTATION

Nurses' Notes

- Document dispensing a controlled substance and the reason it was given (e.g., pain, sedation, etc.).

- Note the results of the medication and any unusual effects that might be attributed to the medication.
- Note if the client refuses the controlled substance. Indicate that the client refused the medication. If the medication was prepared, note that the substance was wasted.
- Document any change in the amount of controlled substances in the safe on the Controlled Substance Record.
- Note the date, time, and disposition of controlled substances. The Controlled Substance Record must always agree with the physical contents of the safe.

Document on appropriate flow sheet or electronic medical record (EMR).

Medical Administration Record (MAR)

- Record the amount and dosage.
- Record date and time the controlled substance was administered.
- Note if the client refuses the controlled substance. Indicate that the client refused the medication. If

the medication was prepared, note that the substance was wasted.

▶ CRITICAL THINKING SKILL

Introduction
Theft of controlled substances occurs.

Possible Scenario
You are working nights in a small intensive care unit. The client beds and nurses' desk are all in the same room so the lights are kept low to promote client comfort. The nurse you are working with seems to be very clumsy tonight and is dropping things. Several times she has dropped a prefilled syringe of morphine with the needle uncapped, contaminating the contents. You are quite busy with your clients and watch from the far side of the room while the nurse wastes the medication. You sign the Controlled Substance Record when you have time.

Possible Outcome
When you count the controlled substances at the change of shift you notice that 90 mg of morphine have been signed out by the other nurse. All but 5 mg have been marked as wasted. You are stunned by the amount of morphine that has been used. You certainly do not remember seeing the other nurse waste anything close to that amount during the night. Before you can leave you must check the client medication records to confirm the morphine that was given, as well as check the controlled substance safe and the record. You also open up the sharps box to determine the number, size, and dosage strength of the morphine syringes present to confirm that they were actually wasted.

Prevention
Do not assume that abuse of controlled substances cannot happen on your floor, unit, or wing. Just as in all walks of life, some nurses may steal and some nurses are addicted to controlled substances. For your protection, as well as the protection of your clients, do not give these nurses a chance to break the law. Watch when a coworker asks you to cosign a wasted substance. Check for possible tampering with containers. If a coworker's behavior seems suspicious, follow up through the appropriate channels. This protects you, your clients, and allows your coworker to get needed help if indeed help is warranted.

▶ VARIATIONS

Geriatric Variations:
- *Not applicable*

Pediatric Variations:
- *Not applicable*

Home Care Variations:
- *If controlled substances are being dispensed in the client's home, the nurse must teach the client or the caregiver about the abuse and addiction potential of these substances.*
- *Teach the client or caregiver not to give extra doses if the medication does not seem to be working. Have them call the health care provider for advice. Extra doses can lead to psychological or physical addiction.*

Long-Term Care Variations:
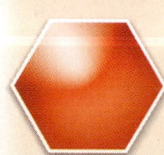
- *In long-term care settings, do not become complacent about controlled substances that a client routinely takes. Follow all Standard Precautions.*
- *Do not leave a controlled substance at the client's bedside for the client to take later.*
- *Be sure to witness the client taking the medication.*

► COMMON ERRORS

Possible Error:

Putting partial doses back in the safe or in the client's drawer for later use.

Prevention:

Unused narcotics must be wasted, not saved. Never keep or reuse partial doses of controlled substances. If a prefilled syringe only comes in a 50-mg dose and the order is for 25 mg, waste the extra 25 mg prior to administering the medication. This helps prevent errors in dosage as well as preventing confusion and diversion of wasted controlled substances. You are accountable for the narcotics you use.

► NURSING TIPS

- Count all controlled substances with a nurse on the opposite shift.
- Check packaging for signs of tampering. Be sure the seals on the top and bottom of boxes are intact. Check unit dose packages to be sure the foil is intact. If the controlled substance is dispensed in a numbered roll of pills, check the other end of the roll to be sure numbers 1, 2, and 3 are there.
- Report discrepancies immediately according to your institutional policy.

- Be sure all sets of keys to the safe are accounted for at all times.
- Do not leave the keys to the safe in the drawer of the medication cart for convenience.
- If you are not using a controlled substance regularly, return it to the pharmacy so you do not have to keep counting it.
- If someone tries to forcibly steal the controlled substances, give them the keys. No drug is worth your life.

► SPECIAL CONSIDERATIONS

- *Never administer a controlled substance without an order or if the order is outdated.*
- *Never leave a controlled substance unattended. Never administer a controlled substance that was prepared by another health care provider unless the label clearly identifies the medication and the seal is intact.*
- *Nurses have the right to decline administering a controlled substance if it will put the client in harm.*

Nutrition and Elimination

Inserting and Maintaining a Nasogastric Tube

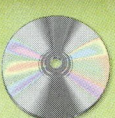

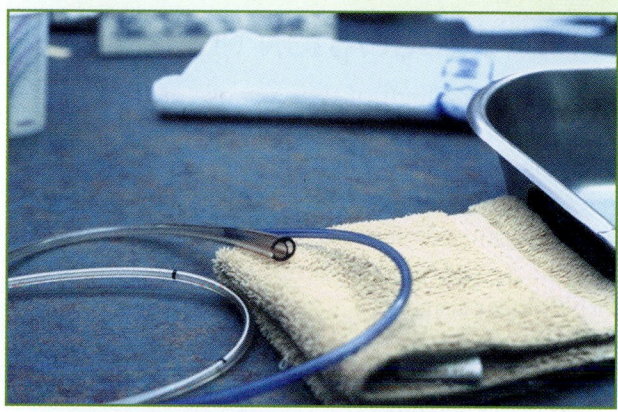

▶ OVERVIEW OF THE SKILL

Nasogastric (NG) tubes are used for several purposes, including feeding for nutrition when the client is comatose, semiconscious, or unable to consume sufficient nutrition orally. Nasogastric suction tubes are used for decompression of gastric content after gastrointestinal surgery and to obtain gastric specimens for diagnosis of peptic ulcer. Tubes are used for irrigation to clean and flush the stomach after oral ingestion of poisonous substances. Finally, NG tubes are used to document the presence of blood in the stomach, monitor the amount of bleeding from the stomach, and identify the recurrence of bleeding in the stomach. The two most commonly used NG tubes are the single-lumen Levin's tube and the double-lumen Salem sump tube. The gastrointestinal tract is considered to be a clean area rather than a sterile one. The procedure to place an NG tube is performed using clean technique unless it is performed in conjunction with gastrointestinal surgery.

▶ ASSESSMENT

1. Assess client's consciousness level **to determine the ability of the client to cooperate during the procedure.**
2. Check the client's chart for any previous medical history of nostril surgery or injury or unusual nostril bleeding. **Reduces risk of injury from the tube.**
3. Use a penlight to assess nostrils for a deviated septum. **Facilitates choice of nostril and size of tube.**

4. Ask the client to breathe through each nostril occluding the other with a finger. **Facilitates choice of nostril and decreases chance that tube will interfere with respirations.**
5. Assess for latex allergy. **Prevents reaction to latex and determines need to use latex-free tubes and gloves.**

▶ DIAGNOSIS

Acute Pain

Imbalanced Nutrition: Less Than Body Requirements

Impaired Oral Mucous Membrane

Impaired Swallowing

Risk for Aspiration

Risk for Deficient Fluid Volume

Risk for Diarrhea

Risk for Impaired Skin Integrity

▶ PLANNING

Expected Outcomes:

1. Client's nutritional status will improve, as indicated by increased body weight, physical strength, and mental status.
2. Client's nutritional needs will be met with the assistance of tube feeding.
3. Client will maintain a patent airway, as evident by absence of coughing, no shortness of breath, and no aspiration.

4. Client will not have diarrhea caused by NG feeding.
5. The mucous membranes in the client's mouth will remain moist and intact.
6. Client will maintain a normal fluid volume, as evident by good skin texture, muscle tone, and blood volume.
7. Client's comfort level will increase.
8. Skin around the tube will remain intact, with no redness or blisters.

Equipment Needed:

- Nasogastric tube: adult, 14 to 18 French; child/infant, 5 to 10 French; single-lumen (Levin's sump): feeding; double-lumen (Salem sump tube): feeding, suction, irrigation (see Figure 6-1-1)
- Water-soluble lubricant
- Syringe with catheter tip or adapter, 50 mL
- Glass of tap water with straw, or ice
- Towel or tissue
- Emesis basin with ice chips
- Tongue blade
- pH chemstrip
- Stethoscope
- Disposable, nonsterile latex-free gloves, goggles

- Hypoallergenic tape, rubber band, and safety pin
- Penlight or flashlight
- Disposable irrigation set (if needed)
- Wall mount or portable suction equipment (if needed)
- Administration set with pump or controller for feeding tube

▶ CLIENT EDUCATION NEEDED:

1. Inform the client of the purpose of the NG tube.
2. Explain the procedure of insertion and any expected discomfort.
3. Establish and clarify a "hand signal" to indicate the need to temporarily stop the NG insertion.
4. Explain how the client can cooperate during tube insertion, especially by swallowing water when asked to do so.
5. Explain potential complications, such as diarrhea, mouth dryness, and nostril irritation.
6. Review the skills and procedures of maintaining the tube.
7. Instruct the client to chew on ice chips to satisfy the basic need to eat (if there is no fluid intake restriction).
8. Encourage physical activity to enhance gastrointestinal mobility (if there is no activity restriction).
9. If a client with dentures is conscious, encourage client to wear the dentures to maintain the normal shape of the oral cavity.

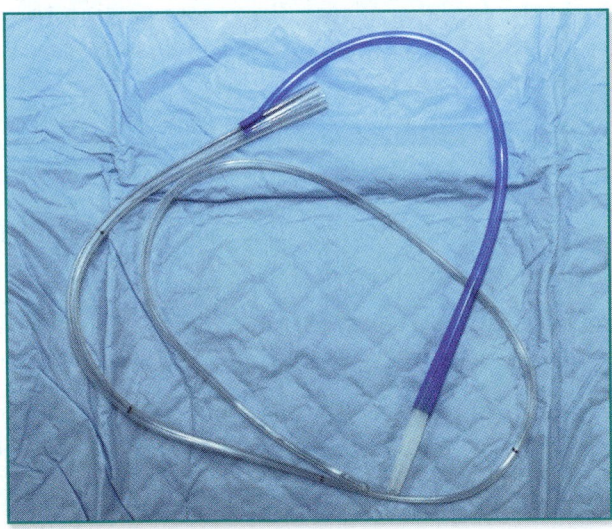

Figure 6-1-1   Double-lumen nasogastric tube

Estimated time to complete the skill: **5–20 minutes**

▶ DELEGATION TIPS

Inserting and maintaining a nasogastric tube is the responsibility of a nurse. Oral hygiene for the client may be delegated.

IMPLEMENTATION—Action/Rationale

Action	Rationale
1. Review client's medical history. Review medical history for conditions that may have resulted in a loss of the gag reflex.	1. To assess for any nostril surgery and abnormal bleeding. A client without a gag reflex is at risk for aspiration.
2. Check client's armband. Assess client's consciousness and ability to understand. Explain the procedure and develop a hand signal.	2. Verifies correct client. Decreases anxiety and promotes cooperation.
3. Close client's door and draw curtains around client's bed.	3. Provides privacy
4. Prepare the equipment, putting tissues, a cup of water, and an emesis basin nearby (see Figure 6-1-2).	4. Facilitates an efficient procedure.
5. Prepare the environment; raise the bed and place it in a high Fowler's position (45 to 60 degrees). Cover the chest with a towel.	5. Facilitates insertion and prevents back strain.
6. Wash hands and then put on gloves.	6. Practices clean technique.
7. Use a penlight to view the client's nostrils. Assess client's nostrils with penlight and have the client blow nose one nostril at a time (see Figure 6-1-3).	7. Choosing the more patent nostril for insertion decreases discomfort and unnecessary trauma.
8. Using the NG tube, measure the distance from the tip of the nose to the earlobe and then to the xiphoid process of the sternum and mark this distance on the tube with a piece of tape (see Figure 6-1-4).	8. Determines the approximate amount of tube needed to reach the stomach.
9. Lubricate first 4 inches of the tube with water-soluble lubricant.	9. Facilitates passage into the naris.
10. Ask the client to slightly flex the neck backward.	10. Makes insertion easier.
11. Gently insert the tube into a naris (see Figure 6-1-5).	11. Promotes passage of tube with minimal trauma to mucosa.

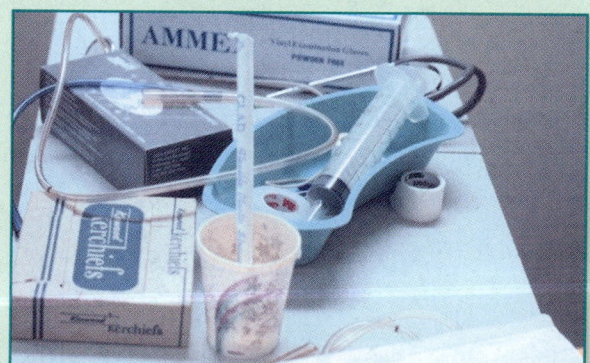

Figure 6-1-2 Put an emesis basin, cup with straw, and tissues nearby.

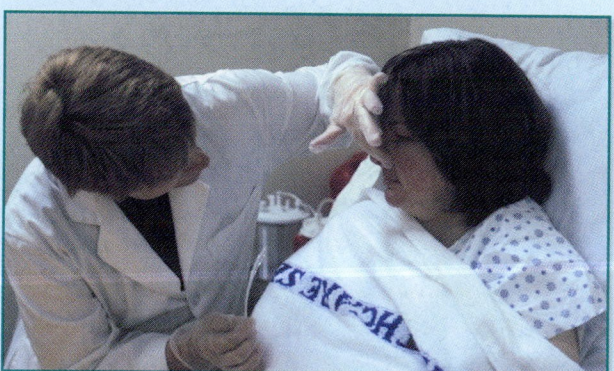

Figure 6-1-3 Assess the client's nostrils before introducing the nasogastric tube.

continues

Action	Rationale

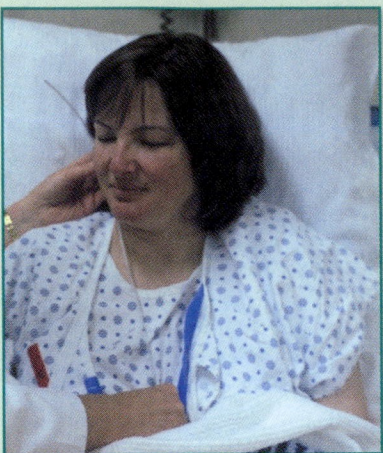

Figure 6-1-4 Measure the distance from nose to earlobe to the xiphoid process to determine how much tube will need to be inserted to reach the stomach.

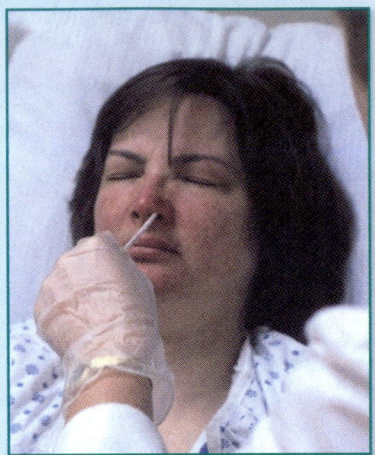

Figure 6-1-5 Gently insert the tube into the naris.

12. Ask the client to tip the head forward once the tube reaches the nasopharynx—this is usually where the client starts to gag. If the client continues to gag, stop a moment (see Figure 6-1-6).

13. Advance the tube several inches at a time as the client swallows. If gag reflex is present, have the client swallow water or ice chips as tube is advanced (see Figure 6-1-7).

14. Withdraw the tube immediately if there are signs of respiratory distress.

12. Tipping the head forward facilitates passage of the tube into the esophagus instead of the trachea. Tube may stimulate gag reflex. Allows the client to rest, reduces anxiety, and prevents vomiting.

13. Assists in advancing the tube past the oropharynx. The action of swallowing facilitates the insertion process. With each swallow, the tracheal opening is closed to prevent inspiration. Clients who do not have a gag reflex are at risk for aspiration.

14. Prevents trauma to bronchus or lung.

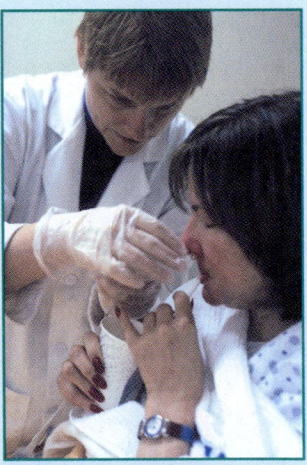

Figure 6-1-7 Advance the tube slowly. The client swallows small sips of water to assist in pushing the tube past the oropharynx.

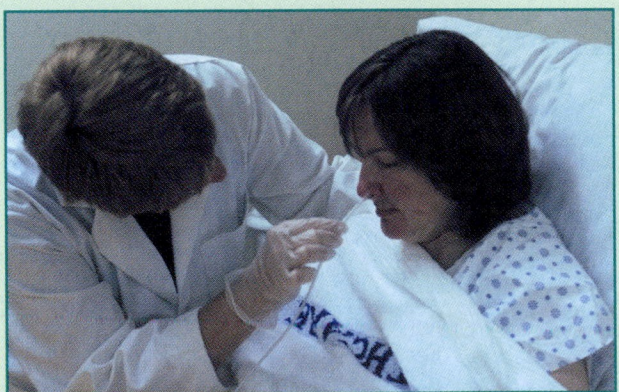

Figure 6-1-6 Tip head forward once tube reaches nasopharynx.

continues

Action	Rationale

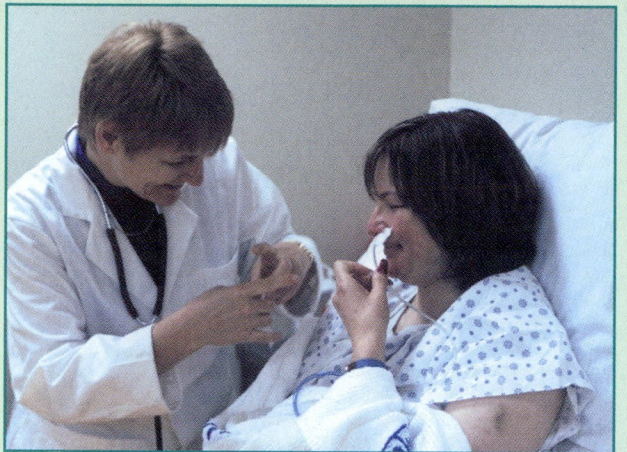

Figure 6-1-8   Advance the tube until the taped mark is at the opening of the naris.

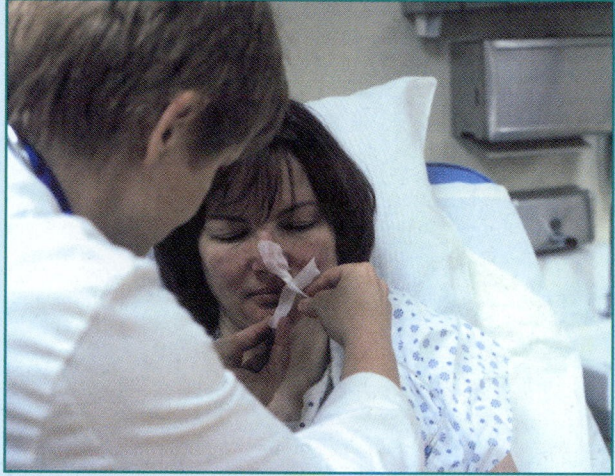

Figure 6-1-9   Secure the tube to the nose.

15. Advance the tube until the taped mark is reached (see Figure 6-1-8).

15. Enables the tube to reach the stomach.

16. Wipe or wash body oils off tip of nose and allow it to dry. Split a 4-inch strip of tape lengthwise 2 inches. Secure the tube with the tape by placing the wide portion of the tape on the bridge of the nose and wrapping the split ends around the tube (see Figure 6-1-9). Tape to cheek as well, if desired (see Figure 6-1-10).

16. Prevents tube displacement.

17. Check the placement of the tube:
- Aspirate for gastric content, assess the color and quality of the content. If required, measure with pH indicator strip (see Figure 6-1-11). Follow protocol regarding reinsertion of contents versus discarding.
- Prepare the client for X-ray check-up, if prescribed.

17. Ensures correct placement. A pH of 5 or less indicates that the tube is in the stomach.

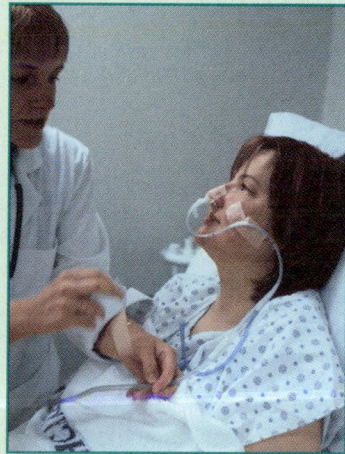

Figure 6-1-10   Tape the tube to the cheek as well, if desired, to provide extra support.

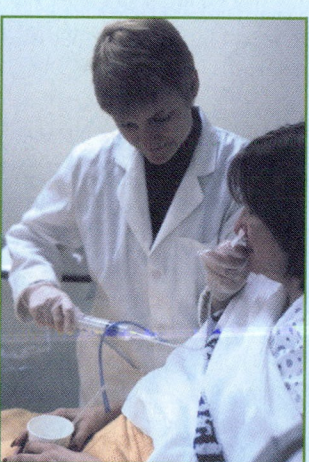

Figure 6-1-11   Aspirate a sample of gastric content to check for pH.

continues

Action	Rationale

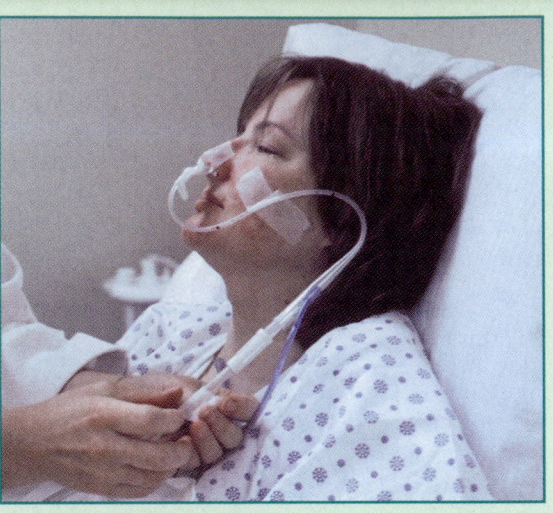

Figure 6-1-12 Connect the distal end of the tube to suction or drainage to complete the procedure.

18. Connect the distal end of the tube to suction, draining bag, or adapter according to the purpose of this nursing intervention (see Figure 6-1-12).

18. Establishes an appropriate pathway for intervention.

19. Secure the tube with tape, or with rubber band and safety pin, to client's gown or bed sheet.

19. Enhances the level of comfort and secures the tubing system.

20. Remove gloves, dispose of contaminated materials in proper container, and wash hands.

20. Implements the principles of infection control.

21. Position client comfortably and place the call light in easy reach.

21. Decreases client's anxiety and provides access to help, if needed.

22. Document procedure.

22. Records implementation of intervention and promotes continuity of care.

Maintaining a Nasogastric Tube

23. Wash hands and apply gloves.

23. Reduces the transmission of microorganisms.

24. Follow the steps in Action 17 to check the proper tubing position before instilling anything per NG tube or at least every 8 hours.

24. Prevents complications from dislocation of the tube.

25. Assess for signs that the tube has become blocked, including epigastric pain and vomiting, and/or the inability to pass medications or feedings through the tube.

25. Prevents complications from the loss of beneficial effects from the tube.

26. Remember never to irrigate or rotate a tube that has been placed by the health care provider during gastric or esophageal surgery.

26. Rotation or irrigation may disturb incisions.

27. Provide oral hygiene and assist client to clean nares daily.

27. Enhances client's comfort and the integrity of skin and nose mucosa.

28. Dispose of contaminated materials in proper container, and wash hands.

28. Reduces the transmission of microorganisms.

► **REAL WORLD ANECDOTES**

Mr. Klotz had just been admitted to the hospital with severe abdominal distention. NG tube placement was ordered for abdominal decompression. Mr. Klotz was not to have any fluids by mouth, but he could have ice chips. The nurse provided Mr. Klotz with ice chips and instructed him to suck on a few chips and swallow as she inserted the NG tube. The nurse inserted the NG tube into Mr. Klotz's right naris but was unable to advance the tube any farther than an inch. After several attempts to advance the tube, the nurse tried Mr. Klotz's left naris. It required several gentle attempts and lots of lubricant to pass the tube into the nasopharynx, but the nurse was finally able to advance the tube into Mr. Klotz's stomach. After Mr. Klotz had received some relief from his distention, he did mention to the nurse that he had broken his nose many years earlier.

► **EVALUATION**

• Client's nutritional status improves, as indicated by increased body weight, physical strength, and mental status.
• Client's nutritional needs are met with the assistance of tube feeding.
• Client maintains a patent airway, as evident by absence of coughing, no shortness of breath, and no aspiration.
• Client does not have diarrhea caused by nasogastric feeding.
• Mouth mucous membranes remain moist and intact.
• Client maintains a normal fluid volume, as evident by good skin texture, muscle tone, and blood-volume.
• Client's comfort level increases.
• Skin around the tube remains intact, with no redness or blisters.

► **DOCUMENTATION**

Nurses' Notes

• Document the type of NG tube inserted, the naris used, how the client tolerated the procedure, and the methods used to verify placement.
• Document care provided to the client to increase comfort of the NG insertion naris.
• Note any unusual findings.

Document on appropriate flow sheet or electronic medical record (EMR).

Intake and Output Record

• Note the amount of fluid the client drank to aid insertion of the NG tube.
• Note the amount of gastric contents removed for testing.

► **CRITICAL THINKING SKILL**

Introduction

Nurses must be able to evaluate the effectiveness of NG tube insertion, maintenance, or removal.

Possible Scenario

The family of your home care client has been assisting in her care, including the care of her feeding tube. You have educated them on the tube and its placement. Although they state they secured the tube in a proper place and the end of the tube is currently positioned higher than the stomach, you observe the tube is filled with gastric content.

Possible Outcome

Client has a continuous risk for infection, electrolyte imbalance, and potential aspiration.

Prevention

Assess that the caregiver is properly securing the end of the tube at a level higher than the stomach. Assess the client's vital signs and respiratory pattern for infection, electrolyte imbalance, or aspiration. Reeducate the caregivers on assessing for correct tube placement, and review with them common situations where the tube might move.

► **VARIATIONS**

Geriatric Variation:

• For elderly clients who wear dentures, oral hygiene and denture care should not be overlooked simply because an NG tube is in place.

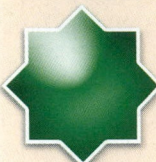

Pediatric Variations:

• Dispose of or securely tape any small parts such as plastic connectors or plugs, to prevent small children from accidentally aspirating or swallowing them.
• Amount of air needed to assess placement is proportionate to client's size.

Home Care Variation:

• Periodically assess the family member's ability to check the placement of the tube, check residual gastric contents, administer tube feedings, or connect the tube properly with suction.

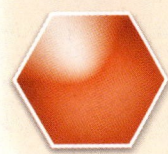

Long-Term Care Variation:

• Teach family members or caregivers to assess the client's nutritional status and assess for any sign of complications related to the NG tube.

► **COMMON ERRORS**

Possible Error:

The nurse is unable to auscultate air bubbles but assumes the NG tube is in place.

Prevention:

If you are unable to verify NG tube position by auscultating air, use another method of verification. Attempt to aspirate gastric contents. If you are unable to verify NG tube placement, do not instill anything through the tube. Notify the client's health care provider. Send the client for an X-ray to verify placement if this is within institutional guidelines.

► **NURSING TIPS**

• Adjust the height of the bed to eliminate back strain.
• Prepare the split tape before putting on gloves.
• This can be an anxiety-provoking procedure. Good communication skills decrease anxiety and promote the client's cooperation.
• The size of the NG tube used depends on client size, client history of damage to the structure of the nose, and the purpose of the procedure.

• Tincture of benzoin (if iodine allergy is not present) may be used to prep the skin on the bridge of the nose. This acts as an adhesive as well as a skin prep.
• Carefully observe client's verbal and nonverbal responses during the entire procedure.
• When feasible, engage family members or caregivers to assist in NG tube insertion.
• Remove air used to check tube placement if NG tube is not connected to suction.

▶ **SPECIAL CONSIDERATIONS**

- *Cold water with ice chips can be used to stiffen the tip of single-lumen Levin's tube to smooth the insertion process.*
- *Avoid using safety pins with psychiatric clients; self-harm behavior could be initiated by leaving a harmful object by the bedside. Use tape instead to secure the nasogastric tube in this case.*
- *Tube placement must be assessed every time anything will be placed down the nasogastric tube to prevent insertion of foreign products into the lungs.*

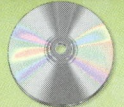

SKILL 6-2

Assessing Placement of a Large-Bore Feeding Tube and Administering an Intermittent Feeding

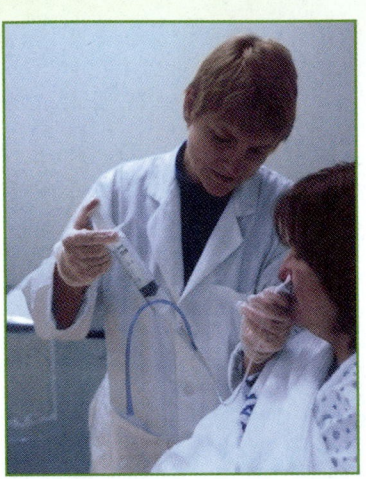

▶ OVERVIEW OF THE SKILL

Clients who cannot take food or fluids orally may require the placement of a feeding tube for enteral nutrition. These clients may be unconscious, unable to respond to the thirst reflex, unable to swallow, or receiving a hyperosmotic enteral preparation. The large-bore nasogastric feeding tube requires a health care provider's order to be placed. The tube can be a firm, polyvinyl large-bore tube or a soft, flexible polyurethane or silicone tube. After insertion, the placement should be checked by X-ray to determine that it is in the stomach or in the intestine as ordered and not in an airway. After the initial X-ray for placement, it is the nurse's responsibility to verify the tube's position before each intermittent feeding or medication, or once a shift if the client is receiving continuous feedings.

There are several types of large-bore feeding tubes. A nasogastric tube is for short-term use; the major complication of its use is aspiration pneumonia. The nasoduodenal tube is also used short-term. There is less risk of aspiration with this tube, as the tip is weighted and rests in the duodenum. However, it is also more difficult to place, and some institutions require that a health care provider insert this type of tube. The gastrostomy tube (GT) is placed surgically by laparoscopy for long-term use. The more common percutaneous endoscopic gastrostomy (PEG) tube is placed under local anesthesia and conscious sedation. A PEG tube is used for long-term feedings. The percutaneous

endoscopic jejunostomy (PEJ) tube may also be placed by the health care provider. It is more comfortable for the client and carries minimal risk of aspiration.

▶ ASSESSMENT

1. Check the health care provider's order for the type and size of feeding tube **to ensure accurate placement of the correct tube.**
2. Review the client's medical record for a history of prior tube use or displacement **as recurring tube displacement may increase the risk of pulmonary placement.**
3. Assess the client for signs and symptoms of inadvertent respiratory placement **as coughing, choking, and cyanosis may indicate placement of the tube in an airway.**
4. Assess the client for signs and symptoms that increase the client's risk of tube dislocation. **Coughing, retching, and nasotracheal suctioning may cause the tube to become dislodged.**

▶ DIAGNOSIS

Imbalanced Nutrition: Less Than Body Requirements

Imbalanced Nutrition: More Than Body Requirements

Impaired Oral Mucous Membrane

Impaired Swallowing

710

Risk for Aspiration

Risk for Deficient Fluid Volume

Risk for Impaired Skin Integrity

▶ PLANNING

Expected Outcomes:

1. The tube will remain in place and intact.
2. The tube feeding or medication will infuse into the client's gastrointestinal (GI) tract.
3. The client will not experience any respiratory distress.
4. The client will not experience any pain.
5. The client will be able to describe the reason for checking the tube's placement.

Equipment Needed (see Figure 6-2-1):

- Catheter tip syringe, 50 mL
- Stethoscope
- Gloves
- pH indicator strip
- Emesis basin
- Towel

▶ CLIENT EDUCATION NEEDED:

1. Tell the client the rationale for checking the placement of the feeding tube.
2. Ask the client to tell you if he or she is having respiratory difficulties.

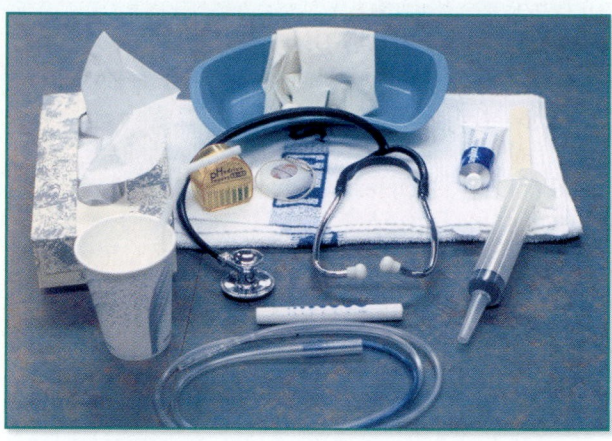

Figure 6-2-1 Stethoscope, syringe, and pH strips are used to assess placement of the tube.

3. Teach the caregiver how to check the tube for correct placement before each feeding or medication.
4. Provide written and oral instructions about how to check for correct tube placement.
5. Tell the client and caregiver not to proceed with a feeding if there is any doubt about the tube's proper placement.

 Estimated time to complete the skill: **5 minutes**

▶ DELEGATION TIPS

Assessment of the proper placement of a large-bore feeding tube may not be delegated to ancillary personnel who may be performing a feeding. The nurse should perform the placement assessment and ancillary personnel should be instructed to properly position the client and to report any conditions that may arise as a result of the tube or the feeding.

IMPLEMENTATION—Action/Rationale

Action	Rationale
1. Review health care provider's order.	1. Confirms prescription and equipment needed.
2. Close client's door and draw curtains around client's bed. Check client's armband.	2. Provides privacy. Verifies correct client.
3. Wash hands (see Figure 6-2-2). Don gloves.	3. Reduces the transmission of microorganisms.

continues

Action	Rationale
4. Assess placement of the tube: • Attach syringe to free end of tube and aspirate 10 mL of gastrointestinal contents with a 50-mL syring (see Figure 6-2-3). • If unable to aspirate, reposition client on side and try again. • Measure pH of GI contents with indicator strip.	**4.** Verify correct placement. • Obtain gastric aspirate. • The tube opening may be lying against the gastric wall. • Ensures proper placement. Gastric contents have a pH of 5 of less. In clients who are receiving an acid-inhibiting drug, gastric content pH may be between 4 and 6. Intestinal contents have a pH of 6 to 7.
Intermittent Bolus Feeding **5.** Position client in high Fowlers.	**5.** Reduces the risk of pulmonary aspiration.
6. Determine gastric residual contents: • Insert syringe into nasogastric tube and aspirate gastric contents. Measure amount. If greater than 50–100 mL (or accordance with agency protocol) hold feeding until residual diminishes. • Instill aspirated contents back into feeding tube.	**6.** Indicates if gastric emptying is delayed. • Reduces the risk of pulmonary aspiration related to gastric distention. • Prevents electrolyte imbalances.
7. Pinch the nasogastric tubing and remove syringe.	**7.** Prevents air from entering the stomach.
8. Remove plunger from syringe and attach syringe to nasogastric tubing.	**8.** Provides a system to deliver the feeding.
9. Fill syringe with formula (see Figure 6-2-4). Unpinch tubing and allow formula to infuse slowly by gravity by adjusting the height of the syringe.	**9.** Slow infusion prevents gastric distention. The higher the syringe, the faster the infusion.
10. Continue to add formula to syringe until prescribed amount has been administered.	**10.** Prevents air from entering the stomach.

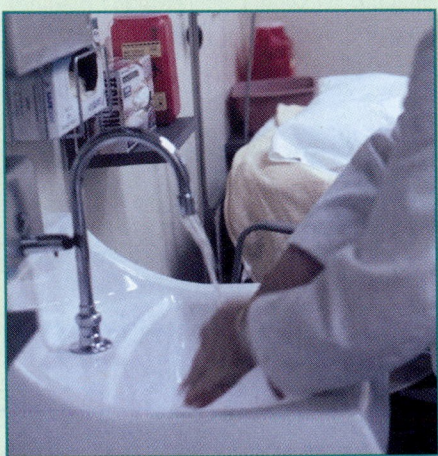

Figure 6-2-2 Wash hands prior to beginning procedure.

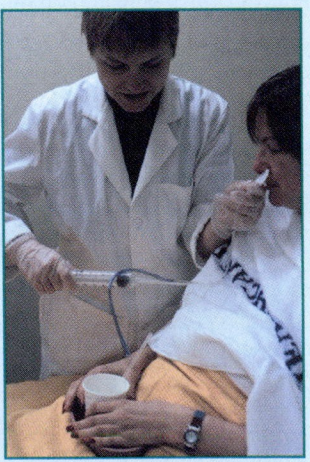

Figure 6-2-3 Aspirate 10 mL of gastric contents to check pH.

continues

Action	Rationale
11. Flush tubing with 30–60 mL of water or prescribed amount (see Figure 6-2-5).	**11.** Flushes formula remaining in tubing and maintains patency of the tube.
12. Remove the syringe and clamp the tubing.	**12.** Prevents air from entering the stomach.
13. Keep head of bed elevated at lease 30 degrees for 1 hour after feeding.	**13.** Prevents pulmonary aspiration.
14. Remove gloves and wash hands.	**14.** Reduces the transmission of microorganisms.

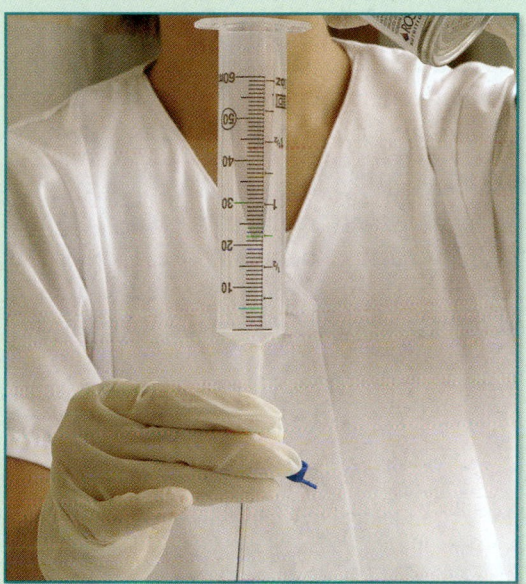

Figure 6-2-4 Fill syringe with prescribed formula.

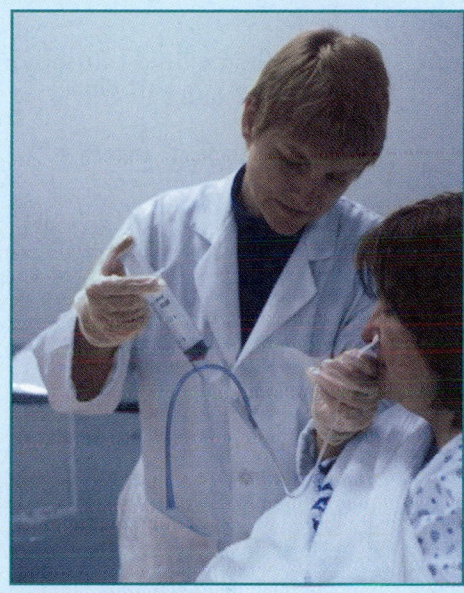

Figure 6-2-5 After feeding, flush the tube with 30–60 mL of warm water to rinse out residue.

▶ REAL WORLD ANECDOTES

Claudia, an 18-year-old girl, was comatose after a motor vehicle accident. She had a head injury and broken clavicle, radius, and pelvis. After the accident she had been in the intensive care unit on a ventilator for 5 days but later was transferred to a medical floor. She was breathing on her own but had not regained consciousness. A large-bore nasogastric feeding tube had been placed for enteral feedings and medication administration. The feedings were intermittent so the nurse began her assessment of its placement before starting the feeding. When the nurse injected air, she heard the characteristic gurgle, but when she started the feeding, Claudia started coughing. The nurse immediately stopped the feeding and assessed her for respiratory distress. She notified the physician, who ordered an X-ray. The tube was found to be looped with the end near Claudia's bronchus. The physician repositioned the tube and obtained another X-ray, which showed it was in good position and the feeding was restarted.

▶ EVALUATION

- The tube remains in place and intact.
- The tube feeding or medication is infusing into the client's GI tract.
- The client has not experienced any respiratory distress.
- The client is not experiencing any pain.
- The client is able to describe the reason for checking the tube's placement.

▶ DOCUMENTATION

Nurses' Notes

- Document the type of tube placed.
- Note the character of GI contents.
- Record the pH measurement.
- Document the assessment of air injected into the stomach.
- Note any client complaints or unusual findings.

Document on appropriate flow sheet or electronic medical record (EMR).

Intake and Output Record

- Record the amount of any fluid infused or removed in the appropriate category.

▶ CRITICAL THINKING SKILL

Introduction

Displacement of a large-bore feeding tube may occur when a client coughs, gags, or vomits. The nurse needs to assess the client for any symptoms that may cause a tube displacement and always reassess placement before injecting anything into tube.

Possible Scenario

Brian was 16 years old when he needed to have a tube placed for feeding. He hated the feeling of the tube in his throat and could not get used to it. He gagged and coughed, sometimes so vigorously that he vomited. When the nurse came to assess the tube placement, she noted that the end of the tube was visible in the back of Brian's throat.

Possible Outcome

The nurse could see the tube was not in its proper position and knew that it could not be repositioned, so she gently removed the entire tube and notified the physician. He reevaluated Brian's need for the tube, considered the risk of aspiration and Brian's difficulty with the tube, and decided to stop the tube feedings and let Brian try to eat on his own.

Prevention

Client teaching and reassurance are an important part of maintaining a large-bore feeding tube in place. Antiemetic or antianxiety medications may be needed to help clients tolerate the tube if it is placed orally or nasally.

▶ VARIATIONS

Geriatric Variations:
- *Elderly clients may have more fragile tissue that could be damaged with a large-bore feeding tube.*
- *Older clients with other respiratory conditions are at increased risk for respiratory complications if the feeding tube migrates to the pulmonary tree.*

Pediatric Variations:
- *Inject only 0.5–1.0 mL of air into a pediatric feeding tube (varies with size of client).*
- *Be sure the child is quiet and calm while checking for placement so you can hear the air being injected.*

Home Care Variations:
- *Assess the sanitation of the home to determine the client's risk for infection.*
- *Teach the caregiver the normal range of pH for GI contents.*
- *Teach the caregiver the signs and symptoms of feeding tube displacement and what to do if displacement is suspected.*

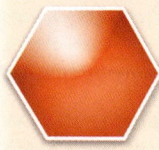

Long-Term Care Variations:
- *Teach staff members the normal range of pH for GI contents.*
- *Equipment for verifying tube placement should be at the client's bedside at all times.*
- *Teach staff members the signs and symptoms of tube displacement and to whom to report the symptoms.*
- *Teach staff members how to discontinue a feeding if they suspect tube displacement.*

▶ COMMON ERRORS

Possible Error:

You do not wait 1 hour after the last tube feeding has finished to check for tube placement so the pH of the aspirated GI contents is inaccurate.

Prevention:

Plan a schedule for feeding, medications, and checking for tube placement so that an accurate measurement will be obtained. Write this plan into the client's plan of care so all staff can comply. If this error does occur, flush the tube with 30 mL warm water. Wait 1 hour. Begin tube placement assessment again.

▶ NURSING TIPS

- A muffled or faint sound of injected air may signal that the tube is in the lungs.
- It may be necessary to inject air two or three times in obese clients as the sound of injected air may be faint. Remove air to prevent distention and discomfort.

- Do not withdraw or advance the tube into clients who have had gastric resections or other abdominal surgery as it could damage the suture lines and cause hemorrhage.
- Assess tube placement routinely if client is on continuous feeding because tubes may become dislodged with movement and coughing.

▶ SPECIAL CONSIDERATIONS

- *As aspirating the gastric or intestinal content is part of tube placement checking, the quality of the aspirated content should be observed and documented. For clients whose insertion purpose is for feeding, the gastric content should be returned to maintain the electrolyte balance whereas the gastric content should be discarded if the insertion purpose is for irrigation or suction (bleeding or poisoning cases).*
- *Use nonlatex tubes and gloves if there is a history of latex allergy.*
- *Reassess tube placement after coughing, vomiting, increased movement, seizures, or upon returning to unit after diagnostic test. Always reassess tube placement before putting anything into an NG tube.*

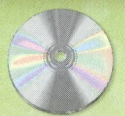

Assessing Placement of a Small-Bore Feeding Tube

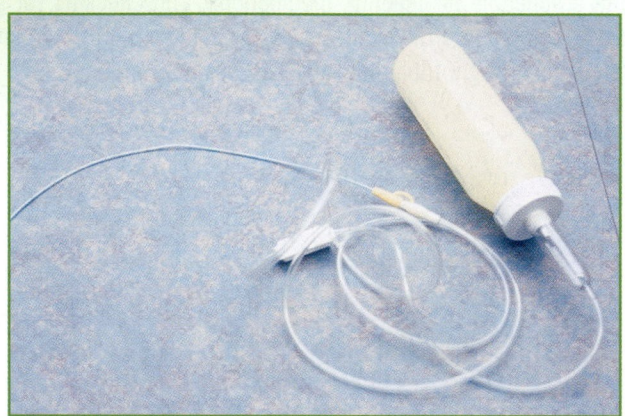

▶ OVERVIEW OF THE SKILL

Clients with a small-bore feeding tube must have placement of the tube verified at time of insertion and every shift to prevent insertion/migration of the tube into the esophagus, trachea, or lungs and aspiration of feeding. Placement of a feeding tube is easy to disrupt because the tubes are small, flexible, and secured only with tape on the nose. There are two effective methods of verifying placement. The first method is to aspirate a sample of gastric contents and check pH levels. The second method to verify placement is to obtain an abdominal X-ray.

▶ ASSESSMENT

1. Assess client for any signs of respiratory distress such as choking, coughing, shallow breathing, or decreasing oxygen saturations. **These symptoms could be indicative of aspiration of the feeding tube.**
2. Check for a tape marker on the tube, near the nose, **which indicates the length of tube inserted. If tube has become displaced, marker will be farther away from nose.**
3. Assess sputum for distinguishing features that would indicate aspiration, such as blue color (tube feeding formula is mixed with blue food coloring to distinguish feeding from normal white sputum). **Blue sputum could signify aspiration of feeding, which could lead to pneumonia.**

4. Assess for latex allergy. **Determines need for latex-free tube.**

▶ DIAGNOSIS

Imbalanced Nutrition: Less Than Body Requirements

Impaired Oral Mucous Membrane

Risk for Aspiration

Risk for Deficient Fluid Volume

Risk for Impaired Skin Integrity

▶ PLANNING

Expected Outcomes:

1. The client's feeding tube will be intact in the ordered area of the gastrointestinal (GI) tract.
2. The client will not experience aspiration secondary to tube feedings.

Equipment Needed:

- Syringe: 30 or 50 mL for adults, 5 or 10 mL for pediatric clients (varies with size)
- Stethoscope
- pH testing equipment (see Figure 6-3-1)
- Progress notes/flow sheets

▶ CLIENT EDUCATION NEEDED:

1. Explain reason for verifying placement.
2. Explain steps of procedure.

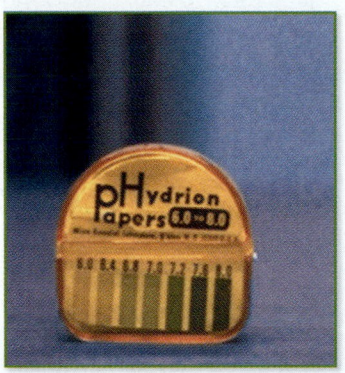

Figure 6-3-1   Equipment used to test pH.

3. Answer questions from client/family.
4. Instruct client to notify staff immediately if experiencing respiratory distress or blue sputum.
5. Explain purpose of X-rays, if needed.

Estimated time to complete the skill: **5–10 minutes**

► DELEGATION TIPS

Obtaining placement sounds or aspirant from small-bore feeding tubes requires the skill and problem solving ability of a nurse; therefore, this task cannot be delegated.

IMPLEMENTATION—Action/Rationale

Action	Rationale
1. Wash hands and apply clean gloves.	1. Practices clean technique.
2. Prepare equipment; put pH testing equipment nearby.	2. Promotes efficiency.
3. Clamp the tube feeding infusion if it has already been running (see Figure 6-3-2).	3. Prevents wasting of feeding.
4. Locate the connection between the feeding tube and feeding bag tubing.	4. To disconnect the tubing.
5. Disconnect infusion tubing from feeding tube and attach a cap to tubing and feeding tube.	5. Prevents contamination of tubing.

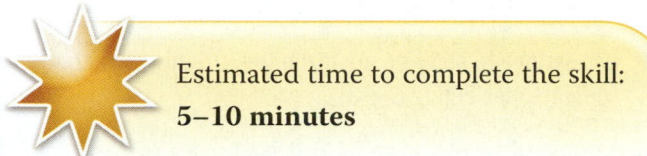

Figure 6-3-2   Clamp the tube feeding infusion.

continues

Action	Rationale
6. Draw 10–20 mL of air into syringe and attach syringe to proximal end of feeding tube.	6. Allows for insertion of air.
7. Inject air into feeding tube.	7. Clears feeding tube of feeding formula.
8. Use syringe to aspirate approximately 10 mL of gastric contents (see Figure 6-3-3).	8. To provide gastric contents for visual inspection and pH testing.
9. Assess the color of aspirate (see Figure 6-3-6).	9. Gastric contents may be green, tan, off-white, bloody, or brown. Intestinal contents may be clear yellow or bile-colored. Pleural contents may be tan, off-white, or pale yellow.
10. Obtain pH level of the gastric contents (see Figures 6-3-4 and 6-3-5). • pH of 4–6 if client is receiving acid-inhibiting medication.	10. The pH of the fluid aspirate can help to verify tube placement. • The pH reading can be altered by the presence of medication or formula, so pH should be tested after the client's stomach has been empty for approximately 1 hour.
11. If unable to aspirate contents or unsure of results of visualization, call health care provider and consider confirmation with X-ray.	11. X-ray is the most precise method of verifying placement of tube in stomach. Keep health care provider informed of progress.

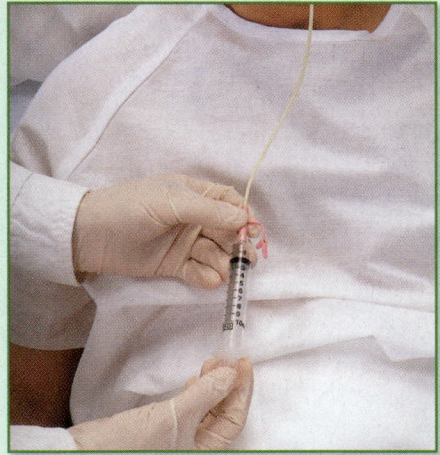

Figure 6-3-3   Aspirate gastric contents.

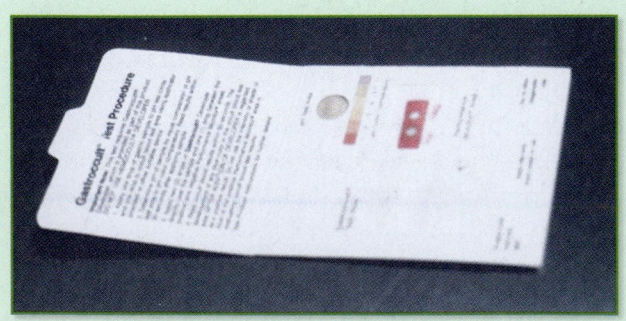

Figure 6-3-5   Read and record the results of the gastric pH test.

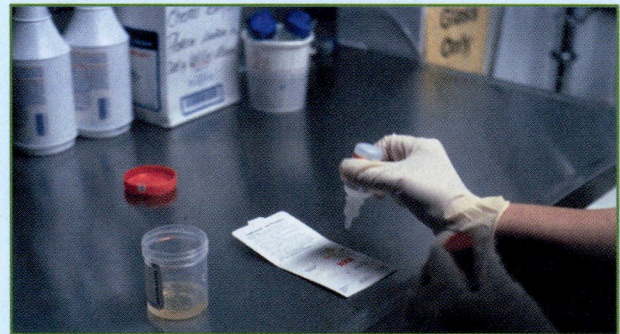

Figure 6-3-4   Check the pH of gastric contents.

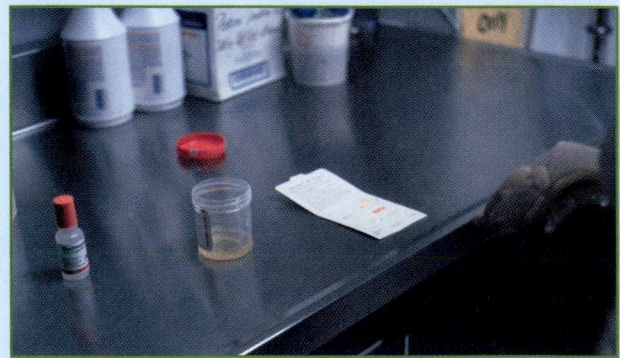

Figure 6-3-6   Assess the color of the gastric aspirate.

continues

Action	Rationale
12. If placement in stomach is verified, flush tube with water as prescribed and reattach feeding tubing and resume tube feedings (see Figure 6-3-7). Recheck placement in 4 hours if feeding is continuous.	12. Ensures adequate nutrition and consistent prevention of aspiration. Water provides hydration and maintains patency of tube.
13. Remove gloves and wash hands.	13. Reduces transmission of microorganisms.
14. Record method of verification and results of placement in flow sheets/progress notes.	14. Provides continuity for other staff and legal documentation.

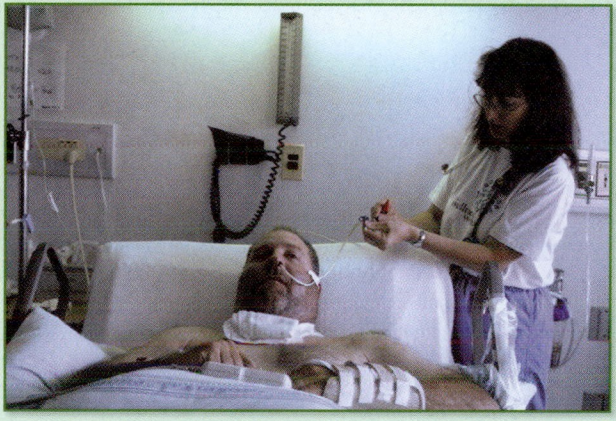

Figure 6-3-7   Once placement is verified, reattach the feeding tube and resume the feeding.

► **REAL WORLD ANECDOTES**

After inserting a small-bore feeding tube in a comatose client, the nurse attempted to verify the tube placement by aspirating gastric contents. She was unable to aspirate any fluid through the tube and thought that perhaps the tube was collapsing under the vacuum of the aspiration. The policy in this institution was to verify all new tube placements with abdominal X-rays as well as measuring the pH of gastric contents, and a portable flat abdominal X-ray was performed. When the X-ray was read, there was no sign of the feeding tube in the abdomen or the lungs. The nurse had inserted nearly 2 feet of tubing, and she was concerned about where that tubing might have gone. Finally it occurred to her to check the back of the client's mouth. There, curled up tightly, was the entire length of the feeding tube. The nurse removed the tube and successfully reinserted a new small-bore feeding tube.

► **EVALUATION**

- The client's feeding tube continues to be intact in the ordered area of the GI tract.
- The client has not experienced aspiration secondary to the tube feedings.

► **DOCUMENTATION**

Nurses' Notes

- Document the time and method of verification of tube placement.

- Note the color of any aspirate and the pH if it was tested.
- Note any unusual findings or suspicion of migration.
- If migration is suspected or placement cannot be verified, note the interventions implemented.
- Record the client's condition and responses to tube; be especially alert for signs and symptoms of possible aspiration.

Document on appropriate flow sheet or electronic medical record (EMR).

▶ CRITICAL THINKING SKILL

Introduction

Feeding tubes are generally secured only by tape to the nose and face. It is easy to disconnect or completely remove a tube.

Possible Scenario

Clara is an 80-year-old woman who is now disoriented and restless at midnight. Upon arrival, her nurse discovers Clara with a respiratory rate of 35, productive cough of blue-tinged sputum, and the tape marker on her feeding tube pulling a fair distance away from her nose. The tape, which secured the tube to her nose, has been pulled off.

Possible Outcome

When the nurse tries to verify placement, she is unable to hear the air rush. The nurse removes the feeding tube and pages the doctor to the room immediately. She assesses for additional signs and symptoms of aspiration.

Prevention

Secure the tube well with tape to the nose, a transparent dressing over the tube on the cheek or forehead, and tape around the tubing secured to the gown. Observe confused clients very closely and restrain as needed to prevent injury and aspiration.

▶ VARIATIONS

Geriatric Variation:
- *Older clients may have problems with confusion. Secure the tubing well and monitor the client closely.*

Pediatric Variations:
- *Infants will require less air for the injection into the stomach. Use a pediatric stethoscope and a smaller syringe.*
- *Because of the much smaller anatomy of a child, a feeding tube has a much shorter distance to migrate before it is in the trachea or lungs. Be sure to assess the feeding tube placement prior to instilling anything into the feeding tube or at least every 4 hours during a continuous feeding.*

Home Care Variations:
- *Teach family members to verify tube placement when administering tube feedings.*
- *Teach the client or caregivers what to do if tube migration is suspected.*

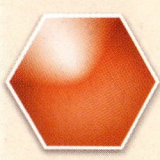

Long-Term Care Variations:
- *Clients with long-term respiratory conditions may cough intensely enough to dislodge a feeding tube. Be sure to assess tube placement regularly.*
- *Be sure the staff members caring for a feeding tube client are aware of the signs and symptoms of aspiration and tube migration.*
- *Teach the staff what to do and whom to notify if they believe a feeding tube has migrated into the pulmonary tree.*

► COMMON ERRORS

Possible Error:

The nurse is not able to aspirate gastric contents.

Prevention:

Keep the stethoscope firmly in place over the epigastric region. If you are unable to hear air rush, always reassess or ask a coworker to assist. Use one hand for the syringe and one hand to hold the diaphragm of the stethoscope. Use a smaller syringe (20 cc) and inject air into the feeding tube prior to aspirating for gastric content.

► NURSING TIPS

- Elevate the bed to a height that is good for you.
- A 50-mL syringe works best if you expect a large amount of aspirate.
- Involve the client; ask client to hold the tubing if you need help.
- Remove tube and replace if unable to verify placement in stomach or small intestine.
- Reevaluate placement before starting a new feeding or giving boluses, every 4 hours while continuously feeding, or every shift when the tube is not in use.
- Keep the client's head elevated at 30 degrees while receiving feeding to prevent aspiration.
- Small, thin feeding tubes may collapse with attempted aspiration. The inability to aspirate anything via the feeding tube is not necessarily an indication of a misplaced tube. Use a second method to verify placement.
- Always check placement before anything is injected into the tube.

► SPECIAL CONSIDERATIONS

- *Tube placement checking should be performed prior to each feeding. As aspirating the gastric or intestinal content is part of the placement checking, the quality of the aspirated content should be observed and documented. In the prefeeding assessment, if the aspirated content is more than 60 to 80 mL, it could be a sign of indigestion. Withholding the feeding may be considered. The amount of residual and the nursing intervention followed should be clearly documented.*
- *Use nonlatex tube and gloves if there is a history of latex allergy.*
- *Reassess placement if client is restless, coughs, vomits, has seizures, and upon returning to unit.*

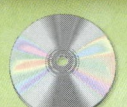

Removing a Nasogastric Tube

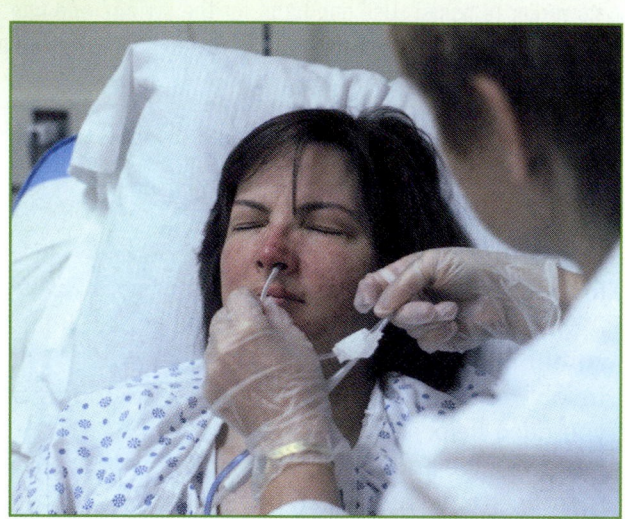

▶ OVERVIEW OF THE SKILL

Once the reason for the nasogastric tube (NG) has been resolved, the health care provider will order the tube removed. Before its removal, the nurse should check the orders and assess the client. If the tube was placed to keep the stomach empty during and after surgery, auscultate all four quadrants of the abdomen to verify that peristalsis is present. Ask the client if he or she is passing gas or flatus. If the tube was in place to measure and monitor gastric bleeding, make sure that little or no blood is being produced. Make sure the tube is not draining large amounts of gastric secretions, which could indicate poor gastric emptying, obstruction, or ileus.

If any problems are noted, report these findings and verify the order to remove the tube before proceeding. After the removal, the nurse should monitor the client's condition, watching especially for signs that the tube may need to be reinserted. Nausea, vomiting, abdominal distention, vomiting blood, and complaints of pain or gastric distress are all signs that should be reported.

If the tube has been in place for more than a few days, the potential for complications from the tube arises. Gastric ulceration occurs when the suction from the tube erodes the gastric wall. Sinusitis and esophagitis can occur from irritation from the NG tube.

▶ ASSESSMENT

1. Assess client's consciousness level **to determine the ability of the client to cooperate during the NG tube removal.**
2. Check the client's chart for orders to remove the tube. **Reduces the risk for a nursing error and the need to reinsert the tube.**
3. Use a penlight to assess nostrils for irritation and dryness. **Establishes a baseline and identifies the risk for nasal irritation and bleeding.**

▶ DIAGNOSIS

Acute Pain

Anxiety

Impaired Oral Mucous Membranes

Risk for Aspiration

Risk for Impaired Skin Integrity

▶ PLANNING

Expected Outcomes:

1. Client will be able to tolerate the removal of the tube without undue anxiety, nausea, pain, or distress.
2. Client will understand the reasons for tube removal.

3. Skin around the tube will remain intact, with no redness or blisters.
4. Client will understand signs and symptoms to report of potential complications.

Equipment Needed (see Figure 6-4-1):
- Syringe with catheter tip or adapter, 20–50 mL
- Towel and tissue, or disposable waterproof pad
- Emesis basin
- Tongue blade
- Stethoscope
- Disposable gloves (nonsterile)
- Penlight or flashlight

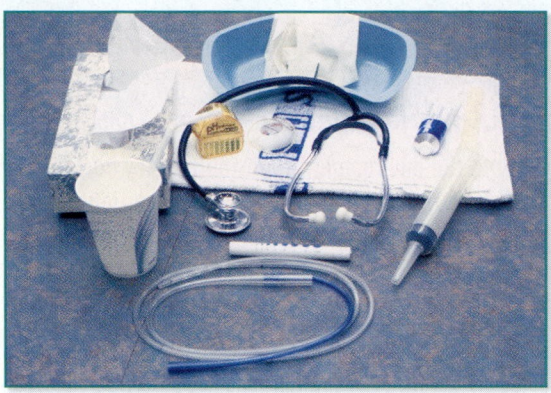

Figure 6-4-1 Stethoscope, syringe, and penlight are used to assess placement of the tube.

▶ **CLIENT EDUCATION NEEDED:**

1. Inform the client of the reason the NG tube is being removed.
2. Explain the procedure and any expected discomfort. Tell the client removing the tube will not be nearly as uncomfortable or lengthy a procedure as the NG tube insertion.
3. Establish and clarify a "hand signal" to indicate the need to temporarily stop the NG tube removal.
4. Explain how the client can cooperate during tube removal.

5. Explain potential complications, such as gastric distention or vomiting, if there is a possibility that the tube might need to be reinserted.

Estimated time to complete the skill:
15–20 minutes

▶ **DELEGATION TIPS**

Removing a nasogastric tube is not a skill the nurse would delegate because of the assessment and airway protection techniques required.

IMPLEMENTATION—Action/Rationale

Action	Rationale
Removing a Nasogastric Tube	
1. Check the qualified health care provider's order for tube removal.	1. Reduces the risk of removing the tube prematurely.
2. Wash hands.	2. Reduces the transmission of microorganisms.
3. Identify client by checking armband; assess client's consciousness and explain the procedure.	3. Verifies correct client; decreases client's anxiety level and promotes cooperation.
4. Prepare the equipment: goggles, tissue, 20- to 50-mL syringe, emesis basin.	4. Facilitates an efficient procedure.

continues

Action	Rationale
Removing a Nasogastric Tube *continued*	
5. Prepare the environment; pull the privacy curtain closed, and place the client in high Fowler's position (see Figure 6-4-2).	5. Elevated position helps removal of the tube and prevents the chance of aspiration if the client vomits. Prevents strain on the nurse's back.
6. Put on gloves.	6. Practices clean technique.
7. Place a clean towel over client's chest.	7. Enhances cleanliness and the comfort of the client.
8. Have the client hold emesis basin and a towel or tissue while the tube is removed.	8. Keeps these items handy for the client in case of vomiting when the tube is removed.
9. Disconnect suction or feeding pump, if any. Remove the tape and safety pin.	9. Prevents the spillage of gastric secretions or tube feeding solution. Protects the esophageal tissue from suction pressure damage.
10. Check placement of the tube.	10. Ensures correct placement before flushing.
11. Inject 30–50 mL of air into the tube.	11. Clears the tube of gastric drainage, which could irritate the esophagus and nasal mucosa or be aspirated into the lungs during removal.
12. Pinch the tubing with your thumb and forefinger. Ask the client to take a deep breath and hold still while you are pulling the tube out (coil the tube around your hand as you are pulling). Remove the tube slowly but evenly over the course of 3 to 6 seconds (see Figure 6-4-3).	12. Facilitates removal of the tube. Pinching the tube prevents spillage of gastric contents.
13. Cover or wrap the tube in a towel or double glove, and remove from the client's bedside. Tube should be handled with biohazard precaution.	13. Seeing the tube can cause nausea or distress, removing it quickly minimizes this risk. Follows biohazard precautions.

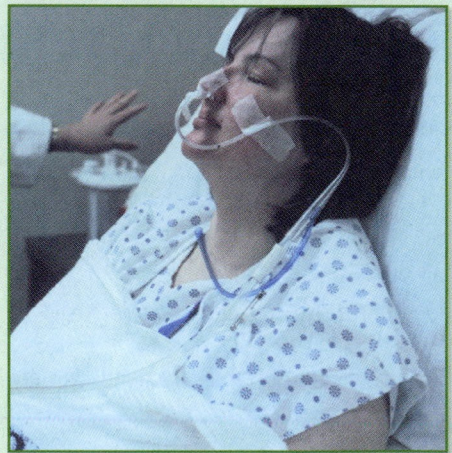

Figure 6-4-2 Position the client in high Fowler's position to help facilitate removal of the tube.

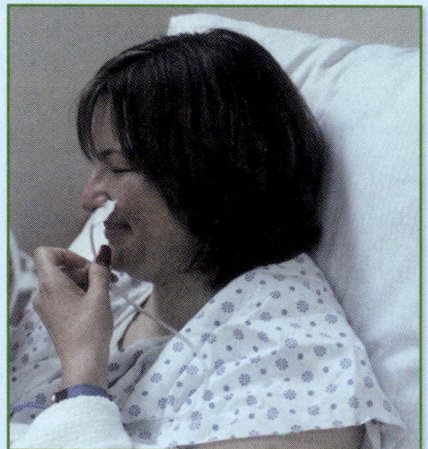

Figure 6-4-3 Remove the tube slowly but evenly.

continues

Action	Rationale
14. Provide oral hygiene and assist the client to clean the nares.	14. Promotes the client's comfort.
15. Dispose of contaminated materials in proper container, remove gloves, and wash hands.	15. Reduces the transmission of microorganisms.
16. Document the NG tube removal, amount of drainage, and client's responses.	16. Records implementation of intervention and promotes continuity of care.
17. Review the original purpose of the tube. Assess for signs that the tube may need to be reinserted.	17. Allows the nurse to provide the health care provider with feedback regarding the client's tolerance of the tube removal.

▶ REAL WORLD ANECDOTES

A nurse addressed the client's anxiety by giving her a hand signal to use when she wanted the removal procedure paused. However, the nurse did not address the client's anxiety directly with support and education about the procedure. The client was so frightened that she used the hand signal every time she felt the tube moving. It took a long time to get the tube out, and the procedure was made more complicated and traumatic for an already upset client. The nurse should have taken the time to carefully address the client's fears by explaining the procedure and what the client would feel during the process.

▶ EVALUATION

- The client was able to tolerate the removal of the tube without undue anxiety, nausea, pain, or distress.
- The client understands the reasons for tube removal.
- Skin around the tube remained intact, with no redness or blisters.
- Client understands signs or symptoms to report complications.

▶ DOCUMENTATION

Nurses' Notes

- Document NG tube removal and the client's responses.
- Document any signs of irritation around the nares or complaints of nose or throat pain.

Document on appropriate flow sheet or electronic medical record (EMR).

Intake and Output Record

- If the NG tube was attached to suction or a feeding pump, record the amount of drainage or intake.

▶ CRITICAL THINKING SKILL

Introduction

The nurse must continuously reassess the client's condition and symptoms.

Possible Scenario

Mrs. Marino is a very demanding client. Everything the nurses do seems to cause her pain, and nothing is ever quite right. The NG tube that has been in place for approximately 1 week has been a major source of complaint, and the nurses are finding it difficult to listen and respond with much compassion. As predicted, removing the tube causes screams of anguish. The nurse quickly wipes Mrs. Marino's nose, offers a tissue, and leaves the room with the tube.

Possible Outcome

Upon discarding the tube, the nurse notices it has blood on the outside. Reassessing the client, she discovers a very red and eroded area just inside the nostril. She reports her findings, and upon further assessment, another ulcerated area at the back of her throat is discovered. The client requires additional treatment for complications from the NG tube.

Prevention

Nurses caring for this client needed to conduct daily assessments of the condition of the nares, look for signs of developing pressure sores from the tube, reposition the tube if needed, and listen to complaints of pain from the client.

▶ VARIATIONS

Geriatric Variations:
- *Make sure the elderly client can hear and understand your instructions and education regarding removal of the tube.*
- *Elderly skin is more delicate and fragile. After tube removal, be especially careful to assess for skin breakdown around the nares and to provide good cleaning and care of the nares.*

Pediatric Variations:
- *A parent may need to assist to hold the child while the tube is being removed. A toddler especially will find the procedure frightening. Sitting on a parent's lap will help the child feel a sense of trust and security.*
- *An older child can help by holding the emesis basin and tissue. An older child will feel less anxiety if provided choices and information about the procedure.*
- *The child may prefer to close his or her eyes while the tube is being removed.*

Home Care Variation:
- *Make sure the home care provider knows what signs and symptoms to assess for after the tube is removed.*

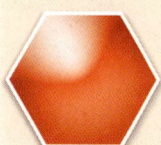

Long-Term Care Variations:
- *Long-term NG tube placement increases the risk of complications such as sinusitis, esophagitis, and gastric ulceration. Make sure staff members in a long-term care facility understand how to assess for these complications even after the tube is removed.*

▶ COMMON ERRORS

Possible Error:

Forgetting to coil the tube around your hand while removing the tube may cause the spillage of gastric content.

Prevention:

Remove the towel and the tube immediately. Change the client's gown and any soiled bed linen to remove the spill.

Possible Error:

Forgetting to clear the tube of gastric secretions or feeding solution could cause these liquids to be aspirated into the lungs as the tube is being removed.

Prevention:

Clear out the tube by flushing 30–50 mL of air before removing the tube. Assess the client for signs of choking or coughing. Notify the health care provider immediately if aspiration is suspected.

▶ **NURSING TIPS**

- Adjust the height of the bed to eliminate back strain when removing the tube.
- This can be an anxiety-provoking procedure. Remind the client that tube removal is quick and painless compared to tube insertion.
- Carefully observe the client's verbal and nonverbal responses during the entire procedure.

- Assess the lungs and breathing carefully after an NG tube has been removed. There is a risk for aspiration. Also, the presence of the tube may suppress the client's coughing and attempts to clear secretions from the throat, which could cause respiratory complications. These complications may not appear until after the tube is removed.

▶ **SPECIAL CONSIDERATIONS**

- *Sore throat or difficulty in swallowing may present as a symptom of inflammation of the insertion area. This symptom should subside in 1–2 days. Lozenges or ice chips can be used to minimize discomfort.*

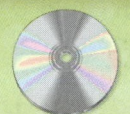

SKILL 6-5

Feeding and Medicating via a Gastrostomy Tube

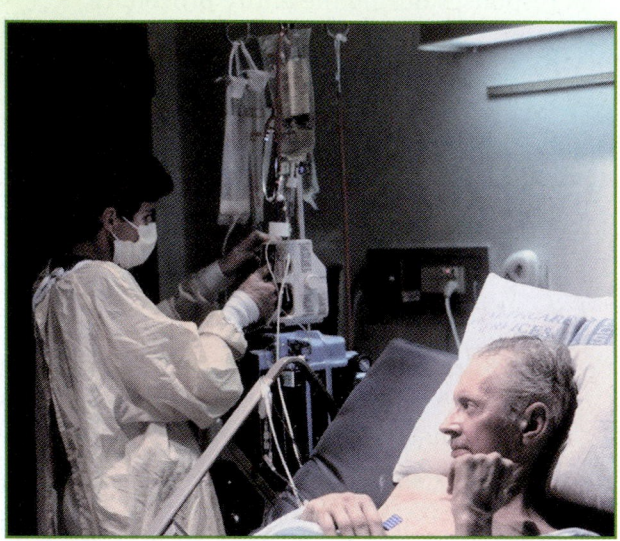

▶ OVERVIEW OF THE SKILL

Enteral nutrition is a procedure whereby liquid food (formula) is instilled directly into the stomach or small intestines using a tube. Other names for this procedure are tube feedings and gastric gavage. Candidates for tube feedings are clients who have a functional gastrointestinal (GI) tract and will not, should not, or cannot eat. Tube feedings are used for clients who are (or may become) malnourished and in whom oral feedings are insufficient to maintain adequate nutritional status.

Enteral tube feedings maintain the structural and functional integrity of the GI tract, enhance the utilization of nutrients, and provide a safe and economic method of feeding. Enteral tube feedings are contraindicated in clients with the following:

- Diffused peritonitis
- Intestinal obstruction that prohibits normal bowel functioning
- Intractable vomiting; paralytic ileus
- Severe diarrhea

Enteral tube feedings are used with caution in clients with the following:

- Severe pancreatitis
- Enterocutaneous fistulae
- GI ischemia

Feeding Tubes

Most feeding tubes are made of silicone or polyurethane, which are durable and biocompatible with formulas. They vary in diameter (8–12 French) and length in accord with the route and formula. The health care provider selects the route and type of feeding tube on the basis of the anticipated duration of feeding, the condition of the GI tract, and the potential for aspiration.

The gastrostomy tube is placed through an opening in the abdominal wall into the intestines. This is done via an enterostomy, the surgical creation of an artificial fistula into the intestines. Tube enterostomies can be placed at various points along the GI tract and are performed when long-term tube feeding is anticipated or when obstruction makes nasoenteral tube feeding impossible.

Percutaneous endoscopic gastrostomy (PEG) tube placement is performed by the health care provider at the bedside or in the endoscopy room; insertion of a PEG tube does not require general anesthesia surgery. This method of enteral feeding is more common than conventional enterostomies; it is less risky because surgery is not required, and it is more economic.

Administration of Enteral Feedings

Once feeding tube position has been radiographically verified, the formula can be administered as prescribed. There are two typical methods of administering tube feedings. Intermittent feeding is given four to six times a day in the form of a bolus. Intermittent feedings are generally given through a large-bore tube. The bolus (generally 250–400 mL of formula for adult clients) can be given using a large syringe fit into the end of the feeding tube or using a gravity drip over 20–30 minutes. The intermittent method is generally practiced in the home care setting because of its ease and need for minimal equipment. It is not the preferred method, however, because the large amount of food it places in the stomach at one time often causes cramping, vomiting, aspiration, flatus, or diarrhea. This method works best with clients who have normal gastrointestinal function. Continuous feeding delivers formula with a pump to regulate the rate. Most clients with a small-bore tube receive continuous feeding. One of the advantages of continuous feeding is that it keeps gastric volume small, minimizing residual volume and reducing the risk of aspiration pneumonia; the client is less likely to experience bloating, nausea, abdominal distention, and diarrhea. Continuous feeding is recommended for the seriously ill or comatose client.

Safety Considerations

Clients receiving enteral nutrition through a tube feeding are at risk for aspiration. Tube feeding aspiration can result from several factors: displacement of the tube into the esophagus, large amounts of gastric residual and lowered intestinal motility, and delayed gastric emptying, which may occur in clients who are on bed rest or receiving narcotics for pain relief. Auscultate for bowel sounds to determine gastric motility. If the bowel sounds are hypoactive or absent, stop or withhold additional feeding and notify the health care provider. Always assess placement of the feeding tube before administering any liquids. Clients who are receiving continuous gastric feeding should be assessed every 4 hours for tube placement and residual gastric contents. Aspirate gastric contents with a syringe. This is done more easily with a large-bore tube. The lumen of a small-bore tube collapses easily, making aspiration difficult and sometimes impossible. Observe and check the pH of the aspirate. Replace stomach contents after checking the residual to prevent fluid and electrolyte imbalance.

Client safety and comfort require daily cleansing of the feeding tube exit site. Cleanse the skin with a clean washcloth, soap, and water. Enterostomy tubes require surgical asepsis of the exit site until the incision heals; rotate the tubes within the stoma

to promote healing. Report any observations of redness, irritation, or gastric leakage at the site. Between feedings, a prosthetic device may be used to cover the ostomy opening.

The PEG tubes require daily rotation to relieve pressure on the skin. Notify the health care provider if you are unable to rotate the PEG; it may be an indication of internal embedding of the tube into the gastric wall. When the tube is internally embedded, it can cause gastric acid reflux, which results in skin breakdown, sepsis, and cellulitis. Care must be taken to avoid dislodgment of the tube. Keep it secured to the client's abdomen with tape, being careful not to use excessive tension. The PEG tubes require frequent flushing to prevent clogging. These tubes have small lumens. If a tube becomes clogged, flush it with 60 mL of lukewarm tap water.

▶ ASSESSMENT

1. Assess the client for signs of gastric distress, such as nausea, vomiting, and cramping, **to determine the client's tolerance for the tube feeding.**
2. Assess the feeding tube placement every 4 hours **to confirm tube placement in the intestines.**
3. Assess the client's respiratory status **to evaluate for pulmonary aspiration of gastric contents.**
4. Assess the client's ongoing nutritional status **to evaluate the effectiveness of the tube feeding.**
5. Assess the client's intake and output **to evaluate for fluid deficit or excess.**

▶ DIAGNOSIS

Imbalanced Nutrition: Less Than Body Requirements

Risk for Deficient Fluid Volume

Risk for Aspiration

Impaired Oral Mucous Membranes

Risk for Impaired Skin Integrity

▶ PLANNING

Expected Outcomes:

1. The client will receive the correct feeding formula and the correct volume of formula over the correct time period.
2. The client will not experience any undesirable effects: aspiration, nausea, vomiting, abdominal distention, cramping, diarrhea, or constipation.
3. The client's weight and nutritional status will remain stable or improve.

4. The client will not experience any adverse skin or gastrointestinal effects from the gastrostomy or PEG tube.

Equipment Needed:

- Asepto syringe or 20- to 50-mL syringe
- Emesis basin
- Clean towel
- Disposable gavage bag and tubing (see Figure 6-5-1)
- Formula (see Figure 6-5-2)
- Infusion pump for feeding tube (see Figure 6-5-3)
- Water to follow feeding
- Nonsterile gloves

► CLIENT EDUCATION NEEDED:

1. If the client will be receiving feedings at home, the client or caregiver must be trained to administer the feeding and care for the tube insertion site.

2. Teach the client the importance of reporting any adverse effects from the tube feeding.

3. Teach the client to keep head or head of the bed elevated during and after tube feedings to avoid aspiration. High Fowler's position, a minimum of 30 degrees elevation, is recommended for the feeding. The client should remain in this position for 30 minutes after the feeding, if possible.

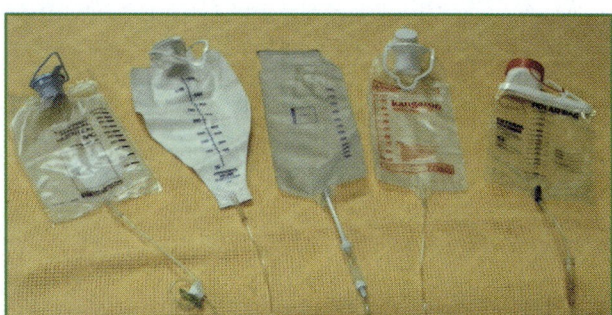

Figure 6-5-1 Gavage bags

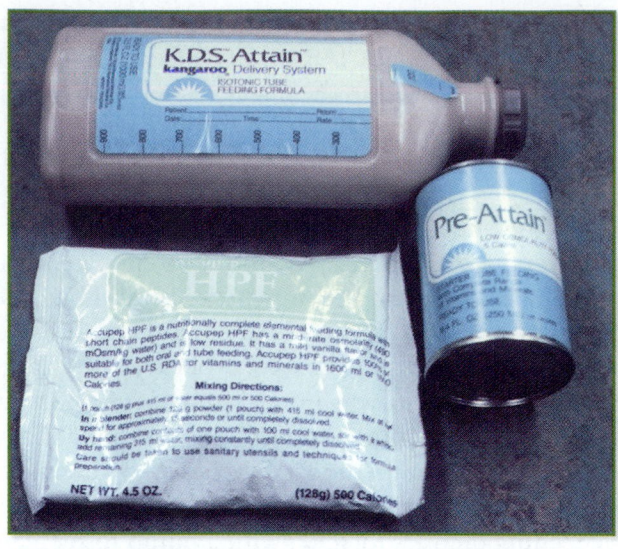

Figure 6-5-2 Feeding formulas

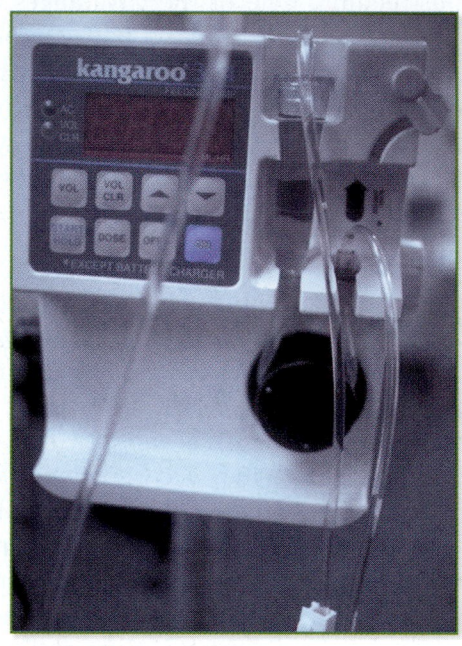

Figure 6-5-3 Feeding pump

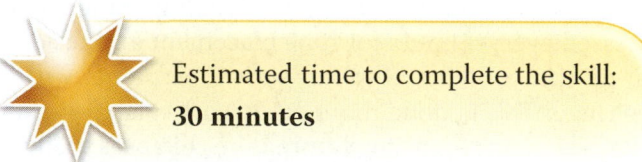

Estimated time to complete the skill: **30 minutes**

► DELEGATION TIPS

Feedings via gastrostomy tubes may be given by properly trained ancillary personnel if the facility and the state permit. The ancillary personnel must be properly trained in assessing tube placement, proper positioning of the client, and in the administration of the correct type and rate of feeding. All medications must be administered by a nurse.

IMPLEMENTATION—Action/Rationale

Action	Rationale
1. Identify client and review medical record for formula, amount, and time.	1. Verifies health care provider's prescription for appropriate formula and amount.
2. Wash hands and gather equipment and formula.	2. Reduces transmission of microorganisms and promotes efficiency during procedure.
3. Check client's armband.	3. Verifies correct client.
4. Explain procedure to client.	4. Reduces anxiety and increases client cooperation.
5. Assemble equipment. Add color to formula per institutional policy. If using a bag, fill with prescribed amount of formula (see Figure 6-5-4).	5. Ensures efficiency when initiating feeding. Color will distinguish formula aspirate.
6. Place client on right side in high Fowler's position.	6. Reduces risk of pulmonary aspiration in the event client vomits or regurgitates formula.
7. Wash hands and don nonsterile gloves.	7. Reduces transmission of pathogens from gastric contents.
8. Provide for privacy.	8. Places client at ease.
9. Observe for abdominal distention; auscultate for bowel sounds.	9. Assesses for delayed gastric emptying; indicates presence of peristalsis and ability of GI tract to digest nutrients.
10. Check feeding residuals (see Figure 6-5-5). Insert syringe into adapter port, aspirate stomach contents, and determine amount of gastric residual. If residual is greater than 50–100 mL (or in accordance with agency protocol), hold feeding until residual diminishes. Instill aspirated contents back into feeding tube.	10. Indicates whether gastric emptying is delayed. Reduces risk of regurgitation and pulmonary aspiration related to gastric distention. Prevents electrolyte imbalance.
11. Administer the tube feeding.	11. Provides nutrients as prescribed.

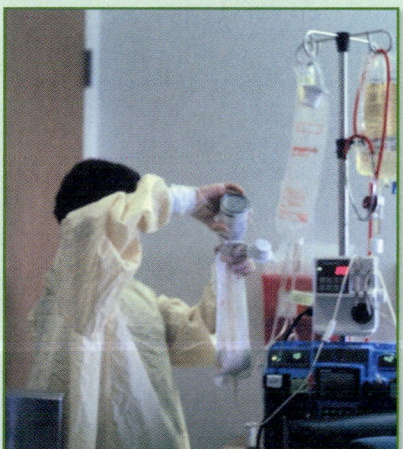

Figure 6-5-4   Fill the bag with the prescribed amount of formula.

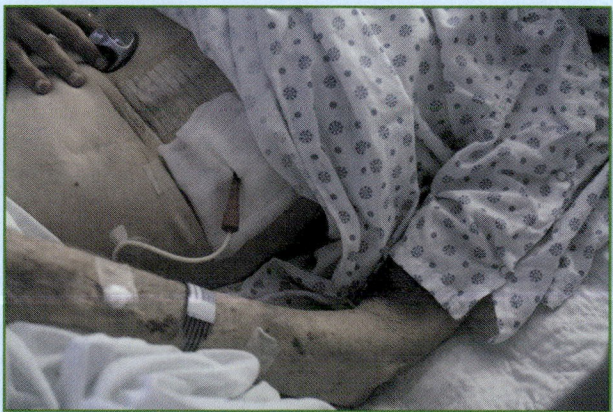

Figure 6-5-5   Check that the feeding tube is intact and in place, auscultate for bowel sounds, and look for abdominal distention.

continues

Action	Rationale
Intermittent Bolus	
12. Pinch the tubing.	12. Prevents air from entering tubing.
13. Remove plunger from barrel of syringe and attach syringe to adapter port.	13. Provides system to deliver feeding.
14. Fill syringe with formula (see Figure 6-5-6).	14. Allows gravity to control flow rate, reducing risk of diarrhea from bolus feeding.
15. Allow formula to infuse slowly; continue adding formula to syringe until prescribed amount has been administered.	15. Prevents air from entering stomach. Decreases risk of diarrhea.
16. Flush tubing with 30–60 mL, or prescribed amount, of water.	16. Ensures that remaining formula in tubing is administered and maintains patency of tube; prevents air from entering the stomach.
17. Remove syringe and place cap into adaptor port.	17. Prevents air from entering stomach and prevents gastric contents from leaving the stomach.
Intermittent Gavage Feeding	
18. Hang bag on IV pole so that it is 18 inches above the client's head (see Figure 6-5-7).	18. Allows gravity to promote infusion of formula.
19. Fill bag with ordered amount of feeding. Remove air from tubing by opening clamp on tubing and allow feeding to flow through tubing	19. Prevents air from entering stomach. Decreases risk of diarrhea.

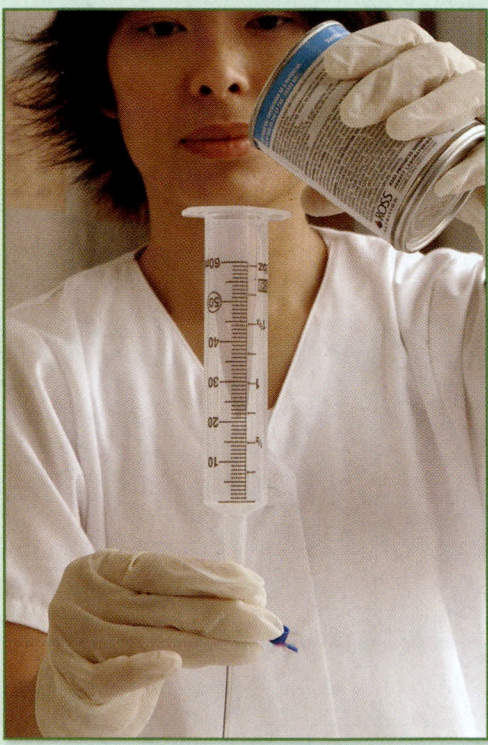

Figure 6-5-6 Fill syringe with formula.

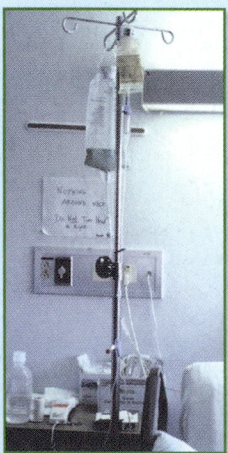

Figure 6-5-7 Hang the formula bag on an IV pole approximately 18 inches above the client's head.

continues

Action	Rationale
20. Attach distal end of tubing to feeding tube adapter and adjust drip to infuse over prescribed time.	**20.** Allows gravity to control flow rate, reducing risk of diarrhea from bolus feeding.
21. When bag empties of formula, infuse 30–60 mL, or prescribed amount, of water.	**21.** Prevents air from entering stomach and reduces risk for gas accumulation. Maintains patency of feeding tube.
22. Remove tubing from adaptor port and cap adaptor port.	**22.** Prevents air from entering stomach and prevents gastric contents from leaving the stomach.
23. Change bags every 24 hours.	**23.** Decreases risk of multiplication of microorganisms in bag and tubing.

Continuous Gavage

Action	Rationale
24. Check tube placement at least every 4 hours.	**24.** Ensures that feeding tube remains in stomach.
25. Check residual at least every 4 hours.	**25.** Indicates ability of GI tract to digest and absorb nutrients.
26. If residual is greater than 100 mL, stop feeding.	**26.** Reduces risk of regurgitation and pulmonary aspiration related to gastric distention.
27. Add prescribed amount of formula to bag for a 4-hour period; dilute with water if prescribed.	**27.** Provides client with prescribed nutrients and prevents bacterial growth (formula is easily contaminated).
28. Hang gavage bag on IV pole. Prime tubing.	**28.** Removes air from tubing.
29. Thread tubing through feeding pump (see Figure 6-5-8) and attach distal end of tubing to feeding tube adapter; keep tubing straight between bag and pump.	**29.** Provides for controlled flow rate; prevents loops in tubing.
30. Program rate.	**30.** Infuses formula over prescribed time.
31. Monitor infusion rate and signs of respiratory distress or diarrhea.	**31.** Prevents complications associated with continuous gavage.

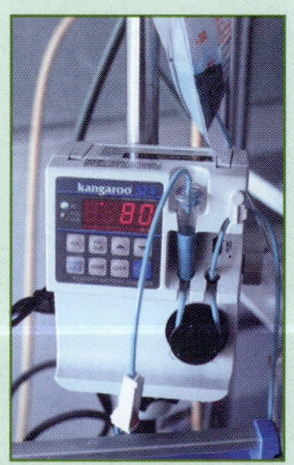

Figure 6-5-8 Thread the gavage bag tubing through the feeding pump.

continues

Action	Rationale
Continuous Gavage *continued*	
32. Flush tube with water every 4 hours as prescribed or following administration of medications.	**32.** Maintains patency of tube.
33. Replace disposable feeding bag at least every 24 hours, in accord with institution protocol.	**33.** Decreases transmission of microorganisms.
34. Elevate head of bed at least 30 degrees at all times and turn client every 2 hours.	**34.** Prevents aspiration and promotes digestion and reduces skin breakdown.
35. Provide oral hygiene every 2–4 hours.	**35.** Provides comfort and maintains the integrity of buccal cavity.
36. Administer water as prescribed with and between feedings.	**36.** Ensures adequate hydration.
37. Remove gloves and wash hands.	**37.** Reduces transmission of microorganisms.
38. Record total amount of formula and water administered on intake and output (I&O) form and client's response to feeding.	**38.** Documents administration of feeding and achievement of expected outcome; for example, client tolerates feeding and weight is maintained or increased.

▶ REAL WORLD ANECDOTES

Penny was a long-term care client in a nursing facility. She was an elderly frail woman with a long-term gastrostomy tube. She had shared this room with the same roommate for several years. Shortly after her roommate died, Penny began to be confused and lethargic. Most of the nurses felt this was because of the loss of her roommate and advised understanding and waiting to see whether she improved. However, one of the younger, newly graduated nurses noted that these same symptoms could be caused by an electrolyte imbalance from Penny's tube feeding. After checking Penny's chart, she found that shortly before the death of Penny's roommate the doctor had changed the formula of Penny's feeding, hoping to help her gain some weight. The nurse informed Penny's doctor of her symptoms and when they had started. The doctor ordered laboratory tests to check Penny's electrolyte balance, and he found that her electrolytes were, in fact, out of balance. He ordered a return to Penny's previous feeding formula, and the staff noted a gradual improvement in Penny's mental and physical condition.

▶ EVALUATION

- Client received the correct feeding formula and the correct volume of formula over the correct time period.
- Client did not experience any undesirable effects such as aspiration, nausea, vomiting, abdominal distention, cramping, diarrhea, or constipation.
- Client's weight and nutritional status remained stable or improved.
- Client did not experience any adverse skin or gastrointestinal effects from the gastrostomy or PEG tube.

▶ DOCUMENTATION

Nurses' Notes

- Document time, date, formula, and amount of feeding, and client's response.

- Note and document the amount of residual that was aspirated prior to the feeding.
- Note that tube placement was checked and what method was used.
- Note if the dressing at the tube insertion site was changed and the condition of the client's skin.
- Note if the tube was rotated or adjusted.
- Note any client complaints or adverse effects such as bloating, nausea, vomiting, diarrhea, or constipation.

Document on appropriate flow sheet or electronic medical record (EMR).

Medication Administration Record

- Note the date and time the feeding was instilled (per institution specifications).

Intake and Output Record

- Record the amount of tube feeding instilled and the amount of water used to flush the feeding tube.

▶ CRITICAL THINKING SKILL

Introduction

Be aware of the effects tube feeding can have on the client.

Possible Scenario

You are giving Mrs. Takai her scheduled tube feeding. She receives 400 mL in an intermittent bolus. Immediately after infusing the tube feeding Mrs. Takai complains of abdominal discomfort. You check her abdomen and note that it is distended and bloated.

Possible Outcome

If Mrs. Takai's stomach remains bloated, she is at risk for nausea, vomiting, and potential aspiration of stomach contents.

Prevention

Several things can cause bloating. If the bolus feeding is given too quickly or if it is cold, the client can become distended. Check for bowel sounds. If the client does not have bowel tones, she may be distended because of lack of peristalsis. What was the residual prior to this feeding? Did she already have a large amount of residual from her previous feeding? Perhaps the feedings are too closely spaced or too large.

Raise the client's head, if possible, to avoid vomiting and possible aspiration. Be sure to have suction ready in case the client does vomit. If the client continues to have trouble with bloating, her physician should be informed.

▶ VARIATIONS

Geriatric Variations:
- *Elderly people often have delicate skin. The gastrostomy insertion site should be checked carefully for breakdown.*
- *Diarrhea can cause skin breakdown quickly in the elderly, so measures to control it should be taken if the tube feedings cause diarrhea.*
- *If the elderly client cannot take anything by mouth, be sure to perform frequent oral care to prevent drying and cracking of the mucous membranes.*
- *The elderly client may feel particularly deprived at not being able to "really eat." It is important to present the feeding as a meal time rather than as a procedure.*

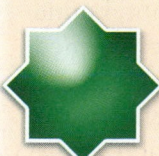

Pediatric Variations:
- *Because of smaller body mass, children are at a greater risk of electrolyte imbalance, dehydration, or fluid overload. When assessing a child with a feeding tube, be aware that a little diarrhea or a little too much water to flush the feeding tube can seriously compromise a small child's health.*
- *Children with feeding tubes can have concerns that adults consider silly. Be sure to talk to the child and find out if they have any misconceptions regarding their tube feeding or illness.*
- *Infants and toddlers may need to be restrained from pulling on the gastrostomy tube and displacing it.*
- *Children in the home care setting may feel deprived when everyone else can eat and they cannot. It is important for the caregiver to remind the child that this is not a punishment and to encourage the child to see the tube feeding as a special kind of meal.*

continues

Home Care Variations:
- The client's caregiver and/or the client must be taught how to administer the tube feeding and then supervised until the nurse is confident that the caregiver can perform the procedure independently.
- The client's health care provider may allow the caregiver to use a homemade formula as a cost-cutting measure. If so, the nurse must be sure the formula is being prepared correctly and in a clean environment.
- The client's caregiver must be taught how to assess the insertion site for signs of infection or skin breakdown and how to tape and rotate the tube to prevent pressure at the insertion site.
- If clients reuse bags, these should be washed with soap and water every 24 hours.

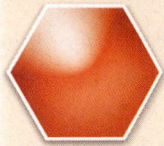

Long-Term Care Variations:
- Feeding tubes can crack and wear when used long-term. The nurse should be sure to check for damage and wear to the tube and alert the health care provider if it shows signs of damage.
- Tube feeding infusion sets should be changed at set intervals, every 24 hours, or the facility policy or the client's health care provider will determine how often the tube feeding set should be changed. The nurse is responsible to track when the infusion set was last changed.

► COMMON ERRORS

Possible Error:
Not using enough water to flush the tube.

Prevention:
Be sure to use enough water to completely clean the inside lumen of the feeding tube. Unless the client is on fluid restriction, the nurse should be able to use up to 100 cc of water to flush the tube after a feeding. If the tube is not adequately flushed following a feeding, the residual formula provides an ideal breeding ground for bacteria. The tube is also much more likely to become occluded by formula and medication particles, leaving the nurse with the problem of unclogging the feeding tube for the next feeding.

► NURSING TIPS

- If a feeding tube becomes plugged or seems to be running slowly, water, a carbonated beverage, or cranberry juice instilled into the tube will sometimes help clean out the inside of the tube. Be sure this is compatible with the client's diet and orders.
- Be sure to warm the formula to at least room temperature before using it for feeding. The temperature of formula can be judged the same way an infant's formula is, that is, on the inside of the wrist.
- If the client's head can be elevated, do so after the feeding to prevent vomiting and possible aspiration of formula. If the client's head cannot be elevated, then it is crucial to turn the head to the side to allow any emesis to drain from the mouth.
- Remember, formulas can spoil. This is especially true in non–air-conditioned areas in hot, humid weather. Discard them if they have been opened and unused per manufacturers' specifications.
- The social aspect of eating should be emphasized. All gastric feedings should have a friendly atmosphere and should be treated as a meal rather than a procedure.
- Assess for skin reaction to tube including latex allergy.
- Discard formula that is outdated, not labeled properly, or not stored correctly.

▶ **SPECIAL CONSIDERATIONS**

- If using food coloring to identify formula in pulmonary aspirate, be sure to use a small amount. It only needs a tinge of color to be identifiable. Some food colorings, such as methylene blue, can deposit in the client's tissues and mucous membranes and cause a blue tinge in the skin. In some facilities, it is now prohibited to use methylene blue or other food coloring as it could be fatal to a client with poor circulation or sepsis.

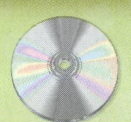

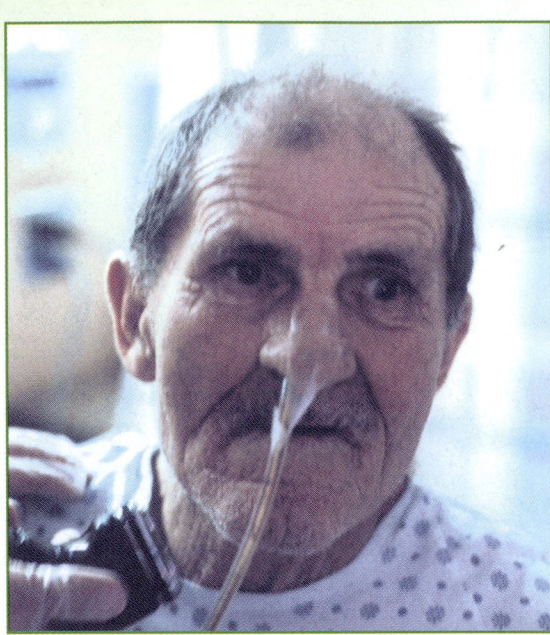

▶ OVERVIEW OF THE SKILL

Gastrointestinal (GI) suctioning is the process of attaching a nasogastric tube (NG) to a portable or in-wall suction device. Gastrointestinal suctioning is used for several reasons, including decompression and drainage of the stomach, to allow the GI system to rest and heal, and to measure and monitor gastric bleeding.

The Salem sump tube is most frequently used for GI suctioning (see Figure 6-6-1). It is a double-lumen tube. The larger lumen is clear and collects drainage. The smaller lumen is blue and is an air vent. The air vent must remain open at all times to provide safe suctioning of the stomach. The air vent prevents the suction catheter tip from sticking the tube to the gastric wall.

The nursing care of GI suctioning devices is a clean procedure. The nurse should always wear clean gloves and dispose of the suction drainage containers as outlined by institution procedure.

▶ ASSESSMENT

1. Review the chart to understand the client's diagnosis and the need for suctioning **to evaluate the need for suctioning.**

2. Assess the client's ability to cooperate with the suctioning setup and continuous suctioning **to evaluate how suctioning will be set up and monitored to prevent client from pulling NG tube out or disconnecting the suction.**

3. Assess for proper placement of the NG tube **to prevent damage to the lung or air passages.**

4. Assess for patency of the NG tube **to establish the effectiveness of suctioning.**

5. Monitor gastric contents for amount, color, consistency, and odor **to assess for evidence**

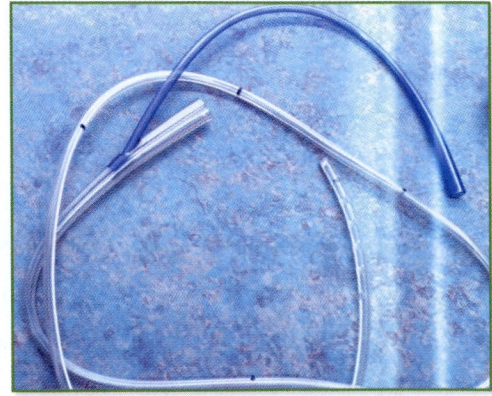

Figure 6-6-1 Salem sump nasogastric tubes

of bleeding or infection and the need for suctioning.

6. Assess the client's understanding of the suctioning procedure. **The suctioning procedure can be distressing for clients. With proper instruction, the client's anxiety may be decreased.**

▶ **DIAGNOSIS**

Impaired Oral Mucous Membrane

Risk for Aspiration

Risk for Deficient Fluid Volume

Risk for Impaired Skin Integrity

▶ **PLANNING**

Expected Outcomes:

1. The client will have a patent NG tube with effective suctioning of the gastric contents.
2. The client will understand the need for suctioning.
3. The client will not experience pain or discomfort from the suctioning or the NG tube.
4. The client will not experience trauma to the gastric wall or the nares from the suction or the NG tube.

Equipment Needed (see Figures 6-6-2A and B):

- Source of negative pressure (wall suction or portable suction machine)
- NG tube in place: 12 to 18 French for adults, 8 to 12 French for children, 5 to 10 French for infants
- Connecting tubing with adapter
- Clean gloves
- Suction canister

▶ **CLIENT EDUCATION NEEDED:**

1. Explain procedure to client, including rationale for performing the procedure.
2. Inform client that the procedure may produce sucking noises, gastric content, and the movement of gastric content through the tubing.

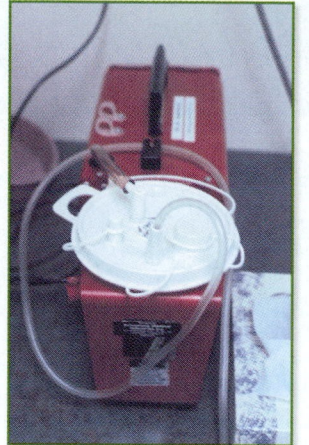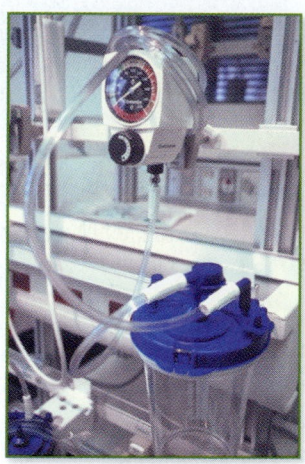

Figure 6-6-2 A. Portable suction device; B. Wall suction device.

3. Prepare the client for the sights and sounds he or she will encounter. Review the suction setup with the client.
4. Teach client and family how to recognize signs of ineffective suction and to report any signs and symptoms to the nurse.
5. Remind the client to reposition frequently to avoid the catheter sticking to one place in the stomach.
6. Explain the action of the system and the importance of alerting someone if the system has failed.
7. Advise the client of comfort measures that can be taken to minimize stress on the nares, mouth, and throat.
8. The best position for the client to sit in is semi-Fowler's position to avoid the chance of aspiration and to allow the catheter tip to move freely.

 Estimated time to complete the skill: **5 minutes**

▶ **DELEGATION TIPS**

Properly trained ancillary personnel may monitor and measure output from a nasogastric tube as well as provide nasal and oral hygiene. The assessment of the suction pressure and gastric drainage appearance and volume should not be delegated by the nurse.

IMPLEMENTATION—Action/Rationale

Action	Rationale
1. Review the health care provider's order.	1. Determine what equipment will be needed and what client evaluations will be required.
2. Gather the equipment needed. Check client's armband.	2. Promotes organization and efficiency. Verifies correct client.
3. Explain the reason for the suction to the client. Reassure the client regarding the appearance of the gastric contents.	3. Helps allay client's fears. Clients often are unfamiliar with the appearance of bodily fluids and may be disturbed by the appearance of the gastric contents.
4. Wash hands and apply gloves.	4. Reduces the transmission of microorganisms.
5. Set up the suction source. If using wall suction, insert the suction regulator into the suction port. If using portable suction, plug the machine into the power source.	5. Provides a suction source.
6. Attach the suction tubing and canister to the suction head. Turn the suction on and test the equipment. Turn the suction off.	6. Evaluates the functionality of the equipment.
7. Remove syringe or plug, if present, from the free end of tube. Connect the NG tube to the suction tubing; set the suction control on type of suction and pressure as prescribed.	7. Provides for decompression as prescribed by health care provider; intermittent or continuous suctioning is determined by type of tube inserted. Single-lumen tubes are connected to intermittent low pressure. Double-lumen tubes are connected to continuous low-suction.
8. Upon instituting suction and at least every 4 hours thereafter: • Observe nature and amount of gastric tube drainage (see Figure 6-6-3). Empty drainage container every 8 hours or when it passes three-quarters full. • Assess client for nausea, vomiting, and abdominal distention.	8. • Provides information about patency of tube and gastric contents. • Nausea, vomiting, and abdominal distention may indicate that the tube is clogged or that suction is not working.

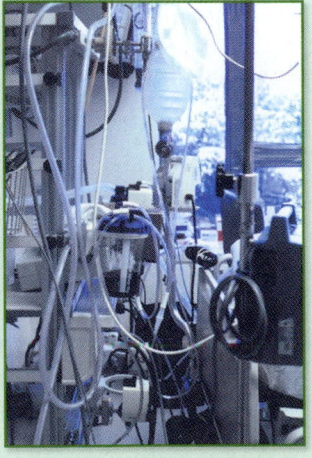

Figure 6-6-3 Observe the nature and amount of gastric drainage and empty the container every 8 hours or when it passes three-quarters full.

continues

Action	Rationale
• Assess the nares and the skin around the nares for signs of irritation or skin breakdown (see Figure 6-6-4).	• Indicates need for skin care.
9. Dispose of contaminated materials in proper container, remove gloves, and wash hands.	9. Reduces transmission of microorganisms.
10. Position client for comfort, in a semi-Fowler's position, and place the call light within easy reach.	10. Promotes comfort and safety.
11. Document the procedure.	11. Promotes continuity of care and shows implementation of intervention.

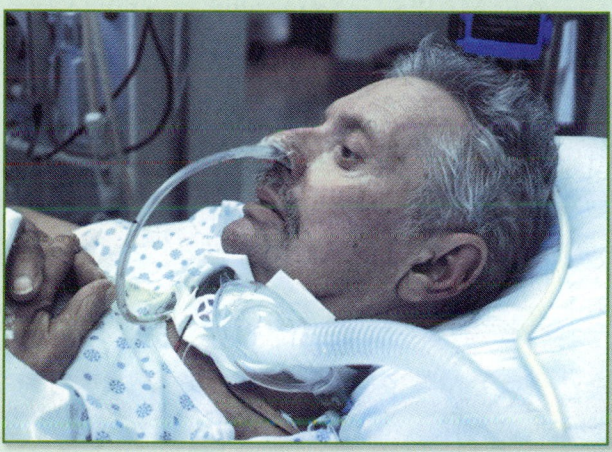

Figure 6-6-4 Assess the client. Check the nares for signs of irritation. Assess for nausea, vomiting, or abdominal distention.

▶ REAL WORLD ANECDOTES

While caring for Mr. Baranski, the student nurse assembled and set up the equipment needed to decompress Mr. Baranski's stomach. Mr. Baranski had a Salem sump tube in place and the student turned the suction on to continuous. However, she did not check the suction level, which was set at high suction. After the student observed that gastric contents were being suctioned through the NG tube, she provided for Mr. Baranski's comfort and went on to other duties. About an hour later Mr. Baranski turned on his call light. When the student answered the light, Mr. Baranski was panicked, pointing out that the fluid being suctioned through the NG tube appeared to be blood. The student turned the suction off and requested another nurse to evaluate the suction return. The nurse quickly realized that Mr. Baranski was bleeding. As the student evaluated Mr. Baranski's vital signs the nurse contacted his physician. Mr. Baranski had to be taken in for emergency surgery, where it was discovered that the high suction had caused the NG tube to erode a hole in Mr. Baranski's stomach, nearly causing him to bleed to death.

▶ EVALUATION

• The client will have a patent NG tube with effective suctioning of the gastric contents.
• The client understands the need for suctioning.
• The client did not experience pain or discomfort from the suctioning or the NG tube.
• The client did not experience trauma to the gastric wall or the nares from the suction or the NG tube.

▶ DOCUMENTATION

Nurses' Notes
Document:
• The reason for the tube insertion.
• The type of tube inserted.
• The type (intermittent or continuous) of suctioning and pressure setting.

- The nature and amount of aspirate and drainage.
- The client's tolerance of the procedure.
- The effectiveness of the intervention, such as nausea relieved.

Document on appropriate flow sheet or electronic medical record (EMR).

Intake and Output Record

- Record the amount of drainage.

► CRITICAL THINKING SKILL

Introduction

Fluid in the drainage container does not guarantee that the suction is working properly.

Possible Scenario

Mr. Ross is a large man who has just undergone abdominal surgery. The nurse enters his room to check the IV line. After surgery, he is attached to continuous GI suction. He complains of fullness in his midsection and nausea. The nurse sees that the GI suction is turned on and there is drainage in the container. He reassures Mr. Ross that it is normal to feel "woozy" after surgery and leaves the room.

Possible Outcome

Mr. Ross calls again. More concerned, the nurse checks the surgical site. As the nurse removes the dressing, Mr. Ross forcefully vomits approximately 250 mL of gastric contents. The force of the vomiting dislodges his stitches and reopens the wound. There is gastric content all over the bed, the client, and in the gaping wound. The wound starts to bleed profusely. Mr. Ross is returned to surgery to explore and repair the damage and to clean the contaminated surgical site.

Prevention

The nurse should have assessed the patency of the tube, as well as the suction. The presence of drainage in the collection chamber does not indicate that a tube is currently patent.

► VARIATIONS

Geriatric Variations:

- *Make sure the elderly client can hear and understand the importance of maintaining the suctioning system.*
- *The client needs to know that a soft hissing noise is normal and an indication the system is working correctly.*

Pediatric Variations:

- *The size of the tubing and the amount of pressure used will be adjusted according to the age and the size of the client.*
- *The parents should be instructed on the actions and purpose for suctioning.*
- *If the child pulls at the tubing, or is restless and might dislodge the tubing, the health care provider may need to order soft restraints.*

Home Care Variation:

- *Gastric suctioning is a short-term procedure and rarely seen in the home. If used as a temporary home procedure, the client would need to be instructed on troubleshooting the portable system.*

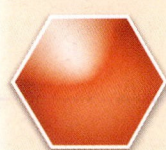

Long-Term Care Variation:

- *GI suctioning is never used as a long-term care option because of the trauma to the esophagus and gastric lining. Long-term care for these clients is based on assessing the client for complications well after the tube has been removed. The damage may be subtle at first and become more pronounced after the client is discharged.*

> ▶ **COMMON ERRORS**

Possible Error:

The tip of the suction catheter becomes plugged.

Prevention:

Check for movement in the tubing and check the container for increased drainage. If policy permits, irrigate the NG tube with 30 mL of normal saline.

▶ **NURSING TIPS**

- Assess all the connections in the system.
- Reposition the client frequently to prevent the catheter from adhering to the stomach wall and causing tissue damage.
- Gently milk the connecting tubing to break up thick drainage.
- If you have a concern about the suction machine, disconnect the NG from the connection tubing. Test the tubing with your gloved finger to see if the suction is working. (You can also put the suction tubing in a small glass of water to see if the water is sucked up.) If the machine is not working, replace it with a new system.
- If irrigation is allowed, gently irrigate the NG tube with 30 cc of normal saline and then draw the solution back out.
- Empty and record the drainage every 8 hours or when the container is at three-quarters full.
- Gastric suction should be set on low suction unless specifically ordered otherwise.
- Do not irrigate the NG tube in clients who have had gastric surgery unless specifically ordered.
- Avoid latex tubes if there is a history of latex allergy.

▶ **SPECIAL CONSIDERATIONS**

- *The double-lumen Salem pump nasogastric tube (see Figure 6-6-1) is usually used for suctioning purposes. The double-lumen tube is designed to have one opening to be connected to a suctioning, feeding, or irrigation device while the other opening remains patent for an air vent. The air vent opening (blue tube as seen in Figure 6-6-1) should remain patent and uncapped at all times to maintain the pressure balancing between the gastrointestinal system and the atmosphere. The blue air vent should be placed upright at a position higher than the stomach to prevent gastric contents from dripping via gravity.*

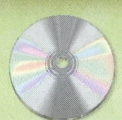

Applying a Condom Catheter

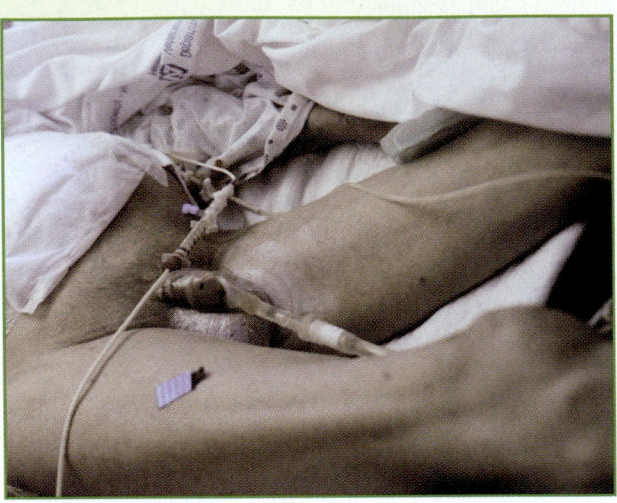

▶ OVERVIEW OF THE SKILL

The condom catheter is an external drainage system to collect urine from male clients who have incontinence. It is less invasive than a retention catheter and allows less contact of the skin with urine than a diaper or blue pad. Condom catheters require an order from an appropriate health care provider.

▶ ASSESSMENT

1. Assess skin integrity around the penis and perineal area **to look for signs of irritation and skin breakdown.**
2. Assess the client for ability to cooperate with the application and retention of the condom catheter **to determine what type of teaching will be necessary.**
3. Assess the amount and pattern of urinary incontinence **to determine whether the condom catheter is the best continence method for the client.**
4. Assess for latex allergy.

▶ DIAGNOSIS

Functional Urinary Incontinence

Impaired Urinary Elimination

Risk for Impaired Skin Integrity

Toileting Self-Care Deficit

Total Urinary Incontinence

▶ PLANNING

Expected Outcomes:

1. The client will have a condom catheter in place without leakage or discomfort.
2. The client will have no skin irritation from the condom catheter.
3. The client will understand the reason for, and cooperate with, the placement and retention of the condom catheter.

Equipment Needed (see Figure 6-7-1):

- Condom catheter kit with adhesive strip
- Urinary drainage bag
- Clean gloves

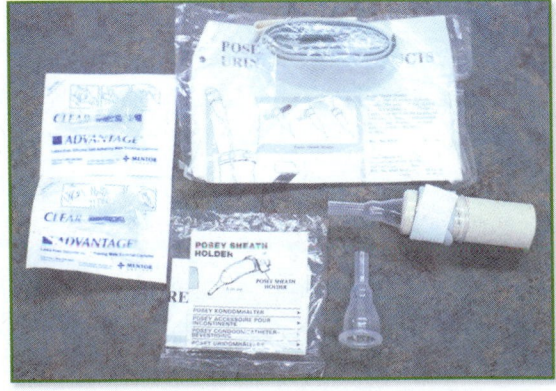

Figure 6-7-1 Condom catheters

- Basin with warm water and soap
- Towel and washcloth

▶ **CLIENT EDUCATION NEEDED:**

1. Explain the need for the catheter carefully so as not to embarrass client.
2. If the client gets an erection, assure him that it is not unusual when applying a condom catheter. Your calm reassurance and matter-of-fact attitude will help decrease client embarrassment and provide guidance for his coping responses.

3. Instruct the client to make sure the bag is carried with him lower than the level of the bladder if he ambulates.
4. Instruct the client to inform the nurse if irritation occurs.

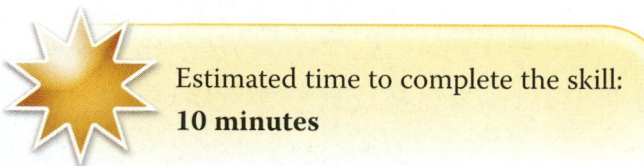

Estimated time to complete the skill:
10 minutes

▶ **DELEGATION TIPS**

Application of a condom catheter may be delegated to properly trained ancillary personnel. The need for condom drainage and the ongoing assessment of the client's skin condition should be followed up by the nurse.

IMPLEMENTATION—Action/Rationale

Action	Rationale
1. Wash hands.	1. Reduces the transmission of microorganisms.
2. Protect the client's privacy by closing the door and pulling curtains around the bed.	2. Allows privacy for the client.
3. Position the client in a comfortable position, preferably a supine position, if tolerated by the client. Raise the bed to a comfortable height for the nurse.	3. The client will be more comfortable and tolerate the procedure more readily; a supine position facilitates the cleaning and application of the catheter. Raising the bed to a comfortable height promotes good body mechanics.
4. Apply gloves (use latex-free gloves if client has a latex allergy).	4. Gloves should be worn to prevent the possible transmission of microorganisms when there is a chance of coming into contact with any body fluid. Avoids an allergic reaction if client has a latex allergy.
5. Fold the client's gown across the abdomen and pull the sheet up over the client's legs.	5. Provides minimal exposure of the client, thereby reducing the client's embarrassment.
6. Assess the client's penis for any signs of redness, irritation, or skin breakdown.	6. The client may require an indwelling catheter if there is a significant amount of skin breakdown. Assessment will give baseline data for comparison with future assessments.
7. Clean the client's penis with warm soapy water. Retract the foreskin on the uncircumcised male and clean thoroughly in folds.	7. Removes microorganisms present in any drainage or feces that could enter the urinary meatus and cause a urinary tract infection. Avoids trapping microorganisms in folds around the meatus.

continues

Action	Rationale
8. Return the client's foreskin to its normal position (see Figure 6-7-2).	8. Failure to return the foreskin to a normal position can lead to swelling of the penis and possible constriction.
9. Shave any excess hair around the base of the penis if required by institutional policy.	9. Prevents additional discomfort from the adhesive strip when the condom catheter is removed. Also prevents hair from catching onto the adhesive strip, causing discomfort.
10. Rinse and dry the area.	10. Moist warm environment can lead to the growth of microorganisms.
11. If a condom kit is used, open the package containing the skin preparation (see Figure 6-7-3). Wipe and apply skin preparation solution to the shaft of the penis. If the client has an erection, wait for termination of erection before applying the catheter.	11. Preparation solutions protect the client's skin from irritation. An erection may occur from manipulation of the penis while cleaning the area. This is a normal reaction and will terminate in a few minutes.
12. Apply the double-sided adhesive strip around the base of the client's penis in a spiral fashion. The strip is applied 1 inch from the proximal end of the penis. Do not completely encircle the penis or tightly encompass penis.	12. Applying the adhesive in a spiral fashion does not compromise circulation of the penis. Encircling the penis can constrict the penis, impair circulation, and cause edema.
13. Grasp the penis with your nondominant hand. With your nondominant hand, position the rolled condom at the distal portion of the penis and unroll it, covering the penis and the double-sided strip of adhesive. Leave a 1- to 2-inch space between the tip of the penis and the end of the condom (see Figure 6-7-4).	13. The condom sticks to the adhesive and remains in place. The extra spacing prevents pressure and erosion of the tip of the penis.
14. Gently press the condom to the adhesive strip.	14. Enables the condom to adhere evenly to the adhesive strip.
15. Attach the drainage bag tubing to the catheter tubing. Make sure the tubing lays over the client's legs, not under. Secure the drainage bag to the side of the bed below the level of the client's bladder or to the drainage bag attached to the leg (see Figures 6-7-5 and 6-7-6).	15. The drainage bag is positioned below the level of the client's bladder to prevent reflux of the urine onto the penis and microorganisms from entering the penis. The tubing is placed over the leg to promote urine flow away from the client. Constant exposure to urine and moisture can irritate the penis.

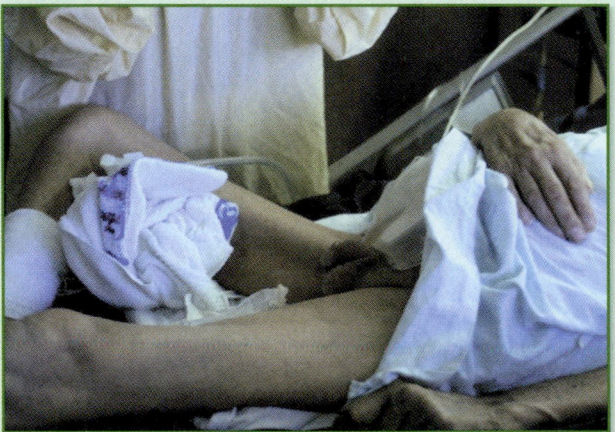

Figure 6-7-2   After cleaning the client's penis, return the foreskin to its normal position.

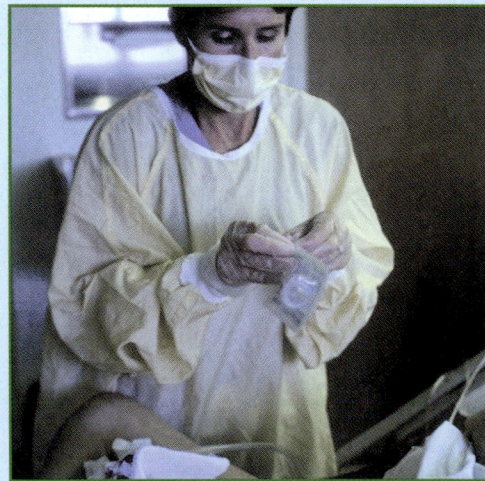

Figure 6-7-3   After preparing the penis, open the condom kit. Apply the skin preparation solution.

continues

Action	Rationale

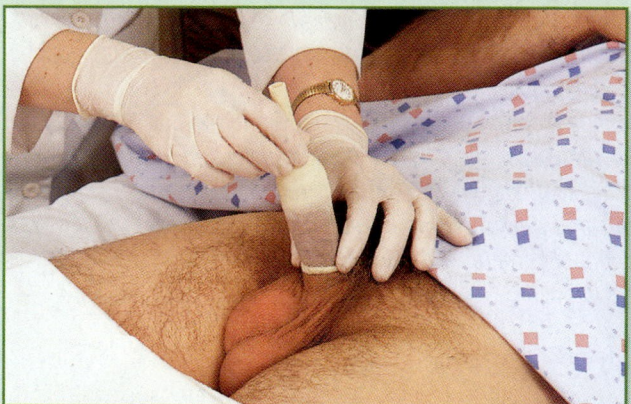

Figure 6-7-4 Unroll the condom from the distal portion of the penis upward to the base.

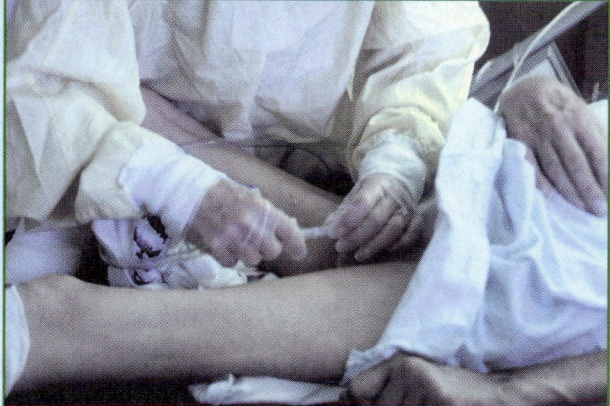

Figure 6-7-5 Attach the drainage bag tubing to the catheter tubing.

16. Determine that the condom and tubing are not twisted.

16. If the condom or tubing is twisted, the urine cannot flow out and the condom will leak or fall off.

17. Cover the client.

17. Maintains privacy of the client.

18. Dispose of the used equipment in appropriate receptacle and wash hands.

18. Reduces the transmission of microorganisms.

19. Return the client's bed to the lowest position and reposition client to comfortable or appropriate position.

19. Reduces potential injury from falls.

20. Empty the bag, measure the client's urinary output, and record every 4 hours. Remove gloves and wash hands after procedure.

20. Records output and prevents bag from becoming overly full and/or too heavy. Reduces transmission of microorganisms.

21. Remove the condom once a day to clean the area and assess the skin for signs of impaired skin integrity.

21. Promotes hygiene and reduces the possibility of skin breakdown.

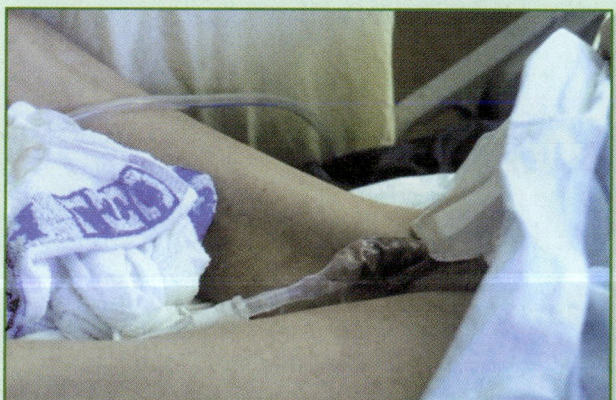

Figure 6-7-6 Make sure the drainage bag tubing lies over the client's leg.

► **REAL WORLD ANECDOTES**

Nurse Griniv was making a home health visit to evaluate Mr. Rodygin's condition. Mr. Rodygin was a confused, bedridden client. His elderly wife was his primary caregiver. While performing an assessment, the nurse noticed that Mr. Rodygin's condom catheter was leaking. When she removed the condom she discovered the skin beneath it was excoriated and inflamed. When asked about the condom catheter, Mrs. Rodygin stammered and was evasive. She finally admitted that she had not changed it in several weeks. She noted that she always had difficulty getting the condom to adhere to the skin so she had decided not to change it as long as it remained in place. The nurse called Mr. Rodygin's doctor requesting orders for skin care ointment and an indwelling catheter until Mr. Rodygin's skin was healed. She then gently reinforced the instructions for applying a condom catheter with Mrs. Rodygin.

► **EVALUATION**

* The client's condom catheter is in place without leakage or discomfort.
* The client does not have any skin irritation from the condom catheter.
* The client understands the reason for, and cooperates with, the placement and retention of the condom catheter.

► **DOCUMENTATION**

Nurses' Notes

* Document the time the procedure was performed.
* Note the condition of the client's skin, recording any irritation, rashes, or open areas.
* Record any client teaching performed.

Document on appropriate flow sheet or electronic medical record (EMR).

Intake and Output Record

* Record the amount of urine emptied from the urine drainage bag.

► **CRITICAL THINKING SKILL**

Introduction

The client complains that the condom catheter is painful.

Possible Scenario

While making rounds, Mr. Zgonc complains that he hurts "down there." Upon examination, the nurse notes that the adhesive strip for Mr. Zgonc's condom catheter completely encircles the shaft of his penis. The area below the adhesive strip is reddened and edematous.

Possible Outcome

The constriction of blood flow could cause tissue and nerve damage, perhaps even necrosis of the penis.

Prevention

It is important to always check that the catheter is not constricting the penis and causing skin breakdown. Wrap the adhesive strip in a spiral. Do not wrap it in a rubber band/tourniquet fashion. Inspect the catheter at least every 4 hours, or more frequently if the client is restless or confused.

► **VARIATIONS**

Geriatric Variations:
* *Elderly clients have thinner skin, which may more readily break down.*
* *Clients may be embarrassed by an erection. Inform clients that this is normal.*

continues

▶ VARIATIONS (continued)

Pediatric Variations:
- *Use a size appropriate to the child.*
- *Other means such as diapers can be used for younger children; however, if output measurements are needed, a condom catheter may be necessary.*
- *This procedure can be extremely embarrassing to children. If the use of a condom catheter is absolutely necessary, the procedure may be best performed by a male staff member.*
- *If the child has an erection, inform him that this can occur naturally.*

Home Care Variations:
- *Change the catheter often as the adhesive and the condom can lead to skin breakdown. Diapers, incontinence pads, or Attends may be more useful or may be used periodically to give the skin on the penis a chance to heal.*
- *Instruct the home caregiver on how to clean, use, apply, and remove the condom catheter.*
- *Discuss signs and symptoms of irritation or skin breakdown.*
- *Discuss alternatives to the condom should it need to be removed.*

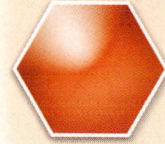

Long-Term Care Variation:
- *If irritation occurs, remove the condom and clean the area more frequently, three times a day if possible.*

▶ COMMON ERRORS

Possible Error:
Condom placed too tight or too loose.

Prevention:
Do not place catheter when client has an erection. Make sure the adhesive strip is snug but do not pull tightly when applying.

Possible Error:
Skin not prepared appropriately. Skin oils not removed and adhesive will not stick.

Prevention:
Take the time to cleanse the skin properly prior to placing the adhesive strip.

Possible Error:
Condom catheter becomes twisted and urine leaks out.

Prevention:
Position the tubing and bag to allow the client maximum mobility without undue tugging or twisting of the tubing or catheter. Teach the ambulatory client wearing a condom catheter to detach the bag from the bed and position it where it will not be twisted when he gets up.

▶ NURSING TIPS

- Use skin preparation solution if available to remove skin oils. This will help condom catheter stay in place.
- Do not reattach a condom catheter if it falls off. It will not stick any better the second try. Start over with a new strip and catheter.

- If client has excessive hair, this can be quite uncomfortable to client and may require partial shaving.
- In an unconscious or confused client, one may need to either position tubing where the client will not pull on the catheter or tubing, or use restraints.

▶ SPECIAL CONSIDERATIONS

- *Assess the skin integrity and blood circulation every 2 to 4 hours as the skin may become irritated or break down after prolonged immersion in urine or fluid. Monitor for signs and symptoms of irritation or skin breakdown. If the skin breakdown worsens, the affected areas should be kept clean and dry. In this case, a condom catheter should not be used until the skin heals.*
- *Clients may have latex allergy and require latex-free condoms. Assess history for latex allergy and assess skin for reactions to latex.*

Inserting an Indwelling Catheter: Male

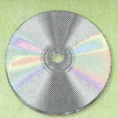

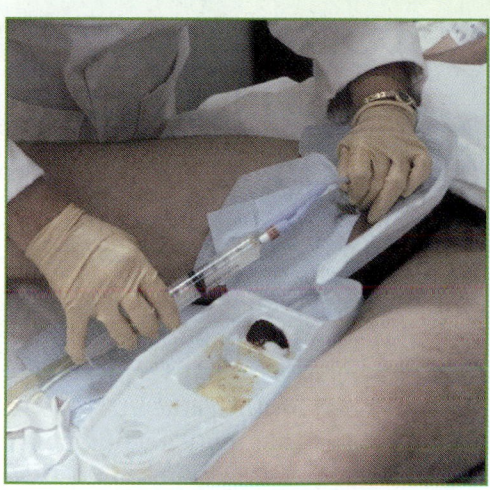

▶ OVERVIEW OF THE SKILL

Catheterization involves passing a rubber or plastic tube into the bladder via the urethra to drain urine from the bladder or to obtain a urine specimen. Intermittent catheterization may be used to obtain a sample or to relieve bladder distention. Indwelling catheters may be used short-term to keep the bladder empty, prevent urinary retention, or allow precise measurement of urine. Long-term indwelling, or retention, catheters are used to control incontinence, prevent retention, or prevent the leakage of urine (see Figure 6-8-1). Catheterization is a sterile procedure.

▶ ASSESSMENT

1. Assess the need for catheterization and the type of catheterization ordered **to ensure the proper procedure is performed.** Use latex-free catheter if client has a history of latex allergy.
2. Assess for the need for genital and perineal care before catheterization **to reduce the transmission of microorganisms.**
3. Assess the urinary meatus for signs of infection or inflammation. Ask the client for any history of difficulty with prior catheterizations, anxiety, or urinary strictures. **Allows detection of potential complications.**
4. Assess the client's ability to assist with the procedure. Can he maintain the proper position while you perform the procedure? Is the client agitated, and could he contaminate the sterile field? Will you need assistance to hold the client's legs in position? **Determines how the procedure is carried out.**
5. Assess the light. Will you be able to see well enough to place the catheter, or do you need a secondary light source? **Determines what preparation needs to be done to ensure a successful procedure.**
6. Assess for an allergy to povidone-iodine and/or latex **to avoid an allergic reaction.**
7. Watch for indications of distress or embarrassment, especially if the nurse is the opposite gender, **to determine what teaching and support are needed. Explore further if indicated.**

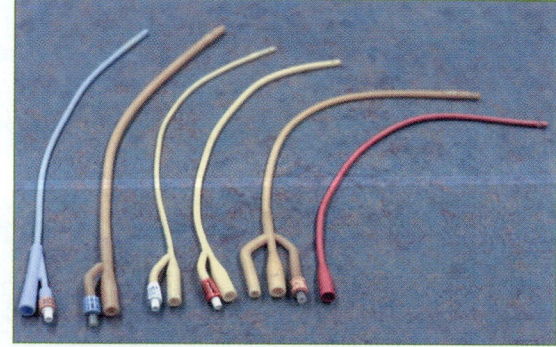

Figure 6-8-1 Indwelling and straight catheters

▶ DIAGNOSIS

Impaired Urinary Retention

Overflow Urinary Incontinence

Reflex Urinary Incontinence

Risk for Infection

Risk for Impaired Skin Integrity

Total Urinary Incontinence

Urinary Retention

▶ PLANNING

Expected Outcomes:

1. The catheter will be inserted without pain, trauma, or injury to the client.
2. The client's bladder will be emptied without complication.
3. The nurse will maintain the sterility of the catheter during insertion.

Equipment Needed (see Figure 6-8-2):

* Indwelling or straight catheter with drainage system
* Sterile catheterization kit
* Adequate lighting source
* Disposable gloves
* Blanket or drape
* Soap and washcloth
* Warm water
* Towel

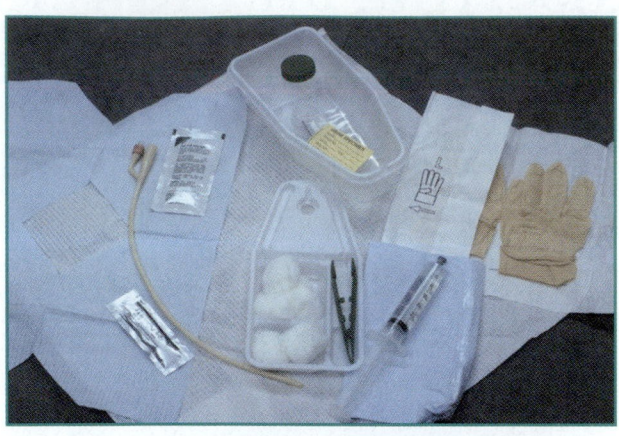

Figure 6-8-2   Catheterization kit

▶ CLIENT EDUCATION NEEDED:

1. Explain the procedure to client and describe anticipated sensations of burning and urgency that occur when the catheter is placed.
2. Explain the need for the catheter.
3. Explain the basics of aseptic technique and the need not to touch or contaminate the sterile field.

Estimated time to complete the skill:
20 minutes

▶ DELEGATION TIPS

The skill of male urinary catheterization may be delegated to properly trained ancillary personnel depending on institution policies. The nurse is responsible to evaluate the client for contraindications to delegating this procedure, such as the risk for a difficult or traumatic insertion. The nurse may then decide to perform the procedure or to defer to the health care practitioner.

IMPLEMENTATION—Action/Rationale

Action	Rationale
Performing Urinary Catheterization: Male Client	
1. Gather the equipment needed. Read the label on the catheterization kit. Note if the catheter is included in the kit and, if so, what type it is. Gather any supplies you will need that are not in the prepackaged kit.	1. Promotes efficiency in the procedure. Kits from various manufacturers come with different equipment. The catheter may or may not be packaged in the kit. Sterile gloves and the urine drainage bag may also need to be gathered separately.

continues

Action	Rationale
2. Identify client by reading armband. Close client's door and draw curtains. Explain procedure to client.	2. Verifies correct client. Provides privacy. Explaining the procedure promotes client cooperation.
3. Set the bed to a comfortable height to work, and raise the side rail on the side opposite you.	3. Promotes proper body mechanics and ensures client safety.
4. Assist the client to a supine position with legs slightly spread.	4. Relaxes muscle and allows visualization of the area to facilitate insertion of the catheter.
5. Drape the client's abdomen and thighs, if needed.	5. Promotes client comfort and warmth.
6. Ensure adequate lighting of the penis and perineal area.	6. Facilitates proper execution of technique.
7. Wash hands, apply latex-free disposable gloves, and wash the genital and perineal area.	7. Reduces transfer of microorganisms. Avoids reaction to latex.
8. Remove gloves and wash hands.	8. Reduces transfer of microorganisms.
9. Remove plastic wrap from catheterization kit and place near work area. Place catheterization kit between client's legs and open using aseptic technique(see Figure 6-8-3):	9. Plastic wrap is a receptacle for used supplies.
a. Unfold the top flap by grasping the corner of the outer surface between your thumb and finger only. Open the top flap away from your body .	a. Outer surface is considered contaminated.
b. Grasp the outer surface of the left and right flaps and open.	b. Maintains sterile technique.
c. Grasp the proximal (closest) flap and open toward you. Avoid touching the inside of the flap or inside of the package with your hands or clothing.	c. Opening the proximal flap last and toward you prevents you from reaching over the sterile field.
10. If the catheter is not included in the kit, carefully drop the sterile catheter onto the field using aseptic technique. Add any other items needed.	10. Prevents contamination of the sterile equipment and the sterile field.
11. Apply sterile gloves. These may be included in the kit.	11. Prevents contamination of the sterile equipment.
12. Place the drape from the catheterization kit between client's thighs, close to the perineum being careful not to touch nonsterile surfaces with the gloves.	12. Provides a sterile field at the procedural site. Prevents accidental contamination from adjacent areas.

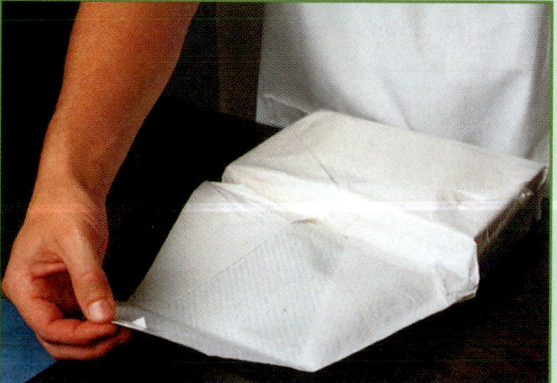

Figure 6-8-3   Touching only the corner, open the distal (top) flap away from your body.

continues

Action	Rationale

Performing Urinary Catheterization: Male Client *continued*

13. Place the fenestrated drape from the catheterization kit over the client's perineal area with the penis extending through the opening, being careful not to touch non-sterile surfaces with gloves.

13. Provides a sterile field at the procedural site.

14. If inserting a retention catheter, test the patency of the catheter balloon. Attach the syringe filled with sterile water to the Luer-lock tail of the catheter. Inflate the balloon by injecting the appropriate amount of fluid (see Figure 6-8-4). Assess for leaks. Deflate the balloon. Keep water-filled syringe attached to the port.

14. Tests the patency of the catheter balloon. A new catheter must be obtained if the balloon does not inflate or if it leaks.

15. Attach the catheter to the urine drainage bag if it is not preconnected.

15. The catheter and drainage system may be preconnected; otherwise it is connected before catheterization to avoid exposing the client to ascending infection from an open-ended catheter.

16. Open the povidone-iodine or other antimicrobial solution and pour over cotton balls. Remove the cap from the water-soluble lubricant syringe.

16. Maintains sterile technique.

17. With your nondominant hand, gently grasp the penis and retract the foreskin (if present). With your dominant hand, use the forceps to pick up a saturated cotton ball. Place the cotton ball on the meatus. Use a circular motion and cleanse from the meatus toward the base of the penis. Discard cotton ball. Clean the meatus three times, using a new saturated cotton ball each time (see Figure 6-8-5).

17. Removes microorganisms and minimizes the risk of urinary tract infection.

18. Hold the penis perpendicular to the body and pull up gently.

18. Facilitates catheter insertion by straightening urethra.

19. Inject 10-mL sterile, water-soluble lubricant (use a 2% Xylocaine lubricant whenever feasible) into the urethra.

19. Avoids urethral trauma and discomfort during catheter insertion and facilitates insertion.

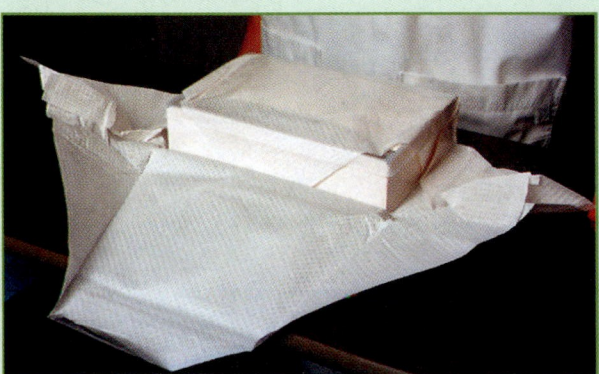

Figure 6-8-4 Carefully grab the wrapper, opening the right and left side of the package.

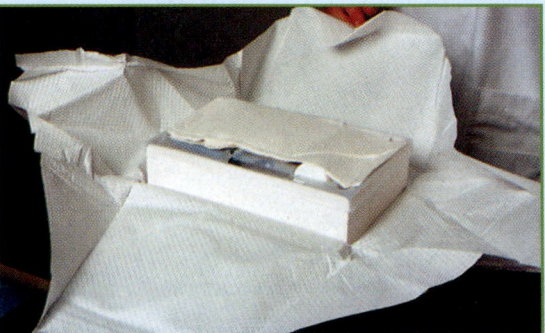

Figure 6-8-5 Open the proximal (closest) flap toward you. Avoid touching the flap or inside of the package with your hands or clothing.

continues

Action	Rationale
20. Holding the catheter in the dominant hand, steadily insert the catheter about 8 inches, until urine is noted in the drainage bag or tubing (see Figure 6-8-6).	**20.** Provides a visual confirmation that the catheter tip is in the bladder.
21. If the catheter will be removed as soon as the client's bladder is empty, insert the catheter another inch, place the penis in a comfortable position, and hold the catheter in place as the bladder drains.	**21.** The catheter needs to be inserted far enough to allow complete bladder drainage, but not so far as to possibly irritate the bladder, causing spasms.
22. If the catheter will be indwelling with a retention balloon, continue inserting the catheter until the bifurcation (where drainage port and retention balloon arm meet) reaches the end of the penis (see Figure 6-8-7).	**22.** Ensures adequate catheter insertion before retention balloon is inflated.
23. Inflate the retention balloon with sterile water per manufacturer's recommendations or the health care provider's orders (see Figure 6-8-8).	**23.** Ensures retention of the catheter in the bladder. Retention catheters are available with a variety of balloon sizes. Use a catheter with the appropriate size balloon.
24. Instruct the client to immediately report discomfort or pressure during balloon inflation; if pain occurs, discontinue the procedure, deflate the balloon, and insert the catheter farther into the bladder. If the client continues to complain of pain with balloon inflation, remove the catheter and notify the client's health care provider.	**24.** Pain or pressure indicates inflation of the balloon in the urethra; further insertion will prevent misplacement and further pain or bleeding.
25. Once the balloon has been inflated, gently pull the catheter until the retention balloon is resting snug against the bladder neck (resistance will be felt when the balloon is properly seated).	**25.** Maximizes continuous bladder drainage and ensures that the catheter is in the bladder.

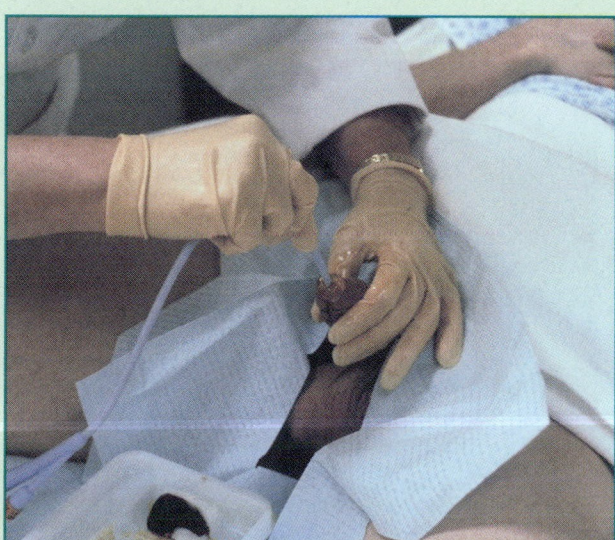

Figure 6-8-6 Steadily insert the catheter.

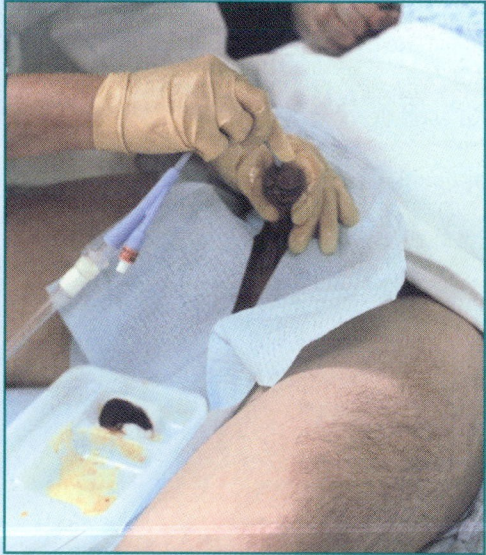

Figure 6-8-7 Continue inserting the catheter until the bifurcation (where the drainage port and the retention balloon arm meet) reaches the end of the penis. This ensures the retention balloon will be fully in the bladder prior to inflation.

continues

Action	Rationale

**Performing Urinary Catheterization:
Male Client** *continued*

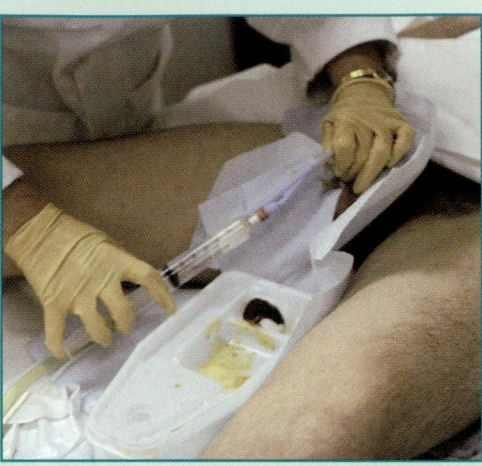

Figure 6-8-8   Inflate the retention balloon.

26. Secure the catheter according to institutional policy. Securing it to either the client's thigh or abdomen is generally acceptable. Be sure to allow slack in the catheter so that the catheter does not pull when the client moves.

26. Prevents excessive traction from the balloon rubbing against the bladder neck, inadvertent catheter removal, or urethral erosion.

27. Place the drainage bag below the level of the bladder. Do not let it rest on the floor (see Figures 6-8-9 and 6-8-10). Secure the drainage tubing to prevent pulling on the tubing and the catheter.

27. Maximizes continuous drainage of urine from the bladder (drainage is prevented when the drainage bag is placed above the abdomen).

28. Clean perineal area with soap and water. Dry the area.

28. Removes antiseptic solution to prevent skin irritation.

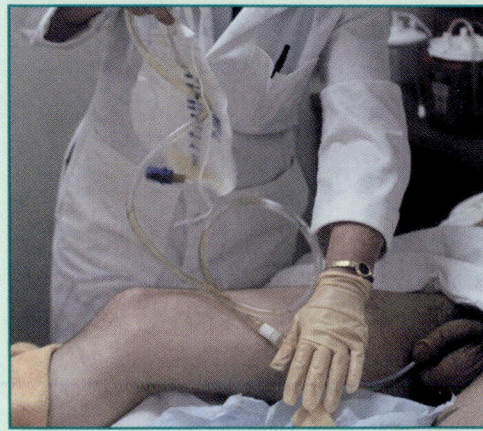

Figure 6-8-9   Place the drainage bag tubing over the leg.

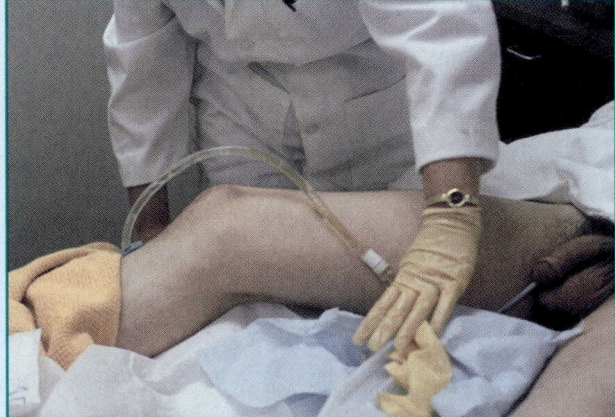

Figure 6-8-10   Place the drainage bag below the level of the bladder, but do not rest it on the floor.

continues

Action	Rationale
29. Dispose of equipment, remove gloves, and wash hands.	**29.** Reduces the transmission of microorganisms.
30. Assist client to a comfortable position. Lower the bed.	**30.** Promotes client comfort and safety.
31. Wash hands.	**31.** Reduces the transmission of microorganisms
32. Assess and document the amount, color, odor, and quality of urine.	**32.** Monitors urinary status.

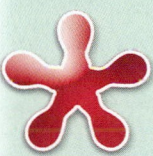

► **REAL WORLD ANECDOTES**

Scenario 1
A nurse is checking on an elderly nursing home client late at night. She found him sitting in the dark, in a chair, complaining that he has to urinate. She knows he has a Foley catheter in place and decides to investigate. Turning on the lights, she sees the client has pulled out his catheter with the 35-mL retention balloon still inflated. She notes that he is bleeding from the urethra and there is blood in the bathroom. This client required several hours of bladder irrigation to stop the bleeding, a new catheter with a 45-mL retention balloon, and increased supervision.

Scenario 2
Mr. Muon was an elderly client in a long-term care facility. His indwelling urinary catheter was due to be changed. As the nurse prepared Mr. Muon for the catheter, she noted that he had bilateral inguinal hernias that had severely distended his scrotum. She prepped Mr. Muon and started inserting the catheter. As the catheter was inserted, the nurse noted that she could see the catheter tip within the client's scrotum. She was concerned that the catheter was no longer in the client's urethra but the client was not in pain and there did not appear to be any obvious trauma. She continued to gently insert the catheter. She started to become concerned when she noted that she had inserted the catheter almost to its hub without a urine return. Just as she was ready to remove the catheter and call Mr. Muon's physician, she noted a urine return. She slid the catheter into the urethra a little further and inflated the retention balloon. The client tolerated the procedure well, despite his obvious urethral displacement. The catheter had been inserted almost to the hub in order to reach Mr. Muon's bladder. After seeing to Mr. Muon's comfort and recording her findings, the nurse reported her observations to Mr. Muon's physician.

Evaluation
- The catheter was inserted without pain, trauma, or injury to the client.
- The client's bladder was emptied without complication.
- The nurse maintained the sterility of the catheter during insertion.

► **DOCUMENTATION**

Nurses' Notes
- Record the time and date the catheter was inserted.

- Note the size and type of catheter used, including the size of the retention balloon and the amount of sterile water used to inflate the balloon.
- Record the client's response to the procedure and the amount, color, and quality of urine returned.

Document on appropriate flow sheet or electronic medical record (EMR).

Intake and Output Record
Record the amount of urine returned.

► CRITICAL THINKING SKILL

Introduction

Each client is different. Complete assessment, including a client history, will help avoid mistakes.

Possible Scenario

You are working in the emergency room. A 27-year-old coworker comes in complaining of not being able to void. Not wanting to get too personal with a coworker, you skip lightly through your assessment. The physician orders you to catheterize this client. As you begin to insert the catheter, the client suddenly complains of sharp pain and pulls back away from the catheter.

Possible Outcome

You stop and notify the physician. This client has urethral strictures, scar tissue from an earlier procedure that would have been torn if you had forced the catheter into the urethra.

Prevention

Assess every client for any history of difficulty with catheterization. Always stop the procedure immediately if resistance or excess pain occurs.

► VARIATIONS

Geriatric Variations:
- *Geriatric clients may need help holding the correct position.*
- *Anatomic landmarks may be more difficult to visualize in an older client.*

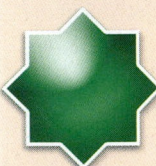

Pediatric Variation:
- *Children need the support of a parent, who can also help the child hold the position and provide distraction during the procedure.*

Home Care Variations:
- *If the client will be catheterized at home, go over the catheterization technique step by step to determine how it will be accomplished in the home setting. For example, will the procedure be done in bed, on a couch, or in the bathroom? Where will clean supplies be obtained and stored? How will the procedure be assessed and documented. Is urine testing needed?*
- *Emphasize the need for good handwashing, cleaning of the catheter, and adequate lubrication of the catheter to reduce the frequency of infection and urethral trauma.*

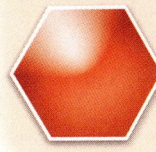

Long-Term Care Variation:
- *Clients who practice long-term self-catheterization may use clean, instead of sterile, technique to catheterize themselves. Reinforce the need for good handwashing and cleaning of the catheter and adequate lubrication of the catheter to reduce the frequency of infection and urethral trauma.*

▶ COMMON ERRORS

Possible Error:

The client moves his foot and contaminates the edge of the sterile field.

Prevention:

If the client has touched a sterile item, such as the catheter or your gloves, you need to replace the item and start over. If the contamination is on the sterile field and you can avoid contact with the area, you may proceed with caution. Make sure the client understands the need to protect the sterile area. Remind him as needed during the procedure, and get assistance holding the client's legs in position during the procedure if you have doubts.

▶ NURSING TIPS

- Make sure a drainage system is in place prior to inserting the catheter, to prevent the spill of urine.
- Consider taping connections closed if you are concerned the client might become confused and pull them apart, thereby breaking the sterility of the closed-system drainage.
- Hold the sides of the penis with gentle pressure to help the meatus stay open as you prepare to insert the catheter.

- If you feel resistance, try gently twisting the catheter one-quarter turn. Try holding the penis at a 90-degree angle to the body, and pull very slightly as you advance the catheter.
- If 700–800 mL of urine has drained right away, clamp the catheter for 20 minutes. Then unclamp and let urine flow. This helps prevent bladder spasms.
- Up to twice the recommended volume of fluid may be inserted safely into the retention balloon, if needed.

▶ SPECIAL CONSIDERATIONS

- *If the area (male: front thigh or lower abdomen) for taping to secure the urinary catheter is hairy, prepare and shave the area to prevent any discomfort. Allow enough space between penis and the taped area to allow for the client's mobilization, and possible erection during sleep.*
- *If the foreskin was retracted during insertion, be sure to put back the foreskin upon completion of the procedure. Prolonged foreskin retraction causes poor blood circulation around the area, and may result in tissue necrosis.*
- *Erection may occur as a normal physical response during the catheterization. This can be an embarrassing moment for the client. Deal with the situation professionally. Withhold the procedure and leave the room; come back in 10 to 15 minutes to finish the procedure.*
- *Use latex-free gloves and catheter if the client has a history of latex allergy.*

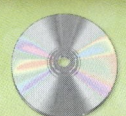

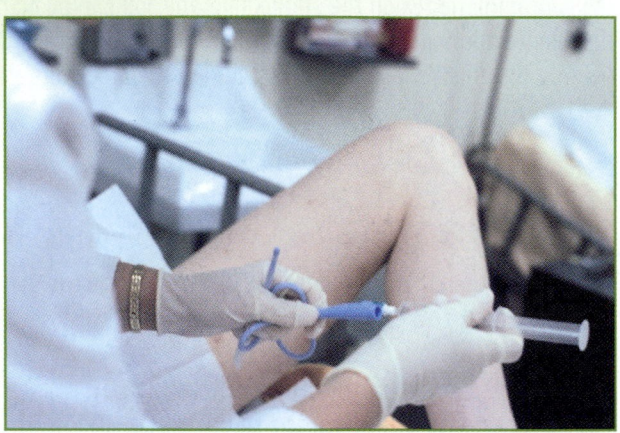

▶ OVERVIEW OF THE SKILL

Catheterization involves passing a rubber or plastic tube into the bladder via the urethra to drain urine from the bladder or to obtain a urine specimen. Intermittent catheterization may be used to obtain a sample or to relieve bladder distention. Indwelling catheters may be used short-term to keep the bladder empty, prevent urinary retention, or allow precise measurement of urine. Long-term indwelling, or retention, catheters are used to control incontinence, prevent retention, or prevent the leakage of urine. Catheterization is a sterile procedure.

▶ ASSESSMENT

1. Assess the need for catheterization and the type of catheterization ordered **to ensure the proper procedure is carried out.**
2. Assess for the need for perineal care prior to catheterization **to reduce the transmission of microorganisms.**
3. Assess the urinary meatus for signs of infection or inflammation. Ask the client for any history of latex allergy, difficulty with prior catheterizations, anxiety, or urinary strictures. **Allows detection of potential complications.**
4. Assess the client's ability to assist with the procedure. Can she maintain the proper position while you perform the procedure? Is the client agitated, and could she contaminate the sterile field? Will you need assistance to hold her legs in position? **Determines how the procedure is to be carried out.**
5. Assess the light. Will you be able to see well enough to place the catheter, or do you need a secondary light source? **Determines what preparation needs to be done to ensure a successful procedure.**
6. Assess for an allergy to povidone-iodine and/or latex **to avoid an allergic reaction.**
7. Watch for indications of distress or embarrassment, especially if the nurse is of the opposite gender, **to determine what teaching and support are needed. Explore further if indicated.**

▶ DIAGNOSIS

Impaired Urinary Retention

Overflow Urinary Incontinence

Reflex Urinary Incontinence

Risk for Infection

Risk for Impaired Skin Integrity

Total Urinary Incontinence

Urinary Retention

▶ PLANNING

Expected Outcomes:

1. A catheter will be inserted without pain, trauma, or injury to the client.
2. The client's bladder will be emptied without complication.

3. The nurse will maintain the sterility of the catheter during insertion.

Equipment Needed (**see Figure 6-9-1**):

- Indwelling or straight catheter with drainage system
- Sterile catheterization kit
- Adequate lighting source
- Disposable clean gloves
- Blanket or drape
- Soap and washcloth
- Warm water
- Towel

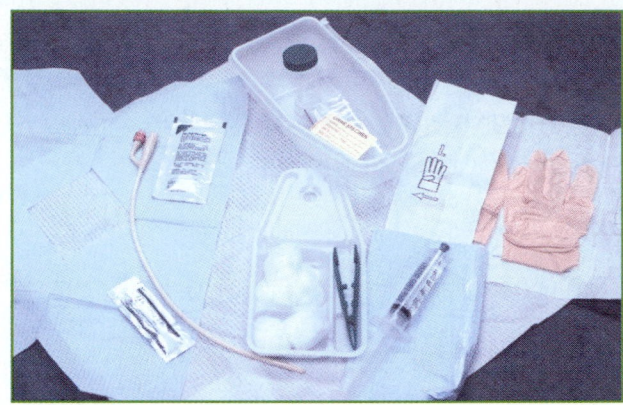

Figure 6-9-1   Catheterization kit

▶ **CLIENT EDUCATION NEEDED:**

1. Explain the procedure to the client, and describe anticipated sensations of burning or urgency that occur when the catheter is placed.
2. Explain the need for the catheter.
3. Explain the basics of aseptic technique and the need not to touch or contaminate the sterile field.

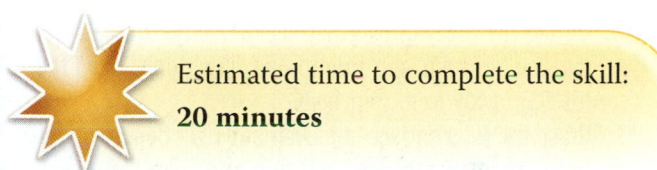

Estimated time to complete the skill:
20 minutes

▶ **DELEGATION TIPS**

The skill of female urinary catheterization may be delegated to properly trained ancillary personnel depending on institution policies. The nurse is responsible to evaluate the client for contraindications to delegating this procedure, such as the risk for a difficult or traumatic insertion. The nurse may then decide to perform the procedure or to defer to the health care practitioner.

IMPLEMENTATION—Action/Rationale

Action	Rationale
Performing Urinary Catheterization	
1. Gather the equipment needed. Read the label on the catheterization kit. Note if the catheter is included in the kit and, if so, what type it is. Gather any supplies you will need that are not in the prepackaged kit.	1. Promotes efficiency in the procedure. Kits from various manufacturers come with different equipment. The catheter may or may not be packaged in the kit. Sterile gloves and the urine drainage bag may also need to be gathered separately.
2. Identify client by reading armband. Close client's door and draw curtains. Explain procedure to client.	2. Verifies correct client. Provides privacy. Explaining the procedure promotes client cooperation.
3. Set the bed to a comfortable height to work, and raise the side rail on the side opposite you.	3. Promotes proper body mechanics and ensures client safety.
4. Assist the client to a supine position with legs spread and feet together or to a side-lying position with upper leg flexed (see Figure 6-9-2).	4. Relaxes muscles and allows visualization of the area to facilitate insertion of the catheter.
5. Drape the client's abdomen and thighs for warmth if needed.	5. Promotes client comfort and warmth.

continues

Action	Rationale
Performing Urinary Catheterization *continued*	
6. Ensure adequate lighting of the perineal area.	6. Facilitates proper execution of technique.
7. Wash hands and apply disposable gloves.	7. Reduces transfer of microorganisms.
8. Wash perineal area.	8. Reduces transfer of microorganisms.
9. Remove gloves and wash hands.	9. Reduces transfer of microorganisms.
10. Remove plastic wrap from catheterization kit and place near work area. Place catheterization kit between client's legs and open the catheterization kit, using aseptic technique (see Figure 6-9-3). a. Unfold the top flap by grasping the corner of the outer surface between your thumb and finger only. Open the top flap away from your body. b. Grasp the outer surface of the left and right flaps and open. c. Grasp the proximal (closest) flap and open toward you. Avoid touching the inside of the flap or inside of the package with your hands or clothing.	10. Plastic wrap is a receptacle for contaminated supplies. a. Outer surface is considered contaminated. b. Maintains sterile technique c. Opening the proximal flap last and towards you, prevents reaching over the sterile field.
11. If the catheter is not included in the kit, drop the sterile catheter onto the field using aseptic technique. Add any other items needed.	11. Prevents contamination of the sterile equipment and the sterile field.
12. Apply sterile gloves. These may be included in the kit.	12. Prevents contamination of the sterile equipment and the sterile field.
13. Place drape from catheterization kit between client's thighs, close to the perineum being careful not to touch nonsterile surfaces with gloves.	13. Provides a sterile field at the procedural site. Prevents accidental contamination from adjacent areas.
14. Place fenestrated drape over the client's perineal area with the labia visible through the opening, being careful not to touch nonsterile surfaces with gloves.	14. Provides a sterile field at the procedural site.

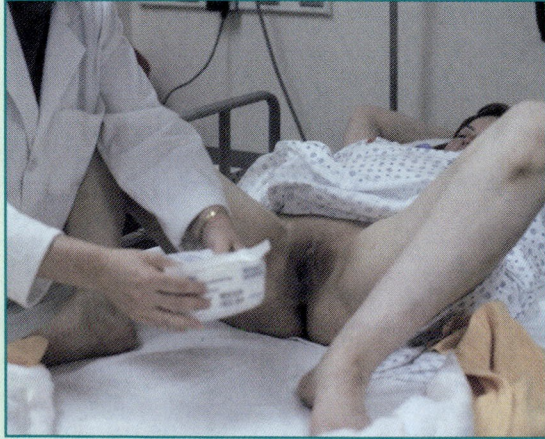

Figure 6-9-2 Position the client supine with legs spread.

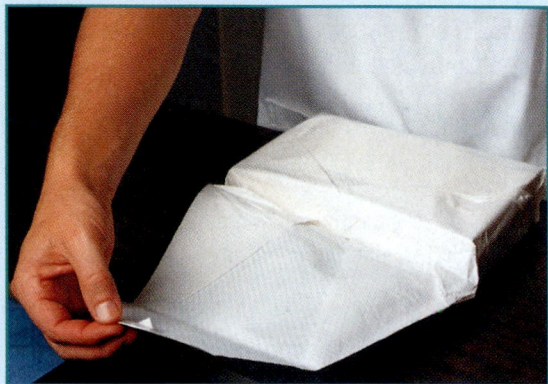

Figure 6-9-3 Touching only the corner, open the distal (top) flap away from your body.

continues

Action	Rationale

15. Open supplies:
    a. Open povidone-iodine or other antimicrobial solution and pour over cotton balls.
    b. Squeeze lubrication package onto sterile field.
	15. Maintains sterile technique and facilitates execution of the skill.

16. If inserting an indwelling catheter, test the patency of the catheter balloon. Attach the syringe filled with sterile water to the Luer-lock port of the catheter. Inflate the balloon by injecting the appropriate amount of fluid. Assess for leaks. Deflate the balloon. Keep water filled syringe attached to port.	**16.** Tests the patency of the retention balloon.
17. Attach the catheter to the urine drainage bag if it is not preconnected.	**17.** The catheter and drainage system may be preconnected; otherwise connect it before catheterization to avoid exposing the client to ascending infection from an open-ended catheter.
18. Generously coat the distal portion of the catheter with water-soluble, sterile lubricant and place it nearby on the sterile field (see Figure 6-9-4).	**18.** Facilitates insertion. Maintains sterile technique by keeping sterile field in sight of vision.
19. Gently spread the labia minora with the fingers of your nondominant hand and visualize the urinary meatus (see Figure 6-9-5).	**19.** Helps locate the meatus, so the catheter can be placed in the correct spot.
20. Holding the labia apart with your nondominant hand, use the forceps to pick up a cotton ball soaked in povidone-iodine, and cleanse the periurethral mucosa (see Figure 6-9-6). Use one downward stroke for each cotton ball and discard. Keep the labia separated with your nondominant hand until you insert the catheter.	**20.** Cleans the area and minimizes the risk of urinary tract infection by removing surface microorganisms.

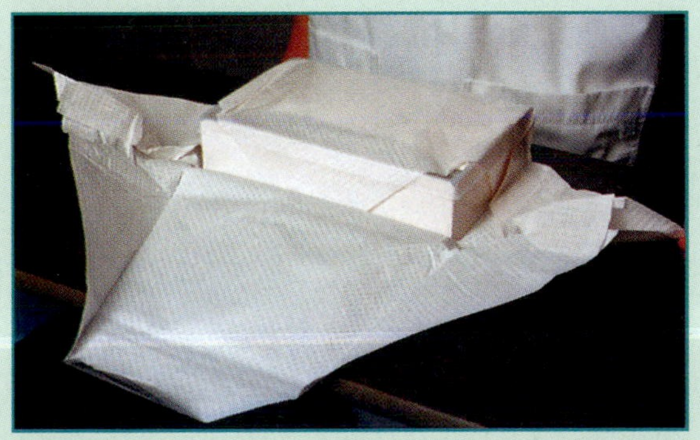

Figure 6-9-4 Carefully grasp the wrapper and open the right and left side of the package.

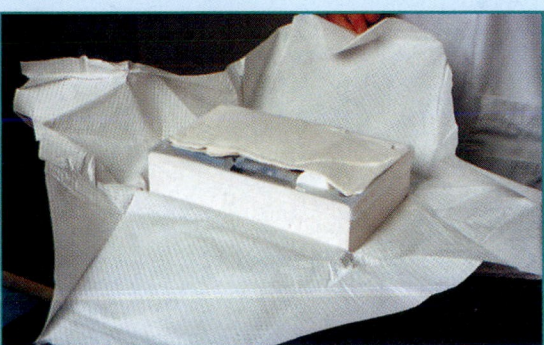

Figure 6-9-5 Open the proximal (closest) flap toward you. Avoid touching the flap or inside of the package with your hands or clothing.

continues

Action	Rationale

Performing Urinary Catheterization *continued*

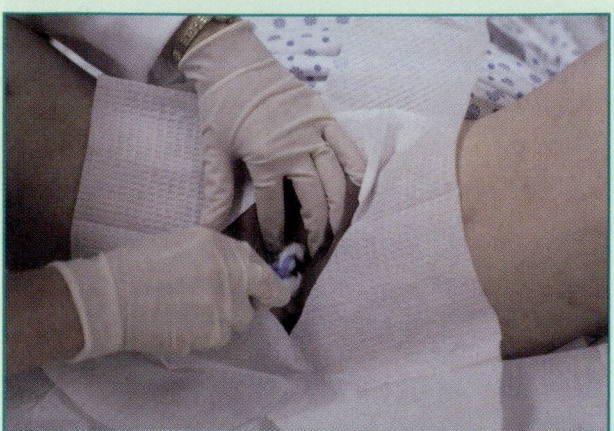

Figure 6-9-6 Using forceps, pick up a cotton ball soaked in povidone-iodine. Cleanse the periurethral mucosa.

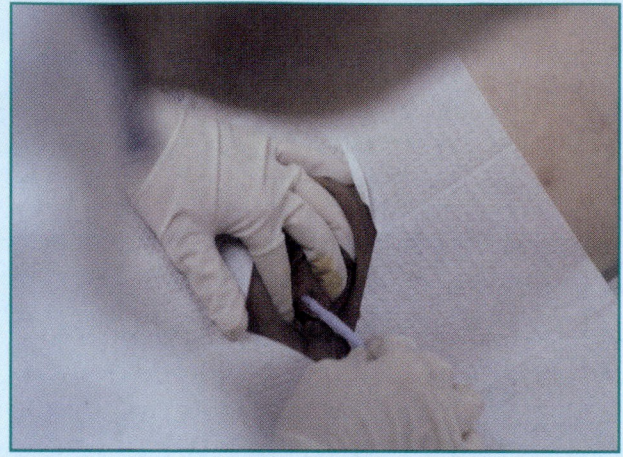

Figure 6-9-7 Steadily insert the catheter into the meatus.

21. Holding the catheter in the dominant hand, steadily insert the catheter into the meatus until urine is noted in the drainage bag or tubing (see Figure 6-9-7).

21. Provides a visual confirmation that the catheter tip is in the bladder.

22. If the catheter will be removed as soon as the client's bladder is empty, insert the catheter another inch and hold the catheter in place as the bladder drains.

22. The catheter needs to be inserted far enough to allow complete bladder drainage, but not so far as to possibly irritate the bladder, causing spasms.

23. If the catheter will be indwelling with a retention balloon, continue inserting another 1–3 inches.

23. Ensures adequate catheter insertion before retention balloon is inflated.

24. Inflate the retention balloon using manufacturer's recommendations or according to the health care provider's orders (see Figure 6-9-8).

24. Ensures retention of the balloon. Retention catheters are available with a variety of balloon sizes. Use a catheter with the appropriate size balloon.

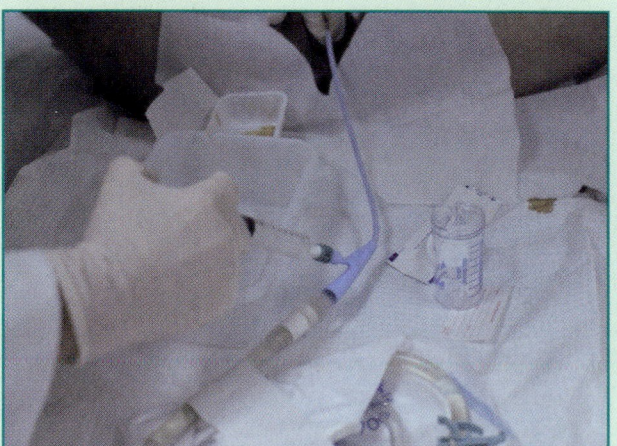

Figure 6-9-8 Inflate the retention balloon.

continues

Action	Rationale
25. Instruct the client to immediately report discomfort or pressure during balloon inflation; if pain occurs, discontinue the procedure, deflate the balloon, and insert the catheter farther into the bladder. If the client continues to complain of pain with balloon inflation, remove the catheter and notify the client's health care provider.	**25.** Pain or pressure indicates inflation of the balloon in the urethra; further insertion will prevent misplacement and further pain or bleeding.
26. Once the balloon has been inflated, gently pull the catheter until the retention balloon is resting snugly against the bladder neck (resistance will be felt when the balloon is properly seated).	**26.** Maximizes continuous bladder drainage and prevents urine leakage around the catheter.
27. Secure the catheter according to institutional policy. Securing it to the client's thigh is generally accepted. Be sure to leave enough slack so it will not pull on the bladder (see Figure 6-9-9).	**27.** Prevents excessive traction from the balloon rubbing against the bladder neck, inadvertent catheter removal, or urethral erosion.
28. Place the drainage bag below the level of the bladder. Do not let it rest on the floor. Make sure the tubing lies over, not under, the leg.	**28.** Maximizes continuous drainage of urine from the bladder.
29. Clean perineal area with soap and water.	**29.** Removes antiseptic solution to prevent skin irritation.
30. Dispose of equipment, remove gloves, and wash hands.	**30.** Prevents transfer of microorganisms.
31. Help client adjust position. Lower the bed.	**31.** Promotes client comfort and safety.
32. Assess and document the amount, color, odor, and quality of urine (see Figure 6-9-10).	**32.** Monitors urinary status.
33. Wash hands.	**33.** Reduces transmission of microorganisms.

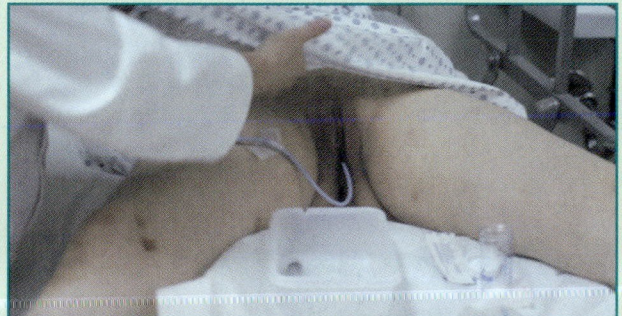

Figure 6-9-9 Tape the catheter to the client's thigh.

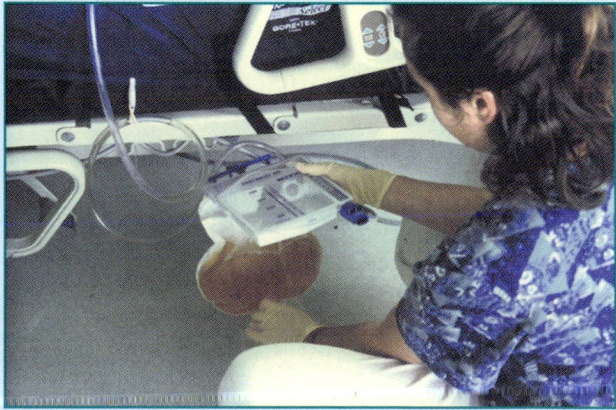

Figure 6-9-10 Monitor the urinary status. Assess and document the amount, color, and quality of urine.

▶ REAL WORLD ANECDOTES

Scenario 1

Entering a room to check a client, the nurse notes that the client's family is visiting. The client's husband has pulled a chair up close to the side of the bed and, not wanting to kick the catheter bag, has rehung the bag from the IV stand adjustment knob. The bag is higher than the bladder. The nurse lowers the bag and provides client and caregiver education about the need to keep the bag lower than the bladder. She documents the incident.

Scenario 2

The nurse caring for a client undergoing a catheter ablation procedure forgot to include the possibility that a retention catheter would be placed during the procedure. She returned to the client's room and informed the client, but preprocedure antianxiety medication and a sedative had already been given. The client woke up after 3 hours of conscious sedation with a retention catheter in place but could not remember what it was and why it was there.

▶ EVALUATION

- The catheter was inserted without pain, trauma, or injury to the client.
- The client's bladder was emptied without complication.
- The nurse maintained the sterility of the catheter during insertion.

▶ DOCUMENTATION

Nurses' Notes

- Record the time and date the catheter was inserted.
- Note the size and type of catheter used, including the size of the retention balloon and the amount of sterile water used to inflate the balloon.
- Record the client's response to the procedure and the amount, color, and quality of urine returned.

Document on appropriate flow sheet or electronic medical record (EMR).

Intake and Output Record

- Record the amount of urine returned.

▶ CRITICAL THINKING SKILL

Introduction

You should always ask for assistance when necessary.

Possible Scenario

A nurse is catheterizing a client in the emergency department to obtain a sterile urine sample as per the physician's request. She notes the perineal area is very swollen, and the client, who is obese, is restless. As this is a busy night shift, she does not seek assistance but attempts to insert the catheter. The nurse cannot clearly see the urinary meatus but has "some idea" where it is.

Possible Outcome

On her first and second attempts, the nurse inserts the catheter into the vagina. She has to stop the procedure twice and obtain a new catheter, thus prolonging the procedure and increasing its expense.

Prevention

This nurse needed to look carefully and be sure she knew where the meatus was. Sometimes it is very difficult to spot. She needed to seek assistance in positioning the client and/or locating the meatus.

▶ VARIATIONS

Geriatric Variations:
- *Geriatric clients may need help holding the position.*
- *Anatomic landmarks may be more difficult to visualize.*
- *It is important to clearly explain the procedure and check that the client understands.*

continues

▶ VARIATIONS *(continued)*

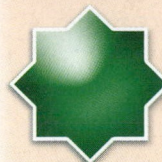

Pediatric Variations:
- When a catheter is used with a child or adolescent, provide simple explanations.
- Allow for privacy and respect the child's or adolescent's wishes regarding the presence of a parent during catheter insertion and care.
- Children or adolescents may be more tempted to pull or tug on the catheter. Children and adolescents may be more active in or out of bed, so the catheter must be taped securely to the thigh to prevent it from being pulled out.

Home Care Variation:
- Clients who practice long-term self-catheterization may use clean, instead of sterile, technique to catheterize themselves. Reinforce the need for good handwashing, cleaning of the catheter, and adequate lubrication of the catheter to reduce the frequency of infection and urethral trauma.

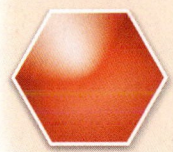

Long-Term Care Variation:
- Follow institutional policy regarding the long-term use and replacement schedule for an indwelling catheter..

▶ COMMON ERRORS

Possible Error:
The catheter is inserted into the vagina instead of the urethra.

Prevention:
Be sure to visually locate the urinary meatus before attempting to insert the catheter. In some women the meatus may be located very near the vagina. If unable to visualize the urinary meatus, gentle upward traction on the perineal floor may expose the meatus.

▶ NURSING TIPS

- If you miss and insert the catheter in the vagina, leave it there so you can use it as a landmark to find the meatus on the next try.
- Consider taping connections closed if you are concerned the client might become confused, pull them apart, and break the sterility of the closed-system drainage.
- If 700–800 mL of urine has drained right away, clamp the catheter for 20 minutes. Then unclamp and let urine flow. This helps prevent bladder spasms.
- Make sure a drainage system is in place prior to inserting the catheter to prevent the spill of urine.

- If the client is unable to tolerate lying supine with her legs spread, attempt to visualize the meatus with the client in the side-lying position.
- If you feel resistance, try gently twisting the catheter one-quarter turn.
- Up to twice the recommended volume of fluid may be inserted safely into the retention balloon, if needed.
- Be aware that a client with a history of sexual assault or trauma may be anxious or apprehensive about the procedure.
- The lithotomy position can be used for women with a history of knee or hip disease or surgery.

▶ **SPECIAL CONSIDERATIONS**

- Sometimes a cotton ball is placed at the opening of the vagina as a landmark to prevent inserting in the wrong pathway. Be sure to remove the cotton ball upon completion of the skill to prevent unnecessary infection.
- If client is in the menstrual cycle when being placed with a urinary catheter, perineal care should be administered daily to prevent urinary tract infection.
- Use latex-free gloves and catheters if the client has a history of latex allergy.

Routine Catheter Care

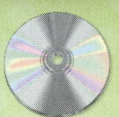

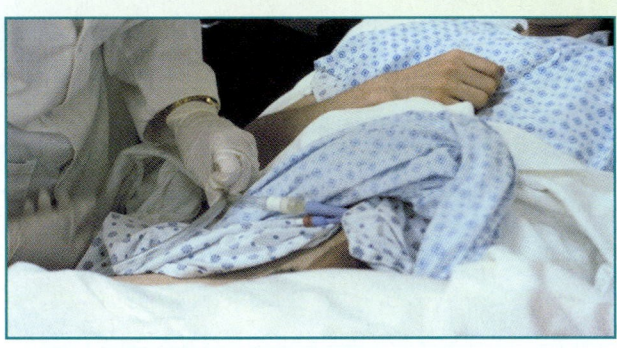

▶ OVERVIEW OF THE SKILL

An indwelling catheter is used to provide continuous drainage of urine from the bladder. The catheter, which is attached to a drainage bag, may be used for episodic or long-term urinary drainage. As the catheter is in the bladder through the urethra, bacteria may enter the urinary system; therefore, care must be taken to ensure that the surrounding area is clean to decrease contamination of the catheter by bacterial flora. Clients may be embarrassed or frightened by the catheter and related care and, therefore, require emotional support.

▶ ASSESSMENT

1. Assess catheter patency and urine color, consistency, and amount while performing the care **to determine if catheter and drainage system are functioning correctly.**
2. Determine the condition of the urinary meatus and perineal area **to monitor for redness, swelling, drainage, or signs of infection. Monitor vaginal discharge and diarrhea as microorganisms may migrate up the catheter and lead to urinary tract infections.**
3. Determine the client's emotional reaction and feelings related to the catheter. **This may prevent untoward reactions to the care and allow the nurse to help the client deal with some deeper emotional issues.**

▶ DIAGNOSIS

Risk for Infection

Risk for Impaired Skin Integrity

Risk for Disturbed Body Image

▶ PLANNING

Expected Outcomes:

1. The client will be free of signs and symptoms of urinary tract infection.
2. The client will understand the reason for the catheter and related cares.
3. The meatus and surrounding area will be clean and free of drainage.

Equipment Needed:

- Antiseptic solution, if indicated
- Sterile swabs
- Clean gloves
- Wash cloth, soap, and water

▶ CLIENT EDUCATION NEEDED:

1. Explain that catheter care is done to keep the catheter and the area surrounding it clean.
2. Teach the client not to pull on the catheter.
3. Teach that it is normal to feel the urge to void while a catheter is in place.

Estimated time to complete the skill:
10 minutes

IMPLEMENTATION—Action/Rationale

Action	Rationale
1. Wash hands.	1. Reduces the transmission of microorganisms.
2. Check institutional protocol or care plan.	2. Ensures proper procedure.
3. Identify client and explain procedure.	3. Prepares client.
4. Provide privacy.	4. Protects client dignity.
5. Place client in supine position and expose perineal area and catheter.	5. Allows for visualization of field. If unable to visualize the perineal area with the client supine, try placing the client in a side-lying position.
6. Put on clean gloves.	6. Reduces transmission of microorganisms.
7. Cleanse perineal area with soap and water	7. Soap has antibacterial qualities adequate to clean the area and will not usually irritate the skin or mucous membranes.
8. For a male client (see Figure 6-10-1): a. gently grasp the penis, retract foreskin (if present); b. using a circular motion, cleanse from the meatus toward the shaft; c. use a new section of the wash cloth for each cleansing; d. if there is drainage, use a non-irritating antiseptic solution on a cotton ball or cotton swab (see Figure 6-10-2); e. return foreskin to natural position.	8. Cleaning from most clean to least clean decreases the risk of urinary tract infections.

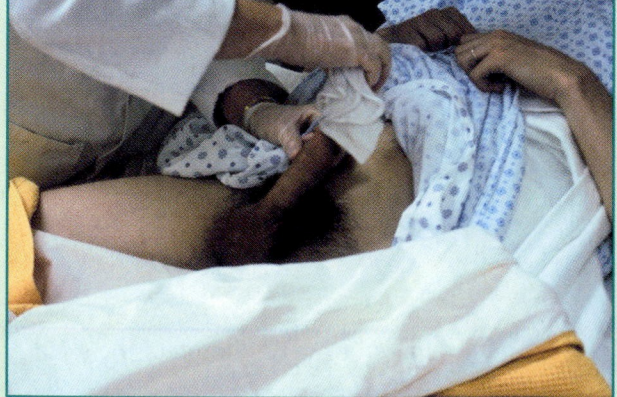

Figure 6-10-1   Using a washcloth, cleanse the penis and perineal area with soap and warm water.

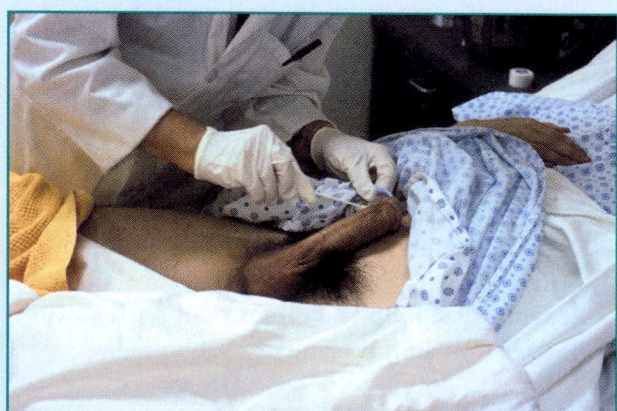

Figure 6-10-2   Cleanse the meatus. An antiseptic solution on a cotton ball or cotton swab may be used if there is excessive drainage.

continues

Action	Rationale

9. For a female client:
  a. separate the labia, cleans from front to back;
  b. begin in the center, then cleanse each side;
  c. use a new section of washcloth for each stroke;
  d. if there is drainage, use a nonirritating antiseptic solution on a cotton ball or cotton swab.
	9. Cleaning from most clean to least clean decreases the risk of urinary tract infections.

10. Cleanse the catheter. Hold the catheter tubing, taking care not to pull on the catheter, begin at the meatus and cleanse toward the end of the catheter (see Figure 6-10-3).	10. Cleaning from most clean to least clean decreases the risk of a urinary tract infection. Trauma to the urethra and bladder are decreased when the catheter tubing is not pulled.
11. Be sure to repeat catheter care anytime it becomes soiled with stool or other drainage (see Figure 6-10-4).	11. Prevents infection.
12. Rinse and dry genitals and perineum.	12. Soap can irritate the skin. Residual moisture provides an ideal environment for microorganisms to grow.
13. Place linen or cotton balls in proper receptacle for laundry or disposal.	13. Reduces transmission of microorganisms.
14. Remove gloves and wash hands.	14. Reduces transmission of microorganisms.

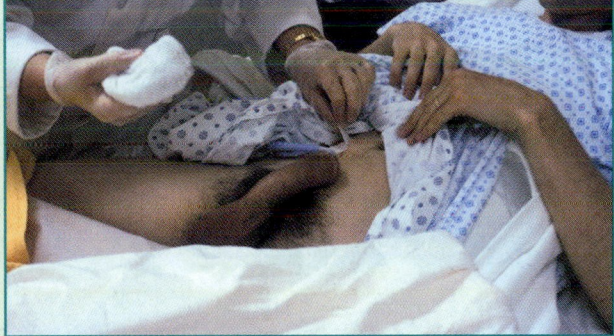

Figure 6-10-3   While cleaning, take care not to pull on the catheter.

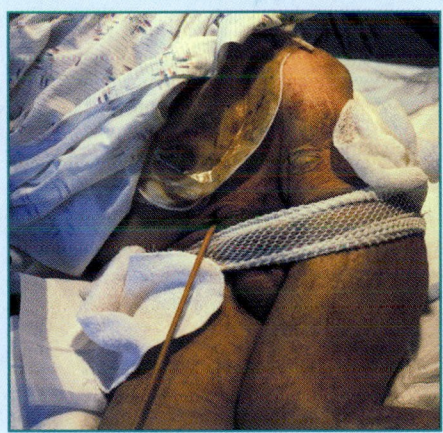

Figure 6-10-4   Meticulous catheter care is important, especially if the perineal area becomes soiled with stool or other drainage.

▶ REAL WORLD ANECDOTES

Mr. Qadri, a confused, long-term care client, required routine care of his indwelling catheter. Mr. Qadri's catheter care was performed irregularly because of his tendency to behave inappropriately during catheter care. Caregivers complained of being groped and pinched. All Mr. Qadri's caregivers met to work out a plan that would allow them to provide catheter care without the inappropriate behavior. The suggestions ranged from diverting Mr. Qadri's attention to restraining him during care. The plan of care that finally worked was to have one caregiver firmly hold Mr. Qadri's hands while talking to him and distracting his attention, while a second caregiver provided catheter and perineal care. As it required a second caregiver, Mr. Qadri's catheter care took a bit more staff time, but this method resulted in a happier staff and consistent catheter care for Mr. Qadri.

▶ EVALUATION

- The client is free of signs and symptoms of urinary tract infection.
- The client understands the reason for the catheter and related care.
- The meatus and surrounding area are clean, intact, and free of drainage.

▶ DOCUMENTATION

Nurses' Notes

- Document the time the procedure was performed and the condition of the area surrounding the catheter.

Document on appropriate flow sheet or electronic medical record (EMR).

▶ CRITICAL THINKING SKILL

Introduction

Some clients have contractures, casts, or surgical dressings that may impede catheter care.

Possible Scenario

A handicapped client who has been on long-term bed rest and has developed contractures has an indwelling catheter and needs care. Her legs are contracted together so that she cannot lie supine.

Possible Outcome

Client will not receive adequate care and may develop bacterial or yeast infection in the area surrounding the catheter.

Prevention

Position client on the side and perform care from behind the client with the assistance of two people to help support the client and allow access to the area surrounding the catheter so that proper care can be done.

▶ VARIATIONS

Geriatric Variation:
- *Contractures, arthritis, and other conditions causing stiffness and pain may make it difficult to position the client for the care.*

Pediatric Variation:
- *Use a doll to demonstrate care first. If the child has a history of abuse, you may need to involve the child's therapist.*

Home Care Variation:
- *Teach family members to provide catheter care.*

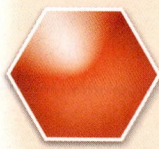

Long-Term Care Variation:
- *Clients with long-term indwelling catheters are at high risk of skin breakdown and infection. Catheter care must be performed regularly and thoroughly.*

► **COMMON ERRORS**

Possible Error:

Not cleaning from the most clean area out to the most dirty area and contaminating the catheter or the area surrounding it.

Prevention:

Clean area from the urinary meatus outward to avoid contamination.

► **NURSING TIPS**

- When doing catheter care do not allow urine to drain back into the bladder.

- If your institution's policy dictates the use of alcohol swabs to clean any part of the catheter system, remember to keep them away from the urinary meatus.

► **SPECIAL CONSIDERATIONS**

- *Most often soap and water are used for catheter care as clients may be allergic to povidone-iodine or other antiseptic solutions. Refer to institution policy for proper protocol and recommended solutions.*
- *If the client has local inflammation to the catheter, assess for latex allergy, and remove if positive history and reinsert a latex-free catheter.*
- *If the catheter slips out from the urethra, never reinsert the catheter. If the client still needs a catheter, see Skill 6-9.*

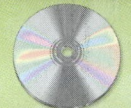

Obtaining a Urine Specimen from an Indwelling Catheter

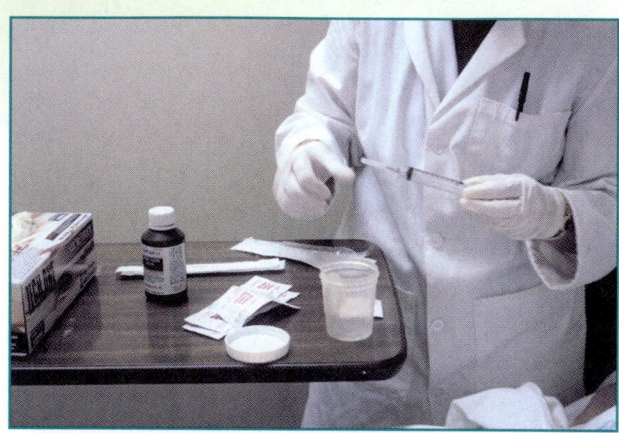

▶ OVERVIEW OF THE SKILL

Indwelling catheters are used frequently in acute care settings for episodic or continuous drainage of urine. Specimens may be required to evaluate urine content, such as electrolytes, dilution, hormones, glucose, or abnormal factors, or renal function. Bacteria can be identified in urine specimens to determine if the catheter needs to be removed or if antibiotic therapy is indicated. Catheter tubing is generally designed to allow for easy access to obtain specimens without disconnecting the catheter from the tubing. Careful technique should prevent contamination of the system, and, hence, risk for infection.

▶ ASSESSMENT

1. Identify the purpose of the urine test **to determine the amount of urine needed and the proper container to collect it in.**
2. Assess the client's understanding of the test **to determine amount of instruction needed.**
3. Identify the type of collecting tubing attached to the indwelling catheter **to determine whether you need to disconnect the catheter from the system or can obtain the specimen from a closed system.**

▶ DIAGNOSIS

Risk for Infection

▶ PLANNING

Expected Outcomes:

1. Client understands the reason for the specimen.
2. Specimen is obtained in the proper container in a timely manner.
3. Specimen will remain uncontaminated.

Equipment Needed (see Figure 6-11-1):

- Nonserrated clamp or rubber band
- Nonsterile gloves
- Syringe with needle (1-inch), 10-mL
- Specimen container, plastic bag, and labels
- Povidone-iodine swabs

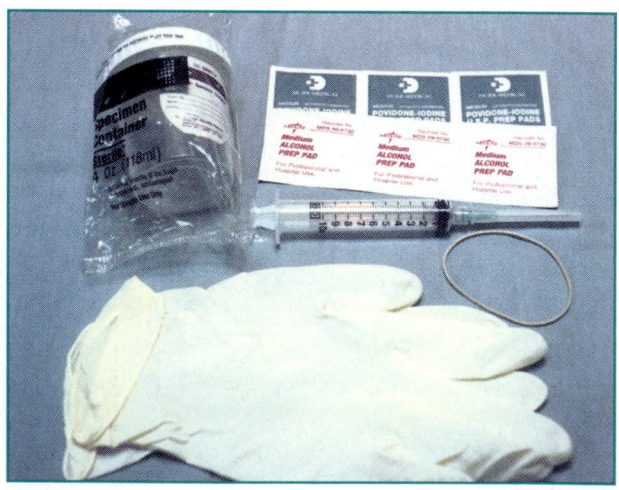

Figure 6-11-1 Specimen container, syringe, nonsterile gloves, and a rubber band are used to obtain a urine specimen from an indwelling catheter.

► **CLIENT EDUCATION NEEDED:**

1. Explain the reason for urine specimen and possible changes in therapy based on results of the test.
2. Explain steps of procedure so client knows what to expect.
3. Explain the reason for the test in terms the client will understand.

4. Make sure the client holds still during specimen collection to prevent contamination of specimen or injury to the client.

Estimated time to complete the skill: **10 minutes**

► **DELEGATION TIPS**

Obtaining a urine specimen from an indwelling catheter requires the skill and problem-solving ability of a nurse. This task cannot be delegated to ancillary personnel.

IMPLEMENTATION—Action/Rationale

Action	Rationale
1. Wash hands.	1. Reduces transmission of microorganisms.
2. Check health care provider's order.	2. Determines test and container needed for the specimen.
3. Explain procedure to the client and provide privacy.	3. Informs client and maintains client dignity.
4. Check for urine in the tubing.	4. Determines if there is sufficient urine in the collecting tubing for a specimen. Urine from the collection bag should not be used for sterile specimens.
5. If more urine is needed, clamp the tubing using a nonserrated clamp or a rubber band for 10 to 15 minutes (see Figure 6-11-2).	5. Collects 10 mL of urine, which is needed for most urinalyses.
6. Put on clean gloves.	6. Practices Standard Precautions.
7. Clean sample port with a povidone-iodine swab.	7. Prevents entrance of microorganisms into the system.
8. Insert sterile needle and syringe into the sample port or catheter at a 45-degree angle and withdraw 10 mL of urine (see Figure 6-11-3).	8. Obtains specimen with sufficient volume for most urine tests.
9. Put urine into sterile container and close tightly, taking care not to contaminate the lid of the container.	9. Prevents contamination of specimen and spill of urine.
10. Remove clamp and rearrange tubing avoiding dependent loops.	10. Re-establishes urine flow and drainage into the system.
11. Label specimen container, put it in a plastic bag, and send to the laboratory.	11. Ensures right test and controls transfer of pathogens.

continues

Action	Rationale

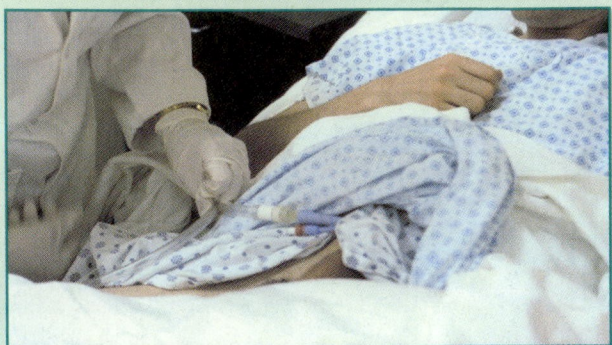

Figure 6-11-2   Clamp the tubing by folding it over and securing it with a rubber band to collect an adequate sample.

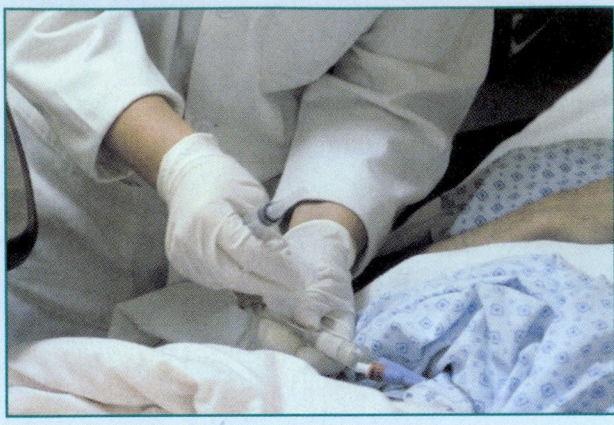

Figure 6-11-3   Cleanse the sample port and insert a sterile needle and syringe into the sample port.

12. Remove gloves and wash hands.

12. Reduces transmission of microorganisms.

▶ REAL WORLD ANECDOTES

During change of shift report, Doris the oncoming nurse, noted that Mr. Clovis's urinalysis laboratory requisition had not been sent. When Doris asked Olga, who was completing her shift, about the urinalysis, Olga realized that she had clamped Mr. Clovis's catheter several hours earlier and then forgotten to return and collect a specimen. When Doris and Olga arrived in Mr. Clovis's room they found him to be quite uncomfortable with a distended bladder. After 30 minutes, Doris reassessed Mr. Clovis before clamping the catheter and obtaining the urine specimen.

▶ EVALUATION

- Client understands the reason for the specimen.
- Specimen was obtained in the proper container in a timely manner.
- Specimen remained uncontaminated.

▶ DOCUMENTATION

Nurses' Notes

- Document the date and time the specimen was sent to the laboratory.
- Note the test(s) ordered.
- Document the date, time, client name and room number, and the test(s) ordered on the laboratory requisition.

Document on appropriate flow sheet or electronic medical record (EMR).

Intake and Output Record

- Record the amount of urine collected for the specimen.

▶ CRITICAL THINKING SKILL

Introduction

This is generally a simple procedure without difficulty. Clients with low urine volume may present a challenge.

Possible Scenario

You are running late, and you follow the correct procedure for obtaining a specimen. No urine is obtained when withdrawing from the port.

Possible Outcome

The laboratory is unable to perform the test and the procedure must be repeated.

Prevention

Make sure the client has had adequate fluid intake and is having sufficient urinary flow before clamping the tubing. You may need to leave the tubing clamped for a longer period of time to obtain the specimen, but be sure to check the client every 15 minutes.

▶ VARIATIONS

Geriatric Variation:
- *The elderly are particularly prone to urinary tract infections and sepsis. Avoid prolonged use of indwelling catheters and keep the system closed.*

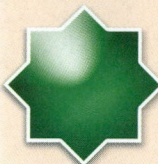

Pediatric Variations:
- *Enlist the parent's help, if needed.*
- *Use pictures or dolls to explain the procedure to the child.*
- *Before the child sees the syringe and needle, reassure the child that he or she will not be poked with the needle. The simple sight of a needle may frighten the child too much to listen to instructions and reassurances.*

Home Care Variations:
- *The catheter may be a suprapubic catheter at home. Care will have to be taken not to break the sterility of the system. Take precautions to prevent contamination.*
- *Take extra care to avoid needle-stick injuries when working in an unfamiliar home environment, especially when using a needle at a crowded bedside.*

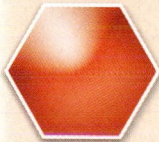

Long-Term Care Variation:
- *Catheters can crack and break down over the long-term. If drawing samples frequently, vary the sample site to prevent breakdown of the rubber.*

▶ COMMON ERRORS

Possible Error:
The nurse forgets to check on the client in 15 minutes and leaves the catheter clamped.

Prevention:
Write a note to yourself, reminding you to check the client in 15 minutes. If the client is alert, ask client to turn on the call light in 15 minutes.

▶ NURSING TIPS

- Open the urine container before starting to aspirate the urine from the port so that you can inject it into the container without having to cap the needle.

- Make sure not to contaminate the inside of the container lid if you are collecting urine for culture and sensitivity.
- Be sure to have adequate help with the confused or combative client so you are able to obtain the specimen safely.

▶ **SPECIAL CONSIDERATIONS**

- After collecting the specimen from an indwelling catheter, observe for any sign of leakage from the catheter tubing. Make sure that the catheter is patent and not clamped or folded from the sample collecting procedure.
- The collected sample should be sent to the laboratory as soon as possible. When this is not possible, a sample can be stored up to 2 hours in a refrigerated environment.

Irrigating a Urinary Catheter

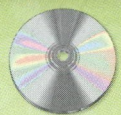

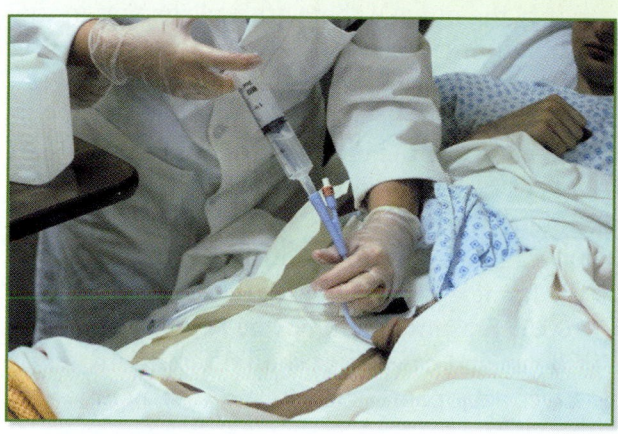

▶ OVERVIEW OF THE SKILL

Open intermittent irrigation of a urinary catheter is generally done for one of two reasons: either to instill medication into the bladder or to irrigate the catheter itself, which may be blocked by either blood clots or urinary sediment. This irrigation is referred to as "open" because the closed bladder drainage system is opened where the drainage tubing inserts into the urinary catheter; the catheter is generally indwelling. Maintaining sterility of the system is paramount in this type of irrigation.

▶ ASSESSMENT

1. Identify the following items in the health care provider's orders: type of irrigation (bladder or catheter); purpose of the irrigation; type and amount of solution to irrigate with; any premedication ordered; and any other details of the order. **This allows the nurse to anticipate responses to the procedure and assess pertinent features of the client's condition.**
2. Assess the condition of the client as it relates to the procedure: patency of the catheter, characteristics of urinary drainage, and total intake and output status of the client. **This establishes a baseline of the client's condition as it relates to elimination and in the case of prn catheterization, which may indicate whether there is a need for the procedure.**
3. Assess for current pain or bladder spasms. **Even when medication is not specifically ordered,**

medicating for pain before the procedure can increase client comfort, and if irrigation does not relieve spasms, the client may need medication afterward.
4. Assess client's knowledge about the procedure **to determine need for education and reduce anxiety about the procedure.**
5. If this is a repeat of the procedure, read the charting from previous nurses. **This provides the nurse with a history of how this client tolerates the procedure and of any teaching done.**

▶ DIAGNOSIS

Acute Pain

Impaired Urinary Elimination

Risk for Infection

Urinary Retention

▶ PLANNING

Expected Outcomes:

1. Urinary catheter will be patent.
2. Sediment/blood clots will be passed through the catheter.
3. Bladder will be free of sources of local irritation.
4. Urinary pH will be lowered to a more acidic state.

Equipment Needed (see Figure 6-12-1):

- Sterile gloves
- Clean gloves
- Sterile cover for the end of the drainage tubing

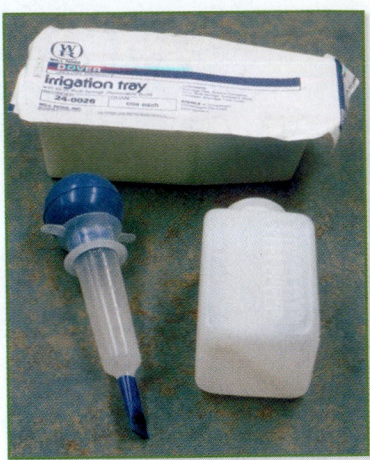

Figure 6-12-1 Irrigation kit

- Disposable, water-resistant drape or towel
- Sterile Asepto or Toomey syringe with container for irrigant
- Sterile antiseptic swabs
- Sterile irrigating solution (labeled with date and time of opening, if opened)

▶ **CLIENT EDUCATION NEEDED:**

1. Carefully explain the purpose of the procedure and the steps of the procedure as it has been ordered.
2. Explain to the client that the nurse must be notified of any unusual pain or pressure as the procedure is performed.

3. If pain medications are needed, carefully explain the role of pain medication in easing discomfort with the procedure.
4. Irrigation setups (syringes and containers) can be washed in very hot water or boiled for 20 minutes if sterility is desired to reduce costs for the home care client.
5. Teach clients who perform the irrigation to notify the nurse if there are any changes in the amount or character of returns when irrigating, as it can indicate bladder or systemic changes. Clients should be able to identify the usual color and clarity of the urine and should realize that mucus or sediment can be found in urine.
6. Be sure that caretakers are able to correctly take a temperature, and instruct them to call the home care nurse for oral temperatures over 100.5° F, as infection may be beginning.
7. Clients and caretakers should report any severe lower back pain, as it may indicate a kidney infection.

Estimated time to complete the skill: **15–20 minutes**

▶ **DELEGATION TIPS**

The skill of irrigating a urinary catheter cannot be delegated, as it requires the skills and problem-solving abilities of a nurse.

IMPLEMENTATION—Action/Rationale

Action	Rationale
1. Verify the need for bladder or catheter irrigation.	1. Ensures that procedure is being applied correctly, to reduce unnecessary opening of the system and risk of infection.
2. For prn catheter irrigation, palpate for full bladder and check current output against previous totals.	2. If irrigation is on a prn basis, it may not be needed currently.
3. Verify health care provider's orders for type of irrigation and irrigant as well as amount.	3. Ensures accuracy in the provision of treatment.
4. If repeat procedure, read previous documentation in the record.	4. Establishes prior client responses to prior teaching done by staff.

continues

Action	Rationale
5. Assemble all supplies.	**5.** Having all supplies in room enables the nurse to maintain sterility of supplies once they are opened and laid out.
6. Premedicate client if ordered or needed.	**6.** Increases comfort for the procedure.
7. Provide teaching to the client as needed, based on what client already knows.	**7.** Knowledge will increase client cooperation and decrease anxiety.
8. Assist the client to a dorsal recumbent position.	**8.** Facilitates the flow of irrigant into the bladder.
9. Wash your hands.	**9.** Decreases transmission of microorganisms.
10. Provide for client privacy with a closed door or curtain.	**10.** Decreases client anxiety.
11. Apply clean gloves and empty the collection bag of urine.	**11.** Starting with an empty collection bag makes it easier to identify clots or sediment passed as a result of irrigation.
12. Remove gloves and wash hands.	**12.** Reduces the transmission of microorganisms.
13. Expose the indwelling catheter and place the water resistant drape underneath it (see Figures 6-12-2 and 6-12-3).	**13.** Protects the bedclothes and client from urine and body fluids.
14. Open the sterile cover for drainage tube.	**14.** Enables nurse to maintain sterility of gloves once they are applied.
15. Open the end of the antiseptic swab package, exposing the swab sticks.	**15.** Enables nurse to maintain sterility of gloves once they are applied.
16. Open the sterile syringe and container. Apply sterile glove to nondominant hand. Use gloved hand to stand container up. Use dominant hand (ungloved) and add 100–200 mL of sterile irrigation solution to container without touching the inside of the receptacle.	**16.** Maintains sterility of the procedure.

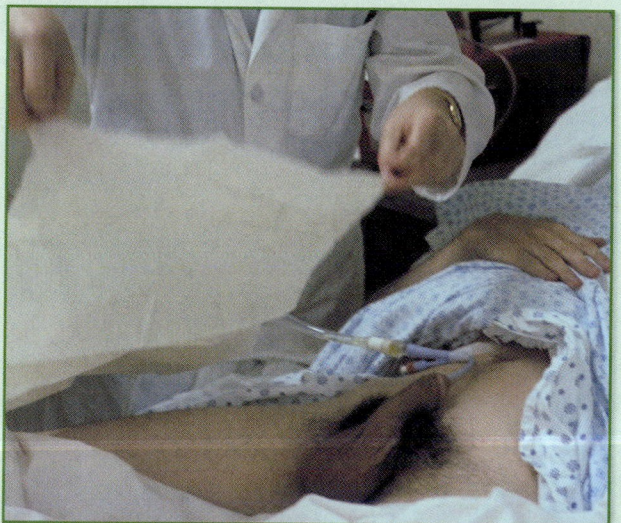

Figure 6-12-2   Expose the retention catheter.

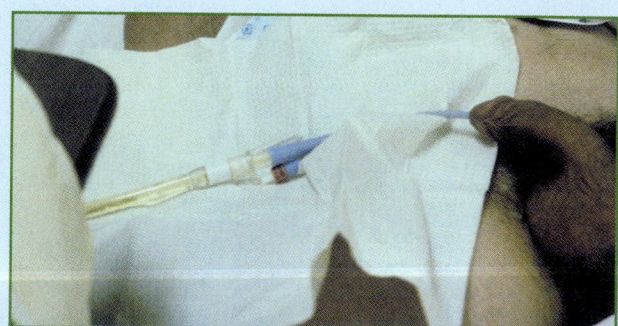

Figure 6-12-3   Place a water-resistant drape under the retention catheter.

continues

Action	Rationale
17. Apply the sterile gloves to dominant hand.	**17.** Maintains sterility of the procedure.
18. Using the antiseptic swab sticks, disinfect the connection between the catheter and the drainage tubing.	**18.** Minimizes risk of contaminating the system.
19. After the disinfectant dries, loosen the ends of the connection.	**19.** Enables the nurse to open the connection without accidentally contaminating either end.
20. Grasp the catheter and tubing 1 to 2 inches from their ends, with catheter in the nondominant hand.	**20.** Maintains sterility of the procedure and allows the nurse to be positioned to use the dominant hand for the syringe.
21. Fold the catheter to pinch it closed between the palm and last three fingers; use the thumb and first finger to hold the sterile cap for the drainage tube.	**21.** Allows for one nurse to handle all equipment simultaneously, thus maintaining sterility.
22. Separate the catheter and tube, covering the tube tightly with the sterile cap.	**22.** Maintains sterility of equipment.
23. Fill the syringe with 30 mL for catheter irrigation, 60 mL for bladder irrigation. Insert the tip of the syringe into the catheter and gently instill the solution into the catheter (see Figures 6-12-4 and 6-12-5).	**23.** Catheter can be irrigated with 30 mL of solution, minimizing bladder discomfort, while irrigating a bladder takes 60 mL.
24. Clamp catheter if ordered (medicated solution). If not clamped, irrigant may be released into a collection container or aspirated back into the syringe (see Figure 6-12-6).	**24.** Fine sediment or clear irrigant with medication can run freely; material with more solids (sediment or clots) may need gentle aspiration.
25. If the bladder or catheter is being irrigated to clear solid material, repeat irrigation until return is clear.	**25.** Clearing the catheter completely in this irrigation means a lower total number of irrigations and less opening of the system, thus decreasing the risk of infection.

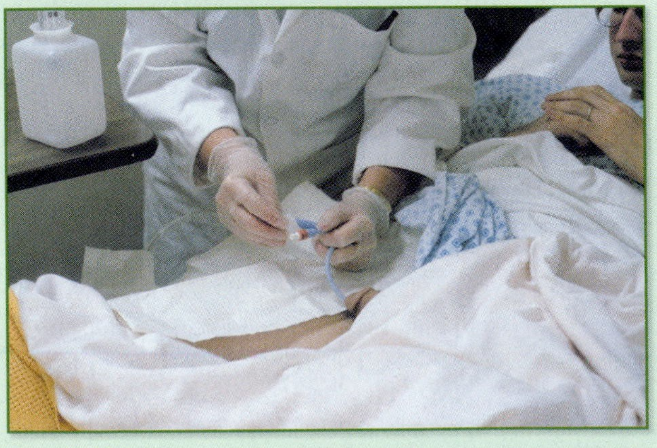

Figure 6-12-4 Separate the catheter and tube.

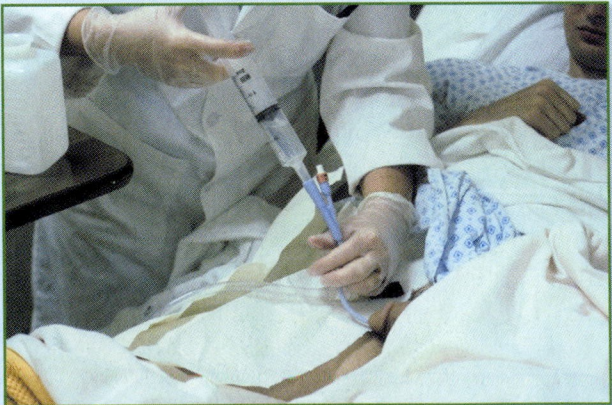

Figure 6-12-5 Insert the tip of the syringe into the catheter and gently instill the solution.

continues

Action	Rationale

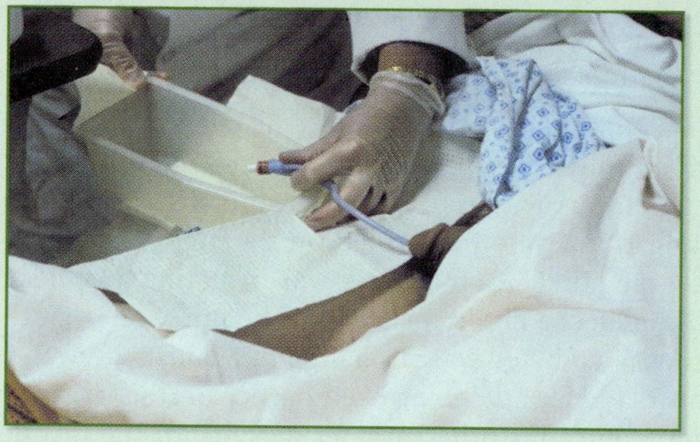

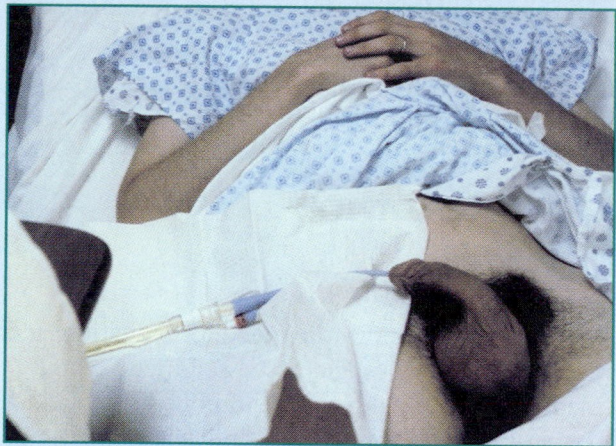

Figure 6-12-6 Irrigant is released into a collection container.

Figure 6-12-7 Reconnect the tubing to the catheter.

26. Reconnect system dispose of equipment and remove sterile gloves. Wash your hands (see Figure 6-12-7).

26. Maintains sterility of system and reduces transmission of microorganisms.

27. When irrigation is finished, record type of returns and total amount of irrigation fluid used.

27. This information can be compared to evaluate status of the urinary tract and catheter. A catheter that is being frequently irrigated for sediment, for instance, may need to be changed, or medications may need to be adjusted.

28. Monitor client for pain, urine color and clarity, any solid material passed, and total intake and output.

28. Monitoring output after irrigation evaluates the efficacy of the treatment.

29. Wash hands.

29. Reduces the transmission of microorganisms.

▶ REAL WORLD ANECDOTES

Deciding to use open or closed irrigation for post-TURP (transurethral resection of the prostate) clients is a matter of physician preference. A TURP client whose physician preferred open prn irrigation was cared for on the 7:00 a.m. to 3:30 p.m. shift by an agency nurse unfamiliar with the care of TURP clients using open irrigation. When the 3:00 p.m. to 11:30 p.m. nurse inquired about when this client had last been irrigated, the day nurse said, "Oh, I didn't want to open the system, so the last irrigation was about 10:00 a.m., when the charge nurse did it for me." When the evening nurse went in, the bladder was full and the output was scanty. This client needed 45 minutes of irrigation to remove an amount equal to approximately three 60-mL syringes full of blood clots as well as medication for pain. This placed the client at risk for bladder rupture or kidney infection as well as causing the client a great deal of pain.

► EVALUATION

- Urinary catheter remains patent.
- Any sediment/blood clots were passed through the catheter.
- Bladder is free of local irritation.
- Urinary pH was more acidic.

► DOCUMENTATION

Nurses' Notes

Document:

- Any assessment indicating need for irrigation, such as decreased output, increased sediment, clots, bladder spasms/pain, or palpation of a full bladder
- Type of irrigant and amount in each instillation
- Amount and quality of returns (returns often include urine trapped in the bladder)
- Any medication given before or after the procedure and response to same
- Urine output, color, and clarity and any solids passed 30–60 minutes after procedure
- Client response, especially changes in pain, spasms, or discomfort

Document on appropriate flow sheet or electronic medical record (EMR).

Medication Administration Record

Document:

- Type of irrigant, if medicated, and amount in each instillation
- Any medication given before or after the procedure

Intake and Output Record

Document:

- Amount of urine emptied from the drainage bag before and after the procedure
- Amount of irrigant instilled

► CRITICAL THINKING SKILL

Introduction

Never try to force irrigation of any tube.

Possible Scenario

In a long-term care facility, all clients with long-term indwelling catheters had orders for a daily catheter irrigation to prevent catheter blockage. The irrigations were performed on the night shift by the charge nurse. As the nurse was irrigating the client's catheter, she noted resistance. The nurse felt that the client's catheter was probably up against the wall of his bladder and she pressed harder on the irrigation syringe to push the catheter away from the bladder wall. As she did this, the client began to complain of severe abdominal pain. The nurse stopped irrigating the catheter to assess the client's condition. The nurse noted that the catheter was not being held in place by the balloon and seemed to be partially dislodged.

Possible Outcome

The client continued to complain of severe abdominal pain and began to be pale and diaphoretic. His abdomen was swollen and hard. The nurse notified the client's physician regarding his change in condition. The physician ordered the client to be transported to the hospital. After being admitted to the hospital, it was determined that the client's prostate had been traumatized by the force of the nurse's irrigation and he was bleeding internally.

Prevention

Never try to force irrigation of any tube. If the tube does not irrigate smoothly, especially if this is a change from previous experience, stop and assess the situation. If you cannot determine the cause of the difficulty, ask for another opinion. Do not force the irrigant into the bladder.

► VARIATIONS

Geriatric Variations:
- *Geriatric clients are most likely to have poor oral intakes; assess intake and output carefully, especially if the bladder is not palpable, before deciding to irrigate.*
- *Be very slow and clear about discussing the procedure with older clients to facilitate their understanding of what will be done. Bring another nurse if the older client is confused.*
- *Use smaller volumes to irrigate as bladder capacity and sphincter tone are decreased.*

continues

▶ VARIATIONS *(continued)*

Pediatric Variations:
- *Use very small volumes, as children's bladders are smaller than adults.*
- *Use plain language that young children can understand ("pee," not urinate, for instance). A demonstration doll is useful to explain the procedure to young children.*

Home Care Variations:
- *Irrigation setups (syringes and containers) can be washed in very hot water and boiled for 20 minutes if sterility is desired to reduce costs for the home care client.*
- *The person performing the irrigation must notify the nurse if there are any changes in the amount or character of returns when irrigating, as they can indicate bladder or systemic changes.*
- *Caretakers must be able to correctly take a temperature and should call the home care nurse for temperatures over 100.5° F, as infection may be beginning.*
- *Any severe lower back pain should be reported, as it may indicate a kidney infection.*

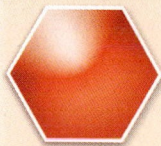

Long-Term Care Variations:
- *Agitation in the elderly can be associated with bladder pressure, so irrigation may help open the catheter.*
- *Another possible cause of agitation in the elderly can be infection, which may have resulted from poor technique.*
- *Remember to offer fluids that the client likes to facilitate proper intake; do not use irrigation as a substitute for proper hydration.*

▶ COMMON ERRORS

Possible Error:
The tip of the irrigation syringe becomes contaminated.

Prevention:
Have all equipment at bedside before exposing the tip of the syringe. Drape the area properly. Never leave client unattended with the setup. Ask for the help of another nurse, in the form of an extra pair of hands, if you cannot handle the catheter, tubing, and syringe without contaminating them. If the syringe has not touched the irrigant, you need a sterile syringe. Call the desk to ask someone to bring it to you, so the rest of the setup does not become contaminated. Have them open the package so you can remove it and maintain sterility.

▶ NURSING TIPS

- If the client has a surgically inserted suprapubic catheter, you may need to use a syringe with a smaller tip to irrigate it. Match the tip of the syringe to the size of the opening of the catheter.
- If a bladder has been surgically repaired, irrigate with 10 mL of solution very gently to avoid disturbing sutures.
- Tell the client that he or she may feel pressure when irrigation begins; if the client complains, cease instilling irrigant, as client's bladder may be full.
- Confused or agitated clients may become increasingly agitated as bladder fills; use the behavior as an indicator to stop instilling fluid.

► **SPECIAL CONSIDERATIONS**

- *Difficulties when irrigating a urinary catheter often happen because of a blood clot obstructing the lumen opening of the catheter. The clot may be removed with "pull back pressure" by gently aspirating the drainage from the catheter.*
- *A client may experience bladder spasms during catheter irrigation. If spasms persist, notify the health care provider. A heating pad or antispasmodic medication may be prescribed.*

Irrigating the Bladder Using a Closed-System Catheter

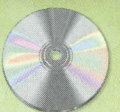

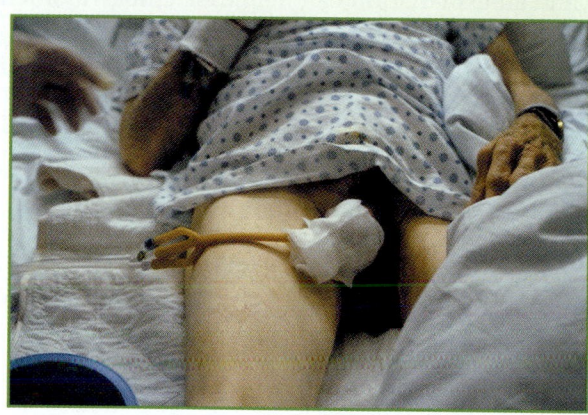

▶ OVERVIEW OF THE SKILL

Surgical procedures such as prostate resections and bladder surgery or traumatic injury may require frequent or continuous bladder irrigation. To prevent the potential introduction of infectious organisms and as a practical matter, open bladder irrigation is not used in these cases. A closed bladder irrigation system is preferable under these circumstances. Closed bladder irrigation may be used to instill medication, encourage hemostasis, or flush clots and debris out of the catheter and bladder.

A three-way catheter is used for closed bladder irrigation. If the client will require closed irrigation following surgery, the surgeon often places the three-way catheter during the operation. If the decision to perform closed bladder irrigation is made after a standard retention catheter has been placed, a Y adapter can be used for intermittent irrigation. If continuous irrigation is ordered, a three-way catheter must be placed. A standard catheter has two ports: one for inflation of the retention balloon and one for urine drainage. A three-way catheter has three ports: one for inflation of the retention balloon, one for urine drainage, and one for instilling irrigant.

As with open bladder irrigation, closed bladder irrigation is a sterile procedure. The irrigant, tubing, and drainage systems must be maintained as a closed sterile system to decrease the risk of infection. Because of the risk of blockage from clots and debris, the system must also be monitored closely for equal amounts of irrigant instilled and irrigant returned.

▶ ASSESSMENT

1. Assess the client for bladder distention or complaints of fullness or discomfort **to assess the patency of the drainage system.**
2. Assess the drainage system for equal or larger amounts of drainage versus infused irrigant **to assess the patency of the system.**
3. Assess the color, consistency, and clarity of the bladder drainage as well as noting any clots or debris present **to assess the effectiveness of the irrigation.**

▶ DIAGNOSIS

Acute Pain

Risk for Infection

Impaired Urinary Elimination

Urinary Retention

▶ PLANNING

Expected Outcomes:

1. The client will not exhibit signs or symptoms of bladder or urinary tract infection.
2. The client will not experience pain or discomfort as a result of the bladder irrigation.
3. The catheter will remain patent, and the client's bladder will not be distended.

Equipment Needed (see Figure 6-13-1):

- Three-way indwelling catheter or Y adapter
- IV pole

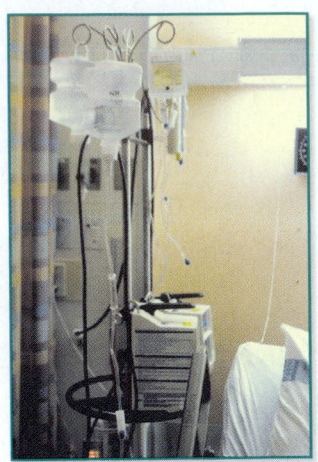

Figure 6-13-1 IV pole, irrigating solution, and irrigation tubing are used to irrigate the bladder using a closed-system catheter.

- Ordered irrigation solution
- Sterile gloves
- Closed-irrigation tubing

- Large urine collection bag
- Antiseptic swabs

▶ **CLIENT EDUCATION NEEDED:**

1. Explain the procedure to the client and the reason it is being performed. This can be an embarrassing procedure because of the area being irrigated, and an explanation can help ease embarrassment.
2. Teach the client the signs and symptoms of bladder distention. Have client notify a nurse if any of these signs and symptoms are noted.
3. Explain to the client the reason for the bladder irrigation and the need to assess for bladder distention or bleeding around the meatus.

Estimated time to complete the skill:
10 minutes

▶ **DELEGATION TIPS**

This skill cannot be delegated. Bladder irrigation using a closed-system catheter requires the skills of a nurse.

IMPLEMENTATION—Action/Rationale

Action	Rationale
Intermittent Bladder Irrigation Using a Standard Retention Catheter and a Y Adapter	
1. Wash hands.	1. Prevents the spread of microorganisms.
2. Close privacy curtain or door.	2. Provides privacy.
3. Hang the prescribed irrigation solution from an IV pole.	3. Different solutions may be ordered depending on the results the health care provider desires. Bladder irrigant is generally packaged in 2,000- to 4,000-mL bottles.
4. Insert the clamped irrigation tubing into the bottle of irrigant and prime the tubing with fluid, expelling all air and reclamping the tube.	4. Prevents introduction of air into the bladder.
5. Prepare sterile antiseptic swabs and sterile Y connector, if one will be used.	5. Prevents contamination of sterile gloves and field.
6. Apply sterile gloves.	6. Minimizes the client's risk of infection when connecting the irrigant to the catheter and drainage system.

continues

Action	Rationale
7. Clamp the urinary catheter.	7. Prevents urine leakage onto the bed linens.
8. Unhook the drainage bag from the retention catheter.	8. Allows the Y adapter to be inserted into the system.
9. While holding the drainage tubing and the drainage port of the catheter in your nondominant hand, cleanse both the tubing and the port with antiseptic swabs.	9. Reduces risk of contamination and infections.
10. Connect one port of the Y connector to the drainage port of the retention catheter.	10. Provides a bifurcation for irrigant to instill as well as urine to drain.
11. Connect another port of the Y adapter to the drainage tubing and bag.	11. Collects the urine and drained irrigant. This may be the established urine collection bag or a new, sterile bag that is large enough to hold the increased volume of drainage.
12. Attach the third port of the Y adapter to the irrigant tubing.	12. Instills the irrigant into the closed system.
13. Unclamp the urinary catheter and establish that urine is draining through the catheter into the drainage bag.	13. If the urine does not flow freely after unclamping, the catheter may have become clogged with a clot or debris. Notify the client's health care provider of the lack of urine drainage.
14. To irrigate the catheter and bladder, clamp the drainage tubing distal to the Y adapter.	14. Prevents the irrigant from by-passing the bladder and flowing directly into the drainage bag.
15. Instill the prescribed amount of irrigant.	15. The bladder normally feels full when it contains approximately 300 cc of urine. If a prescribed amount of irrigant was not ordered, do not instill more than 150 cc of irrigant. If the client has undergone bladder surgery, do not instill irrigant without knowing the specific amount ordered.
16. Clamp the irrigant tubing (see Figure 6-13-2).	16. Prevents further instillation of irrigant.
17. If the health care provider has ordered the irrigant to remain in the bladder for a measured length of time, wait the prescribed length of time.	17. Some irrigation solutions contain medication and are meant to remain in contact with the bladder wall for a prescribed length of time.
18. Unclamp the drainage tubing and monitor the drainage as it flows into the drainage bag.	18. Assess the drainage for volume, color, clarity, and the presence of any clots or debris.

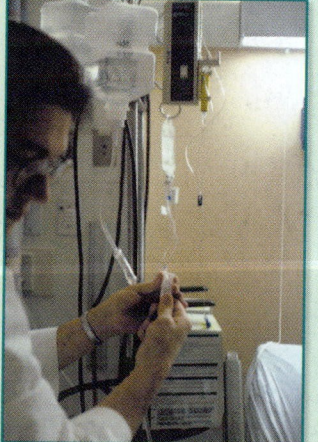

Figure 6-13-2 Clamp the irrigant tubing.

continues

Action	Rationale
Closed Bladder Irrigation Using a Three-Way Catheter	
19. Wash hands.	19. Reduces the transmission of microorganisms.
20. Close privacy curtain or door.	20. Provides privacy.
21. Explain the procedure to the client. Answer questions and provide support.	21. Reduces anxiety and uncertainty associated with the procedure.
22. Hang the prescribed irrigation solution from an IV pole.	22. Different solutions may be ordered depending on the results desired. Bladder irrigant is generally packaged in 2,000- to 4,000-mL bottles.
23. Insert the clamped irrigation tubing into the bottle of irrigant and prime the tubing with fluid, expelling all air and reclamping the tube (see Figure 6-13-3).	23. Prevents introduction of air into the bladder.
24. Prepare sterile antiseptic swabs and any other sterile equipment needed.	24. Prevents contamination of sterile gloves and field.
25. Apply sterile gloves (see Figure 6-13-4).	25. Minimizes the client's risk of infection when connecting the irrigant to the catheter and drainage system.
26. Clamp the urinary catheter.	26. Prevents leakage of urine onto the bedclothes.
27. Remove the cap from the irrigation port of the three-way catheter (see Figure 6-13-5).	27. Allows access for the irrigant tubing.

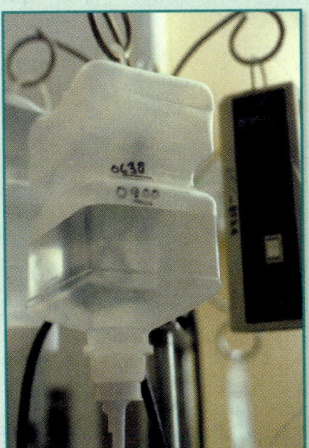

Figure 6-13-3 Insert the clamped irrigation tubing into the bottle of irrigant.

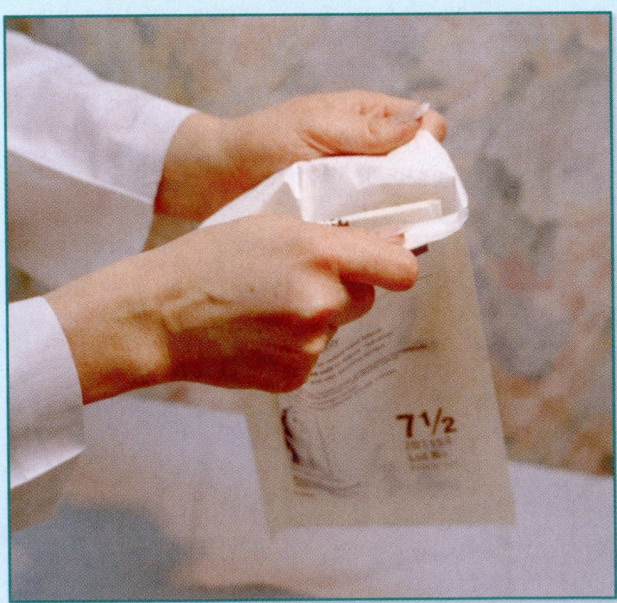

Figure 6-13-4 Apply sterile gloves.

continues

Action	Rationale

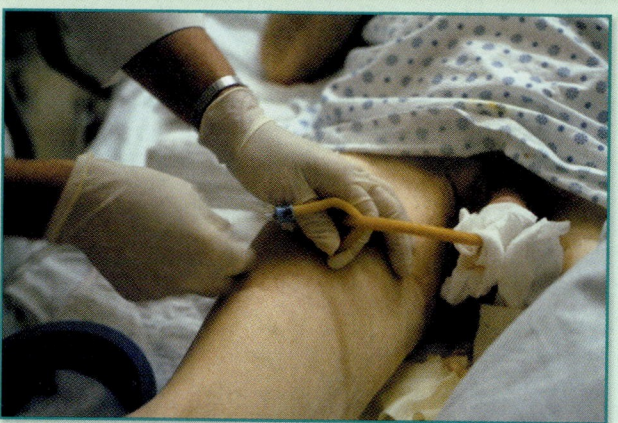

Figure 6-13-5 Remove the cap from the irrigation port of the three-way catheter.

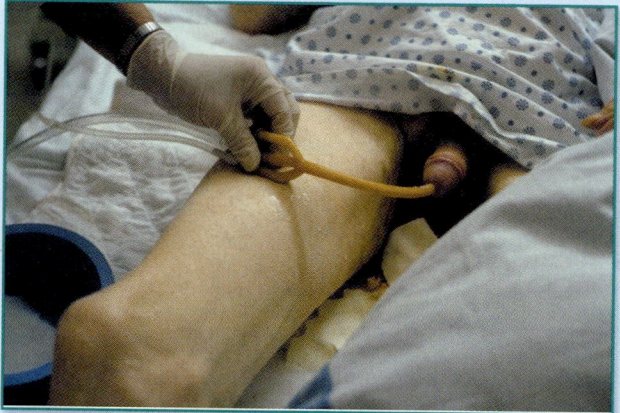

Figure 6-13-6 Attach the irrigation tubing, remove the clamp from the catheter, and observe for urine drainage. Carefully observe the drainage for color, clarity, and the presence of debris.

Action	Rationale
28. Cleanse the irrigation port with the sterile antiseptic swabs.	28. Minimizes the risk of infection.
29. Attach the irrigation tubing to the irrigation port of the three-way catheter.	29. Introduces the irrigant into the system.
30. Remove the clamp from the catheter and observe for urine drainage (see Figure 6-13-6). If intermittent irrigation has been ordered:	30. Ensures catheter remains patent after being clamped. Some surgical procedures can cause bleeding and clotting of the catheter.
31. Instill the prescribed amount of irrigant.	31. The bladder normally feels full when it contains approximately 300 mL of urine. If a prescribed amount of irrigant was not ordered, do not instill more than 150 mL of irrigant. If the client has undergone bladder surgery, do not instill irrigant without knowing the specific amount ordered.
32. Clamp the irrigant tubing.	32. Prevents further instillation of irrigant.
33. If the health care provider has ordered the irrigant to remain in the bladder for a measured length of time, clamp the drainage tube prior to instilling the irrigant and wait the prescribed length of time.	33. Some irrigation solutions contain medication and are meant to remain in contact with the bladder wall for a prescribed length of time.
34. Monitor the drainage as it flows into the drainage bag. If continuous bladder irrigation has been ordered:	34. Assesses the drainage for volume, color, clarity, and the presence of any clots or debris.
35. Adjust the clamp on the irrigation tubing to allow the prescribed rate of irrigant to flow into the catheter and bladder.	35. Regulates the amount of irrigant flowing in and out of the bladder to prevent distention or damage to any surgical site.

continues

Action	Rationale

Closed Bladder Irrigation Using a Three-Way Catheter *continued*

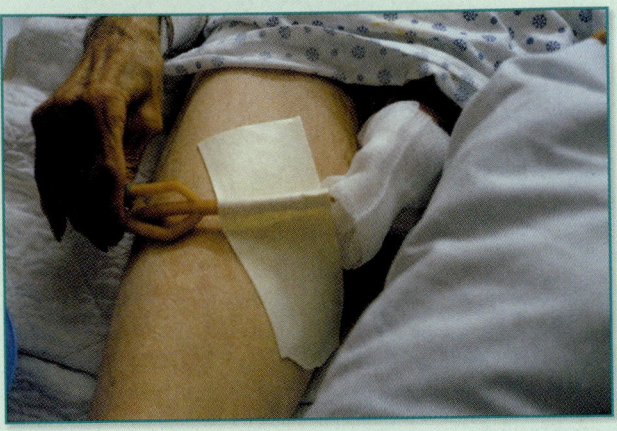

Figure 6-13-7 Securely tape the catheter to the thigh to prevent it from becoming dislodged.

36. Monitor the drainage for color, clarity, debris, and volume as it flows back into the drainage bag.

37. Tape the catheter securely to the thigh (see Figure 6-13-7).

38. Remove gloves and wash hands.

36. Assesses for bleeding, clotting, and blockage of urine drainage or other complications.

37. Prevents the catheter from becoming dislodged.

38. Reduces the transmission of microorganisms.

▶ REAL WORLD ANECDOTES

Mr. Elizondo was 1 day postoperative. His physician had ordered constant closed bladder irrigation. Mr. Elizondo's nurse checked his irrigant periodically throughout his shift and noted that it was instilling well. He did not, however, note that the urine drainage bag was becoming quite full. About 5 hours into the shift, Mr. Elizondo turned on his call light and started to call out for help. When help arrived, Mr. Elizondo was very agitated. He reported hearing an explosion and was concerned that something inside him had ruptured. While one nurse took Mr. Elizondo's vital signs and calmed and assessed him, a second nurse noted that the floor was wet. Upon closer investigation she discovered that Mr. Elizondo's urine drainage bag had overfilled to the breaking point, causing the loud explosive sound that he had heard.

▶ EVALUATION

- The client does not exhibit signs or symptoms of bladder or urinary tract infection.
- The client has not experienced pain or discomfort as a result of the bladder irrigation.
- The catheter remains patent, and the client's bladder is not distended.

▶ DOCUMENTATION

Nurses' Notes

- Describe client's tolerance for the procedure.

- Note the color, clarity, volume, and debris in the drainage.

Document on appropriate flow sheet or electronic medical record (EMR).

Intake and Output Record

- Record amount of irrigant instilled and amount of drainage measured. Subtracting the used irrigant from the drainage total will leave the amount of the client's urine output.

▶ **CRITICAL THINKING SKILL**

Introduction
Standard descriptions are needed for continuity of care.

Possible Scenario
You are starting your shift and have been assigned to care for Mr. Turner, who had a transurethral prostatectomy the day before. During reporting you were told that Mr. Turner's urine/irrigant output was dark tea colored with small clots. When you are making rounds after reporting, you note that Mr. Turner's urine/irrigant output looks more burgundy-colored than tea-colored.

Possible Outcome
You assume that the color difference is simply a difference in reporting, noting that the urine could possibly be described as dark tea colored. You check the continuous irrigation setup and assess Mr. Turner's vital signs. Four hours into your shift, when you return to reassess Mr. Turner's vital signs, his urine/irrigant is frankly bloody and Mr. Turner's skin is pale and moist. You notify Mr. Turner's surgeon, who urgently returns Mr. Turner to surgery. Because of a large blood loss, Mr. Turner requires transfusions and spends 2 days in surgical intensive care.

Prevention
You wonder if this is the color that the previous nurse reported as dark tea. As it seems darker than the report you received, you decide to monitor Mr. Turner more closely for a while. You return in 1 hour to check Mr. Turner's bladder irrigation and note that it continues to be burgundy and seems to actually be darker than earlier. You assess Mr. Turner's vital signs and update his physician regarding Mr. Turner's progress. The physician orders an increase in the rate of continuous irrigation and vital signs every 2 hours for the next 8 hours. Within 2 hours Mr. Turner's output has lightened considerably and he no longer seems to be bleeding.

▶ **VARIATIONS**

Geriatric Variation:
* *Elderly clients may have a larger amount of debris in their urine. Their urine/irrigant output must be monitored closely for potential blockages or retention.*

Pediatric Variations:
* *Children have smaller bladders and require smaller amounts of irrigant.*
* *Children have smaller bladders and a catheter is more prone to plug with mucus or clots. The patency of the catheter and the first signs of bladder distention must be carefully watched for.*
* *Children may be very embarrassed regarding bladder irrigation and monitoring for clots or distention. Be sure to provide privacy and explanations to allay their fears and embarrassment.*

Home Care Variation:
* *Closed bladder irrigation is not commonly used in the home care setting.*

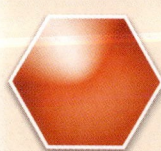

Long-Term Care Variation:
* *Closed bladder irrigation is not commonly used in the long-term care setting.*

► COMMON ERRORS

Possible Error:

Slowing the irrigation rate if a new bottle of irrigant is not readily available.

Prevention:

Continuous irrigation is often ordered to flush clots and debris out of the bladder and the catheter. Slowing the irrigation rate could allow clots and debris to build in the bladder or plug the catheter, leading to bladder distention. Be sure to have the supplies needed before the critical moment when they are needed.

► NURSING TIPS

- Do not slow a continuous irrigation without specific orders from the client's health care provider, obvious signs of bladder distention, or a plugged catheter.
- Be sure to track the amount of irrigant instilled and the amount of drainage. The drainage must always equal or exceed the amount instilled.
- Be sure to note the amount of irrigant instilled in the intake and output record so the amount instilled can be subtracted from the output to determine the urine output. Negative amounts must be reported.

- Confused clients may interpret the feeling of bladder irrigation as the need to urinate. Attempt to reorient the client regarding the presence of the catheter and not to try to pull it out. It may be necessary to restrain the client's hands while the catheter is in place.
- Try to maintain as much privacy as possible for the client. This procedure can be embarrassing for the client.
- Be sure the irrigant is at least at room temperature to avoid bladder spasms. Body temperature is preferable.
- The solution can be soaked in a water bath prior to use. Sterility must be maintained at all times.

► SPECIAL CONSIDERATIONS

- *If the purpose of the intervention is to stop postoperative bleeding, urine output should eventually become light pink or straw-colored. If a bright red drainage continues, closely monitor vital signs and notify the health care provider.*

Removing an Indwelling Catheter

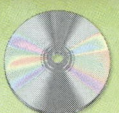

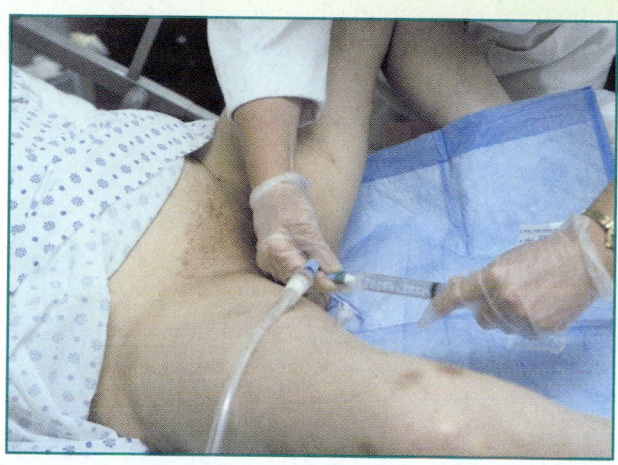

▶ OVERVIEW OF THE SKILL

Indwelling catheters may be placed during surgery for a few days postoperatively or for months if the client has long-term incontinence. Even if the catheter is considered permanent, it is changed every 1 to 2 months depending on the institution's policy. Therefore, the nurse may be removing the catheter in a variety of situations, for example, postanesthesia recovery, acute care, or long-term care.

▶ ASSESSMENT

1. Determine previous history of incontinence, infection, urinary patterns, fluid intake, and rationale for current treatment **to prepare for potential problems after the catheter is removed and to understand reasons for procedure.**
2. Assess client for temperature, current condition of urinary meatus and perineal area, and urine color, consistency, and clarity **to determine skin condition and assess for potential urinary tract infection, dehydration, or breakdown.**
3. Assess client for understanding of the procedure and ability to cooperate with positioning **to encourage client to participate in care to the best of his or her ability.**
4. Assess room setup to determine ability of client to get to the bathroom and/or need for bedside commode or urinal **to facilitate client's easy**

return to normal voiding patterns if catheter will remain out.

▶ DIAGNOSIS

Impaired Urinary Elimination

Risk for Infection

Risk for Impaired Skin Integrity

Urge Urinary Incontinence

Urinary Retention

▶ PLANNING

Expected Outcomes:

1. Catheter will be removed intact.
2. Clients will void within 8 hours of removal without burning, urgency, or incontinence.
3. Client will not develop any bleeding, pain, or other complications related to removal.
4. Client will verbalize understanding of the procedure and the need to notify staff when they void or if they have any difficulty with voiding.

Equipment Needed (see Figure 6-14-1):

- Syringe, Luer-Lock, 10 mL
- Nonsterile latex-free gloves
- Protective pad
- Soap, towel, and washcloth
- Container for waste disposal
- Urinal or bedpan in room if client is nonambulatory

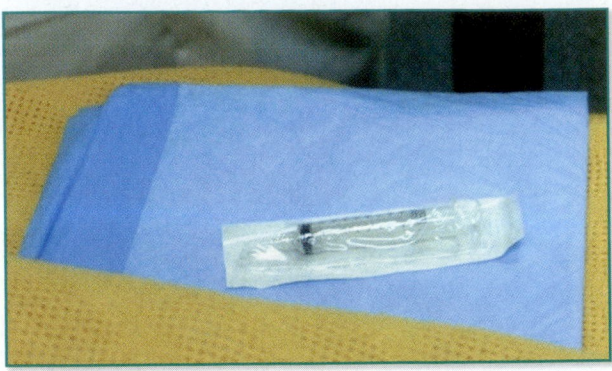

Figure 6-14-1   A syringe and a protective pad are used in removing an indwelling catheter.

- Sterile specimen cup and sterile scissors for catheter tip culture, if needed

▶ **CLIENT EDUCATION NEEDED:**

1. Provide rationale for changing or removing catheter.

2. Instruct the client to notify the nurse when he or she first voids after the catheter is removed.
3. Instruct client to inform health care team if he or she has any difficulty voiding or incontinence.
4. Teach the client the symptoms of bladder infection and bladder irritation. Instruct client to inform the nurse if experiencing any pain or symptoms after the catheter is removed.
5. Instruct client to perform Kegel exercises (contract and tighten perineal muscles for a count of five; then relax muscles) 10 to 20 times qid and increase duration for a longer count.

Estimated time to complete the skill: **6–10 minutes**

▶ **DELEGATION TIPS**

Removing an indwelling catheter is a skill that can be delegated to ancillary personnel after they have been given proper training and supervision. Ancillary personnel should know how to properly deflate the balloon and monitor the frequency and amount of urine voided after the catheter is removed.

IMPLEMENTATION—Action/Rationale

Action	Rationale
1. Wash hands.	1. Decreases the transmission of microorganisms.
2. Check health care provider's order and unit protocol.	2. Ensures correct client and treatment.
3. Identify client and explain procedure.	3. Verifies correct client and elicits client cooperation.
4. Provide privacy and position client on back.	4. Providing privacy demonstrates respect for client dignity.
5. Remove covers and drape so as to expose catheter.	5. Protects client privacy and reduces embarrassment.
6. Put on nonsterile gloves.	6. Practices Standard Precautions.
7. Place protective pad under client's thighs (see Figure 6-14-2).	7. Prevents bed from becoming soiled.
8. Empty urine in tubing into catheter bag.	8. Prevents leakage from catheter onto client when the catheter is removed.
9. Remove any tape that may be holding the catheter to the leg (see Figure 6-14-3).	9. Allows for easy removal of catheter.

continues

Action	Rationale

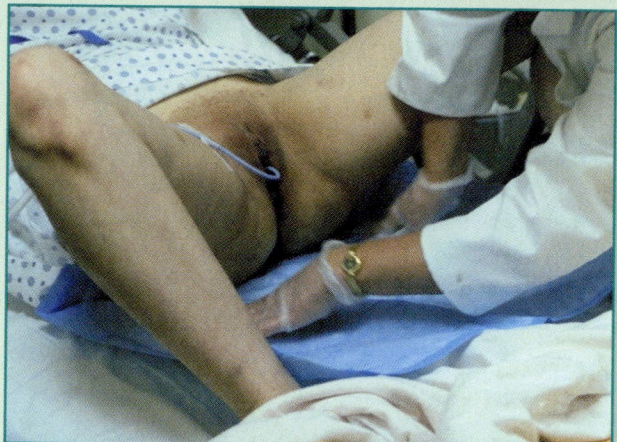

Figure 6-14-2   Place a protective pad under the client's thighs and perineal area.

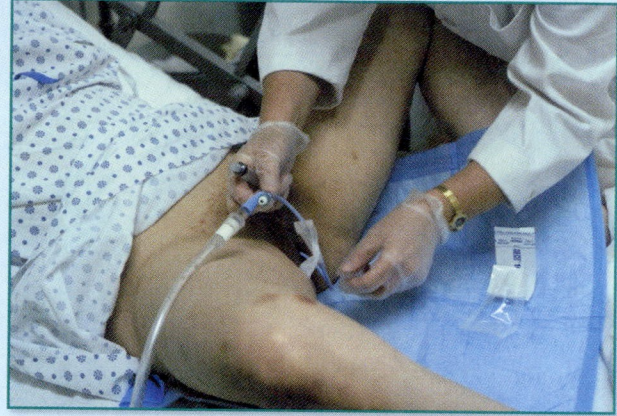

Figure 6-14-3   Remove the tape holding the catheter to the thigh.

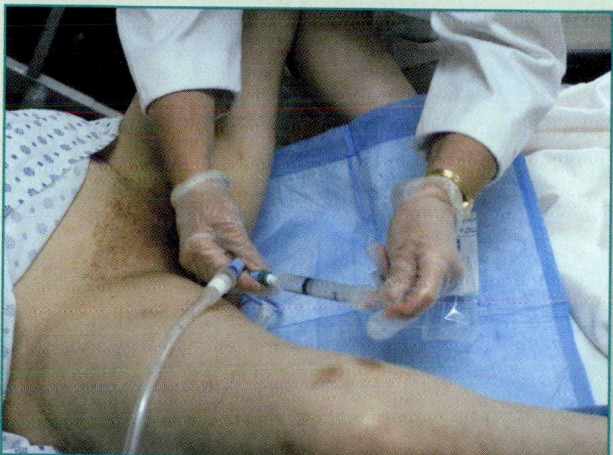

Figure 6-14-4   Insert the syringe into the balloon port and remove all the air or fluid from the retention balloon.

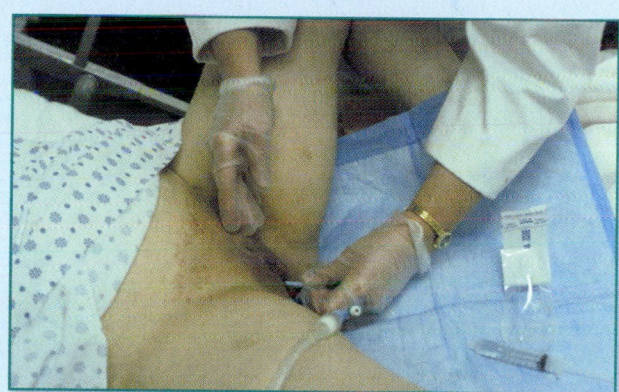

Figure 6-14-5   Gently remove the catheter.

10. Insert syringe end into balloon port and remove all the air or fluid from the balloon, generally 5–10 mL. Do not cut the port. On some systems, the port should flatten out as all contents are evacuated (see Figure 6-14-4).

11. Ask the client to take a deep breath if able and gently and smoothly remove the catheter on expiration. Stop if you meet resistance and recheck the balloon port (see Figure 6-14-5).

12. Note any sediment, mucus, or blood that may be on the catheter. If needed, culture tip of catheter by cutting it off with sterile scissors and placing in appropriate container.

13. Cleanse the client's perineal area or provide a warm, moist cloth with instructions for self-cleaning. Remove and dispose of materials (see Figure 6-14-6). Remove gloves and wash hands. Cover client and put in position of comfort (unless you will be replacing the catheter).

10. Keeping port intact ensures the ability to drain the contents of the balloon. Cutting the port does not always drain the balloon, and once the port is cut, there is no other way to drain the balloon contents.

11. Damage to the urethra may occur if the balloon is not fully deflated.

12. Assesses for any indications of infection or trauma related to the catheter.

13. Provides for privacy and comfort. Reduces transmission of microorganisms.

continues

Action	Rationale

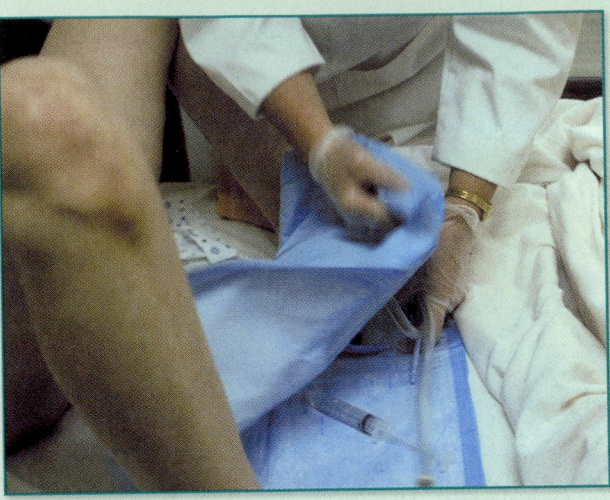

Figure 6-14-6   Remove used materials and make the client comfortable.

14. Instruct the client to drink oral fluids as tolerated and to call when needing to void. Record time and amount of first voiding. If needed, offer bedpan/urinal q 2–4 h until client is able to void.

15. If the client is unable to void within 8 hours, report to the health care provider.

14. It is important to determine that client has returned to usual voiding pattern or other interventions will need to be implemented.

15. Allows assessment and intervention to determine the cause of the client's inability to void after the catheter is removed.

▶ REAL WORLD ANECDOTES

A nurse is removing an indwelling catheter. She deflates the balloon and removes 10 cc of fluid from the balloon. As she removes the catheter, she encounters resistance, and the client cries out in pain. She then reinserts the syringe and draws out another 7 mL of fluid from the retention balloon. The nurse who inserted the catheter added the extra fluid because this client had a history of indwelling catheters pulling out. The nurse who inserted the catheter had documented the amount of fluid used to inflate the balloon, but the nurse removing the catheter had failed to check the nursing notes.

▶ EVALUATION

- Catheter was removed intact.
- Client voided within 8 hours of removal without burning, urgency, or incontinence.
- Client did not develop any bleeding, pain, or other complications related to removal.
- Client verbalized understanding of the procedure and the need to notify staff when voiding or if having any difficulty with voiding.

▶ DOCUMENTATION

Nurses' Notes

- Record the time the catheter was removed and the condition of the catheter and client.
- Note the time and amount of first voiding, if applicable.

Document on appropriate flow sheet or electronic medical record (EMR).

Intake and Output Record

- Record the amount of urine in the collection bag.

► CRITICAL THINKING SKILL

Introduction

Physicians may write to have a catheter discontinued but may not be aware of all the other orders the client has. Being aware of the interactions of different orders may help a client.

Possible Scenario

A postoperative cardiac surgical client had an order to have the indwelling catheter removed and also an order for Lasix (furosemide) 80 mg IV.

Possible Outcome

The client would need to get up frequently as a result of the diuretic effects of the Lasix, thereby causing fatigue and possible undue strain on the heart.

Prevention

The nurse prevented this by looking at all the client's orders and determining priorities. She then discussed her concerns with the client's physician, who agreed that the catheter could be discontinued after the effects of the Lasix had worn off. The nurse discussed it with the client, explaining the reason for waiting to discontinue the catheter. The client was reassured and saved the stress of frequent trips to the bathroom.

► VARIATIONS

Geriatric Variations:
- An elderly client may need incontinence pads after catheter removal.
- The client may need to perform Kegel exercises to regain urinary continence.
- The client may need more skin care to maintain perineal and perianal areas and skin free of irritation and breakdown.

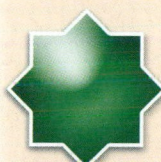

Pediatric Variation:
- Children may be very frightened. Demonstration on a doll along with much reassurance and step-by-step instructions will help to allay some of their fears. Focus on the positive effects of removal. Two people may be needed to complete the task.

Home Care Variations:
- Indwelling catheters are a last resort for incontinence at home.
- A nurse may remove the catheter in the home setting to change it.
- Make sure to take all the equipment needed to remove the catheter in the home setting.
- Make sure to educate the home caregiver to report if the client has not voided within 8 hours of catheter removal.
- Discuss how to continue to measure intake and output using a urinal, bedpan, or toilet if intake and output are to be measured.

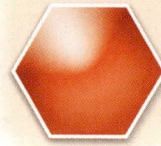

Long-Term Care Variations:
- The nurse will probably replace the catheter if it is being used for incontinence.
- Long-term care facilities are using straight catheters more frequently as indwelling catheters provide a good route for infections and urosepsis.

▶ COMMON ERRORS

Possible Error:

Not removing all the air or water in the balloon.

Prevention:

Be sure to remove the catheter slowly and note any resistance. If resistance is felt, check to make sure the balloon is completely deflated. If resistance is still felt, do not force or pull on the catheter. Stop the procedure and report findings to the health care provider.

▶ NURSING TIPS

- Remember to measure output in the collection bag prior to disposing of the bag.

▶ SPECIAL CONSIDERATIONS

- *Voiding difficulty usually occurs after removal of an indwelling catheter, especially if the catheter has been in place for a period of time. Encourage sufficient fluid intake (at least 2,000 to 3,000 cc if it is not restricted). Perineal care with warm water may help the client to void.*
- *The client may complain about irritation in the urethra after the catheter has been removed. If the condition persists, monitor for signs of a urinary tract infection and notify the health care provider if necessary.*

Catheterizing a Noncontinent Urinary Diversion

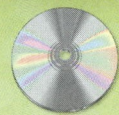

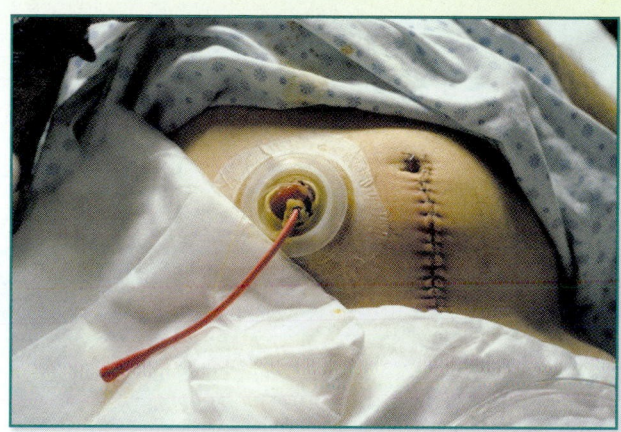

▶ OVERVIEW OF THE SKILL

Catheterizing a noncontinent urinary diversion is done in order to obtain a sterile urine sample for culture and sensitivity. Clients with urinary diversions are at increased risk for urinary tract infections; therefore, proper technique is employed to prevent introducing bacteria into the system when collecting specimens.

▶ ASSESSMENT

1. Inspect the stoma for color and texture. Allows the nurse **to determine the viability and turgor of the stoma.**
2. Observe the color and odor of the urine. **Provides clues to the nurse of the possibility of a urinary tract infection.**

▶ DIAGNOSIS

Disturbed Body Image

Impaired Urinary Elimination

Risk for Impaired Skin Integrity

▶ PLANNING

Expected Outcomes:

1. Client will express positive feelings about self.
2. Client will voice understanding of the procedure.
3. The stoma and peristomal skin will not be traumatized by the procedure.
4. The client will not suffer infection secondary to this procedure.

Equipment Needed:

- Clean and sterile gloves
- 4 × 4 gauze pads
- Povidone-iodine solution
- Sterile straight catheter (size is dependent on stoma orifice; 14 French is usually used) (see Figure 6-15-1)
- 50-mL tapered-tip syringe
- Sterile container (see Figure 6-15-2)
- Straight catheter specimen kit (if available, replaces gloves, gauze, povidone-iodine, and catheter above)
- Appropriate urinary ostomy equipment

▶ CLIENT EDUCATION NEEDED:

1. Explain rationale for obtaining a sterile urine specimen.
2. Explain need to replace current ostomy appliance with a clean system if only obtaining a clean specimen.

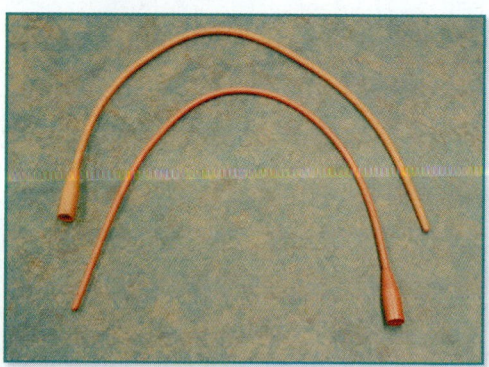

Figure 6-15-1   Straight catheters

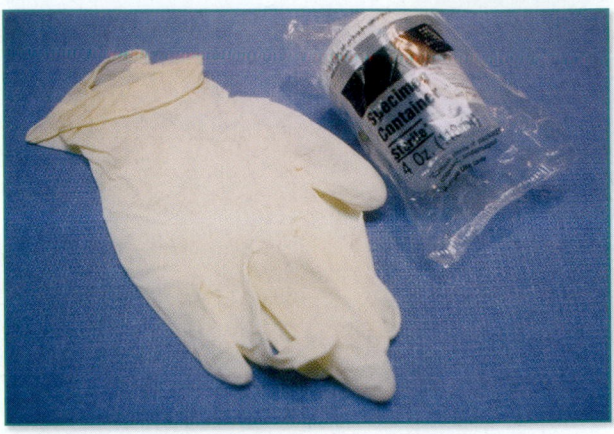

Figure 6-15-2   Sterile specimen container and gloves

3. Instruct client to increase fluid intake (if no restrictions) to prevent occurrences of urinary tract infection.

4. Instruct client on the signs and symptoms of a urinary tract infection. Instruct client to inform nurse and/or health care provider whenever there are signs and symptoms of a possible urinary tract infection.

Estimated time to complete the skill: **15–20 minutes**

▶ DELEGATION TIPS

This skill cannot be delegated to ancillary personnel. Catheterizing a noncontinent urinary diversion requires the skills and problem-solving abilities of a nurse.

IMPLEMENTATION—Action/Rationale

Action	Rationale
1. Wash hands.	1. Reduces transmission of microorganisms.
2. Assemble equipment (straight catheter, sterile container, gauze, and povidone-iodine OR straight catheter specimen kit).	2. Ensures that all equipment is ready to use.
3. Apply clean gloves.	3. Practices clean technique.
4. Remove current ostomy appliance (see Figure 6-15-3).	4. This system cannot be used to collect a clean urine sample as it is already contaminated with microorganisms.

Figure 6-15-3   Remove the ostomy appliance.

continues

Action	Rationale
5. Dispose of appliance in appropriate waste container.	5. Practices infection control policies.
6. Wash hands.	6. Reduces the transmission of microorganisms.
7. Open all sterile equipment.	7. Ensures that all equipment is ready to use.
8. Squeeze a moderate amount of water-soluble jelly onto sterile field of one of the opened packages.	8. Water-soluble jelly will be used on tip of catheter to facilitate insertion into stoma.
9. Apply sterile gloves.	9. Practices aseptic technique.
10. Cleanse stoma with povidone-iodine (if no allergy to iodine) on gauze or cotton ball. Pat dry with dry sterile gauze.	10. Gentle care of the stoma prevents injury to the mucosa, which has no nerve endings and is very friable.
11. Wipe excess povidone-iodine off stoma.	11. Prevents destruction of any microorganisms in urine sample.
12. Holding catheter, lubricate tip with water-soluble jelly.	12. Facilitates insertion of catheter into stoma.
13. Gently insert catheter into orifice of stoma (see Figure 6-15-4).	13. Prevents trauma to the mucosa and conduit.
14. Place other end of catheter into sterile container, if not using a closed specimen system, to collect urine.	14. Collects urine sample.
15. If urine does not readily drain from catheter, apply slight suction to end of catheter using a syringe (see Figure 6-15-5).	15. Facilitates obtaining a urine sample.
16. After collecting an adequate sample, remove catheter and dispose in an appropriate waste container.	16. Practices infection control policies.
17. Label container, place in biohazard bag, and send to laboratory. Remove gloves.	17. Appropriate labeling of specimen ensures that client is treated correctly following results of laboratory test.

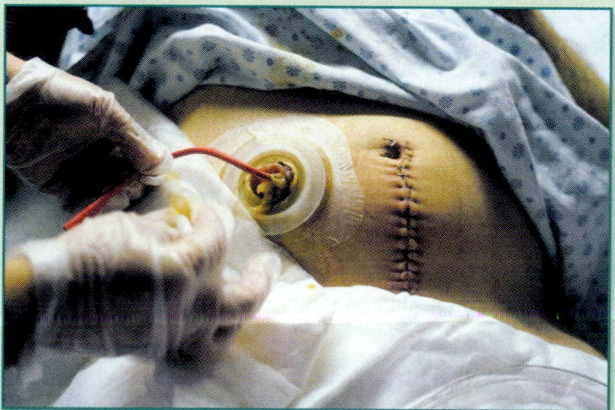

Figure 6-15-4   Gently insert the straight catheter into the stoma.

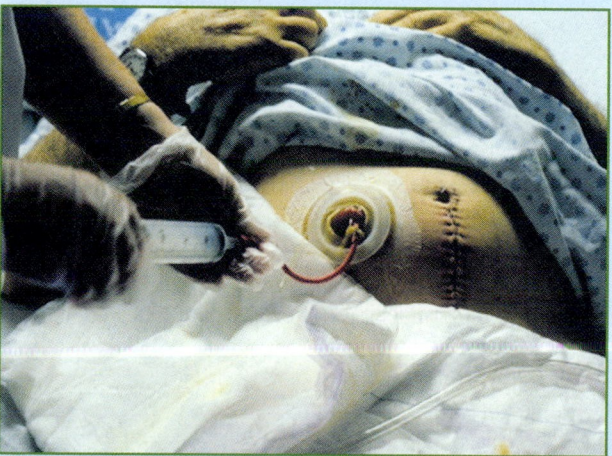

Figure 6-15-5   If urine does not drain freely, apply mild suction.

continues

Action	Rationale

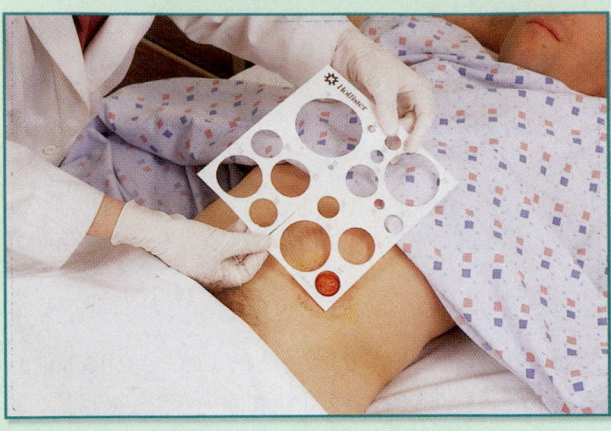

Figure 6-15-6   Measuring the stoma

18. Apply clean gloves. Cleanse stoma and skin with warm tap water. Pat dry.

18. Gentle care of the stoma prevents injury to the mucosa, which has no nerve endings and is very friable.

19. If replacing the entire appliance, measure stoma using a measuring guide for appropriate length and width of stoma at base (where skin meets stoma) (see Figure 6-15-6).

19. Correct measurement of the stoma's dimensions ensures a good fit of the ostomy appliance without excess skin at the base of the stoma exposed to urine.

20. Place wick of gauze over orifice of stoma to wick urine while you are preparing the wafer and pouch for application.

20. Using something to wick urine away from the skin ensures a good seal of the wafer to the client's skin.

21. Trace pattern onto paper backing of wafer.

21. It is important to trace the measurements of the stoma and not "eyeball" the stoma measurements. Inaccurate pattern size results in either laceration of the stoma by the wafer or maceration of peristomal skin from constant contact with urine.

22. Cut wafer as traced.

22. Accurately cutting the traced pattern ensures a snug fit.

23. Attach clean pouch to wafer. Make sure port is closed.

23. Preattaching the pouch to the wafer saves time and prevents urine from leaking underneath the wafer during the application process.

24. Remove guaze from orifice of stoma.

24. Allows visualization of the stroma and accurate placement of the water.

25. Remove paper backing from wafer and place on skin with stoma centered in cutout opening of wafer.

25. Paper backing needs to be removed from wafer in order for wafer to become adherent to skin.

26. Remove gloves. Wash hands.

26. Reduces transmission of microorganisms.

▶ REAL WORLD ANECDOTES

A woman with a primary history of myelomeningocele comes to clinic complaining of her urine being thick and foul smelling. She has had an ileal conduit for the past 20 years secondary to neurogenic bladder. The client is known to have a history of noncompliance in regard to maintaining adequate fluid intake to prevent possible urinary tract infection. While catheterizing the stoma, the nurse notes that the client is crying and refuses to watch the procedure. When questioned by the nurse, the young woman explains, "I'm just so tired of dealing with all of this. I hate to even drink a glass of water because it just pours out the other end." The nurse determines that the client has not been taking in an adequate amount of fluids for some time secondary to not wanting to care for her stoma. The urine sample shows a urinary tract infection. The young woman is treated for the infection and counseled regarding the care of her stoma and acceptance of the continued need for it.

▶ EVALUATION

- Client expressed positive feelings about self and the procedure.
- Client voiced understanding of procedure.
- The stoma and peristomal skin were not traumatized by the procedure.
- The client did not suffer infection secondary to this procedure.

▶ DOCUMENTATION

Nurses' Notes

Document:
- Time and date of urine specimen collection
- Size and type of catheter used
- Condition of stoma and peristomal skin before and after specimen collection
- Amount, color, and odor of urine collected
- How client tolerated procedure.
- If there is a stoma care checklist, note if the pouch was changed, the condition of the peristomal skin, and the condition of the stoma.

Document on appropriate flow sheet or electronic medical record (EMR).

Intake and Output Record

- If the client is on intake and output measurements, note the amount of urine collected in the output record.

▶ CRITICAL THINKING SKILL

Introduction

A client with a urinary diversion is experiencing signs and symptoms of possible urinary tract infection.

Possible Scenario

A 63-year-old white man, status post–ileal conduit for bladder cancer, is seen in clinic by the ostomy nurse specialist for complaints of foul odor from urine and increased amount of mucus in urine. Assessments of stoma and peristomal skin are not remarkable. Urine is dark yellow with thick mucus threads and a very strong odor. Client responds to questions on self-care by stating, "I don't have the time during the day to empty my pouch of urine, so I limit how much I drink." Further questioning reveals that the client is only drinking approximately 32 oz. of fluid every 24 hours for the past week. The ostomy nurse specialist obtains two urine samples. One is a clean catch and the other is a sterile sample.

Possible Outcome

If the nurse is not astute enough to pick up the correlation between increased color tone of urine, mucus threads, and a very strong odor, the client is at potential risk for a silent infection and possible extension of infection to the kidneys.

Prevention

The nurse should immediately notify the physician regarding the change in the client's status. The second nursing action is to obtain a urine sample. This action allows the physician to appropriately treat the client's urinary tract infection. The nurse also needs to provide client education on the importance of preventing future episodes of urinary tract infection, which is a normal complication in urinary diversion surgeries.

▶ VARIATIONS

Geriatric Variation:
- *Be especially alert for signs of infection in older or debilitated clients who may not be able to easily maintain adequate fluid intake.*

Pediatric Variations:
- *The nurse will need to use a smaller-sized catheter to obtain a specimen in a child. The size of the catheter is dependent on the size of the orifice at the fascia level.*
- *Explain to the child, if appropriate, what you will be doing and why. Describe any sensations the child might experience, and reassure the child that the procedure will not hurt.*
- *Obtain assistance of a parent to distract and, if necessary, briefly restrain the child to avoid contaminating the sterile catheter.*

Home Care Variations:
- *When obtaining a sterile specimen using a catheter in the home care setting, make sure to plan in advance and bring along the necessary equipment. This may include a small portable table to lay out supplies, extra catheters in case of contamination, and wafers and pouches to reapply after the procedure.*
- *Explain to the client the difference between a clean catch and a sterile specimen so they understand why the extra "hassle" is necessary in the home setting.*

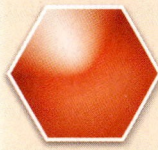

Long-Term Care Variations:
- *Be especially alert for signs of infection in older or debilitated clients who may not be able to easily maintain adequate fluid intake.*
- *Staff in long-term care settings may not have much experience working with clients who have noncontinent urinary diversions. Make sure a resource person is available on the phone and in person, if needed, to provide staff education and answer questions. Informed care will help reduce the risk of infection for the client and allow the staff to feel more comfortable performing unfamiliar procedures on the client.*

▶ COMMON ERRORS

Possible Error:
Urine is not easily obtained using the catheter method.

Prevention:
Slowly rotate catheter in conduit and apply suction using a syringe. Use of suction with syringe will facilitate obtaining a sample. Also, encourage client to hydrate self prior to obtaining a urine sample. A dehydrated client will not produce adequate amounts of urine to sample for cultures.

▶ NURSING TIPS
- Recognize that all urinary stomas are not the same. Each stoma needs to be assessed for the appropriate catheter size to be used for obtaining a sterile urine sample.
- Client teaching is easily incorporated into the procedure of obtaining a urine sample by encouraging the client to express knowledge on urinary tract infections.

- Use of a clean, new urinary pouching system is the simplest way to obtain a urine sample and is accurate as the bowel used for urinary diversions is already contaminated with microorganisms.

- Costs to the client and the health care institution are reduced when using a clean, new urinary pouching system to obtain a clean urine sample for culture.

▶ **SPECIAL CONSIDERATIONS**

- *Before the catheterization, cleanse the stoma with povidone-iodine using a circular motion from inside to outside. If the client is allergic to povidone-iodine, use sterile saline, sterile water, or other solutions based on the institution's policy.*
- *Use latex-free gloves and catheters if client has a history of latex allergy.*

Maintaining a Continent Urinary Diversion

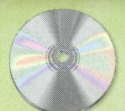

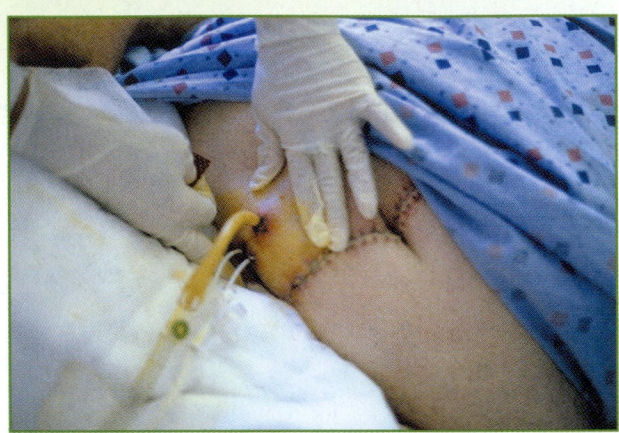

▶ OVERVIEW OF THE SKILL

A continent urinary diversion is cared for initially by irrigating the various tubes and stents to maintain patency. The client does not begin to learn catheterization of the "new bladder" until 3 weeks after surgery. A client with an orthotopic bladder will learn intermittent catheterization as a safety measure in case of mucus plug obstruction. All clients will learn how to perform irrigation of tubes before discharge home from the hospital.

▶ ASSESSMENT

1. Inspect the stoma for color and texture, if present. **Allows the nurse to determine the viability and turgor of the stoma.**
2. Inspect the condition of the skin surrounding the stoma, if present. **Alterations in skin integrity will prohibit a closed drainage system from adhering to the skin.**
3. Inspect all tubes and drains (immediate postoperative period). **Allows the nurse to ascertain that all tubes and drains are functioning appropriately.**

▶ DIAGNOSIS

Deficient Knowledge

Disturbed Body Image

Impaired Urinary Elimination

Risk for Impaired Skin Integrity

Social Isolation

808

▶ PLANNING

Expected Outcomes:

1. Peristomal skin integrity will remain intact if stoma is present.
2. Irritated or denuded peristomal skin integrity will heal if stoma is present.
3. Client will acknowledge the change in body image and express positive feelings about self.
4. Client will maintain fluid balance.
5. Client will express understanding regarding the need for a urinary diversion and how to maintain it.
6. Instruct client to report changes in urine flow or difficulty catheterizing and/or flushing neobladder to wound/ostomy care nurse.

Equipment Needed (see Figure 6-16-1):

Irrigation of Tubes/Drains

- Normal saline
- Water-soluble lubricant
- Piston syringe
- Sterile gloves
- Sterile basin

Catheterization of Continent Urinary Diversion

- Urinary catheter (Do not use rubber catheter if client is allergic or sensitive to latex.)
- Water-soluble lubricant
- Sterile gloves
- Povidone-iodine solution or other antimicrobial solution
- Gauze pads (4 × 4)

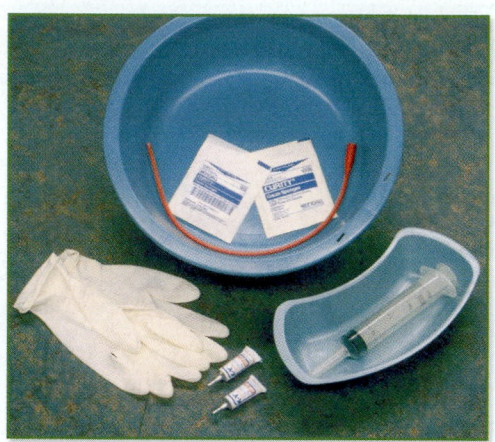

Figure 6-16-1   Straight catheter, emesis basis, syringe, gloves, lubricant, and gauze sponges

▶ CLIENT EDUCATION NEEDED:

1. Instruct client to flush tubes and drains every 2 to 4 hours.
2. Instruct client to catheterize neobladder (with stoma) initially every 2 hours and increasing time frame by 1 hour until an every-4-hours schedule is reached.
3. Instruct client to clean catheter after use with soap and water, rinse, and pat dry. Clean catheter is stored in a closed sealable plastic bag.
4. Instruct the client to replace the catheter every 3 months or when the catheter begins to look worn.
5. Provide the client with a list of equipment and product numbers and a list of retailers where supplies can be purchased.
6. Instruct client with a continent urinary stoma to obtain a Medic-Alert tag, which identifies the type of urinary diversion that requires catheterization.
7. Instruct client to report changes in urine flow or difficulty catheterizing and/or flushing neobladder to wound/ostomy care nurse.

Estimated time to complete the skill:
10–15 minutes

▶ DELEGATION TIPS

This skill cannot be delegated to ancillary personnel. Maintaining a continent urinary diversion requires the skills and problem-solving abilities of a nurse.

IMPLEMENTATION—Action/Rationale

Action	Rationale
Irrigating Tubes	
1. Wash hands.	1. Reduces the transmission of microorganisms.
2. Assemble equipment.	2. Ensures that all equipment is ready to use.
3. Pour sterile normal saline into a sterile basin.	3. Ensures that all equipment is ready to use.
4. Open remaining sterile packages.	4. Ensures that all equipment is ready to use.
5. Apply sterile gloves.	5. Practices aseptic technique.
6. Draw up 30 mL of sterile normal saline into piston syringe.	6. Prepares irrigant for use.
7. Disconnect the tube into the stoma from the drainage system (see Figure 6-16-2).	7. Facilitates flushing of tube.
8. Attach syringe to catheter (see Figure 6-16-3).	8. Catheter is flushed to remove clumps of mucus.

continues

Action	Rationale

Irrigating Tubes *continued*

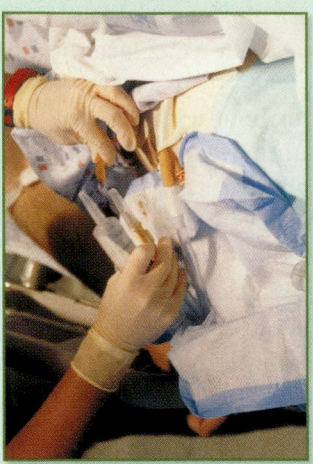

Figure 6-16-2 Disconnect the catheter that leads into the stoma from the drainage system.

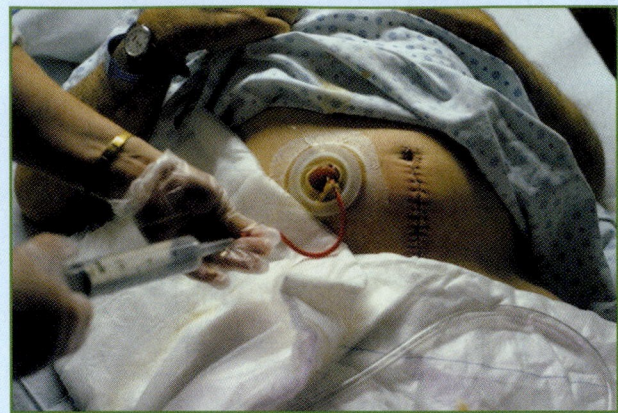

Figure 6-16-3 Attach the syringe to the catheter.

9. Flush catheter until irrigant is free of mucus strands (see Figures 6-16-4 and 6-16-5).

10. Reconnect Foley catheter/tube to drainage system (see Figures 6-16-6 and 6-16-7).

11. Repeat the procedure if ordered for additional catheters or stents using a new sterile syringe for each catheter.

12. Remove gloves and wash hands.

Catheterizing Continent Urinary Diversion

13. Wash hands.

14. Assemble equipment.

15. Open packages and apply povidone-iodine to gauze pads.

9. Prevents possible plugging of the tubes by mucus strands.

10. Facilitates continuous drainage of urine.

11. A new sterile syringe prevents cross contamination.

12. Reduces transmission of microorganisms.

13. Reduces transmission of microorganisms.

14. Ensures that all equipment is ready to use.

15. Ensures that all equipment is ready to use.

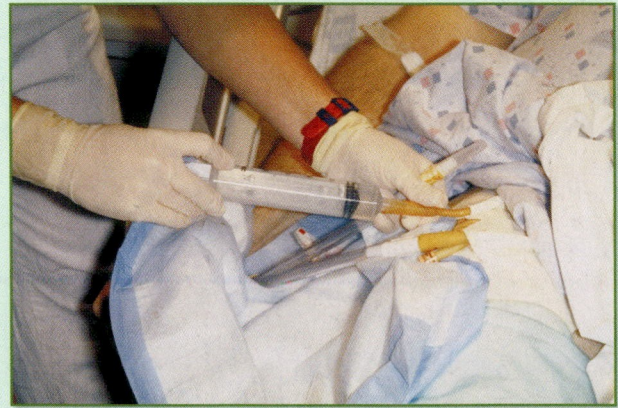

Figure 6-16-4 Flush the catheter with irrigant.

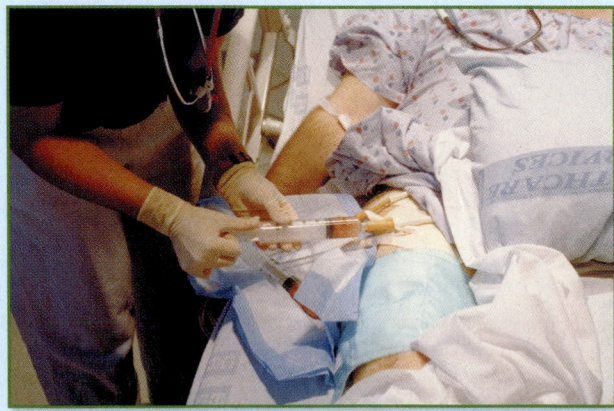

Figure 6-16-5 Flush the catheter until returning irrigant is free of mucus strands.

Action	Rationale
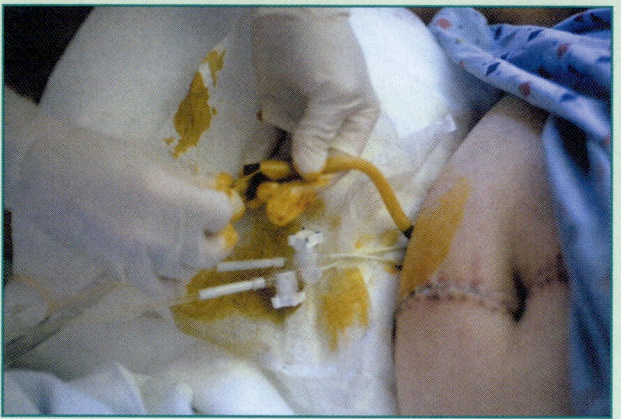 **Figure 6-16-6** Reconnect the catheter to the drainage system.	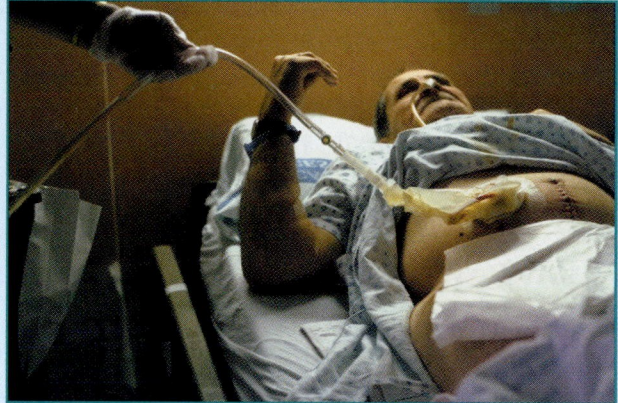 **Figure 6-16-7** Make sure all connections are secure.

16. Apply sterile gloves.	**16.** Practices aseptic technique.
17. Draw up 30 mL of sterile normal saline into piston syringe.	**17.** Ensures that all equipment is ready to use.
18. Cleanse stoma with povidone-iodine solution or other antimicrobial solution gauze pads.	**18.** Removes microorganisms and minimizes the risk of a urinary tract infection.
19. Coat the distal end of the catheter with water-soluble sterile lubricant and gently insert catheter into the stoma.	**19.** Facilitates catheter insertion. Mucosa is friable and rough insertion may cause trauma.
20. Place other end of catheter into container.	**20.** Allows for measurement of urine.
21. After all urine has drained out, insert piston syringe into catheter and irrigate bladder with sterile normal saline. Irrigate until irrigant is free of mucus strands.	**21.** Irrigating the bladder prevents possible plugging by mucus strands.
22. Remove catheter.	**22.** Irrigation is complete.
23. Apply a gauze over stoma.	**23.** Protects the stoma.
24. In hospital, dispose of catheter. At home, client can reuse catheters by washing in soap and water, rinsing, and drying. Once cleaned, catheter is placed in a sealable plastic bag.	**24.** In hospital, prevents possible nosocomial infection. At home, reduces client cost. There is less risk of nosocomial infection in the client's home setting.
25. Dispose of equipment, remove gloves and wash hands.	**25.** Reduces transmission of microorganisms.

► **REAL WORLD ANECDOTES**

The home health nurse is visiting Mrs. Hanson, a 63-year-old woman, at home to evaluate her continent urinary diversion. The nurse asks to watch Mrs. Hanson perform a catheterization and the care she would normally use at that time. Agreeing to do so, Mrs. Hanson walks to the kitchen sink, opens a drawer next to the sink, and pulls a red rubber catheter out of the drawer. She then opens up the front of her smock and proceeds to catheterize her urinary stoma, draining the urine into the sink. After the urine has stopped flowing, Mrs. Hanson wipes her stoma

continues

▶ EVALUATION

- Peristomal skin integrity remains intact if stoma is present.
- Irritated or denuded peristomal skin integrity has healed if stoma is present.
- Client acknowledges the change in body image and expresses positive feelings about self.
- Client has maintained fluid balance.
- Client expresses understanding regarding the need for a urinary diversion and how to maintain it.

▶ DOCUMENTATION

Nurses' Notes

- Document the condition of the stoma if one is present and the peristomal skin if appropriate.
- Note the color, amount, and odor of the urinary drainage.
- Note any mucus plugs or unusual findings.
- If skin care was performed, note what was done and the client's response to the care.
- Record any client teaching performed.

Document on appropriate flow sheet or electronic medical record (EMR).

Intake and Output Record

- Note the amount of irrigant instilled and the amount of urine/drainage evacuated.

▶ CRITICAL THINKING SKILL

Introduction

Look at a scenario in which the client has an Indiana pouch for treatment of bladder cancer following cystectomy.

Possible Scenario

A 35-year-old man is diagnosed with recurrent bladder cancer and chooses to have an Indiana pouch as the urinary diversion. His recovery is uneventful and he is discharged home in 7 days. He is able to perform all aspects of self-care within 2 weeks. The client is readmitted to the hospital 1 year following surgery with recurrence of the cancer. He is admitted to begin receiving chemotherapy.

Possible Outcome

As chemotherapy is administered, the client will need to be hydrated and his urine output monitored. The astute nurse will insert a Foley catheter into the Indiana Pouch and attach the catheter to bedside bag to facilitate accurate recording of urinary output and to reduce the possibility of toxicity.

Prevention

Insertion of a Foley catheter into a neobladder will ensure that the client's possible complications to receiving chemotherapy are lessened.

▶ **VARIATIONS**

Geriatric Variations:
- *Elderly clients often have delicate skin and extra care must be taken to prevent peristomal irritation and breakdown.*
- *Elderly clients may not respond to thirst appropriately and may become dehydrated. Elderly clients with urinary diversion require adequate fluids to maintain good urinary function.*

continues

▶ **VARIATIONS** *(continued)*

Pediatric Variations:
- *If the continent stoma requires catheterization, use a catheter of the appropriate size.*
- *Only insert the catheter until urine flows.*
- *Teenagers may be embarrassed or have body image and self-esteem problems regarding their urinary diversion. Provide a safe, nonjudgmental environment for the teenager to vent any anger and frustration.*
- *When irrigating a neobladder in children, use smaller amounts of normal saline and irrigate gently.*

Home Care Variation:
- *Clients in the home care setting may become careless regarding hygiene and catheter care. This increases the risk of urinary tract infections and other complications. Reinforce teaching regarding diversion care and hygiene.*

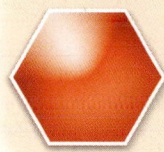

Long-Term Care Variation:
- *Long-term care clients who are unable to care for themselves may be at risk of dehydration. Ensure that all clients with urinary diversion receive adequate hydration to prevent urinary complications.*

▶ **COMMON ERRORS**

Possible Error:

Urine is not flowing when the neobladder is catheterized.

Prevention:

Slowly rotate catheter in conduit and apply suction using a syringe. Flush neobladder with normal saline to dislodge possible mucous plugs for conduit lumen. Use of gentle suction with syringe will facilitate flow of urine through catheter. Also, encourage client to hydrate self throughout the day.

▶ **NURSING TIPS**

- Recognize that all continent urinary diversions are not the same. Each continent urinary diversion must be treated individually, which requires that the nurse assess the stoma (if present), the peristomal skin condition, and ability of client to void (orthotopic neobladder).

- Client teaching can be incorporated into the care of the continent urinary diversion by encouraging the client to assist during the application process.
- Catheters and irrigation equipment that are easy to use increase the client's comfort level and thereby their participation in self-care activities.

▶ **SPECIAL CONSIDERATIONS**

- *Taking vitamin C and drinking cranberry juice help to keep the urine acidic and reduce the ammonia-like odor. To help prevent a possible urinary tract infection, increased fluid intake (2,000 to 3,000 mL) is encouraged if it is not restricted.*

Pouching a Noncontinent Urinary Diversion

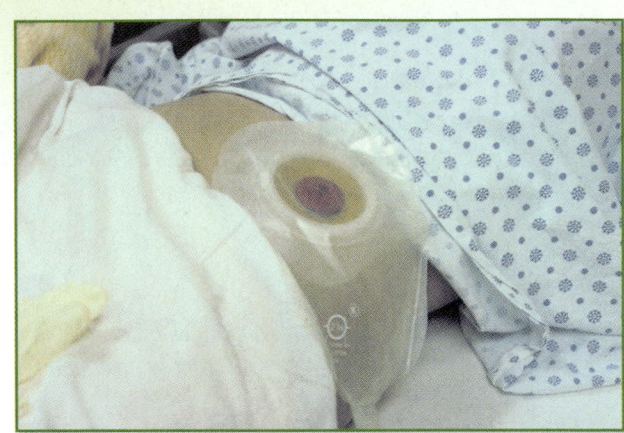

► OVERVIEW OF THE SKILL

Noncontinent urinary diversions are surgical procedures that allow urine to drain from the body. This can be done by creating openings directly from the ureters to the abdominal surface (cutaneous ureterostomy) or by connecting the ureters to an internal pouch formed using a portion of the ileum. The pouch then drains to the abdominal wall. Finally, a continent urostomy, or Koch's pouch, collects urine inside the body in a pouch made from a portion of the ileum. Urine is periodically drained by inserting a catheter into the pouch via a nipple opening in the abdominal wall. Pouching a noncontinent urinary diversion ensures that the client's peristomal skin remains intact and provides the client with artificial continence.

► ASSESSMENT

1. Inspect the stoma for color and texture. **This allows the nurse to determine the viability and turgor of the stoma.**
2. Inspect the condition of the skin surrounding the stoma. **Alterations in skin integrity prohibit a closed drainage system from adhering to the skin.**
3. Measure the dimensions of the stoma before obtaining an ostomy appliance system from central supply. **This alleviates the problem of obtaining the wrong size equipment.**
4. Inspect stents for appropriate placement and drainage. **The stents are placed intraoperatively**

to ensure that urine drains from the kidneys through the edematous ureters. The stents are removed 7–21 days post-op (depending on the surgeon's preference).

► DIAGNOSIS

Deficient Knowledge

Disturbed Body Image

Risk for Impaired Skin Integrity

Impaired Urinary Elimination

Social Isolation

► PLANNING

Expected Outcomes:

1. Peristomal skin integrity will remain intact.
2. Irritated or denuded peristomal skin integrity will heal.
3. Client will acknowledge the change in body image.
4. Client will express positive feelings about self.
5. Client will maintain fluid balance.

Equipment Needed (see Figure 6-17-1):

- Clean washcloth or 4 × 4 gauze sponges
- Warm tap water
- Appropriate urinary ostomy appliance
- Stoma measuring guide
- Scissors
- Pen or pencil
- Bedside drainage bag (optional)

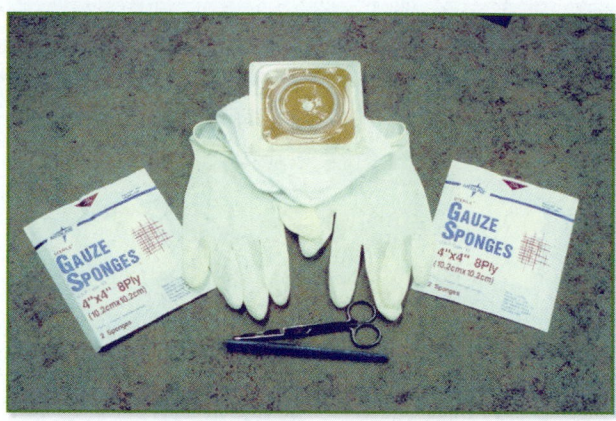

Figure 6-17-1 Gloves, scissors, pen or pencil, and sponges are used when pouching a noncontinent urinary diversion.

- Clean gloves
- 4 × 4 gauze sponges

▶ CLIENT EDUCATION NEEDED:

1. Explain care of the ostomy appliance.
2. Provide instruction on how to empty and measure contents of urinary appliance.
3. Provide list of equipment and product numbers.
4. Provide list of retailers where supplies can be purchased.

5. Provide list of reasons and situations to call health care provider, or enterostomal/ostomy care nurse.
6. Instruct the client to initially change ostomy appliance every 3 days, and after 2 changes to increase change time by 1 day until client reaches maximum change time (5 to 71 days).
7. Instruct client to keep appliance change procedure simple. Do not use pectin paste or powder or skin sealant unless there has been a problem with leakage and skin irritation.
8. Instruct client to empty urinary appliance every 2–4 hours while awake.
9. Instruct client to attach urinary appliance to a bedside drainage bag at night. This will facilitate a good night's sleep and prevent possible overflow of urine into the pouch and subsequent leakage.
10. Arrange an appointment for follow-up care with the enterostomal/ostomy nurse.

Estimated time to complete the skill:
10–20 minutes

▶ DELEGATION TIPS

This skill requires the skills and problem-solving ability of a nurse. Pouching a noncontinent urinary diversion cannot be delegated to ancillary personnel.

IMPLEMENTATION—Action/Rationale

Action	Rationale
1. Wash hands.	1. Reduces the transmission of microorganisms.
2. Assemble clean urinary pouch and wafer.	2. Ensures that all equipment is ready to use.
3. Apply clean gloves.	3. Practices clean technique.
4. Remove current ostomy appliance after emptying pouch of urine, if present (see Figure 6-17-2).	4. Regular pouch changes help prevent urinary infections.
5. Dispose of appliance and contaminated gloves in appropriate waste container.	5. Practices infection control.
6. Wash hands.	6. Reduces the transmission of microorganisms.

continues

Action	Rationale

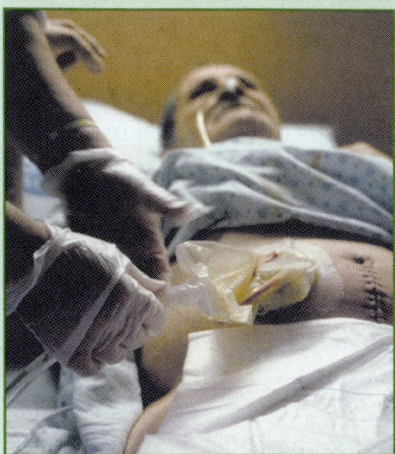

Figure 6-17-2 Remove current ostomy appliance.

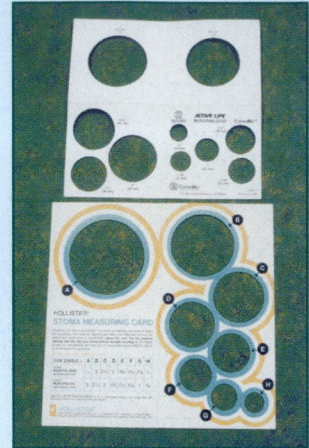

Figure 6-17-3 Measure the stoma using a stoma measuring card to ensure the best fit for the ostomy appliance.

Action	Rationale
7. Apply clean gloves.	7. Practices clean technique.
8. Cleanse stoma and skin with warm tap water. Pat dry.	8. Gentle care of the stoma prevents injury to the mucosa, which has no nerve endings and is very friable.
9. Measure stoma using a measuring guide for appropriate length and width of stoma at base (where skin meets stoma) (see Figure 6-17-3).	9. Correct measurement of the stoma's dimensions ensures a good fit of the ostomy appliance without excess skin at the base of the stoma exposed to urine.
10. Place gauze over stoma to wick urine while you are preparing the wafer and pouch for application.	10. Ensures a good seal of the wafer to the client's skin.
11. Trace pattern onto paper backing of wafer.	11. It is important to trace the measurements of the stoma and not "eyeball" the stoma measurements. Inaccurate pattern size will result in either laceration of the stoma by the wafer or maceration of peristomal skin from constant contact with urine.
12. Cut wafer as traced.	12. Accurately cutting the traced pattern will ensure a snug fit.
14. Remove paper backing from wafer. Dry peristomal skin if wet. Place wafer on skin with stoma centered on opening of wafer.	14. Paper backing needs to be removed from wafer in order for wafer to adhere to skin. Dry skin helps the wafer to adhere to the skin.
13. Remove wick from orifice of stoma.	13. Allows visualization of the stoma and accurate placement of the wafer.
15. Attach clean pouch to wafer. Make sure drainage port is closed.	15. Saves time and prevents urine from leaking underneath the wafer during application process.
16. Remove gloves and wash hands.	16. Reduces the transmission of microorganisms.

▶ EVALUATION

- Peristomal skin integrity remains intact.
- Irritated or denuded peristomal skin integrity healed.
- Client acknowledges the change in body image.
- Client expresses positive feelings about self.
- Client maintains fluid balance.

▶ DOCUMENTATION

Nurses' Notes

Document:
- Assessment of peristomal skin

- Assessment of stoma
- Stoma measurements (length, width, height)
- Color and amount of drainage
- Peristomal skin care if alteration in skin integrity was noted
- Type of ostomy pouch applied

Document on appropriate flow sheet or electronic medical record (EMR).

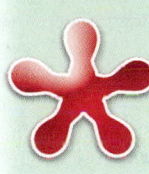

▶ REAL WORLD ANECDOTES

A 45-year-old man is diagnosed with bladder cancer and decides to have a noncontinent urinary diversion (ileal conduit) rather than a continent surgical procedure (neobladder) that would require an additional 8–10 hours of surgical time. The usual operative time for a total cystectomy and creation of an ileal conduit is 3–4 hours. There is no difference in length of hospitalization (7–10 days). Clients may make decisions based on priorities different from yours. In this instance, the client is more concerned about the length of the surgery than the postoperative outcome. It is important to listen to the client's priorities and to make sure he has enough information on which to base a decision.

▶ CRITICAL THINKING SKILL

Introduction

The client is postoperative from removal of bladder and re-creation of an ileal conduit or urostomy.

Possible Scenario

A 60-year-old man is 4 days postoperative for a total cystectomy and creation of an ileal conduit. He complains that his skin is itching under the wafer of his ostomy appliance. Inspection of the ostomy appliance reveals that urine is leaking below the wafer. The nurse removes the current appliance, which has not been changed since the surgery 4 days previously. This would be the client's first learning opportunity. The nurse takes the time to include the client in a learning process as she changes the appliance. An assessment of the peristomal skin reveals mild maceration from

constant urine contact. Stoma is viable and measures 1 inch × 1.5 inches with a height of 0.5 inches. There are no noted creases or crevices at the base of the stoma.

Possible Outcome

If the astute nurse did not pick up on the clue offered by the client ("My skin itches under this thing"), the appliance would have continued to leak and cause further peristomal skin damage.

Prevention

Assessment of a new urinary ostomy appliance should be done every shift until the client is independent in care. Most ostomy appliances should be changed by the third day postoperative to begin client teaching. Also, by this time the stoma has decreased in size because of loss of edema. A change in stoma size results in increased exposure of the peristomal skin to urine.

▶ VARIATIONS

Geriatric Variations:

- *If a client has arthritic hands it is best to use either a one-piece appliance that is precut or a two-piece appliance that is adaptable to decreases in hand dexterity.*
- *Make sure the client can see and hear your teaching instructions. Ask for feedback to assess if the client heard and understood the procedure.*
- *If the client needs assistance, instruct a willing family member or caregiver on the procedure.*

Pediatric Variation:

- *An ostomy located near a child's groin will need an appliance that is very flexible and can bend with the client's movement and play without becoming nonadherent.*

Home Care Variations:

- *Make sure the client has the necessary supplies and facilities to clean and change his or her urinary diversion.*
- *Changes in body image could cause the client to withdraw from social situations or even become house-bound. As the home care nurse entering the home, you are in a unique position to assess psychosocial needs and changes resulting from alterations in body image.*

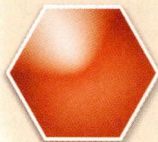

Long-Term Care Variation:

- *Consider the ongoing cost of supplies, and discuss any concerns with the client. Connect the client with community resources, support groups, or further assessment, if needed.*

▶ COMMON ERRORS

Possible Error:

The appliance chosen is too small or too large for the stoma's dimensions.

Prevention:

Measure the dimensions of the stoma prior to obtaining and preparing a pouch for application. If the error occurs, remove the leaking appliance and remeasure the stoma dimensions before reapplying the ostomy appliance.

▶ NURSING TIPS

- Recognize that all stomas are not the same. Each stoma must be treated individually, requiring the nurse to assess the dimensions and location in relation to the client's body movements (e.g., sitting, bending) and the peristomal skin's condition.
- Client teaching is easily incorporated into the care of the ostomy by encouraging the client to be your assistant during the application process.
- Use of an ostomy appliance that is intact, comfortable, and easy to use will increase the client's comfort level and thereby increase participation in self-care activities.
- Costs to the client and the health care institution are reduced when simplistic ostomy care is provided. Simplistic ostomy care excludes the daily use of pectin powder, pectin paste, and skin sealant.

▶ **SPECIAL CONSIDERATIONS**

- *Assess skin integrity when performing stoma care. Assess stoma site. It should be red and moist. Document any sign of skin breakdown.*
- *Frequently change the stoma pouch if the skin underneath the appliance appears irritated. Chemical or scented wipes are usually irritating to the skin and should be avoided.*

Administering Peritoneal Dialysis

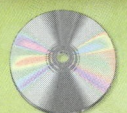

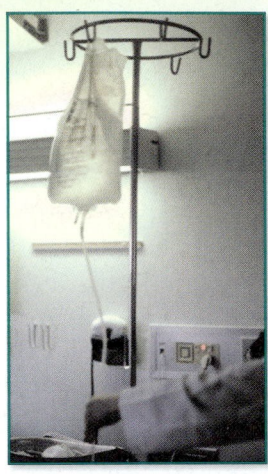

▶ OVERVIEW OF THE SKILL

Peritoneal dialysis is a method of removing waste products of metabolism, excess fluids, drugs, or chemicals from the body and restoring proper fluid and electrolyte balance by diffusion and osmosis through the client's peritoneal membrane. A concentrated dialysate is instilled into the peritoneal cavity by a catheter inserted into the peritoneum through the abdomen. It is left in the abdomen for a prescribed period of time. The fluid is then drained, and the process is repeated. The process is similar to paracentesis, except a catheter is left in place for dialysis. As this is an invasive procedure, surgical aseptic technique is required to place the catheter.

While the dialysate is in place, products (nitrogenous waste products, chemicals, and electrolytes) in the blood flowing through the rich capillary system of the peritoneal membrane diffuse into the dialysate. Water also moves from the blood into the fluid. This is accomplished by adding concentrations of glucose in varying degrees to the dialysate, which makes the solution hypertonic and allows osmosis to occur.

Peritoneal dialysis can be used in clients who cannot tolerate hemodialysis or in situations where hemodialysis is not readily available. After the dialysis catheter is placed, the wound requires dressings for approximately 8 weeks until it heals.

There are two main types of peritoneal dialysis: continuous and intermittent. Continuous ambulatory peritoneal dialysis (CAPD) is ongoing. The dialysate remains in the peritoneal cavity between 4 and 8 hours, then the cycle is repeated. During intermittent peritoneal dialysis, the dialysate remains in the abdomen for 20 minutes. Then the cycle is repeated a prescribed number of times or interrupted until the next session.

▶ ASSESSMENT

1. Assess the client's cardiovascular and respiratory status **to establish a baseline for future comparisons to detect increasing shortness of breath, rales, atelectasis, or elevated pulse.**
2. Measure the client's abdominal girth **to establish a baseline for future comparisons to detect if fluid has been retained (see Figure 6-18-1).**

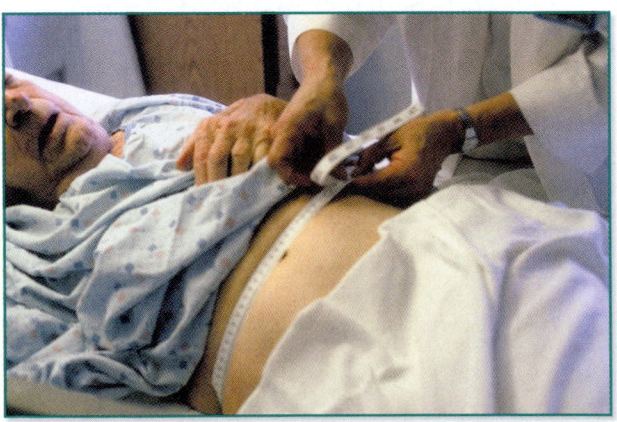

Figure 6-18-1 Measuring the abdominal girth before and after the procedure helps detect if fluid has been retained.

3. Assess the client's abdomen **to establish the state of skin integrity before the procedure and to look for signs of abdominal distention and infection.**

▶ DIAGNOSIS

Acute Pain

Deficient Knowledge

Ineffective Tissue Perfusion

Risk for Fluid Volume Excess

Risk for Ineffective Breathing Pattern

Risk for Ineffective Coping

Risk for Impaired Skin Integrity

Risk for Infection

▶ PLANNING

Expected Outcomes:

1. Client will experience relief of respiratory symptoms related to pressure from fluid on the diaphragm.
2. Client will experience relief of symptoms related to nitrogenous waste products.
3. Client will not suffer from fluid volume overload.
4. Client will not exhibit any signs or symptoms of infection following the dialysis.
5. The skin at the catheter entry site will remain intact without infection or excoriation.
6. Client will not experience pain or discomfort related to the procedure.

Equipment Needed (see Figure 6-18-2):

- Dialysate
- Sterile drape
- Sterile basin
- Povidone-iodine swabs or sterile 4 × 4 dressings and povidone-iodine liquid

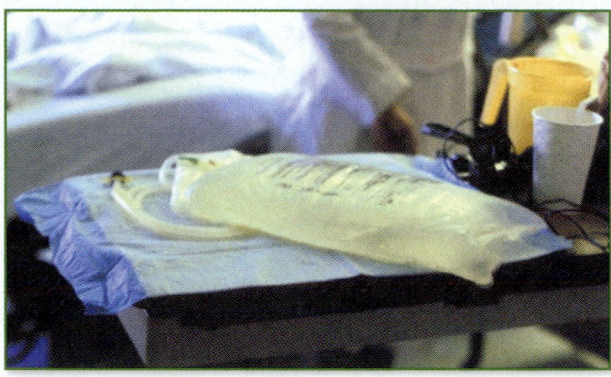

Figure 6-18-2 Dialysate

- Sterile gloves
- Masks
- Biohazard bag
- Clean gloves

▶ CLIENT EDUCATION NEEDED:

1. Explain the purpose of the procedure to the client.
2. Explain the need for the low Fowler's position during the procedure.
3. Teach the client the need for aseptic technique in caring for the catheter and the insertion site. This will reduce the risk of infection in the peritoneal cavity.
4. If the client will be performing this procedure at home, have client return-demonstrate the procedure.
5. Clients can participate as much as possible in the procedure, especially if performing it at home.

Estimated time to complete the skill: **15–30 minutes to infuse the dialysate; 15–30 minutes to drain the dialysate**

▶ DELEGATION TIPS

Administering peritoneal dialysis requires the skills and problem-solving abilities of a nurse. This skill cannot be delegated.

IMPLEMENTATION—Action/Rationale

Action	Rationale
1. Gather equipment needed at the bedside. Warm the dialysate to body temperature and bring it to the bedside.	1. Smoothes the performance of the procedure. Warming the dialysate prevents shock in the client from infusing cold fluid directly into the abdomen.

continues

Action	Rationale

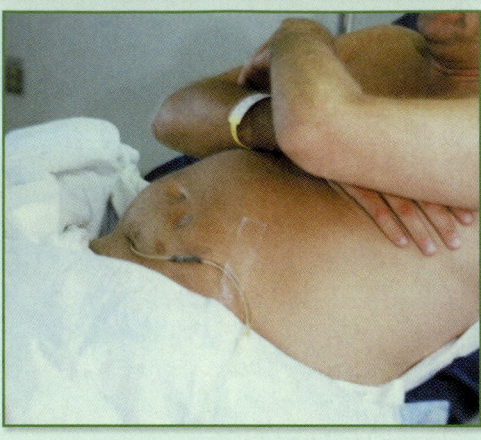

Figure 6-18-3   Position the client in a semi-Fowler's position.

Action	Rationale
2. Wash hands.	2. Reduces the transmission of microorganisms.
3. Position the client in a comfortable position, usually semi-Fowler's position (see Figure 6-18-3).	3. Positioning for comfort allows the client to tolerate the dialysis for longer periods of time. Semi-Fowler's position ensures that there is room for peritoneal expansion.
4. Weigh the dialysate.	4. Establishes a baseline to compare with returned fluid weight.
5. Apply mask to client and nurse.	5. Masks prevent the transmission of microorganisms.
6. Spike the dialysate bag with the tubing, hang the bag from an IV pole and prime the tubing. Clamp the tubing once it is primed.	6. Prepares the equipment for use as soon as the connector has been cleaned.
7. Establish a sterile field under the end of the peritoneal catheter, using the sterile drape.	7. Provides a sterile surface for cleaning the catheter and reducing the transmission of microorganisms.
8. Open the povidone-iodine swabs using aseptic technique and drop them onto the sterile field. If using sterile 4 × 4 pads, open the sterile basin and, using aseptic technique, pour povidone-iodine into the basin. Taking care not to contaminate the 4 × 4 pads, drop them into the povidone-iodine in the basin.	8. Provides a sterile bacteriocide to cleanse the catheter.
9. Apply sterile gloves.	9. Prevents contamination of the sterile materials.
10. Using the povidone-iodine swabs or the soaked 4 × 3-4 pads, cleanse the proximal end of the catheter. Allow the povidone-iodine to dry prior to connecting the tubing.	10. Povidone-iodine must be allowed to dry to provide a bacteriocidal action.
11. Attach the infusion tubing and dialysate to the dialysis catheter (see Figure 6-18-4). The dialysate is hung on a pole and administered by gravity. The type and amount of dialysate of each bag will be determined by the client's laboratory results, the purpose of the dialysis, and orders.	11. Because peritoneal dialysis is a process of osmosis, concentrations of dialysate are determined by the amount of waste products and amount of fluid desired to be removed by the process of gradients.
12. Remove mask from client and nurse.	12. Promote client comfort. Masks are not needed after the infusion tubing is attached to the dialysis catheter.

continues

Action	Rationale

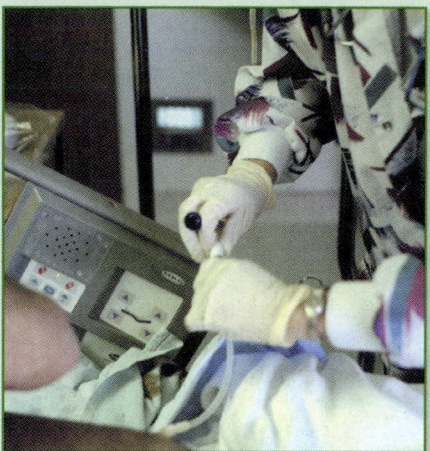

Figure 6-18-4 Attach the infusion tubing to the dialysis catheter.

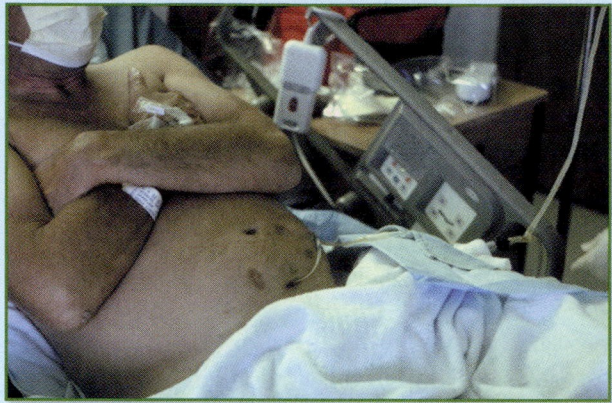

Figure 6-18-5 Allow the dialysate to enter the abdomen and remain the appropriate time.

13. Unclamp the tubing and allow dialysate to enter the abdomen and remain the appropriate time as ordered. Dialysate takes approximately 5–15 minutes to infuse (see Figure 6-18-5).

13. Dialysate must remain in the abdomen for osmosis to occur and for waste products to be pulled out of the system.

14. Assess the client for pain or discomfort. Pain sometimes occurs with the procedure, especially while the fluid is being infused. It is very important to assess the pain accurately.

14. If the pain is accompanied by signs of peritonitis or bleeding, follow up immediately.

15. When the ordered amount of dialysate has been infused, clamp the dialysis tubing for the ordered amount of dwell time.

15. Allows the dialysate to remain in contact with the peritoneum. If the dwell time of the dialysate will be hours, the client can fold the empty bag and carry it along, tucked into clothing, until it is time to drain the dialysate.

16. Dispose of equipment, remove gloves, and wash hands.

16. Reduces the transmission of microorganisms.

17. After the dialysate has remained in the abdomen a specified time (usually 20 minutes for intermittent dialysis, 4–8 hours for continuous dialysis) and is ready to be drained, wash hands, apply gloves, and remove the empty bag from the pole and place it below the level of the peritoneum. Unclamp the tubing leading to the bag and allow drainage of the effluent into the empty bag.

17. The level of the bag must be placed well below the abdomen to facilitate drainage by gravity.

18. Periodically weigh the bag of effluent as the abdomen drains. When the weight of the effluent bag has been stable for 10 to 15 minutes, clamp the drainage tubing. This usually takes approximately 30 minutes.

18. When the weight of the bag no longer changes, the abdomen should be fully drained. At this point the bag of effluent should weigh more than it did prior to instillation as it will also contain waste products and wastewater. If the stable weight of the effluent bag is less than the preinfusion weight, unclamp the tubing and reposition the client from side to side to allow any trapped effluent to drain.

19. Hold the full bag up to the light and inspect the fluid. The color should be light to medium yellow or amber and clear. If it is red-tinged, dark, or cloudy, consult the health care provider and report findings.

19. Red-tinged, dark, or cloudy effluent could indicate bleeding, infection, or perforation.

continues

Action	Rationale
20. Compare the weight of the returned fluid with the preinfusion weight. If there is substantially less fluid returned than was administered, report findings to health care provider.	20. The amount of drainage generally exceeds the amount of fluid entering the abdominal cavity as the process of dialysis also removes excess fluid. If the amount of returned fluid is less than the amount instilled, report this finding since this could indicate that the client is retaining dialysate fluid related to dehydration or occlusion of the catheter by tissue or kinking.
21. Remove gloves and wash hands.	21. Reduces the transmission of microorganisms.
22. Ensure that any laboratory tests ordered are performed to track the client's fluid and electrolyte balance. Notify the health care provider of any significant changes in the laboratory results.	22. Determines how much dialysis is required and what concentrations of dialysate are required.
23. Warm the next bag of dialysate to be exchanged, if ordered. Repeat the above process. Use new tubing for each bag of dialysate.	23. Ensures the procedure continues as ordered.

▶ EVALUATION

- Client experienced relief of respiratory symptoms related to pressure from fluid on the diaphragm.
- Client experienced relief of symptoms related to nitrogenous waste products.
- Client did not suffer from fluid volume overload.
- Client has not exhibited any signs or symptoms of infection following the dialysis.
- The skin at the catheter entry site remained intact without infection or excoriation.
- Client did not experience pain or discomfort related to the procedure.

▶ DOCUMENTATION

Nurses' Notes

- Document the client's response to dialysis, such as any change in vital signs or general cardiovascular or respiratory symptoms.

- Document the color and clarity of effluent.
- Document any symptoms that may be associated with peritonitis or internal bleeding, including rebound tenderness, cloudy outflow, blood in the outflow, fever, or abdominal rigidity.
- Document the time the procedure was started and how long it took.
- If the procedure was repeated, document how many repetitions were completed.
- If the health care provider was notified, document the time, reason, and any orders that were received.

Document on appropriate flow sheet or electronic medical record (EMR).

Intake and Output Record

- Record the amount of dialysate infused and the amount returned.

▶ REAL WORLD ANECDOTES

Mr. Ybarra was due for three rounds of peritoneal dialysis. As the nurse infused the first bagful of dialysate, Mr. Ybarra complained of abdominal pain. The nurse's assessment did not reveal any other symptoms of infection or internal bleeding, and slowing the dialysate's infusion rate seemed to help ease Mr. Ybarra's pain. Mr. Ybarra tolerated the 30-minute dwell time and the nurse proceeded to drain the dialysate. As the fluid return flowed into the bag, the nurse noticed it was cloudy with sediment in it. The nurse assessed Mr. Ybarra and noted that he had abdominal tenderness and rigidity. His temperature was slightly elevated and his pulse was rapid. The nurse continued to drain the dialysate and notified Mr. Ybarra's physician. The physician determined that Mr. Ybarra had developed peritonitis and instituted antibiotic therapy.

▶ CRITICAL THINKING SKILL

Introduction
Monitor carefully to detect and intervene in the complications of peritoneal dialysis.

Possible Scenario
Mary is undergoing peritoneal dialysis this morning. The catheter was placed about an hour ago, and this is the end of the outflow segment of her first cycle of dialysis. You note that Mary has peripheral edema. She complained of mild pain during the infusion segment. Now she has dizziness and apprehension and is sweating. Her pulse is 120, and her respirations are 25 and shallow. She is pale.

Possible Outcome
Your client has developed orthostatic hypotension. Fluid was removed too rapidly. Her intravascular volume is decreased. The physician orders intravenous fluids even though the client has an extravascular fluid excess.

Prevention
Assess sodium levels prior to dialysis; assess for postural changes in blood pressure before procedure.

▶ VARIATIONS

Geriatric Variations:
- *Elderly clients may not tolerate rapid changes in volume.*
- *Elderly clients may have multiple other conditions, such as diabetes, hypertension, or chronic skin conditions. Assess how these conditions, and the medications the client takes for them, may interact with the dialysis.*

Pediatric Variation:
- *While it is important to encourage the child to be as active as possible, discourage activities that involve close physical contact, especially to the abdominal area.*

Home Care Variations:
- *Peritoneal dialysis can be performed in the home setting, by the family, the client, or home-based caregivers. Assess the caregiver for willingness to undertake the commitment to learn and perform the procedure daily.*
- *Assess the home environment to determine if cleanliness and safety can be maintained.*
- *Determine whether a "backup" person is willing to be trained to provide relief to the primary caregiver. The dialysis procedure can be complex to learn. When teaching home care prior to hospital discharge, establish follow-up contacts and emergency contacts so the client or caregiver knows whom to call for help with troubleshooting the dialysis routine in the home environment. Scheduling the procedure, preparation, storage and warming of the dialysate, operation of dialysis equipment (if automated equipment is used), comfort, and caregiver burnout are all issues that need to be discussed. Teaching must include information on site care, nutrition, the basics of fluid and electrolyte balance, and signs of infection, bleeding, or perforation.*

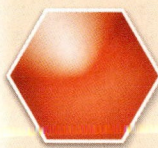

Long-Term Care Variations:
- *Long-term fluid restriction and immobility could lead to constipation. Assess the client for signs and symptoms of constipation.*
- *Assess for signs of depression or helplessness related to the long-term need for dialysis and the food, activity, and fluid restrictions involved.*

▶ COMMON ERRORS

Possible Error:

The dialysate is cold and causes pain on inflow.

Prevention:

Remember to warm the dialysate to body temperature prior to administering the procedure.

Possible Error:

Leaving the dialysate in the abdomen too long.

Prevention:

Set a timer; set your watch alarm if you have one. If the client is alert and cooperative, have the client remind you when the time is up.

▶ NURSING TIPS

- Carefully assess cardiovascular and respiratory status prior to procedure. Accurate assessment is crucial to detect often subtle changes in the client's status.
- Assess laboratory values prior to procedure. Changes in laboratory values help determine if the procedure is working and can help explain symptoms that occur.

- Be cognizant of systemic symptoms caused by laboratory value changes. Tremors or weakness, for example, can be caused by low levels of potassium.
- Remember that fluid shifts, symptoms, or complications can arise well after the dialysis procedure is completed.

▶ SPECIAL CONSIDERATIONS

- *If the returned dialysate solution is not clear, it may be a sign of peritonitis. Watch for signs such as abdominal rigidity, palpation tenderness, increased body temperature, or cloudy output of the dialysate solution. Document the assessment and notify the health care provider.*
- *Limit the dialysis cycle to the designated length (usually less than an hour). Prolonged fluid in the peritoneal cavity may decrease the effectiveness of dialysis as the BUN and creatinine on either side of the membrane equilibrate.*
- *When the returned fluid is less than expected, higher concentration of dialysate solution may be prescribed by the health care provider to improve the effectiveness. Hypertonic fluid (usually 1.5–4.25% dextrose) attracts more body fluid across the peritoneal membrane.*

Administering an Enema

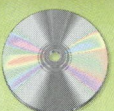

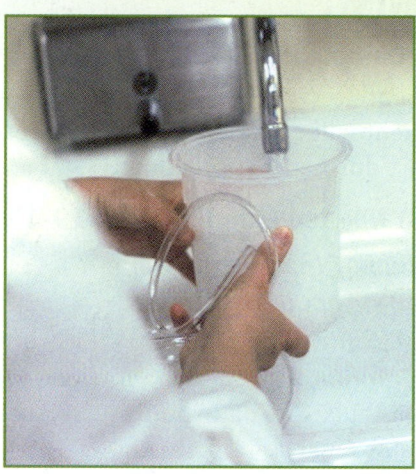

▶ OVERVIEW OF THE SKILL

An enema is a solution inserted into the rectum and sigmoid colon for the purpose of removing feces and/or flatus. Enemas can also be used to instill medications or nutrition. A cleansing enema is probably the most common type of enema. This type of enema stimulates peristalsis via irritation of the colon/rectum and by causing intestinal distention with fluid. The solution used in a cleansing enema must be chosen with care. Some solutions, such as tap-water-based solutions, draw fluid and electrolytes out of the body. They should not be used in clients with preexisting fluid and electrolyte imbalances. There are two general types of cleansing enemas: the large-volume enema and the small-volume enema.

A large-volume enema is designed to clean the colon of as much feces as possible. In a large-volume enema, between 500 and 1000 mL of fluid are instilled into the rectum/colon and the client is asked to retain the fluid as long as possible. This action allows the fluid to soften and loosen the feces. The large volume of fluid also distends the bowel, stimulating peristalsis. Large-volume enemas are the traditional intervention for constipation. Traditionally soapsuds enemas were used, and many large-volume enema kits still come with a small packet of liquid soap to be dissolved in the enema solution. Soapsuds enemas are very irritating to the colon and are rarely ordered anymore. Large-volume enemas are often ordered prior to procedures

or surgeries that require visualization of the colon. When used for this reason, the health care provider will often order "enemas until clear." This indicates that large-volume enemas are to be given until the fluid returned is clear of fecal matter. Most institutions have guidelines regarding the maximum number of large-volume enemas that can be administered to a client.

Small-volume enemas are designed to clear the rectum and the sigmoid colon of fecal matter. Small-volume enemas can be delivered with the traditional enema kit using 50–200 mL of solution, but most frequently they are administered using a prepackaged disposable enema. There are a number of prepackaged small enemas available. These enemas work by using a hypertonic rectal stimulant that stimulates peristalsis and draws fluid from the intestinal walls to soften the feces. Because these enemas use the body's own fluid to lubricate the stool, this type of enema is contraindicated in clients who are dehydrated. Prepackaged enemas are easily administered and available over-the-counter in most drug stores. This makes them ideal for home care use.

There are several types of enemas used for purposes other than cleansing. An oil retention enema is a small-volume enema that instills oil into the rectum. The oil is retained for up to an hour and is designed to soften very hard stool. It is often followed by a large-volume cleansing enema. Medications can be administered by enema as well. A small-volume enema can deliver a medicated solution directly to the rectal mucosa. This method of medication administration is useful when the rectum is the area to be medicated if the client is unable to take oral medications or if rapid absorption of the medication is required. The return-flow enema is used to remove flatus and stimulate peristalsis. It is frequently used following abdominal surgery to reduce intestinal distention and to stimulate the resumption of bowel function.

Many different solutions are used for enemas, including tap water, normal saline, hypertonic solutions, soap solutions, oil, and carminative solutions. Tap water is a hypotonic solution. Because it is a less concentrated solution than the body's cells, it is drawn into the body and may cause water toxicity, electrolyte imbalance, or circulatory overload. Normal saline is an isotonic solution. It is the same concentration as the body's own fluids and is considered to be a safe enema solution. It is important that children and infants only be given normal saline enemas as their small size predisposes them to fluid imbalances. Prepackaged small-volume enemas use hypertonic solutions to draw fluid from the body to lubricate the stool and distend the rectum. Hypertonic solutions are contraindicated in dehydrated clients and small children. Carminative solutions are used to provide relief from gas. An example of a carminative enema is MGW solution, which is 30 mL of magnesium, 60 mL of glycerin, and 90 mL of water.

Enemas are contraindicated in clients with bowel obstruction, inflammation, or infection of the abdomen or if the client has had recent rectal or anal surgery. If the nurse has any question regarding the advisability of administering an enema, he or she should consult the client's health care provider.

▶ ASSESSMENT

1. Identify the type of enema ordered as well as the rationale for the enema. **Allows the nurse to verify the appropriateness of the type of enema ordered.**
2. Assess the physical condition of the client. Determine whether the client has bowel sounds. Assess for a history of constipation, hemorrhoids, or diverticulitis. Determine whether the client will be able to hold a side-lying or knee-chest position or be able to retain the enema solution. **Allows the nurse to plan the procedure with the client's limitations in mind.**
3. Assess the client's mental state, including ability to understand and cooperate with the procedure, the client's knowledge level regarding the procedure, and any pre-existing fears the client may have regarding the procedure. Knowing if the client can comprehend and cooperate with the

procedure will help the nurse plan ahead. **Many clients have pre-existing fears and beliefs regarding enemas and their administration.**

▶ DIAGNOSIS

Constipation

Deficient Knowledge

▶ PLANNING

Expected Outcomes:

1. The client's rectum will be free of feces and flatus.
2. The client will experience a minimum of discomfort during the procedure.

Equipment Needed (see Figure 6-19-1):

Large-Volume Cleansing Enema

- Absorbent pad for the bed
- Disposable gloves
- Bedside commode or bedpan if client will not be able to ambulate to bathroom (see Figure 6-19-2)
- Lubricant
- Enema container
- Tubing with clamp and nozzle

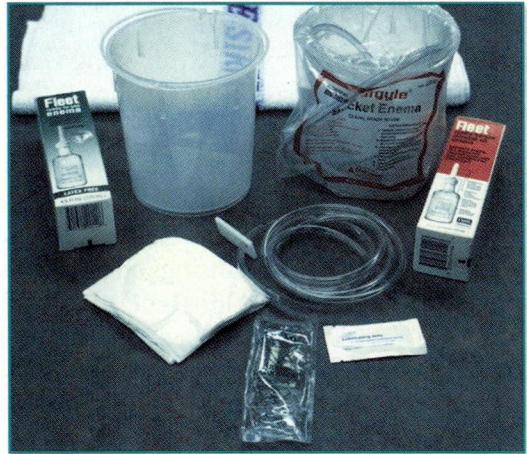

Figure 6-19-1 Various types of enema equipment and solutions are available.

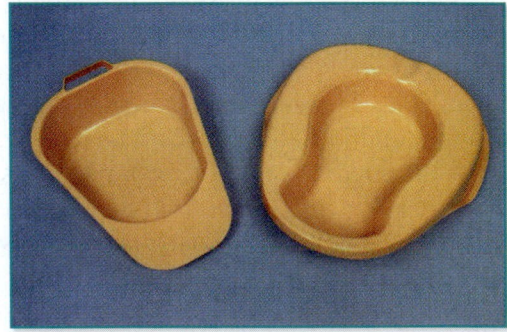

Figure 6-19-2 Bedpans are used when administering an enema if the client cannot ambulate to the bathroom or use a bedside commode.

- Thermometer for enema solution
- Toilet tissue
- IV pole
- Washcloth, towel, and basin

Small-Volume Prepackaged Enema (see Figure 6-19-3)
- Prescribed prepackaged enema
- Lubricant, if the tip is not prelubricated
- Toilet tissue
- Bedpan or commode if the client cannot use the bathroom
- Absorbent pad for bed
- Gloves

Return-Flow Enema

- Absorbent pad for the bed
- Disposable gloves
- Bedside commode or bedpan if client will not be able to ambulate to bathroom

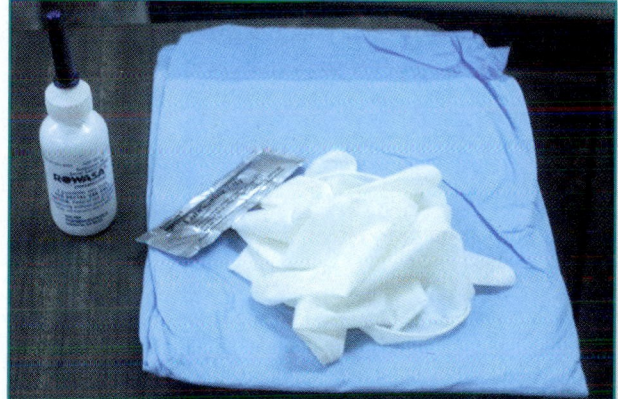

Figure 6-19-3 Small-volume prepackaged enema, gloves, protective pad, and lubricant

- Prescribed solution
- Lubricant
- Enema container
- Tubing with clamp and nozzle
- Thermometer
- Toilet tissue

► CLIENT EDUCATION NEEDED:

1. Explain rationale for enema (to clear the bowel of feces).
2. Explain the procedure and steps involved.
3. Explain need to retain enema solution for prescribed time period to ensure success.
4. Clients should be taught that enemas should not be used to treat constipation on a routine basis.
5. Clients should be instructed not to flush the toilet until the nurse can observe the contents.
6. Clients who are unfamiliar with enema administration should be warned about the feeling of fullness or need to evacuate as the enema is administered.
7. Clients should be instructed to inform the nurse if cramps or abdominal pain occurs.
8. Clients should be instructed that lying on the back with knees and hips flexed toward the chest may make it easier to self-administer an enema.

Estimated time to complete the skill: **Depending on the type of enema ordered, approximately 15 minutes to prepare client and administer solution.**

► DELEGATION TIPS

Administering an enema is a procedure that ancillary personnel are able to perform after proper instruction and supervision. Instruct ancillary personnel to notify the nurse if any difficulties in administering or negative reactions such as severe cramping or inability to retain the enema occur. Results should be documented and reported to the nurse.

IMPLEMENTATION—Action/Rationale

Action	Rationale
Large-Volume Cleansing Enema	
1. Wash hands.	1. Reduces the transmission of microorganisms.
2. Assess client's understanding of procedure and provide privacy.	2. Prepares client for procedure.

continues

Action	Rationale
Large-Volume Cleansing Enema *continued*	
3. Apply gloves.	3. Prevents contact with feces.
4. Prepare equipment (see Figure 6-19-4).	4. Ensures a smooth procedure.
5. If specified, heat solution to desired temperature using thermometer to measure. Enemas administered to adults are usually given at 105° to 110° F (40.5° to 43° C), and those administered to children are usually administered at 100° F (37.7° C). Solution should be at least body temperature to prevent cramping and discomfort.	5. Enemas work best when solution is warm. If enemas are too hot, damage can be done to the bowel mucosa. If enemas are too cold, spasms may occur.
6. Fill the bucket or bag with warm water, add solution if ordered. Mix the solution gently (see Figure 6-19-5). Open the clamp and allow solution to prime the tubing. Clamp the tubing when primed.	6. Adding solution to the water prevents suds from forming. Priming the tubing expels air from the tubing, which could cause the client intestinal distention and discomfort.
7. Place absorbent pad on bed under client. Assist client in attaining left lateral position with right leg flexed as sharply as possible. If there is a question regarding the client's ability to hold the solution, place a bedpan on the bed nearby (see Figure 6-19-5).	7. Facilitates flow of solution into the rectum and colon. The flexed leg provides the best exposure of the anus.
8. Lubricate 5 cm (2 inches) of the rectal tube unless the tube is part of a prelubricated enema set (see Figure 6-19-6).	8. Minimizes trauma to the anal sphincter during insertion of the rectal tube.
9. Have the client take a deep breath. Simultaneously, slowly and smoothly insert rectal tube into rectum approximately 7–10 cm in an adult (3–4 inches). Aim the rectal tube toward the client's umbilicus (see Figure 6-19-7).	9. A deep breath helps to relax the sphincter. The rectum of an adult is usually 10–20 cm (4–6 inches). The tube should be inserted beyond the internal sphincter. Insertion of rectal tube toward the umbilicus guides tube along rectum.

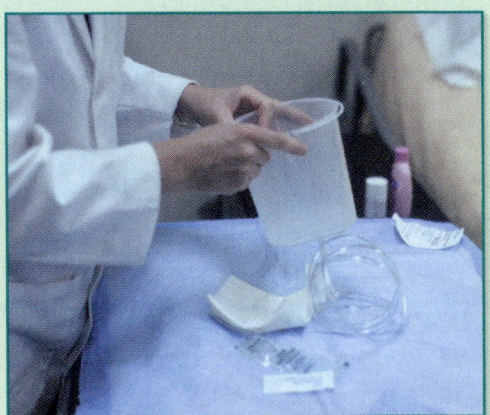

Figure 6-19-4   Assemble equipment at the bedside.

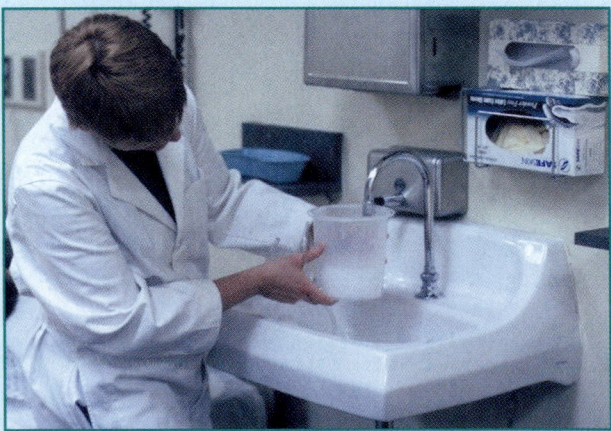

Figure 6-19-5   Place solution into the bucket and add water as needed.

continues

Action	Rationale

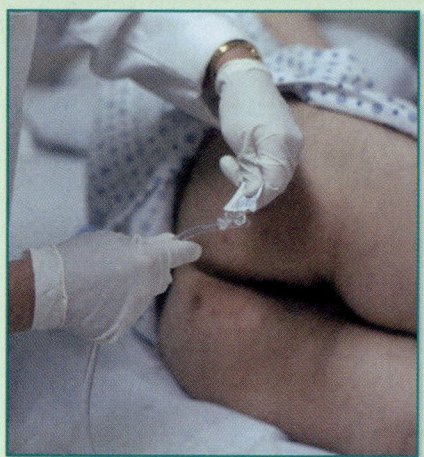

Figure 6-19-6 Lubricate 2 inches of the rectal tube with lubricant.

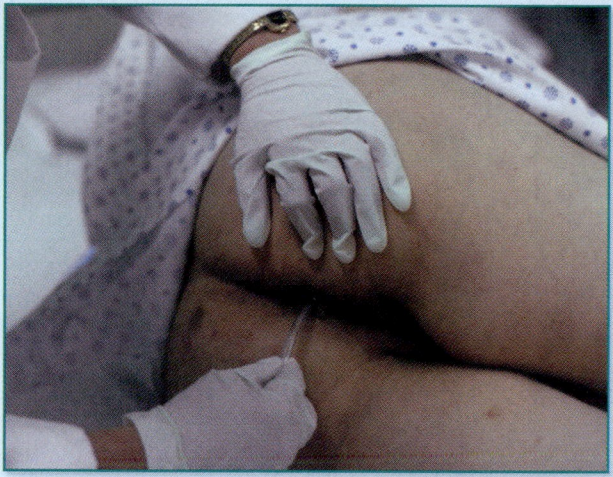

Figure 6-19-7 Gently and smoothly insert the rectal tube into the rectum.

10. Raise the container holding the solution and open clamp. (If using an enema set, squeeze the container holding solution). The solution should be 30–45 cm (12–18 inches) above the rectum for an adult, and 7.5 cm (3 inches) above the rectum for an infant. The solution may be placed on an IV pole at the proper height.

11. Slowly administer the fluid.
   a. If the client complains of cramping, clamp the tubing and instruct the client to take slow breaths. When cramping has decreased, unclamp the tubing to continue fluid flow.

12. When solution has been completely administered or when the client cannot hold any more fluid, clamp the tubing, remove the rectal tube, and dispose of it properly.

13. Clean lubricant, any solution, and any feces from the anus with toilet tissue (see Figure 6-19-8).

14. Have the client continue to lie on the left side for the prescribed length of time.

15. When the client has retained the enema for the prescribed amount of time, assist to the bedside commode or toilet or onto the bedpan. If the client is using the bathroom, instruct not to flush the toilet when finished.

10. Solution should be at a height above rectum that allows gravity flow of solution into the rectum, but does not cause damage to the rectal lining because of a too rapid increase in rectal pressure.

11. Administering enema slowly with momentary pauses decreases the incidence of intestinal spasms and cramps.

12. The urge to defecate indicates that a sufficient amount of fluid has been administered.

13. Minimizes skin irritation.

14. Certain types of enemas are more effective when retained for a specified amount of time. It is easier for the client to retain the enema in a lying position, where gravity can be resisted.

15. Client will be prepared to expel fluid and feces.

continues

Action	Rationale

Large-Volume Cleansing Enema *continued*

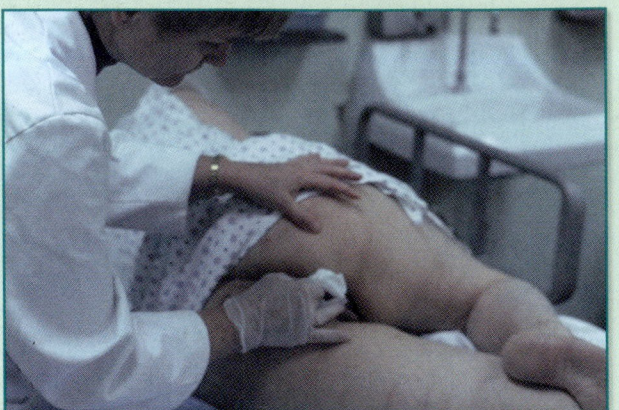

Figure 6-19-8 Clean the anal area to remove excess lubricant.

16. When the client is finished expelling the enema, assist to clean the perineal area, if needed.

17. Return the client to a comfortable position. Place a clean, dry protective pad under the client to catch any solution or feces that may continue to be expelled.

18. Observe feces.

19. Remove gloves and wash hands.

Small-Volume Prepackaged Enema

20. Wash hands.

21. Remove prepackaged enema from packaging. Be familiar with any special instructions included with the enema. The packaged enema may be stood in a basin of warm water to warm the fluid prior to use (see Figure 6-19-9).

22. Apply gloves.

23. Place absorbent pad on bed under client. Assist client in attaining left lateral position with right leg flexed as sharply as possible (see Figure 6-19-10), or you may use the knee-chest position (see Figure 6-19-11). If there is a question regarding the client's ability to hold the solution, place a bedpan on the bed nearby.

24. Remove the protective cap from the nozzle and inspect the nozzle for lubrication. If the lubrication is not adequate, add more.

25. Squeeze the container gently to remove any air and prime the nozzle.

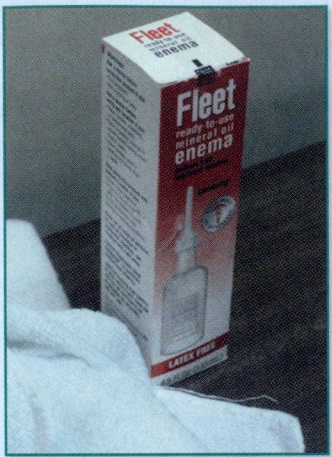

Figure 6-19-9 A commercial enema

16. Prevents skin breakdown and excoriation.

17. Provides comfort for the client and protects the linen from potential soiling.

18. Results can be documented.

19. Reduces transmission of microorganisms.

20. Reduces transmission of microorganisms.

21. Prepares the enema for use.

22. Protects hands from exposure to feces.

23. Facilitates flow of solution into the rectum and colon. The flexed leg provides the best exposure of the anus. The knee-chest position provides good exposure and allows gravity to aid in retention of the enema.

24. Prevents trauma to the rectal mucosa.

25. Reduces introduction of air into the rectum.

continues

Action	Rationale

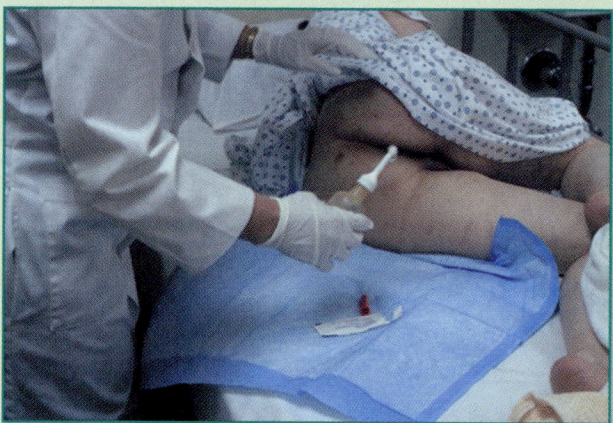

Figure 6-19-10 Position the client in the left lateral position with the right leg sharply flexed.

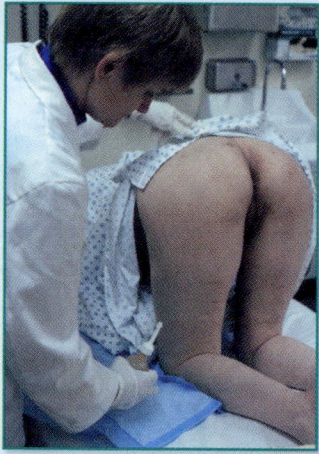

Figure 6-19-11 Alternately, you may position the client in the knee-chest position.

26. Have the client take a deep breath. Simultaneously gently insert the enema nozzle into the anus, pointing the nozzle toward the umbilicus.

26. Relaxes the rectal sphincter. Pointing the nozzle toward the umbilicus positions the nozzle away from the rectal walls.

27. Squeeze the container until all the solution is instilled (see Figure 6-19-12).

27. Allows the client to get the full benefit of the solution.

28. Remove the nozzle from the anus and dispose of the empty container in a trash receptacle (see Figure 6-19-13).

28. Prevents the spread of microorganisms.

29. Clean lubricant, any solution, and any feces from the anus with toilet tissue.

29. Minimizes skin irritation.

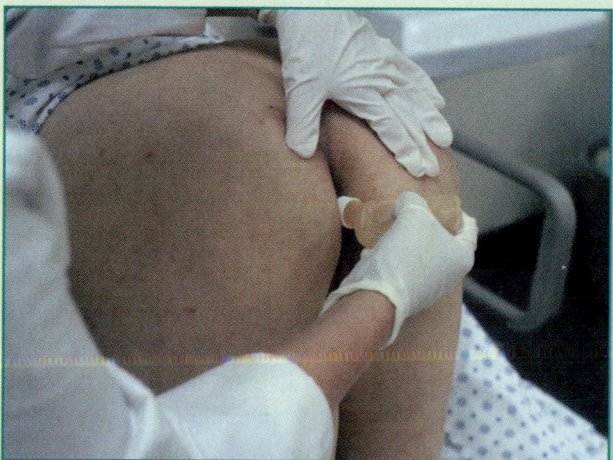

Figure 6-19-12 After inserting the nozzle into the anus, squeeze the container until all the solution is instilled.

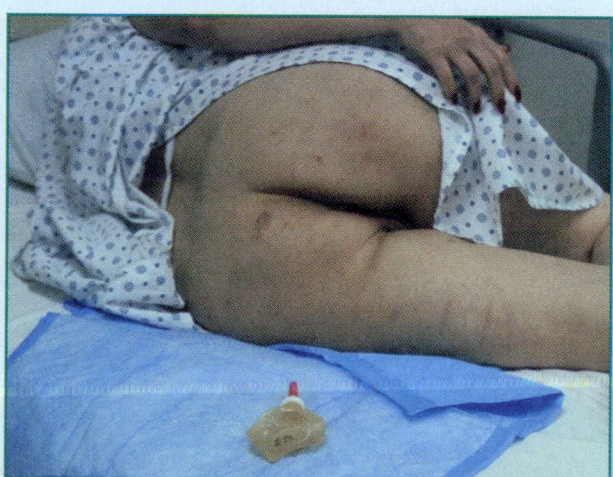

Figure 6-19-13 Remove the nozzle and container and have the client continue to lie on the left side for the prescribed length of time. Dispose of the empty container in a trash receptacle.

continues

Action	Rationale
Small-Volume Prepackaged Enema *continued*	
30. Have the client continue to lie on the left side for the prescribed length of time.	30. Certain types of enemas are more effective when retained for a specified amount of time. It is easier for the client to retain the enema in a lying position, where gravity can be resisted.
31. When the client has retained the enema for the prescribed amount of time, assist to the bedside commode or toilet or onto the bedpan. If the client is using the bathroom, instruct not to flush the toilet when finished.	31. Client will be prepared to expel fluid and feces.
32. When the client is finished expelling the enema, assist to clean the perineal area, if needed.	32. Prevents skin breakdown and excoriation.
33. Return the client to a comfortable position. Place a clean, dry protective pad under the client to catch any solution or feces that may continue to be expelled.	33. Provides comfort for the client and protects the linen from potential soiling.
34. Observe feces.	34. Results can be documented.
35. Remove gloves and wash hands.	35. Reduces transmission of microorganisms.
Return-Flow Enema	
36. Wash hands.	36. Practices clean technique.
37. Assess if client understands procedure.	37. Prepares client for procedure.
38. Apply gloves.	38. Prevents contact with feces.
39. Place absorbent pad on bed under client. Assist client in attaining left lateral position with right leg flexed as sharply as possible.	39. Facilitates flow of solution into the rectum and colon. The flexed leg provides the best exposure of the anus.
40. If specified, heat solution to desired temperature using thermometer to measure. Enemas administered to adults are usually given at 105° to 110° F (40.5° to 43° C) and those administered to children are usually administered at 100° F (37.7° C). Solution should be at least body temperature to prevent cramping and discomfort.	40. Enemas work best when solution is warm. If enemas are too hot, damage can be done to the bowel mucosa. If enemas are too cold, spasms may occur.
41. Pour solution into the bag or bucket, open clamp, and allow solution to prime tubing. Clamp tubing when primed.	41. Expels air from the tubing that could cause intestinal distention and discomfort.
42. Lubricate 5 cm (2 inches) of the rectal tube unless the tube is part of a prelubricated enema set.	42. Minimizes trauma to the anal sphincter during insertion of the rectal tube.
43. Have the client take a deep breath. Simultaneously, slowly and smoothly insert rectal tube into rectum approximately 7–10 cm (3–4 inches). Aim the rectal tube toward the client's umbilicus.	43. A deep breath helps to relax the sphincter. The rectum of an adult is usually 10–20 cm (4–6 inches). The tube should be inserted beyond the internal sphincter. Insertion of rectal tube toward the umbilicus guides tube along rectum.

continues

Action	Rationale

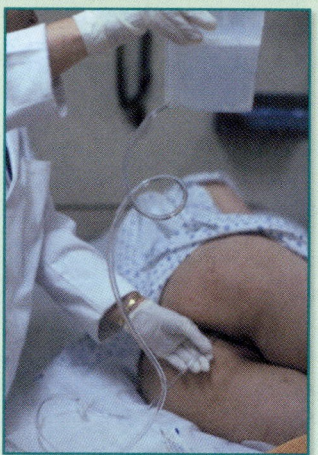

Figure 6-19-14   Raise the container 12–18 inches above the rectum and instill 200 mL of solution.

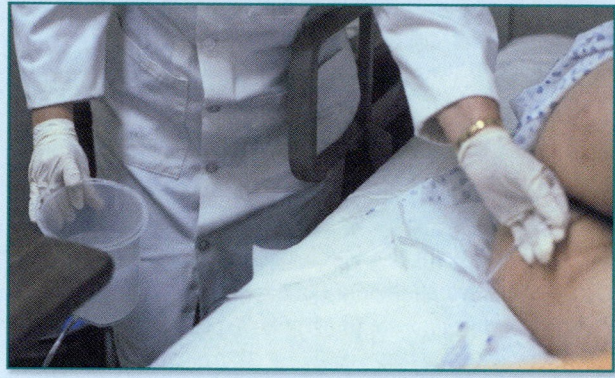

Figure 6-19-15   Lower the container 12–18 inches below the client's rectum. Observe for air bubbles as the solution returns.

44. Raise the container holding the solution and open clamp. The solution should be 30–45 cm (12–18 inches) above the rectum for an adult and 7.5 cm (3 inches) above the rectum for an infant (see Figure 6-19-14).

44. Solution should be at a height that allows gravity flow of solution into the rectum, but does not cause damage to the rectal lining because of a too-rapid increase in rectal pressure.

45. Slowly administer approximately 200 mL of solution.

45. Administering enema slowly with momentary pauses decreases the incidence of intestinal spasms and cramps.

46. Clamp the tubing and lower the enema container 12–18 inches below the client's rectum. Open the clamp (see Figure 6-19-15).

46. Allows the solution to flow back out of the rectum.

47. Observe the solution container for air bubbles as the solution returns. Note any fecal particles that may be returned.

47. Assesses the effectiveness of the procedure. Air bubbles in the container indicate flatus being passed from the rectum.

48. When no further solution is returned to the container, clamp the tubing and raise the enema container 12 to 18 inches above the client's rectum. Open the clamp and instill approximately 200 mL of fluid.

48. Continues to stimulate peristalsis and remove flatus.

49. Repeat raising and lowering the solution container until no further flatus is seen. Most institutions have guidelines regarding the number of returns to perform. A good rule of thumb is not more than 3 times.

49. Limiting the number of returns prevents unduly tiring or stressing the client.

50. After the final return of fluid, clamp the tubing and gently remove it from the client's anus. Clean the anus with tissue to remove any lubricant or solution.

50. Prevents skin irritation.

continues

Action	Rationale
Return-Flow Enema *continued*	
51. If the client feels the need to empty his rectum, assist onto the bedpan or up to the bathroom or commode.	51. Allows any retained solution to be expelled.
52. When the client is finished expelling any retained solution, assist to clean the perineal area if needed.	52. Prevents skin breakdown and excoriation.
53. Return the client to a comfortable position. Place a clean, dry protective pad under the client to catch any solution or feces that may continue to be expelled.	53. Provides comfort for the client and protects the linen from potential soiling.
54. Observe any expelled solution.	54. Results can be documented.
55. Remove gloves and wash hands.	55. Reduces transmission of microorganisms.

▶ REAL WORLD ANECDOTES

Scenario 1

Mrs. Delorenzo is a 45-year-old woman who has been complaining of constipation for 5 days. She noted that the constipation had started when she began taking acetaminophen with codeine to ease the pain from recent colorectal cancer surgery. After unsuccessfully attempting to increase peristalsis by administering suppositories, the nurse was preparing Mrs. Delorenzo for a cleansing enema. The nurse was explaining the procedure when Mrs. Delorenzo interrupted her, saying, "Oh, I know all about them. I had lots of enemas before my cancer surgery."
When questioned regarding her cancer surgery, Mrs. Delorenzo explained that she had been discharged from the hospital 5 days earlier after abdominal surgery for colorectal cancer. She was taking the acetaminophen with codeine for postoperative pain relief. Upon discovering this, the nurse set aside the prepared enema and called Mrs. Delorenzo's doctor. The doctor who had ordered the enema was not Mrs. Delorenzo's regular physician. When he was notified of the recent surgery, he told the nurse not to give the enema and he would be in to see Mrs. Delorenzo and re-evaluate her condition. Because her nurse understood the dangers of administering an enema shortly after abdominal surgery, Mrs. Delorenzo was spared a procedure that could have caused serious complications.

Scenario 2

Three days ago, Mrs. Faezi had a baby by cesarean section. On this day, her third postoperative day, she was complaining of abdominal pain and bloating. Upon evaluation, the nurse noted that she did not have any bowel sounds and her abdomen was tympanic. Upon reporting this to Mrs. Faezi's nurse practitioner, a return-flow enema was ordered. When the nurse approached Mrs. Faezi and explained the procedure and the reason for it, Mrs. Faezi became quite distressed and refused to allow the procedure. When the nurse asked Mrs. Faezi why she was upset, Mrs. Faezi explained that she was sure she would not be able to hold all that fluid without soiling herself. She would rather suffer with the distention than be embarrassed by soiling herself. The nurse explained in detail that this would be only a small amount of liquid and the liquid would be drained back out. She explained that Mrs. Faezi would not have to retain any fluid. After the more detailed explanation and assurances by the nurse that the return-flow enema would make her feel much better, Mrs. Faezi agreed to the procedure. Following the return-flow enema, which had returned a large amount of flatus, Mrs. Faezi did indeed feel much better and she thanked the nurse for her kindness and patience.

► **EVALUATION**

- The client's rectum is free of feces or flatus.
- The client experienced a minimum of discomfort from the procedure.

► **DOCUMENTATION**

Nurses' Notes

- Record the time and date of the procedure.
- Document the type of enema given, the amount of fluid infused and returned, and the amount and description of the feces expelled.
- Note the client's tolerance for the procedure and any complaints or unusual findings.

Medication Administration Record (MAR)

- If this is a medicated enema be sure to note it on the MAR.

Intake and Output Record

- If the amount of fluid returned is significantly less than the amount infused, note this on the I&O record.

Document on appropriate flow sheet or electronic medical record (EMR).

► **CRITICAL THINKING SKILL**

Introduction

A client's preconceptions may obstruct good care. Education is essential when assisting the client with independent care.

Possible Scenario

You are evaluating a new home health client. She is an elderly woman who recently fell and broke her ankle. Because of the injury, she is not as mobile as she was previously. She is complaining of constipation and reports that she has been giving herself prepackaged, small-volume enemas daily to relieve this.

Possible Outcome

The nurse explains that frequent enemas decrease bowel tone rather than increase it, but is unable to offer any acceptable alternatives. The client continues to give herself daily enemas. When she is finally able to resume her previous activity level, the client finds that she is unable to stop using the daily enemas because of rebound constipation.

Prevention

The nurse questions the client regarding her need to use enemas daily, explaining that bowel movements every 2 or 3 days is "normal" and daily bowel movements are not required. They discuss the client's reduced activity level and talk about ways to increase her activity without stressing her ankle. They discuss stool softeners and bulk-producing products as ways to improve her bowel function without the use of enemas. The nurse asks about the nature of the client's "constipated" stools and discovers that they are soft and formed. The nurse reassures the client that she is not constipated, but that her reduced activity has reduced the frequency of her bowel movements. The nurse makes a note to herself to follow up with the client regarding her "constipation." Many people believe that they must have daily bowel movements to be normal. They need to be educated that as long as their stools are soft and formed they are not constipated even if their bowel movements occur every 2 or 3 days. If a client is concerned or truly suffering from occasional constipation, there are lifestyle changes they can make that are far superior to frequent enemas, which can damage the bowel. Some lifestyle changes include drinking at least 8 glasses of water a day, going for daily walks, and increasing the amount of fiber in the diet.

► **VARIATIONS**

Geriatric Variations:

- *Elderly clients may have impaired mobility, thus having difficulty maintaining an acutely flexed right leg as well as having difficulty quickly walking to the bathroom.*
- *The client may need encouragement to maintain the position desired, and a bedside commode or bedpan may be required.*
- *Elderly clients may not be able to hear instructions well, especially if you are facing away from the client or have a soft voice. Make sure to communicate at eye level and allow the client to see your lips as you speak. Establish hand signals prior to the procedure to use if the client cannot hear you while you are administering the enema.*

continues

▶ VARIATIONS *(continued)*

- Take extra precautions to protect privacy and dignity if you must speak in a loud voice to communicate with the client.

Pediatric Variations:
- The child may be too young to understand why an enema is being administered, which may cause increased anxiety on the child's part.
- Have a parent administer the enema if reasonable, or have the parent present to comfort the child and facilitate cooperation.
- Care must be taken to ensure that the temperature of the solution is maintained to prevent damaging the child or make the child uncomfortable.
- It is important that the enema nozzle be well lubricated and that it is inserted only 7.5 cm (2–3 inches) in children and 2.5–3.75 cm (1–1.5 inches) in infants.
- Be aware of the volumes required for different body sizes in infants and children.
- Only isotonic solutions should be used in infants and children.
- Children who are not toilet trained will not be able to retain the enema solution. Give the enema on an absorbent pad or while the child is on the bedpan.

Home Care Variations:
- Clients can be taught to administer the enemas to themselves, if needed.
- Enema kits are easily available and may be easier for the client to use without assistance.
- Clients may find that lying on the back with the knees flexed and legs raised or using the knee-chest position is an easier position for self-administration of the enema.
- Clients should be instructed not to use the same nozzle for douching and enemas. Douche bags often come with an enema tip and the bag can be used for either purpose; however, the tips are not interchangeable.
- Clients should not use enema/douche bags that hold the solution under pressure and forcefully expel the fluid into the rectum.

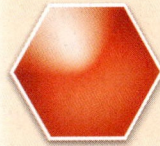

Long-Term Care Variations:
- Constipation is a common concern in the long-term setting. Clients at risk must be monitored regarding their bowel habits.
- Long-term care clients may develop rituals regarding their bowel habits. As long as the rituals are not unhealthy, a client should be allowed to perform any ritual that will help maintain bowel regularity.

▶ COMMON ERRORS

Possible Error:
Giving a prepackaged enema that is cooler than body temperature.

Prevention:
Think about what happens when cooler than body temperature fluid is infused into the rectum. Be sure to warm all fluids infused into the rectum. An enema is an unpleasant procedure for most clients, and the cramping caused by fluids that are too cool only increases the client's discomfort. Since many prepackaged enemas are designed to stimulate peristalsis, the client may experience severe cramping from the cool fluid. If this is a medicated enema that the client should retain, the cramping induced by the cool water may cause the client to expel the fluid and the medication.

► **NURSING TIPS**

- Assess the client's room to ensure that there is a clear, easy path to the bathroom.
- The order "Enemas until clear" means that enemas are to be repeated until the client passes fluid that contains no fecal matter, not until the fluid returned is not cloudy.
- Although disposable enema kits may come with prelubricated tips, additional lubricant may be needed (see Figure 6-19-16).
- The enema should be stopped immediately if severe cramping or sudden abdominal pain occurs. In the event this happens, the client should be assessed for possible bowel perforation and bleeding.
- An enema should be used as a last resort for the treatment of constipation. Oral medication, suppositories, increased fluids, and exercise, if appropriate, should be attempted first.
- If the client is unable to retain the enema solution during the procedure, the enema can be given with the client lying on the back on the bedpan.

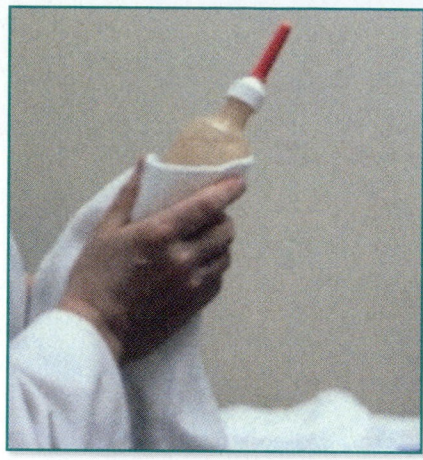

Figure 6-19-16   Many prepackaged enemas come with prelubricated tips. Check the enema for this type of tip. Bring additional lubricant to the bedside.

This method is not as effective as retaining the solution, but it may be enough to stimulate peristalsis and flush the stool out of the client's rectum.

► **SPECIAL CONSIDERATIONS**

- *Clients with hemorrhoids may experience discomfort or bleeding from an enema. A warm sitz bath can be given to relieve discomfort. Be observant for persistent rectal bleeding.*
- *Barium sometimes is used prior to the radiograph testing as an image enhancer. Inform the client that white or gray stool may present for the next 2–3 days. Increased water intake (3000–4000 mL per day if not restricted) should be encouraged to eliminate the barium substance.*

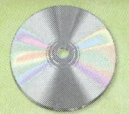
Digital Removal of Fecal Impaction

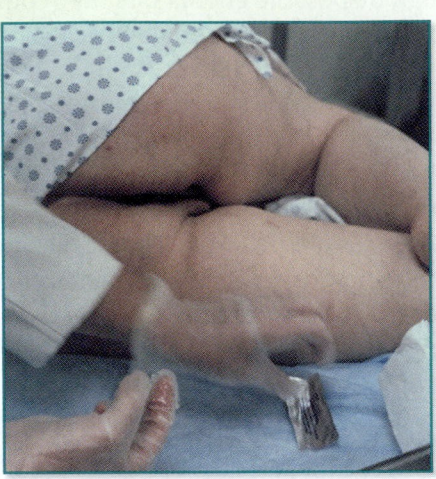

▶ OVERVIEW OF THE SKILL

Sometimes, because of severe constipation from immobility, surgery, medications, or neurologic deficit, the feces becomes so hard and large that it will not pass through the anus without tissue damage. When this happens, the nurse is called upon to remove the fecal mass manually. This is done by inserting one or two gloved fingers into the rectum and manually breaking up the fecal impaction. The nurse then removes the hard stool and disposes of it appropriately.

This procedure can be uncomfortable and embarrassing for the client. Manipulating the rectal mucosa can cause local trauma and possibly bleeding. The vagus nerve is easily stimulated rectally and may cause the client's heart rate to decrease. This procedure should be performed with caution in clients with a history of cardiac disease, dysrhythmias, or recent rectal or pelvic surgery.

▶ ASSESSMENT

1. Assess the date and quality of client's last bowel movement **to avoid procedure if it is not necessary.**
2. Assess the client for signs of fecal impaction. These signs include complaints of nausea or anorexia, abdominal fullness, abdominal pain or cramps, an absence of formed stool for 3 days or longer, and incontinence of liquid stool. **This helps to differentiate between the need for**

manual disimpaction and a cleansing enema.

3. Assess the condition of the client's perianal area. Check for anal irritation, hemorrhoids, fissures, or breaks in skin integrity. **This allows the nurse to determine whether there is a pre-existing alteration in skin integrity.**
4. Auscultate bowel sounds. This allows the nurse **to determine whether the client is experiencing an alteration in gastrointestinal function other than severe constipation.**

▶ DIAGNOSIS

Acute Pain

Constipation

Risk for Impaired Skin Integrity

Deficient Knowledge

▶ PLANNING

Expected Outcomes:

1. The client's rectum will be free of feces.
2. The client will experience a minimum of discomfort during the procedure.
3. The client will not experience any adverse side effects during or as a result of this procedure.

Equipment Needed:

- Disposable absorbent pads
- Bed pan
- Clean gloves

- Water-soluble lubricant
- Washcloth, towel
- Basin of water or perianal cleanser
- Odor eliminator spray (optional to decrease odor, which may increase client embarrassment over procedure)
- Toilet tissue

▶ **CLIENT EDUCATION NEEDED:**

1. Teach the client the importance of proper dietary intake and bulk to prevent constipation.

2. Note the importance of exercise in promoting peristalsis.
3. Teach the importance of responding to the urge to defecate when it occurs.
4. Teach the client that drinking plenty of fluids will help reduce the possibility of constipation.

Estimated time to complete the skill: **10–20 minutes**

▶ **DELEGATION TIPS**

Removing a fecal impaction requires the assessment and skills of a nurse. The risk of vagal stimulation and pain requires nursing intervention.

IMPLEMENTATION—Action/Rationale

Action	Rationale
1. Wash hands.	1. Reduces transmission of microorganisms.
2. Assemble equipment.	2. Ensures that all equipment is ready to use.
3. Explain procedure to client.	3. Decreases client's anxiety in relation to an unnatural process of removing stool from the rectum.
4. Position client in the left lateral position (Sims') with upper leg bent over lower leg (see Figure 6-20-1).	4. Facilitates easy access to anal canal.
5. Place disposable pads (if not available, use towels) underneath client. Position a bedpan near the client.	5. Protects bed linen. Allows for a receptacle to place stool into once removed.
6. Use odor eliminator per manufacturer (optional).	6. Decreases odor, which may increase client embarrassment over procedure.
7. Apply gloves (see Figure 6-20-2).	7. Practices Standard Precautions.
8. Apply lubricant to a gloved finger.	8. Protects fragile mucosa from injury.
9. Insert lubricated finger into rectum to check for fecal impaction.	9. Prevents possible injury to bowel mucosa.
10. Gently probe for stool by moving finger upward toward the umbilicus, moving finger back and forth to dislodge stool (see Figure 6-20-3).	10. Stimulates peristalsis in lower colon to facilitate removal of stool.

continues

Action	Rationale

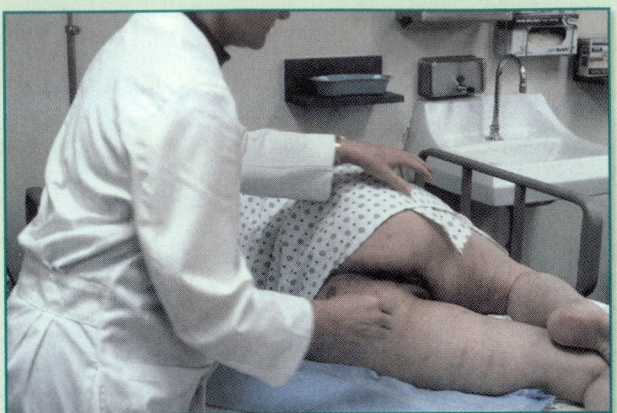

Figure 6-20-1 Position the client in the left lateral position with the right leg sharply flexed.

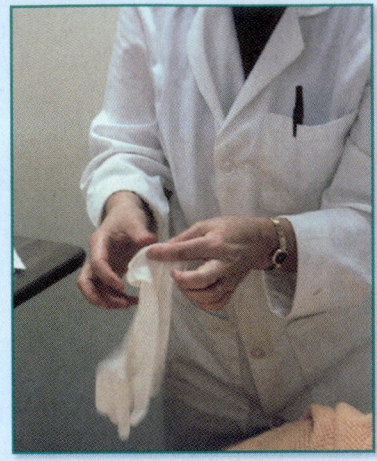

Figure 6-20-2 Apply gloves.

11. Manipulate the stool mass with the finger, breaking it up into small pieces.

11. Allows removal of the stool without traumatizing the anus.

12. Move the stool pieces toward the anus and remove them. Place removed stool into appropriate receptacle (i.e. , bedpan or disposable bed pad).

12. Preserves cleanliness.

13. Monitor the client for complications such as rectal bleeding or slowed heart rate. If heart rate decreases, stop the procedure, assess heart rate and blood pressure, and notify the physician.

13. Rectal bleeding may be caused by trauma to internal or external hemorrhoids Rectal manipulation stimulates the vagus nerve, which decreases heart rate.

14. Assist client to use the bedpan or commode if he or she needs to defecate.

14. Digital stimulation of the rectum can stimulate peristalsis.

15. With clean gloves, provide pericare (see Figure 6-20-4).

15. Provides client with personal hygiene and protects healthy perianal tissue.

16. Dispose of stool in appropriate receptacle.

16. Practices infection control standards.

17. Remove gloves and wash hands.

17. Reduces transmission of microorganisms.

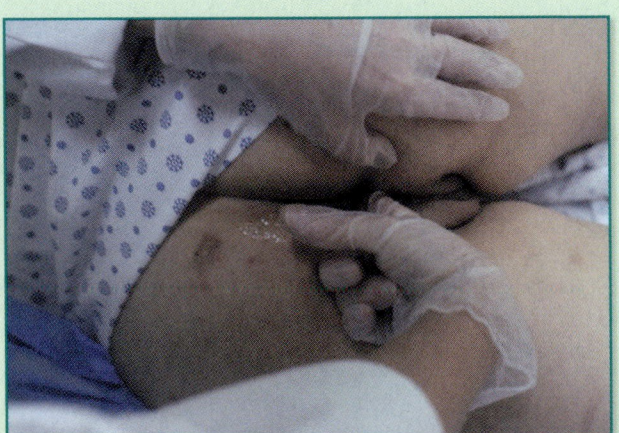

Figure 6-20-3 Gently probe for stool and gently move finger to dislodge stool.

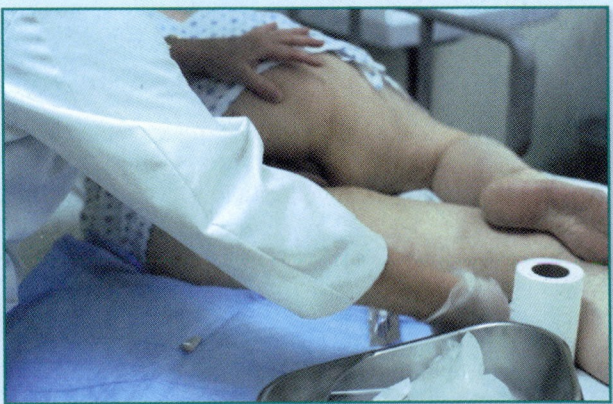

Figure 6-20-4 Change gloves and clean anal area, removing excess lubricant and stool.

> ## REAL WORLD ANECDOTES

An 80-year-old woman with a recent history of cerebrovascular accident (CVA) was admitted to the hospital from a long-term care facility. Her admitting notes indicated that her food and fluid intake had been poor for the last week. When the nurse attempted to perform an abdominal assessment, the client began to moan and grimace. The records that accompanied the client did not indicate when she had last had a bowel movement. During her admission assessment her nurse noted that the client was passing liquid stool. The nurse put on gloves and performed a rectal exam. She found a large mass of hard stool in the client's rectum. The client moaned and was in obvious pain throughout the examination. The nurse reported her findings to the client's physician and a manual removal of the fecal impaction was ordered. When the client's nursing home record finally arrived at the hospital, the nurse noted that her client had not had a recorded bowel movement for 7 days before her hospital admission.

> ## EVALUATION

- The client's rectum is free of feces.
- The client experienced a minimum of discomfort during the procedure.
- The client did not experience any adverse side effects during or as a result of the procedure.

> ## DOCUMENTATION

Nurses' Notes

- Document the procedure. Indicate the date and time the procedure was performed.
- Note the client's tolerance of the procedure; indicate if the client had any significant complications from the procedure, such as slowing of heart rate or rectal bleeding.
- Indicate the color, consistency, odor, and amount of stool removed. Note any alterations in perianal skin integrity that were found.

Document on appropriate flow sheet or electronic medical record (EMR).

> ## CRITICAL THINKING SKILL

Introduction
Client teaching is an essential part of nursing care.

Possible Scenario
Mr. Jeanperre was admitted to the hospital after an automobile accident. He was in skeletal traction secondary to several fractures. After 2 days of hospitalization Mr. Jeanperre's nurse became concerned that he had not had a bowel movement. She offered him the bedpan, but he politely refused. By his fourth day of hospitalization, Mr. Jeanperre's nurse started to insist that he try to use the bedpan. He allowed her to place the bedpan but it was apparent that he would not use it. After 5 days without a bowel movement,

Mr. Jeanperre's nurse discussed this issue with his physician. His physician performed a rectal exam and discovered a large hard mass of stool in Mr. Jeanperre's rectum. He noted that it was too large for Mr. Jeanperre to pass without damage to the sphincter so he ordered manual removal of the hardened stool.

Possible Outcome
When the nurse approached Mr. Jeanperre and explained the procedure and the reason it was needed, he was visibly upset. He explained that he had not used the bedpan earlier because of his intense embarrassment and to have to undergo this procedure would be much more humiliating. The nurse was empathetic and assured Mr. Jeanperre that his privacy would be respected as much as possible, but she was insistent that this was a necessary procedure. Mr. Jeanperre finally consented to the procedure. He tolerated the procedure well despite tightly clenched teeth. After the nurse had finished, he thanked her for her patience and gentleness and noted that in the future he would use the bedpan in a timely manner.

Prevention
Client teaching and timely intervention could have saved Mr. Jeanperre discomfort. If the nurse had discussed the need for regular bowel movements with Mr. Jeanperre when she first became concerned, this incident may have been avoided. She could have offered alternatives that may have been more acceptable to the client. He might have been more comfortable with a male nurse assisting him. He might have accepted a family member assisting him rather than a staff member. The nurse needs to take an active role in problem solving to provide the best care possible for clients.

▶ VARIATIONS

Geriatric Variations:

- *Elderly clients may have a very fragile rectal mucosa. Be sure to use an adequate amount of lubrication and perform this task gently.*
- *Elderly clients may be confused and unable to understand what you are doing and why.*
- *You may need assistance to safely complete the procedure.*

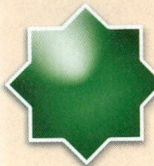

Pediatric Variations:

- *Do not explain too much in advance to a younger child, as this will only cause needless fear. Explain each step as you start to perform it.*
- *Be aware of the child's smaller anatomy. Break the pieces of stool up very small to prevent trauma to the anal sphincter. Use your little finger to protect the small child or infant from injury.*
- *Be aware that a younger child may see this invasive procedure as punishment. Reassure the child that he or she has not done anything wrong, and that this procedure will help him or her feel better.*

Home Care Variations:

- *If fecal impaction is a frequent problem for the home care client, a caregiver or the client may need to be taught the procedure.*
- *Encourage the home care client to develop a bowel routine to prevent fecal impaction. Find out what cues and rituals help stimulate the urge to defecate and encourage to incorporate them into the daily routine.*

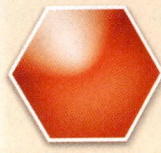

Long-Term Care Variations:

- *Long-term care clients are at a high risk for impaction. If their mobility is impaired, impaction may be a frequent problem. Frequent monitoring of the client's bowel status and ongoing client teaching regarding the importance of regular bowel movements are important in this setting.*
- *Long-term care clients may simply resign themselves to having this procedure done on a regular basis rather than try to maintain a regular schedule of bowel movements. Be sure to encourage these clients to develop as normal a pattern of elimination as possible.*

▶ COMMON ERRORS

Possible Error:

Missing the cues of extended period of time without a bowel movement.

Prevention:

Read the client's medical record if client is unable to provide accurate history of bowel habits.

▶ NURSING TIPS

- Manual stimulation of rectum may cause excessive vagal nerve stimulation and subsequent cardiac arrhythmia; monitor for signs of vasovagal reaction.
- If the client's anal skin integrity is impaired prior to the procedure, care must be taken not to contaminate the open area with stool.
- This procedure must be done gently. The rectal mucosa is thin and easily damaged. Tearing the rectal mucosa can introduce *Escherichia coli* into the client's bloodstream.
- Use of Xylocaine gel to lubricate fingers will help decrease pain. Beware that it may impair the client's ability to perceive and report injury to the tissues.

► **SPECIAL CONSIDERATIONS**

- A well-balanced diet, adequate water intake, and sufficient exercise may help prevent the recurrence of a fecal impaction.
- Clients with special sexual habits or with mental illness may perceive the procedure as pleasurable. A response such as "Oh, this feels good" could be a sign. Nursing staff should be aware of the variety of clients, keep calm, and maintain a professional attitude throughout the nursing intervention. Document the observation and intervention.

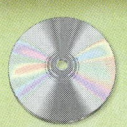

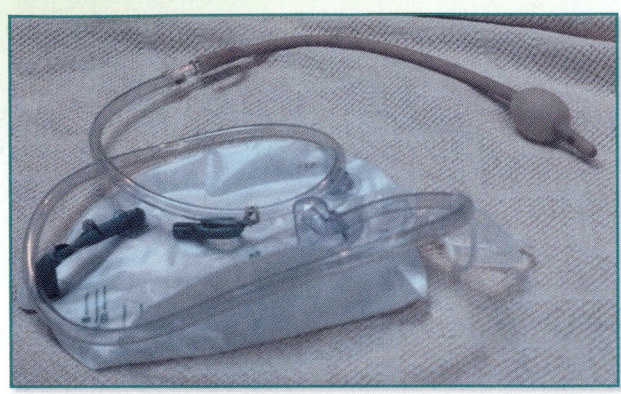

▶ OVERVIEW OF THE SKILL

The insertion of a rectal tube is done to manage flatulence (gas) after abdominal surgery and/or reduce abdominal distention caused by flatulence. It is also used to control diarrhea that cannot be medically managed or with the use of rectal pouches, pads, or diapers because of extensive skin breakdown. The use of a rectal tube is a short-term solution.

▶ ASSESSMENT

1. Auscultate bowel sounds. **Allows the nurse to determine whether the client is experiencing reduced or increased peristalsis and establishes a baseline for comparisons after the procedure.**
2. Assess fluid intake and output status. **Enables the nurse to determine possible changes in the client's oral intake that need to be addressed.**
3. Assess nutritional intake. **Enables the nurse to determine possible changes in the client's food intake that need to be addressed.**
4. Inspect the perianal skin. **Allows the nurse to determine whether there is a pre-existing alteration in skin integrity.**
5. Assess for complaints of cramping, pain, or abdominal distention, **which may indicate the presence of gas and reduced peristalsis.**

▶ DIAGNOSIS

Acute Pain

Risk for Impaired Skin Integrity

Bowel Incontinence

Risk for Infection

Risk for Injury

▶ PLANNING

Expected Outcomes:

1. Elimination pattern returns to normal.
2. Client's abdominal girth will return to a size within normal limits for client's body type.
3. Client's skin integrity will not be damaged by the procedure.

Equipment Needed (see Figure 6-21-1):

- Rectal tube or catheter, 22 to 30 French (latex-free if history of latex allergy)

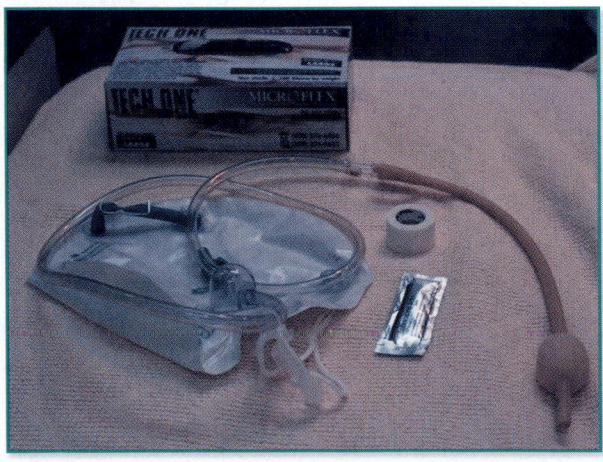

Figure 6-21-1 Rectal tube, drainage bag, lubricant, and gloves

- Water-soluble lubricant
- Bedside drainage bag (optional, if rectal tube used to manage diarrhea)
- Ostomy odor eliminator or similar product (optional)
- Clean latex-free gloves
- Disposable pads or towels

▶ **CLIENT EDUCATION NEEDED:**

1. Explain rationale regarding need of tube and its short duration of use.

Estimated time to complete the skill: **3–5 minutes**

▶ **DELEGATION TIPS**

Insertion of a rectal tube requires the assessment and evaluation of the client by a nurse; it cannot be delegated. Ancillary personnel may monitor and measure the output from the tube, if required. Any medication inserted through the tube must be given by a nurse.

IMPLEMENTATION—Action/Rationale

Action	Rationale
1. Wash hands.	1. Reduces transmission of microorganisms.
2. Assemble equipment.	2. Ensures that all equipment is ready to use.
3. Explain procedure to client.	3. Decreases client's anxiety in relation to an unnatural process of removing stool from the rectum.
4. Position client in left lateral position with upper leg bent over lower leg (see Figure 6-21-2).	4. Facilitates easy access to anal canal.
5. Place disposable pads (if not available, use towels).	5. Protects bed linen. Allows for a receptacle for diarrhea until rectal tube is inserted.
6. Use odor eliminator per manufacturer (optional).	6. Decreases odor, which may cause client embarrassment over procedure.
7. Apply gloves.	7. Practices clean technique.
8. Apply lubricant to a gloved finger.	8. Protects fragile mucosa from injury.
9. Insert lubricated finger into rectum to check for possible impactions before insertion of rectal tube (see Figure 6-21-3).	9. Prevents possible injury to bowel mucosa from a blind entry.
10. Change gloves if soiled from rectal exam.	10. Avoids spreading feces to external parts of the tube, the client, and the surrounding area.

continues

Action	Rationale

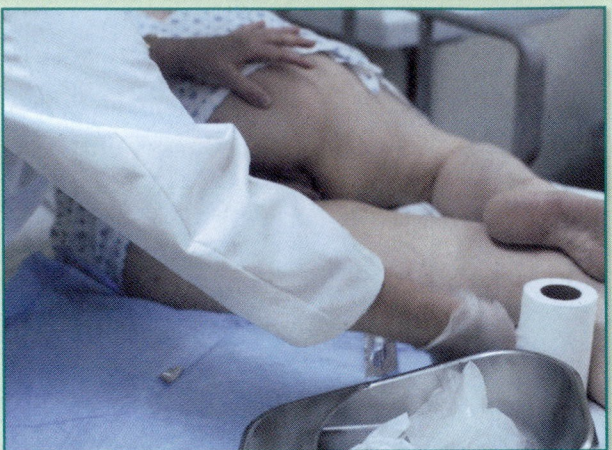

Figure 6-21-2 Position the client in the left lateral position with the right leg sharply flexed.

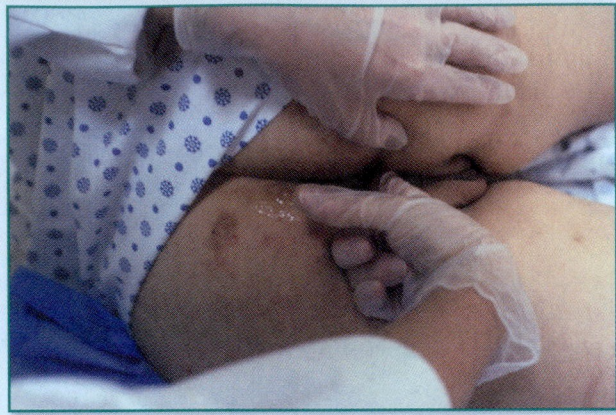

Figure 6-21-3 Gently probe for stool and gently move finger to dislodge stool.

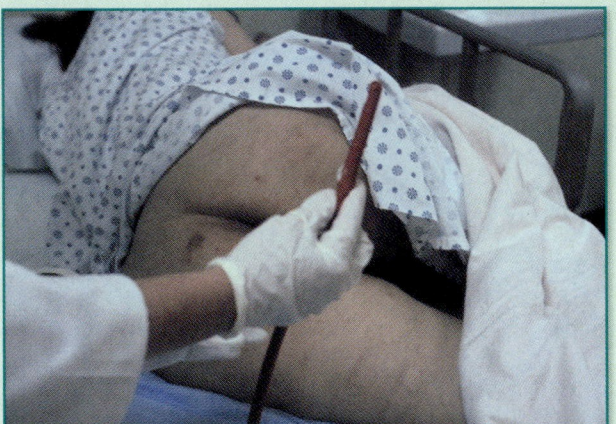

Figure 6-21-4 Lubricate the end of the catheter to facilitate entry into the anal canal.

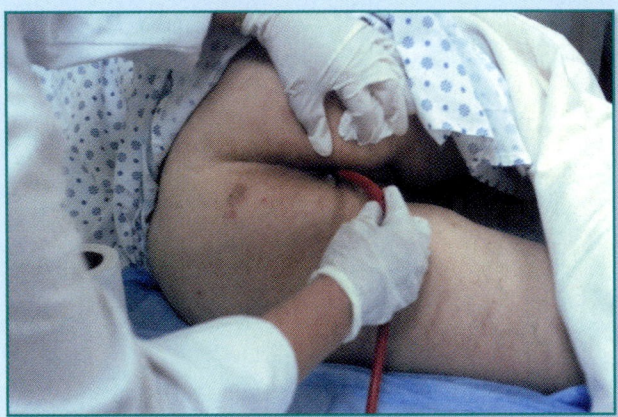

Figure 6-21-5 Insert the catheter into the anal canal 4–6 inches.

11. Lubricate end of catheter (see Figure 6-21-4).

12. Gently insert catheter into anal canal approximately 10–15 cm (4–6 inches) (see Figure 6-21-5).

13. Inflate balloon of catheter and tape tube to the lower buttock (see Figure 6-21-6).

14. Attach plastic bag or drainage bag to end of catheter if needed to control odor or stool (see Figure 6-21-7).

11. Facilitates entry of catheter into anal canal.

12. Facilitates entry of catheter into anal canal.

13. Stabilizes catheter if it is not immediately removed.

14. Controls odor and contains any liquid stool that might be passed through the catheter.

continues

Action	Rationale

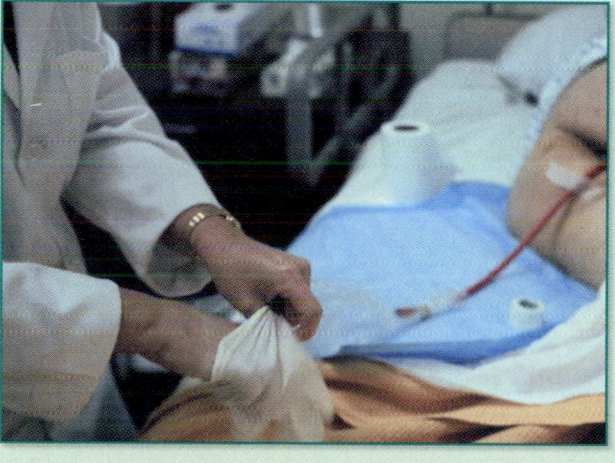

Figure 6-21-6 Tape the tube to the lower buttock.

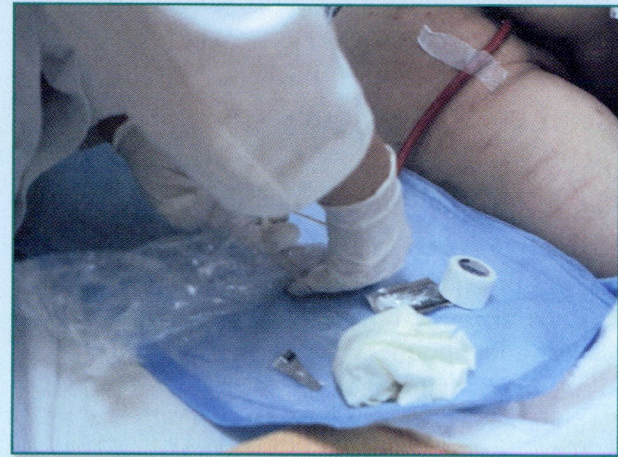

Figure 6-21-7 Attach a plastic bag to the end of the catheter to control odor or contain liquid stool.

Figure 6-21-8 Remove soiled gloves.

15. Dispose of pad. Remove soiled gloves (see Figure 6-21-8) and place in appropriate receptacle.

16. Wash hands.

15. Practices infection control standards.

16. Reduces transmission of microorganisms.

▶ **REAL WORLD ANECDOTES**

Mr. Goodman was admitted to the intensive care unit with severe pancreatitis. He was NPO for several weeks and was receiving parenteral nutrition. By the time Mr. Goodman was able to tolerate oral feedings, his gag and swallow reflexes had been damaged secondary to prolonged intubation. His physician ordered a feeding tube placed to provide Mr. Goodman with nutrition and fluids. After 2 days of tube feedings Mr. Goodman started to suffer with incontinent liquid diarrhea. His perianal area was becoming excoriated from contact with stool and from frequent cleansing. Mr. Goodman's doctor ordered a rectal tube placed to drain the liquid stool. The rectal tube saved Mr. Goodman from further perianal irritation while allowing his stool to drain.

▶ EVALUATION

- Elimination pattern returned to normal.
- Client's abdominal girth returned to a size within normal limits for client's body type.
- Client's skin was not damaged by the procedure.

▶ DOCUMENTATION

Nurses' Notes

Document:
- Description of bowel sounds
- Abdominal girth
- Insertion and removal of rectal tube
- Color and amount of diarrhea, if present
- Presence of flatus release
- Appearance of perianal skin
- Client tolerance of the procedure

Document on appropriate flow sheet or electronic medical record (EMR).

▶ CRITICAL THINKING SKILL

Introduction

A client is unable to evacuate flatus in the normal manner because of physiologic disease.

Possible Scenario

A 70-year-old man is 3 days status post repair of ruptured abdominal aortic aneurysm. He complains of increasing respiratory difficulty, and the nursing notes indicated that his abdomen appears distended. He has not passed flatus or stool since 48 hours before admission and surgery. Examination of the abdomen reveals diminished bowel sounds.

Possible Outcome

An astute nurse would realize that the client has a possible partial ileus, which could result in retaining flatulence, increased abdominal girth, and possible bowel obstruction. The physician should be immediately informed of the client's condition. Temporary placement of a rectal tube may be indicated.

Prevention

Early ambulating of client facilitates peristalsis. The client should be observed frequently and gastrointestinal and respiratory status assessed.

▶ VARIATIONS

Geriatric Variations:
- *Elderly clients may have more friable rectal mucosa. If a balloon is used to hold the rectal tube in place, deflate the balloon and reposition the catheter frequently.*
- *Confused clients may become agitated by the presence of the tube, believing they need to move their bowels.*

Pediatric Variations:
- *Use a tube that is the appropriate size for the child.*
- *Leaving a rectal tube in place may not be appropriate for very small children.*
- *Teenagers may be acutely embarrassed by passing flatus. Be sensitive to their developing body image.*

Home Care Variation:
- *Rectal tubes are not generally used in the home care setting.*

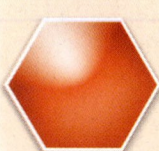

Long-Term Care Variation:
- *Rectal tubes are not generally used in the long-term care setting.*

► COMMON ERRORS

Possible Error:

Missing the cues of decreased bowel sounds and increased abdominal distention.

Prevention:

Assess gastrointestinal system (auscultation of bowel sounds) and include abdominal girth in the case of diminished or absent bowel sounds. Ask client questions appropriate to ascertaining status of gastrointestinal tract (e.g., "Have you passed any gas today or belched?" "Are you having any cramping in your stomach/abdomen?"). Also, always do an accurate review of client's medical record, including assessment of gastrointestinal status.

► NURSING TIPS

- Rectal tube may be reinserted every 2–3 hours.
- Discontinue rectal tube when stool is no longer liquid or when gas is relieved.
- Use of an external collection system is preferred, particularly if client's integument is intact.

- Odor and noise are good ways to determine if flatulence is being removed. Be aware, however, that these may be acutely embarrassing to the client.
- A rectal tube is contraindicated for clients with rectal disease or neutropenia, and for those who are immunocompromised or receiving anticoagulation therapy.

► SPECIAL CONSIDERATIONS

- *Deflate the tube's balloon every hour for 5–10 minutes to decrease possible bowel wall necrosis from compression of microvasculature.*
- *Use of latex-free gloves and tubes if client has a history of latex allergy.*

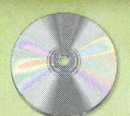

Irrigating and Cleaning a Stoma

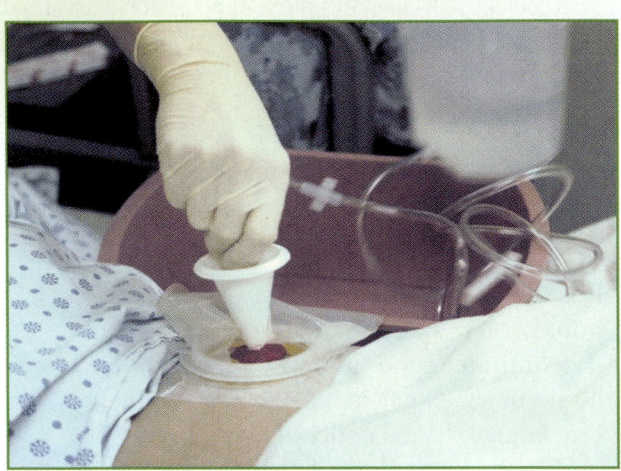

▶ OVERVIEW OF THE SKILL

The purpose of a colostomy irrigation is to empty the large colon of stool. The colostomy irrigation can be performed at the bedside or in the bathroom. This process is similar to performing an enema. This procedure is not commonly done in many facilities. Check with the health care provider, facility procedure manual, or nursing supervisor if you are uncertain.

▶ ASSESSMENT

1. Inspect the stoma for color and texture. **This allows the nurse to determine the viability and turgor of the stoma.**
2. Inspect the condition of the skin surrounding the stoma. **Alterations in skin integrity prohibit a closed drainage system from adhering to the skin.**
3. Determine the direction of the intestine by digitalization of the stoma. **This allows the nurse to know the direction of the intestinal tract before beginning the irrigation, which will prevent possible perforation of the bowel.**
4. Measure the dimensions of the stoma before obtaining an ostomy appliance system from central supply. **This alleviates the problem of obtaining the wrong size equipment.**

▶ DIAGNOSIS

Bowel Incontinence

Deficient Knowledge

Disturbed Body Image

Risk for Impaired Skin Integrity

▶ PLANNING

Expected Outcomes:

1. Client will experience bowel movement after irrigation of colon (colostomy).
2. Client and/or caregiver will demonstrate skill in performing irrigation of colon (colostomy).
3. Periostomal skin integrity will remain intact.
4. Irritated or denuded periostomal skin integrity will heal.
5. Client will acknowledge the change in body image.
6. Client will express positive feelings about self.
7. Client will maintain fluid balance.

Equipment Needed (see Figure 6-22-1):

- Colostomy irrigation kit
- 4 × 4 gauze or stoma cover
- Tape, if gauze is used
- Clean gloves
- Bedpan, toilet, or basin

▶ CLIENT EDUCATION NEEDED:

1. Instruct the client on the frequency of colostomy irrigation. Most clients irrigate their colostomy every day to every other day.

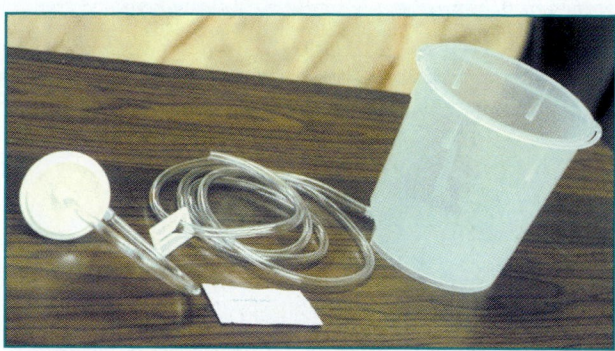

Figure 6-22-1 Colostomy irrigation kit

2. Clients with a normal bowel habit of movements every 2 to 3 days are more easily regulated with colostomy irrigation than those individuals with 2 to 3 bowel movements per day.
3. Instruct the client on changes in skin condition or stoma to report to enterostomal/ostomy care nurse.

Estimated time to complete the skill:
45 minutes

▶ **DELEGATION TIPS**

This skill cannot be delegated to ancillary personnel. Colostomy irrigation and cleaning require the skills of a nurse.

IMPLEMENTATION—Action/Rationale

Action	Rationale
1. Wash hands.	1. Reduces the transmission of microorganisms.
2. Apply clean gloves.	2. Practices clean technique.
3. Assemble irrigation kit: Attach cone to irrigation bag tubing.	3. Ensures that all equipment is ready to use.
4. Fill irrigation bag with 1000 mL of tepid tap water (see Figure 6-22-2).	4. The colon is already filled with microorganisms so the use of sterile water is not necessary.
5. Open clamp and let water from the irrigation bag fill the tubing.	5. This eliminates any air bubbles, which can cause intestinal cramping.
6. Hang bottom of irrigation bag at height of client's shoulder, or 18 inches above the stoma if the client is supine.	6. Hanging the irrigation bag too high will cause increased intestinal cramping, and hanging the irrigation bag below shoulder level will cause poor results. This height provides resistance of back pressure from flatus.
7. Remove existing ostomy appliance. Place irrigation sleeve over stoma and hold in place with belt (see Figure 6-22-3).	7. Provides a means for irrigant and stool to drain.
8. Place end of irrigation sleeve into toilet bowl (if client is in bathroom) or bed pan (if client is in bed or chair (see Figure 6-22-4).	8. Facilitates drainage of water and stool.

continues

Action	Rationale

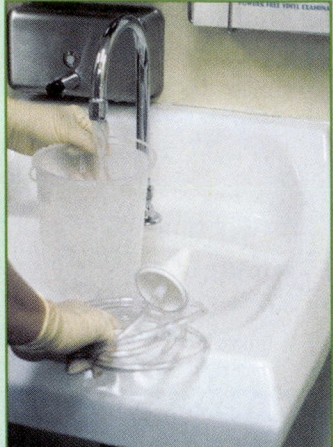

Figure 6-22-2 Colostomy irrigation solution may be administered using a bag or bucket. Fill with tepid tap water.

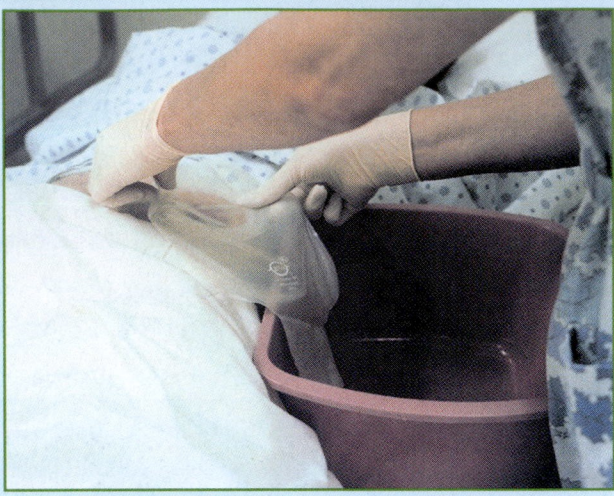

Figure 6-22-3 Place the irrigation sleeve over the stoma.

9. Check the direction of intestine by inserting a lubricated gloved finger into orifice of stoma.

9. Determines the direction of stoma prior to irrigation of colostomy prevents trauma to mucosa.

10. Generously lubricate the cone at the end of the irrigation tubing (see Figure 6-22-5) and insert into orifice of stoma through the top opening of irrigation sleeve (see Figure 6-22-6). Hold the cone in place.

10. Lubricating the cone prevents trauma to intestinal lumen. Holding the cone prevents the cone from coming out of stoma.

11. Close top of irrigation sleeve over the tubing.

11. Prevents water and stool from splashing outside the irrigation sleeve.

12. Open the clamp on the tubing and slowly run water into colon (see Figure 6-22-7). If cramping occurs, stop the infusion and have the client take deep breaths. Resume instilling the water when cramps have subsided.

12. Slow administration of the water decreases the incidence of intestinal spasms and cramps.

13. Slowly run water through tubing into colon (see Figure 6-22-7).

13. This will alleviate intestinal cramping. If cramping should start, immediately stop and allow client to rest for a few minutes.

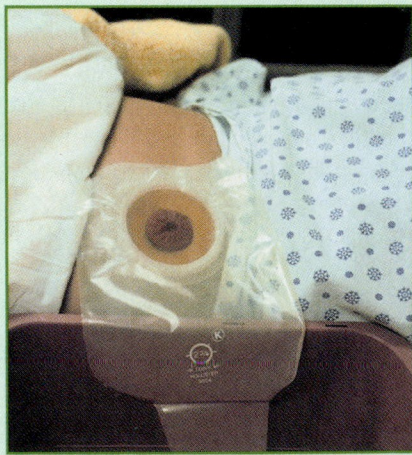

Figure 6-22-4 Place the end of the irrigation sleeve into a basin, bedpan, or toilet bowl.

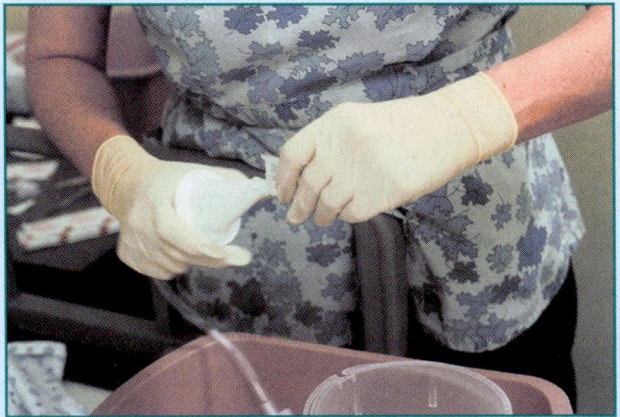

Figure 6-22-5 Lubricate the cone end of the irrigation tubing.

continues

Action	Rationale

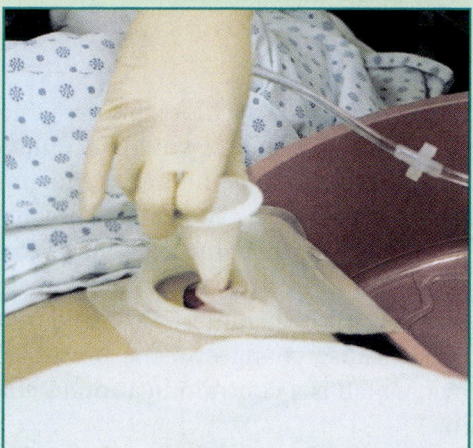

Figure 6-22-6   Insert the cone into the orifice of the stoma.

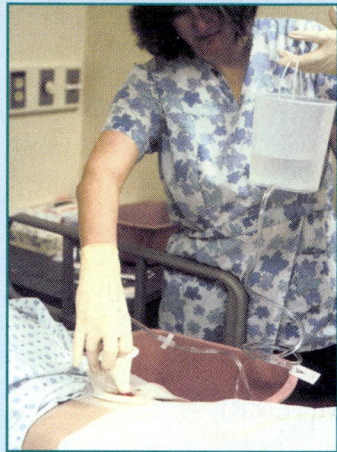

Figure 6-22-7   Gently instill 500–1000 mL of tepid water.

14. Remove cone after all water has emptied out of irrigation bag.

14. Irrigation of colostomy has been completed.

15. Close the top and the end of the irrigation sleeve with clamps.

15. This maintains a closed system for any remaining stool and irrigant to empty into.

16. Encourage client to ambulate to facilitate emptying of remaining stool from colon.

16. Ambulating influences peristalsis.

17. Remove irrigation sleeve after 20–30 minutes or when stool is no longer emptying from colon.

17. Ensures that fluid and feces have been expelled.

18. Cleanse stoma and skin with warm tap water. Pat dry.

18. Gentle care of the stoma prevents injury to the mucosa, which has no nerve endings and is very friable.

19. Apply ostomy appliance. See skill 6-23.

19. Provides a reservoir for drainage and protects the client's skin.

20. Remove gloves and wash hands.

20. Reduces the transmission of microorganisms.

▶ REAL WORLD ANECDOTES

A 78-year-old woman has had her colostomy for 20 years because of rectal cancer. After a short recovery room stay after surgery, she had radiation therapy. She has irrigated her own colostomy for the past 20 years. She is now complaining of severe intestinal cramping that is not relieved by colostomy irrigation and is having persistent diarrhea. The client continued to irrigate the colostomy until seen by the enterostomy/ostomy nurse who reviewed the basic guidelines for performing colostomy irrigation with the client. The client discontinued irrigation of the colostomy after learning that it is not appropriate to irrigate when experiencing diarrhea.

▶ EVALUATION

- Client experiences a bowel movement after irrigation of colon (colostomy).
- Client or caregiver is able to demonstrate skill in performing irrigation of colon (colostomy).

- Peristomal skin integrity remains intact.
- Irritated or denuded peristomal skin integrity is healed.
- Client acknowledges the change in body image.
- Client expresses positive feelings about self.
- Client maintains fluid balance.

► DOCUMENTATION

Nurses' Notes

Document:

- Assessment of peristomal skin
- Assessment of stoma
- Stoma measurements (length, width, height)
- Amount of water used for irrigation
- Amount of stool flushed from colon
- Peristomal skin care if alteration in skin integrity was noted
- Type of dressing or ostomy pouch applied following irrigation

Document on appropriate flow sheet or electronic medical record (EMR).

► CRITICAL THINKING SKILL

Introduction

The client with a colostomy is in need of a colostomy irrigation.

Possible Scenario

A 54-year-old man is recovering from an abdominal perineal resection and is requesting information on colostomy irrigation. He is 5 days postsurgery and is scheduled to begin chemotherapy and radiation therapy within the next 6 weeks.

Possible Outcome

If the client were to start colostomy irrigation now, there is the possibility that he would become discouraged with the process once he began chemotherapy and radiation therapy. It takes approximately 6–12 weeks for the bowel to become acclimated to the irrigation process, and this is when the client would be receiving his cancer therapies. Both chemotherapy and radiation cause changes in the bowel, resulting in diarrhea, which is a contraindication to colostomy irrigation.

Prevention

The nurse should provide the client with information on colostomy irrigation and the rationale for waiting to begin the learning process after completion of cancer therapies. A second nursing action is to consult the enterostomal/ostomy care nurse.

► VARIATIONS

Geriatric Variation:

- *A client who is too old to do the cleaning and maintenance of a colostomy without assistance will need regular help from a caregiver. Instruct the caregiver, and "backup" caregivers if available, how to do the procedure.*

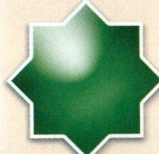

Pediatric Variation:

- *A client who is too younger (i.e., younger than 5 years of age) to do the procedure without assistance will need help from a parent. Instruct the parents how to do the procedure.*

Home Care Variation:

- *If the client performs the procedure at home, assess the environment for safety. In the event the client feels weak or faint during the procedure, he or she should know how to stop the procedure and lie down.*

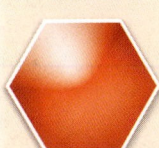

Long-Term Care Variations:

- *Make periodic assessments of the condition of the colostomy.*
- *Provide periodic refreshers on the procedures and technique for the cleaning and maintenance of a colostomy.*
- *When reviewing the colostomy procedures with the client, reinforce the need to maintain good hygiene.*

▶ COMMON ERRORS

Possible Error:

Client complains of severe cramping during irrigation of colostomy.

Prevention:

Slowly infuse tepid water into colostomy and hang irrigation bag no higher than 12 to 18 inches above the stomach.

▶ NURSING TIPS

- Client teaching is easily incorporated into the care of the ostomy by encouraging the client to be your assistant during the irrigation process.

- Clients who irrigate their colostomy still need to learn how to apply an ostomy appliance.
- Clients should always be instructed to use the cone adapter for irrigation and not a catheter, so as to avoid possible bowel perforation.

▶ SPECIAL CONSIDERATIONS

- *Assess skin integrity when performing stoma care. Document any sign of skin breakdown. An ischemic stoma usually appears dark red or black.*
- *Change the stoma pouch frequently if the skin underneath the appliance appears irritated.*

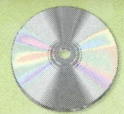

Changing a Bowel Diversion Ostomy Appliance: Pouching a Stoma

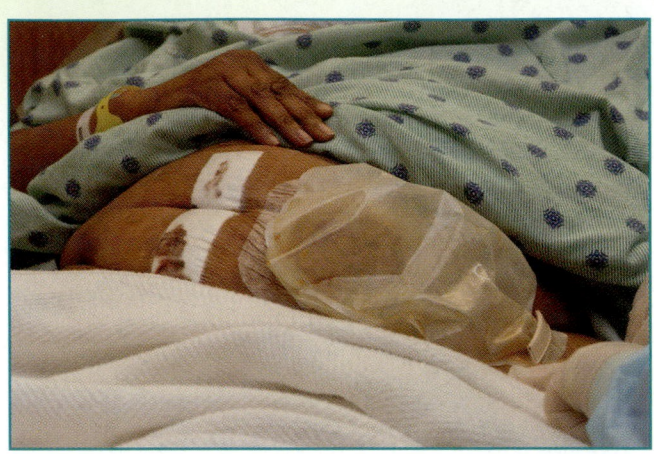

▶ OVERVIEW OF THE SKILL

A colostomy is an opening surgically created from the ascending, transverse, or descending colon to the abdominal wall. An ileostomy is an opening from the ileum to the abdominal wall. Colostomies and ileostomies function to discharge waste (liquids, solids, and gases) to the outside of the body. Pouching a fecal diversion ensures that the client's peristomal skin remains intact and provides the client with artificial continence.

The purpose of creating ileostomies and colostomies is to improve survival and the quality of life. Anger, grief, body image disturbances, socialization disturbances, depression, and helplessness often accompany these procedures.

▶ ASSESSMENT

1. Inspect the stoma for color and texture. **Allows the nurse to determine the viability and turgor of the stoma.**
2. Inspect the condition of the skin surrounding the stoma. **Alterations in skin integrity prohibit a closed drainage system from adhering to the skin.**
3. Measure the dimensions of the stoma prior to obtaining an ostomy appliance system from central supply. **Alleviates the problem of obtaining the wrong size equipment.**

▶ DIAGNOSIS

Risk for Impaired Skin Integrity

Deficient Knowledge

Disturbed Body Image

Risk for Deficient Fluid Volume

▶ PLANNING

Expected Outcomes:
1. Peristomal skin integrity will remain intact.
2. Irritated or denuded peristomal skin will heal.
3. Client will acknowledge the change in body image.
4. Client will express positive feelings about self.
5. Client will maintain fluid balance.

Equipment Needed (see Figures 6-23-1 to 6-23-3):
- Clean washcloth or 4 × 4 gauze pads
- Warm tap water

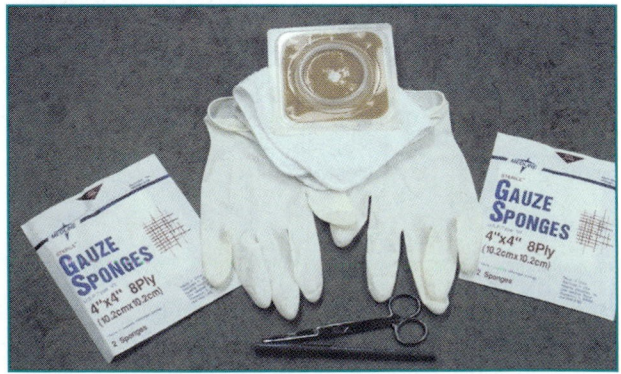

Figure 6-23-1 Ostomy water, gloves, scissors, pen or pencil, and sponges are used when pouching a stoma.

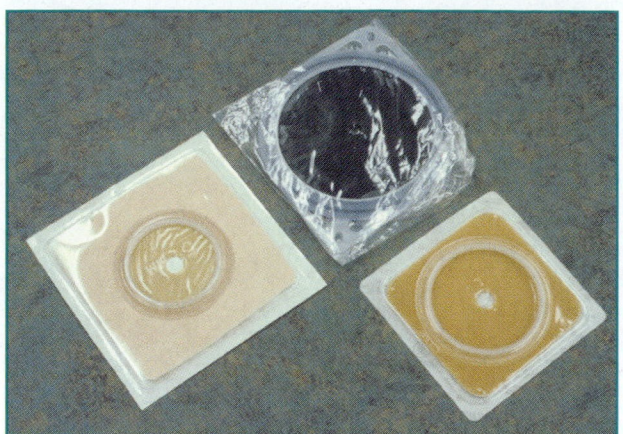

Figure 6-23-2 Ostomy skin barriers, also called wafers.

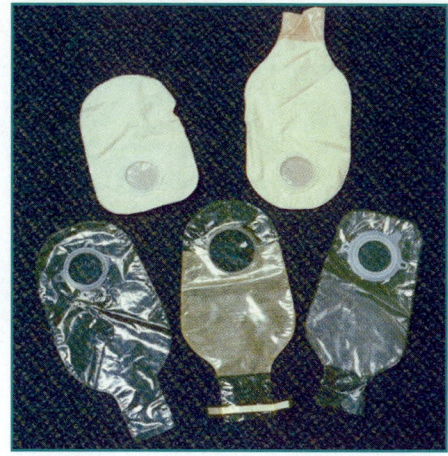

Figure 6-23-3 Ostomy drainage bags.

- Appropriate drainable ostomy appliance
- Scissors
- Pen or pencil
- Clean gloves

▶ **CLIENT EDUCATION NEEDED:**

1. Instruct client on pouch application, including frequency of change. Most pouching systems can be maintained for a minimum of 3 days to a maximum of 7 days.
2. Instruct client on changes in skin condition to report to wound/ostomy care nurse.

3. Provide the client with a list of equipment and product numbers as well as a list of retailers where supplies can be purchased.
4. Provide a list of reasons and situations on when to call the health care provider.

Estimated time to complete the skill:
10–20 minutes

▶ **DELEGATION TIPS**

This skill cannot be delegated to ancillary personnel. Changing an ostomy appliance requires the skills and problem-solving ability of a nurse.

IMPLEMENTATION—Action/Rationale

Action	Rationale
1. Wash hands.	1. Practices aseptic technique.
2. Assemble drainable pouch and wafer.	2. Ensures that all equipment is ready to use.
3. Apply clean gloves.	3. Practices clean technique.
4. Remove current ostomy appliance after emptying pouch of stool, if present.	4. Prevents contamination of surrounding environment if stool accidentally leaks from appliance when removed from client's skin.
5. Dispose of appliance in appropriate waste container.	5. Practices infection control.

continues

Action	Rationale

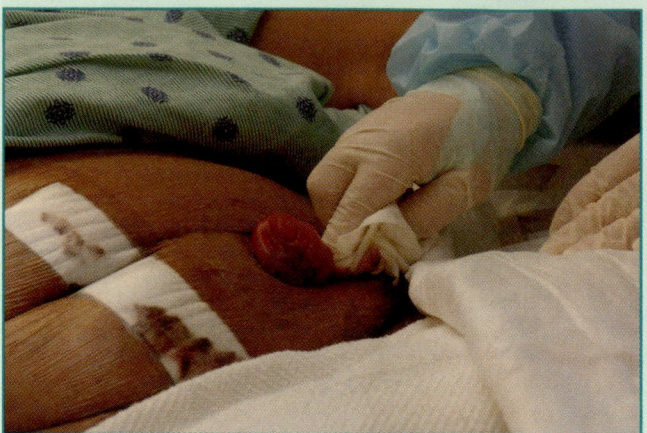

Figure 6-23-4 Cleanse the stoma and surrounding skin with warm tap water.

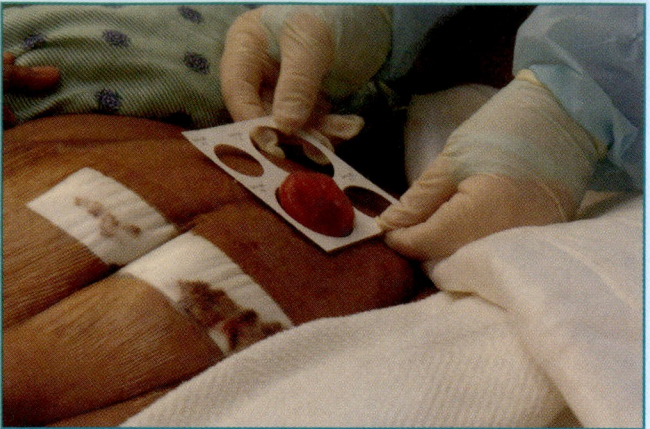

Figure 6-23-5 Measure stoma using a measuring guide.

6. Remove gloves and wash hands.

7. Apply clean gloves.

8. Cleanse stoma and skin with warm tap water. Pat dry (see Figure 6-23-4).

9. Measure stoma using a measuring guide for appropriate length and width of stoma at base (where skin meets stoma) (see Figure 6-23-5).

10. Place gauze pad over orifice of stoma to wick stool while you are preparing the wafer and pouch for application.

11. Trace pattern onto paper backing of wafer (see Figure 6-23-6).

6. Practices aseptic technique.

7. Practices clean technique.

8. Gentle care of the stoma prevents injury to the mucosa, which has no nerve endings and is very friable.

9. Correct measurement of the stoma's dimensions ensures a good fit of the ostomy appliance without excess skin at the base of the stoma exposed to stool.

10. Using something to wick stool away from the skin ensures a good seal of the wafer to the client's skin.

11. It is important to trace the measurements of the stoma and not "eyeball" the stoma measurements. Inaccurate pattern size results in either laceration of the stoma by the wafer or maceration of peristomal skin from constant contact with stool.

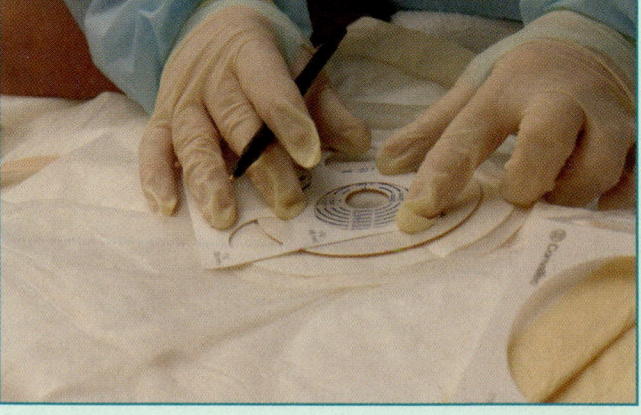

Figure 6-23-6 Trace pattern onto paper backing of wafer.

continues

Action	Rationale
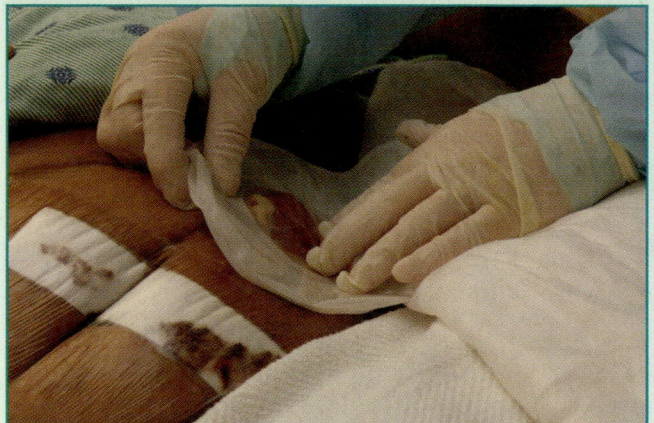 **Figure 6-23-7** Place the wafer and pouch with the stoma centered in the cutout opening of the wafer.	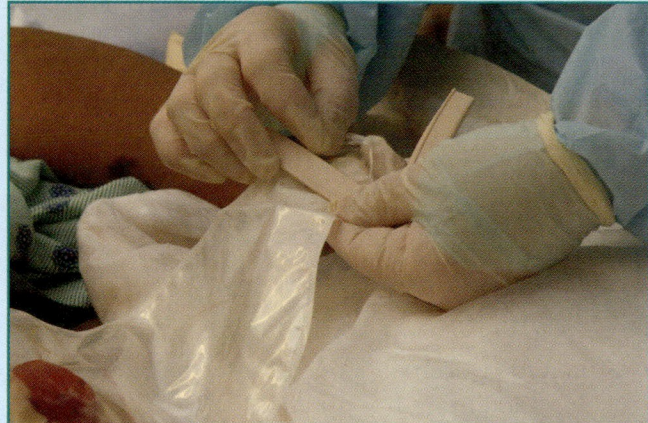 **Figure 6-23-8** Apply closure clamp to pouch.

Action	Rationale
12. Cut wafer as traced.	12. Accurately cutting the traced pattern ensures a snug fit.
13. Attach clean pouch to wafer.	13. Preattaching the pouch to the wafer saves time and prevents stool from leaking underneath the wafer during application process.
14. Remove gauze pad from orifice of stoma.	14. It is easier to visualize the stoma.
15. Remove paper backing from wafer and place on skin with stomac centered in cutout opening of wafer (see Figures 6-23-7).	15. Paper backing needs to be removed from wafer in order for wafer to become adherent to skin.
16. Tape the wafer edges down with hypoallergenic tape (optional).	16. Ensures that the edges of the wafer will not adhere to client's clothing.
17. Apply closure clamp to pouch (see Figure 6-23-8).	17. Keeps intestinal contents in pouch.
18. Dispose of used materials, remove gloves and wash hands.	18. Reduces transmission of microorganisms.

▶ REAL WORLD ANECDOTES

A 65-year-old woman with a history of Crohn's disease was admitted for bowel obstruction. An exploratory laparotomy, a total colectomy with removal of 18 inches of small bowel, and an ileostomy were performed. The client's postoperative course was uneventful. Output from the ileostomy averaged 2000 mL per 24 hours. The client was instructed in ostomy care using a two-piece system. This enabled the client to use a drainable pouch during waking hours and switch to a urinary pouch at night, which could be attached to a bedside drainage bag.

▶ EVALUATION

- Peristomal skin integrity remains intact.
- Irritated or denuded peristomal skin integrity is healed.
- Client acknowledges the change in body image.
- Client expresses positive feelings about self.
- Client maintains fluid balance.

▶ DOCUMENTATION

Nurses' Notes

Document:

- Assessment of peristomal skin
- Assessment of stoma
- Stoma measurements (length, width, height)
- Color and amount of drainage
- Peristomal skin care if alteration in skin integrity was noted
- Type of ostomy pouch applied

Document on appropriate flow sheet or electronic medical record (EMR).

▶ CRITICAL THINKING SKILL

Introduction

A client is postoperative abdominal perineal surgery with a permanent colostomy for rectal cancer.

Possible Scenario

A 78-year-old man is recovering from an abdominal perineal resection with a permanent colostomy for rectal cancer. He asks his nurse, "When will the surgeon remove this?" pointing to the colostomy. Upon further conversation with the client, the nurse learns that the client had been told an ostomy might not be needed if the surgeon "got everything" during the surgery.

Possible Outcome

The astute nurse will recognize the client's clue that he is not aware of the permanence of the colostomy given the surgical procedure he recently underwent. It is possible that the client has not fully recovered from the anesthetic agents used during surgery or the client is experiencing some confusion regarding details of the surgery.

Prevention

Review with the client the type of surgery he had and the permanence of the ostomy. Report any of your concerns regarding the client's understanding of the surgery and ostomy to the physician.

▶ VARIATIONS

Geriatric Variation:

- If a client has arthritic hands, it is best to use either a one-piece appliance that is precut or a two-piece appliance that is adaptable to decreases in hand dexterity.

Pediatric Variations:

- A child's ostomy bag needs to be very flexible so it can bend with the client's movement without becoming nonadherent.
- Adolescents need careful assessment and intervention to help them adjust to changes in body images related to the stoma and appliance.

Home Care Variation:

- Assess the client's home for an appropriate setting in which to change the ostomy appliance and proper means to dispose of the contaminated items.

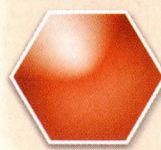

Long-Term Care Variation:

- Consider the ongoing stress of a slowly healing colostomy and the potential changes to body image large scars and marks will cause even after they have healed. Connect the client with support groups or further assessment if needed.

▶ COMMON ERRORS

Possible Error:

The appliance chosen is too small for the stoma's dimensions.

Prevention:

Measure the dimensions of the stoma prior to obtaining and preparing a pouch for application. If the error has occurred, remove the leaking appliance and remeasure the stoma dimensions before reapplying the ostomy appliance.

Possible Error:

The ostomy pouch is always full of liquid stool and the pouch has come unsnapped from the wafer several times.

Prevention:

Increase the frequency of checking and emptying the pouch. If increasing the frequency of emptying the pouch is impractical, it is best to change the pouch from a drainable system to a urinary pouch, which can be attached to bedside drainage.

▶ NURSING TIPS

- Recognize that all stomas are not the same. Each stoma must be treated individually, which requires that the nurse assess the dimensions, the location in relation to the client's body movements (i.e., sitting, bending), and the peristomal skin's condition.
- Client teaching is easily incorporated into the care of the ostomy by encouraging the client to assist the nurse during the application process.

- Use of an ostomy appliance that is intact, comfortable, and easy to use will increase the client's comfort level and thereby participation in self-care activities and socialization.
- Costs to the client and the health care institution are reduced when simplistic ostomy care is provided. Simplistic ostomy care excludes the daily use of pectin powder, pectin, paste, and skin sealant.

▶ SPECIAL CONSIDERATIONS

- *Assess skin integrity when performing stoma care. Document any sign of skin breakdown. An ischemic stoma usually appears dark red or black.*
- *Change the stoma pouch frequently if the skin underneath the appliance appears irritated.*
- *Use latex-free gloves and pouches if client has a history of allergy or contact dermatitis.*

Oxygenation

Administering Oxygen Therapy

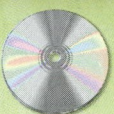

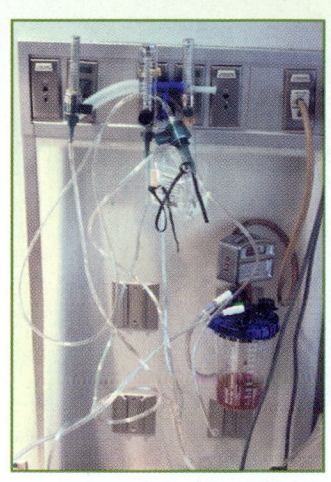

▶ OVERVIEW OF THE SKILL

Administration of oxygen must be ordered by the physician or qualified practitioner. Some hospitals and health care facilities will have protocols that govern oxygen therapy and allow the nurse to begin therapy independently. Oxygen is a drug, so medication administration criteria are followed in addition to the steps unique to oxygen therapy. Clients unable to maintain adequate PaO_2 and O_2 saturation levels on room air are candidates for oxygen therapy. An adequate airway is essential to effectiveness of the treatment. It is best to treat the hypoxia with the lowest oxygen dose possible. Some clients with normal oxygen levels are also given oxygen if they are at risk for complications related to hypoxia; for example, the myocardial infarction client often receives oxygen therapy to prevent dysrhythmias.

The health care provider will order the oxygen delivery system and flow rate, and the nurse will monitor response to the therapy. The dosage of oxygen may be ordered as an FIO_2 (fraction of inspired oxygen), which is expressed as a percentage or as liters per minute (lpm). Respiratory therapists may be available to assist in the administration and client assessment of oxygen therapy.

▶ ASSESSMENT

1. Determine client history and acute and chronic health problems. **Clients with carbon dioxide retaining chronic obstructive pulmonary disease (COPD) will need lower amounts of oxygen so as not to obliterate their hypoxic respiratory drive. They may already be on oxygen and need long-term continuous therapy.**

2. Assess the client's baseline respiratory signs, including airway, respiratory pattern, rate, depth, and rhythm, noting indications of increased work of breathing. **This will help determine the client's need for oxygen as well as response to the therapy.**

3. Check the extremities and mucous membranes closely for color. **This gives some indication of oxygenation, although problems with circulation and tissue perfusion can alter these factors also.**

4. Review arterial blood gas (ABG) and pulse oximetry results. **These are the most important determinants of the effectiveness of the pulmonary system and determine the need for therapy as well as changes in therapy.**

5. Note lung sounds for rales/crackles. **Secretions will interfere with airway patency and diffusion of oxygen and carbon dioxide across the alveolar-capillary bed.**

6. Assess the nares, behind the earlobes, cheek, tracheostomy site, or other places where oxygen tubing or equipment is in constant contact with the skin **to look for signs of skin irritation or breakdown.**

▶ DIAGNOSIS

Impaired Gas Exchange

Ineffective Breathing Pattern

Risk for Injury

Ineffective Airway Clearance

Risk for Impaired Skin Integrity

Activity Intolerance

Impaired Spontaneous Ventilation

▶ PLANNING

Expected Outcomes:

1. Oxygen levels will return to normal in blood and tissues as evident by oxygen saturation ≥ 92%; skin color normal.
2. Respiratory rate, pattern, and depth will be within the normal range for client.
3. The client will not develop any skin or tissue irritation or breakdown.
4. The client will demonstrate methods to clear secretions and maintain optimal oxygenation.
5. Breathing efficiency and activity tolerance will be increased.
6. The client will understand the rationale for the therapy.

Equipment Needed (see Figures 7-1-1A, 7-1-1B, and 7-1-1C):

• Stethoscope
• Oxygen source—portable or in-line
• Oxygen flow meter
• Oxygen delivery device: nasal cannula, mask, tent, or T-tube with adapter for artificial airway
• Oxygen tubing
• Pulse oximetry

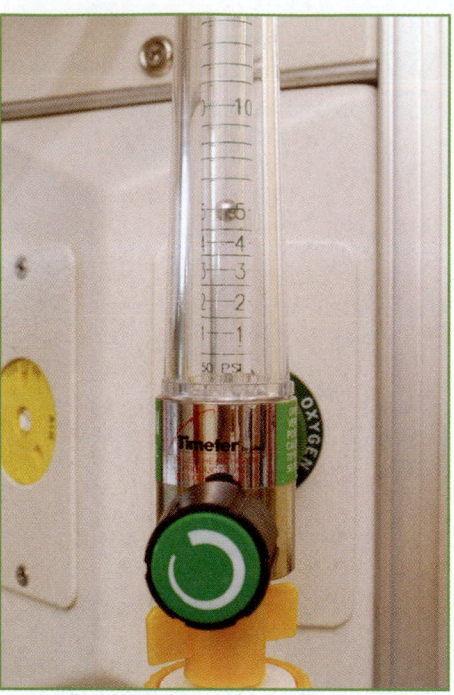

Figure 7-1-1B   In-line oxygen and flow meter

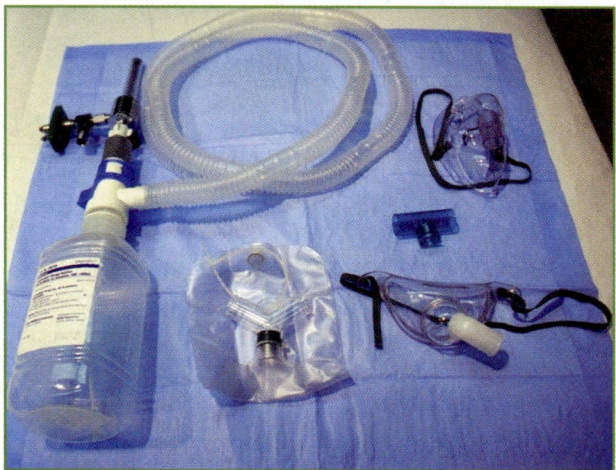

Figure 7-1-1C   Humidifier, reservoir bag, tracheostomy mask, T-tube, and a simple face mask are used when administering oxygen therapy.

• Humidifier and distilled or sterile water (not needed with low flow rates per nasal cannula)

▶ CLIENT EDUCATION NEEDED:

1. Clearly explain to the client the reason for oxygen therapy.
2. Help the client understand the importance of leaving the delivery system on.
3. Use pictures to help clients understand their lungs and airway so they will be more likely to cooperate with the therapy.
4. Make sure clients know what signs and symptoms to report that indicate therapy is not effective and needs to be changed.

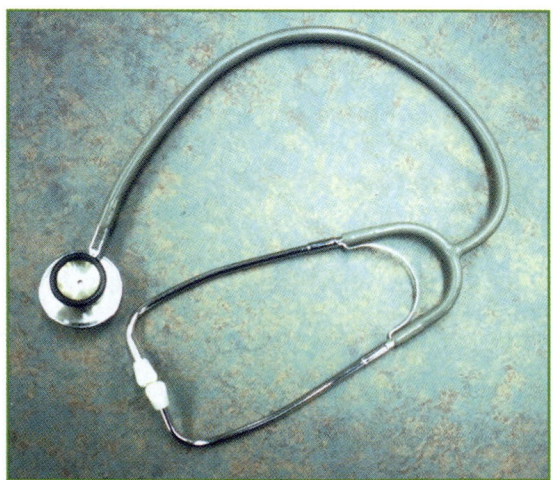

Figure 7-1-1A   Stethoscope

5. Reinforce safety issues—do not make clients overly afraid of a fire, but make sure they understand that oxygen supports combustion.
6. Show clients methods to increase oxygenation such as pursed-lip breathing, deep breathing, coughing, and changes in positioning.

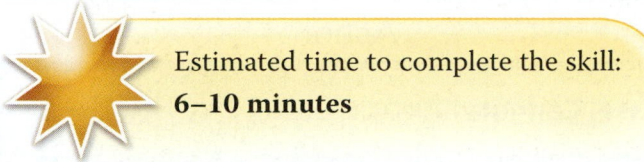

Estimated time to complete the skill:
6–10 minutes

> ► **DELEGATION TIPS**

The initiation of oxygen therapy requires assessment by a nurse or respiratory care practitioner. All personnel are responsible to maintain fire/safety precautions when oxygen is in use. Ancillary personnel should be instructed to report dyspnea, tachycardia, any changes in the client's activity tolerance, a respiratory rate less than 12 or greater than 20 breaths per minute in the adult client, or changes in mental status. Ancillary personnel should be instructed how to properly reapply respiratory therapy equipment, how to initiate assistance with activities of daily living for the client requiring oxygen therapy, and to report any abnormal client responses.

IMPLEMENTATION—Action/Rationale

Action	Rationale
Nasal Cannula (see Figure 7-1-2)	
1. Wash hands.	1. Reduces the transmission of microorganisms.
2. Verify the health care provider's order.	2. Ensures correct dosage and route.
3. Explain procedure and hazards to the client. Remind clients who smoke of the reasons for not smoking while O_2 is in use.	3. Increases compliance with procedures. Oxygen supports combustion.
4. If using humidity, fill humidifier to fill line with distilled water and close container.	4. Prevents drying of the client's airway and thins any secretions.

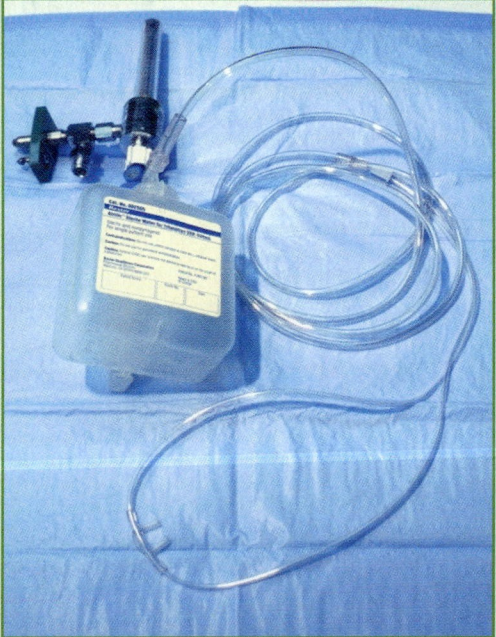

Figure 7-1-2 Nasal cannula and oxygen tubing attached to a humidifier

continues

Action	Rationale

Nasal Cannula *continued*

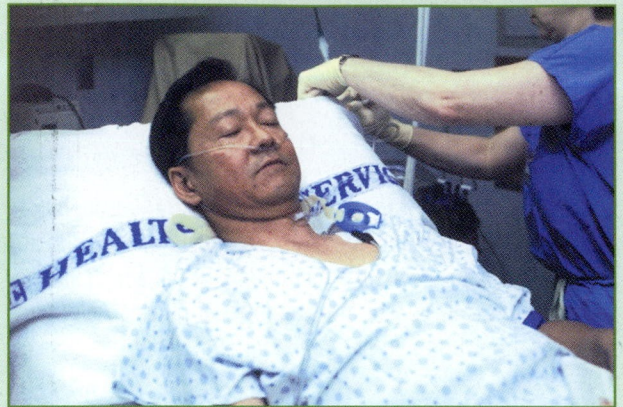

Figure 7-1-3   Oxygen being delivered via a nasal cannula.

5. Attach humidifier to oxygen flow meter.

6. Insert humidifier and flow meter into oxygen source in wall or portable unit.

7. Attach the oxygen tubing and nasal cannula to the flow meter and turn it on to the prescribed flow rate (1 to 5 liters/min). Use extension tubing for ambulatory clients so they can get up to go to the bathroom (see Figure 7-1-3).

8. Check for bubbling in the humidifier.

9. Place the nasal prongs in the client's nostrils. Secure the cannula in place by adjusting the tubing around the client's ears and using the slip ring to stabilize it under the client's chin (see Figure 7-1-4).

10. Check for proper flow rate every 4 hours and when the client returns from procedures.

11. Assess client's nostrils every 8 hours. If the client complains of dryness or has signs of irritation, use sterile lubricant to keep mucous membranes moist. Add humidifier if not already in place.

12. Monitor vital signs, oxygen saturation, and client condition every 4 to 8 hours (or as indicated or ordered) for signs and symptoms of hypoxia.

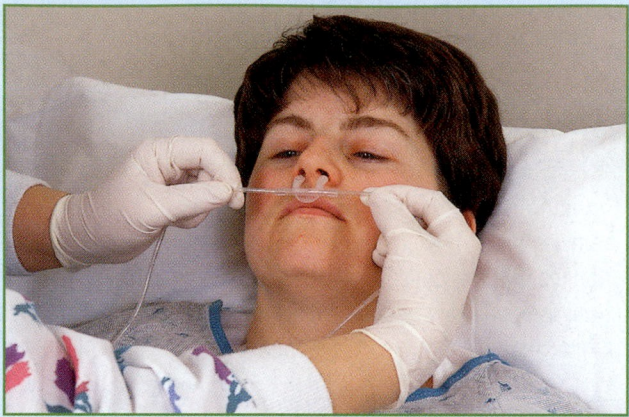

Figure 7-1-4   Insert nasal cannula prongs into nostrils.

5. Allows the oxygen to pass through the water and become humidified.

6. For access to oxygen. Many institutions also have compressed air available from outlets very similar in appearance to oxygen outlets. Green always stands for oxygen. Be sure to plug the flow meter into the green outlet.

7. Rates above 6 liters/min are not efficacious and can dry the nasal mucosa.

8. Ensures proper functioning.

9. Keeps delivery system in place so client receives the amount of oxygen ordered.

10. Ensures that client receives proper dose. The nasal cannula is a low flow system because it administers oxygen while the client also inspires room air. The actual dose of oxygen received by the client will vary depending on the client's respiratory pattern. The delivery rate may be changed during procedures.

11. Dry membranes are more prone to breakdown by friction or pressure from nasal cannula.

12. Detects any untoward effects from therapy.

continues

Action	Rationale
13. Wean client from oxygen as soon as possible using standard protocols. Mask: Venturi (high flow device), simple mask (low flow), partial rebreather mask, nonrebreather mask, and face tent	**13.** Oxygen is not without side effects and should be used only as long as needed. Problems with reimbursement may develop if criteria for therapy are not met.
14. Wash hands.	**14.** Reduces the transmission of microorganisms.
15. Repeat Actions 2–6.	**15.** See Rationales 2–6.
16. Attach appropriately sized mask (see Figure 7-1-5) or face tent to oxygen tubing and turn on flow meter to prescribed flow rate. The Venturi mask will have color-coded inserts that list the flow rate necessary to obtain the desired percentage of oxygen. Allow the reservoir bag of the nonrebreathing or partial rebreathing mask to fill completely. Figure 7-1-6 shows several types of oxygen masks.	**16.** Ensures proper fit; size needed is based on the client's size. Checks the oxygen source and primes the tubing and mask or tent.
17. Check for bubbling in the humidifier.	**17.** Ensures proper functioning.
18. Place the mask or tent on the client's face, fasten the elastic band around the client's ears and tighten until the mask fits snugly.	**18.** Prevents loss of oxygen from the sides of the mask.
19. Check for proper flow rate every 4 hours.	**19.** Ensures that client is receiving the proper dose.
20. Ensure that the ports of the Venturi mask are not under covers or impeded by any other source.	**20.** Air must be entrained to mix room air and oxygen coming from source to ensure proper oxygen percentage (FIO_2).
21. Assess client's face and ears for pressure from the mask and use padding as needed.	**21.** Provides client comfort and prevents skin breakdown.

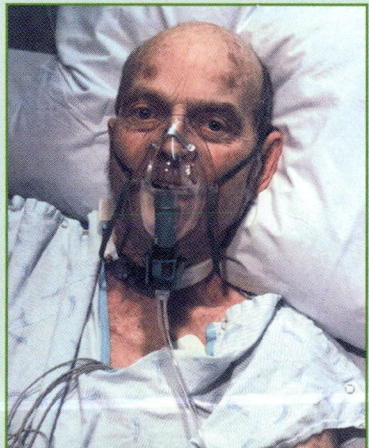

Figure 7-1-5 Make sure the mask used is the appropriate size for the client.

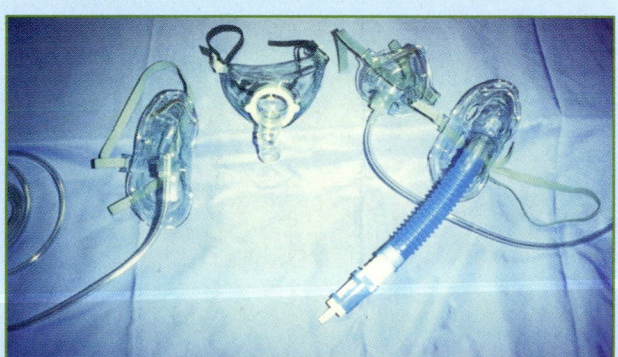

Figure 7-1-6 Different types of oxygen masks are available: simple oxygen mask, tracheostomy mask, pediatric mask, and Venturi mask.

continues

Action	Rationale
Nasal Cannula *continued*	
22. Wean client to nasal cannula and then wean off oxygen per protocol.	22. Oxygen is not without side effects and should be used only as long as needed. The nasal cannula provides a lower FIO_2 than the mask. Problems with reimbursement may develop if criteria for therapy are not met.
Oxygen via an Artificial Airway (tracheostomy or endotracheal tube)	
23. Wash hands.	23. Reduces the transmission of microorganisms.
24. Verify the physician's or qualified practitioner's order.	24. Ensures correct dosage and time.
25. Fill the humidifier with sterile water and close the container.	25. Avoids contamination of the water.
26. Attach humidifier and warmer to the oxygen flow meter (see Figure 7-1-7).	26. Humidification and warming of the air are essential with an artificial airway because the upper airway is bypassed by the tube.
27. Attach the wide bore oxygen tubing and T-tube adapter or tracheostomy mask to the flow meter and turn the meter to the flow rate needed to achieve the prescribed oxygen concentration. An oxygen analyzer may be used to check the actual oxygen percentage being delivered.	27. Checks the oxygen source and primes the tubing and adapter.
28. Check for bubbling in the humidifier and a fine mist from the adapter.	28. Ensures proper functioning.
29. Attach the T-piece to the client's artificial airway or place the mask over the client's airway. Be sure the T-piece is firmly attached to the airway (see Figure 7-1-8).	29. Ensures that client will not develop complications related to an interrupted oxygen supply.

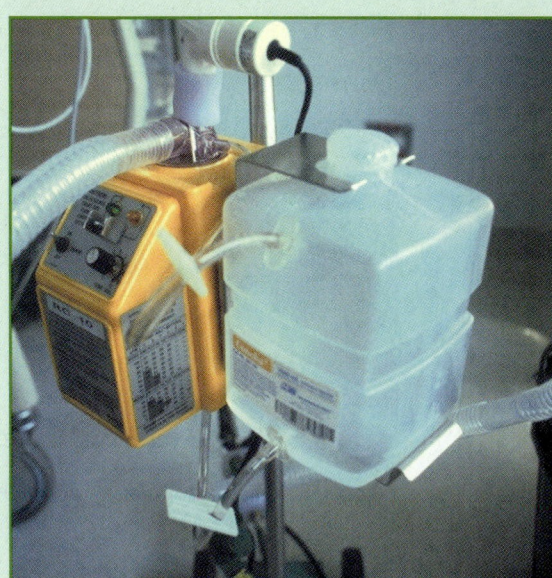

Figure 7-1-7 Oxygen humidifier and warmer

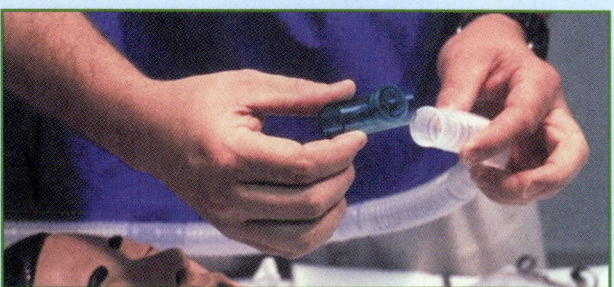

Figure 7-1-8 Attach the T-piece to the oxygen tubing.

continues

Action	Rationale
30. Position tubing so that it is not pulling client's airway.	**30.** Provides for client comfort and prevents dislodgment of the artificial airway.
31. Check for proper flow rate and patency of the system every 1 to 2 hours depending on the acuity of the client. Suction as needed to maintain a patent airway.	**31.** Ensures that client is receiving proper dose.
32. Monitor airway patency, vital signs, oxygen saturation, and for signs and symptoms of hypoxia every 2 hours, or more frequently as necessary or as ordered. Additionally, monitor breath sounds and tube position every 4 hours.	**32.** Detects response to or any untoward effects from therapy. Determines whether tube is in place.
33. Wean client from therapy as ordered by physician or qualified practitioner. The client will probably receive oxygen via another route once the tube is removed. Some clients have tracheotomies permanently.	**33.** Prevents untoward effects of oxygen.

▶ **REAL WORLD ANECDOTES**

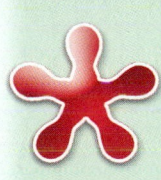

A client came to the unit with an extremely low arterial oxygen level and a slightly high arterial carbon dioxide level. He was at risk for needing mechanical ventilation, but because he had chronic obstructive lung disease and there was a good chance that he would become dependent on the ventilator, the physician elected to treat him with oxygen therapy and bronchodilator aerosol treatments only. An antibiotic was also started until pneumonia could be ruled out. The client was continuously monitored with pulse oximetry, and his oxygen saturation levels slowly rose and stayed around 90%. Everyone was pleased, but as the day went on, the client became less and less responsive. When arterial blood gases were drawn mid-afternoon, his arterial carbon dioxide levels had risen above 100 mm Hg. The health care team was reminded of two major effects. First, pulse oximetry is not the panacea in monitoring. In clients who are prone to CO_2 retention, more frequent ABG analysis is necessary to detect changes before levels get too high. Additionally, the nurse needs to assess other indicators of PCO_2, including decreased sensorium, headache, and flushing. Second, the nurse was reminded of the changes that occur in the ventilatory drive of clients with COPD. Because their respiratory center is "numbed" to elevations in CO_2, it is the hypoxic drive that stimulates respirations. Because the oxygen satisfied his hypoxic drive, the client began to hypoventilate and to retain carbon dioxide. COPD clients need low oxygen concentrations, usually 1 to 2 liters/min or ≤24% and astute monitoring of their respiratory rate and sensorium.

▶ **EVALUATION**

- Oxygen levels returned to normal in blood and tissues as evident by oxygen saturation ≥92%; skin color normal for client.
- Respiratory rate, pattern, and depth are within the normal range.
- The client did not develop any skin or tissue irritation or breakdown.

- Breathing efficiency and activity tolerance are increased.
- The client understands the rationale for the therapy.

▶ **DOCUMENTATION**

Nurses' Notes

- Record O_2 saturation and respiratory status.
- Note method of oxygen delivery and rate.

- Document client's assessment parameters and response to treatment.
- Note and record changes in mental status.

Document on appropriate flow sheet or electronic medical record (EMR).

▶ CRITICAL THINKING SKILL

Introduction

Look at an example in which the nurse prevents potential cardiac arrest in a client receiving oxygen via a tracheostomy.

Possible Scenario

The client is receiving oxygen at 40% via a tracheostomy mask. The client's respirations are increased with intercostal retractions and tachycardia, and are very flushed to cyanotic color. The nurse quickly checks to make sure the oxygen is hooked up to the wall and connected to the client properly. The oxygen source is attached correctly, but the humidification bottle is dry. There are no visible secretions in the tracheostomy or T-tube adapter. When assessing the client's breath sounds, the nurse notices very diminished sounds and observes that the client is in more and more distress. While calling for help, the nurse tries to pass a suction catheter down the tracheostomy, but is unable to pass the catheter or ventilate with a manual resuscitation bag (Ambu®-bag). Finally, the nurse removes the inner cannula and finds a large, solid mucus plug attached to the cannula. The client's respiratory distress subsides and the cannula is cleaned and replaced.

Possible Outcome

Cardiopulmonary arrest and death of the client resulting from an obstructed airway, could result.

Prevention

Ensure that clients with tracheostomies receive humidification to prevent secretions from thickening and obstructing the airway.

▶ VARIATIONS

Geriatric Variation:
- *Clients may pull at tubes; they need frequent reorientation and explanation.*

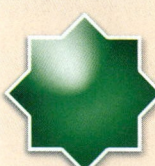

Pediatric Variation:
- *Clients may be frightened and pull off the O₂ mask and increase respiratory effort with crying. Try putting the mask on yourself and make a game out of it so the child is less frightened.*

Home Care Variations:
- *Oxygen may be provided by a high pressure cylinder, an oxygen concentrator, or a liquid oxygen system. Spare tanks and a backup power source are recommended. Compressed oxygen gas in a cylinder is available in sizes H or K for large stationary tanks and sizes D and E for travel and in the event of a power failure. Portable carts and carrying shoulder cases are also available. The company supplying the equipment will usually have personnel that will help with the setup and specific cleaning needs of the oxygen source.*
- *While any delivery system may be used in the home, nasal cannulas and tracheostomy tents/masks are the most commonly used. Home care clients may receive oxygen via a Spofford Christopher Oxygen Optimizing Prosthesis transtracheal system (SCOOP) catheter placed down into the trachea via a small stoma. It is held in place by a bead chain necklace and needs regular cleaning. Tubing, delivery system, and humidifier container should be washed regularly every 2 to 7 days with soap and water, disinfected, and dried before reuse, so an alternate setup should be available. Post safety precautions in the home. Oxygen sources should be kept from heating units, walls, drapes, and combustible substances such as hair spray.*

continues

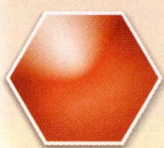

▶ **VARIATIONS** (continued)

Long-Term Care Variation:
- *Long-term clients are more likely to develop skin irritation and mucous membrane dryness from oxygen therapy. Padding may be needed at friction sites. Humidity may be needed to reduce dryness.*

▶ **COMMON ERRORS**

Possible Error:

The wrong flow rates are used.

Prevention:

Be sure to administer the flow rate ordered. Be aware of client history of lung disease. Clients with lung disease cannot tolerate high flow rates of oxygen.

Possible Error:

The wrong delivery system is used.

Prevention:

Double-check the order. Assess the client's needs. Is the client a mouth breather? Does the client have an artificial airway in place? Does the client need humidified oxygen?

Possible Error:

The wrong client receives treatment.

Prevention:

Double-check the wristband, or ask the client to tell you his or her name. Double-check written orders.

▶ **NURSING TIPS**

- Recognize which equipment to use; keep a chart on the unit that gives information on flow rates and settings of different devices.
- Promote client comfort by adjusting tubing or padding so that clients are more likely to leave oxygen therapy equipment on.

- Water will often collect in the corrugated tubing used for masks, T-tubes, and tracheostomy tents, and creates pulls on the devices and bubbling noises. Try to avoid dependent loops and empty the water from the tubing into the appropriate container. Do not empty water back into the humidifier container because this can cause contamination of the humidifier.

> **SPECIAL CONSIDERATIONS**

- When clients with lung disease or serious medical conditions are considering air travel, they should be encouraged to consult their health care provider. Clients at risk may need supplemental oxygen during the flight as flying at high altitudes can induce significant hypoxia.
- The goal of oxygen supplementation is to use the lowest concentration of oxygen required to meet oxygenation goals. Clients requiring oxygen should be monitored with pulse oximetry and arterial blood gas analysis. The nurse should be aware that clients may experience oxygen toxicity as evident by substernal heaviness, pleuritic chest pain, cough, and dyspnea within 24 hours of breathing pure oxygen. The nurse must understand how each mask works and not rely solely on respiratory therapy personnel.
- The nurse should be cognizant of the potential for decreased respiratory drive and CO_2 retention in clients with COPD as exhibited by tachycardia, tachypnea, increased BP, lack of mental alertness, or confusion. Clients with COPD may be maintained at low levels of PaO_2 (65–80 mm Hg) to protect their respiratory drive and receive only minimal levels of oxygen delivery (usually less than 2 liters/minute).
- Oxygen toxicity, which causes damage to the hyaline membrane lining in the lungs, can occur when a high concentration of oxygen (greater than 50%) is administered for more than 48 hours. The symptoms are restlessness, dyspnea, paresthesia, fatigue, malaise, and progressive respiratory distress and may culminate in pulmonary disease.

Assisting a Client with Controlled Coughing and Deep Breathing

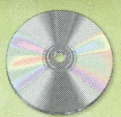

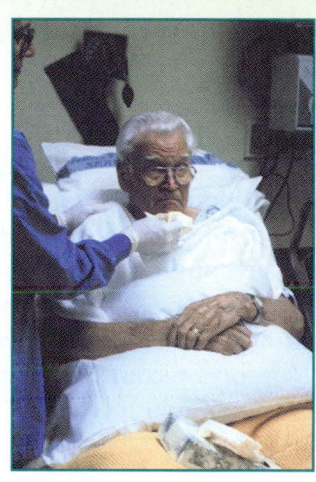

▶ OVERVIEW OF THE SKILL

Teaching clients controlled, effective coughing techniques is essential in the management of bronchial secretions. It should be taught to all clients undergoing surgery and is essential for the management of excessive respiratory secretions in clients with lung conditions from acute to chronic. Secretions must be removed to prevent atelectasis and pneumonia. Furthermore, immobility causes the pooling of bronchial secretions in the gravity-dependent areas of the lungs and blocks off small airways, and leads to trapping of secretions or closure of these airways. As a result, less surface area of the lung is available for ventilation, which leads to hypercapnia and hypoxemia. Deep, controlled breathing reopens small airways, and coughing promotes the removal of secretions.

▶ ASSESSMENT

1. Identify need for controlled coughing such as thick, tenacious secretions; weak or ineffective cough; abnormal breath sounds; or inability to take a deep breath **because these conditions may increase the client's risk for impaired respiratory function.**
2. Assess breath sounds by auscultation throughout lung fields, especially in dependent areas so comparison **can be made to baseline assessment after coughing and deep breathing.**

3. Assess by percussion, if necessary, **to verify ausculatory sounds.**
4. Assess by tactile means for fremitus **to verify presence of secretions.**
5. Assess the client for understanding, ability, and cooperation to perform a controlled cough **so the nurse can tailor client education needs.**

▶ DIAGNOSIS

Ineffective Airway Clearance

Altered Tissue Perfusion

Ineffective Breathing Pattern

Deficient Knowledge Regarding Controlled Coughing Technique

▶ PLANNING

Expected Outcomes:

1. The client will be able to breathe deeply and clearly.
2. The client will be able to use effective breathing techniques.
3. The client will be able to cough productively if secretions are present on assessment.
4. The lung fields will be clear to auscultation; that is, there is absence of atelectasis, or adventitious sounds (rales/crackles, or rhonchi).

877

5. The client's respiratory rate will be normal.
6. The client will have good skin color (for race) and mentation.

Equipment Needed (see Figure 7-2-1):

- Tissues
- Water pitcher and glass
- Emesis basin
- Stethoscope
- Pillows for splinting the client's chest and abdomen
- Gloves

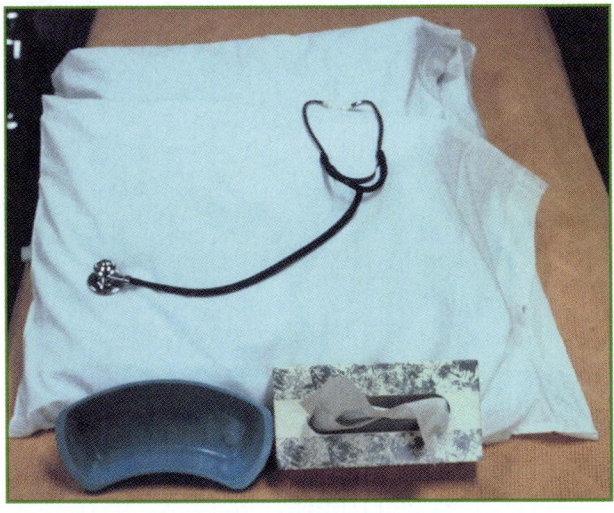

Figure 7-2-1 Stethoscope, pillow, tissues, and emesis basin are used to assist the client with coughing and deep breathing.

▶ CLIENT EDUCATION NEEDED:

1. Teach the client the rationale for effective deep breathing and coughing.
2. Show the client how to hold a pillow to the chest to support the chest and abdominal muscles.
3. Instruct the caregiver how to assist the client with coughing and deep breathing.
4. Teach the caregiver how to recognize changes in the client's respiratory pattern.
5. Ask clients to turn their head away from the nurse when coughing.
6. Instruct clients to cover their mouth with tissue paper while coughing.
7. Tell the client to hold the inspiration for 1–2 seconds before coughing for it to be effective.
8. Teach clients with lung disease to huff cough to clear central airways: Take a slow, deep breath; hold it for 2 seconds; contract expiratory muscles; and open mouth and say "huff" several times while exhaling.

Estimated time to complete the skill:
10 minutes

▶ DELEGATION TIPS

Ancillary personnel may assist the client to perform coughing and deep breathing exercises. It is the nurse's responsibility to initiate the client teaching after completing an assessment validating the need for this intervention. Follow-up assessment regarding the effectiveness of the coughing and deep breathing exercises is the nurse's responsibility but ancillary personnel should be instructed to encourage this activity, to assist the client into proper position, and to report the results, for example, increased sputum production and the color and amount of expectorant.

IMPLEMENTATION—Action/Rationale

Action	Rationale
1. Wash hands.	1. Reduces the transmission of microorganisms.
2. Assess the client's pain status.	2. If pain is not controlled in clients with abdominal or thoracic surgery, they will not be able to cooperate.

continues

Action	Rationale

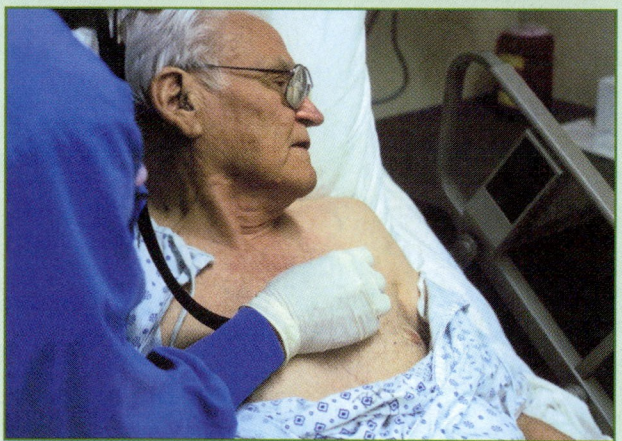

Figure 7-2-2   Auscultate the lungs prior to beginning the procedure.

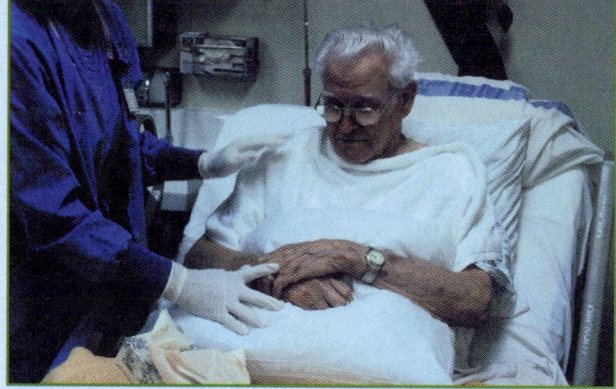

Figure 7-2-3   The client holds a pillow over the chest or abdomen while coughing.

3. Explain the purpose and importance of the procedure.

4. Help the client sit in a high Fowler's position if able.

5. Auscultate lungs before procedure (see Figure 7-2-2).

6. Place the palms of your hands on the client's rib cage.

7. Use pillow or folded towels to splint the abdomen or chest if client has had surgery (see Figure 7-2-3).

8. Practice deep breathing with client:
   • Instruct the client to cover the mouth with tissue (use mask, gloves, and gown for staff as needed).
   • Take a deep breath in and exhale slowly and repeat 2–3 times.
   • Repeat 10 times every 1–2 hours as needed.

9. Reassess lung fields after procedure.

10. Assist the client to cough as follows:
   • Follow the procedure for deep breathing and have the client hold breath for 1 to 2 seconds.
   • Contract abdominal muscles, cough forcefully, and expectorate secretions into tissue or basin as nurse splints incision areas as appropriate (see Figure 7-2-4).
   • Splint the client's abdomen and chest as he or she coughs by pressing on lower chest wall and abdomen with your hands.

3. Elicits client's cooperation.

4. An upright posture allows for maximal lung expansion.

5. Allows nurse to know which areas of the lungs need more effective coughing, deep breathing, and repositioning.

6. Assesses effective expansion of chest.

7. Decreases pain with deep expansion in postoperative clients and promotes effective deep breathing and coughing.

8. Promotes loosening of secretions.
   • Repetition is necessary to cough up secretions.

9. Evaluation of procedure is necessary to know whether procedure should be repeated.

10. Even though deep inspirations may clear the airways of clients with atelectasis, coughing is essential to clear bronchial secretions, especially from lower airways.
   • After a deep inspiration, the force of the air will be behind the mucus and propel it upward. The force of the air after the deep inspiration and the muscle contractions enable more effective coughing.
   • The nurse can also use splinting at this time to help with force of abdominal contraction.

continues

Action	Rationale

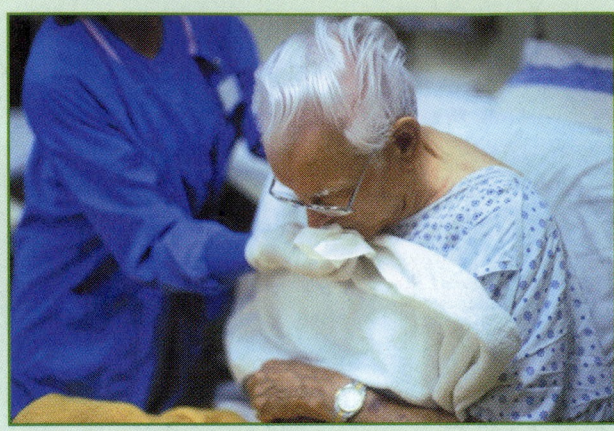

Figure 7-2-4   The client expectorates secretions into a tissue.

11. Repeat as necessary to clear lung fields; however, be aware that excessive coughing can irritate the trachea and bronchial tree. Clients with chronic respiratory problems may need to repeat the procedure at more frequent intervals but with fewer coughs with each procedure. Adjunct therapy may be necessary.

11. It is essential to clear airways to prevent atelectasis and pneumonia. If excessive coughing happens, the client may cause irritation and compromise respiratory status.

12. Observe for dizziness, shortness of breath, or other respiratory problems.

12. May indicate hyperventilation.

13. Dispose of all tissues and wash hands.

13. Reduces the transmission of microorganisms.

► **REAL WORLD ANECDOTES**

Harry had abdominal surgery 2 days ago and had been taught the importance of deep breathing and coughing. While the nurse was helping him take deep breaths and cough, he had a coughing spasm. The nurse held in place the pillow that she used to splint his abdomen until the episode stopped. She offered Harry sips of warm water to help soothe the trachea. He said that his incisional pain was worse so he used his PCA button. The nurse took off her gloves and gown and told Harry to rest for 30 minutes. When she returned, his pain had decreased and he felt ready to try the procedure again. After assessing his lung fields, the nurse held the pillow firmly against Harry's abdomen, and he was able to take deep breaths and cough up a moderate amount of thick, yellowish mucus. When she listened to his lungs again, they were clear where she had heard rhonchi before.

► **EVALUATION**

- The client is able to breathe deeply and clearly.
- The client is able to use effective breathing techniques.
- The client is able to cough productively if secretions are present on assessment.

- The lung fields are clear to auscultation, that is, there is absence of atelectasis, rales/crackles, or rhonchi.
- The client's respiratory rate is normal.
- The client has good skin color and mentation.

▶ **DOCUMENTATION**

Nurses' Notes

• Record date and time of procedure.
• Include description of secretions and amount expectorated.
• Record results of auscultation before and after procedure.

Document on appropriate flow sheet or electronic medical record (EMR).

▶ **CRITICAL THINKING SKILL**

Introduction

If a client continues to have crackles and decreased breath sounds after controlled breathing and coughing, there may be cardiovascular involvement.

Possible Scenario

A 58-year-old smoker with a history of mild congestive heart failure has a hernia repair. After surgery he continues to have a moist cough and crackles in the lower bases of the lungs.

Possible Outcome

This client's nurse knows that the presence of fluid in the lungs may be related to pulmonary edema. He or she has the client cough to determine if post-tusic rales are present. The nurse instructs him to change positions and assesses whether the areas of crackles/rales or rhonchi change. They do not. The nurse checks the client's weight and assesses for edema. He or she listens for a third heart sound and reviews the intake and output information. Finally, he or she checks vital signs and notifies the physician of signs and symptoms indicative of congestive heart failure.

Prevention

Monitor fluid status and risk status of client each shift and be cognizant of any early signs of change in cardiac and respiratory status.

▶ **VARIATIONS**

Geriatric Variations:

• *Elderly clients may not effectively use deep breathing and may need more instruction from the nurse.*
• *The tracheal tissue may be more fragile and at risk for bleeding if coughing is too vigorous.*
• *Elderly clients may need more support during the procedure such as help splinting the chest or abdomen with a pillow.*

Pediatric Variations:

• *Crying may occur with coughing and pain after surgery and may be appropriate in clearing airways of children.*
• *Children may benefit from hugging their favorite stuffed animal instead of a pillow.*
• *Play therapy can be used in performing the procedure so it is like a game.*
• *Children will need to have pain medication 30 minutes before the procedure to help them cooperate.*

Home Care Variations:

• *Long-term immobility will lead to increased secretions.*
• *Ask family members to assist with routine coughing and deep breathing procedures.*
• *Assess the home for ventilation or air conditioning and the client's reaction to the environment.*
• *Provide instruction on the proper disposal of secretions and used tissues to decrease the risk of transmission of microorganisms.*

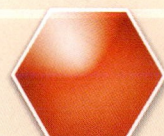

Long-Term Care Variations:

• *Immobility may lead to increased secretions.*
• *Encourage clients to walk in the halls.*
• *Increasing fluid intake will decrease viscosity of secretions.*

▶ COMMON ERRORS

Possible Error:

The client is not able to take a deep breath because you did not allow enough time for pain control before starting the controlled breathing and coughing procedure.

Prevention:

Plan the pain medication dose for at least 30 minutes before the time of the procedure. If not enough time was allowed for pain control, stop the breathing exercise and allow the pain medication to take effect. Assess the client for pain. Ask whether client is ready to do the deep breathing and coughing. When client is ready, proceed.

▶ NURSING TIPS

- As clients take deep inspirations, breathe with them to help with timing.
- Use gown, gloves, and mask with clients who have copious secretions or clients who expectorate vigorously.
- Abdominal binders may be necessary for clients with major abdominal surgery to avoid dehiscence.
- If clients complain of severe abdominal pain with the procedure, evaluate the wound site and pain status.

▶ SPECIAL CONSIDERATIONS

- *Clients are often noncompliant with deep breathing and coughing every hour, which greatly increases their risk of postoperative pneumonia or atelectasis. The creative nurse might involve the family members and delegate the responsibility of engaging the client in breathing activities every hour. Of course, the nurse is still responsible to assess the client's lungs and encourage turning, coughing, and deep breathing.*
- *Often clients get reliant on the incentive spirometer (Skill 7-3) and neglect deep breathing if the spirometer is not within reach. Explain to the client that the goal of lung expansion is accomplished with either deep breathing or incentive spirometry.*

Assisting a Client with an Incentive Spirometer

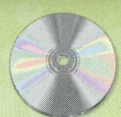

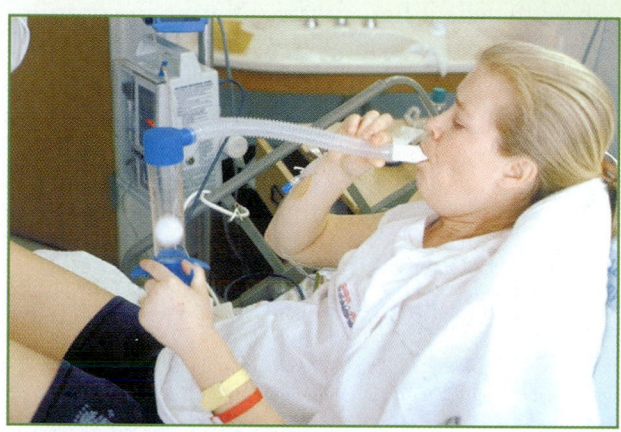

► OVERVIEW OF THE SKILL

Incentive spirometers (IS) encourage clients to sustain deep voluntary breathing and maximum inspiration to open airways, encourage coughing, and prevent or reduce atelectasis. Incentive spirometers provide visual feedback to clients and, therefore, enhance deep voluntary breathing and sustained inspiration. Incentive spirometers are used for postoperative clients, chest trauma victims, and clients with respiratory disorders. Clients who have had abdominal or thoracic surgery and elderly clients are especially at risk for atelectasis and consolidation. Incentive spirometers may be used as adjunct treatment in other high risk clients such as those on long-term bed rest, clients with chronic and restrictive lung diseases, or clients on medications that depress respiration.

► ASSESSMENT

1. Assess need for incentive spirometry. Clients who are postsurgery, or clients with pneumonia or postchest trauma **are at increased risk for respiratory complications.**
2. Assess the client's respiratory status by general observation, auscultation of breath sounds, and percussion of thorax to be able **to compare future assessments with a baseline evaluation.**
3. Review medical record for recent arterial blood gases **to determine need for using incentive spirometer.**

► DIAGNOSIS

Altered Tissue Perfusion

Ineffective Airway Clearance

Ineffective Breathing Pattern

Impaired Gas Exchange

Acute Pain

► PLANNING

Expected Outcomes:

1. The client will have clear breath sounds throughout lung fields, especially at the bases of the lungs.
2. The client will have normal depth and rate of respiration.
3. The inspiratory lung expansion will return to client's preevent status.
4. The client's arterial blood gases will be normal.
5. There will be an absence of consolidation or atelectasis.
6. Respirations will not be labored.

Equipment Needed (see Figure 7-3-1):

- Stethoscope
- Incentive spirometer with appropriate mouthpiece
  a. Flow-oriented
  b. Volume-oriented
- Tissue

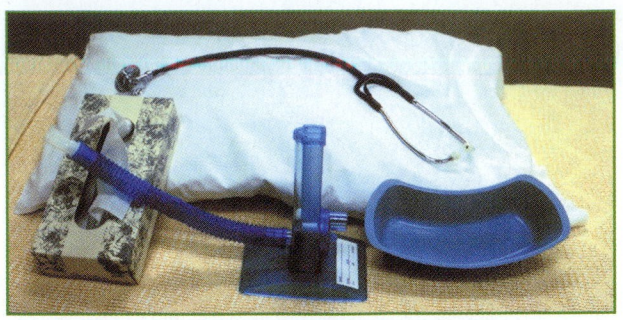

Figure 7-3-1 Stethoscope, tissue, pillow, and emesis basin are all used with the incentive spirometer to open airways and encourage coughing.

- Emesis basin
- Pillow, if needed

► **CLIENT EDUCATION NEEDED:**

1. Teach the client the purpose of IS.
2. Show the client how to seal the mouthpiece and use the spirometer.

3. Teach the client that the goal of sustained inspiration and expansion of the lungs is to prevent atelectasis and consolidation.
4. Tell the client that inspiration must be sustained for the treatment to be effective.
5. Teach the client how to use diaphragmatic breathing.
6. Teach the client how to build up depth of inspiration.
7. Show the client how to use splinting to control incisional pain during IS use.
8. Teach the client to use tissues to dispose of expectorated secretions.

Estimated time to complete the skill: **5–20 minutes**

► **DELEGATION TIPS**

Ancillary personnel may assist the client to perform incentive spirometry exercises. It is the nurse's responsibility to initiate client teaching after completing an assessment that validates the need for this intervention. Follow-up assessment regarding the effectiveness of the exercises is the nurse's responsibility but ancillary personnel should be instructed to encourage this activity, to assist the client into proper position, and to report the results, for example, increased sputum production and the color and amount of expectorant.

IMPLEMENTATION—Action/Rationale

Action	Rationale
1. Wash hands.	1. Reduces the transmission of microorganisms.
2. Check chart for previous respiratory assessment.	2. Establishes a baseline for comparison.
3. Gather equipment.	3. Ensures preparation.
4. Explain procedure to client.	4. Encourages client's cooperation.
5. Demonstrate deep, sustained inspiration.	5. Demonstration is a reliable teaching technique.
6. Instruct client to assume a semi-Fowler's or high-Fowler's position.	6. Promotes optimal lung expansion.
7. Set pointer on IS at appropriate level or point to level where disk or ball should reach.	7. Encourages client to reach appropriate goal.

continues

Action	Rationale
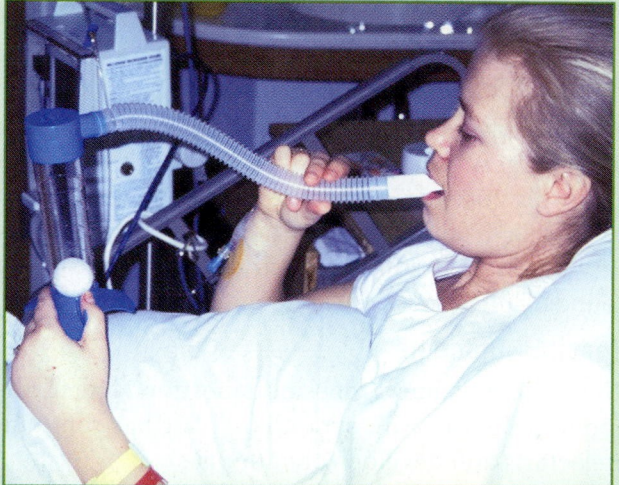	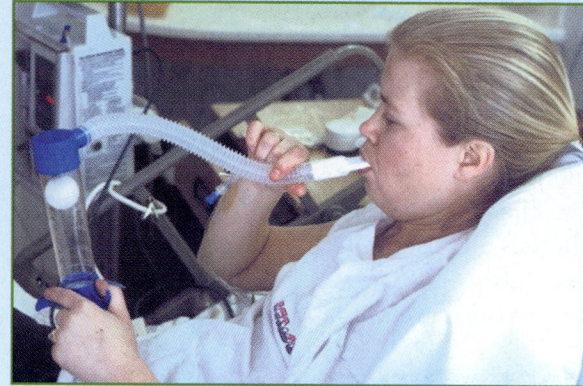

Figure 7-3-2 Have the client seal his or her lips around the mouthpiece.

Figure 7-3-3 Inhale slowly and deeply for at least three seconds.

Action	Rationale
8. Use incentive spirometer: • Have client breathe in and exhale completely before using IS. • Hold unit upright. • Have client seal lips around mouthpiece and inhale slowly and deeply until desired volume is attained (see Figure 7-3-2). • Sustain inspiration for at least 3 seconds (see Figure 7-3-3). • Exhale slowly.	8. • Promotes clearing of secretions before using the IS. • Prevents ineffective use of the spirometer. • Allows gauge to register effective inspiration. • Allows the alveolar sacs to open and remain open and discourages atelectasis.
9. Repeat 10–20 times every 1–2 hours while awake for 72 hours and as needed.	9. Ensures airways remain open and prevents atelectasis. May be required longer than 72 hours.
10. Teach client to perform IS every hour and verify that the client is compliant.	10. Encourages clients to take responsibility for their health care.
11. Dispose of soiled equipment or tissues and wash hands.	11. Reduces the transmission of microorganisms.

 ► **REAL WORLD ANECDOTES**

Mrs. Hoang, a 37-year-old Asian woman, was recovering from abdominal surgery. Because she spoke very little English, the nurse showed her how to use the incentive spirometer (IS). She asked Mrs. Hoang's daughter to tell her why she needed to use the IS and she seemed to understand. The nurse demonstrated first and then the client returned the demonstration with a very low volume. The nurse then showed her how hugging a pillow would splint her incision, and the client felt more comfortable attaining larger and larger volumes. The client seemed pleased when the nurse applauded her good efforts at reaching the goal volume. Then the nurse showed her the times on the wall clock when she should repeat the procedure. At the appointed hour, the nurse noted that Mrs. Hoang was already preparing to use her IS when she went into her room to check on her.

▶ EVALUATION

- The client has clear breath sounds throughout lung fields, especially at the base of the lungs.
- The client has normal depth and rate of respiration.
- The inspiratory lung expansion returned to client's preevent status.
- The client's arterial blood gases are normal.
- There is an absence of consolidation or atelectasis.
- Respirations are not labored.

▶ DOCUMENTATION

Nurses' Notes

- Record lung volume in cubic centimeters (cc).
- Record respiratory assessment, including auscultation of breath sounds and rate and depth of respiration.
- Note the type and amount of secretions expectorated.

Document on appropriate flow sheet or electronic medical record (EMR).

▶ CRITICAL THINKING SKILL

Introduction

Nurses must be able to evaluate effectiveness of IS by auscultation of the lung fields.

Possible Scenario

Nate is recovering at home from cardiac-valve replacement surgery. The nurse caring for him is concerned about his postsurgical progress. He states he continues to use IS faithfully every hour and yet his respiratory assessment still demonstrates decreased breath sounds, dull percussion, and increased temperature.

Possible Outcome

The nurse, in a hurry, does not question Nate further about his IS use or his symptoms. Nate has continued atelectasis and develops pneumonia.

Prevention

Assessing that the client is properly using IS and on a regular basis by observing the client is important. Include assessing for tactile fremitus and voice sounds to note the development of consolidation. Report an increase in temperature because it may be a sign of a lung infection.

▶ VARIATIONS

Geriatric Variations:

- *Elderly clients with dentures or dry mouth may have difficulty sealing their mouth around the mouthpiece.*
- *Respiratory rates vary with age, and elderly clients may have more difficulty sustaining deep inspirations.*
- *Elderly clients frequently have abdominal, cardiac, or orthopedic surgery that requires IS use.*
- *Elderly clients with chronic respiratory disease or a history of smoking will be at higher risk of respiratory compromise.*

Pediatric Variations:

- *Respiratory rate and volume vary with age.*
- *Younger children have increased activity and crying and may not be cooperative with IS use.*
- *Making a game out of the IS can promote more compliance in young children.*

Home Care Variations:

- *Remind clients to clean the mouthpiece with soap and water every 24 hours.*
- *Ask the client to return-demonstrate the correct use of the IS before discharge.*
- *Assess the home for ventilation and air conditioning as well as proper disposal of soiled respiratory material.*
- *Teach family members to hold their hands on the client's chest to watch expansion of the chest.*
- *Tell the caregiver to breathe with the client during the procedure.*

continues

▶ VARIATIONS *(continued)*

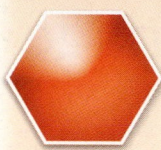

Long-Term Care Variations:
- *Clients with chronic obstructive disease should be taught the pursed-lip technique after deep inspiration and slow exhalation to allow airways to stay open and to avoid air trapping.*
- *Use oral pharyngeal suctioning or ask the client to cough before attempting IS use in clients with chronic bronchitis or those with excessive secretions.*

▶ COMMON ERRORS

Possible Error:

You note that the client is not sealing his or her lips around the mouthpiece, so the ball does not rise to the desired level.

Prevention:

Ask the client to demonstrate the ability to maintain a seal around the mouthpiece before the procedure. If the error does occur, set the IS aside. Ask the client whether he or she would like to remove his or her dentures, if applicable. Give the client a drink of water or apply a lip balm to moisten the lips. Ask the client to try making a seal around the mouthpiece. If successful, go ahead with the procedure.

▶ NURSING TIPS

- Have client practice deep breathing before IS so coughing will clear secretions in upper airways, reducing the risk of secretions entering lower airways.
- Increase depth of inspirations with each use of IS.
- Avoid hyperventilation by allowing pauses between breaths.
- Assess for adequate pain control for clients having undergone abdominal or thoracic surgery so the client can effectively use IS.

- Have tissues available so clients will not cough on staff. Staff may use masks if clients have copious secretions.
- If clients are unable to sit up while using IS, ask them to turn from side to side between the use of IS to hyperinflate all areas of the lung.
- Slowly build up respirations from shallow to deep to prevent clients from vomiting due to excessive coughing during spirometry use.

▶ SPECIAL CONSIDERATIONS

- *It is important to set realistic goals for the client with regard to the gauge of mL per second noted on the spirometer. If the client has a disability, such as one lung or severe chronic obstructive pulmonary disease, then his or her inspired measurement may never meet that of an otherwise healthy individual.*
- *Often clients get reliant on the incentive spirometer and neglect deep breathing (Skill 7-2) if the spirometer is not within reach. Explain to the client that the goal of lung expansion is accomplished with either deep breathing or incentive spirometry.*

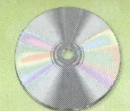

Administering Pulmonary Therapy and Postural Drainage

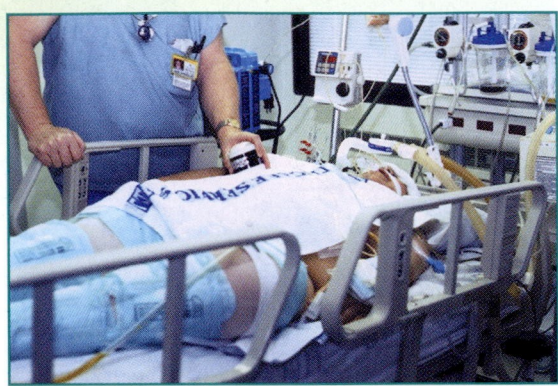

▶ OVERVIEW OF THE SKILL

Chest pulmonary therapy and postural drainage (CPPD), also known as chest physiotherapy (CPT), may, through proper positioning and chest wall percussion, facilitate airway clearance and be effective in mobilizing pulmonary secretions in the postoperative client and those suffering pneumonitis, emphysema, asthma, chronic bronchitis, bronchiectasis, and cystic fibrosis.

▶ ASSESSMENT

1. Assess the client's breath sounds via auscultation and the ability to clear secretions. **Determines the amount of congestion present.**
2. Determine the client's rhythm, depth of breathing, and rate. **Determines whether the client will tolerate the procedure.**
3. Observe the quality of the secretions. **Humidification therapy may be necessary if secretions are thick and tenacious.**
4. Take note of any complicating conditions. **Look for symptoms or history of congestive heart failure (CHF), cerebral edema, head trauma, abdominal distention, arrhythmias, hypertension, or end-stage chronic obstructive pulmonary disease (COPD).**

▶ DIAGNOSIS

Ineffective Airway Clearance

Ineffective Breathing Pattern

Impaired Gas Exchange

▶ PLANNING

Expected Outcomes:

1. Clearance of pulmonary secretions will be improved.
2. Ventilation will be improved.
3. Potential complications will be minimized.
4. Client will experience an improved sense of well-being.

Equipment Needed:

- Electric or pneumatic percussors, the Thairapy Vest, or manual percussion (see Figure 7-4-1)
- Tissues or suction equipment and manual ventilator when appropriate

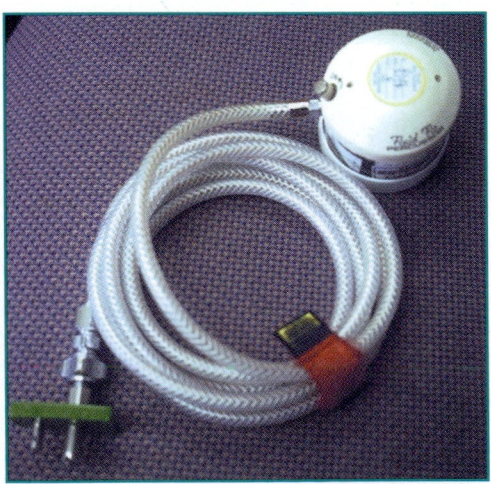

Figure 7-4-1 Pneumatic percussor

► **CLIENT EDUCATION NEEDED:**

1. Explain the procedure and rationale to the client.
2. Teach coughing and breathing mechanics.

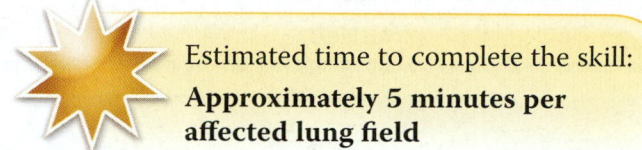

Estimated time to complete the skill:
Approximately 5 minutes per affected lung field

► **DELEGATION TIPS**

The initiation of pulmonary therapy requires the assessment of a nurse or respiratory care practitioner. Ancillary personnel should be instructed to report dyspnea, any changes in the client's activity tolerance, or an increase in the client's secretions. The actual percussion and clapping should be performed by trained respiratory care or nursing staff.

IMPLEMENTATION—Action/Rationale

Action	Rationale
1. Wash hands.	1. Reduces the transmission of microorganisms.
2. Auscultate.	2. Establishes baseline and confirms areas of concentration.
3. Confirm presence of appropriate equipment.	3. Ensures thorough and safe therapy.
4. Turn off tube feeding, if appropriate.	4. Prevents aspiration.
5. Position client properly.	5. Allows drainage of affected segments.
6. Initiate CPT (see Figure 7-4-2).	6. Delivers therapy.
7. Move the percussor around the chest area where CPT has been ordered (see Figures 7-4-3 and 7-4-4).	7. CPT provided to the designated area promotes effective treatment.
8. Monitor the client during the therapy for signs of discomfort, difficulty breathing, or distress.	8. Allows early intervention for the effects of the treatment.

Figure 7-4-2 Initiate chest pulmonary therapy.

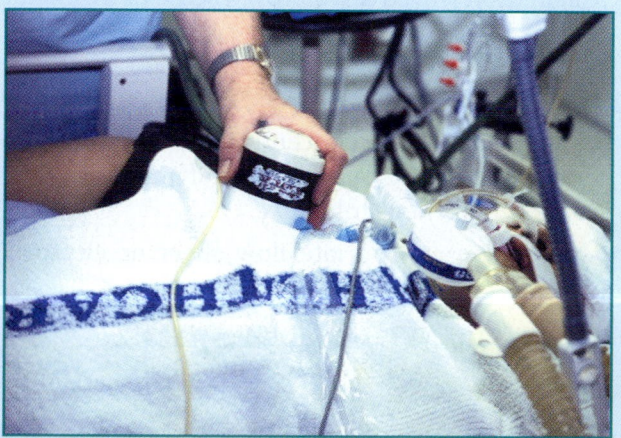

Figure 7-4-3 Slowly move the percussor around the target chest area.

continues

Action	Rationale
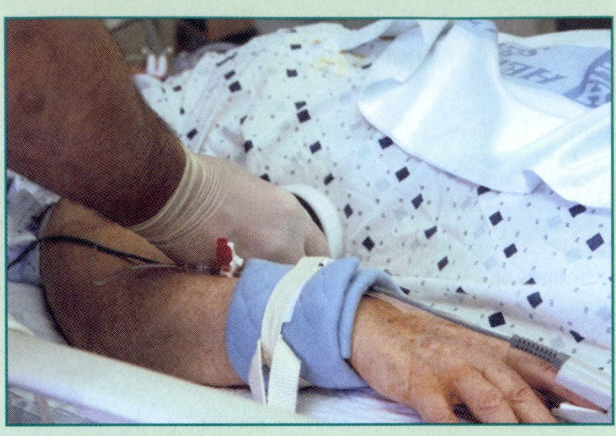	 Figure 7-4-4 Cover all parts of the target chest area.
9. Auscultate after the therapy is completed.	**9.** Checks for changes in breath sounds.
10. Suction secretions as necessary.	**10.** Keeps the airway clear.
11. Wash hands.	**11.** Reduces the transmission of microorganisms.

▶ REAL WORLD ANECDOTES

A 57-year-old postoperative female client with a history of COPD presented with low oxygen saturation on a 50% mask and diminished right lower and middle lobe breath sounds. A chest film showed right lower and middle lobe atelectasis. CPT to the right lower and middle lobes every 4 hours was ordered. After the third treatment, the client, through strong coughing, produced a large mucus plug. Breath sounds and oxygen saturation improved, and a subsequent chest X-ray indicated improved ventilation.

▶ EVALUATION

- Clearance of pulmonary secretions was improved.
- Ventilation was improved.
- Potential complications were minimized.
- Client experienced an improved sense of well-being.

▶ DOCUMENTATION

Nurses' Notes

- Document areas of concentration; duration of treatment; nature of secretions, if any; breath sounds; and client tolerance.

Document on appropriate flow sheet or electronic medical record (EMR).

▶ CRITICAL THINKING SKILL

Introduction

A 47-year-old man postliver transplant client was ordered to receive CPT every 4 hours to both lower lobes. The client was 48 hours postoperative, on a nasal cannula, with a nasal feeding tube in place.

Possible Scenario

The client was placed in the Trendelenburg position, and CPT was initiated.

Possible Outcome

The feeding tube could become dislodged, leading to aspiration.

Prevention

Halting flow to the feeding tube prior to positioning the client in the Trendelenburg position will reduce the risk of aspiration.

▶ VARIATIONS

Geriatric Variation:
- *Elderly clients may not be able to assume and hold positions needed for postural drainage. Modifications may be needed.*

Pediatric Variation:
- *Small vibrators are available for neonatal use, or neonatal resuscitation masks may be used for manual percussion.*

Home Care Variations:
- *Not applicable.*

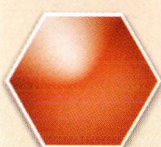

Long-Term Care Variations:
- *Not applicable.*

▶ COMMON ERRORS

Possible Error:

A variety of tubes and lines may be in place and at risk when positioning the postoperative client, including endotracheal tubes, chest tubes, IV and arterial lines, Swan-Ganz catheters, and Foley catheters.

Prevention:

Be aware of placement of tubes. Get assistance if needed.

▶ NURSING TIPS

- Maintain adequate client oxygenation during the treatment.
- Prevent aspiration.
- Provide adequate pain control.
- Be aware of all client tubes, lines, and catheters.
- Assess effectiveness of CPT by listening to lungs before and after treatment.

▶ SPECIAL CONSIDERATIONS

- *When using electric or pneumatic percussors on the client monitored by telemetry or any ECG monitoring, the rhythm displayed will be altered and, therefore, not indicative of the client's normal rhythm. Carefully assess the client's rhythm before and after the procedure and alert the staff member who is responsible for observing the centrally located cardiac monitors.*

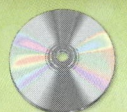

Administering Pulse Oximetry

SKILL 7-5

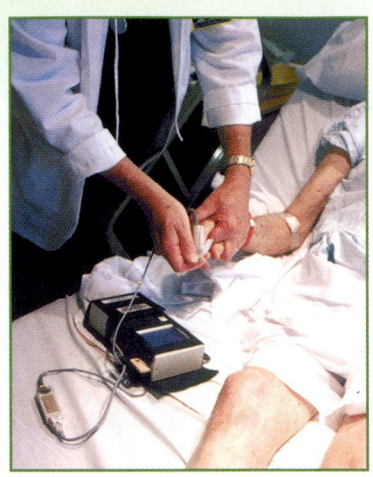

► OVERVIEW OF THE SKILL

Pulse oximetry is a quick, easy, noninvasive method to assess the arterial blood oxygen saturation of a client by using an external sensor. There are several types of sensors; however, the most common for adult use is a finger sensor. The finger is placed between a clip mechanism. On one side of the clip are light-emitting diodes (a red and an infrared); a photon detector is on the other side. The beam of light goes through the tissue and blood vessels, and the photon detector receives the light and measures the amount of light absorbed by oxygenated and unoxygenated hemoglobin. Unoxygenated hemoglobin absorbs more red light and oxygenated hemoglobin absorbs more infrared light. The amount of each light and, hence, the arterial blood oxygen saturation (SaO_2) is determined by the spectrum of light. Other types of sensors can be used on the toe, nose, ear, forehead, or around the hand or foot and use this same principle of spectrometry. Special sensors are available for the neonatal hand and pediatric toe. Reusable sensors include two sensor heads that are secured with y-strip tapes. The center strip aids placement into 25-mm tapes. The appropriate sensor should be determined by the measurement site.

► ASSESSMENT

1. Assess the client's hemoglobin level. **Because pulse oximetry measures the percent of SaO_2,**
the results of the oxygenation status will be affected. The results may appear normal if the hemoglobin level is low because all hemoglobin available to carry O_2 is completely saturated; therefore, it is important to know the hemoglobin level.
2. Assess the client's color. **If the client has vasoconstriction of the extremities, an inaccurate recording may be obtained.**
3. Assess the client's mental status **because this will assist in general evaluation of oxygen delivery to the brain and be indicative of high levels of CO_2.**
4. Assess the client's pulse rate. The pulse oximeter measures pulse rate. **Manually assessing pulse can be used as a cross-reference to indicate functioning of the oximeter.**
5. Assess the area where the sensors will be placed **to determine whether it is an area with adequate circulation (no scars or thickened nails).**
6. Remove nail polish and/or acrylic nails, **which interfere with sensor measurements.**

► DIAGNOSIS

Impaired Gas Exchange

Ineffective Tissue Perfusion

Risk for Impaired Skin Integrity

892

▶ PLANNING

Expected Outcomes:

1. The SaO$_2$ will be in a normal range for the client (95%–100% in the absence of chronic respiratory disease).
2. The client will be alert and oriented.
3. The client's color will remain normal.
4. The client will tolerate the placement of sensors.
5. There will not be any skin irritation or pressure at area of sensors.

Equipment Needed:

- Pulse oximeter (see Figure 7-5-1)
- Proper sensor
- Alcohol wipe or soap and water
- Nail polish remover, if necessary

▶ CLIENT EDUCATION NEEDED:

1. Explain the purpose of oximetry.
2. Explain selection of site and necessity for a clean site.

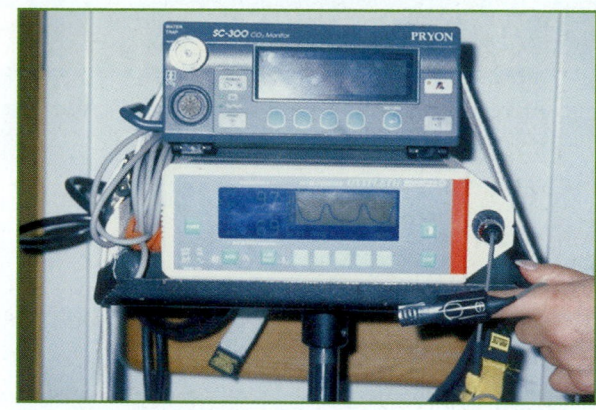

Figure 7-5-1 Pulse oximeter

3. If using oximeter for monitoring purposes, explain the need to keep sensors in place.

Estimated time to complete the skill:
5 minutes

▶ DELEGATION TIPS

Ancillary personnel routinely perform pulse oximetry. They should be instructed on acceptable parameters and to report any abnormal findings to the nurse.

IMPLEMENTATION—Action/Rationale

Action	Rationale
1. Wash hands.	1. Reduces the transmission of microorganisms.
2. Select an appropriate sensor. Sensors are commonly used for the fingertips.	2. The sensor should be selected based on the size of the person and the site to be used.
3. Select an appropriate site for the sensor. Fingers are most commonly used; however, toes (see Figure 7-5-2), ear lobes, nose, forehead (see Figure 7-5-3), hands, and feet can be used. Assess for capillary refill and proximal pulse. If the client has poor circulation, use an earlobe, forehead, or nasal sensor instead. In children, sensors may be used on the hand, foot, or trunk. If elderly clients have thickened nails, pick another site.	3. Decreased circulation alters the O$_2$ saturation measurement.
4. Clean the site with an alcohol wipe. Remove artificial nails or nail polish if present or select another site. Clean any tape adhesive. Use soap and water if necessary to clean the site.	4. Polish and artificial fingernails alter the results.

continues

Action	Rationale

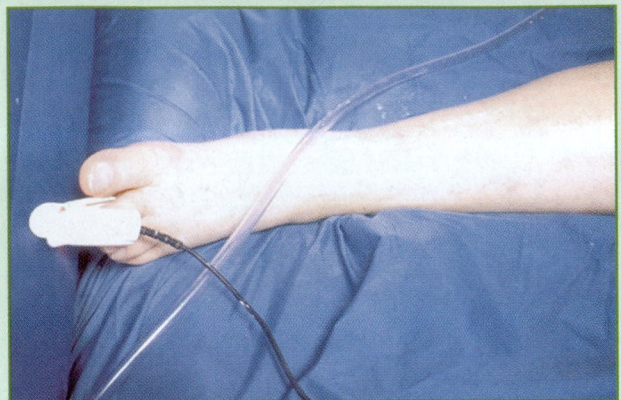

Figure 7-5-2 Pulse oximeter sensor placed on a toe

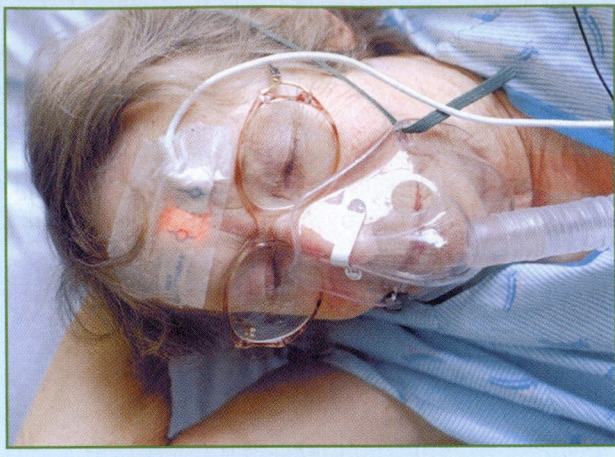

Figure 7-5-3 Pulse oximeter sensor placed on the forehead

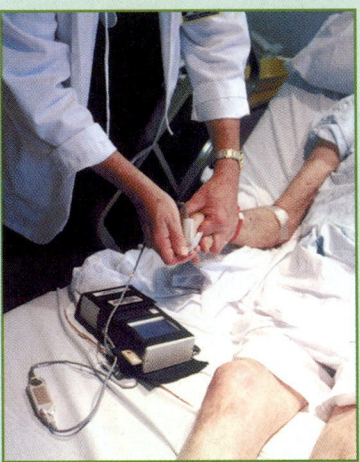

Figure 7-5-4 Apply the sensor to the selected site.

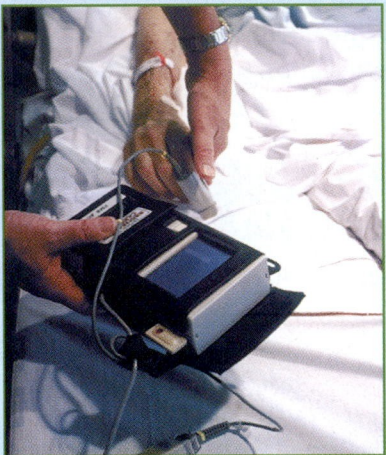

Figure 7-5-5 Follow the manufacturer's instructions when taking an oximetry reading.

5. Apply the sensor. Make sure the photon detectors are aligned on opposite sides of the selected site (see Figure 7-5-4).

5. Proper application is necessary for accurate results.

6. Connect the sensor to the oximeter with a sensor cable. Turn on the machine. Initially a tone can be heard, followed by an arterial wave-form fluctuation with each arterial pulse. In most oximeters if the battery is low, a low-battery light illuminates when 15 minutes of battery life are remaining. Oximeters should remain plugged in even when not in use (see Figure 7-5-5).

6. The tone and wave-form fluctuation indicate that the machine is detecting blood flow with each arterial pulsation.

7. Adjust the alarm limits for high and low O_2 saturation levels according to the manufacturer's directions. Pulse rate limits most often can also be set. Adjust volume.

7. The alarms indicate that the saturation levels or pulse rates are outside the designated levels and alert the nurse of abnormal O_2 saturation levels and pulse rates.

8. If taking a reading, note the results (see Figure 7-5-6). If the oximeter is being used for constant monitoring, move the site of spring sensors every 2 hours and adhesive sensors every 4 hours.

8. Prevents skin breakdown from pressure and skin irritation from the adhesive.

continues

Action	Rationale

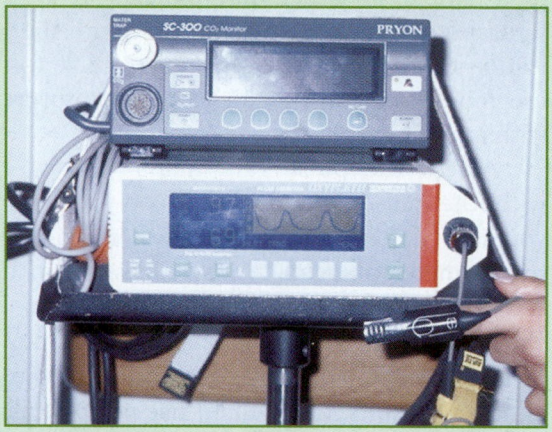

Figure 7-5-6 Note the results on the oximeter.

9. Cover the sensor with a sheet or towel to protect it from exposure to bright light.

9. Ambient light sources such as sunlight or warming lights may interfere with the sensor and alter the SaO_2 results.

10. Notify the health care provider of abnormal results.

10. Low SaO_2 levels require medical attention because permanent tissue damage may result from low oxygen saturation.

11. Record the results of O_2 saturation measurements according to health care provider's order or protocol. Include in the documentation the type of sensor used, the site of application, the hemoglobin levels, and your assessment of the client's skin at the sensor site.

11. Communicates the findings to the other members of the health care team and contributes to the legal record by documenting the care given to the client.

▶ **REAL WORLD ANECDOTES**

Scenario 1
Brian is an active 8-year-old boy who thinks the pulse oximeter sensor is fun to squeeze. He frequently reaches over and squeezes. The nurse comes in with some coloring pens and a coloring book so Brian's mom can distract him. He quickly forgets about the sensor.

Scenario 2
Chin has come to the outpatient clinic for tachycardia. The physician has medicated him but wants him to be monitored for 1 hour before he leaves the clinic. Left in the observation room with nothing to do for an hour, he is afraid to move for fear of setting off one of the many alarms on the ECG, IV, or oximetry machines attached to him. When the nurse returns to check on him, he is extremely anxious and stiff from remaining in one position on the gurney. The nurse should have shown him how to move and summon help if he was uncertain.

▶ **EVALUATION**

- The SaO_2 is in the normal range for the client (95–100% in the absence of chronic respiratory disease).
- The client is alert and oriented.
- The client's color is normal.
- The client tolerates the placement of sensors.
- There is not any skin irritation or pressure at area of sensors.

▶ **DOCUMENTATION**

Nurses' Notes

- Document when pulse oximetry was placed, the location of the sensor, and the baseline readings.

Flow Sheet

- Document pulse, oxygen, flow rate, and saturation readings.

► CRITICAL THINKING SKILL

Introduction

Things are not always as they appear.

Possible Scenario

In response to an alarm, the nurse enters the room of a client who has an oximetry sensor on her right index finger. The nurse observes a reading of 85 on the pulse oximeter. She immediately summons the nurse practitioner. The practitioner and several staff members come into the room. A nursing student who is working with the nurse practitioner notes that the client has nail polish on her fingers and toes.

Possible Outcome

The nursing student brings in nail polish remover and cleans the fingernail. She reapplies the sensor probe and resets the alarm. Subsequent readings are within normal limits.

Prevention

Improper readings may lead to improper treatment; for example, an order may indicate to keep oxygen saturation between a certain range with the administration of oxygen. The client may receive too little or too much oxygen. This could be harmful in a client with chronic respiratory diseases.

Assess the pulse rate manually and compare with the pulse rate indicated on the oximeter. If you find inaccuracies, use another machine. Keep the oximeter plugged in when it is not in use. Protect sensors from ambient light sources. Properly check the location of the sensor. Improper sensors or improper location or preparation of the site can affect the results. If the client has peripheral vascular disease and poor peripheral circulation, use ear lobes or the nose with the proper sensor. If a signal bar is available, check the signal bar. The signal bar reflects pulsatile signal strength. Strong signals produce a tall bar; a weak signal a short bar. Typical signals are 25–75% of signal bar height.

► VARIATIONS

Geriatric Variations:
- *Elderly clients may have poor peripheral circulation and require other than finger sensors.*
- *Elderly clients may have thickened nails, which can lead to inaccurate readings if finger sensors are used.*

Pediatric Variations:
- *Finger sensors are generally not sized appropriately for children and are not intended for neonatal or pediatric use. Adhesive sensors can be used on the hand or feet of children or on the hand of the neonate.*
- *Children may pull off sensors and activate alarms.*

Home Care Variation:
- *Pulse oximeters are available for home health nurses; however, oximeters are expensive and may be used infrequently in home settings. If used, teach the family members how to use the equipment and rotate sensors to avoid skin breakdown.*

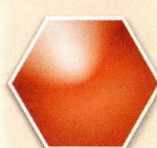

Long-Term Care Variation:
- *If a pulse oximeter is available and necessary in the long-term setting, make sure staff, who may be unfamiliar with the equipment, are given a refresher course in how to use it. Make sure they understand how to interpret the results.*

▶ COMMON ERRORS

Possible Error:

Sensor is not protected from ambient light source.

Prevention:

Place a towel over the sensor to block the light.

Possible Error:

Oximeter is not plugged in between use and battery is low.

Prevention:

Place the task of checking the oximeter on the list of routine equipment and stocking checks that are done on a regular basis. Make sure the responsibility for checking the oximeter is assigned to a specific person or a specific time of day.

Possible Error:

Poor perfusion in finger or toe leads to an inaccurate reading of systemic saturation.

Prevention:

Put the sensor somewhere else. Experiment, if necessary, until you find a location that gives accurate readings.

▶ NURSING TIPS

- Clean nails or skin properly before applying sensors.
- Always plug in the oximeter between uses.
- Do not use oximeter if light indicates low battery.
- Compare previous results and especially compare pulse of oximeter reading with palpable or auditory pulse.
- Use an appropriate site. If there is inadequate perfusion, try another site.

▶ SPECIAL CONSIDERATIONS

- *If the client has a chronic lung disease (COPD) then the highest attainable value might be 90% (or even lower [65–80%]) instead of 92% to 100%. Know the client's normal values and carefully evaluate changes in respiratory, cardiac, and mental status. The monitor needs to be set accordingly or alarms will constantly sound and frighten or annoy the client.*
- *The client with diabetes, peripheral vascular disease, or hypothyroidism may have thickened or discolored nail beds. Assess the client and move the sensor to an alternate site if required.*
- *Always remember to treat the client and not the machine. If the alarm goes off frequently, yet the client is asymptomatic, then move or, better yet, secure the sensor or change the machine.*
- *Frequently, unnecessary alarms are heard from the pulse oximeter. Never turn the machine off because the client looks fine and the machine is a bother. Reassess the client and update the health care provider with a suggestion of oximeter removal if appropriate.*

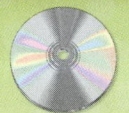

SKILL 7-6

Measuring Peak Expiratory Flow Rates

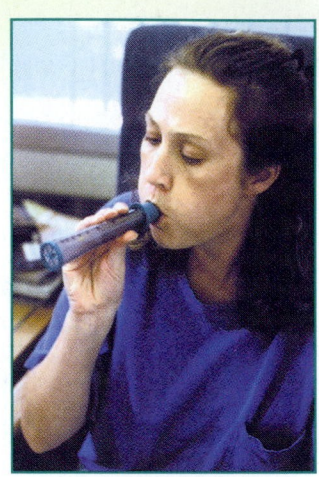

▶ OVERVIEW OF THE SKILL

A peak flow meter is a device that measures how well air moves out of the lungs. Peak expiratory flow rate measures the rate of air expired at the beginning of respiration, which correlates with the large airway status. This test can be performed on children as young as 3–4 years of age; other pulmonary function tests usually require more maturity (i.e., older than 5 years of age). It is a simple measure of the airflow and can determine how well one is breathing. If a client has a breathing problem such as asthma, the physician or qualified practitioner may recommend that the client use a peak flow meter. The health care provider can provide a treatment plan that will tell what actions to take when there is a change in the airflow. A written record (peak flow monitoring chart) should be kept. Reviewing the daily record can help the client and the health care provider check closely on the asthma to provide the best treatment plan.

The peak flow meter should be used for the following:

1. When a client with asthma has an attack, the lungs are blocked and air cannot move easily. Therefore, the peak flow meter will help determine for a client with asthma how much the lungs are blocked.
2. The peak flow meter should be used when the client is experiencing breathing problems to let the health care provider and client know how

serious the problem is and how well the asthma treatment is working.
3. The peak flow meter can provide an objective measure of the severity of the disease; response to treatment permits detection of airway obstruction before wheezing can be heard through a stethoscope or symptoms can be felt. Thus, the client can begin treatment of episodes earlier and the likelihood of serious episodes decreases.
4. During an asthma episode, the airways of the lungs begin to narrow slowly. The use of a peak flow meter can help determine whether there is a narrowing hours before symptoms of asthma appear. By taking the medication(s) early (before the symptoms), the asthma exacerbation can be stopped quickly and a serious episode avoided.

▶ ASSESSMENT

1. Take a complete history from the client, or a reliable informant, about the signs and symptoms of the attack, and the frequency of the attacks. **Evaluates the frequency and severity of the episodes.**
2. Ask about all medications the client takes on a regular basis, or as needed, including over-the-counter drugs. **If the client uses medication frequently, regular measurement with a peak flow meter may be required.**

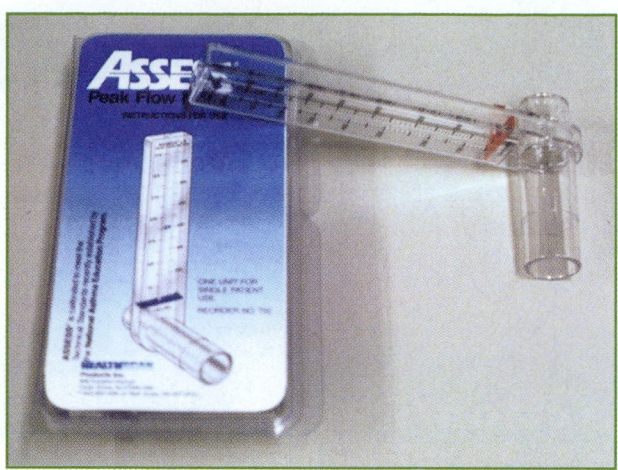

Figure 7-6-1A Peak flow meter

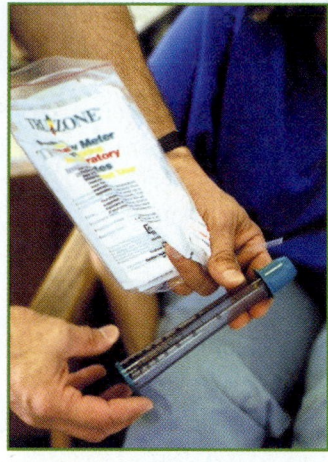

Figure 7-6-1B Remember that there are many types of peak flow meters available on the market so you should be familiar with all types.

3. Assess the client's ability to cooperate with testing. **A client who is unable to reliably perform a spirometry or pulmonary function test may not be able to provide an accurate peak flow meter reading.**

► DIAGNOSIS

Ineffective Breathing Pattern

Risk for Suffocation

Impaired Gas Exchange

► PLANNING

Expected Outcomes:

1. The client will use the peak flow monitor to monitor the course of asthma and response to treatment using objective criteria to add or decrease medication.
2. The client will detect early stages of airway obstruction.
3. The client will have an accurate perception of the severity of the obstruction.
4. The client will accurately determine when emergency medication care is needed.
5. The client will be able to distinguish between airway obstruction (e.g., asthma) and other causes of breathlessness (e.g., hyperventilation).
6. The effectiveness of client communication will be improved by providing objective assessment of asthma severity.

Equipment Needed:

- Peak flow meter with mouthpiece (see Figures 7-6-1A and 7-6-1B)
- Peak flow record or chart
- Calculator

► CLIENT EDUCATION NEEDED:

1. Show the client the peak flow meter. It has a mouthpiece with a needle or pointer that corresponds to a particular number or reading.
2. Describe the advantages of using a peak flow meter.
3. Explain how it works.
4. Demonstrate to the client the correct use of a peak flow meter.
5. Explain the peak flow zone system for using the peak flow meter to manage asthma.
6. Calculate the client's three zones (green/yellow/red) based on predicted values. "Predicted or usual" value is an average peak flow value based on the peak flow reading of a large number of people grouped by height and age. An individual peak flow reading may vary widely and may be consistently higher or lower than such average values. Therefore, each client will have his or her own "personal best" value—the peak flow value established by the client during a 2- to 3-week period in which the client records peak flow measurements at least two times a day. The personal best is the best number a client has ever achieved with or without medications. Remind the client that many clients have peak flow scores that are either higher or lower than the predicted value. Emphasize that it is important to find the client's true personal best in order to develop the best treatment to manage asthma for the individual client.

Estimated time to complete the skill: **2–3 minutes**

► **DELEGATION TIPS**

The assessment and teaching required to perform peak flow measurements require the nurse or respiratory care practitioner to initiate and evaluate the client's competency. Reporting client results and use of a peak flow meter may be delegated to ancillary personnel once client competency is established. Reportable conditions should be specifically explained to ancillary personnel, such as the client's use of "prn" (as needed) medication or a peak flow at or below 50%.

IMPLEMENTATION—Action/Rationale

Action	Rationale
1. Set up all the equipment needed such as the peak flow meter with mouthpiece, record/chart, and calculator before going to the client's room.	1. Promotes efficiency, thus gains the client's confidence in the nurse.
2. Identify the client and confirm the height, age, and gender of the client.	2. Promotes accuracy in teaching the use of a peak flow meter.
3. Explain and demonstrate the procedure to the client.	3. Promotes client's compliance.
4. Have the client stand up or sit in high-Fowler's position with the chin slightly up.	4. Expands the lungs to their maximum.
5. Show the client how to place the indicator/pointer at the base of the numbered scale.	5. Ensures accuracy in the reading.
6. Have the client take a deep breath through the mouth.	6. Maximizes expansion of the lungs.
7. Teach the client to hold the peak flow meter without touching the pointer or needle.	7. Promotes accuracy in the reading.
8. Have the client place the peak flow meter in the mouth and close the lips and teeth around the mouthpiece without putting the tongue inside the tube (see Figure 7-6-2).	8. Promotes a good seal and reflects the actual flow.
9. Have the client blow out as hard and as fast as possible over a period of about a second (not a prolonged expiration).	9. Reflects the actual flow in the lungs.
10. Teach the client how to read the number on the meter and where to record the number (see Figure 7-6-3).	10. Ensures accurate documentation of the results.
11. Show the client how to slide the pointer down to 0 and have the client repeat Actions 5–10 two more times.	11. Permits choosing the best value among the three tries.
12. Allow the client to rest between attempts, if necessary.	12. Ensures that each test is the maximum possible value.
13. Write down the highest of the three numbers achieved on the client's chart/record.	13. The highest number is used to identify the client's best peak expiratory flow rate. Subsequent rates are compared to the client's best rate in order to identify the client's zone.

continues

Action	Rationale

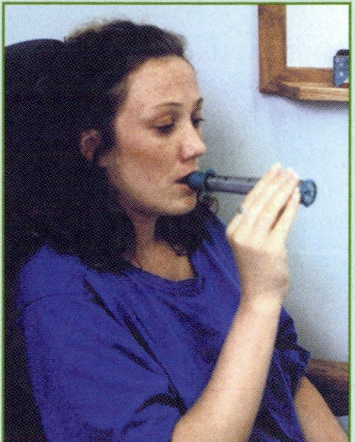

Figure 7-6-2 Place the flow meter in the client's mouth and have her close her lips around it.

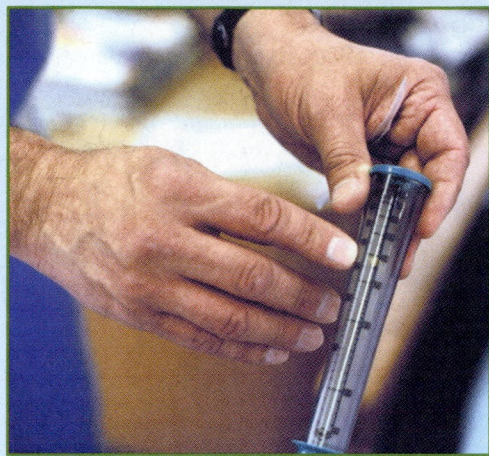

Figure 7-6-3 Read and record the number on the meter.

14. Use the zone determination to evaluate what course of treatment should be followed.
   - A peak flow reading between 80% and 100% of the predicted value or personal best is the green zone. The client should continue using the regular asthma medications.
   - A peak flow reading between 50% and 80% of the predicted value or personal best is the yellow zone. The client should use the "as needed" medication ordered by the physician or qualified practitioner. The peak flow reading should be checked again 10 minutes after medication usage to evaluate medication effectiveness. If no improvement is observed, the client may call the physician or qualified practitioner, or wait another 4 hours to do another peak flow reading and see whether the value has gone up to the green zone.
   - A peak flow reading of less than 50% of the predicted value or personal best is the red zone. The client should use the "as needed" medication ordered and call the health care provider right away.

14. Zone determination provides an accurate, understandable indicator of the course of treatment to follow.
   - The green zone indicates that the asthma is under control.

   - The yellow zone indicates some increase in inflammation and airway obstruction.

   - The red zone indicates a severe amount of inflammation and reactivity.

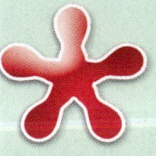

▶ **REAL WORLD ANECDOTES**

Scenario 1

A mother calls the clinic complaining of her 5-year-old son having shortness of breath and wheezing with a peak flow reading of 68% of the boy's personal best of 200 (yellow zone). Albuterol inhaler was given already but to no avail. The parent wanted advice because her son had never been in the yellow zone before—his asthma was in control most of the time. The parent was advised by the triage nurse to give the client another albuterol treatment. Assuming that the client's peak flow technique is correct, albuterol treatment every 4 hours can be given as needed. If the client's numbers/values have been consistently in the yellow zone after a series of 4 treatments during the day or if the parent thinks the client needs a treatment more frequently than every 4 hours, the child may need to be brought in to the clinic or emergency room.

continues

▶ **REAL WORLD ANECDOTES** (continued)

Scenario 2

A 30-year-old female client had been diagnosed as having asthma and was advised to use a peak flow meter at home. She awoke in the middle of the night coughing and having shortness of breath. She checked her peak flow reading, and it was in the yellow zone. She used an albuterol inhaler, but her numbers were still in the yellow zone. Four hours later, the number on her reading was down to the red zone. She took an albuterol inhaler and called the physician right away. She was advised to go to the clinic immediately where she was given an albuterol nebulization with oxygen and injectable steroids. Another nebulization was given and then her values increased to the upper limit of the yellow zone. She stabilized, and was not sent to the hospital; she was given oral steroids to take home. She was reminded to take her asthma medications on a regular basis. Three days later on a follow-up visit, she was much better and the peak flow readings were back to normal in the green zone.

▶ **EVALUATION**

- The client uses the peak flow meter to monitor the course of asthma and response to treatment, using objective criteria to increase or decrease the medication.
- The client can detect early stages of airway obstruction.
- The client has an accurate perception of the severity of the obstruction.
- The client accurately determines when emergency medical care is needed.
- The client is able to distinguish between airway obstruction (e.g., asthma) and other causes of breathlessness (e.g., hyperventilation).
- The effectiveness of client communication is improved by providing objective assessment of asthma severity.

▶ **DOCUMENTATION**

Peak Flow Meter Record/Chart

- Record the best reading.
- Note any symptoms the client may have.
- Record any interventions required.

Document on appropriate flow sheet or electronic medical record (EMR).

Medication Administration Record

- If a client will be given a treatment such as albuterol, document the amount, dosage, manner, and time the medication was given.

▶ **CRITICAL THINKING SKILL**

Introduction

It is important that the client understands the necessity of doing peak flow readings and monitoring the results.

Possible Scenario

A mother and a 7-year-old daughter came to the clinic with the latter referred for an evaluation of asthma. The client was taught how to use the inhalers and peak flow meter. The mother was uncooperative and thought that doing the peak flow readings was just a waste of time and plotting the numbers was too complicated.

Possible Outcome

The client's mother calls a week later complaining that her daughter has some chest tightness and coughing. Now the peak flow reading is about 100 (lower limit of the yellow zone). The mother is not sure of the significance of that number and does not know what to do next. She also does not know the client's personal best. The peak flow measurement had only been taken once because they "did not have time to do it."

Prevention

Explain the importance of peak flow monitoring. Demonstrate to the client the correct way of using a peak flow meter and let the client demonstrate it to you. Correct the client's technique if needed. Explain the peak flow zone system to manage asthma. Have a practice and let the client/parent plot the reading/value on the chart. Do a possible scenario, such as giving a value, and then let them decide what to do next by using the asthma action plan.

► VARIATIONS

Geriatric Variations:

- Peak expiratory flow rate is based on age, height, and gender. The numbers usually decrease in the geriatric age group compared with adults as a whole because lung capacity decreases as people age.
- When using the peak flow meter, the client should be in a standing position if possible; otherwise, an upright sitting position is preferred.
- Make sure that the client understands how to plot and interpret the numbers and zones.
- Have a sample practice for better client compliance.
- Enlarged-print versions of charts will let the client see the readings/values more easily.

Pediatric Variations:

- It takes some maturity to use the peak flow meter and usually 3- to 4-year-olds can start doing it.
- Some kids treat it as a game and have an incentive to do it correctly.
- Some nurses or parents instruct the client to do it just like blowing out birthday candles or use a tissue paper, hold it about a foot away, and have the client blow as hard as possible to move it.
- The nurse should convey the instructions so that the child can understand it at his or her own level.
- Use colored graphs (green, yellow, and red) to let the child participate in the task. Remind parents that they need to bring in the child's peak flow meter, including the colored graphs, every time they come in for the recheck appointments.
- As the child grows taller, the predicted values should also increase. Therefore, regular physician's visits should be kept.

Home Care Variations:

- Demonstrate to the client the correct use of a peak flow meter and have the client practice. Correct the client's technique as needed. Write the instructions step-by-step.
- It is important to keep the peak flow meter clean and dust-free. The removable mouthpiece can be cleaned by washing it in warm soapy water and then rinsing thoroughly.
- Use the predicted peak flow value until the client's personal best value is determined. Explain the difference between the predicted and personal best values as well as the zone system in managing asthma.
- Calculate the client's three zones (green, yellow, and red) based on the predicted value. Develop a schedule to establish the client's true personal best value. Emphasize that identifying the client's personal best peak flow value by filling out a diary for 2 to 3 weeks will help ensure that the client receives the right amount and type of medication. It may also lead to a reduction in the number and severity of asthma episodes. Instruct the client to take peak flow readings every day for 2 to 3 weeks, morning and afternoon before medication(s).
- Schedule a follow-up appointment to determine the true personal best score that will be used instead of the predicted value. Remind the client to bring the sheets on the return visit.

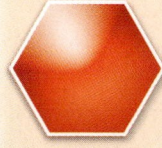

Long-Term Care Variations:

- Continue daily monitoring of peak flow if more data are needed to establish a pattern or if the peak flow reading is consistently in the yellow or red zone.
- There are clients who are on daily medications such as inhaled corticosteroids and/or long-acting beta-2 agonists, and these clients are also advised to check the peak flow rate twice a day before the medications.
- Clients should bring their peak flow meter to the physician's or qualified practitioner's office to check the accuracy of the unit and to review the proper use of the peak flow meter as well as the charts to check client compliance.
- Use the colored peak flow diary to keep track of the peak flow readings.
- Clients should find the personal best peak flow number per instructions of the nurse and follow the asthma control plan on the peak flow zone system as explained previously. A decrease of 20% or greater of the client's personal best may mean the start of an asthma episode. Indicate if any symptoms are present.

▶ COMMON ERRORS

Possible Error:

The client is getting very low values even though the client seems to be doing well and is not having symptoms.

Prevention:

Give proper instructions and a demonstration to the client prior to the test and observe and correct the technique to get a reliable and accurate result. Instruct the client not to put the tongue into the tube. The client should stand up straight, take a deep breath, and blow as fast and as hard as possible in just 1 second.

Possible Error:

An 8-year-old boy has a 3-year-old peak flow meter and the numbers are always low.

Prevention:

Change the peak flow meter about once a year. Make sure that the needle or pointer works well. The metallic spring inside the peak flow meter might develop some rust over time, thus skewing the results. There is a pediatric or low range meter, which goes up to 300, and an adult or standard range meter, which goes up to 800. However, if a client is in the pediatric age group but can blow close to or as high as 300, the standard range peak flow meter should be used.

▶ NURSING TIPS

- Demonstrate the technique and explain the purpose of using the peak flow meter. Avoid using technical jargon when teaching the client or the parent.
- Make sure the clients/parents are well informed before you let them go home. Let the client demonstrate to you the technique in using the peak flow meter.
- Practice plotting the numbers on the chart and give a sample scenario to check whether the client understands the instructions. Ask the client what to do based on the peak flow zoning system and asthma action plan.
- Make sure the client's effort is valid and technique correct. The client should stand up straight, take a deep breath, and blow into the mouthpiece very hard and fast. The tongue should not be in the tube while blowing. The nurse should distinguish between coughing and a real blow.
- Be aware of the client's predicted value, which is based on height, age, and gender. Find out the ranges or zones based on the predicted value. Plot the numbers on the chart.
- The peak flow reading can be repeated 5 to 10 minutes after the treatment is done (post-blow) to see whether the reading will go back to the green zone. If the reading is still in the yellow or red zone, the peak flow can be checked again after 4 hours to see whether the numbers have improved (green zone). If not, another albuterol treatment can be given, followed by another post blow in 5 to 10 minutes. If the reading continues to be in the yellow or red zone, the health care provider should be consulted.

▶ SPECIAL CONSIDERATIONS

- *The client with asthma should be encouraged to keep an asthma diary to record peak flow monitor readings done at home as well as any symptoms or asthma attacks.*
- *When the peak expiratory flow rate (PEFR) is done at home, the results should be compared to office spirometry results at least once a year, or any time there is a question about its validity.*

Administering Intermittent Positive-Pressure Breathing (IPPB)

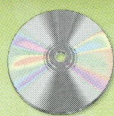

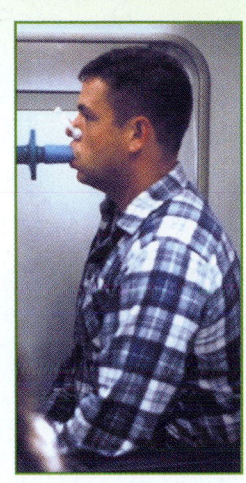

▶ OVERVIEW OF THE SKILL

Intermittent positive-pressure breathing (IPPB) is a form of intermittent mechanical ventilation that may be used to provide hyperinflation therapy and improve the distribution of ventilation, prevent or treat atelectasis, provide intermittent ventilation for clients with hypoventilation, and improve airway secretion clearance in clients who cannot cough or clear secretions effectively. IPPB may be used to deliver aerosol medication to clients with muscle weakness affecting the ability to inhale and exhale the medication, for example, clients with underlying spinal cord injury, trauma, or neuromuscular disease. IPPB can be used in intubated or nonintubated clients. Indications for IPPB include the following conditions:

- Atelectasis
- Decreased pulmonary function:
  Vital capacity (VC) of less than 10 to 15 mL/kg

  Forced vital capacity (FVC) of less than 70% of predicted rate

  Forced expiratory volume in 1 second ($FEV1$) of less than 65% of predicted rate
- Neuromuscular disorders associated with fatigue and decreased lung volumes
- Bronchospasm that has failed to respond to other medication delivery systems

IPPB is effective when an increase in alveolar distending pressure is generated. IPPB creates a positive pressure at the airway (mouth), causing gas to flow into the lungs, with a resultant increase in tidal volume, decreased work of breathing, and increased minute ventilation.

Complications of IPPB therapy include nosocomial infection, gastric distention, overdistended alveoli, pneumothorax, and other changes in oxygenation.

Once a popular mode of therapy, IPPB is infrequently used today. Less expensive and less invasive therapies, such as incentive spirometry, deep breathing, chest physiotherapy, and early mobilization are considered to be more effective in managing the postoperative client. Nebulizers are more effective for delivering medications.

IPPB is given for short time periods, typically 10–20 minutes four times per day, or every 4 hours with daily assessments.

▶ ASSESSMENT

1. Assess the ability of the client to understand instructions and cooperate with the procedure **to determine how to structure the procedure and what type of teaching to provide.**
2. Assess the orders for IPPB **to make sure the orders are clear and seem appropriate for the client.**
3. Assess the equipment being used **to review the proper operation of the equipment.**

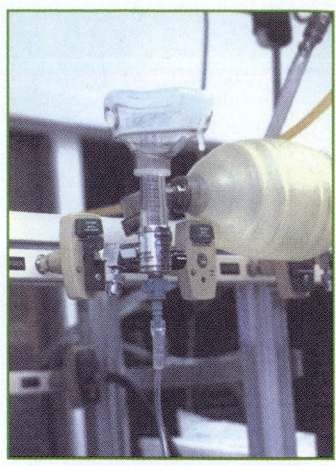

Figure 7-7-1A   Compressed oxygen source

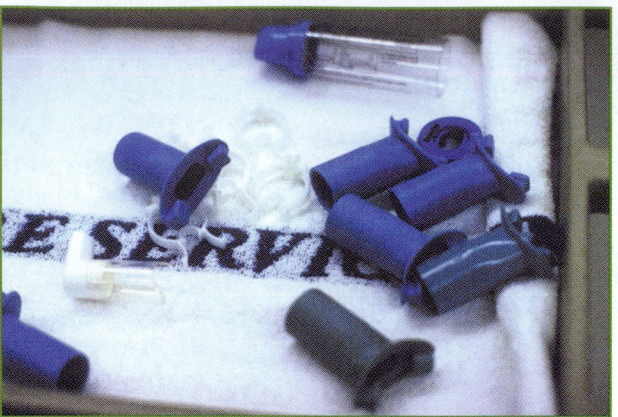

Figure 7-7-1B   Mouthpieces and nose clips are used when administering IPPB therapy.

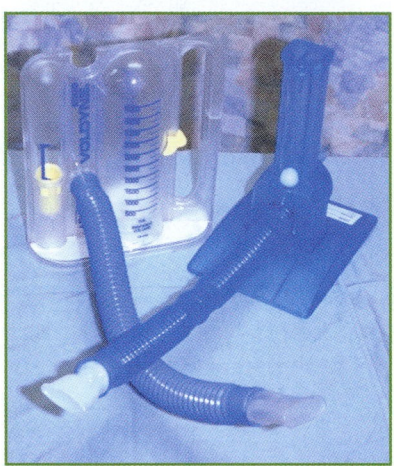

Figure 7-7-1C   Incentive spirometer

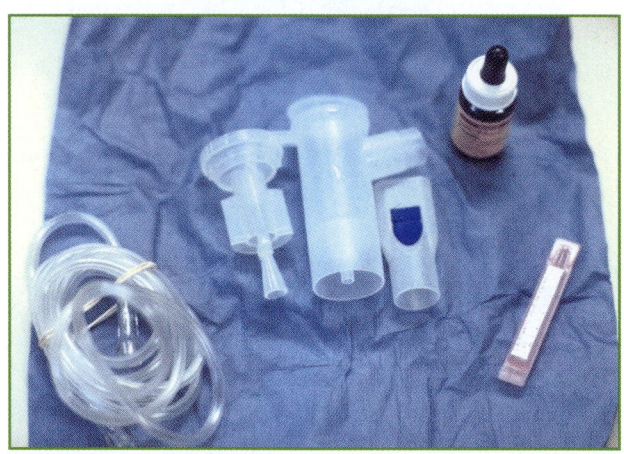

Figure 7-7-1D   Nebulizer and tubing

▶ DIAGNOSIS

Altered Tissue Perfusion

Impaired Gas Exchange

Ineffective Breathing Pattern

Deficient Knowledge, Related to Procedure

▶ PLANNING

Expected Outcomes:

1. The client will have improved tidal breathing, as measured by a tidal volume during IPPB of at least 25% greater than taken in during a regular breath.
2. The client will have a more effective cough.
3. The client will have increased sputum production.
4. The client will have improved breath sounds and an improved chest X-ray.

Equipment Needed (see Figures 7-7-1A–D):

- IPPB device, available from a variety of manufacturers; the most common are made by Bird Products

Corporation and Nellcor Puritan Bennett

- Obtain circuit to the IPPB with mouthpiece or appropriately sized face mask
- Nebulizer (usually included with the circuit)
- Compressed gas source
- Mouthpiece, mouth seal, nose clips, mask, or endotracheal tube adapter
- Tissues or container for expectorated sputum
- Suction equipment if the client is intubated or trached
- Spirometer
- Gloves, goggles, gown, and mask as indicated
- Saline or appropriate medication in nebulizer

▶ CLIENT EDUCATION NEEDED:

1. Explain the procedure to the client, why the client is receiving the therapy, and the expected outcome.
2. Explain technique; for example, initiate the breath and passively allow the IPPB to inflate the lungs until the machine terminates inspiration. Exhalation is through the mouthpiece.

3. Explain the name and purpose of any medication to be nebulized.
4. Remind the client to keep a tight seal with the lips around the mouthpiece.

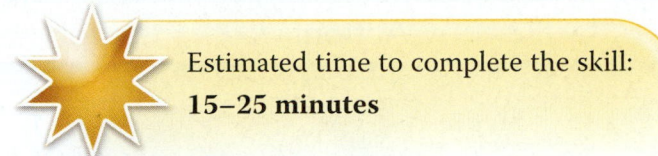

Estimated time to complete the skill:
15–25 minutes

► DELEGATION TIPS

The initiation of IPPB therapy requires the assessment of the nurse or a respiratory care practitioner. Typically this treatment is performed by respiratory therapists but a nurse with proper training may perform this procedure. It is not performed by ancillary personnel.

IMPLEMENTATION—Action/Rationale

Action	Rationale
1. Review and verify health care provider's order.	1. Ensures application of appropriate therapy.
2. Wash hands. Apply protective clothing as needed (see Figure 7-7-2).	2. Reduces the transmission of microorganisms.
3. Explain treatment and technique to client.	3. Encourages client cooperation and ensures effective treatment.
4. Set up equipment and connect to gas source.	4. Prepares mechanics.
5. Set parameters on IPPB device: flow setting, trigger sensitivity, and inspiratory pressure.	5. Parameters must be set to meet orders and meet individual client's requirements.
6. Fill nebulizer with sterile normal saline or medication.	6. Decreases the drying effect of the gas during the treatment.
7. Assist the client to an upright sitting position.	7. Optimizes ventilation distribution.
8. Assess client's breath sounds, respiratory rate, and pulse and obtain inspiratory capacity.	8. Establishes baseline status.

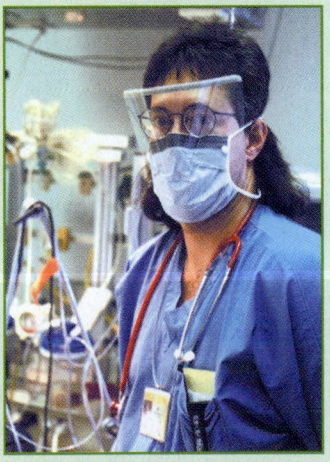

Figure 7-7-2 Wear a protective mask and other protective gear as needed when performing IPPB.

continues

Action	Rationale

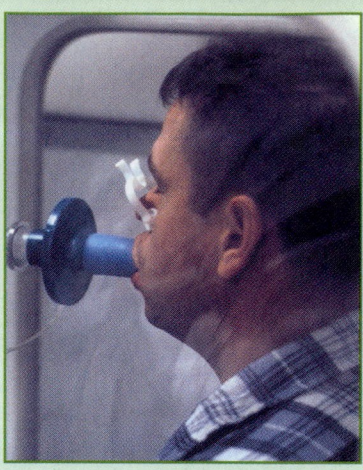

Figure 7-7-3 Have the client use a nose clip if there is leakage through the nose during treatment.

9. Initiate therapy and monitor effectiveness of treatment, measuring exhaled volumes. Use a nose clip if there is air leakage through the nose (see Figure 7-7-3).	9. If exhaled volumes are not greater or equal to inspiratory capacity, incentive spirometry may be of greater therapeutic value.
10. Discontinue treatment when medication is administered or time limit is reached.	10. IPPB is given typically for 10 to 20 minutes.
11. Assess breath sounds, respiratory rate, pulse, and inspiratory capacity.	11. Determines effectiveness.
12. Disconnect IPPB from gas source.	12. Prevents autocycling.
13. Rinse nebulizer with sterile water or sterile saline and air dry.	13. Cleans equipment between treatments.
14. Wash hands.	14. Reduces the transmission of microorganisms.

► REAL WORLD ANECDOTES

A 43-year-old male client with myasthenia gravis developed bilateral lobar atelectasis. Tidal volumes were 250–300 mL. The client had a weak cough and an inspiratory capacity of 500 mL. IPPB was administered every 4 hours over 14 days until the client had significantly regained respiratory strength secondary to medical treatment. Lobar atelectasis was adequately reversed to prevent intubation and mechanical ventilation. Weak respiratory muscles would make alternative therapies less effective. This is an example of an IPPB procedure as an effective treatment. The nurse was able to provide education on the need to clean the equipment with sterile water or saline only.

► EVALUATION

- The client has improved tidal breathing, as measured by a tidal volume, during IPPB, of at least 25% greater than taken in during a regular breath.
- The client has a more effective cough.
- The client has increased sputum production.
- The client has improved breath sounds and an improved chest X-ray.

▶ DOCUMENTATION

Nurses' Notes

- Document IPPB device parameters (flow setting and inspiratory pressure).
- Record pretest and posttest breath sounds, tidal volumes, respiratory rate, inspiratory capacity, pulse, and sputum production.

Document on appropriate flow sheet or electronic medical record (EMR).

Medication Administration Record

- Document medication administered.
- Record adverse reactions, if any.

▶ CRITICAL THINKING SKILL

Introduction

Monitor the client on IPPB therapy carefully for problems.

Possible Scenario

A 57-year-old male client was given IPPB via face mask when he had difficulty using a mouthpiece.

Possible Outcome

During 10 minutes of IPPB, he suffered gastric distention from air being pushed into his stomach. This caused him to vomit. His panic, confusion, and the tight face mask caused him to aspirate the vomitus.

Prevention

With careful observation of the client, the nurse would have recognized this developing problem. IPPB should be discontinued or not initiated with a client at risk for aspiration.

▶ VARIATIONS

Geriatric Variation:
- *A face mask may be appropriate for clients lacking the strength to effect a tight seal around a mouthpiece.*

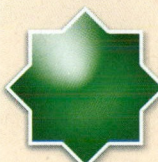

Pediatric Variations:
- *Lower pressures may be required.*
- *Use an appropriately sized face mask.*

Home Care Variations:
- *Explain the importance of cleaning the equipment with sterile saline or sterile water.*
- *Review the medication dosage with the client.*

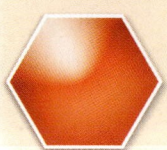

Long-Term Care Variations:
- *Periodically review techniques for using the equipment.*
- *Review with the client the importance of cleaning the equipment with sterile saline or sterile water.*
- *Explain the medication dosage to the client.*

▶ COMMON ERRORS

Possible Error:

The IPPB cycles off before the client is able to obtain adequate breath.

Prevention:

The pressure limit is set too low. You should consult the physician or qualified practitioner, or if you are qualified, increase the pressure setting.

Possible Error:

The client is stopping flow with the tongue or by exhaling prematurely instead of allowing a passive inspiratory phase to occur.

Prevention:

Instruct the client to allow a passive inflation and automatic cycling of the IPPB device after initiating inspiration.

Possible Error:

The flow rate is set too high, causing a pressure spike and early termination of inspiration.

Prevention:

Decrease the flow rate.

▶ NURSING TIPS

- Help the client relax.
- Discuss the treatment before introducing the client to the equipment.
- Adjust flow rate in conjunction with the pressure limit to achieve the best tidal breath.
- Remember contraindications to IPPB use, including increased intracranial pressure (greater than 15 mm Hg); facial, skull, or esophageal surgery; nausea; hiccups; or hemoptysis.

▶ SPECIAL CONSIDERATIONS

- *IPPB is more expensive than other methods of encouraging lung expansion and is infrequently used today. Because of its association with gastric distention it is recommended that it be done with an empty stomach.*
- *IPPB, although infrequently used in respiratory units or general medical care, is still of benefit to clients with underlying spinal cord injury, head trauma, or neurologic disorders, such as myasthenia gravis or muscular dystrophy.*

Assisting with Continuous Positive Airway Pressure (CPAP)

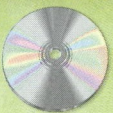

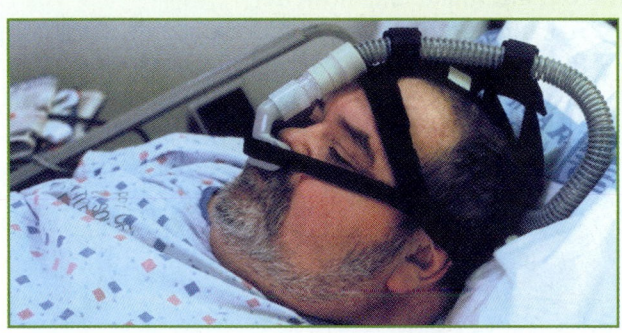

▶ OVERVIEW OF THE SKILL

Continuous positive airway pressure (CPAP) is the application of positive pressure to the airways of the spontaneously breathing client throughout the respiratory cycle. During CPAP therapy, the client breathes from pressurized tubing that maintains positive, consistent airway pressures during both inspiration and expiration. CPAP maintains inspiratory and expiratory pressure above atmospheric pressure, which should result in an increased functional residual capacity (FRC), an improvement in static lung compliance, and decreased airway resistance. Because CPAP increases mean airway pressure, the associated FRC should improve ventilation-perfusion relationships and potentially reduce oxygen requirements.

CPAP is used for respiratory distress syndrome, pulmonary edema, atelectasis, apnea, or recent extubation. There are no absolute contraindications to the use of CPAP therapy; however, clients with the following conditions should be carefully evaluated before the initiation of CPAP therapy: nausea; esophageal surgery; recent facial, oral, or skull surgery or trauma; intracranial pressure greater than 20 mm Hg; hemodynamic instability; and untreated pneumothorax.

▶ ASSESSMENT

1. Assess for breath sounds. **With effective therapy, breath sounds may clear up or the movement of secretions into larger airways may cause an increase in adventitious breath sounds. Improved ease of clearing secretions during and after treatments supports continuation of the treatments.**

2. Assess clients for their response to therapy before, during, and after. **Feelings of pain, discomfort, shortness of breath, dizziness, and nausea should be considered in modifying and stopping therapy.**

3. Assess changes in vital signs. **Moderate changes in respiratory rate and/or pulse rate are expected. Bradycardia, tachycardia, increasingly irregular pulse, or a decrease or dramatic increase in blood pressure are indications for stopping therapy.**

4. Assess changes in arterial blood gas values or oxygen saturation as per orders if applicable. **Normal oxygenation should return as atelectasis or other obstruction resolves.**

5. Assess changes in chest X-rays as per orders. **Improvement or resolution of atelectasis and localized infiltrates may be slow or dramatic.**

▶ DIAGNOSIS

Impaired Gas Exchange

Ineffective Breathing Pattern

Ineffective Tissue Perfusion

Risk for Impaired Skin Integrity

▶ PLANNING

Expected Outcomes:

1. The client will have a reduction in the work of breathing as indicated by a decrease in respiratory rate by 30%. The apneic client will have a decrease in the number and duration of apneic episodes.

2. The client will have a decrease in the severity of retractions, grunting, and nasal flaring.

3. The client will have improvement in lung volumes and appearance of lung as indicated by chest X-ray.
4. The client will have increased comfort in breathing as assessed by the nurse.
5. The client will have an improvement in oxygen saturation.

Equipment Needed:

- CPAP machine capable of delivering 5–20 cm of pressure during passive expiration, with one-way valves allowing unobstructed inspiration
- Continuous noninvasive oxygenation monitoring by pulse oximetry
- Transparent mask or mouthpiece
- Tissues and emesis basin for collecting expectorated sputum
- Gloves, goggles, gown, mask, if needed

▶ CLIENT EDUCATION NEEDED:

1. Teach the client the rationale for the use of the CPAP machine.
2. Tell the client what possible side effects there are and what to report to the nurse.
3. Have clients try on a CPAP mask before applying the mask for treatment so they can get used to it and make adjustments.
4. Ask clients to tell you the reason they are having the CPAP treatment.
5. Teach clients the symptoms they should report such as discomfort, dyspnea, headache, rapid pulse or palpitations, and dizziness.

Estimated time to complete the skill:
10–20 minutes

▶ DELEGATION TIPS

The initiation of CPAP therapy requires the assessment of the nurse or a respiratory care practitioner. Typically this treatment is performed by a respiratory therapist but a nurse with proper training may perform this procedure. It is not performed by ancillary personnel.

IMPLEMENTATION—Action/Rationale

Action	Rationale
1. Wash hands.	1. Reduces the transmission of microorganisms.
2. Check orders regarding CPAP administration.	2. Ensures CPAP administration is appropriate and the correct settings are used.
3. Assess breath sounds, vital sounds, and oxygen saturation.	3. Determine baseline respiratory assessment.
4. Assist client into position of comfort.	4. Ensures client is more comfortable during CPAP application.
5. Secure mask over the nose and/or mouth of the client (see Figure 7-8-1 and Figure 7-8-2). Check connections.	5. An airtight seal is required for proper functioning of the CPAP machine.
6. Turn CPAP machine on and check settings.	6. Settings should be checked with each application.
7. Maintain CPAP for prescribed length of time (see Figure 7-8-3).	7. Prevents hyperventilation and fatigue.
8. Assess breath sounds, vital signs, and oxygen saturation.	8. Determine changes in respiratory status.

continues

Action	Rationale

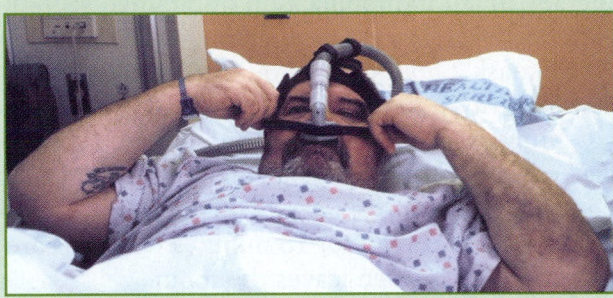

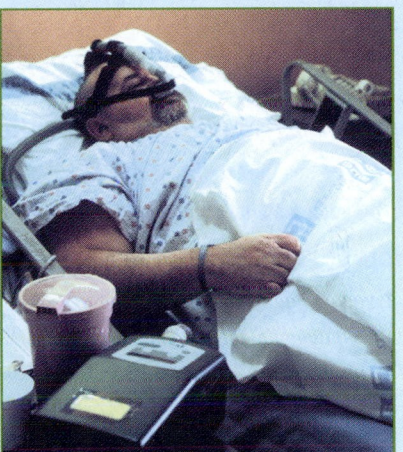

Figure 7-8-1   Place the mask over the nose.

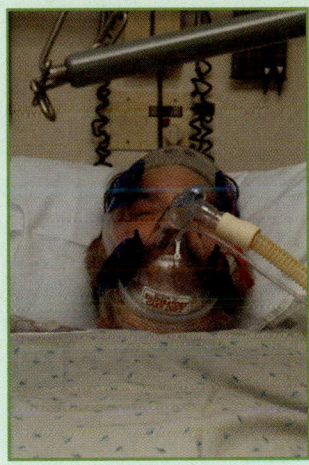

Figure 7-8-2   Place the mask over the mouth and nose. Make sure the mask forms a tight seal over the face.

Figure 7-8-3   Assist the client in continuing the CPAP therapy for the prescribed length of time.

9. Observe the client for side effects.

10. Wash hands.

9. Assess for potential problems related to CPAP administration.

10. Reduces the transmission of microorganisms.

▶ **REAL WORLD ANECDOTES**

After carefully applying Bill's CPAP mask, the nurse turned on the CPAP machine and stood at the side of the bed to observe his response as well as his oxygen saturation. His oxygen saturation started to slowly drop but stabilized at 84%. His nurse, concerned with the drop, began to check all the connections to the CPAP machine. She discovered that the oxygen source had been disconnected. After reconnecting the oxygen source, Bill's oxygen saturation stabilized at 98%. She was reminded that the connections should be checked before initiating CPAP therapy.

The nurse entered Bill's room later that shift after noting a decrease in his oxygen saturation from 98% to 90%. She checked all the connections as well as the seal on the mask over Bill's face and was unable to find anything wrong. She asked Bill to remove the CPAP mask momentarily and noticed that the tubing was almost completely occluded with a mucus plug. She cleaned out the tubing, reapplied the CPAP mask, checked all the connections, and once again, Bill's oxygen saturation stabilized at 98%.

▶ EVALUATION

- Evaluate the effectiveness of CPAP administration 20–30 minutes after the treatment.
- The client had a reduction in the work of breathing as indicated by a decrease in respiratory rate by 30%. The apneic client had a decrease in the number and duration of apneic episodes.
- The client had a decrease in the severity of retractions, grunting, and nasal flaring.
- The client had improvement in lung volumes and appearance of the lungs as indicated by chest X-ray.
- The client has increased comfort in breathing as assessed by the nurse.
- The client has an improvement in oxygen saturation.
- The client has no impairment of skin integrity.

▶ DOCUMENTATION

Nurses' Notes

- Record time CPAP was applied.
- Record settings.
- Note breath sounds before and after the procedure.
- Record vital signs, oxygen saturation.
- Note client's response to application of CPAP machine.
- Include signature of nurse applying CPAP machine.

Document on appropriate flow sheet or electronic medical record (EMR).

▶ CRITICAL THINKING SKILL

Introduction

Because of the airtight seal that must be obtained when applying a CPAP mask, the potential for skin breakdown on the nose, cheeks, and chin is high. It is important that the nurse be aware of this and observe for early signs of breakdown so that she or he can intervene before the breakdown is significant.

Possible Scenario

Jim is a 44-year-old man who has started on CPAP therapy to aid in mobilization of retained secretions secondary to chronic bronchitis. He is to wear the CPAP mask 2 hours on, 2 hours off while awake, and continuously at night. This is his third day of therapy. His nurse applies the mask and checks for any air leaking around the mask. She then checks all the connections and settings and turns the CPAP machine on. She monitors Jim for 15 minutes to make sure he is in no distress, then leaves the room.

When his nurse returns to remove the mask after Jim has been on CPAP therapy for 2 hours, she notices areas of redness on his nose and chin. She leaves the mask off for the prescribed 2 hours, then returns at 10:00 PM to apply the mask for the night. Jim notices that it is uncomfortable when the mask is applied; however, he knows he must have this therapy and does not say anything to the nurse. At 4:00 AM Jim puts his light on and the nurse enters his room to find that he has removed the mask. He tells her that the discomfort became unbearable, so he had to remove the mask. The nurse notices that there are small blisters on his nose and a 1-cm open area on his chin.

Possible Outcome

CPAP therapy must be discontinued because of the skin breakdown on Jim's nose and chin. Other methods must be used to aid in mobilization of Jim's secretions, and he recovers from his chronic bronchitis more slowly than expected.

Prevention

Upon noticing the reddened area on Jim's nose, the nurse could have adjusted the mask, avoiding this area if possible. She may have needed to decrease the duration of time that he was to wear the mask that night, knowing that skin breakdown was likely. The use of an acceptable skin barrier (no petroleum products or powders, which could be aspirated) when the redness was noted might have helped to prevent further breakdown.

▶ VARIATIONS

Geriatric Variations:

- *Skin in the elderly is thinner and more prone to breakdown. Care must be taken to assess the skin frequently to prevent breakdown from occurring.*
- *Caregivers must be taught the importance of monitoring the client during CPAP treatment.*

continues

► VARIATIONS *(continued)*

Pediatric Variations:
- *Claustrophobia is common with CPAP therapy in young children. Education about the mask and what CPAP therapy will feel like is important.*
- *Starting therapy for short intervals and slowly increasing the time can be helpful in overcoming fear and the confinement of the mask.*
- *Distraction with TV, books, or games may enhance the cooperation of the child when using the CPAP mask.*

Home Care Variations:
- *Make sure the client demonstrates proper technique for administration, proper use of equipment, appropriate breathing patterns and cough techniques, and the ability to modify technique in response to adverse reactions.*
- *Teach caregivers in the home to use the CPAP machine and to care for the equipment.*
- *Teach caregivers the signs and symptoms of respiratory infection.*
- *Medicare may reimburse for the CPAP machine used at home.*

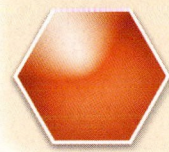

Long-Term Care Variations:
- *CPAP equipment needs to be maintained for each client use.*
- *Medicare may not reimburse for the CPAP machine in a long-term care facility.*

► COMMON ERRORS

Possible Error:

The oxygen source is disconnected from the CPAP machine.

Prevention:

Make sure the connections are secure. Be sure the CPAP machine and the oxygen source are close enough so the connection is not being stressed.

Possible Error:

A mucus plug forms in the tubing of the CPAP machine, occluding it.

Prevention:

Assess tubing before and after application of the CPAP mask. Clean the tubing or replace it with new tubing prn.

► NURSING TIPS

- Familiarize yourself with the CPAP equipment so you will feel comfortable when using it with a client.
- Determine the policy in your hospital regarding who performs the initial assessment of the client, who administers CPAP therapy, and who is responsible for ongoing assessment and care of stable and unstable clients.
- Claustrophobic or anxious clients will need you to stay at their bedside during the treatment.
- Demonstrating the mask on yourself may allay the fear and anxiety a client may have about the treatment.

SPECIAL CONSIDERATIONS

- *CPAP may be used for primary atelectasis prevention in less cooperative clients who are unable to perform regular deep breathing exercises or incentive spirometry.*
- *Intermittent CPAP may be associated with complications, including client discomfort, gastric distension, hypoventilation, and pneumothorax. If these occur the client should be encouraged to turn, cough, and breathe deeply to prevent further respiratory complications.*
- *Coughing devices, such as Mechanical In-Exsufflation, are available for clients who have muscle weakness and are unable to cough and breathe deeply.*

Preparing the Chest Drainage System

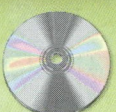

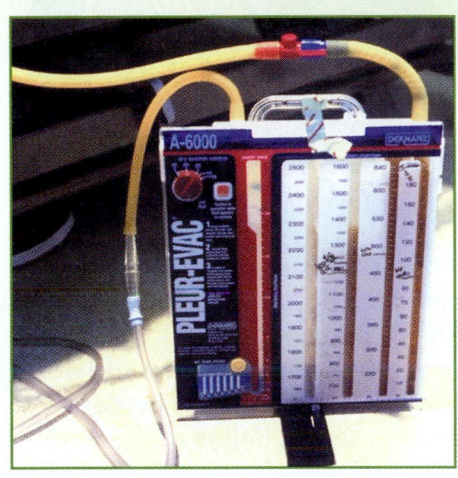

▶ OVERVIEW OF THE SKILL

The chest drainage system is a closed system designed to drain air or fluid from the pleural cavity while restoring or maintaining the negative intrapleural pressure needed to keep the lungs properly expanded. The space between the lungs and chest wall is called the pleural cavity and it normally contains only a small amount of fluid for lubrication between the lungs and the chest wall. Negative intrapleural pressure between the lungs, chest wall, and diaphragm allows the movement of the chest and diaphragm to expand and contract the lungs.

Large amounts of fluid or air in the pleural cavity impede the expansion of the lungs, causing respiratory distress or "collapse" of the lung. Excess fluid or air can enter the pleural cavity by several means. Thoracic surgery breaks the vacuum seal in the pleural cavity, allowing fluid and air to enter. Trauma to the chest wall can lead to bleeding into the pleural cavity (hemothorax) or air entering the pleural cavity (pneumothorax). Occasionally, spontaneous pneumothorax occurs, without apparent cause.

The chest drainage system is designed to help restore the vacuum seal in the pleural cavity by draining excess fluid or air while keeping the pleural cavity sealed. Occlusive dressings, water seals, gravity, and additional suction, if necessary, work together to create a sealed system with slight negative pressure to draw fluids away from the chest.

The drainage system uses a water seal to prevent air return into the pleural cavity. Once pleural air passes through the water seal, it cannot return to the chest and is vented to the atmosphere. Occlusive dressings at the puncture site prevent air from entering the pleural space. All connections between the tubing are airtight.

The chest drainage system can be attached to suction to increase the negative pressure between the pleural space and the drainage system, which improves drainage. The amount of suction is controlled by a dial in some chest drainage setups and by the amount of saline added to the suction control container in other setups.

When setting up a chest drainage system, it is important to understand why the system works. Read the manufacturer's instructions for commercial chest drainage setups.

▶ ASSESSMENT

1. Assess the physician's or qualified practitioner's orders **to determine what kind of chest drainage system is required.**
2. Assess the available equipment **to determine what kind of drainage system setups are available.**
3. Assess the client's environment **to determine what kind of equipment will be required and what drainage system would be optimal for the client.**

▶ DIAGNOSIS

Risk for Infection

Impaired Gas Exchange

▶ PLANNING

Expected Outcomes:

1. The chest drainage system will be appropriate for the client as well as consistent with the system ordered by the physician or qualified practitioner.
2. The chest drainage system will be set up in accordance with institutional policy.
3. The chest drainage system will not pose a hazard for infection or loss of air seal to the client.

Equipment Needed:

Disposable Chest Tube Drainage System

- Sterile water or saline
- Disposable chest tube drainage system (see Figure 7-9-1)
- Suction tubing if the drainage system will be connected to suction
- Tape

Reusable Bottle Chest Drainage System

- Sterile glass bottles—1 to 3 depending on the physician's or qualified practitioner's order
- Sterile water or saline
- Glass tubes—2 to 7 depending on the physician's or qualified practitioner's order
- Rubber tubing

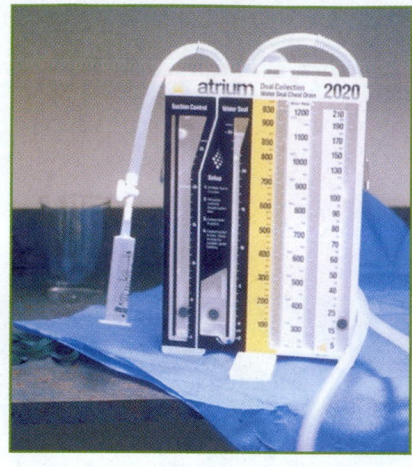

Figure 7-9-1 Disposable chest tube drainage system

- Suction tubing if the drainage system will be connected to suction
- Rubber stoppers with holes the size of the glass tubes to be used on the glass bottles—2 with 2 holes and 1 with 3 holes
- Tape
- Sterile gloves

▶ CLIENT EDUCATION NEEDED:

1. Teach the client that some bubbling in the water seal container and the suction container is normal.
2. Instruct the client regarding the need to keep the drainage system below the level of the chest tube insertion site.

IMPLEMENTATION—Action/Rationale

Action	Rationale
Disposable Chest Tube Drainage System	
1. Gather equipment in a clean area or at the client's bedside.	1. Helps maintain sterility while assembling the chest drainage system.
2. Wash hands.	2. Reduces the transmission of microorganisms.
3. Open the prepackaged disposable chest tube system using aseptic technique (see Figure 7-9-2).	3. Maintains sterility while assembling the chest drainage system. Most prepackaged disposable chest tube systems are basically a three-bottle system packaged in one disposable container.
4. Set the unit upright (see Figure 7-9-3).	4. Allows the unit to be filled.
5. If only a water seal has been ordered, pour the measured amount of sterile water or saline into the funnel provided (see Figures 7-9-4 and 7-9-5).	5. This provides a water seal to prevent air from entering the pleural cavity.

continues

Action	Rationale

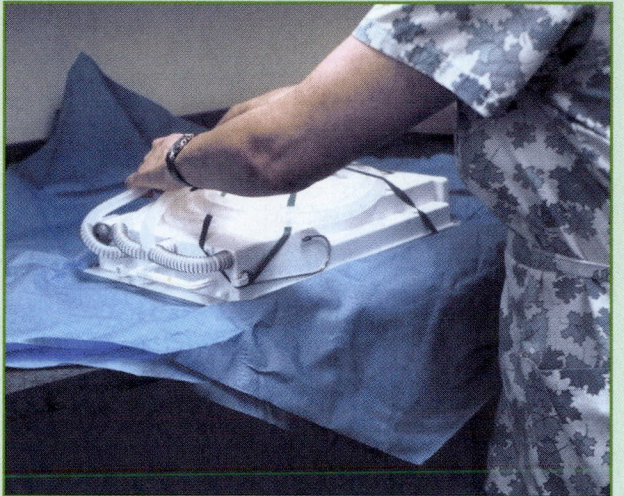

Figure 7-9-2   Open the chest tube system package using aseptic technique.

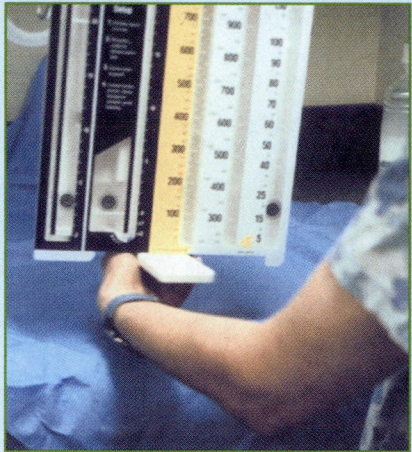

Figure 7-9-3   Set the unit upright.

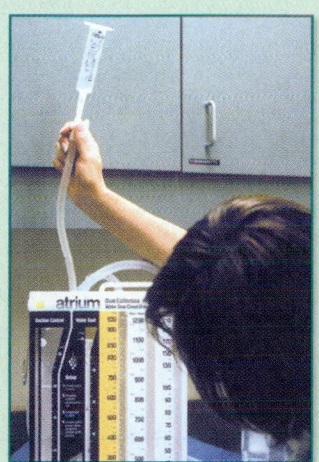

Figure 7-9-4   Fill the appropriate chambers with sterile water or saline.

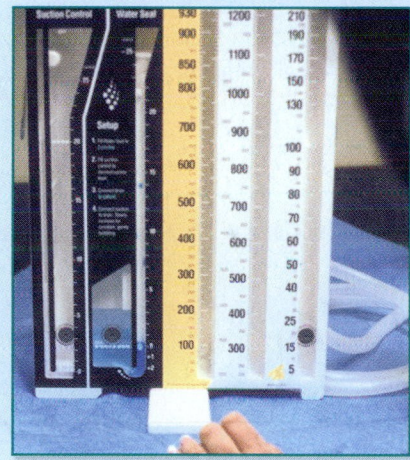

Figure 7-9-5   Fill the appropriate chamber with the amount of fluid indicated in the manufacturer's instructions.

6. If suction has been ordered, fill the suction control chamber to the ordered level of fluid, usually 20 cm of water (see Figures 7-9-6 and 7-9-7).

6. This provides extra suction to increase the drainage of fluid or air from the pleural cavity.

7. If suction has been ordered, attach suction tubing to the marked suction port and to the suction source.

7. Provides suction to the system.

8. Turn the suction up until there is gentle bubbling in the suction control section of the system.

8. The level of suction is determined by the air flow through the water in the suction chamber. This is indicated by the bubbling of the suction control chamber.

continues

Action	Rationale

Disposable Chest Tube Drainage System *continued*

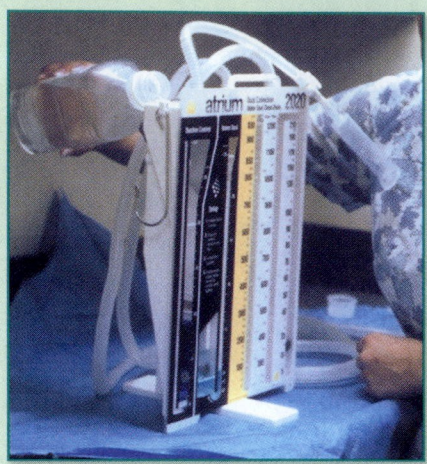

Figure 7-9-6 If suction has been ordered, fill the suction control chamber to the ordered level of fluid.

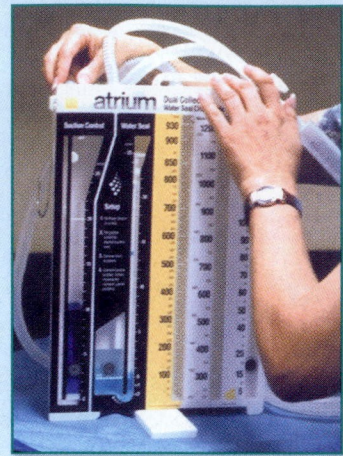

Figure 7-9-7 Make sure the tubing connections are attached and secure.

9. Set the system up at the client's bedside. Keep the drainage system below the level of the client (see Figure 7-9-8).

9. Prevents backflow of air or fluid into the pleural cavity.

10. Wash hands.

10. Reduces the transmission of microorganisms.

Reusable Bottle Chest Drainage System

11. Repeat Actions 1–3.

11. See Rationales 1–3.

12. Apply sterile gloves.

12. Maintains sterility while assembling the chest drainage system.

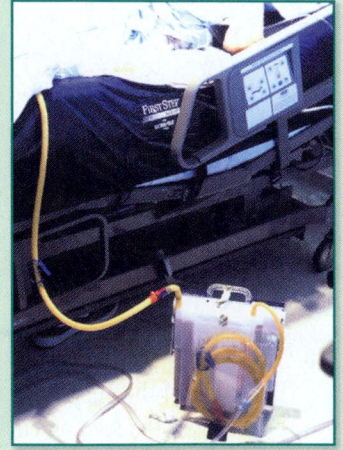

Figure 7-9-8 Set the system upright at the bedside below the level of the client.

continues

Action	Rationale
13. One-bottle water seal:	**13.** This system is generally used only for pneumothorax as one bottle is required to act as a water seal and a drainage bottle.
• Insert a long glass tube through one hole of a two-hole rubber stopper. Insert a short glass tube through the other hole in the stopper.	• The long tube will provide a water seal, and the shorter tube will work as an air vent to prevent the buildup of pressure in the bottle as fluid and air drain out of the pleural cavity and into the bottle.
• Pour sterile saline or sterile water into the glass bottle, filling it to a depth of at least 4 cm.	• Provides a sterile water seal to prevent air return into the pleural cavity.
• Being careful not to contaminate the inside of the rubber stopper or the portion of the glass tubes that will be inside the bottle, put the rubber stopper onto the bottle.	• Maintains sterility while assembling the chest drainage system.
• Be sure the end of the long glass tube is submerged 2 cm into the water in the bottle. If the tube does not extend deeply enough, add more water to the bottle. Do not fill the bottle more than one-third full.	• Provides a water seal that prevents the return of air into the pleural cavity. The higher water level creates increased resistance to drainage.
• Attach rubber tubing to the outside end of the long glass tube for drainage from the client's chest tube.	• The long glass tube is sealed, providing a sealed drainage system.
• Place a measuring guide on the side of the bottle, marking the water level before connection to the client.	• Documents the amount of drainage from the chest tube.
14. Two-bottle drainage and water seal:	**14.** This system is used when gravity drainage is adequate but a separate drainage container is desired for accurate assessment of the drainage and to prevent increased resistance as the drainage bottle fills.
• Insert two short glass tubes into a two-hole rubber stopper. Place this rubber stopper onto the drainage bottle.	• This allows drainage to flow into the bottle without creating a water seal in this container.
• Insert one long glass tube and one short glass tube into a second two-hole rubber stopper.	• The long tube will provide a water seal, and the shorter tube will work as an air vent to prevent the buildup of pressure in the bottle as fluid and air drain out of the pleural cavity and into the bottle.
• Pour sterile water or sterile saline into the water seal bottle to a depth of about 4 cm. Do not fill the bottle more than one-third full.	• Provides a sterile water seal to prevent air return into the pleural cavity.
• Place the rubber stopper with the long glass tube onto the water seal bottle, being careful not to contaminate the inside of the bottle or the glass tubes.	• Maintains sterility while assembling the chest drainage system.
• Be sure the end of the long glass tube is submerged 2 cm into the water in the bottle. If the tube does not extend deeply enough, add more water to the bottle. Do not fill the bottle more than one-third full.	• Provides a water seal that prevents the return of air into the pleural cavity. The higher water level creates increased resistance to drainage.
• Place a length of rubber tubing between the outer end of one of the short glass tubes on the drainage bottle and the outer end of the long glass tube on the water seal bottle.	• The long glass tube is sealed by water, providing a sealed drainage system.

continues

Action	Rationale
Reusable Bottle Chest Drainage System *continued*	
• Place a length of rubber tubing on the outer end of the second short glass tube in the drainage bottle. This tube is for connecting to the client for drainage.	• This will provide a continuous sealed system for drainage without allowing air or fluid to return to the pleural cavity.
• Place a measuring guide on the side of the drainage collection bottle before connection to the client.	• Documents the amount of drainage from the client's chest tube.
15. Two-bottle drainage and suction control:	15. This system is used when additional suction is required to remove air from the pleural cavity. Because the drainage and the water seal occupy the same bottle, it is not desirable for situations in which significant amounts of drainage are expected.
• Insert a long glass tube through one hole of a two-hole rubber stopper. Insert a short glass tube through the other hole in the stopper.	• The long tube will provide a water seal, and the shorter tube will connect to the suction control bottle.
• Insert a long glass tube through the middle hole of a three-hole rubber stopper and short glass tubes through the other two holes in the three-hole stopper.	• The long tube will remain open to the air as a vent. The two shorter tubes are connectors to the water seal/drainage bottle and to the suction source.
• Pour sterile saline or sterile water into the water seal/drainage bottle, filling it to a depth of at least 4 cm.	• Provides a sterile water seal to prevent air return into the pleural cavity.
• Pour sterile saline or sterile water into the suction control bottle to the ordered depth, usually 20 cm of water.	• Provides a measured amount of suction. The depth of the water controls the amount of suction applied to the pleural cavity.
• Place the two-hole rubber stopper with the long glass tube onto the water seal/drainage bottle, being careful not to contaminate the inside of the bottle or the glass tubes.	• Maintains sterility while assembling the chest drainage system.
• Be sure the end of the long glass tube is submerged 2 cm into the water in the bottle. If the tube does not extend deeply enough, add more water to the bottle. Do not fill the bottle more than one-third full.	• Provides a water seal that prevents the return of air into the pleural cavity. The higher water level creates increased resistance to drainage.
• Place the three-hole rubber stopper with the long glass tube and two short glass tubes onto the suction control bottle, being careful not to contaminate the inside of the bottle or the glass tubes.	• Maintains sterility while assembling the chest drainage system.
• Be sure the long glass tube extends well into the water but does not touch the bottom of the bottle.	• If the long tube touches the bottom of the suction control bottle, it will be unable to vent outside air, and the suction to the pleural cavity will be infinite.
• Attach a length of rubber tubing to the outer end of the short glass tube in the water seal/drainage bottle and connect it to the outer end of one of the short glass tubes in the suction control bottle.	• Connects the water seal/drainage bottle into the suction system.
• Attach the suction tubing to the outer end of the second short glass tube in the suction control bottle.	• Attaches the system to suction.
• Do not attach any tubing to the outer end of the long glass tube in the suction control bottle.	• Maintains a vent to the air. This allows control of the amount of suction inside the system.

continues

Action	Rationale
• Attach the drainage tubing from the client to the outer end of the long glass tube in the water seal/drainage bottle.	• The amount of suction is controlled by the air being pulled from the outside, through the long glass tube and the water. The amount of water the air has to be pulled through determines the amount of suction in the system.
• Turn the suction source up until a gentle bubbling is noted in the suction control bottle. To increase the suction, add more water to the suction control bottle. To decrease the suction, remove water from the suction control bottle.	• Accurately documents the amount of drainage from the pleural cavity.
• Place a measuring guide on the side of the water seal/drainage bottle, marking the water level before connection to the client.	• Completes the closed drainage system and allows drainage, water seal, and suction to work to heal the pleural cavity.
16. Three-bottle drainage, water seal, and suction control:	16. This method is used when significant amounts of drainage are expected and the client requires suction to the chest tubes.
• Insert short glass tubes through the holes in one of the two-hole rubber stoppers.	• Allows drainage to empty into the drainage bottle while keeping the bottle open to the water seal.
• Insert a long glass tube through one hole of a two-hole rubber stopper. Insert a short glass tube through the other hole in the stopper.	• The long tube will provide a water seal, and the shorter tube will connect to the suction control bottle.
• Insert a long glass tube through the middle hole of a three-hole rubber stopper and short glass tubes through the other two holes in the three-hole stopper.	• The long tube will remain open to the air as a vent. The two shorter tubes are connectors to the water seal bottle and to the suction source.
• Pour sterile saline or sterile water into the water seal bottle, filling it to a depth of at least 4 cm.	• Provides a sterile water seal to prevent air return into the pleural cavity.
• Pour sterile saline or sterile water into the suction control bottle to the ordered depth, usually 20 cm of water.	• Provides a measured amount of suction. The depth of the water controls the amount of suction applied to the pleural cavity.
• Being careful not to contaminate the inside of the rubber stopper or the portion of the glass tubes that will be inside the bottle, put the rubber stopper with the two short glass tubes onto the drainage collection bottle.	• Maintains sterility while assembling the chest drainage system.
• Place the two-hole rubber stopper with the long glass tube onto the water seal bottle, being careful not to contaminate the inside of the bottle or the glass tubes.	• Maintains sterility while assembling the chest drainage system.
• Be sure the end of the long glass tube is submerged 2 cm into the water in the bottle. If the tube does not extend deeply enough, add more water to the bottle. Do not fill the bottle more than one-third full.	• Provides a water seal that prevents the return of air into the pleural cavity. The higher water level creates increased resistance to drainage.
• Place the three-hole rubber stopper with the long glass tube and two short glass tubes onto the suction control bottle, being careful not to contaminate the inside of the bottle or the glass tubes.	• Maintains sterility while assembling the chest drainage system.
• Be sure the long glass tube extends well into the water but does not touch the bottom of the bottle.	• If the long tube touches the bottom of the suction control bottle, it will be unable to vent outside air, and the suction to the pleural cavity will be infinite.

continues

Action	Rationale
Reusable Bottle Chest Drainage System *continued*	
• Attach rubber tubing to the outside end of one of the short glass tubes extending from the drainage collection bottle to attach to the client's chest tube.	• Entrains the pleural cavity into the closed drainage system.
• Attach a length of rubber tubing from the second short glass tube in the drainage collection bottle to the long glass tube in the water seal bottle.	• Entrains the drainage collection bottle to the water seal.
• Attach a length of rubber tubing from the short glass tube in the water seal bottle to one of the short glass tubes in the suction control bottle.	• Entrains the water seal to the suction control bottle.
• Attach the suction tubing to the second short glass tube in the suction control bottle and to the suction source.	• Entrains the system to suction.
• Do not attach any tubing to the outer end of the long glass tube in the suction control bottle.	• Maintains a vent to the air. This allows control of the amount of suction inside the system.
• Turn the suction source up until a gentle bubbling is noted in the suction control bottle. To increase the suction, add more water to the suction control bottle. To decrease the suction, remove water from the suction control bottle.	• The amount of suction is controlled by the air being pulled from the outside, through the long glass tube and the water. The amount of water the air has to be pulled through determines the amount of suction in the system.
• Place a measuring guide on the side of the drainage bottle before connection to the client.	• Accurately documents the amount of drainage from the pleural cavity.
17. Tape all connections.	17. Prevents accidental breakage of the sealed system.
18. Dispose of gloves in the proper container.	18. Maintains standard precautions.
19. Arrange the drainage system at the client's bedside. Keep the drainage system below the level of the client.	19. Prevents backflow of water or drainage into the pleural cavity.
20. Wash hands.	20. Reduces the transmission of microorganisms.

► REAL WORLD ANECDOTES

Rachel Knik, a temporary registry nurse, was working a 12-hour shift in a small rural hospital. Her client's physician ordered a closed chest drainage system to be ready at the client's bedside when the client returned from surgery. Ms. Knik went to the supply room to look for a pleur-evac to set up. She was unable to find any disposable chest drainage systems and became quite confused about how to proceed. After she had asked several other staff members, one of them took her aside and explained that they did not use those fancy disposable systems, they used the old reliable three-bottle system. When Ms. Knik admitted that she had never heard of the three-bottle system, the staff nurse showed her how to set it up using three sterile bottles, glass tubes, and rubber tubing.

▶ EVALUATION

- The chest drainage system is appropriate for the client and consistent with the system ordered by the health care provider.
- The chest drainage system was set up in accordance with institutional policy.
- The chest drainage system did not pose a hazard for infection or loss of air seal to the client.

▶ DOCUMENTATION

Nurses' Notes

- Indicate the type of chest drainage system used.
- If suction control was ordered, indicate the centimeter level of fluid in the suction control bottle.

Document on appropriate flow sheet or electronic medical record (EMR).

▶ CRITICAL THINKING SKILL

Introduction

Understand the physics underlying the chest tube setup.

Possible Scenario

The nurse is assembling the chest tube drainage system using the bottle system. The order is for two bottles, a drainage collection bottle, and a water seal bottle. As she is setting up the system, she remembers that it is important that the system be closed to prevent air leakage back into the pleural cavity. While setting up the water seal bottle, she notices that the short glass tube is open to the air. She is concerned that this will leave the system open, so she plugs the short glass tube in the water seal bottle.

Possible Outcome

The chest tube is placed and hooked up to the drainage system. The physician had expected a large amount of drainage immediately following the chest tube insertion, but there is no drainage. The client's condition does not improve. The physician is concerned that she might have misplaced the chest tube and orders a chest X-ray. The nurse on hand first checks the chest tube drainage system and notices that the short glass tube is plugged. She unplugs the vent tube in the water seal bottle to equalize with the atmospheric pressure. The nurse notifies the physician and the X-ray is delayed while the client is monitored with the correct setup. There is substantial drainage through the chest tube and the client's condition improves. The X-ray is cancelled.

Prevention

Be aware of the physics involved in the closed chest drainage system. Understand what each chamber of the system is for and how it works. Despite the name, the system requires one port to be open to the air. Knowing where in the system the air vent is placed and why it will prevent serious, if not life-threatening, errors.

▶ VARIATIONS

Geriatric Variation:
- *Explain sounds and sensations associated with the chest tube that the elderly client may not be able to see or hear clearly.*

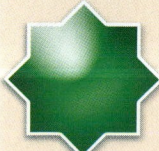

Pediatric Variations:
- *Keep a demonstration (clean and empty) system to teach the child how it works. Match your explanations to the age of the child.*
- *Explain the sounds that the child will be hearing.*
- *If the system is attached to suction, reassure the child that the suction cannot be inadvertently turned up high enough to hurt him or her.*

continues

▶ VARIATIONS *(continued)*

Home Care Variation:
- *Chest tubes are not used in the home care setting.*

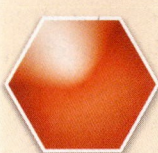

Long-Term Care Variation:
- *Chest tubes are not used in the long-term care setting.*

▶ COMMON ERRORS

Possible Error:

The nurse tries to adjust the amount of suction in the system by turning up the suction at the source.

Prevention:

Know how the system works. The suction is regulated by the depth of fluid in the suction control chamber, not by the amount of external suction applied. Increasing the suction source only increases the noise level in the suction control chamber, not the amount of suction in the system.

▶ NURSING TIPS

- Set up the closed drainage system below the level of the chest tube insertion site.
- Keep the closed drainage system on a flat, sturdy surface so it is not tipped over. If the system is knocked over, the water seal may be lost, causing the introduction of air into the client's chest.
- If the water seal container is irretrievably compromised, a stopgap water seal can be devised by placing the end of the chest tube itself about 2 cm deep in sterile water or saline.

▶ SPECIAL CONSIDERATIONS

- *In the wet suction system, the intensity of suction is controlled by the height of fluid water in the suction chamber. Always follow the instruction manual and use the amount of solution recommended for the desired suction. Sterile procedure, especially the instilled solution, is required when setting up the drainage system.*
- *Latex-free products are available for clients who are allergic to latex. A well-documented health history serves as a great reference in selecting the appropriate drainage system.*

Maintaining the Chest Tube and Chest Drainage System

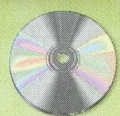

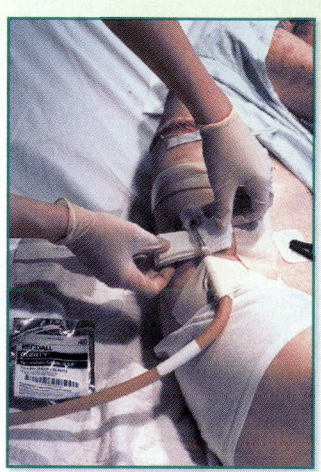

▶ OVERVIEW OF THE SKILL

This nursing skill involves the care of a client with a chest tube in place. Skills to be assessed include monitoring and maintaining the chest tube and the disposable drainage system; there are also specific safety issues to be aware of when caring for a client with a chest tube in place.

▶ ASSESSMENT

1. Assess that the chest tube is set to the appropriate amount of suction as ordered by the health care provider. **Suction is what draws the air or fluid from the pleural space, and it is essential that the appropriate amount is applied.**

2. Assess that the water level in the water seal chamber is maintained at the marked line. **If the level drops below the marked level, there is a chance that air could be drawn into the pleural cavity and cause or increase a pneumothorax.**

3. Assess for an air leak in the water seal chamber. **An air leak indicates a persistent or new pneumothorax.**

4. Assess that all connections are taped. **The presence of a loose connection could allow air to be drawn into the pleural cavity and cause a pneumothorax.**

5. Assess the chest tube dressing and change every 24 to 48 hours. **The dressing provides an occlusive covering to prevent any air from entering the pleural cavity and also to prevent infection at the insertion site.**

6. Assess the drainage system and note the amount and color of the drainage. **The output is closely monitored to note bleeding and also to know when output has decreased enough for the tube to be removed.**

7. Assess that the tubing is free of kinks and dependent loops and is not pinned to the bed. **The presence of kinks or loops prevents adequate drainage of the chest tube, and pinning the chest tube to the bed increases the risk that the tube could become accidentally dislodged.**

8. Ensure that the drainage system has not been tipped over, dropped, or crushed. **Any trauma to the collection system could cause damage and increase the risk of air being drawn into the pleural cavity.**

9. Identify risk factors for a tension pneumothorax in the client with a chest tube. **A tension pneumothorax is a life-threatening condition and prevention is important.**

▶ DIAGNOSIS

Impaired Gas Exchange

Pain

Risk for Infection

Risk for Impaired Skin Integrity

► **PLANNING**

Expected Outcomes:

1. Client will have chest tube and drainage system maintained without increase of the pneumothorax.
2. Client will be free of infection related to the chest tube.
3. Chest tube and drainage system will be maintained in a safe manner.

Equipment Needed (see Figure 7-10-1):

- Orders from physician or qualified practitioner
- Sterile water or normal saline
- Silk tape, 1-inch roll
- 3 packages of 4 × 4 pads
- Vaseline, gauze, 1 package for each chest tube to be dressed
- Foam tape, 2-inch roll
- Chest tube clamps

► **CLIENT EDUCATION NEEDED:**

1. Explain the rationale for the dressing change or drainage system change.
2. Explain the rationale for the assessment of an air leak.

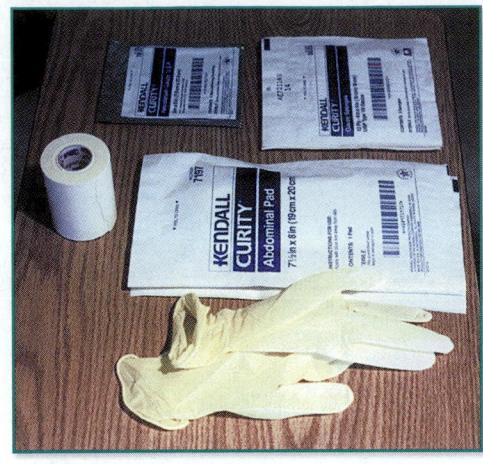

Figure 7-10-1   Clean gloves, dressing, and tape are used to maintain the chest tube.

3. Teach the client to be aware of the drainage system and to avoid tipping or kicking it over.

Estimated time to complete the skill:
10–20 minutes, depending on whether a dressing or drainage unit needs to be changed

► **DELEGATION TIPS**

Maintaining chest drainage systems is the responsibility of the nurse and is not delegated. Ancillary personnel should report all concerns or client complaints immediately to the nurse.

IMPLEMENTATION—Action/Rationale

Action	Rationale
1. Assess that the drainage system is set to the ordered amount of suction. This is achieved by filling the suction chamber with sterile water to the level of suction ordered, usually 20 cm, and maintaining that level of water at all times. Bubbling in the suction chamber needs to be maintained at a gentle bubbling; vigorous bubbling does not increase the amount of suction being provided. Vigorous bubbling only increases the rate of evaporation of the water in the suction chamber.	1. Suction is removing air and fluid from the pleural cavity to resolve the pneumothorax.
2. Assess that the water seal chamber is filled to the marked level.	2. The water seal chamber prevents air from returning to the pleural cavity; if it is not maintained at the marked level, air could be drawn into the cavity.

continues

Action	Rationale
3. Assess for an air leak by watching for bubbling in the water seal chamber and having the client take a deep breath and cough.	3. An air leak can indicate a new or persistent pneumothorax.
4. If there is a new air leak, the physician or qualified practitioner may have you assess whether the air leak is from within the client or from the chest tube or drainage system. This can be done by briefly clamping the chest tube at the entrance site and assessing again for the air leak; if it is no longer present, it came from the client, and if it is still present, it is coming from the chest tube or the system. This same procedure should be continued down the length of the tube and tubing until the air leak is no longer present. If the leak is still present at the end, the entire drainage chamber should be changed.	4. An air leak from the system indicates that it is not functioning properly and, therefore, appropriate suction may not be provided.
5. Assess that all connections at site are spiral-wrapped with silk tape.	5. The spiral taping prevents the tubing from pulling apart, and the silk tape is a strong adhesive.
6. Assess the chest tube dressing every shift (see Figure 7-10-2) and change the dressing every 24 to 48 hours (see Figure 7-10-3). Record the date and time of the last dressing change directly on the dressing (see Figure 7-10-4).	6. The dressing provides an occlusive seal to the site, preventing air from being drawn in. Changing the dressing every 24–48 hours will prevent infection at the site.
7. Every 1–8 hours, depending upon the orders, assess the drainage output from the chest tube, noting the color and amount (see Figure 7-10-5).	7. The amount and color of the drainage will indicate any bleeding, and monitoring overall output will indicate when the chest tube may be removed.
8. Assess that the drainage system is safely on the floor, lower than the client, or hung off the end of the bed to prevent tipping of the system (see Figure 7-10-6).	8. The drainage system needs to be lower than the client to ensure adequate drainage, and the system needs to be safe from tipping to prevent a disruption in the amount of suction provided.

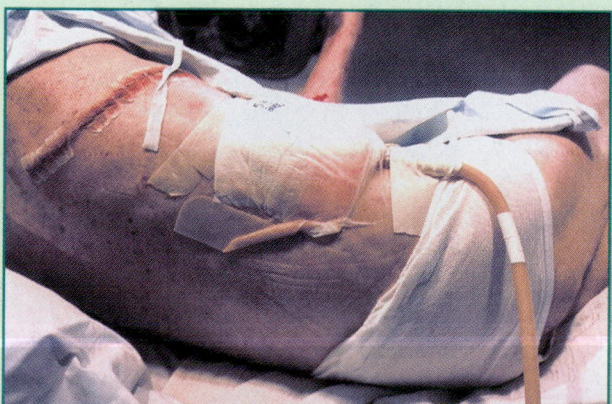

Figure 7-10-2 Assess the chest tube dressing at least once a shift. If the chest tube dressing has become saturated, it needs to be replaced.

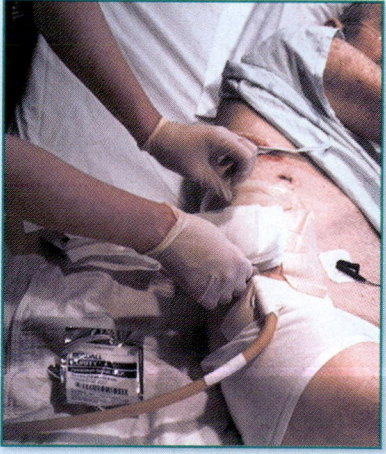

Figure 7-10-3 Change the dressing every 24–48 hours, or more frequently if needed.

continues

Action	Rationale

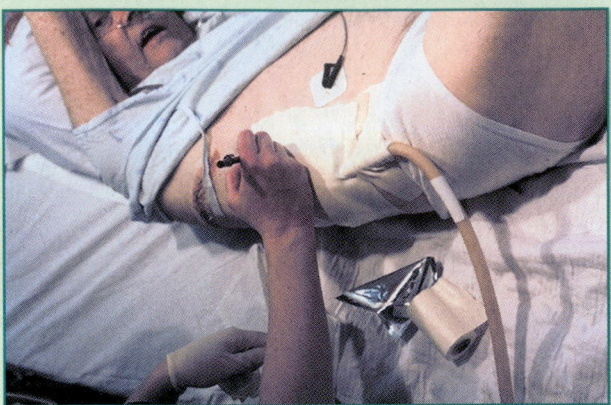

Figure 7-10-4 Write the date and time of the dressing change directly on the dressing.

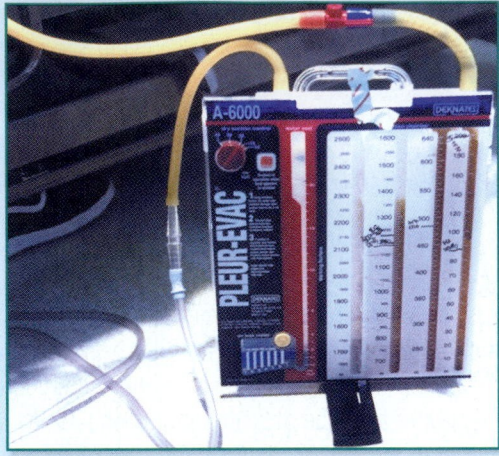

Figure 7-10-5 Assess the color and amount of drainage from the chest tube at least once a shift, or as ordered.

9. Assess that the tubing is free from kinks and dependent loops and is not pinned to the bed linens (see Figure 7-10-7).

10. Ensure that a bottle of sterile water or saline is at the client's bedside (see Figure 7-10-8).

9. Any kinks or dependent loops interfere with the drainage of the chest tube. To prevent accidental dislodging of the chest tube, the tube should never be pinned to the bedding.

10. The bottle of sterile water/saline can be used to refill the water seal and suction chambers as needed, and if the chest tube becomes disconnected from the drainage system, the end of the chest tube should be placed in the bottle of water, creating a temporary water seal until a new drainage system is set up. A chest tube should never be clamped, except on orders from a physician or qualified practitioner.

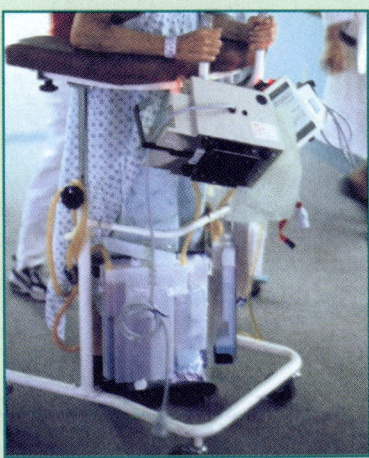

Figure 7-10-6 The drainage system must be lower than the client.

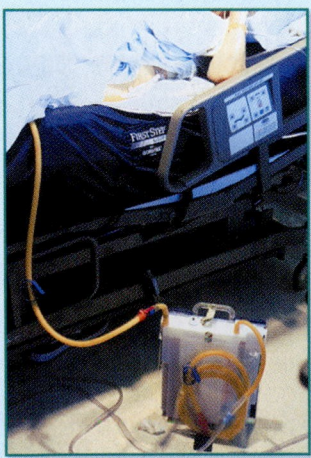

Figure 7-10-7 Check the tubing between the chest tube and the drainage system to make sure it is not pinched or kinked.

continues

Action	Rationale
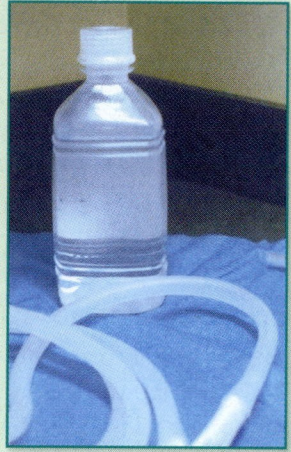 **Figure 7-10-8** Keep replacement fluid at the bedside to refill water seal and/or suction chambers if needed.	
11. Ensure that an occlusive dressing is applied in the event that the chest tube accidentally falls out or is accidentally pulled out.	11. An occlusive dressing can decrease the risk of pneumothorax.
12. Ensure that the chest tube is never milked or stripped to maintain patency.	12. Milking or stripping can cause an increase of pressures up to 400 cm H2O, which can cause damage to lung tissue and vasculature. If a chest tube is clotted, the physician or qualified practitioner should be notified and other methods used.
13. Keep chest tube clamps at the bedside.	13. To clamp chest tube in the event the tubing becomes disconnected.

▶ REAL WORLD ANECDOTES

Scenario 1

An RN is performing assessment on a client who had a chest tube placed 2 days ago because of a spontaneous pneumothorax. The client has been without an air leak for 24 hours, but the RN notices in the assessment that there is now an air leak. After ensuring that the client is not compromised, the RN completes the assessment of the drainage system and finds that the water seal level is well below the marked line. She adds sterile water to the water seal chamber and then notifies the physicians, who request a portable chest X-ray to assess for a pneumothorax. This RN was reminded of the importance of maintaining the water level and assessing the drainage system every shift.

Scenario 2

A client with a chest tube was being transferred from stretcher to bed, and the drainage system was placed on the floor. When the client's bed was returned to a low position, the drainage system became caught beneath the bed, and, although there was no visible damage to the drainage system, the RN replaced the drainage system to prevent any potential adverse effects.

► **EVALUATION**

• Client has a chest tube and drainage system maintained without increase of pneumothorax.
• Client is free of infection related to the chest tube.
• Chest tube and drainage system are maintained in a safe manner.

► **DOCUMENTATION**

Nurses' Notes

• Document chest tube to suction at ordered amount.
• Note presence or absence of air leak.
• Note condition of the dressing and when it was changed.
• If there was a disconnection or dislodgment of the tube, note client condition, physician or qualified practitioner notified, and actions taken.
• Record chest tube drainage amount and color.

Document on appropriate flow sheet or electronic medical record (EMR).

► **CRITICAL THINKING SKILL**

Introduction

Look at an example of the importance of noting the amount and color of chest tube drainage.

Possible Scenario

A client has just been admitted from the emegency department with a chest tube for a hemothorax after a fall from a ladder. On initial assessment, the nurse fails to mark the drainage container at the level of the output and notes the color as a red to dark red bloody drainage. The nurse does no further follow-up on the drainage output until 3 hours later, when "from what she can remember," the client now has had an additional 400 mL of dark red, bloody drainage.

Possible Outcomes

This client is probably just draining the blood that collected from the injury, but because the nurse did not mark the level of the drainage upon admission from the emergency department, it is very hard to accurately assess the amount of output and to assess for continued bleeding.

Prevention

The drainage container should be marked and dated and the time indicated each time it is assessed. The color of the output should be documented in the nurse's notes.

► **VARIATIONS**

Geriatric Variations:

• *It is important to maintain mobility, especially in the elderly client. Make sure the client is not afraid to move about, sit in the chair, or ambulate with the chest tube system.*
• *Explain to the client that the 6 feet of tubing is to allow movement. Explain how the tube is anchored and how the dressings are secured. Encourage the client to move about and change positions in bed or in the chair.*

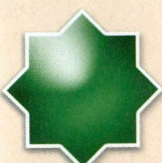

Pediatric Variations:

• *Secure airtight connections with tape and assess the dressing frequently if the child is moving around in bed.*
• *Assist the parent who wishes to hold or rock the child with the chest tube drainage system in place.*
• *Teach parents about the system, showing them normal movement and bubbling in the system.*

Home Care Variation:

• *Chest tubes are not used in the home care setting.*

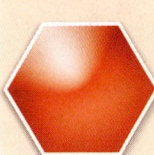

Long-Term Care Variation:

• *Chest tubes are not used in the long-term care setting.*

▶ COMMON ERRORS

Possible Error:

The suction is not at the ordered amount.

Prevention:

Always check orders for the correct suction level and always assess that the suction is being delivered at the ordered amount.

Possible Error:

The water seal chamber is not full.

Prevention:

Always assess the water level and refill as needed with sterile water.

Possible Error:

The chest tube becomes disconnected.

Prevention:

Always check that the connections are spiral-taped.

▶ NURSING TIPS

- If your client has a large and persistent air leak, the water seal level will evaporate quickly and need to be assessed frequently.
- If there is concern that the chest tube has become clotted, the physician or qualified practitioner can suction the chest tube using a small suction catheter.
- If you are not working with a "wet" drainage system, the way to assess the amount of suction being applied is to check the suction dial to see that it is set to the amount ordered, and then check that the suction indicator is present consistently, indicating that the appropriate amount of suction is being applied.
- Evaluate chest tube drainage system and tubing for safe positioning.
- Determine that emergency items are available if the chest tube becomes dislodged or disconnected.

▶ SPECIAL CONSIDERATIONS

- *Know chest tube equipment and functioning. Some chest tubes require water while others do not. Check the health care provider's orders and use the correct system for the client.*
- *Clients of the Jehovah's Witness belief may allow reinfusion of blood from the chest tube if the exchange remains in a closed system. Such a device is available and blood collected from the chest tube may be reinfused into the client via an autotransfusion system.*
- *Precautions must be taken when moving the client or bed to avoid pulling the chest tube.*

Measuring the Output from a Chest Drainage System

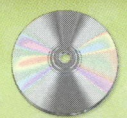

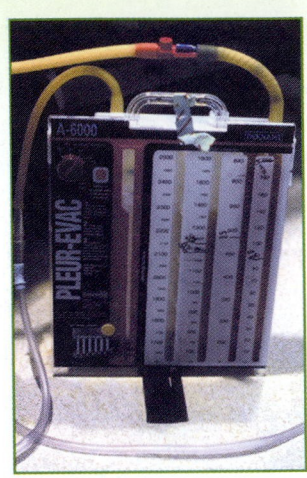

▶ OVERVIEW OF THE SKILL

The chest drainage system is a closed system designed to drain air or fluid from the pleural cavity while restoring or maintaining intrapleural pressure by creating a vacuum seal. The goal of the chest drainage system is to allow the lung to reexpand after surgery or trauma.

One or more chest tubes are inserted and covered with airtight dressings. These tubes are attached to approximately 6 feet of rubber tubing, which terminates in a water seal drainage collection system attached to wall suction. The system draws fluid and air away from the intrapleural space. While the escaping air is not measured, the fluid drained through the chest tube is considered to be output and must be measured at regular intervals. The amount is then added to the intake and output totals.

Because the chest drainage system is a closed system, the drainage is not emptied from the system when the output measurement is taken. The drainage level is marked on the outside of the drainage container at each measurement, and the amount of fluid between the previous mark and the current mark is calculated for the output measurement. Disposable plastic chest drainage systems may have three columns for drainage. If the drainage container has been tipped or moved, the drainage may have run into the other columns, requiring marking and calculating the drainage in all the columns.

▶ ASSESSMENT

1. Assess the chest drainage system **to determine how the drainage will be measured.**
2. Assess the drainage **to determine its color, consistency, and amount.**

▶ DIAGNOSIS

Risk for Deficient Fluid Volume

▶ PLANNING

Expected Outcomes:

The amount of drainage from the chest drainage system will be accurately determined and recorded.

Equipment Needed:

- Intake and output record
- Marker or pen

▶ CLIENT EDUCATION NEEDED:

1. Explain to the client the need for accurate intake and output measurements.
2. Explain the importance of leaving the drainage system below the level of the chest.
3. Tell the client to be careful not to tip over the drainage system or set it on the bedside table.
4. Explain that movement of the drainage in the tube is normal.

5. Explain that, unlike urine and other drains, it is normal not to empty and discard the drainage container regularly.

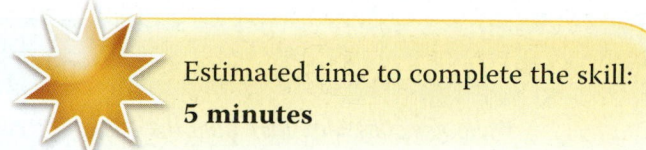

Estimated time to complete the skill:
5 minutes

▶ **DELEGATION TIPS**

Measuring output from chest drainage systems is the responsibility of the nurse and is not delegated. Ancillary personnel should report all concerns or client complaints immediately to the nurse.

IMPLEMENTATION—Action/Rationale

Action	Rationale
1. Wash hands.	1. Reduces the transmission of microorganisms.
2. Determine which bottle or chamber of the chest drainage system contains the drainage (see Figure 7-11-1).	2. Measures the correct fluid level. If the drainage system is a plastic, disposable system, there may be more than one drainage collection column to measure.
3. With the fluid meniscus as close to eye level as possible, note the level of the drainage.	3. For as accurate a reading as possible.
4. Use the pen or marker to mark the current fluid level. Indicate the time and date of the measurement and mark it with your initials.	4. For continuity of care, so the next nurse will know where and when the last measurement was taken.
5. Note the level of drainage marked just prior to this measurement. Subtract the previous drainage total from your current drainage total to obtain an accurate determination of the amount of drainage during that time period.	5. By subtracting the total amount of previous drainage from the total amount of current drainage, the difference will indicate the amount of drainage since the last measurement.
6. Note the amount of drainage since the last measurement on the intake and output record (see Figure 7-11-2). If the drainage is more than 100 mL per hour, notify the health care provider.	6. Provides an accurate record of the client's output.
7. Wash hands.	7. Reduces the transmission of microorganisms.

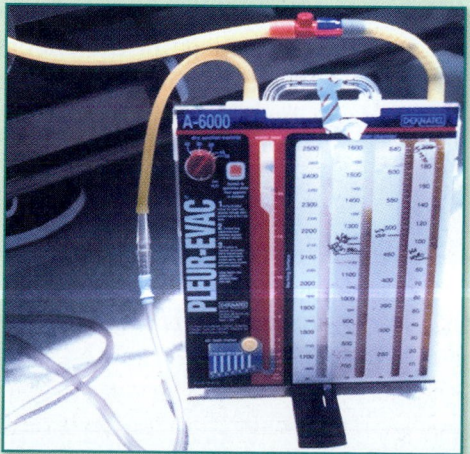

Figure 7-11-1 Check the chest tube drainage system and measure the correct fluid level.

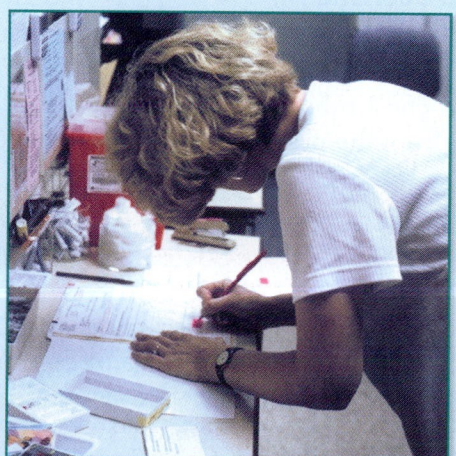

Figure 7-11-2 Record the drainage on the input and output record.

► REAL WORLD ANECDOTES

While assisting Mrs. Rios from the bed to the commode, the nurse accidentally knocked over the plastic chest drainage unit. The water seal was intact, and Mrs. Rios denied any shortness of breath or distress. When righting the unit, the nurse noted that the drainage that had been present only in the first column of the drainage chamber had spilled into the other two columns. As a result, the previous shift's drainage mark was no longer accurate. The nurse didn't know how she would determine the next output reading from Mrs. Rios's chest tube. Rather than take the time and trouble to mark all the columns, add the amounts up from each column, and then subtract the previous total, the nurse estimated the amount of drainage based on the drainage from the previous shift. Because she hadn't marked all the columns, the next nurse caring for Mrs. Rios was unable to obtain an accurate drainage measurement. As a result, it was almost 24 hours before it was discovered that Mrs. Rios had had almost no drainage from her chest tube since the incident when the chest drainage container was tipped over. When the lack of drainage was finally discovered, Mrs. Rios's doctor stripped the chest tube, dislodging a clot. After passing the clot, the chest tube almost immediately drained a large amount of serosanguineous fluid.

► EVALUATION

- The amount of drainage from the chest drainage system was accurately determined and recorded.

► DOCUMENTATION

Input and Output Record

- Note the amount of drainage in the intake and output record. If the amount is significantly different from previous readings, indicate this.

Document on appropriate flow sheet or electronic medical record (EMR).

► CRITICAL THINKING SKILL

Introduction

Subtract the old drainage total from the new drainage total to get the amount of drainage for the shift.

Possible Scenario

You are calculating the intake and output totals at the end of the shift for your client, Mr. Miles. As you check his chest tube drainage, you note that there is no mark from the previous shift's measurement.

Possible Outcome

Without any notation from the previous shift's output, you note the last mark on the drainage container. It was applied 16 hours earlier. As an estimate of the shift output, you divide the amount of drainage following the mark 16 hours earlier in half, estimating that the drainage was probably approximately equal the last two shifts. When you return to duty the next day, you hear in report that Mr. Miles developed a hemothorax in the night from a clot in his chest tube. The clot and lack of drainage went unnoticed for a prolonged period of time because of the incorrect chest tube output you recorded the day before.

Prevention

You mark the current drainage level and note the last marked measurement. You then check the chest tube output recorded in the client's chart by the previous shift. By subtracting the amount of recorded drainage from the amount of current, unmarked drainage, you can obtain an accurate reading for the chest tube drainage on your shift. If the previous shift did not record the amount of drainage in the client's chart, you should record the total unmarked amount and note that this is a 16-hour total.

► VARIATIONS

Geriatric Variation:

- *Elderly clients may be at increased risk of dehydration secondary to large amounts of chest tube drainage. Monitor the elderly client's intake and output closely.*

continues

▶ VARIATIONS *(continued)*

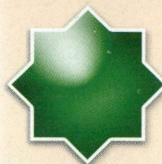

Pediatric Variation:
- *Children are susceptible to dehydration with much smaller fluid losses than adults. Chest tube drainage should be monitored very closely to be sure the volume of drainage is within acceptable fluid loss limits.*

Home Care Variation:
- *Chest tubes are not generally left in place in the home care setting.*

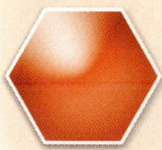

Long-Term Care Variation:
- *Chest tubes are not generally left in place for long-term care.*

▶ COMMON ERRORS

Possible Error:

If the water seal bottle is also the drainage bottle, the baseline amount is not subtracted, and results in an inaccurate reading.

Prevention:

If the water seal bottle will also collect drainage, mark the water level when the chest drainage system is first set up to provide a baseline for drainage calculations.

▶ NURSING TIPS

- Measure the output at the meniscus.
- If the drainage amount seems to be very different from that of the previous shift, investigate possible reasons.
- While measuring the drainage, check lung sounds and assess the wound site.
- Document your findings.

▶ SPECIAL CONSIDERATIONS

- *Secure the drainage system to a steady object such as the bed frame or floor. In some situations the unit is taped to the floor; however, it is critical to be alert to the length of tube and take precautions when moving the client or bed. In most drainage systems, if the container is tipped over and the drainage spilled through the chambers, the output measure is difficult to trace.*
- *When measuring the output, evaluate the quantity and color of the drainage. If the drainage suddenly becomes bright red, and the amount rapidly increases, check vital signs and notify the health care provider.*

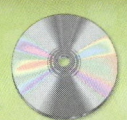

SKILL 7-12

Obtaining a Specimen from a Chest Drainage System

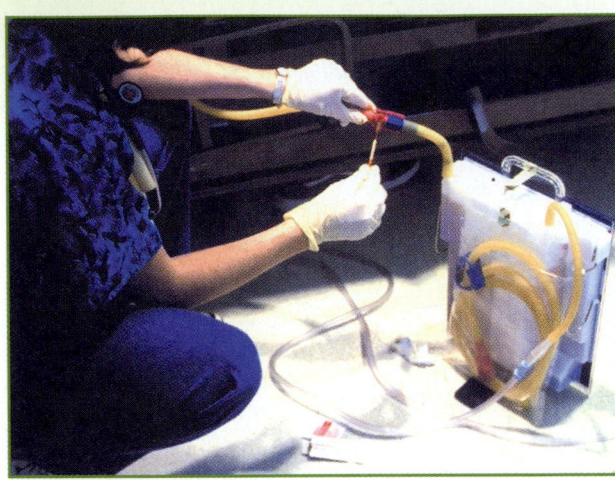

▶ OVERVIEW OF THE SKILL

The chest drainage system is a closed system designed to drain air or fluid from the pleural cavity and help restore its vacuum seal. Occasionally, the drainage will need to be sampled. If the client has signs of infection or if the drainage is copious or an unusual color, a specimen may be obtained for analysis. Because the chest drainage system is closed, the specimen must be obtained using a closed technique.

▶ ASSESSMENT

1. Assess the physician's or qualified practitioner's orders to determine what kind of specimen is required.
2. Assess the available equipment to determine what kind of equipment will be needed for the specimen retrieval.

▶ DIAGNOSIS

Risk for Infection

▶ PLANNING

Expected Outcomes:

The chest drainage specimen will be obtained without increasing the client's risk of infection or loss of air seal.

Equipment Needed (see Figure 7-12-1):

- Povidone-iodine swabs

- Syringe with needle (syringe size determined by the amount of drainage needed for the specimen)
- Specimen container
- Label for specimen container
- Lab slip

▶ CLIENT EDUCATION NEEDED:

Explain to the client the reason for collecting the specimen.

Estimated time to complete the skill: **10 minutes**

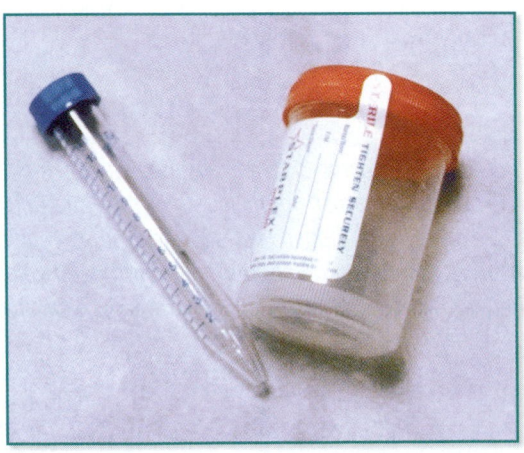

Figure 7-12-1 Two types of sterile specimen containers

938

► DELEGATION TIPS

Obtaining a specimen from chest drainage systems requires sterile technique. It is the responsibility of the nurse and is not delegated to ancillary personnel.

IMPLEMENTATION—Action/Rationale

Action	Rationale
1. Wash hands.	1. Reduces the transmission of microorganisms.
2. Determine if there is drainage in the tubing. If not, curl the tubing on the bed.	2. Obtains fresh drainage for a specimen.
3. Apply clean gloves.	3. Prevents contact with bodily fluids.
4. If an access port is present in the tubing, cleanse it with povidone-iodine if the client is not allergic or sensitive to iodine products (see Figure 7-12-2). If there is no access port, cleanse the rubber tubing, near the drainage pool, with povidone-iodine (see Figure 7-12-3).	4. Prevents the introduction of microorganisms into the closed system. Some institutions may use non-iodine products. Alcohol-based products may cause burning.
5. Puncture the access port or the rubber tubing with the syringe and needle. Puncture at a 45-degree angle (see Figure 7-12-4).	5. Withdraws the drainage specimen without opening the system. Use a 45-degree angle to reduce the possibility of puncturing the opposite side of the tubing and to increase the "seal" of the rubber after the needle has been removed.
6. Gently withdraw the needed amount of drainage from the tubing.	6. Obtains a sterile specimen. Gentle suction avoids increasing the suction in the client's chest to dangerous levels.

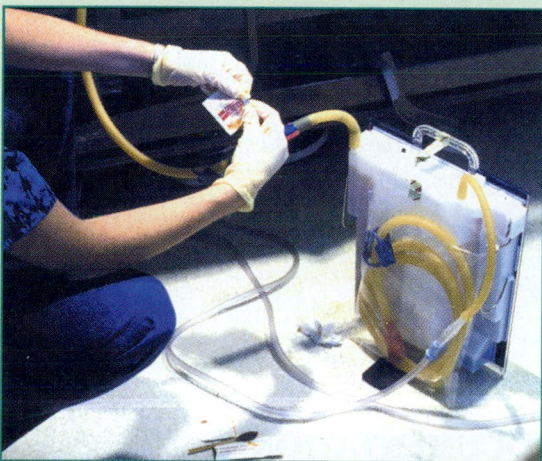

Figure 7-12-2 Use a povidone-iodine swab to clean the access ports in the chest tube tubing (if this is the protocol of the institution).

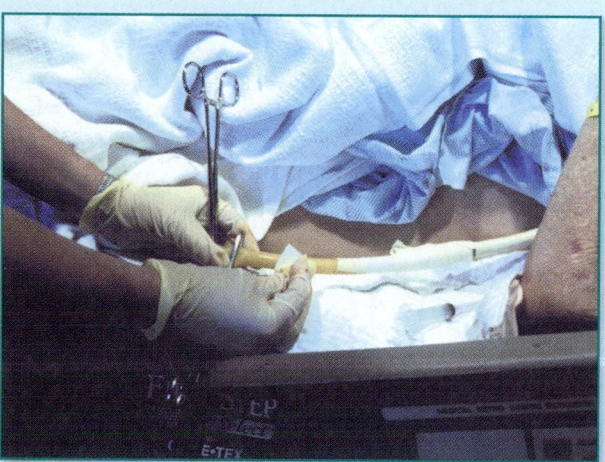

Figure 7-12-3 If there is no access port, clean the rubber tubing itself.

continues

Action	Rationale

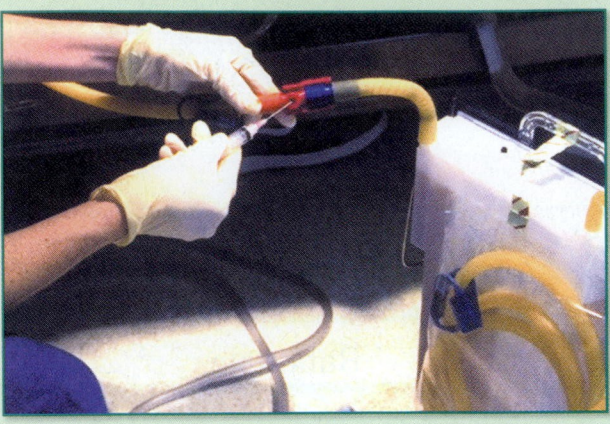

Figure 7-12-4 Puncture the access port at a 45-degree angle.

7. Remove the needle from the port or tubing and place the drainage specimen into a laboratory specimen container, or label the syringe and send it to the laboratory, depending on institutional policy.

7. Allows proper testing of the specimen and prevents possible contamination in the laboratory.

8. Dispose of the syringe and needle in the appropriate container.

8. Observes Standard Precautions.

9. Label the specimen container with the client's name, room number, the date, and the time the specimen was collected.

9. Allows proper identification of the specimen and reduces the opportunity for laboratory error.

10. Remove gloves and dispose of in the proper container.

10. Observes Standard Precautions.

11. Wash hands.

11. Reduces the transmission of microorganisms.

► REAL WORLD ANECDOTES

When a chest drainage specimen was ordered by Mrs. Ipsen's physician, her nurse hastened to comply. It was getting close to the end of her shift and she wanted to get this order taken care of quickly. When the nurse arrived at Mrs. Ipsen's bedside, she noted that there was no drainage in the tubing. She did not want to wait for more drainage to collect, so she gently lifted the drainage collector level with the client and poured some of the collected drainage back into the tubing. She then aspirated the drainage to send to the lab.

When the lab results returned, they indicated a large growth of several pathogens. Luckily, Mrs. Ipsen's physician noted that Mrs. Ipsen's condition did not match the seriousness of the lab results. He personally collected a drainage specimen and had a heated discussion with the charge nurse regarding the proper collection of specimens.

► EVALUATION

- The chest drainage specimen was obtained without increasing the client's risk of infection or loss of air seal.

► DOCUMENTATION

Nurses' Notes

- Indicate the date and time the specimen was collected. Keep a copy of the lab slip in the chart if the lab slip has a chart copy.

Document on appropriate flow sheet or electronic medical record (EMR).

Intake and Output Record

- If the client's chest tube drainage is being monitored closely, indicate the amount of drainage removed.

► CRITICAL THINKING SKILL

Introduction

Understand the physics underlying the chest tube setup.

Possible Scenario

Mr. Rosario's physician ordered a chest tube drainage specimen collected. The nurse assigned to care for Mr. Rosario collected the necessary equipment and took it to Mr. Rosario's bedside. There was no drainage in the tubing when the nurse checked Mr. Rosario's tubing. Thinking she would use the same technique as collecting a urine specimen from a closed system, the nurse clamped the chest tube to allow a drainage specimen to collect.

Possible Outcome

Within 15 minutes Mr. Rosario was in severe respiratory distress. He turned on his call light and started to call for help. His nurse ran to his bedside. As she assessed his condition, she realized that his distress must somehow be related to the clamped chest tube and she quickly unclamped the tube. Within minutes Mr. Rosario's condition stabilized. When the nurse checked the tubing, she noted that there was still no drainage in the tube.

Prevention

If the nurse had understood the physics underlying the chest tube system, she would have realized that clamping the chest tube would block drainage from the chest because the suction was blocked. Also by blocking the suction she had prevented the chest drainage system from reinflating the client's lung, potentially causing a tension pneumothorax. If there is no drainage in the tubing, the nurse should create a dependent loop in the tubing that will collect future drainage that can be used for a specimen.

► VARIATIONS

Geriatric Variation:
- *Elderly clients may be hearing-impaired or confused. Be sure they can hear and understand your instructions.*

Pediatric Variation:
- *Tell the child that obtaining a specimen will not hurt. Remind the child that the needle will not be going into him or her. Let the child watch, if possible, while you collect the specimen. Answer questions about the chest drainage system and how it works.*

Home Care Variation:
- *Not applicable.*

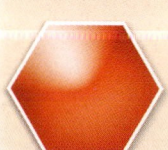

Long-Term Care Variation:
- *Not applicable.*

▶ COMMON ERRORS

Possible Error:

The needle is inserted at a 90-degree angle into the port or rubber tubing.

Prevention:

Insert the needle at a 45-degree angle to help the rubber "heal" itself and to prevent the needle from piercing the far side of the tubing.

▶ NURSING TIPS

- Use gentle suction when withdrawing the specimen to avoid increasing the suction level in the pleural cavity.
- Insert the needle at a 45-degree angle to decrease the chance of puncturing the far side of the tubing as well as to provide a better seal after withdrawing the needle.
- While obtaining a sample, check for leaks in the system and check that connections are secure.
- While obtaining a sample, check for other signs of infection.

▶ SPECIAL CONSIDERATIONS

- *Most chest tube drainage systems have one or two specimen collection ports, which are made with self-sealed materials. The specimen collected at the port closest to the client represents more recent drainage.*

Removing a Chest Tube

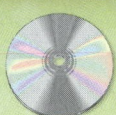

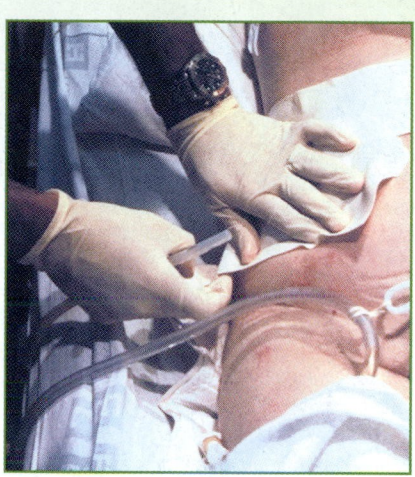

▶ OVERVIEW OF THE SKILL

Chest tubes are removed by the health care provider, with the assistance of the nurse. Generally, a chest tube has been placed during thoracic surgery to remove a collection of fluid or air (a hemothorax or pneumothorax) between the parietal pleura and the visceral pleura, or after cardiac surgery to prevent a collection of fluid or blood in the mediastinum, which could lead to cardiac tamponade. Chest tubes are also placed in the case of spontaneous pneumothorax. The chest tube is removed once the lung has reexpanded and there is minimal drainage, or the risk of fluid collection in the mediastinum is diminished post-cardiac surgery.

▶ ASSESSMENT

1. Assess whether the client has a new or larger air leak present before chest tube removal and notify the health care provider. **A new air leak or a larger air leak may indicate a new or enlarging pneumothorax, and removal may need to be postponed.**
2. Ensure that the client has had a chest X-ray before the removal of the chest tube. **This assesses whether the lung is expanded prior to chest tube removal.**
3. Check that your client has received pain medication before chest tube removal. **Although it is a brief procedure, it can be uncomfortable.**

4. Assess the anxiety level of the client regarding the chest tube removal procedure **to determine what education, support, and/or medication might be needed.**
5. Assess that the client has tolerated the absence of chest tube suction for 1–2 days before chest tube removal **to confirm the appropriate time to remove the tube.**
6. Check when the health care provider is planning to remove the tube **to allow time to gather supplies and prepare the client.**
7. Assess that the client can assist with the chest tube removal by performing the Valsalva's maneuver at the appropriate time **to prevent air from being pulled back into the pleural space at the moment of chest tube removal.**

▶ DIAGNOSIS

Pain

Ineffective Breathing Pattern

▶ PLANNING

Expected Outcomes:

1. Client will have the chest tube removed without complication.
2. The nurse will assist with the procedure while avoiding exposure to bodily fluids.
3. Client will not experience undue pain or anxiety during the chest tube removal.

943

Equipment Needed (see Figures 7-13-1A and 7-13-1B):

- Sterile gloves, (gowns and goggles if needed)
- Vaseline gauze (1 package for each chest tube to be removed)
- Sterile 4 × 4 pads (2 packages for each chest tube to be removed)
- Foam tape, preferably a 2-inch roll
- Disposable waterproof absorbing pads
- Sutures, if requested by health care provider
- Suture removal kit or sterile scissors, if requested by health care provider
- Chest tube clamps
- Pain medication to premedicate the client 15–30 minutes before chest tube removal, if possible
- Requisition for chest X-ray post-chest tube removal

► CLIENT EDUCATION NEEDED:

1. Explain the rationale for the removal of the chest tube.
2. Explain the rationale for taking the pain medication.
3. Explain to clients that they will be asked to help during the removal of the chest tube by taking a deep breath and holding it while bearing down slightly (as if to have a bowel movement). Explain to clients that this exercise will help to prevent them from re-collecting air in their lung space.
4. Explain to clients that the dressing over the site of the chest tube will need to remain in place for at least 24 hours.
5. Teach clients the signs and symptoms of pneumothorax (shortness of breath, chest pain, or pain with inspiration) and instruct clients to notify the nurse if they have any of the symptoms.

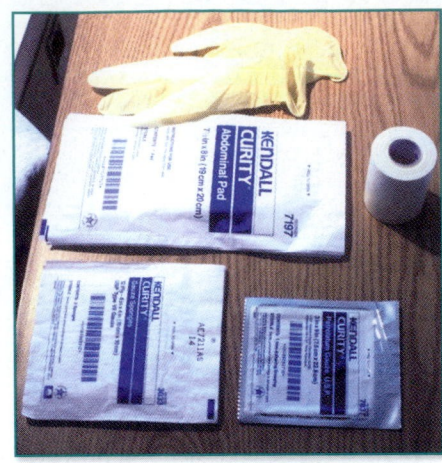

Figure 7-13-1A Vaseline gauze, dressings, rubber gloves, and tape are used when removing a chest tube.

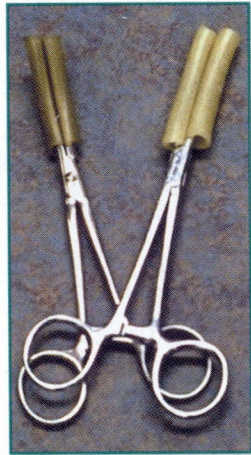

Figure 7-13-1B Chest tube clamp

Estimated time to complete the skill: **15–20 minutes**

► DELEGATION TIPS

Assisting the health care provider in the removal of a chest tube is the responsibility of the nurse and is not delegated. Ancillary personnel should be instructed to report any abnormal responses or complaints of difficulty with breathing postprocedure to the nurse immediately.

IMPLEMENTATION—Action/Rationale

Action	Rationale
1. Gather all equipment in the client's room (see Figure 7-13-2).	1. Ensures that everything is available for the physician or qualified practitioner and does not prolong the procedure.
2. Wash hands.	2. Reduces the transmission of microorganisms.

continues

Action	Rationale

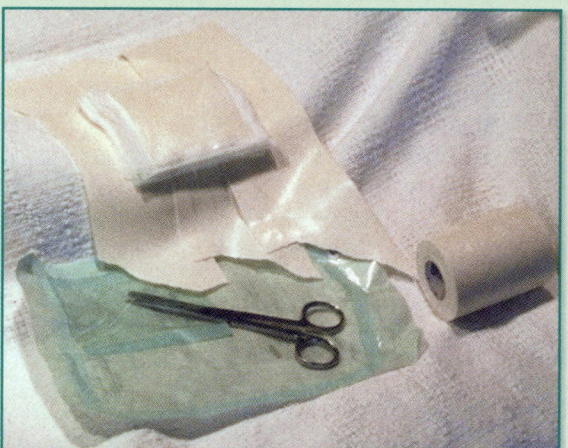

Figure 7-13-2   Gather equipment at the bedside.

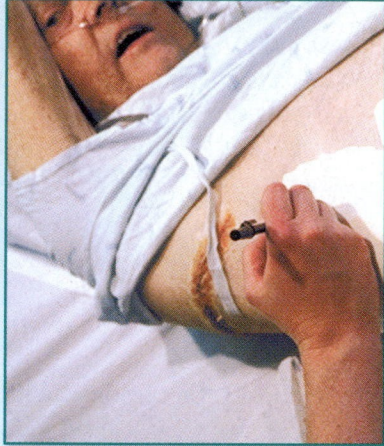

Figure 7-13-3   The dressing applied immediately after the drainage tube is removed should not be changed for at least 24 hours. Mark the current date and time on the dressing.

Action	Rationale
3. Premedicate the client.	3. Decreases the discomfort of chest tube removal.
4. Assist the client into bed and place in accessible and comfortable position for chest tube removal.	4. Ensures safe and comfortable position for chest tube removal.
5. Reassure client and explain what you are doing as you proceed.	5. Decreases anxiety and alleviates fears.
6. Assess for effects of premedication on respiratory status.	6. Monitors for possible respiratory depression.
7. Apply gloves.	7. Decreases risk of exposure to bodily fluids.
8. Assist physician or qualified practitioner as directed.	8. Facilitates safe removal of the chest tube.
9. Once the tube is out and the dressing is applied, check that the dressing is secure and airtight. The dressing should not be removed for 24 hours; if drainage is soaking through, reinforce with 4 × 4 pads and foam tape (see Figure 7-13-3).	9. Reduces risk of pneumothorax post-chest tube removal.
10. Check that the post-chest tube removal X-ray has been ordered.	10. Determines whether a pneumothorax is present post-chest tube removal.
11. Auscultate lung sounds.	11. Determines adequate air movement.
12. Check that the health care provider has properly disposed of the drainage system in the biohazards waste can.	12. Ensures correct handling of biohazards and decreases risk of exposure.
13. Dispose of gloves and wash hands.	13. Reduces the transmission of microorganisms.
14. Assess client in 30 minutes, watching for signs and symptoms of a pneumothorax, including rapid heart rate, decreased breath sounds, increased shortness of breath, decreased oxygen saturation, chest pain, or pain with inspiration. Assess the dressing. Be sure it is dry and intact.	14. Ensures early recognition of a post-chest tube removal pneumothorax.

▶ **EVALUATION**

- Client had the chest tube removed without complication.
- The nurse assisted with the procedure while avoiding exposure to bodily fluids.
- Client did not experience undue pain or anxiety during the chest tube removal.

▶ **DOCUMENTATION**

Nurses' Notes

- Document chest tube removal procedure.
- Note the health care provider performing the procedure.
- Indicate client was premedicated.
- Note client's response to the medication.
- Document outcome of the procedure.
- Note the status of the dressing.
- Document completion of the chest X-ray.
- Document assessment of the client post-chest tube removal.
- Record time procedure was completed.

Document on appropriate flow sheet or electronic medical record (EMR).

Medication Administration Record

- Indicate client was premedicated.
- Document client's response to the medication.

▶ **CRITICAL THINKING SKILL**

Introduction

It is important to reassess the client post-chest tube removal and be able to recognize signs and symptoms of a pneumothorax.

Possible Scenario

A physician removed a pleural chest tube from a client 30 minutes ago. The nurse has just returned to reassess the client and finds the client extremely anxious and in respiratory distress. Upon further assessment, the nurse finds that the airtight dressing has peeled loose, and the chest tube site is exposed.

Possible Outcome

The nurse immediately replaced the airtight dressing to stop more air from being pulled back into the pleural space, and he notified the doctor immediately. A new chest tube was reinserted and attached to suction. If the nurse had not returned promptly to reassess the client, this setback could have evolved to respiratory failure and/or arrest.

Prevention

It is essential to check that the dressing is intact and airtight after a chest tube has been removed. The nurse needed to instruct the client to call for assistance immediately if the client noticed any shortness of breath or if the dressings loosened.

▶ **VARIATIONS**

Geriatric Variation:
- *Older clients may not hear well, so it is important to assess whether they have heard and understood the instructions for breathing during the removal of the chest tube. Allow time to practice the Valsalva's maneuver.*

continues

► **VARIATIONS** *(continued)*

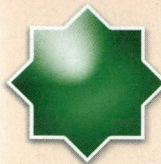

Pediatric Variations:

* *Younger clients may not understand the instructions for breathing or they may not be mature enough to coordinate the breathing. It is important that this is assessed prior to the removal. Allow extra time to teach the child what will be happening and what special kinds of breathing will be necessary. Practice.*
* *Use special hand signals to assist the child, or have a parent in the room do the breathing along with the child. For example, fingers held over the lips indicate it is time to hold the breath.*
* *A younger client may be less anxious with a parent in the room to provide support and distraction during the procedure.*

Home Care Variation:

* *Chest tubes are generally not used in the home care setting.*

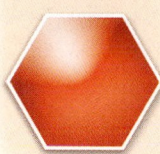

Long-Term Care Variation:

* *Chest tubes are generally not used in the long-term care setting.*

► **COMMON ERRORS**

Possible Error:

The dressing is not intact.

Prevention:

Always assess that the dressing is secure before leaving the client.

Possible Error:

The drainage system is disposed of in the wrong waste can.

Prevention:

Check that the physician or qualified practitioner has disposed of the system in the biohazards waste.

► **NURSING TIPS**

* If your client has a tape allergy or has skin breakdown, DuoDerm can be used around the tube site, and foam tape can be applied to this surface rather than the skin.
* Use water-absorbent pads beneath the client on the side the tube is to be removed. This will absorb any drainage that may leak and prevent a complete bed change.
* Supply the physician or qualified practitioner with two packets of 4 × 4 pads in addition to the Vaseline packet for each chest tube site that is to be dressed. This will allow for enough absorption as this dressing should remain in place for 24 hours.

► SPECIAL CONSIDERATIONS

- *After removing the chest tube, check vital signs and auscultate lung sounds regularly. Monitor for signs of respiratory distress, asymmetry of chest expansion, labored breathing, and level of consciousness.*
- *If the chest tube was in place to remove drainage in the pericardial space following open heart surgery, auscultate and percuss lungs to monitor for hemothorax as well as pericardial tamponade. Assess heart sounds for regularity and quality. Pericardial tamponade may be identified by muffled heart sounds, dull percussion, a paradoxic blood pressure, tachycardia, and/or other signs of decreased cardiac output.*
- *If the chest tube was in place for lung reexpansion, pneumothorax, or drainage, auscultate and percuss the lungs and compare sides of the chest for inequality.*
- *A pneumothorax and even a tension pneumothorax can occur after chest tube removal. Be alert for shortness of breath, decreased breath sounds, tachycardia, anxiety, and hyperresonant percussion sounds over the area of the pneumothorax. If a tension pneumothorax (generally from a flap of tissue creating a one-way valve) ensues, the trachea may deviate to either side, along with a drop in blood pressure as cardiac output is depressed from the pressure on the heart. An acute crisis exists and shock will be encountered. Call the health care provider who will most likely immediately reinsert the chest tube or a chest needle.*

Ventilating the Client with an Ambu®-Bag

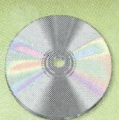

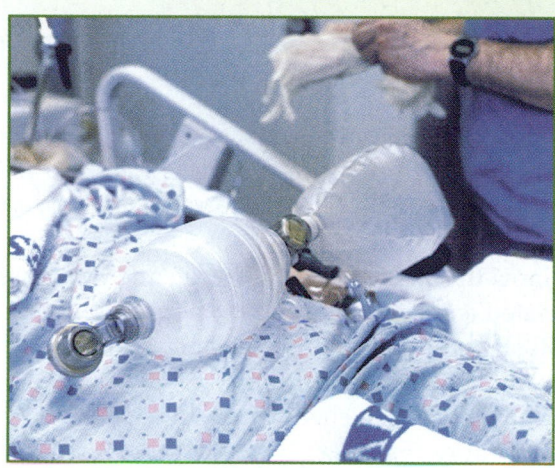

▶ OVERVIEW OF THE SKILL

An Ambu®-bag is an "air mask bag unit" that is used in numerous situations that require manual ventilation. Common uses of the Ambu®-bag include manual ventilation before and after suctioning an endotracheal or tracheostomy tube, emergency resuscitation in the event of respiratory or cardiopulmonary arrest, hyperventilation of the client with increased intracranial pressure (ICP), and maintenance of respiratory support during the transfer of ventilator-dependent clients between care locations.

The Ambu®-bag is manufactured in infant, child, and adult models capable of delivering inspiratory volumes of 240–2000 mL per breath. It is made up of five basic components: a mask, an adapter for endotracheal or tracheostomy tubes, the bag (also referred to as a reservoir), an air control flow system, and an oxygen adapter. Reservoir tubing may also be used to increase oxygen levels.

Operation of the Ambu®-bag is simple; however, incorrect technique may significantly compromise the client's respiratory status. To use the Ambu®-bag, the mask is either placed over the client's nose and mouth, making a seal between the mask and the skin, or is connected to the endotracheal or tracheostomy tube using the adapter. Additional oxygen may be added to the air in the reservoir. The bag, or reservoir, is then compressed with one or two hands, forcing the air into the client's lungs. Once released, the bag automatically reinflates and additional breaths can be delivered as needed.

▶ ASSESSMENT

1. Determine the need to use manual ventilation. There are many situations that require the use of manual ventilation. **Some situations are planned, such as client transfer or suctioning, while others are unexpected emergencies.**

2. Identify signs and symptoms that may indicate the need to provide manual ventilation. **It is imperative that a nurse assess the client for skin color that is dusky or cyanotic in appearance and decreased or absent (apnea) respirations/pulse, which indicate cardiopulmonary arrest. Laboratory results such as arterial blood gas may indicate elevated CO_2 and decreased O_2 levels; client monitoring equipment such as pulse oximetry may set off an alarm with decreasing O_2 saturation; and intracranial pressure monitors may become elevated with increasing CO_2.**

3. Review medical history **to identify factors that could affect respiratory status. This includes a history of central nervous system insult (such as trauma, central nervous system tumor, seizures), alcohol or drug overdose, altered level of consciousness, and respiratory alkalosis or acidosis. It also can occur with pulmonary injury or inability of the thoracic cage to generate pressure gradients needed for ventilation trauma (chest trauma, diaphragmatic hernia, motor vehicle accident).**

4. In assessment of the alert client (such as a ventilator-dependent client requiring transfer to another room), assess the client's knowledge and ability to cooperate with the procedure. **Clients may become anxious when suctioned or moved. It is important to provide an explanation of the planned procedure, length of time, and activities the client can do to assist in a smooth process. Additionally, some alert clients have been ventilator dependent for a long time and have caregivers that have been trained to assist in this process.**

▶ **DIAGNOSIS**

Anxiety

Ineffective Airway Clearance

Ineffective Breathing Pattern

Impaired Gas Exchange

Impaired Spontaneous Ventilation

▶ **PLANNING**

Expected Outcomes:

1. The client will have spontaneous respirations or will be maintained on mechanical ventilation with stable vital signs.
2. Laboratory tests and client monitoring equipment will indicate appropriate CO_2 and O_2 levels.
3. Intracranial pressure will be within normal limits.
4. The client will be able to maintain effective ventilation during transportation.
5. The client will have improved airway clearance as evident by removal of secretions and/or mucus plugs from the endotracheal/tracheostomy tube.
6. The client/caregiver will report minimal anxiety related to the procedure.

Equipment Needed (see Figure 7-14-1):

• Disposable gloves
• Ambu®-bag (appropriate reservoir for client size)
• Appropriate-size mask or endotracheal/tracheostomy tube adapter
• Oxygen source (if indicated)
• Oxygen connecting tubing (if indicated)
• Face shield, goggles, or other eye protection
• Suctioning equipment
• Oropharyngeal airway (for unconscious client in cardiopulmonary arrest)

▶ **CLIENT EDUCATION NEEDED:**

1. Explain the purpose of the procedure.
2. Describe the procedure and length of time.

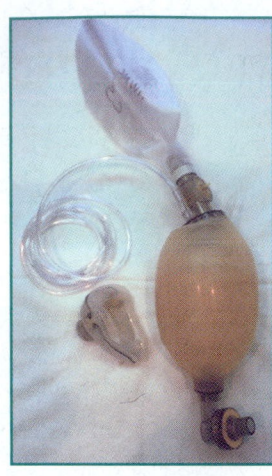

Figure 7-14-1 Manual resuscitator, reservoir bag, tubing, and mask

3. Show the client the Ambu®-bag and other associated equipment.
4. Explain the sensations the client may feel, for example, during suctioning.
5. Explain how the client can help with the procedure.
6. Go over basic messages that the client might need to communicate during the procedure, and assign hand signals.
7. Instruct the alert client to try to breathe with the Ambu®-bag.
8. Teaching relaxation techniques can sometimes minimize the anxiety or restlessness the client may experience during suctioning or transfer.
9. Provide opportunities for a caregiver to practice with the Ambu®-bag on a dummy prior to initial experience on the client.

Estimated time to complete the skill:

1. **In the event of cardiopulmonary arrest, manual ventilation is continued until either spontaneous respiration has returned or the client is placed on mechanical ventilation.**
2. **If a ventilator-dependent client is being transferred between care locations, the length of manual ventilation will correspond to the time required to transfer the client between mechanical ventilation support systems.**
3. **Estimated time to provide hyperinflation before and after suctioning is 5 minutes.**

► **DELEGATION TIPS**

Ventilating a client with an Ambu®-bag may be delegated to ancillary personnel with proper advanced training such as basic life support (BLS) or emergency care. The nurse is still responsible to evaluate the impact and effectiveness of the intervention on the client's clinical status.

IMPLEMENTATION—Action/Rationale

Action	Rationale
1. Obtain baseline assessment of client, including vital signs.	1. Provides a baseline for comparison after procedure to assess tolerance and improvement in clinical status.
2. Prepare, connect, and check functioning of necessary equipment: • Oxygen supply/tubing • Suction equipment/supplies • Correct-size adapter or mask	2. Provides a safe, organized approach to the procedure.
3. Raise or lower bed, table, or transport cart to a comfortable working height.	3. Maintains good body mechanics for the nurse throughout the procedure.
4. Wash hands, apply gloves and face shield.	4. Practices Standard Precautions and reduces the transmission of microorganisms.
5. For the client with an existing endotracheal or tracheostomy tube requiring suctioning or transfer: • Remove the current mechanical ventilation system. • For transfer, attach Ambu®-bag to endotracheal or tracheostomy tube and compress bag to administer one breath every 3–5 seconds. Compress the reservoir 20 times per minute to mimic a normal breathing pattern. • Adjust the flow meter to ensure adequate oxygenation. • The Ambu®-bag may be compressed with two hands if the existing airway tube is stable and the client is not fighting the procedure; otherwise, the nurse may have to use the dominant hand to compress the Ambu®-bag while stabilizing the airway tube during the procedure. It is preferable to have two health care providers perform this skill as Ambu®-bags may be difficult to compress with one hand. • For suction, if the client has thick secretions, some agencies recommend instilling normal saline as per agency protocol (approximately 5–10 mL depending on the health care provider's order). • Suction the client, reattach the Ambu®-bag, and repeat the three preceding steps. • End the procedure with administration of several breaths before reconnecting client to mechanical ventilatory support • The chest is assessed to verify air flow.	5. • Opens airway for Ambu®-bag use. • Provides hyperinflation and increases O_2 levels, which prevents hypoxia, and decreases CO_2 levels prior to suctioning. • Adequate air flow is necessary to fully inflate the lungs. • Maintenance of artificial airway is of paramount importance with the use of an Ambu-bag.® • Normal saline is used to loosen secretions and mucus plugs as well as stimulate coughing. • Removes secretions and mucus plugs, and maintains patency of artificial airway. • Replaces O_2 and prevents atelectasis. • Verification of adequate inspiratory effort.

Action	Rationale
6. For the client who is unconscious and not intubated: • Assess appropriateness of use of Ambu®-bag and need for mask or immediate intervention with intubation. • Clear oral cavity of vomit, mucus, or other debris. • Insert an oropharyngeal airway. • Position client using either the head-tilt/chin-lift method, or in the case of suspected or potential cervical spine injury, use the modified jaw-thrust maneuver. • Position Ambu®-bag over the client's nose and mouth using the nondominant hand. The thumb and index finger are used to stabilize the seal between the mask and the client's face, while the remaining fingers maintain head position. • The dominant hand is used to deliver breaths to the client. Breath rate is administered according to cardiopulmonary resuscitation protocol. • The chest is assessed to verify adequate inspiratory flow. • Assess for the need to insert a nasogastric tube. • Suction as necessary.	**6.** • Some clients presenting with facial injuries will not be appropriate for use of Ambu®-bag with mask, and an endotracheal tube must be placed. • Opens airway; helps prevent aspiration into lungs. • Assists in maintaining airway patency and preventing the tongue from falling back into the oropharynx. • The modified jaw-thrust maneuver maintains the head in a neutral position if a cervical spine injury is suspected. • A proper seal ensures adequate ventilation. • Provides adequate oxygenation per cardiopulmonary resuscitation protocol. • Verifies patent airway and adequacy of manual ventilatory support. • Manual ventilation may force air into the stomach and the client may vomit and aspirate secretions. A nasogastric tube decompresses the air in the stomach. • Suctioning maintains a patent airway and prepares the oropharyngeal cavity for intubation if necessary.
7. Ongoing assessment to determine need to discontinue procedure as evident by: • Endotracheal or tracheostomy secretions minimal and artificial airway patent • Client no longer coughing or "bucking" ventilation • Stable vital signs • Client no longer dusky or cyanotic • Return of spontaneous respirations • Decreased intracranial pressure	**7.** Ongoing assessment is critical in determining improvement or deterioration in the client's clinical status. • Provides information on tolerance of the procedure.
8. Remove Ambu®-bag and reattach client to mechanical ventilation system.	**8.** Maintains ventilatory and oxygen support. Additionally, an unconscious client who required cardiopulmonary resuscitation will probably be intubated and placed on mechanical ventilatory support.
9. Discontinue oxygen flow to the Ambu®-bag.	**9.** Promotes client and staff safety by preventing hyperoxygenation of the room atmosphere.
10. Reposition client and return bed and guard rails to original position.	**10.** Promotes client comfort and safety.
11. Clean supplies per institution protocol (i.e., endotracheal tube adapter).	**11.** Assists in the prevention of infection transmission.

continues

Action	Rationale
12. Dispose of gloves and face shield and disposable supplies used during procedure.	**12.** Promotes adherence to Standard Precautions.
13. Document tolerance of procedure.	**13.** Provides information on airway patency and client knowledge and comfort with procedure.

▶ REAL WORLD ANECDOTES

Scenario 1

The nurse went into Mr. McBride's room and prepared to suction his endotracheal tube. She began the procedure, using an Ambu®-bag to provide hyperinflation and supplemental oxygen to the client during the procedure. While suctioning the client, he became cyanotic and his pulse oximetry suddenly dropped. She began to increase the rate and volume of breaths delivered to the client with no change in his condition. Another nurse who came to the bedside to assist noted that the nurse had failed to check the oxygen tubing connection, which was disconnected, and the client was not receiving oxygen. The nurse was reminded to double-check all equipment prior to starting the procedure.

Scenario 2

An apneic infant is admitted to the emergency room. The nurse grabbed the first Ambu®-bag she saw and attempted to ventilate the client. It was immediately apparent that she had grabbed the child-size Ambu®-bag and not the infant bag. She was unable to make an adequate seal to provide sufficient ventilatory support with the incorrect bag size. Another nurse brought the correct size Ambu®-bag. The infant Ambu®-bag provided the proper equipment for resuscitation.

▶ EVALUATION

- The client has spontaneous respirations or is maintained on mechanical ventilation with stable vital signs.
- Laboratory tests and client monitoring equipment indicate appropriate CO_2 and O_2 levels.
- Intracranial pressure is within normal limits.
- The client is able to maintain effective ventilation during transportation.
- The client has improved airway clearance as evident by removal of secretions, or mucus plugs, from the endotracheal/tracheostomy tube.
- The client experiences minimal anxiety related to the procedure.

▶ DOCUMENTATION

Nurses' Notes

- Document assessments before and after the procedure, including vital signs and other physiologic parameters such as ICP.

- Note length of and tolerance to procedure.
- Record rate of respirations, volume, and amount of supplemental O_2 utilized.
- Describe secretions, including amount and quality.

Document on appropriate flow sheet or electronic medical record (EMR).

▶ CRITICAL THINKING SKILL

Introduction

The use of an Ambu®-bag requires attention to details and continual assessment of the client. Failure to properly assess the client can result in significant adverse outcomes such as loss of airway patency, cardiopulmonary arrest, or paralysis.

Possible Scenario

A ventilator-dependent client, Mr. Ying, needed to be transferred from the intensive care unit to CT scan. This was a multiple trauma client with increased intracranial pressure. The intracranial pressure level was stable and the client was prepared for transfer;

however, the endotracheal tube was not suctioned and portable suction was not taken during the transfer.

Possible Outcome

Failure to ensure that the endotracheal tube was patent and free of secretions prior to transfer of a critically ill, ventilator-dependent client could have resulted in hypoxia, hypercapnia, and increased ICP if the tube became occluded. If portable suction was not available during the transfer, the client could have experienced a prolonged period of insufficient oxygenation and ventilation.

Prevention

Clients who are ventilator dependent and require transfer should have the patency of their artificial airway assessed and be suctioned prior to transfer. In addition, appropriate support supplies should be taken during transfer to help maintain the efficiency of manual ventilation with an Ambu®-bag.

▶ VARIATIONS

Geriatric Variations:

- *Older adults must be assessed for dentures, which need to be removed prior to manual ventilation.*
- *It may be difficult to obtain an occlusive seal in debilitated elderly individuals, and assistance may be necessary to ventilate these clients.*

Pediatric Variations:

- *Appropriate-size (infant or child) Ambu®-bags are essential to provide an occlusive seal and effective air volume. An adult Ambu®-bag mask is never appropriate for use on an infant or child. Many emergency kits or facilities have a single Ambu®-bag with child and infant face mask adapters. Practice quickly removing the adult mask and attaching the child mask.*
- *It is essential to remember that the rate and depth of respirations in children depend on the child's age and correlated lung capacity. Compress the bag only partially with each breath, and deliver breaths more frequently according to the age of the child.*

Home Care Variation:

- *Teach the client (when appropriate) and the caregiver to recognize signs and symptoms of ineffective airway clearance, hypoxia, and abnormal breathing patterns. Because the hand placement is tricky, the caregiver should be given opportunities to practice manual ventilation first with a dummy and then gradually on the client with ample opportunity for return demonstration. Home ventilator-dependent clients or their caregivers are often aware of procedures for suction and care/reinsertion of the tracheostomy tube.*

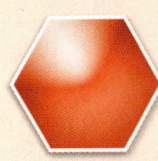

Long-Term Care Variations:

- *Ventilator-dependent clients maintained in long-term care facilities usually have a tracheostomy tube in place as their artificial airway. Care providers need to be aware not only of the use of an Ambu®-bag necessary for suctioning and client transfer but also of the skills needed to maintain a tracheostomy tube.*
- *Additionally, many of the high-tech physiologic assessment tools such as pulse oximetry and arterial blood gases will not be routine practice in long-term care facilities. Careful assessment of airway breathing patterns, lung auscultation, client color, and vital signs will be of tremendous importance in the care of these clients using an Ambu®-bag.*

► COMMON ERRORS

Possible Error:

The nurse does not use Standard Precautions (gloves and face shield) during an emergency situation (cardiopulmonary arrest).

Prevention:

Remember that Standard Precautions can help to prevent life-threatening infections to both the nurse and client, and are just as important in an emergency as in nonemergency procedures. Practice Standard Precautions in every aspect of client care. If the error has already been made, stop and take time to put on gloves and face shield and begin manual ventilation per protocol.

Possible Error:

The correct head position is not used in a client with a potential cervical spine injury.

Prevention:

Gather a history regarding the events that preceded the onset of respiratory arrest. Assess the client fully before intervention with manual ventilation and utilize the appropriate head position in the event of potential cervical spine injury.

► NURSING TIPS

- Check all supplies (oxygen, tubing, and so on) to be sure you are prepared to suction, transfer, or resuscitate a client with functioning equipment.
- Monitor baseline vital signs and maintain continued client assessment throughout the procedure.
- The client should be in a comfortable, relaxed position at a level that is appropriate for the nurse or caregiver to perform manual ventilation.
- Apply pulse oximetry to monitor oxygen saturation.
- The nurse should approach the client with confidence because this will reduce the client's anxiety level.
- Another nurse should be aware of the procedure in progress, and the nurse performing the procedure should be able to obtain assistance in the event of an unexpected outcome.
- Provide comfort measures (e.g., blanket, toy) to the alert child to help reduce anxiety.

► SPECIAL CONSIDERATIONS

- *When providing manual ventilation via Ambu®-bag, the nurse should observe the rise and fall of the client's chest with each squeeze of the bag. If uneven, or one side is rising and not the other, it may indicate atelectasis, collapsed lung, endotracheal tube misplaced, or mucus plug. The trachea may also shift to one side in this situation (tracheal shift).*
- *Know if the Ambu®-bag in your facility is latex-free. Most are latex-free and recommended in emergency situations.*
- *It is sometimes difficult to get a good mask seal over the mouth and nose when ventilating by yourself. If this is the case, ask for additional help so one respondent can hold the seal and the other can ventilate the client by squeezing the bag. When no additional help is available, use both hands to obtain a good mask seal, and position the bag under one arm and squeeze by adducting and abducting the elbow.*

Inserting the Pharyngeal Airway

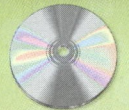

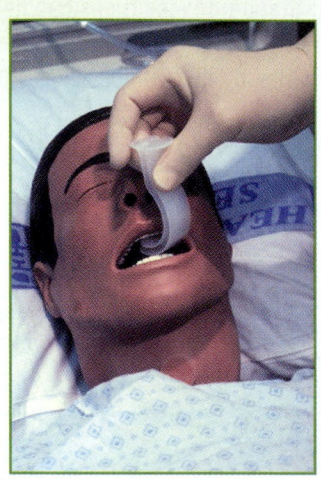

▶ OVERVIEW OF THE SKILL

The pharynx has three anatomic divisions: the nasal pharynx, the oral pharynx, and the laryngeal pharynx. The pharynx functions as a passageway for air into the lungs and for food into the esophagus. It is also involved in filtering, warming, and humidifying the inhaled air. Nasopharyngeal and oropharyngeal artificial airways are used for short-term airway maintenance. They function to hold the tongue forward, away from the posterior wall of the pharynx, and provide an open passageway past the lips and teeth. They are designed to allow airflow around or through them, and they easily accommodate the passage of a suction catheter into the laryngopharynx. These tubes are also used to prevent biting of the endotracheal tube. When properly placed, these airways relieve the rescuer of the necessity for providing continuous chin-lift or jaw-thrust maneuvers. However, even with the airway in place, the head should remain tilted slightly backward. The oropharyngeal tube should be used only in unconscious clients because it may cause gagging, vomiting, or laryngospasm in the client with intact airway reflexes. Nasal airways are more readily tolerated by the semiconscious or stuporous victim and are easier to place. It is important that the nasopharyngeal airway that is used is the correct size. The larger the internal diameter (ID), the longer the tube (see Table 7-15-1).

▶ ASSESSMENT

1. Assess need for pharyngeal intubation. **Indications include apnea or inadequate spontaneous respiratory rate or effort. Client must not have an intact gag reflex.**
2. Assess the age and size of the client **to help select the correct size of pharyngeal tube needed.**
3. Assess response to pharyngeal tube placement. **Monitor for gagging, regurgitation, and need for suctioning.**

▶ DIAGNOSIS

Impaired Gas Exchange

Risk for Trauma

Ineffective Airway Clearance

▶ PLANNING

Expected Outcomes:

1. Airway patency will be established and maintained.

Table 7-15-1 Nasopharyngeal Airway Sizes	
NASOPHARYNGEAL	OROPHARYNGEAL
Large adult: 8.0–9.0 ID	100 mm
Medium adult: 7.0–8.0 ID	90 mm
Small adult: 6.0–7.0 ID	80 mm

2. Suctioning equipment can be passed into the pharyngeal area as needed.

3. The client will not bite the suctioning equipment or the endotracheal tube, if used.

Equipment Needed (see Figure 7-15-1):

- Pharyngeal airway if needed
  a. Large adult—100 mm
  b. Medium adult—90 mm
  c. Small adult—80 mm
- Nasopharyngeal airway if needed—adult size 6.0–9.0 ID
- Suction equipment
- Stethoscope
- Oxygen source
- Water-soluble lubricant

► CLIENT EDUCATION NEEDED:

1. Explain to the client how the tube will feel when placed and that it may produce gagging or regurgitation.

2. Oropharyngeal airway placement is usually performed on the unconscious client, so teaching is not possible.

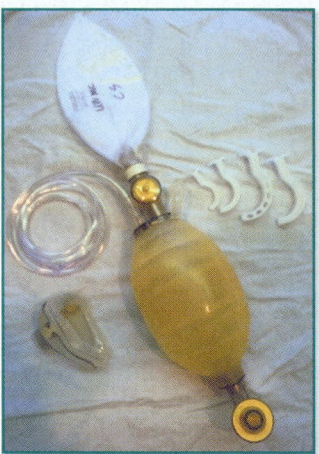

Figure 7-15-1   Resuscitator bag with reservoir, oxygen tubing, face mask, and oral pharyngeal airways

Estimated time to complete the skill: **5–10 minutes**

► DELEGATION TIPS

Inserting a pharyngeal airway may be delegated to ancillary personnel with the proper advanced training such as basic life support or emergency care. The nurse is responsible to evaluate the impact and effectiveness of the intervention on the client's clinical status.

IMPLEMENTATION—Action/Rationale

Action	Rationale
1. Wash hands.	1. Reduces the transmission of microorganisms.
2. Apply clean gloves. Put on mask, eyewear, and gown if there is the risk of vomiting or contact with blood or emesis.	2. Use Standard Precautions when in contact with bodily fluids.
3. Ensure that the mouth and pharynx are cleared of secretions, blood, or vomit using a suctioning catheter. Select appropriate size of pharyngeal airway (Figure 7-15-1).	3. Reduces the potential for aspiration.
4. Nasopharyngeal airway insertion (see Figure 7-15-2): • Lubricate the nasopharyngeal airway with water-soluble lubricant. • Gently insert nasopharyngeal airway close to the midline of the nostril along the floor into the posterior pharynx behind the tongue. Rotate the tube slightly if resistance is encountered.	4. • Ensures smooth introduction of airway past tissues. • Ensures proper placement and minimal trauma to pharynx and surrounding structures.

continues

Action	Rationale

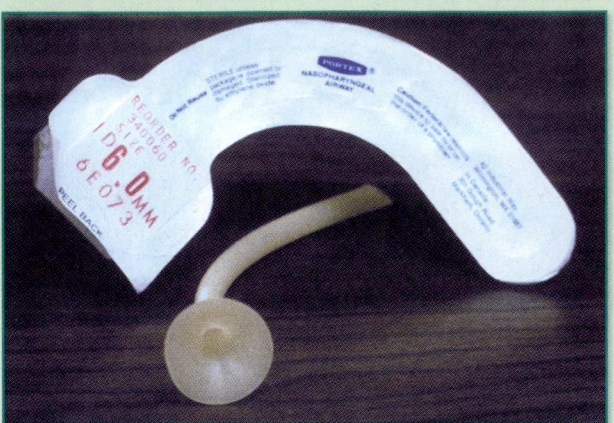

Figure 7-15-2 Nasopharyngeal airway

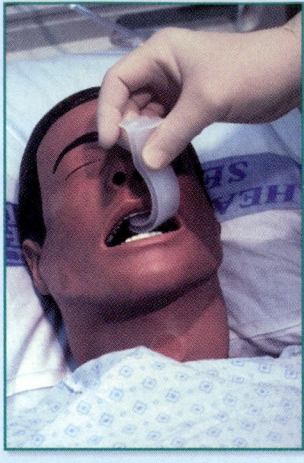

Figure 7-15-3 Turn the oropharyngeal airway upside down and gently slide it into the mouth.

- Reposition the tube to the other nostril per institutional policy.

- Decreases trauma to nostril.

5. Oropharyngeal airway insertion:
   - Gently insert oropharyngeal airway by turning it upside down (into a *U* shape) and sliding it into the mouth (see Figure 7-15-3).
   - As you continue to insert the airway, rotate it so the ends of the *U* turn downward into an arch shape after it transverses the oral cavity and approaches the posterior wall of the pharynx (see Figure 7-15-4).

5. Ensures proper placement and minimal trauma to pharynx and surrounding structures.

6. Maintain head slightly tilted back with chin elevated.

6. Ensures the airway remains patent.

7. Ensure that the airway is in proper position by visually inspecting the mouth and auscultating the lungs.

7. The external part of the airway should be at the entrance to the mouth. The airway should curve over the tongue in alignment with the tongue, in the center of the mouth. Clear breath sounds should be heard on auscultation.

8. Dispose of all soiled material and wash hands.

8. Reduces the transmission of microorganisms.

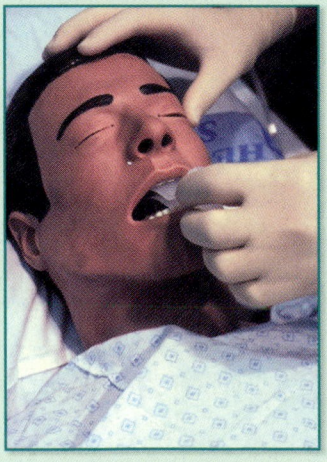

Figure 7-15-4 Rotate the airway until it turns downward and slides into place.

► **REAL WORLD ANECDOTES**

Scenario 1

John is an 88-year-old man admitted to the hospital yesterday for pneumonia. He has had copious secretions and has needed oropharyngeal suctioning occasionally. He is on the medical-surgical floor. His nurse for the day shift enters his room and sees him lying in bed, unresponsive. She attempts to open his airway by lifting his chin and tilting his head, but this is unsuccessful. She decides that she needs to insert a pharyngeal airway and uses a 100-mm tube. After insertion, the airway remains obstructed. A second nurse enters the room and decides that a smaller airway should be inserted (90 mm). The 100-mm airway is removed and replaced with the smaller one. The client is now able to move air into and out of his lungs and the nurse suctions the airway. The nurse learns that if the airway is too long, it may press the epiglottis against the entrance of the larynx and produce complete airway obstruction.

Scenario 2

Miguel needed to have an airway placed to help with suctioning of secretions. The nurse set up the suction equipment and gathered the oropharyngeal airway and other supplies needed. Upon insertion of the oropharyngeal airway, Miguel began to gag and then vomited. The nurse was reminded that an oropharyngeal airway should be placed only in clients who are unconscious. She removed the airway and inserted a nasopharyngeal airway instead. She was able to successfully suction Miguel's secretions through the nasopharyngeal airway.

► **EVALUATION**

- Airway patency was established and maintained.
- Suctioning equipment was passed into the pharyngeal area as needed.
- The client did not bite the suctioning equipment, or the endotracheal tube, if used.

► **DOCUMENTATION**

Nurses' Notes

- Note date and time the airway was inserted.
- Indicate size of pharyngeal airway.
- Document assessment of secretions present and number of times suctioning required.
- Record breath sounds, vital signs, and oxygen saturation.
- Describe client's response to airway placement.
- Include signature of nurse performing this activity.

Document on appropriate flow sheet or electronic medical record (EMR).

► **CRITICAL THINKING SKILL**

Introduction

It is necessary to insert a nasopharyngeal airway into a semiconscious client who is having difficulty clearing secretions and achieving adequate ventilation.

Possible Scenario

The nurse does not have much time to assess a client with increased secretions, and chooses a 90-mm tube and inserts it into the nasal passage.

Possible Outcome

Minutes later, the client experiences hypoventilation. The nurse realizes that the nasopharyngeal tube chosen was too long and it entered the esophagus. The nurse removes the tube and inserts a 70-mm tube instead. The client was successfully suctioned and breath sounds were normal bilaterally.

Prevention

The size of a nasopharyngeal airway is important to assess before insertion. The larger the internal diameter (ID), the longer the tube.

► VARIATIONS

Geriatric Variation:
- *Tissues of elderly clients may be more fragile, so they have increased risk of trauma to the oropharynx or nasopharynx.*

Pediatric Variation:
- *Adult pharyngeal airways are contraindicated in people younger than 16 years of age and those less than 5 feet tall. Child-size airways are available. Make sure you have the right size airway for the size of the child to reduce damage to the tissues and to make sure the airway is effective.*

Home Care Variation:
- *Not applicable.*

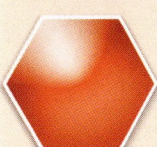

Long-Term Care Variation:
- *Not applicable.*

► COMMON ERRORS

Possible Error:

A water-soluble lubricant was not used when inserting the nasopharyngeal airway.

Prevention:

Always use a lubricant when inserting a nasopharyngeal airway.

Possible Error:

Proper head position was not obtained when inserting the pharyngeal airway with head tilted backward; therefore, it was difficult to insert the airway.

Prevention:

Always tilt the head backward when inserting an oropharyngeal or nasopharyngeal airway and when suctioning the client. Ask for help from an assistant, if available. If unable to insert pharyngeal airway, put head in proper position and attempt reinsertion of pharyngeal airway.

► NURSING TIPS

- Mouth and pharynx should be cleared of secretions, blood, and vomit before pharyngeal airway is inserted.

- A tongue depressor may be useful to move the tongue out of the way when inserting the pharyngeal airway.
- A water-soluble lubricant or anesthetic jelly is helpful when inserting the pharyngeal airway through the nostril.

▶ **SPECIAL CONSIDERATIONS**

- *A nasopharyngeal airway, also called a "trumpet," may accompany a client out of surgery. When asked to remove the "trumpet," the nurse should inform the client and then pull the airway out with a smooth, steady motion. The client should be positioned properly to avoid aspirating in the event of emesis, and may need a tissue for the nose or an emesis basin, as this motion may stimulate the gag reflex.*

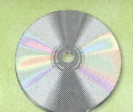

Maintaining Mechanical Ventilation

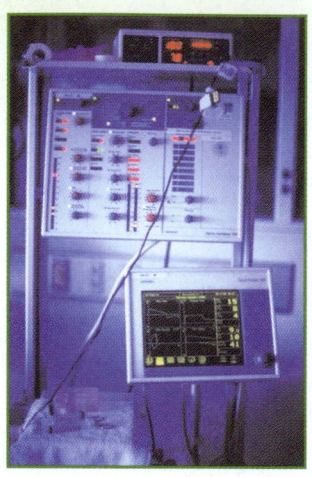

▶ OVERVIEW OF THE SKILL

Mechanical ventilation is used for clients who are in respiratory failure or have chronic obstructive pulmonary disease (COPD), respiratory muscle paralysis, infections involving the pulmonary system such as pneumonia, or neuromuscular diseases. Traditionally, clients requiring mechanical ventilation were managed in the intensive care unit. However, many hospitals care for medically stable ventilator clients on medical-surgical floors and/or step-down units, as well as in the home. There are also facilities that specialize in caring for long-term ventilator clients.

Mechanical ventilation is available via two types of ventilators: positive pressure and negative pressure. Clients who require negative-pressure ventilation are typically those whose illnesses affect respiratory muscle function, such as clients with multiple sclerosis or muscular dystrophy. These clients do not usually need a tracheostomy but are fitted with a shell (or poncho) that is connected to the ventilator. The client is forced to inhale when air is removed from between the interior wall of the shell and the client's chest wall.

Positive-pressure ventilation inflates the lungs using positive pressure. Clients in respiratory failure usually require positive-pressure ventilation. They may require a tracheostomy or may have an endotracheal tube. There are two kinds of positive-pressure ventilators: pressure-cycled ventilators and volume-cycled ventilators. A pressure-cycled ventilator supplies a specified amount of pressure to the client. Clients using pressure-cycled ventilators are at risk for pneumothorax, decreased cardiac output, and hypotension. A volume-cycled ventilator delivers a specified tidal volume to the client. Volume-cycled ventilators are more sensitive to lung compliance and are used more frequently in the acute care clinical setting.

There are many modes of ventilation. These include assist control, control, intermittent mandatory ventilation (IMV), pressure support, and synchronized intermittent mandatory ventilation (SIMV). Positive end expiratory pressure (PEEP) increases oxygenation by allowing more time for gas exchange.

It is essential that the nurses caring for a client on mechanical ventilation have a thorough understanding of the ventilator settings, type of ventilation the client is on, and how to troubleshoot ventilator problems.

▶ ASSESSMENT

1. Understand the rationale for the need for mechanical support for the client, as well as know the ordered settings for the ventilator. **This allows the nurse to compare the ordered settings with the actual settings and also provides the nurse with the information necessary to make accurate nursing judgments about the client.**
2. Assess the client's vital signs, including the most recent arterial blood gas (ABG) results. Also

observe for a patent airway. **This provides the foundation information needed for the nurse to note any change. Also, a patent airway is necessary for the client to receive sufficient oxygenation. Altered vital signs could be an indication of hypoxia.**

3. Assess the client's level of comfort. **Mechanical ventilatory support usually causes some discomfort, and often pain, as well as anxiety. The client should be receiving medication to reduce pain as well as anxiety, particularly if the client is in a drug-induced paralysis, which is often required to assist ventilation.**

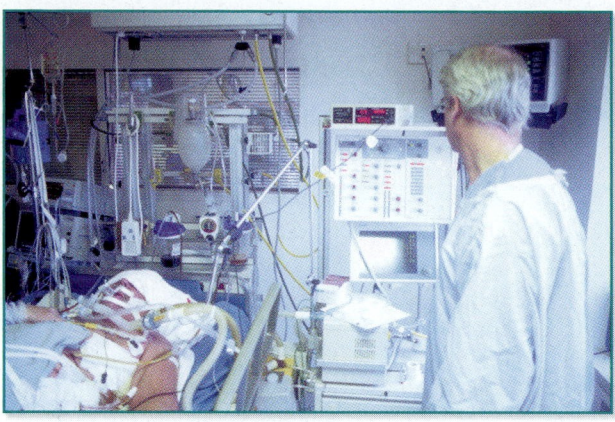

Figure 7-16-1 Mechanical ventilator and tubing

▶ DIAGNOSIS

Impaired Gas Exchange

Ineffective Airway Clearance

Ineffective Breathing

Impaired Spontaneous Ventilation

Deficient Knowledge

Risk for Infection

Anxiety

Impaired Verbal Communication

▶ PLANNING

Expected Outcomes:

1. Client's pain and anxiety will be controlled.
2. Client's ABGs and O_2 saturation levels will be within normal limits, showing adequate oxygen delivery.
3. Client (and family) will understand the need for mechanical oxygenation.

Equipment Needed (see Figure 7-16-1):

• Mechanical ventilator
• Oxygen source
• Humidifier systems
• Gloves
• Ambu®-bag with oxygen connecting tubing
• Tape for supporting endotracheal (ET) tube
• Endotracheal tube or tracheostomy tube

▶ CLIENT EDUCATION NEEDED:

1. Explain the purpose of the ventilation to the client and health care provider/family member.
2. Explain and identify the equipment used in the room because it will be foreign to and may alarm the client.
3. Provide the client with descriptions and explanations of the noises, especially the alarms, the ventilator will emit.
4. Provide the client with an explanation of the health care setting and a description of the immediate environment the client is in (especially if the client is in intensive care or was unconscious before the intubation and placement on mechanical ventilation).
5. Provide constant explanation of what procedures the health care team members are doing as they care for the client.
6. Explain to the client where the nurse is when she is out of eyesight, and give explanations/reassurance of how the client is monitored. Assure the client that assistance is immediately available at all times.

Estimated time to complete the skill:
Maintaining mechanical ventilation is an ongoing process.

▶ DELEGATION TIPS

The initiation and maintenance of mechanical ventilation is not delegated to ancillary personnel. Ancillary personnel may assist the nurse in providing care to clients receiving this treatment and should be instructed to report any abnormal symptoms, such as a change in color, increased blood pressure, tachycardia, anxiety, or the client's breathing against the pattern of the ventilator, to the nurse.

IMPLEMENTATION—Action/Rationale

Action	Rationale
1. Wash hands and apply gloves.	1. Reduces the transmission of microorganisms.
2. Attach the mechanical ventilator to the endotracheal tube (or tracheostomy tube) once the tube is secured.	2. Provides mechanical ventilation.
3. Compare ventilator settings with ordered settings and observe ventilator as it functions (see Figures 7-16-2 and 7-16-3).	3. Ensures equipment is working and that client is receiving oxygen as ordered.

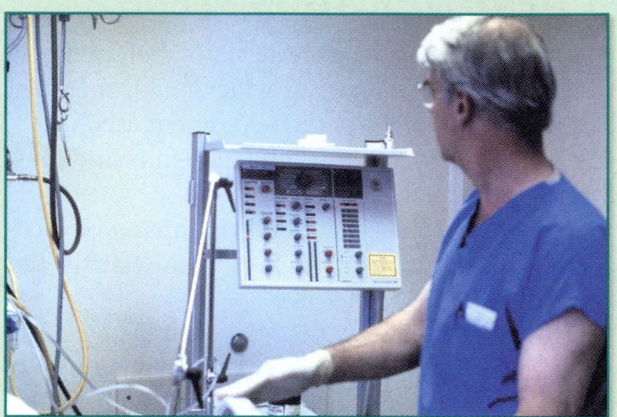

Figure 7-16-2 Check ventilator settings.

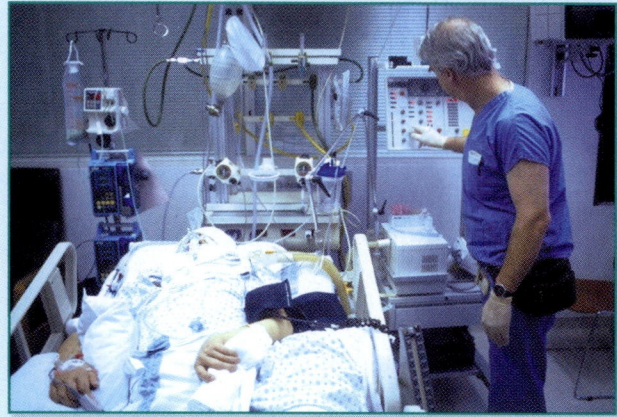

Figure 7-16-3 Observe the ventilator and the client as the ventilator functions.

Action	Rationale
4. Monitor vital signs; observe client for distress and lack of comfort (see Figure 7-16-4).	4. Altered vital signs may indicate that mechanical ventilator settings need to be adjusted. Client may need medication for pain and/or anxiety.
5. Apply pulse oximeter.	5. Monitor oxygen saturation.
6. Set up suction equipment.	6. Suctioning will be required when caring for the client and ensuring the airway is clear.
7. Draw ABGs or assist if the physician or qualified practitioner draws ABGs.	7. Obtains blood sample to verify that adequate oxygenation is being supplied to the client.
8. Remove gloves and wash hands.	8. Reduces the transmission of microorganisms.
9. Periodically empty accumulated water from tubing (see Figure 7-16-5). Make sure there is no water in the tubing prior to turning the client.	9. Prevents a reduction of airflow. Prevents water from moving from the tubing into the lungs.
10. Periodically verify that the Ambu®-bag is at hand where you expect to find it in an emergency.	10. Prevents loss of time searching for manual equipment to maintain airway should the ventilator fail or an emergency arise.

continues

Action	Rationale

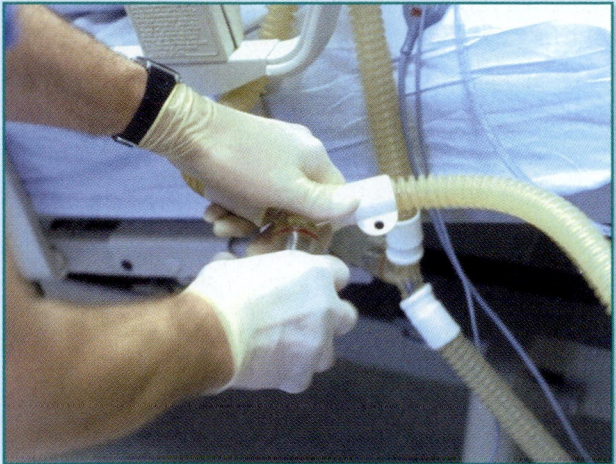

Figure 7-16-5   Periodically empty the accumulated water from the tubing to prevent a reduction of airflow.

Figure 7-16-4   Observe the client for distress and discomfort.

11. Every 2 hours, provide oral care to client, after washing hands and applying gloves.

11. Client with endotracheal tubes will not have oral intake. Clients with tracheostomy tubes can eat and drink. Oral care will be needed to decrease risk of oral cavity infections and dental caries.

12. As needed, provide skin care to client, after washing hands and applying gloves.

12. For clients with endotracheal tubes, the tape on the endotracheal tube will need changing periodically, per institutional policy. Clients with tracheostomy tubes will need skin care around the tube. Overall skin care is especially important with clients on mechanical ventilation because they will most likely be sedated or not able to provide self-care.

13. Document interventions.

13. Provides continuity of care and a record of actions.

▶ REAL WORLD ANECDOTES

Sarah, a 45-year-old woman, had a diagnosis of leukemia. During her admission for induction chemotherapy, she developed a fever of 102° F and became hypotensive and tachycardic. Although she was receiving broad-spectrum antibiotics, after 4 days she was still febrile. Her nurses noted that her respiratory rate was 42 and she was using her accessory muscles to assist in breathing. A chest X-ray showed bilateral patchy infiltrates, and ABGs showed that she was in metabolic acidosis. Sarah was intubated, transferred to the intensive care unit, and put on mechanical ventilation with PEEP. She was also started on dopamine to maintain her blood pressure, as well as a morphine drip at 2 mg/hour for pain. The antibiotics were adjusted, and eventually the infiltrates on the chest X-ray disappeared. After a week, Sarah was weaned off the ventilator and returned to the oncology unit.

► EVALUATION

- Client's pain and anxiety are controlled.
- Client's ABGs and O_2 saturation levels are within normal limits, showing adequate oxygen delivery.
- Client (and family) understand the need for mechanical ventilation.

► DOCUMENTATION

Nurses' Notes

- Document the ventilator settings at the beginning and end of shift, as well as any changes in them throughout the shift.
- Document client responses to the interventions.
- Document vital signs of the client, as well as results of ABGs and any labs drawn, as well as interventions done in response to the results.

Document on appropriate flow sheet or electronic medical record (EMR).

► CRITICAL THINKING SKILL

Introduction

Rapid assessment by a nurse familiar with the equipment and possible equipment errors allowed a timely intervention.

Possible Scenario

The client had been on mechanical ventilation for 48 hours secondary to respiratory failure. His ABGs had improved, and the physician decided to start weaning him from the ventilator. However, the nurse noted that the client had become increasingly agitated and restless.

Possible Outcome

The nurse checked the client's blood vital signs and noted that his blood pressure and heart rate were both elevated. The nurse spoke to the client, trying to ascertain if he was in pain, and when he shook his head to answer no, she started checking the ventilator settings. The alarm button on the ventilator had been pushed to silence the alarm but was flashing, indicating that something was malfunctioning. The nurse noted that the tubing connecting the ventilator to the endotracheal tube had become loosened, probably when the client had been repositioned a few minutes before. The nurse quickly reconnected the tubing and soothed the client, and also increased the FIO_2 for a few seconds to administer an added amount of oxygen to the client until he stabilized, before changing the setting back to the ordered amount. The client's blood pressure and pulse stabilized, and the client calmed down. The nurse explained to the client what had happened and that by taping the connections it would not happen again.

Prevention

Taping the connections could have prevented this from happening. Also, lifting the tubing away from the client and arranging it so that the tension was eased may have eliminated the loosening of the connections. Having another nurse assist with the repositioning of a client helps—one nurse can ensure that there is enough slack in the tubing without it separating, while the other can be away from the ventilator while moving the client.

► VARIATIONS

Geriatric Variations:
- *Geriatric clients may have less flexibility in the lungs because they have had extra years to develop pulmonary damage and changes caused by aging. Care must be taken to ensure that an older client does not develop a pneumothorax.*
- *Geriatric clients are often on a wide variety of medications that may interact with each other, potentially making the client hemodynamically unstable.*
- *It is important to orient the geriatric client to the intensive care unit and assist the client in communication because the environment can cause anxiety and confusion.*

continues

▶ VARIATIONS *(continued)*

Pediatric Variations:
- It will be important to include the family in caring for the child, especially if the child is in the intensive care unit.
- Research has shown that although children respond to pain the same way that adults do, they are often undermedicated. It is important to assess the child for pain and discomfort and medicate accordingly.
- The pediatric client will need to have a means of communicating. If the client is too young to read and write, possibly a board with symbols can be used to assist in communication.

Home Care Variations:
- If the client is stable, very often he or she will be discharged to home on a ventilator.
- Extensive planning and education is required for this to be successful and a teaching plan should be established. The client as well as a caregiver needs to be taught how to use the ventilator, and how to provide oxygen via the Ambu®-bag if the ventilator breaks down.
- It is important that a home care nurse establish a relationship with the client and family and assess the client and caregiver's knowledge level and ability to use the ventilator.
- Make sure the home caregiver and any professional staff in the home know whom to call for emergencies or if the ventilator breaks down.

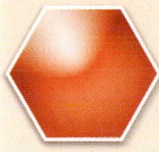

Long-Term Care Variations:
- If a client is to be on mechanical ventilation for a long period of time and is unable to be at home, possibly a facility that specializes in this type of client would be beneficial.
- If the client is to be on a positive-pressure mechanical ventilator for long-term, a tracheostomy should be performed.
- If the client is to be on negative-pressure mechanical ventilation, the client should be encouraged to care for the ventilator him or herself.

▶ COMMON ERRORS

Possible Error:

Water in the tubing is not emptied before turning the client, thus it enters the client's airway as the client is repositioned.

Prevention:

Check tubing carefully before moving a client.

Possible Error:

The high pressure alarm is not audible or is not functioning.

Prevention:

The alarm is often triggered when the client needs to be suctioned. Never disable the alarm.

▶ NURSING TIPS
- Medicate the client for pain before changing the tape on the endotracheal tube and/or repositioning the client.
- Make sure there is no water in the tubing before turning the client.
- Forewarn the family about the equipment and the many intravenous lines and monitors before

they visit the client. Their expression of alarm can frighten the client.

- Help the family and client develop a communication system.
- Do not forget that the client cannot talk but can hear what is being said.
- It should become a habit to check the settings on the ventilator at the beginning and end of each shift, as well as after any manipulation of the ventilator.
- Make sure you understand what each alarm means, how to respond to it, and how to reset the alarm. Request additional education and instruction if you are not familiar with the equipment. Know whom to call if additional assistance is needed.

► SPECIAL CONSIDERATIONS

- *Clients' families may be faced with the decision to remove mechanical ventilation. Many states allow the removal of ventilator support only after three consecutive flat brain waves or electroencephalograms (EEGs) have been obtained. These criteria vary widely among facilities, therefore know policies or laws that govern client and family rights.*
- *Determine if the client has a living will. At times a clinically deceased client will be kept alive via mechanical ventilation for the purpose of harvesting organs. This is done when the client or the family have given consent for organ donation.*

Suctioning Endotracheal and Tracheal Tubes

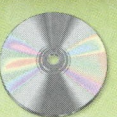

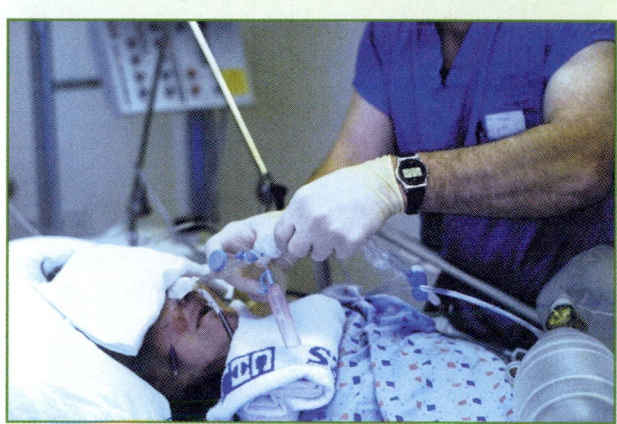

▶ OVERVIEW OF THE SKILL

Suctioning secretions is necessary to maintain the airway of a client who is unable to clear his own secretions by coughing. Some clients may be able to cough but not effectively enough to expel the secretions. Suctioning the client's airway is considered a sterile procedure. Using sterile technique prevents the introduction of contagion into the client's airway and lungs.

Suctioning is performed as often as necessary to remove excess secretions. The procedure may be performed as often as every 5 minutes or as infrequently as every few hours, depending on the amount of secretions the client is generating and the client's ability to clear his or her own airway. The nurse must evaluate the client's airway and oxygenation to determine the need for suctioning. For an adult, wall suction should be set at 100–120 mm Hg (millimeters of mercury); for portable suction, use 8–15 mm Hg. There are variations for children and infants (see Table 7-17-1).

▶ ASSESSMENT

1. Assess respirations for rate, rhythm, and depth **to evaluate airway.**
2. Auscultate lung fields **to evaluate airway and determine need for suctioning.**
3. Monitor arterial blood gas and/or pulse oximetry values **to determine oxygen levels and adequate air exchange.**
4. Assess passage of air through the tracheostomy tube **to determine air exchange and obstruction of the tube.**
5. Monitor tracheal secretions for amount, color, consistency, and odor **to assess for evidence of bleeding or signs of infection and need for suctioning.**
6. Assess for anxiety and restlessness. **Anxiety and restlessness may be signs of airway distress and/or hypoxia.**
7. Assess the client's understanding of the suctioning procedure **to decrease the client's anxiety.**

Table 7-17-1	Amount of Negative Pressure Necessary for Suctioning	
	PORTABLE SUCTION MACHINE	**WALL SUCTION UNIT**
Adult	8–15 mm Hg	100–120 mm Hg
Children	5–8 mm Hg	50–100 mm Hg
Infants	3–5 mm Hg	40–60 mm Hg

▶ DIAGNOSIS

Impaired Gas Exchange

Anxiety

Ineffective Airway Clearance

Risk for Infection

▶ PLANNING

Expected Outcomes:

1. The client will have no crackles or wheezes in large airways and the absence of cyanosis.
2. The client will report breathing comfortably and will have no apparent anxiety or restlessness.
3. The client will have minimal amount of thin, normal-colored secretions.
4. The client will maintain a patent airway.
5. The client will maintain adequate pulse oximetry.

Equipment Needed (see Figures 7-17-1A and B):

- Sterile gloves
- Mask, eye protection, and gown if appropriate
- Source of negative pressure (suction machine or wall suction)
- Sterile suction catheter
- Oxygen or Ambu®-bag
- Equipment for tracheostomy care or tracheostomy care tray

▶ CLIENT EDUCATION NEEDED:

1. Explain procedure to client, including rationale for performing the procedure.
2. Instruct the client in good handwashing technique.
3. Encourage coughing and deep breathing to decrease the need for suctioning.
4. Teach client and family how to suction.

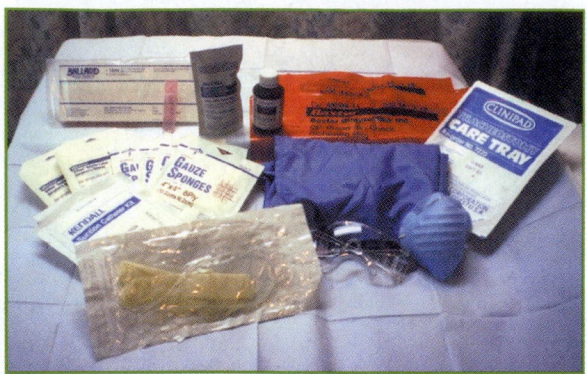

Figure 7-17-1A Protective gear, dressing, and a tracheostomy care tray

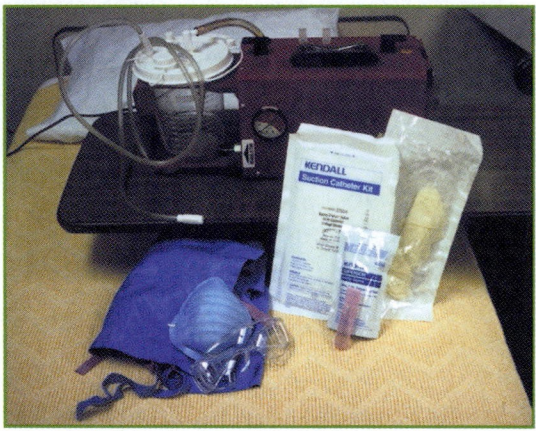

Figure 7-17-1B Protective gear and suction equipment

5. Provide multimedia instructions for the client learning how to suction the tracheostomy tube (videotape, written instructions).

Estimated time to complete the skill: **10–15 minutes**

▶ DELEGATION TIPS

The suctioning of endotracheal and tracheal tubes is not delegated by the nurse. Ancillary personnel may assist the nurse in providing care to clients receiving this treatment and should be instructed to report a client experiencing increased secretions, dyspnea, or the need for suctioning to the nurse.

IMPLEMENTATION—Action/Rationale

Action	Rationale
Suctioning a Tracheal Tube	
1. Assess depth and rate of respirations; auscultate breath sounds (see Figure 7-17-2).	1. Determines need for suctioning.
2. Assemble supplies on bedside table.	2. Organizes work.
3. Wash hands.	3. Reduces the transmission of microorganisms.
4. Connect suction tube to source of negative pressure.	4. Prepares for suctioning procedure.
5. Administer oxygen or use Ambu®-bag before beginning procedure.	5. Hyperoxygenates client and prevents hypoxia during suctioning.
6. Apply sterile glove to your dominant hand.	6. For sterile technique.
7. Open sterile suction catheter or use the reusable closed system catheter. The sterile suction catheter is removed from the package with your dominant, sterile hand. Wrap the catheter tubing around your hand from the tip of the catheter down to the port end. Attach catheter to suction.	7. This maintains catheter sterility and prevents accidental contamination.
8. Insert the catheter into the trachea without suction.	8. Minimizes removal of oxygen and trauma to the tracheal mucosa.
9. Apply suction intermittently while gently rotating the catheter and removing it. • In a disposable catheter, suction is applied by placing the thumb of your dominant hand over the open port of the catheter connector. • In a closed system catheter, suction is applied by depressing the white button at the connector end of the catheter.	9. Increases removal of mucus while minimizing irritation to tracheal mucosa.
10. Wrap the disposable suction catheter around your sterile, dominant hand while withdrawing it from the endotracheal tube.	10. This prevents accidental contamination of the catheter.
11. Suction for no more than 10 seconds.	11. Prevents hypoxia.
12. Administer 100% oxygen using the sigh function on the ventilator or using an Ambu®-bag.	12. Reoxygenates the client.
13. Assess airway and repeat suctioning as necessary.	13. Determines need to continue suctioning.
14. Apply humidified oxygen or compressed air (see Figure 7-17-3).	14. Thins secretions.

continues

Action	Rationale

Suctioning a Tracheal Tube *continued*

15. Remove gloves and discard.

16. Wash hands.

17. Record the procedure and client's tolerance of the procedure, including amount and consistency of secretions.

Suctioning an Endotracheal Tube

18. Repeat Actions 1–13 (see Figures 7-17-4 and 7-17-5).

19. Remove gloves and discard.

20. Wash hands.

21. Record the procedure and client's tolerance of the procedure, including amount and consistency of secretions.

15. Prevents transmission of microorganisms to other clients.

16. Reduces the transmission of microorganisms.

17. Provides documentation of the procedure.

18. See Rationales 1–14.

19. Prevents transmission of microorganisms to other clients.

20. Reduces the transmission of microorganisms.

21. Provides documentation of the procedure.

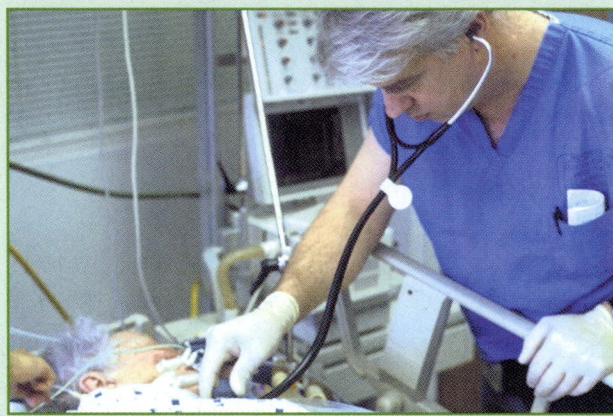

Figure 7-17-2   Assess respirations and auscultate breath sounds.

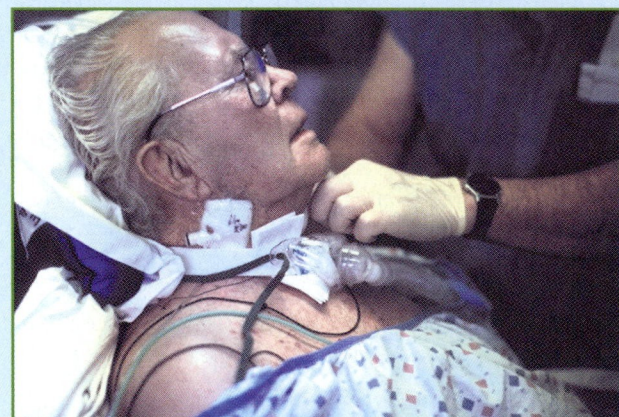

Figure 7-17-3   Attach oxygen.

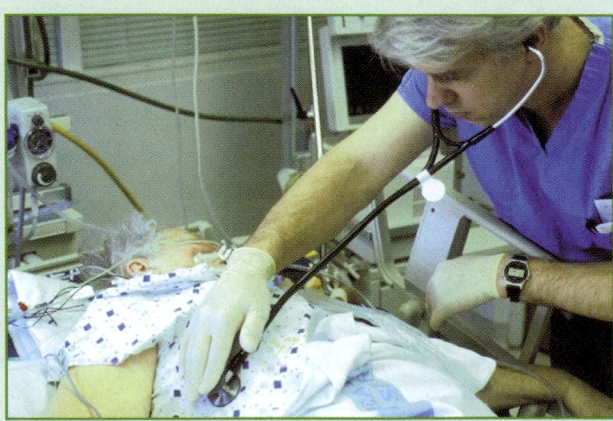

Figure 7-17-4   Assess for respiratory rate and lung sounds. Repeat suctioning if needed.

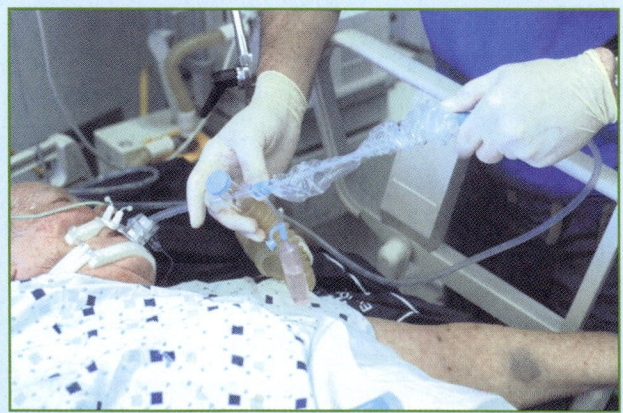

Figure 7-17-5   Endotracheal suctioning. Apply suction while gently rotating the catheter and removing it. Do not suction for more than 10 seconds.

▶ REAL WORLD ANECDOTES

Tina, 6 years old, had a tracheostomy performed after a near-drowning. She is recovering but still unable to breathe on her own. She has copious secretions from the infection that developed within the first week of admission. Tina hates to be suctioned. Early in her stay at the hospital, the nurses would simply hold Tina down while they suctioned her. Because this was traumatic to both Tina and the nurses, the staff and Tina's family worked on a way to help Tina deal with the suctioning. After talking to Tina's family, the nurses placed a tracheostomy tube into Tina's teddy bear, Harvey. They showed Tina how to suction using Harvey as a model and gave Tina a suction catheter to keep. Periodically, Tina suctions Harvey's tracheostomy tube and she insists on holding Harvey whenever she is suctioned. However, she is more cooperative with the procedure now and sometimes she tries to assist with it.

▶ EVALUATION

* Ask client whether breathing is easier.
* Evaluate breath sounds for a patent airway.
* Evaluate arterial blood gas and/or pulse oximetry results.
* Evaluate client for signs of dyspnea.
* Evaluate consistency, color, amount, and odor of secretions.

▶ DOCUMENTATION

Nurses' Notes

* Note date and time of suctioning procedure.
* Describe client's tolerance of the suctioning procedure.
* Note amount, consistency, color, and odor of secretions.
* Record arterial blood gas and/or pulse oximetry readings.

Record on appropriate flow sheet or electronic medical record (EMR).

▶ CRITICAL THINKING SKILL

Introduction

The suctioning procedure removes oxygen as well as mucus.

Possible Scenario

You are suctioning Mr. Halunen, who was intubated after cardiac arrest. He has copious secretions and requires frequent, vigorous suctioning. After the third time you try to clear his airway, he becomes cyanotic and his oximeter indicates a low oxygen saturation.

Possible Outcome

You decide that Mr. Halunen's poor oxygenation is caused by a mucus plug and redouble your efforts at suctioning. His oxygen saturation does not improve, and his heart rhythm begins to deteriorate. Within moments Mr. Halunen is in full respiratory and cardiac arrest and a code is called.

Prevention

The client should be given supplemental oxygen before suctioning and between suction attempts to minimize the incidence of hypoxia and resulting respiratory arrest.

▶ VARIATIONS

Geriatric Variations:

* *The tissues of the trachea and bronchi may be more fragile and need special care when suctioning.*
* *Older clients with decreased levels of consciousness, impaired gag reflex, stroke, chronic obstructive pulmonary disease, congestive heart failure, and pulmonary edema may be at greater risk for retained secretions.*
* *Elderly clients may have lost some properties of elastic recoil and gas exchange.*

continues

► **VARIATIONS** *(continued)*

Pediatric Variations:
- *In infants and young children, airways have smaller diameters, the glottis is higher, the thorax is smaller, and the diaphragm is higher. Be sure to use a suction catheter with the proper diameter, and not to insert it too deeply.*
- *The amount of negative pressure necessary for suctioning an infant or child is much less than the pressure needed for an adult. Refer to Table 7-17-1.*
- *The infant's or child's head should be turned to the right or left to facilitate bronchial suctioning on that side.*
- *The size of the suction catheter used depends upon the age of the client and the size of the tracheostomy tube.*
- *The suction catheter should be of a diameter equal to or less than one-half the inside diameter of the tracheostomy tube.*

Home Care Variations:
- *All self-care instructions need to be reinforced before the client leaves the hospital.*
- *Durable medical equipment must be available in the home prior to hospital discharge.*
- *Specific instructions related to durable medical equipment need to be given to the client and/or family before and after discharge.*

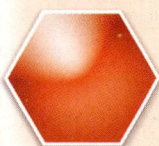

Long-Term Care Variations:
- *A source of humidity and oxygen is needed for clients in long-term care.*
- *Promoting adequate fluid intake may help decrease the client's risk for thick secretions.*

► **COMMON ERRORS**

Possible Error:
An elderly client needs frequent suctioning. After the second time in 30 minutes, the client begins to cough vigorously and you notice blood-tinged mucus in the catheter.

Prevention:
Be very gentle when inserting and withdrawing the catheter. Ask the client to try to relax; take slow, easy breaths; and not cough too strenuously.

►**NURSING TIPS**

- Assemble all equipment before beginning the procedure.
- If the client will be discharged with a tracheostomy tube in place, self-care teaching should begin once the client is awake and alert.
- Suctioning is a sterile technique when performed by professional nursing staff. However, once the procedure is taught to the client, a clean technique can be used by the client in the home setting.
- Normal saline (5–10 mL) may be instilled in clients with thick secretions before suctioning to loosen secretions. Know agency policy and orders as this practice may vary. It may also stimulate coughing.

- Closed system catheters may be left in place and changed every 24 hours.
- In closed system catheters, be sure the tip of the suction catheter is completely pulled back past the ventilator airway when suctioning is finished (see Figure 7-17-6). Leaving the tip of the suction catheter in the air pathway can decrease the air available to the client.
- Unplug a closed system catheter from the suction source to prevent accidental initiation of the suction (see Figure 7-17-7).
- In a closed system catheter, lock the suction button when you are finished suctioning to prevent accidental suctioning (see Figure 7-17-8).

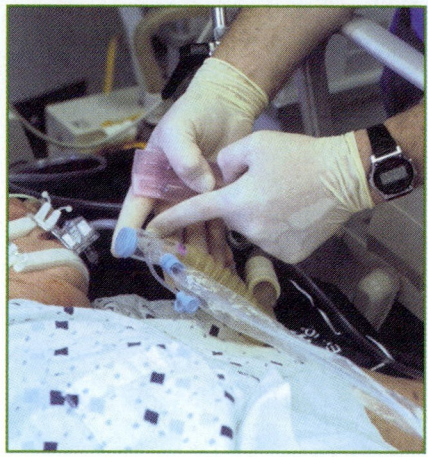

Figure 7-17-6 When suction is finished, be sure the tip of the suction catheter is completely retracted past the ventilator airway.

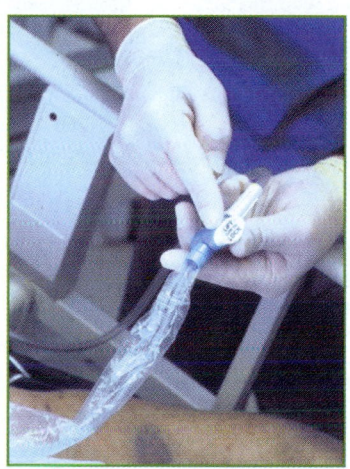

Figure 7-17-7 It is critical to lock the suction button or unplug the suction source to prevent accidental initiation of the suction.

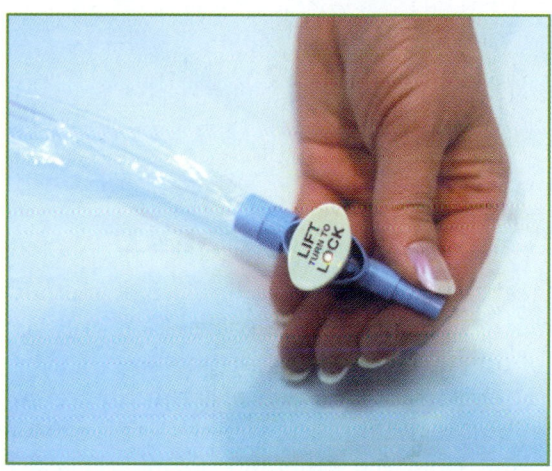

Figure 7-17-8 Locking suction button on a closed system catheter

▶ **SPECIAL CONSIDERATIONS**

- *Correct endotracheal tube position can help to avoid airway leaks. When tubes are placed during an emergency they are often found to be malpositioned.*
- *Clients with persistent hoarseness lasting longer than 7 to 10 days need to be evaluated by the health care provider. They may have developed a laryngeal granuloma that may require surgical removal.*
- *Some nurses worry that they will suction too long and leave the client gasping for a breath. One method to monitor and prevent this from happening is for the nurse to hold his or her breath for the length of time it takes to suction the client. If the nurse becomes out of breath, the client probably is as well.*
- *Avoid use of latex tubes and gloves if positive history.*

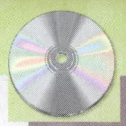

SKILL 7-18

Maintaining and Cleaning Endotracheal Tubes

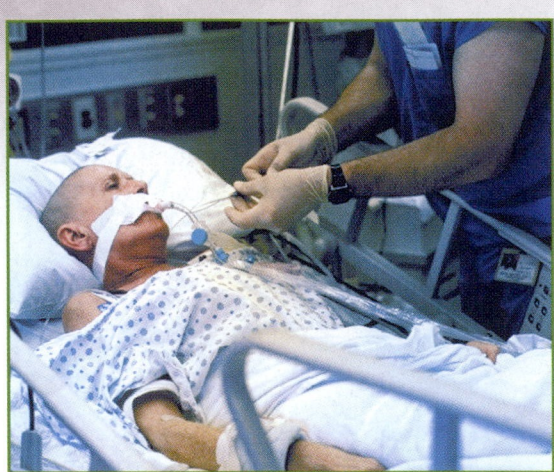

▶ OVERVIEW OF THE SKILL

Tracheal intubation is the preferred method for advanced airway control. Oxygenation and ventilation of the lungs by exhaled air methods usually precede attempts at endotracheal intubation. However, in the absence of a protected airway, gastric distention can result from the generation of pharyngeal pressure. This can increase the potential for aspiration of gastric contents into the lungs. Therefore, the trachea should be intubated as soon as possible during a resuscitative effort. Endotracheal intubation isolates the airway, keeps it patent, reduces the risk of aspiration, permits suctioning of the trachea, ensures delivery of a high concentration of oxygen, provides a route for administration of certain drugs, and ensures delivery of a selected tidal volume to maintain adequate lung inflation. The selected tidal volume is 10–15 mL/kg.

▶ ASSESSMENT

1. Assess the need for endotracheal intubation. **Indications include cardiac arrest with ongoing chest compressions, inability of a conscious client to ventilate adequately, inability of the client to protect the airway, and the inability of the rescuer to ventilate the conscious client with conventional methods.**
2. Assess placement of the endotracheal tube. **Ideally, the tip of the endotracheal tube should be about 3 cm above the carina. In the average adult, the position of the tube usually results in the depth marking on the side of the tube lying between the 19- and 23-cm mark at the front of the teeth. Delivery of the first manual breath by auscultating the epigastrium while observing the chest wall for evidence of thoracic inflation confirms tube placement. If stomach gurgling occurs and chest wall expansion is not evident, inadvertent esophageal intubation should be assumed and no further breaths delivered. Once inserted, the position of the endotracheal tube should be changed from side to side in the mouth every 8 hours to relieve pressure on the lips and tongue.**
3. Assess response to endotracheal tube placement. **During the initial phases after arrest, 12–15 breaths per minute should be provided. Each breath should be delivered to the lungs over a 2-second period using 100% oxygen. Monitor oxygen saturation, blood gases, and exhaled carbon dioxide level.**
4. Assess cuff pressure. **Cuff pressure should be evaluated every 4–8 hours to minimize tracheal damage. Check your individual facility's policy regarding frequency of deflating the cuff.**

▶ DIAGNOSIS

Impaired Gas Exchange
Ineffective Airway Clearance

976

Ineffective Breathing Pattern

Impaired Spontaneous Ventilation

Risk for Trauma

Impaired Verbal Communication

Impaired Skin Integrity

Anxiety

Risk for Infection

▶ PLANNING

Expected Outcomes:

1. Client will have adequate oxygenation of tissues as evident by oxygen saturation level.
2. Cuff will be inflated and deflated at designated intervals to minimize trauma to the trachea. Endotracheal tube will be rotated side to side at regular intervals in an effort to avoid trauma to lips and tongue.
3. Client will be sedated as needed and will be made comfortable while undergoing tracheal intubation.

Equipment Needed (see Figures 7-18-1A and B):

- Tape
- Suction equipment
- Normal saline
- Gauze
- Flashlight
- 10-mL syringe to deflate cuff
- Cuff manometer

▶ CLIENT EDUCATION NEEDED:

1. Alert client that you will be cleaning his or her endotracheal tube, rotating it to the other side, and deflating then inflating the cuff.
2. Establish a system of communication so that the client can give a signal if he or she becomes short of breath or needs a break during this procedure (such as raising a hand).

3. Thoughtful instructions to the client about what you are doing and what to expect will also help to reduce anxiety.
4. Tell the client that he or she may experience some coughing during this procedure.
5. Teaching the client distraction or imagery techniques can also be helpful to reduce anxiety.

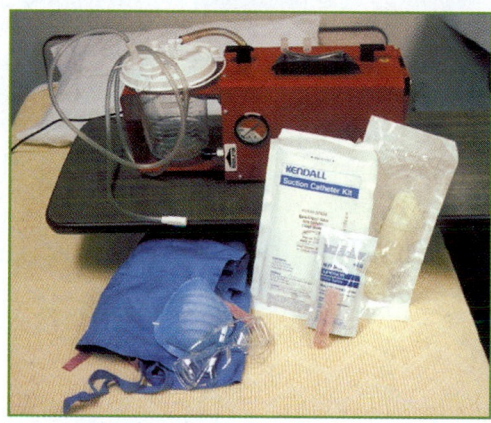

Figure 7-18-1A   Protective gear and suction equipment

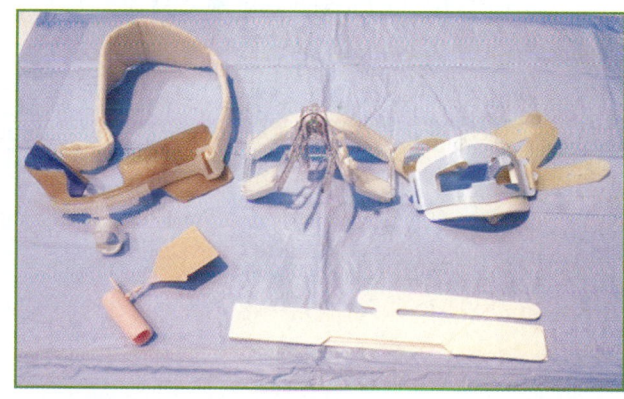

Figure 7-18-1B   Endotracheal tube ties

IMPLEMENTATION—Action/Rationale

Action	Rationale
1. Wash hands.	1. Reduces the transmission of microorganisms.
2. Prepare appropriate amount of tape to be placed when endotracheal tube is rotated to the other side.	2. This should be done ahead of time to minimize the chance that the endotracheal tube could become dislodged during the cleaning process.
3. Apply gloves.	3. Decreases the transmission of microorganisms.

continues

Action	Rationale

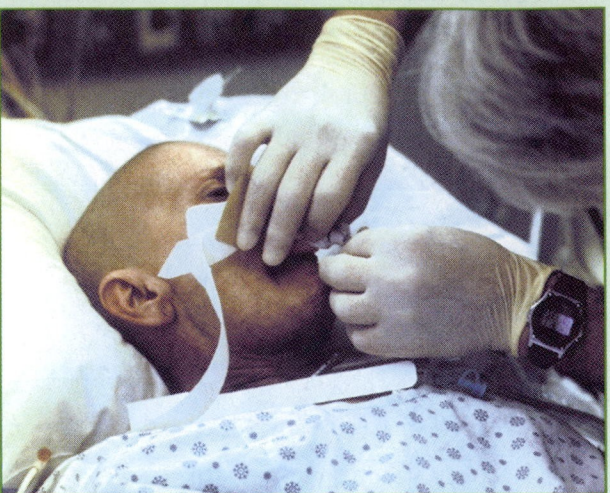

Figure 7-18-2 Clean secretions from the endotracheal tube.

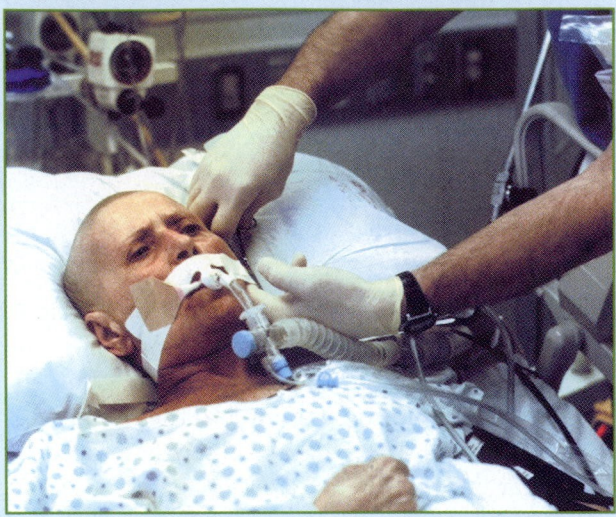

Figure 7-18-3 Remove tape. The nurse is carefully using scissors to remove the tape. Note how the position of the nurse's fingers protects the tube itself from being cut.

4. Using normal saline and gauze, clean any secretions from the endotracheal tube (see Figure 7-18-2). Remove old tape (see Figures 7-18-3 and 7-18-4).

5. Gently bring the endotracheal tube to the other side of the client's mouth (see Figure 7-18-5) and secure with tape (see Figure 7-18-6). Assess inside and outside of mouth for breakdown.

6. Suction oral cavity as needed (see Figure 7-18-7). Deflate the cuff.

4. Decreases risk of infection.

5. Rotating the endotracheal tube will ensure that tongue and lips remain intact. The tube should be securely taped because body movements could lead to accidental extubation.

6. Suctioning is important to avoid aspiration.

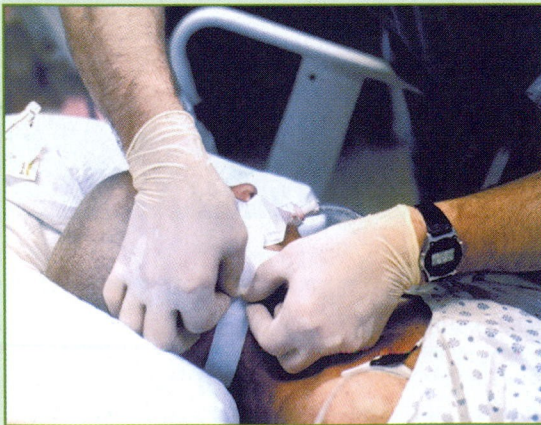

Figure 7-18-4 Remove tape.

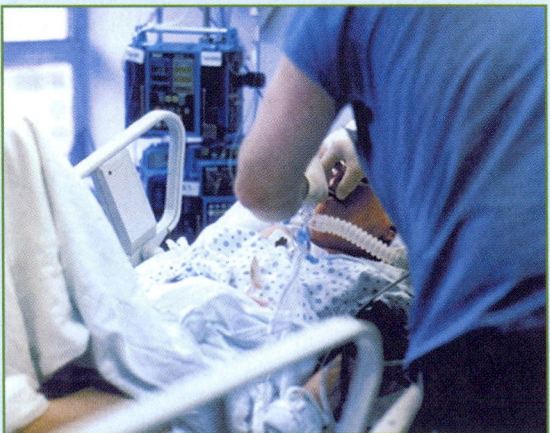

Figure 7-18-5 Gently move the tube to the opposite side of the client's mouth.

continues

Action	Rationale

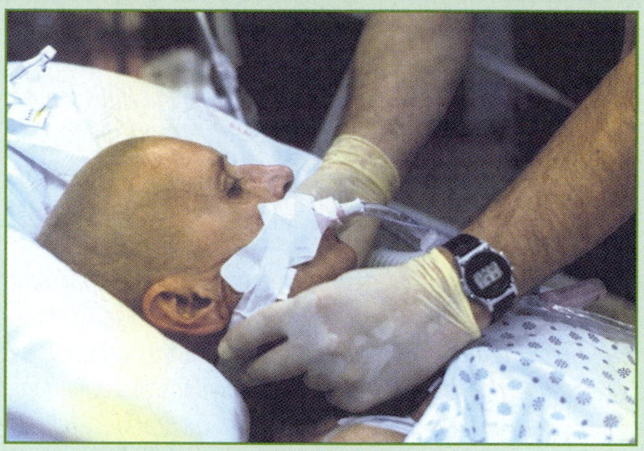

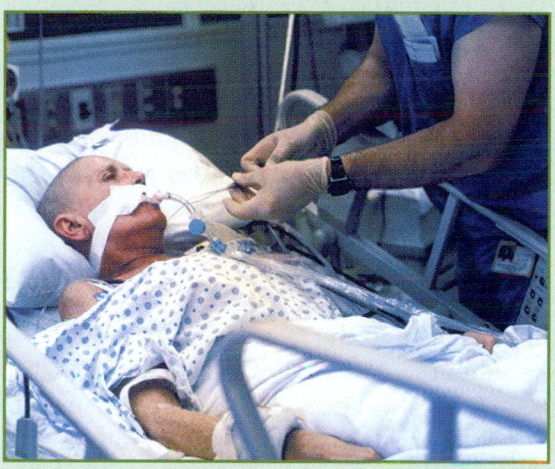

Figure 7-18-6 Secure the tube with tape.

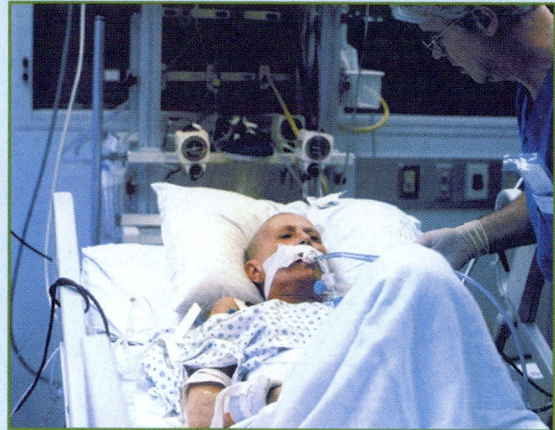

Figure 7-18-7 Suction the oral cavity, if needed.

Figure 7-18-8 Carefully inflate the cuff to the ordered pressure. Do not overinflate.

7. Inflate the cuff to a maximum pressure of 15 to 20 mm Hg (10 to 20 mL of air) as measured by connecting the balloon port to a manometer (see Figure 7-18-8).

7. This low pressure is important to ensure that tracheal damage is avoided. Damage occurs when pressure exerted by the inflated cuff against the tracheal walls exceeds the tracheal capillary pressure (about 25 mm Hg).

8. Remove gloves.

8. Decreases the transmission of microorganisms.

9. Monitor client for adverse effects; place the call light within easy reach.

9. Decreases the risk of complications.

10. Wash hands.

10. Reduces the transmission of microorganisms.

▶ **REAL WORLD ANECDOTES**

Scenario 1

Bill underwent endotracheal intubation 2 days previously, and his nurse enters the room to rotate the tube and deflate the cuff. She removes the old tape and gently slides the endotracheal tube to the other side of Bill's mouth. Realizing that she did not prepare her tape ahead of time, she attempts to hold the tube and tear off the tape at the same time. Bill's body jerks and he accidentally extubates himself. The nurse was reminded to prepare her supplies before beginning this procedure and to have someone else in the room when possible.

Scenario 2

John underwent endotracheal intubation 1 week previously after experiencing respiratory distress. It was decided that John would be extubated at 1:00 pm and John's physician would remove the endotracheal tube. After extubation, John's oxygen saturation level remained 98% and he experienced no distress. John did admit that his throat was sore and his voice was very hoarse. After discussing these symptoms with a colleague, John's nurse was reminded that sore throat and hoarseness are commonly experienced by clients after they are extubated. However, if these symptoms persist for a week or longer, cord ulcerations, polyps, or granulomas must be suspected. John's nurse was reminded that teaching the client about signs and symptoms, both normal and abnormal, is an important part of endotracheal intubation.

▶ EVALUATION

- Client has adequate oxygenation of tissues as evident by oxygen saturation level.
- Cuff is inflated and deflated at designated intervals to minimize trauma to the trachea. Endo-tracheal tube is rotated side to side at regular intervals in an effort to avoid trauma to lips and tongue.
- Client is sedated as needed and made comfortable while undergoing endotracheal care.

▶ DOCUMENTATION

Nurses' Notes

- Indicate the time the endotracheal tube was cleaned and rotated, and the cuff was deflated.
- Detail assessment of oral cavity, noting any areas of breakdown.
- Document breath sounds, vital signs, oxygen saturation.
- Document the depth marking on the side of the tube that is at the level of the mouth.
- Describe the client's response to manipulation of endotracheal tube.
- Include signature of the nurse performing this activity.

Document on appropriate flow sheet or electronic medical record (EMR).

▶ CRITICAL THINKING SKILL

Introduction

The endotracheal tube must remain unplugged and unkinked to ensure that the client receives adequate oxygenation. It is important to check the endotracheal tube for patency every 2–4 hours and prn. When a client has large amounts of secretions, it becomes even more critical to monitor the tube to ensure that it does not become clogged.

Possible Scenario

Jim has been in the intensive care unit and intubated for about 1 week. Jim's oxygen saturation alarm begins to ring—it is 78% and decreasing. The nurse enters Jim's room to find him agitated and restless. She is unable to see his chest rise and fall. She quickly checks the connections to his endotracheal tube and finds none dislodged. She then assesses the endotracheal tube and discovers there is a mucus plug obstructing it.

Possible Outcome

The nurse quickly sets up the suction equipment and clears the mucus plug. She is reminded that frequent assessment of the endotracheal tube is necessary to maintain patency.

Prevention

Assess the client for the likelihood of a mucus plug formation (large amounts of thick and copious secretions). Carefully assess the endotracheal tube every 2 to 4 hours and prn to ensure that it remains clear.

▶ VARIATIONS

Geriatric Variation:
- *Older clients may have dry mouth, teeth in poor condition, or alterations in taste or oral sensations. Check for these conditions when performing an oral assessment. Perform oral care every 2 hours for comfort and to reduce the risk of mucosa breakdown.*

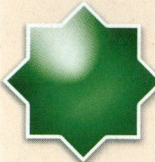

Pediatric Variations:
- *Make sure the parent and the child have a way to communicate. Have the parent use touch to reassure the child.*
- *Monitor or restrain the child if needed to keep the child from pulling on the tube and dislodging it.*

Home Care Variation:
- *Endotracheal tubes are used to manage the airway of clients needing short-term interventions. In the case of the client needing more long-term airway assistance, another type of airway would be chosen.*

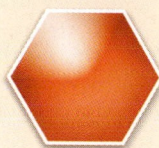

Long-Term Care Variation:
- *Endotracheal tubes are used to manage the airway of clients needing short-term interventions. In the case of the client needing more long-term airway assistance, another type of airway would be chosen.*

▶ COMMON ERRORS

Possible Error:

The client is not suctioned orally before deflating the endotracheal tube, causing aspiration of mucus.

Prevention:

Always suction the area above the cuff before deflating it.

Possible Error:

The endotracheal tube causes trauma to the tongue and cheeks.

Prevention:

Rotate the endotracheal tube at regular intervals to avoid skin breakdown. Remove old tape from the endotracheal tube, gently rotate the endotracheal tube to the other side of the client's mouth, assess for skin breakdown, and apply new tape.

▶ NURSING TIPS

- Having someone to assist, if available, in the rotation of the endotracheal tube can be helpful to ensure that the tube does not become dislodged.
- Premedication of the client may be needed before an endotracheal tube rotation to ensure adequate client comfort.
- Suctioning before deflation of the cuff is critical to avoid aspiration.

- Bend 2 cm of the ends of the tape to function as tabs that will later assist in removal of the tape. If available, use adhesive remover when removing old tape.
- Try to anticipate client concerns and questions so you can provide information. Fears about communicating, choking, not being able to attract the nurse's attention, and having the air supply "cut off" are common concerns.

▶ **SPECIAL CONSIDERATIONS**

- *Clients may experience laryngeal injury from an endotracheal tube. Injury can result in vocal cord or airway edema, mucosal ulcerations, airway granulomas, tracheal stenosis, and/or tracheoesophageal fistula. Most laryngeal lesions heal without intervention.*
- *Endotracheal intubation is associated with nosocomial pneumonia and nosocomial sinusitis. The incidence increases with reintubation and it should be avoided whenever possible.*
- *Successful extubation occurs when the client has the strength for a spontaneous cough and has decreased need for suctioning.*
- *Avoid latex tubes and gloves if positive history.*

Maintaining and Cleaning the Tracheostomy Tube

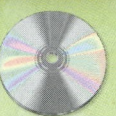

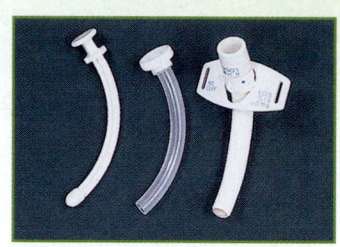

▶ OVERVIEW OF THE SKILL

A tracheotomy is an incision made into the trachea with insertion of a cannula for airway management. A tracheostomy is performed for the client with potential or present airway obstruction, for ventilatory assistance, to provide pulmonary hygiene, to decrease the anatomic dead space in the client with chronic obstructive pulmonary disease, to avoid prolonged endotracheal intubation, and to provide an airway for the client with severe obstructive sleep apnea syndrome. The tracheostomy is performed below the level of the vocal cords, and allows air to enter and exit the tracheostomy rather than through the upper airway. The tracheostomy tube can be plugged to evaluate the client's ability to tolerate removal of the tracheostomy tube (decannulation) and to provide verbal speech to the client with a tracheostomy. During the acute phase after a tracheostomy has been performed, all care must be performed using sterile technique. Once care of the tracheostomy tube becomes a client procedure, a clean technique is used. The tracheostomy becomes a part of the client's body, and hygiene is important to prevent infection and odors.

▶ ASSESSMENT

1. Assess respirations for rate, rhythm, and depth **to evaluate airway.**
2. Auscultate lung fields **to evaluate airway and determine need for suctioning.**
3. Monitor arterial blood gas and/or pulse oximetry values **to determine oxygen levels and adequate air exchange.**
4. Assess passage of air through tracheostomy tube **to determine adequate air exchange and obstruction of the tube.**

5. Evaluate amount and color of tracheal secretions **to assess for evidence of bleeding or infection and need for suctioning.**
6. Assess anxiety, restlessness, and fear because **anxiety and restlessness may be symptoms of airway distress and hypoxia. Anxiety and restlessness can also occur because of the fear associated with the new procedure.**
7. Assess the client's understanding of the tracheostomy procedure **to determine the need for additional education in order for the client to participate in self-care.**
8. Assess the area around the tracheostomy for redness, swelling, and drainage **to evaluate skin integrity.**

▶ DIAGNOSIS

Impaired Skin Integrity

Ineffective Airway Clearance

Anxiety

Impaired Gas Exchange

Deficient Knowledge

Risk for Infection

Impaired Verbal Communication

▶ PLANNING

Expected Outcomes:

1. The tracheostomy site will heal with minimal drainage and erythema.
2. There will be no evidence of infection.
3. The client will maintain a patent airway.
4. The client will have inner and outer cannulas free of secretions, and clean, secure ties.

Equipment Needed (see Figure 7-19-1):

- Gloves
- Hydrogen peroxide
- Sterile water or saline
- Cotton-tip applicators
- Tracheostomy dressing (4 × 4 gauze without cotton lining)
- Tracheostomy ties (twill tape, intravenous tubing, or commercially available Velcro ties)

► CLIENT EDUCATION NEEDED:

1. Explain each step of the procedure to the client as it is being performed.
2. Explain rationale of procedure to the client (to clean the surgical site in order to prevent infection, skin irritation, and odor).
3. Allow the client to observe the procedure in a mirror while the procedure is being performed.
4. Review with the client ways of obtaining durable medical equipment for this procedure.
5. Ask the client to demonstrate the ability to perform the procedure.

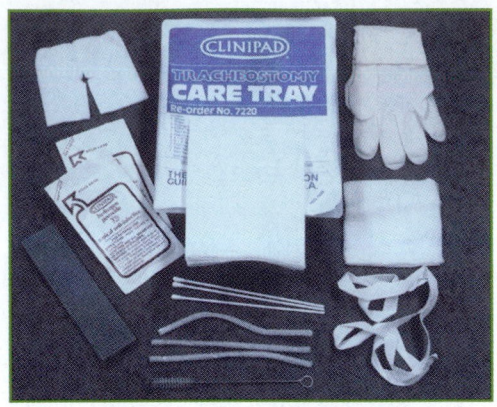

Figure 7-19-1   Tracheostomy care tray, hydrogen peroxide, tape, dressing, and clean gloves

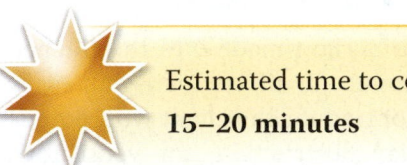

Estimated time to complete the skill:
15–20 minutes

► DELEGATION TIPS

The maintenance and cleaning of tracheal tubes cannot be delegated by the nurse. Ancillary personnel may assist the nurse in providing care to clients receiving this treatment and should be instructed to report a client experiencing increased secretions, dyspnea, or the need for suctioning to the nurse.

IMPLEMENTATION—Action/Rationale

Action	Rationale
Cleaning Trach Tube Site	
1. Wash hands and apply gloves.	1. Reduces the transmission of microorganisms.
2. Remove soiled dressing and discard (see Figure 7-19-2).	2. Prevents contamination of other areas.
3. Cleanse neck plate of tracheostomy tube with cotton applicators moistened with hydrogen peroxide.	3. Removes crusted secretions from neck plate of tracheostomy tube.
4. Rinse neck plate of tracheostomy tube with applicators moistened with sterile water or saline.	4. Removes hydrogen peroxide.
5. Cleanse skin under neck plate of tube with cotton applicator moistened with hydrogen peroxide (see Figure 7-19-3).	5. Removes dried and crusted secretions from under neck plate of tracheostomy tube.

continues

Action	Rationale

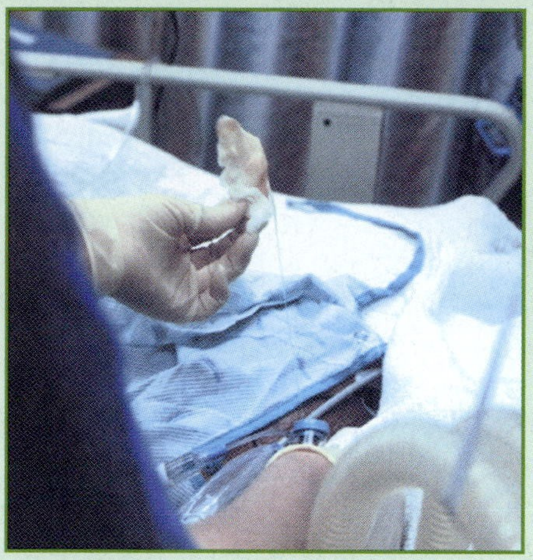

![Figure 7-19-2 Remove old dressings and discard.]

Figure 7-19-2   Remove old dressings and discard.

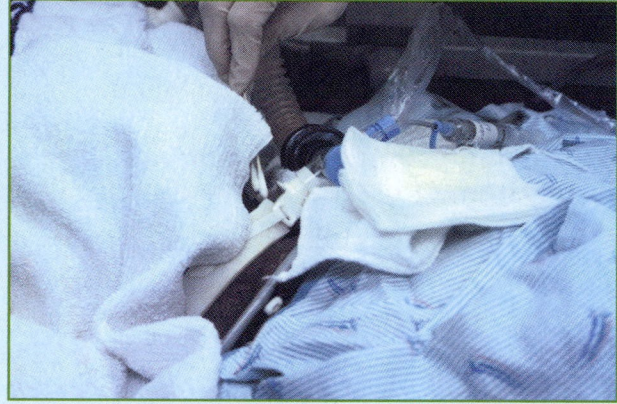

Figure 7-19-3   Cleanse skin under the neck plate with a cotton applicator moistened with hydrogen peroxide. Note: The towel placed over the client's face is for privacy and is not required for the procedure.

6. Rinse skin under neck plate with applicators moistened with sterile water or saline.

6. Removes hydrogen peroxide.

7. Dry skin under neck plate with cotton applicators.

7. Removes moisture, which can result in skin irritation.

One-Person Technique of Changing Tracheostomy Ties

8. Prepare clean tracheostomy ties.
   - Cut a length of twill tape that will fit around the client's neck plus 6 inches. Cut the ends of the twill tape on the diagonal.
   - Open Velcro ties on continuous neck band.

8. To have all equipment prepared before beginning procedure. A diagonal cut will make the tape easier to thread.

9. Leaving the old tracheostomy ties in place, insert one end of the new tracheostomy tie through the hole in the tracheostomy neck plate from back to front. Pull the ends even, and slide both ends of the tape around the back of the head to the other side.

9. Maintains tube security while tapes are changed.

10. Insert one end of tape through the opening on the other side of the tracheostomy tube neck plate from back to front.

10. Secures tracheostomy tube.

11. Tie the two ends of the new tape with a square knot at side of neck. Keep two fingers under the tape as the knot is tied. Without putting pressure on the neck plate or the tape, pull on the knot to make sure it will stay tied.

11. Secures tracheostomy tube. Fingers under tape prevent the tape from being tied too tightly.

12. Untie and remove old tracheostomy tapes and discard. Hold the neck plate firmly with one hand while untying the old tapes.

12. Old tapes can be removed once the tracheostomy tube has been secured. Holding the plate firmly prevents dislodgment if the new tie is accidentally cut.

continues

Action	Rationale
One-Person Technique of Changing Tracheostomy Ties *continued*	
13. Place one finger under tracheostomy ties.	13. Checks for tightness and security.
Two-Person Technique of Changing Tracheostomy Ties	
14. Cut two pieces of twill tape about 12 to 14 inches in length.	14. Prepares equipment before beginning procedure.
15. Make a fold about 1 inch below the end of each piece of twill tape and cut a half-inch slit lengthwise in the center of the fold.	15. Prepares tape for insertion.
16. Have a second person gently hold the tracheostomy tube in place with fingers on both sides of the neck plate.	16. Prevents accidental movement of the tracheostomy tube resulting in coughing and accidental decannulation.
17. Untie old tracheostomy ties and discard.	17. Removes tracheostomy ties.
18. Insert the split end of the tracheostomy tape through the opening on one side of the tracheostomy tube neck plate. Pull the distal end of the tracheostomy tie through the cut end and pull tightly.	18. Secures tracheostomy tie within neck plate.
19. Repeat procedure with second piece of twill tape.	19. Secures tracheostomy tube.
20. Tie tracheostomy tapes with a double knot at the side of the neck.	20. Secures tracheostomy tube.
21. Insert one finger under tracheostomy tapes.	21. Ensures that tube has been tied securely.
22. Insert tracheostomy gauze under neck plate of tube (see Figure 7-19-4).	22. Prevents irritation of skin from secretions and rubbing of tracheostomy tube.
23. Discard all used materials and wash hands.	23. Reduces the transmission of microorganisms.

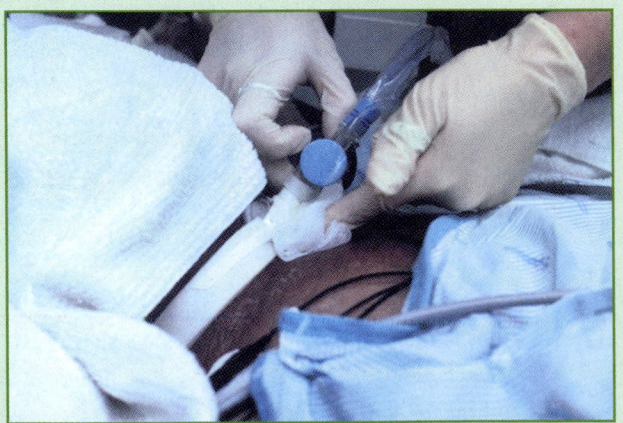

Figure 7-19-4 Insert gauze under the neck plate of the tracheostomy tube.

▶ REAL WORLD ANECDOTES

Mr. Sampson has a long history of smoking and has copious secretions that he coughs through his tracheostomy tube. Because of this, the tracheostomy dressing and ties are always soiled and wet and must be changed frequently. In this situation, intravenous tubing may be used as tracheostomy ties. The tubing can be moved slightly to dry the area under the ties and the tubing will not absorb secretions and become soiled. Although intravenous tubing is more difficult to insert into the openings of the neck plate while the tube is in the client, it is more appropriate for use with a client with increased secretions or for the client at home who cannot change the ties as often.

▶ EVALUATION

- The tracheostomy site healed with minimal drainage and erythema.
- There is no evidence of infection.
- The client maintains a patent airway.
- The client has inner and outer cannulas free of secretions, and clean, secured ties.

▶ DOCUMENTATION

Nurses' Notes

- Record date and time of procedure.
- Note size and type of tracheostomy tube in place.
- Describe client's tolerance of the procedure.
- Record amount and consistency of any secretions.
- Document condition of the client's skin.

Document on appropriate flow sheet or electronic medical record (EMR).

▶ CRITICAL THINKING SKILL

Introduction

A new tracheostomy or a client with increased secretions may be at higher risk of skin irritation because of moisture under the dressing or ties.

Possible Scenario

Thelma had a tracheostomy performed because of upper-airway obstruction. The nurse enters the room and notices the client coughing copious amounts of secretions. Upon evaluating the client's tracheostomy tube site and skin, the nurse notices the tracheostomy ties and dressing are wet and soiled.

Possible Outcome

Moistened and soiled tracheostomy gauze and ties may result in skin irritation and excoriation under the tracheostomy tube and ties. In addition, moistened ties may result in stretching of the material, thus decreasing the security of the tracheostomy tube.

Prevention

To prevent skin irritation, excoriation, and/or infection under the tracheostomy tube and possible accidental decannulation, the nurse should frequently change the tracheostomy gauze. In addition, tracheostomy ties should be assessed at least once per shift to ensure their tightness.

▶ VARIATIONS

Geriatric Variation:
- *Care of the skin at the tracheostomy site is crucial because the integrity of the skin may be impaired.*

Pediatric Variation:
- *Pediatric clients may need two people to clean the tracheostomy tube and change the ties because young clients may be less cooperative or restless, thus increasing the risk of decannulation.*

continues

► **VARIATIONS** *(continued)*

Home Care Variations:
- *The procedure is a clean technique in a home care setting.*
- *Good handwashing technique should be stressed.*
- *Use tap water for rinsing the inner cannula.*
- *Inner cannula care should be performed on a routine basis.*
- *Normal saline can be made by adding 2 teaspoons of table salt to 1 quart of boiled water.*
- *Store normal saline in a quart or pint jar that has been sterilized.*

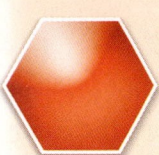

Long-Term Care Variations:
- *Care of the tracheostomy tube may be done by the nursing personnel or the client.*
- *It is a "sterile" procedure if done by the nurse and a "clean" technique if done by the client.*

► **COMMON ERRORS**

Possible Error:

You use gauze with cotton filling under the tracheostomy tube.

Prevention:

Think about why you should avoid using regular gauze under a tracheostomy tube. Gauze with cotton fibers may result in aspiration of the fibers through the tracheostomy opening. Always use specialized tracheostomy gauze dressing or gauze without cotton fibers.

► **NURSING TIPS**

- Assemble all equipment before beginning the procedure.
- Obtain the assistance of a second person to help with tracheostomy tie changes. If a second nurse is not available, review the procedure for a single person changing tracheostomy ties or delay the procedure until a second nurse is available to assist.
- Use sterile equipment and careful technique while performing the procedure to prevent microorganisms from contaminating a new trach wound.

► **SPECIAL CONSIDERATIONS**

- *Methylene blue had been added to enteral feedings for years to determine aspirate of oropharyngeal contents with tracheal tubes. Now, obtaining a glucose oxidase test strip reading >20 mg/dL detects aspirate more readily.*
- *Clients with long-term tracheostomies and mechanical ventilation may develop symptoms of tracheal obstruction related to the development of granulation tissue. This may be treated with a longer tracheostomy tube, surgical intervention, or a tracheal stent.*
- *Avoid latex tubes and gloves if client has a positive history of latex allergy.*

Maintaining a Double Cannula Tracheostomy Tube

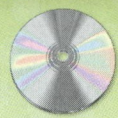

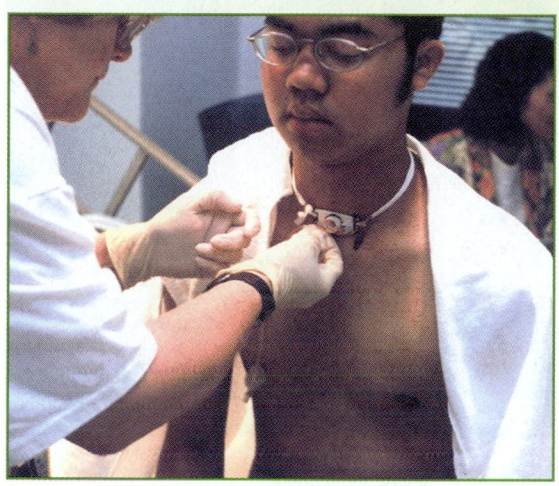

► OVERVIEW OF THE SKILL

A tracheotomy is an incision made into the trachea with insertion of a cannula for airway management. Tracheostomy is the creation of an opening into the trachea through the neck. The two terms can be used interchangeably. The term tracheostomy will be used in this skill. A tracheostomy is performed for the client with potential or present airway obstruction, for ventilatory assistance, to provide pulmonary hygiene, to decrease the anatomic dead space in the client with chronic obstructive pulmonary disease, to avoid prolonged endotracheal intubation, and to provide an airway for clients with severe obstructive sleep apnea syndrome. A tracheostomy is usually performed between the second, third, and fourth tracheal rings. The tracheostomy tube can have a single or double cannula. The determination of the tube design used is based on the needs of the client. Many of the longer tracheostomy tubes are single cannulas because of the curvature of the tube. The double-cannula tube allows for the tube to be cleaned to prevent obstruction caused by dried secretions.

► ASSESSMENT

1. Assess respirations for rate, rhythm, and depth **to evaluate the airway.**
2. Assess the client's lung sounds **to determine the need for suctioning.**

3. Assess the client's arterial blood gases and/or pulse oximetry values **to evaluate air exchange and blood oxygen levels.**
4. Assess the movement of air through the tracheostomy tube **to evaluate the air exchange through the tube and determine whether there is any obstruction.**
5. Assess the amount and color of tracheal secretions **to evaluate for bleeding, infection, and the need for suctioning.**
6. Assess the client's level of consciousness. **Anxiety and restlessness could be symptoms of hypoxia.**
7. Assess the client's understanding of the procedure **to determine client education and support needed.**

► DIAGNOSIS

Ineffective Airway Clearance

Risk for Infection

Risk for Suffocation

Impaired Skin Integrity

Impaired Verbal Communication

Deficient Knowledge

Anxiety

► PLANNING

Expected Outcomes:

1. The client's airway will be free of obstruction.

2. The procedure will be performed with a minimum of client anxiety.

3. The client's skin will remain intact and free of redness and excoriation.

4. The client will remain free of signs and symptoms of infection.

Equipment Needed:

Cleaning the Inner Cannula (see Figure 7-20-1)

- Sterile gloves
- Disposable inner cannula (if available)
- Tracheostomy care kit: 2 basins, tracheostomy brush, tracheostomy ties
- Hydrogen peroxide
- Sterile water or sterile saline

▶ CLIENT EDUCATION NEEDED:

1. Explain to the client that cleaning the inner cannula will promote breathing.

2. Inform the client that the procedure may cause coughing.

3. After performing the procedure and explaining each step to the client, the nurse should supervise the client in self-care. Make a list of the steps the client should follow when performing the procedure.

4. Allow the client to observe the procedure in a mirror. The mirror should be placed at a comfortable level and in a setting similar to that used by the client once discharged from the hospital.

5. Suggest alternative types of equipment. For example, if tracheostomy brushes cannot be purchased once the client is discharged from the hospital, a small percolator brush, gauze, or pipe cleaners can be used to remove crusted secretions.

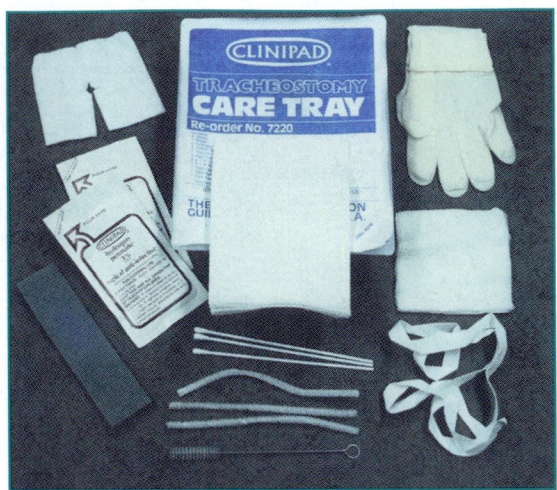

Figure 7-20-1 Tracheostomy care tray, hydrogen peroxide, tape, dressing, and clean gloves

Estimated time to complete the skill: **5–10 minutes**

▶ DELEGATION TIPS

The maintenance of a double cannula tracheal tube cannot be delegated by the nurse. Ancillary personnel may assist the nurse in providing care to clients receiving this treatment and should be instructed to report a client experiencing increased secretions, dyspnea, or the need for suctioning to the nurse.

IMPLEMENTATION—Action/Rationale

Action	Rationale
1. Wash hands.	1. Reduces the transmission of microorganisms.
Conventional/Reusable Inner Cannula	
2. Open tracheostomy care set.	2. Provides sterile equipment for use in the procedure.
3. Place hydrogen peroxide solution in one basin and sterile water or saline in a second basin.	3. Prepare solutions prior to applying gloves.

continues

Action	Rationale

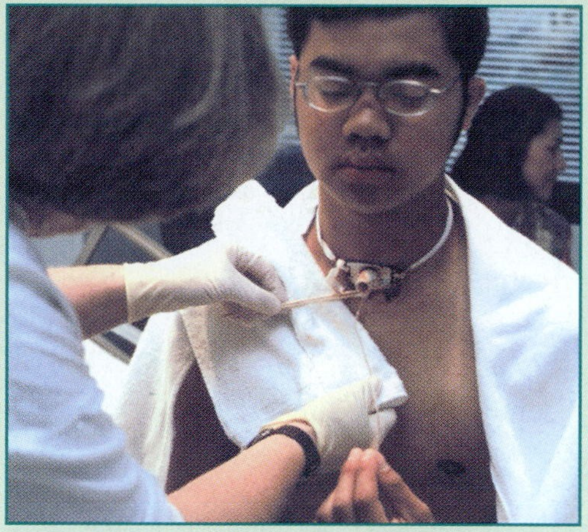

Figure 7-20-2   Clean the area under the neck plate with a cotton applicator moistened with hydrogen peroxide.

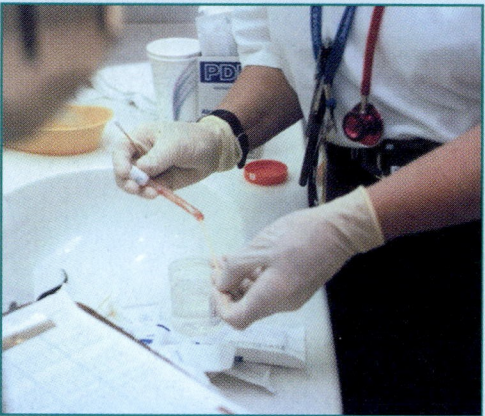

Figure 7-20-3   Use a sterile cotton-tipped applicator to clean the inner cannula area and remove crusted secretions.

Action	Rationale
4. Apply sterile gloves.	4. Uses aseptic technique.
5. Remove inner cannula.	5. To clean tracheostomy double cannula tube.
6. Place inner cannula in basin of hydrogen peroxide.	6. Loosens secretions.
7. Clean the area under the neck plate of the tracheostomy tube using a cotton applicator moistened with hydrogen peroxide (see Figure 7-20-2). Dip the applicator in the basin of hydrogen peroxide before the cannula is added to the basin to prevent contamination of the applicator.	7. Decreases microorganisms and removes crusting.
8. Rinse area under neck plate with cotton applicator moistened with sterile water or saline.	8. Removes hydrogen peroxide from the skin.
9. Dry skin under neck plate with cotton-tip applicator.	9. Prevents skin excoriation from moisture.
10. Apply tracheostomy gauze under neck plate of tube. Note: If using tracheostomy gauze under the neck plate of the tracheostomy tube, change gauze frequently to prevent skin excoriation and infection from a moist environment.	10. Prevents irritation of skin from secretions and rubbing of tracheostomy tube.
11. Use a tracheostomy brush or sterile cotton-tip applicator to clean inner cannula (see Figure 7-20-3).	11. Removes crusted secretions.
12. Rinse inner cannula with sterile water or sterile saline (see Figure 7-20-4).	12. Removes hydrogen peroxide from inner cannula.
13. Dry inner cannula.	13. Prevents introduction of solutions into the trachea.
14. Reinsert inner cannula and lock it into place (see Figures 7-20-5 and 7-20-6).	14. Prevents accidental removal of the inner cannula during coughing.
15. Remove gloves and discard.	15. Prevents transmission of microorganisms to other clients.

continues

Action	Rationale

Conventional/Reusable Inner Cannula *continued*

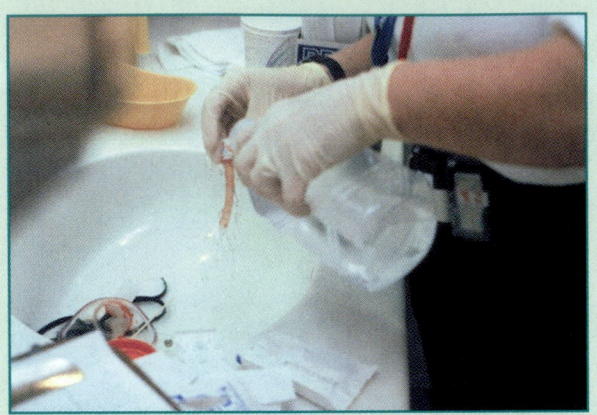

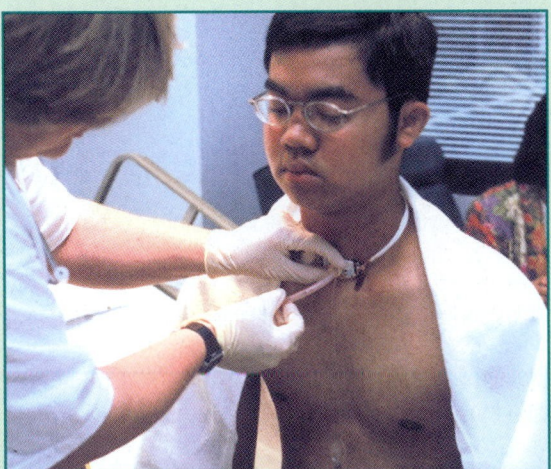

Figure 7-20-4   Rinse inner cannula thoroughly with sterile water or sterile saline.

16. Wash hands.

17. Record the procedure and client's tolerance of the procedure, including amount and consistency of secretions.

Disposable Inner Cannula

18. Wash hands. Open disposable cannula container without touching cannula.

19. Apply sterile gloves.

20. Remove inner cannula and discard.

21. Replace inner cannula with new disposable cannula.

22. Remove gloves and discard.

23. Wash hands.

24. Record the procedure and client's tolerance of the procedure, including amount and consistency of secretions.

16. Reduces the transmission of microorganisms.

17. Provides documentation of the procedure.

18. Reduces the transmission of microorganisms.

19. Uses aseptic technique.

20. Do not reuse disposable inner cannulas.

21. Provides an open cannula.

22. Prevents transmission of microorganisms to other clients.

23. Reduces the transmission of microorganisms.

24. Provides documentation of the procedure.

Figure 7-20-5   Carefully reinsert inner cannula.

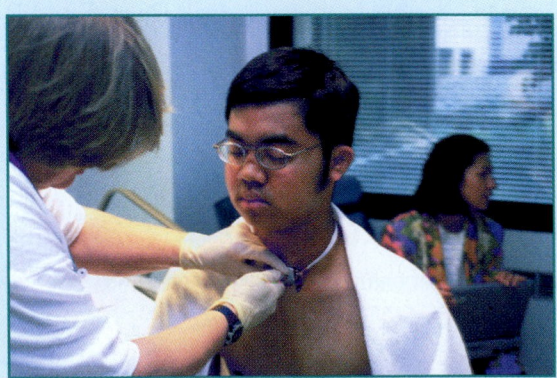

Figure 7-20-6   Lock inner cannula into place.

► **REAL WORLD ANECDOTES**

A student nurse was assigned to care for Mr. Sidik. He had recently had a double cannula tracheostomy tube placed secondary to sleep apnea. The student was unsure how to clean the inner cannula of the tracheostomy. She asked several staff members, but everyone was too busy to do more than tell her to remove the inner cannula, clean it, and soak it in disinfectant. Her instructor was not on the floor at the time and Mr. Sidik had not performed the procedure before and was not yet aware of how it was done. The student decided to give it a try on her own. She removed the inner cannula and placed it in the sink for cleaning. She did not know what was normally used to disinfect the cannula, but there was a bottle of Betadine sitting on the sink. Thinking that this must be what was used, she poured the Betadine over the cannula while she industriously cleaned it. As she was scrubbing at the sink, Mr. Sidik's nurse entered the room.

Seeing the student pouring Betadine over the inner cannula, she immediately informed the student that Betadine was not used for tracheostomy cleaning and discarded the now contaminated inner cannula. The nurse ordered a new inner cannula for Mr. Sidik and cleaned and redressed his tracheostomy site while waiting for the new inner cannula. The student was reminded not to try to bluff her way through things she did not truly understand.

► **EVALUATION**

- The client's airway is free of obstruction.
- The procedure was performed with a minimum of client anxiety.
- The client's skin remains intact and free of redness and excoriation.
- The client remains free of signs and symptoms of infection.

► **DOCUMENTATION**

Nurses' Notes

- Document what procedure was done and the client's tolerance of the procedure.
- Indicate the amount and consistency of any secretions that were noted in the inner cannula.
- Document client teaching and participation.

Document on appropriate flow sheet or electronic medical record (EMR).

► **CRITICAL THINKING SKILL**

Introduction

When cleaning the inner cannula of a double cannula tracheostomy tube, it is important to clean and reinsert the tube in a timely manner before secretions are allowed to dry on the outer cannula.

Possible Scenario

Mr. Jinwon had a tracheostomy performed following surgery in the oral cavity. During routine cleaning of the inner cannula, the nurse removed the inner cannula and placed it in hydrogen peroxide to loosen secretions. During this time, she was called away from the client's bedside.

Possible Outcome

Becoming involved in another procedure, the nurse did not return to Mr. Jinwon's bedside to complete the procedure until several hours later. After cleaning the inner cannula, the nurse found she could not reinsert it. The outer cannula of the tracheostomy was encrusted with dried secretions and the inner cannula could not be reinserted. The entire tracheostomy tube had to be changed to restore the client's airway.

Prevention

Double cannula tracheostomy tubes are used to provide a removable cannula for cleaning. In a double cannula tracheostomy tube, an inner cannula can be removed, cleaned, and replaced. In the anecdote, the double cannula tube became a single cannula tube. Secretions that can normally be removed by removing the inner cannula accumulated in the lumen of the outer cannula and obstructed the airway. In a situation where a single cannula tube is used or in the case study just discussed, supplemental humidification should be applied to the tracheostomy site to moisten secretions and prevent drying, which would result in obstruction.

▶ VARIATIONS

Geriatric Variation:

- *Elderly clients often have thin, fragile skin that is at increased risk of irritation and excoriation. Keep the area around the tracheostomy clean and dry.*

Pediatric Variations:

- *Pediatric tracheostomy tubes are generally single cannula tubes.*
- *Because of the small internal diameter of the lumen of a pediatric tracheostomy tube, double cannula tubes are usually not available in pediatric sizes.*

Home Care Variations:

- *It is essential that the procedure be taught to the client.*
- *Routine cleaning of the inner cannula of a double cannula tracheostomy tube will prevent obstruction and airway distress.*

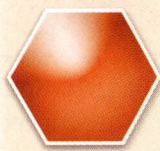

Long-Term Care Variations:

- *Once a client is discharged from the hospital, the procedure is converted from a sterile technique to a clean technique.*
- *When the client is doing self-care, good handwashing technique and clean procedures should be stressed. Instead of using sterile water or sterile saline, tap water can be used for rinsing the inner cannula.*
- *In a home care or long-term care setting, inner cannula care should be performed on a routine basis. It must be remembered that the tracheostomy is the client's only airway. Once obstruction occurs, hypoxia and respiratory arrest can occur quickly.*

▶ COMMON ERRORS

Possible Error:

There is alteration in aseptic technique.

Prevention:

Think about what steps you must follow to prevent contaminating the inner cannula during this procedure. Review the procedure. Arrange your equipment and open the tracheostomy care kit before applying sterile gloves.

Possible Error:

The equipment is inadvertently contaminated.

Prevention:

Think about why this procedure is performed sterilely and what will happen to the client if it is not done that way. The procedure is performed sterilely in the hospital setting for several reasons. The client is generally ill and, therefore, the client's immune system is compromised. The tracheostomy is a direct route to the lungs with no intervening nose and sinuses to filter out bacteria. Hospitals are a breeding ground for germs and disease. Compromising sterile technique endangers your client's health and possibly his or her life.

▶ NURSING TIPS

- Assemble equipment before beginning the procedure. If all the equipment is within reach once sterile gloves are applied, the procedure can proceed with little difficulty.
- While assembling the equipment and performing the procedure, the nurse should use this time to instruct the client. The need to clean the inner cannula will continue as long as the tracheostomy tube is in use. Inner cannula care is one of the first procedures that can be taught to the client in preparation for hospital discharge.

▶ SPECIAL CONSIDERATIONS

- *Methylene blue had been added to enteral feedings for years to determine aspirate of oropharyngeal contents with tracheal tubes. Now, obtaining a glucose oxidase test strip reading ≥20 mg/dL detects aspirate more readily.*
- *Clients with long-term tracheostomies and mechanical ventilation may develop symptoms of tracheal obstruction related to the development of granulation tissue. This may be treated with a longer tracheostomy tube, surgical intervention, or a tracheal stent.*
- *Take time to alleviate the client's anxiety prior to removing the inner cannula. Initiate methods of relaxation that have worked for the client in the past.*
- *Avoid latex tubes and gloves if client has a positive history of latex allergy.*

Plugging the Tracheostomy Tube

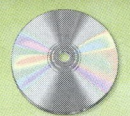

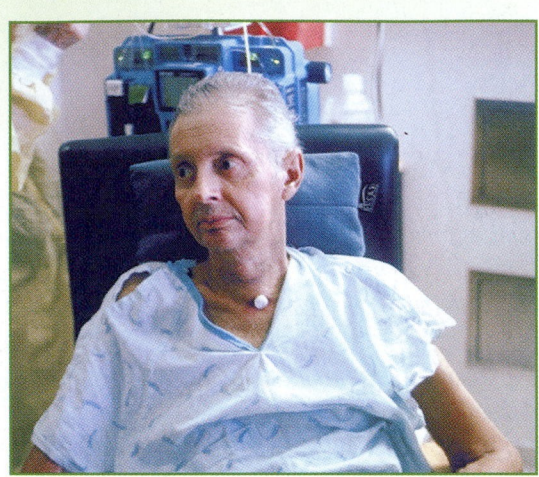

▶ OVERVIEW OF THE SKILL

A tracheostomy is an incision made into the trachea with insertion of a cannula for airway management. A tracheostomy is performed for the client with potential or present airway obstruction, for ventilatory assistance, to provide pulmonary hygiene, to decrease the anatomic dead space in the client with chronic obstructive pulmonary disease, to avoid prolonged endotracheal intubation, and to provide an airway for the client with severe obstructive sleep apnea syndrome. The tracheostomy is performed below the level of the vocal cords, and allows air to enter and exit the tracheostomy rather than through the upper airway. The tracheostomy tube can be plugged to evaluate the client's ability to tolerate removal of the tracheostomy tube (decannulation) and to provide verbal speech to the client with a tracheostomy.

▶ ASSESSMENT

1. Assess respirations for rate, rhythm, and depth, **to evaluate airway.**
2. Assess the client's ability to speak, **to determine whether air is passing around the tracheostomy tube, vibrating the vocal cords.**

▶ DIAGNOSIS

Impaired Verbal Communication

Disturbed Body Image

Powerlessness

Anxiety

▶ PLANNING

Expected Outcomes:

The client will tolerate plugging of the tracheostomy tube while maintaining an adequate airway.

Equipment Needed (see Figure 7-21-1):

- Syringe to deflate cuff of tracheostomy tube
- Smaller uncuffed tracheostomy tube
- Capped inner cannula of tracheostomy tube currently in use

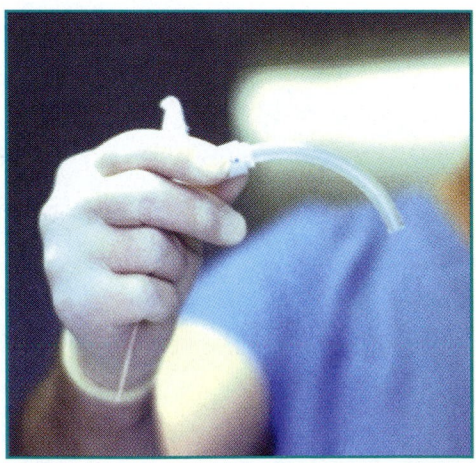

Figure 7-21-1 Capped inner cannula

▶ **CLIENT EDUCATION NEEDED:**

1. Explain the procedure to the client.
2. Reinforce descriptions of airway anatomy using illustrations.
3. Inform the client that capped inner cannula can be removed within seconds if the client exhibits difficulty breathing.

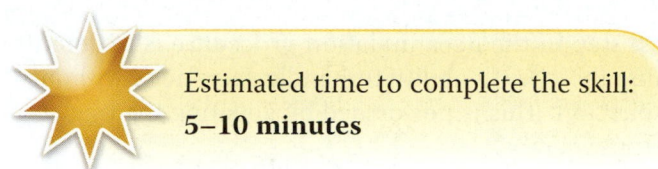

Estimated time to complete the skill:
5–10 minutes

▶ **DELEGATION TIPS**

The insertion of a tracheal tube plug is not delegated by the nurse. Ancillary personnel may assist the nurse in providing care to clients receiving this treatment and should be instructed to report a client experiencing increased secretions, dyspnea, increased respiratory rate, or the need for suctioning to the nurse.

IMPLEMENTATION—Action/Rationale

Action	Rationale
1. Deflate the cuff on a cuffed tracheostomy tube.	1. Determines the client's ability to handle secretions without aspiration.
2. Change the tracheostomy tube to a smaller uncuffed tube.	2. Determines the client's ability to breathe around the tube and through the nose and mouth.
3. Replace the inner cannula with a capped inner cannula.	3. Occludes the opening of the tracheostomy tube and evaluates the client's ability to breathe.

▶ **REAL WORLD ANECDOTES**

Mr. Jacobson has had a tracheostomy for several days. On rounds, it was discussed that decannulation can begin. The cuff of Mr. Jacobson's tracheostomy tube is deflated. As you enter Mr. Jacobson's room later in the day, you notice that he appears to be depressed. While talking to Mr. Jacobson, you learn that he is afraid he will never speak again. By using a gloved finger (or teaching the client to use his finger), you can briefly occlude the opening of the tracheostomy tube. The client can attempt to speak because the air will now exit through the upper airway, causing the vocal cords to vibrate.

▶ **EVALUATION**

• The client tolerated plugging of the tracheostomy tube while maintaining an adequate airway.

▶ **DOCUMENTATION**

Nurses' Notes

Document the client's tolerance of:
• Cuff deflation
• Ability to breathe through a smaller tube
• Ability to breathe with a plugged tracheostomy tube

Document on appropriate flow sheet or electronic medical record (EMR).

▶ **CRITICAL THINKING SKILL**

Introduction

Careful assessment is crucial to good care.

Possible Scenario

Mr. Sinclair had a tracheostomy performed at the time of head and neck surgery. Healing has progressed and an order is written to begin decannulation. The first step in the decannulation procedure is to determine the client's ability to handle secretions without aspiration. This is performed by deflating the tracheostomy cuff.

Possible Outcome

During the next 5–10 minutes, the client continuously coughs, expectorating large amounts of mucus through the tracheostomy tube. The nurse determines that the client is probably aspirating secretions and is unable to tolerate the deflation of the cuff. Because the cuff cannot be deflated, the tracheostomy tube cannot be plugged.

Prevention

Better assessment of the client's airway, presence of secretions, and frequency of coughing and suctioning may have indicated the client is not ready for decannulation (see Figure 7-21-2).

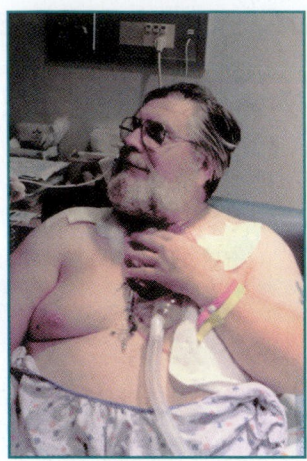

Figure 7-21-2 The client is using his finger to cover the opening of the tracheostomy tube so he can speak.

► **VARIATIONS**

Geriatric Variation:
- *Elderly clients may lack the manual dexterity to place and remove the tracheostomy plug.*

Pediatric Variation:
- *Pediatric tracheostomy tubes are generally single cannula tubes. Because of the small internal diameter of the lumen of the pediatric tracheostomy tube, an inner cannula is usually not available. For short periods of time, a finger can be placed over the opening of the tracheostomy tube, allowing the client to speak. However, pediatric tubes are usually not plugged.*

Home Care Variation:
- *Teach the client or caregiver the signs and symptoms of respiratory distress caused by the plugged tracheostomy tube, and how to respond to these signs and symptoms.*

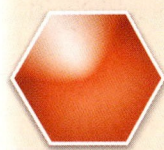

Long-Term Care Variation:
- *Teach the client or caregiver the proper care and handling of the tracheostomy plug. Because it is inserted into the tracheostomy, it must be handled cleanly.*

► COMMON ERRORS

Possible Error:

A plugged tracheostomy tube is inserted in a client with an inflated cuff.

Prevention:

Think about why you can never use a capped tracheostomy inner cannula in a client with an inflated cuff. Once the plugged inner cannula is used, the client will breathe around the tracheostomy through the upper airway. If the cuff is inflated, the client will be unable to pass air around the tube, resulting in an inability to breathe.

► NURSING TIPS

- Assemble all equipment prior to beginning the procedure.
- Explain the procedure to the client to avoid anxiety.
- Review with the client the procedure to remove the inner cannula.
- Suction the client orally to remove any secretions that may have pooled on top of the cuff to prevent aspiration when the cuff is deflated.

► SPECIAL CONSIDERATIONS

- *Weaning clients from tracheostomy tubes can be accomplished in a variety of ways. The size of the tracheostomy tube can be progressively decreased, or a tracheostomy plug or button may be used. The plug is useful when a client demonstrates borderline clearance of secretions and requires a longer period of observation for stoma maintenance.*
- *Successful decannulation, like extubation, occurs when the client has the strength for a spontaneous cough, no upper airway obstruction, and a decreased need for suctioning.*
- *Avoid latex tubes and gloves if positive history.*

Circulatory

Performing Venipuncture (Blood Drawing)

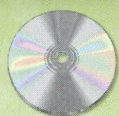

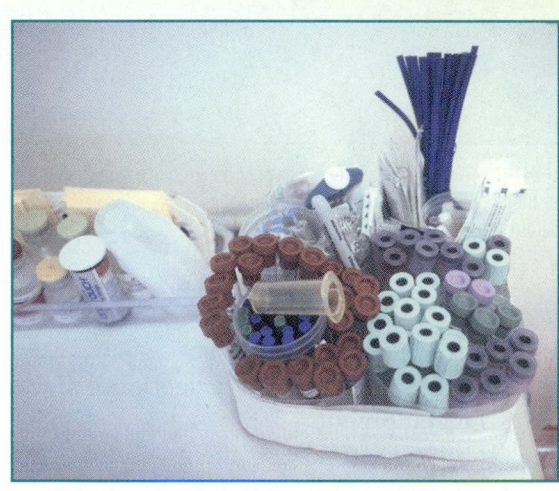

▶ OVERVIEW OF THE SKILL

Obtaining a sample of blood through venipuncture is a commonly used procedure for many diagnostic tests. Blood test results are a source of valuable information to screen clients for disease, to evaluate the progress of therapy, and to monitor the well-being of the client. The nurse is often required to obtain a variety of specimens. As some specimens require special handling, it is important for the nurse to be familiar with the particular test that is ordered.

There are three primary methods of obtaining blood specimens: venipuncture, skin puncture, and arterial stick. Venipuncture is the most common method and involves inserting a large-bore needle into a vein. The nurse attaches either a syringe or a vacutainer tube for the collection of the blood specimen. Skin puncture is the easiest way to obtain a small specimen from the finger, toe, or heel. A lancet is used for the puncture and a drop of blood is collected through a capillary tube. An arterial stick is the most complicated and requires special assessment skills and techniques.

As with any procedure, it is important that nurses review their employer's policies and procedures as well as their state's nurse practice act.

▶ ASSESSMENT

1. Determine which test(s) is ordered and be familiar with any special conditions associated with the timing of the collection or the handling of the specimen. Many specimens may be collected at very specific times, that is, before or after administration of a drug, while the client is nothing per mouth (NPO), or after fasting. Other specimens may require special handling; that is, ice is used to transport ammonia levels; heparinized collection containers are needed for platelet counts; and so on. **Using a damaged vein may cause further injury to the vein. A compromised site may not provide an adequate amount of blood for the specimen and may lead to another venipuncture for the client.**

2. Assess the integrity of the veins that may be used in the procedure. Identify any conditions that may contraindicate venipuncture. Avoid veins injured by infiltration or phlebitis or compromised by surgery (e.g., modified radical mastectomy). In addition, **drawing samples from sites near IV infusion solutions may alter the composition of the blood sample.**

3. Review the client's medical history to determine if there are any expected complications from the venipuncture. **Clients with a history of abnormal clotting disorders, low platelets, or related disorders (hemophilia) may be at risk for increased bleeding at the site or hematoma formation.**

4. Determine the client's ability to cooperate with the procedure. **Many clients are fearful of needles—**

especially children—and additional help may be needed. Very young children may need to have the extremity restrained during the procedure.

5. Review the physician's or qualified practitioner's order. Check for appropriateness of the test as well as the frequency of the test. Critically ill clients may require frequent blood tests and venipuncture. **Combining tests and carefully evaluating frequency may reduce unnecessary blood loss for the client.**

▶ DIAGNOSIS

Deficient Knowledge

Risk for Infection

Risk for Injury

Impaired Tissue Integrity

Anxiety

Fear

▶ PLANNING

Expected Outcomes:

1. Venipuncture site will show no evidence of continued bleeding or hematoma.
2. The venipuncture site will show no evidence of signs and symptoms of infection.
3. The laboratory test will be properly acquired and appropriately handled after collection.
4. The client will be able to discuss the purpose of the test and describe the procedure.
5. The client will report minimal anxiety associated with the procedure.

Equipment Needed (see Figure 8-1-1):

- Disposable gloves
- Alcohol swabs
- Rubber tourniquet
- Sterile 2 × 2 gauze pads
- Band-Aid® or adhesive tape (precut)
- Appropriate blood collection tubes
- Labels for each collection tube with the appropriate client information included
- Completed laboratory requisition forms
- Needle/equipment disposal container
- Small pillow or folded towel to support the extremity, if needed
- Syringe method: sterile needles: 20- to 21-gauge for adults, 23- to 25-gauge butterfly for older adults, 23- to 25-gauge butterfly for children
- Vacutainer method: Vacutainer tube with needle holder; sterile double needles (20- to 21-gauge for adults, 23- to 25-gauge for children)

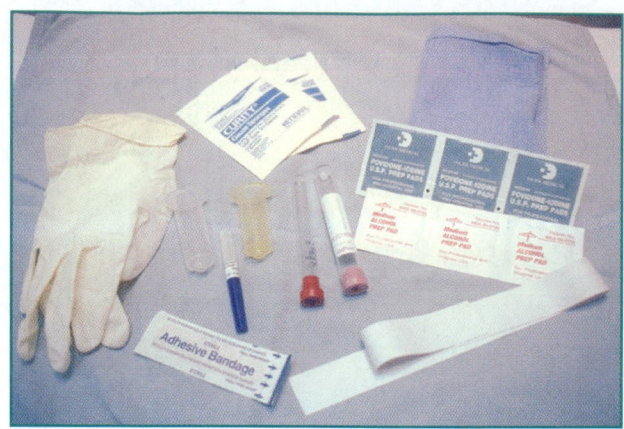

Figure 8-1-1 Nonsterile gloves, sponges, povidone-iodine, alcohol swabs, blood collection tubes, vacutainer tube, vacutainer needle, and rubber tourniquet.

▶ CLIENT EDUCATION NEEDED:

1. Explain the purpose of the test.
2. Describe the procedure for collection. Show the client the equipment.
3. Explain the sensations the client will experience with the tourniquet placement, alcohol swab, and needle stick.
4. Explain when the client may expect results from the diagnostic tests.
5. Instruct the client to apply direct pressure to the venipuncture site postprocedure for 3 to 5 minutes. Clients with bleeding disorders should be instructed to alert health care providers of those specifics prior to any procedures. They should also expect to apply pressure to the site for at least 5 minutes.
6. Teach the client deep-breathing techniques for relaxation prior to any procedure. This will provide the client with some "control" in the situation and also provide the client with some distraction during the procedure.
7. Teach the young child how to "draw blood" on a toy before performing the procedure on the child. Play therapy is commonly used in pediatrics as a way to help reduce anxiety in the child. Including a favorite toy in the action helps the child see what the procedure involves.
8. Explain to the client that the site may be slightly sore for a day or two following the stick. Encourage the client to report any symptoms that may be of concern.

Estimated time to complete the skill: **Approximately 10 minutes**

► **DELEGATION TIPS**

The procedure of performing a venipuncture for the purposes of blood drawing is frequently delegated to properly trained ancillary personnel. Documentation of their competency and skill should be available to the nurse and periodic reevaluation should occur according to agency and state policy. The ancillary personnel should be reminded to not obtain blood specimens from an extremity above the site of infusing fluids and to report to the nurse any complications or concerns the client might express postprocedure.

IMPLEMENTATION—Action/Rationale

Action	Rationale
1. Greet client by name and validate client's identification.	1. Proper client identification ensures safety for the client and the nurse.
2. Explain the procedure to the client (see Client Education Needed).	2. Client rights dictate that any action be explained to the client. The client always has the right to refuse a procedure. Information decreases anxiety.
3. Wash hands.	3. Reduces transmission of microorganisms.
4. Bring equipment to bedside or client exam room. Transfer client to the procedure room, especially for small children, as it is important to keep their hospital room a "safe haven."	4. Provides an organized approach to the procedure.
5. Close curtain or door.	5. Provides privacy.
6. Raise or lower bed/table to comfortable working height.	6. Maintains good body mechanics for the nurse during the procedure.
7. Assess the extremities for the presence of an arteriovnous shunt used for dialysis or history of mastectomy before selecting an appropriate site for the venipuncture.	7. Extremities with a shunt or on the same side as the mastectomy should not be used for a venipuncture site.
8. Position client's arm; extend arm to form a straight line from shoulder to wrist. Place pillow or towel under upper arm to enhance extension. Client should be in a supine or semi-Fowler's position.	8. Helps stabilize the arm. The bed should support the client's body (when possible) in case client should feel faint during the procedure.
9. Apply disposable gloves.	9. Reduces the risk of infection to both the client and the nurse (Standard Precautions).
10. Apply the tourniquet 3 to 4 inches above the venipuncture site. Most often the antecubital fossa site is used. The tourniquet should be able to be removed by pulling the end with a single motion.	10. Tourniquet provides improved visibility of the veins as they dilate in response to decreased venous return of blood flow from the extremity to the heart.

continues

Action	Rationale
11. Check for the distal pulse. If there is no pulse felt, then the tourniquet is applied too tightly and must be reapplied more loosely.	**11.** If the pressure is too tight, it may impede arterial flow to the extremity.
12. Have client open and close fist several times, leaving fist clenched prior to venipuncture.	**12.** Increases the venous distension and enhances visibility of the vein. Vigorous motion, however, may result in hemoconcentration of the specimen.
13. Maintain tourniquet for only 1–2 minutes.	**13.** Prolonged time may increase client discomfort and alter some laboratory results (e.g., falsely elevated serum potassium).
14. Identify the best venipuncture site through palpation; the ideal site is a straight prominent vein that feels firm and slightly rebounds when palpated. Palpate potential site.	**14.** Straight, intact veins are easier to puncture. A thrombosed vein is rigid, or rolls easily, and is difficult to stick.
15. Select the vein for venipuncture. (If the tourniquet has been on too long, release it and let the client rest for 1 to 2 minutes before reapplying the tourniquet.)	**15.** Allowing the client to rest increases client comfort and ensures accurate laboratory results.
16. Prepare to obtain the blood sample. Technique varies depending on equipment used: • Syringe method: Have syringe with appropriate needle attached. • Vacutainer method: Attach double-ended needle to vacutainer tube and have the proper blood specimen tube resting inside the vacutainer. Do not puncture the rubber stopper yet.	**16.** • A needle with a very small bore can damage the red cells as the blood is drawn and lead to inaccurate test results. • The long end of the needle is used to puncture the vein and the short end enters the blood tube.
17. Cleanse the venipuncture site with alcohol swab or chlorhexidine alcohol using a circular method at the site and extending the motion 2 inches beyond the site (see Figure 8-1-2). Allow the alcohol to dry.	**17.** The alcohol solution and mechanical cleaning motion cleans the skin surface of bacteria that may cause infection at the site. Allowing the alcohol to dry reduces the stinging sensation that the client may experience.

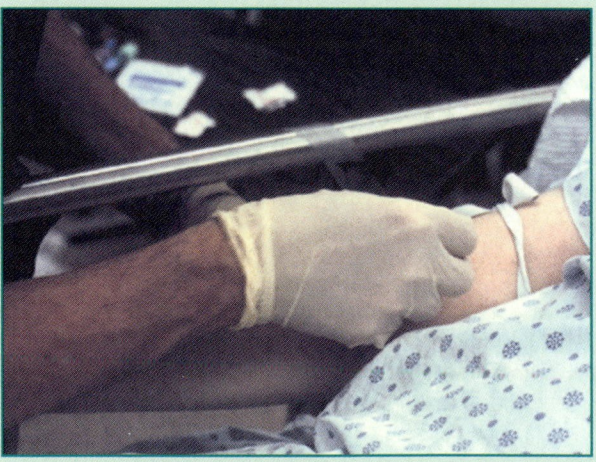

Figure 8-1-2 After applying the tourniquet, cleanse the skin at the venipuncture site. Do not let the tourniquet stay on longer than 2 minutes. If you need more time, remove the tourniquet for a couple of minutes to allow the client to rest, and begin again.

continues

Action	Rationale
18. Remove the needle cover and warn that client will feel the needle stick for a few seconds.	**18.** Clients will be better able to control their reaction if they know what to expect.
19. Place the thumb or forefinger of the nondominant hand 1 inch below the site and pull the skin taut.	**19.** Helps stabilize the vein during insertion.
20. Hold syringe needle or vacutainer at a 15- to 30-degree angle from the skin with the bevel up.	**20.** This angle reduces the chance of penetrating though the vein during insertion. The needle causes less trauma to the skin and vein when the bevel is up during insertion.
21. Slowly insert needle/vacutainer (see Figure 8-1-3).	**21.** Prevents puncture through the other side of the vein.
22. Technique varies depending on equipment used: • Syringe method: Gently pull back on syringe plunger and look for blood return. Obtain desired amount of blood into the syringe. • Vacutainer method: Hold vacutainer securely and advance specimen tube into needle of holder. Be careful not to advance the needle into the vein. The blood should flow into the collection tube. After the collection tube is full, grasp the vacutainer firmly, remove the tube, and insert additional specimen collection tubes as indicated (see Figures 8-1-3 and 8-1-4).	**22.** • If blood does not appear, the needle is not in the vein. • Pushing the needle through the stopper breaks the vacuum and causes the flow of blood into the collection tube. Failure of blood to appear in the collection tube indicates the vacuum in the tube has been lost or the needle is not in the vein.
23. After the specimen collection is completed, release the tourniquet.	**23.** Reduces bleeding from pressure when the needle is removed.
24. Apply 2 × 2 gauze over the puncture site without applying pressure and quickly withdraw the needle from the vein.	**24.** Positions the gauze for removal and helps to gently prevent the skin from pulling with the needle removal.

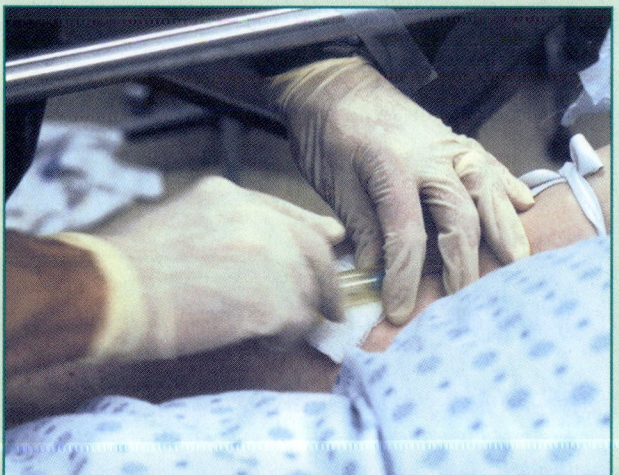

Figure 8-1-3 Hold the vacutainer and needle assembly securely and press the specimen tube into the holder. The needle inside the holder will pierce the specimen tube and blood should begin to flow into the tube.

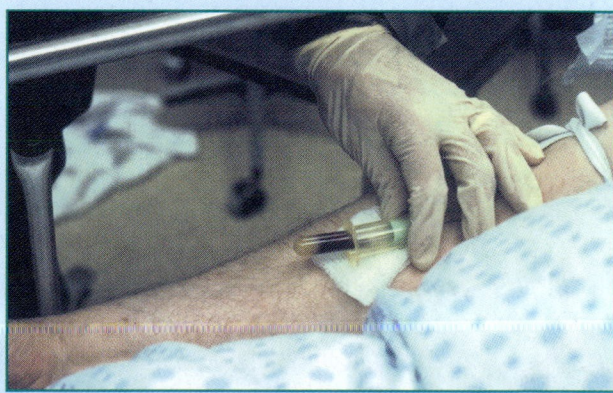

Figure 8-1-4 Allow the tube to fill with blood. When it is full, remove the tube and insert additional tubes, if needed.

continues

Action	Rationale
25. Immediately apply pressure over the venipuncture site with the gauze for 2 to 3 minutes or until the bleeding has stopped. Tape the gauze dressing over the site (or apply the Band-Aid®).	25. Direct pressure stops the bleeding and minimizes formation of a hematoma. You may avoid using tape or a Band-Aid® if, after applying pressure, no bleeding is present. Many clients are sensitive to tape and its removal can be painful.
26. Syringe method: • Using one hand, insert the syringe needle into the appropriate collection tube and allow vacuum to fill. You may also remove the stopper from each vacutainer collection tube, remove the needle from the syringe, fill the tube, and replace the stopper.	26. Using a one-handed method to fill the syringe helps reduce the chance of needle-stick injury. • This alternative method allows you to control the speed and amount of fill in the collection tubes.
27. If any of the blood tubes contain additives, gently rotate back and forth 8–10 times.	27. Ensures that the additive is properly mixed throughout the specimen.
28. Inspect the client's puncture site for bleeding. Reapply clean gauze and tape, if necessary.	28. Keeps site clean and dry.
29. Assist client into a comfortable position. Return bed to low position with side rails up, if appropriate.	29. Provides comfort and safety for the client.
30. Check tubes for any external blood and decontaminate with alcohol as appropriate.	30. Prevents contamination to other equipment and personnel.
31. Check tubes for proper labeling. Place tubes into appropriate bags/containers for transport to the laboratory.	31. Ensures the specimens are properly identified.
32. Dispose of needles, syringe, and soiled equipment into proper container.	32. Prevents spread of disease and needle-stick injury.
33. Remove and dispose of gloves.	33. Reduces transmission of microorganisms.
34. Wash hands after the procedure.	34. Reduces transmission of microorganisms.
35. Send specimens to the laboratory.	35. Facilitates timely handling of specimens and accurate results.

▶ REAL WORLD ANECDOTES

Scenario 1
The nurse went into Mrs. Smith's room, introduced herself, and proceeded to draw a CBC and platelet count. After completing the procedure, the nurse went out to the nurse's station and processed the specimens. The nurse went to cross the orders off the unit laboratory sheet and noticed that there was another client by the name of Smith down the hall. Unfortunately for the client, the nurse had not checked the client's ID band and had obtained the specimen from the wrong client. This could have resulted in the wrong information being posted in the client's record, and inappropriate treatment based on those results.

continues

> **REAL WORLD ANECDOTES** (continued)

Scenario 2

A nurse was helping a busy colleague and offered to draw a specimen of blood from Mr. Van Hook. The client was properly identified and the procedure went very smoothly. The nurse processed the specimens and went back to recheck the venipuncture site on Mr. Van Hook. He reported some tenderness and the nurse noted a large hematoma at the site. The nurse had failed to check the medical record and did not realize that Mr. Van Hook was on heparin therapy. The venipuncture site for Mr. Van Hook would have required direct pressure for at least 5 minutes.

▶ EVALUATION

- Venipuncture site shows no evidence of continued bleeding or hematoma.
- Venipuncture site shows no signs or symptoms of infection.
- The laboratory test is properly acquired and appropriately handled after collection.
- The client is able to discuss the purpose of the test and describe the procedure.
- The client reports minimal anxiety associated with the procedure.

▶ DOCUMENTATION

Nurses' Notes

- Record the date and time of the venipuncture, the site used for the procedure, any complications, the tests obtained, and the disposition of the specimens.
- Note the client's reaction to the procedure and the condition in which the client was left (i.e., bed lowered with side rails up).

Document on appropriate flow sheet or electronic medical record (EMR).

▶ CRITICAL THINKING SKILL

Introduction

Understanding the specific requirements for collection of blood specimens is crucial. Failure to do so may result in inaccurate results, which can lead to errors in treatment of the client or a repeat of the venipuncture test.

Possible Scenario

The home care nurse received orders to draw a cyclosporine level on Mr. Jones. Mr. Jones was day 42 postallogeneic blood cell transplant and receiving infusions of cyclosporine every 12 hours for the prevention of graft-versus-host disease. Mr. Jones was independent with his infusion administration and had scheduled nursing visits for laboratory draws twice a week. The nurse scheduled a visit to draw the blood for 11:00 a.m. The drug level was collected and the specimen dropped off to the transplant center for processing.

Possible Outcome

The home care nurse received the cyclosporine level results the following day and called Mr. Jones's physician with the results. Upon receiving the results, the physician was alarmed that the cyclosporine level was so high and concerned that Mr. Jones might have symptoms of toxicity. During further discussion with the nurse, it was determined that the cyclosporine level was drawn 2 hours *after* Mr. Jones had completed his morning infusion.

Prevention

Cyclosporine levels are drawn *before* the next dose. As with many drug levels, the timing of the blood sample in relation to the dose is essential for accurate results. In this case, the home care nurse should have instructed Mr. Jones to hold his morning dose of cyclosporine until after the blood sample. The home care nurse would then schedule the visit in accordance with the scheduled timing of the dose.

▶ VARIATIONS

Geriatric Variations:

- *Older clients often have very fragile veins or veins that roll. Vein integrity is very important to access and veins need to be secured carefully before venipuncture.*
- *These clients may also need direct pressure post-needle stick for a longer period of time as they are prone to bruising and hematoma development.*

Pediatric Variations:

- *Dorsal surfaces of the hands and feet are the most frequently selected venipuncuture sites in children.*
- *Select a site that requires the least amount of restraint for the child/infant.*
- *Have another nurse (not the parent) assist you with restraint of the child during the procedure as necessary.*
- *Scalp veins may be used for neonates or infants, but this site is often the least desired site by the parent.*
- *Use topical transdermal numbing medications at least 30 minutes prior to the needle stick.*

Home Care Variations:

- *Teach the client/caregiver to recognize signs and symptoms of infection or phlebitis and to report pain, redness, or significant bruising.*
- *Home care clients who have been on infusion therapy for a long period of time will often provide the nurse with information related to which veins are the "best" to use for venipuncture. Evaluate the sites carefully and include the client's preferences when possible.*

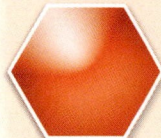

Long-Term Care Variation:

- *These clients may be scheduled for venipuncture on a regular basis and may also have vein preference or poor venous access at some sites. Consider the client's suggestions carefully and listen to what the client tells you; often an experienced client is right.*

▶ COMMON ERRORS

Possible Error:

Piercing through the other side of the vein during venipuncture.

Prevention:

Hold the syringe and needle at a 15- to 30-degree angle from the client's arm with the bevel up. This position should reduce the chance of penetrating both sides of the vein.

Possible Error:

Sample results are diluted from IV fluids near the site of the venipuncture.

Prevention:

Select a site away from the IV infusion site. An alternative may be to stop the infusion during the venipuncture procedure (depending on the therapy and the venous access used).

► **NURSING TIPS**

- Apply warm packs (wet compresses or dry chemical packs) for 10–15 minutes to the site, allowing for venous distension and easier visual location of the site.
- Neonates and infants may need to be wrapped in a warm blanket or placed under an infant warming light for 10 to 15 minutes before attempting venipuncture to facilitate visual location of sites.
- The client should be in a comfortable, relaxed position.

- The nurse should approach the client with confidence, as this will reduce the client's anxiety level.
- For obese clients with difficult veins to locate, create a visual image of venous anatomy and use palpation to guide you through venipuncture.
- With experience the nurse will feel the vein "pop" as the needle enters.
- Avoid any site that pulsates with palpation as this indicates the site is an artery.
- To avoid prolonged use of the tourniquet, release it as you prepare the site and then reapply it before the actual venipuncture.

► **SPECIAL CONSIDERATIONS**

- *Confidence is essential when drawing blood. Approach the task with self-assurance and the client will feel less frightened.*
- *Labeling the lab specimen with the correct client name is the first step to a successful blood draw. If the client is getting a type and cross-match for blood and receives the wrong blood type because of a labeling error, the client can die as a result of incompatible blood. The phlebotomist must always be vigilant when labeling a specimen.*
- *When drawing blood for an HIV test, the phlebotomist must ensure that HIV testing is informed, voluntary, and consented and that counseling and information are provided prior to taking the test. Certain laws at the local, state, and federal levels may regulate how HIV testing is done and it is important for the nurse to become familiar with these laws and mandates (i.e., testing of the minor, the intubated client, etc.).*

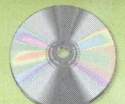
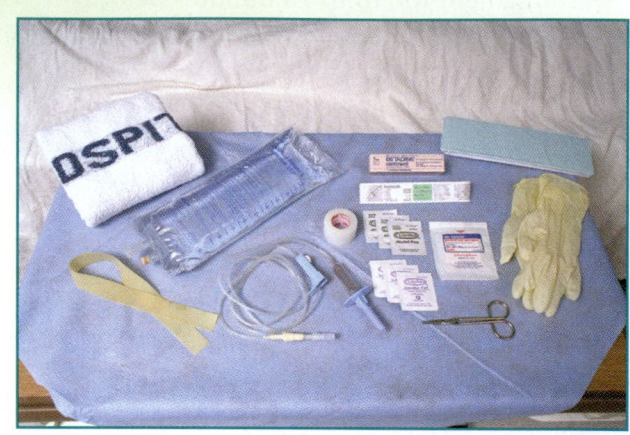

▶ OVERVIEW OF THE SKILL

Performing venipuncture in order to establish venous access is a priority for clients with fluid and electrolyte disturbances, clients who are critically ill, clients who are nothing per mouth (NPO) after surgery, or clients who for other reasons are not able to take fluids or food by mouth. Venous access can be used for infusions of IV fluids, emergency medications, parenteral nutrition, blood products, and routine intravenous (IV) medications.

There are a variety of IV needles and catheters. They vary in gauge from small bore to large bore. A 20- to 22-gauge flexible catheter is used for adults while a 22- to 24-gauge catheter is used for pediatric clients. If large volumes of fluid or blood products are anticipated to be given, a larger bore (e.g., 18- or 19-gauge) is recommended.

A commonly used angiocatheter has an over-the-needle catheter (ONC) made of plastic, Teflon, or other materials. These flexible catheters have a metal stylet that is used to pierce the skin and vein and a plastic catheter that is threaded into the vein and attached to the IV tubing after the stylet has been removed.

The other type of IV needle is a straight, steel needle that is inserted into the vein and secured after being attached to an IV tubing. With an increased emphasis on safety, many health care facilities use a safety-shielded intravenous catheter or retractable needle system when placing a peripheral intravenous line. This consists of a traditional metal stylet used for the skin puncture covered by the plastic or Teflon angiocatheter. Once the intravenous line is successfully placed, the health care provider initiating the IV pushes a button and the stylet retracts completely into a protective casing, thereby reducing the risk of needle-stick injury.

Needle sticks are common among health care workers, so strict care in handling needles while starting an IV is imperative. Centers for Disease Control and Prevention (CDC) guidelines must be followed in order to decrease the risk of infection for the client such as changing the IV solution every 24 hours, changing the IV site and catheter every 48–72 hours, and changing the IV tubing every 72 hours. Occupational Safety and Health Administration (OSHA) standards are necessary to prevent exposure to blood-borne pathogens through the use of gloves, puncture-resistant containers for sharps, and special training for health care workers (see Figure 8-2-1).

▶ ASSESSMENT

1. Check the health care provider's order for the type of therapy planned **to determine the optimal needle size and type to use.**
2. Review information regarding the insertion of the IV **in order to insert the catheter safely.**
3. Know the agency's policy regarding who may start an IV **as many agencies require that nurses have special training before they can perform this procedure.**

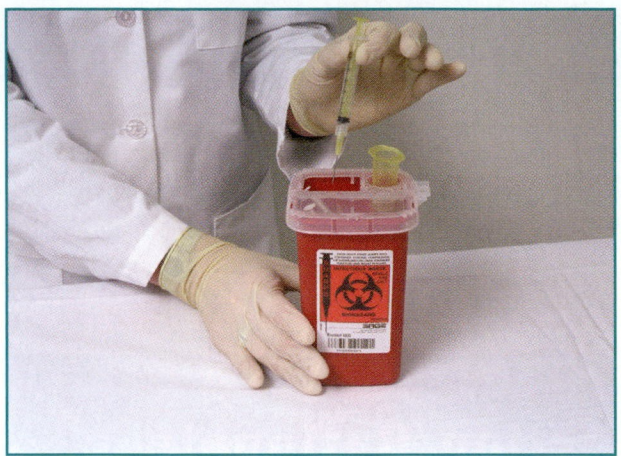

Figure 8-2-1   Needle sticks are common among health care workers. Use proper technique and dispose of all sharp equipment in puncture-resistant containers.

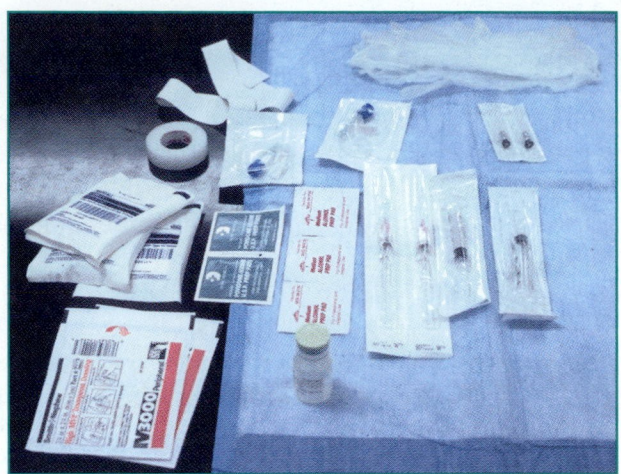

Figure 8-2-2   Povidone-iodine, alcohol pads, various IV needles, tourniquet, tape, and transparent dressings

4. Assess the client's veins **to optimize planning of the IV site.**
5. Check the client's fluid, electrolyte, and nutritional status **to provide baseline data for comparison with the client's response to IV therapy.**
6. Assess the client's understanding of the purpose of the procedure **so that client teaching can be used to decrease anxiety.**

▶ DIAGNOSIS

Deficient Knowledge

Risk for Infection

Excess Fluid Volume

Deficient Fluid Volume

Impaired Skin Integrity

Risk for Injury

▶ PLANNING

Expected Outcomes:

1. The IV will be inserted into the vein without complications and will remain patent.
2. Fluid and electrolyte balance will be restored to the client.
3. Nutrition will be restored or maintained.
4. The IV site will remain free of swelling and inflammation.

Equipment Needed (see Figure 8-2-2):

- Appropriate safety needle or catheter for venipuncture
- Tourniquet
- Povidone-iodine swabs (3) or chlorhexidine alcohol (chloroprep)
- Alcohol swab sticks (3) (not needed if using chlorhexidine alcohol)
- Disposable gloves
- Arm board, if needed
- Towel or absorbent drape
- Povidone-iodine ointment (not used in all institutions)
- Gauze dressing
- Tape
- Scissors
- IV tubing and solution

▶ CLIENT EDUCATION NEEDED:

1. Give the client oral and written instructions about the insertion of an IV.
2. Teach the client to report any signs of inflammation, clotting, leaking, or breaking.
3. Teach the client how to bathe without getting the dressing wet.
4. Instruct the client how to prevent the IV from becoming dislodged.
5. Instruct the client how to properly position the arm to maintain IV flow if the IV is positional.
6. Teach the client how to walk with an IV pole.
7. Suggest client wear clothes with wide sleeves.
8. Discuss with the client what activities he or she engages in to be sure such activities are safe and will not cause damage to the IV.

Estimated time to complete the skill: **15 minutes**

▶ **DELEGATION TIPS**

Initiating IV therapy via venipuncture is a skill involving assessment and the use of medical asepsis. It is an invasive procedure not delegated by the nurse unless other licensed personnel have been trained and certified to perform the procedure. Ancillary personnel who will be caring for the client need to be instructed to handle the extremity with the IV gently and to report any complaints of pain or swelling in the affected extremity to the nurse.

IMPLEMENTATION—Action/Rationale

Action	Rationale
1. Check health care provider's order for an IV and identify client.	1. Ensures accurate insertion of catheter on the correct client.
2. Wash hands and put on mask and gown, if needed.	2. Reduces the transmission of microorganisms.
3. Organize all equipment at bedside.	3. Ensures smooth procedure without accidents or contamination.
4. Explain procedure and reason the catheter is being inserted.	4. Information decreases anxiety.
5. Assess the extremities for the presence of an arteriovenous shunt used for dialysis or history of mastectomy before selecting an appropriate site for the IV.	5. Extremities with a shunt or on the same side as the mastectomy should not be used for an IV site.
6. Inspect potential veins to be used: • Place a tourniquet around the upper arm close to the axilla. • Examine the veins as they dilate. • Palpate the vein to test for firmness (see Figure 8-2-3). • Release the tourniquet.	6. Promotes ease of placement of catheter. • Distends vein to allow visual and tactile examination. • To evaluate the viability of the vein. • To determine the best site for venipuncture and IV placement. • Prevents engorgement of vein.
7. Select vein for venipuncture: • Use most distal part of the vein first. • Avoid bony prominences. • Avoid client's wrist or hand. • Avoid client's dominant hand and arm. • Avoid an extremity with decreased sensation. • Avoid an area of skin affected by a rash or infection.	7. • If the vein is later damaged, the proximal part can be used. • Increases client comfort. • Bending of the wrist or hand increases the risk of infiltration or phlebitis. • Allows freedom of movement. • Promotes earlier detection of infiltration. • Decreases risk of infection.
8. Select safety shield or angiocatheter that is appropriate for ordered IV fluid. Select the correct size of gauge and length of catheter (see Figure 8-2-5).	8. Necessary to puncture vein. Angiocatheter gauge sizes vary widely. Particular intravenous therapies, such as transfusions, require specific sizes of intravenous access. Age and quality or location of veins can affect choice of size.

continues

Action	Rationale

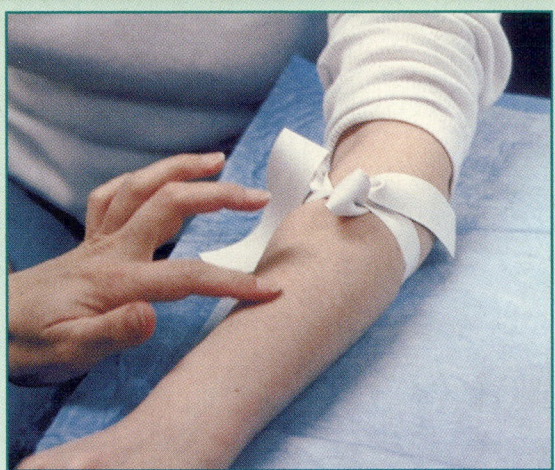

Figure 8-2-3 Inspect the site for potential veins to use, and palpate to further locate a vein and test for firmness.

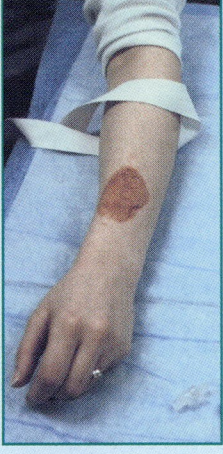

Figure 8-2-4 After scrubbing the insertion site with alcohol and povidone-iodine, allow it to dry. Note: The tourniquet is released while the site is drying.

9. Prepare supplies:
   • Place towel or drape on table for supplies.
   • Place supplies on towel.
   • Open needle adapter end of IV tubing set.

9. Provides a clean working surface for an efficiently performed procedure.

10. Shave hair on skin at site, if necessary.

10. Ensures adherence of dressing and that removal is less painful. Shaving should be avoided as it causes small abrasions that increase the risk of infection.

11. Ask client to rest arm in a dependent position, if possible.

11. Allows better venous dilation and visibility.

12. Put on disposable gloves.

12. Reduces transmission of microorganisms.

13. Prepare insertion site (see Figure 8-2-5):
   • Place absorbent drape under the arm.
   • Scrub the insertion site with 3 alcohol swabs then 3 povidone-iodine swabs.

   • Follow institution protocol. Some facilities use chlorhexidine alcohol instead of iodine.
   • Allow the antiseptic solution to air dry.

13.
   • Reduces transmission of microorganisms.
   • Alcohol removes fat on the skin and vigorous scrubbing in circular motion with povidone-iodine removes bacteria. Using a separate swab and starting in the middle of the site working outward prevents bacteria from being reintroduced to the site.
   • Povidone-iodine or chlorhexidine alcohol must be dry to be effective.

14. Apply tourniquet 5–6 inches above the insertion site.

   • Secure it tightly enough to occlude venous flow, not arterial flow.
   • Check presence of distal pulse.

14. Tourniquet is needed to allow the vein to engorge for easier venipuncture.
   • Decreased arterial flow prevents venous filling.

   • Ensures arterial flow is present.

continues

Action	Rationale

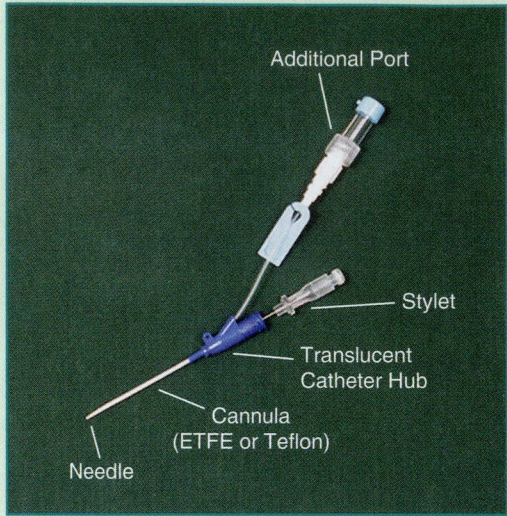

Figure 8-2-5 An angiocatheter type of IV catheter.

Additional Port

Stylet

Translucent
Catheter Hub

Cannula
(ETFE or Teflon)

Needle

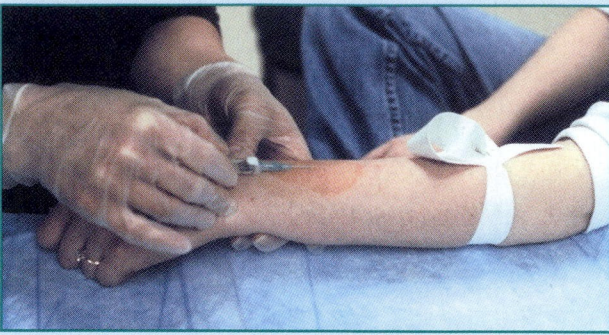

Figure 8-2-6 Insert the needle with the beveled side up. Keep the angle low, 20 to 30 degrees.

15. Perform the venipuncture:
   - Anchor the vein by placing thumb over vein and stretching the skin against the direction of insertion 2 to 3 inches distal to the site.
   - Insert the stylet needle at a 20- to 30-degree angle with the bevel up (see Figure 8-2-6).
   - Watch for a quick blood return through the flashback chamber of the ONC.
   - Verify needle placement in a vein, not artery.

   - Advance ONC ¼ inch into the vein while it is parallel to the skin.
   - Loosen stylet and advance catheter into vein until hub rests at venipuncture site (see Figure 8-2-7).
   - Do not reinsert stylet.

15.
   - Stabilizes the vein for ease of venipuncture.

   - Prevents puncture of posterior wall of vein.

   - Venous pressure from tourniquet causes backflow of blood into catheter or tubing.
   - Some veins are close to an artery. Arterial blood is bright red and pulses.
   - Ensures the catheter is in the vein.

   - Ensures proper placement of the catheter.

   - Prevents the catheter from being punctured by the stylet.

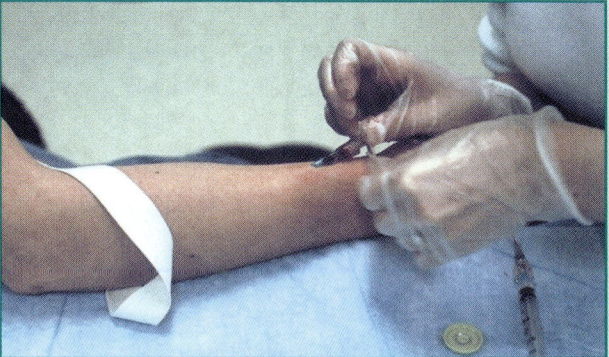

Figure 8-2-7 Loosen the stylet and advance the catheter into the vein until the hub rests on the skin at the venipuncture site.

continues

Action	Rationale
• Hold thumb over vein above catheter tip.	• Prevents blood from leaking out of vein until IV tubing is connected.
• Release the tourniquet.	• Reestablishes venous blood flow.
16. Attach IV tubing to ONC.	**16.**
• Stabilize the catheter with one hand.	• Maintains catheter placement.
• Remove the stylet from ONC or if using a safety catheter push the button on the protective casing and stylet will fully retract into the casing.	• Provides entry portal for IV fluids. Reduces risk of inadvertent needle-stick injury.
• Quickly release pressure over vein and quickly connect needle adapter of IV set to hub of ONC.	• Reduces blood loss.
• Begin infusion at slow rate to keep vein open (see Figure 8-2-8).	• Prompt initiation of infusion maintains patency of IV.
17. Secure catheter in place:	**17.**
• Place tape over the hub of the catheter.	• Ensures catheter's safe position.
• Place transparent dressing over the site and secure (see Figure 8-2-9).	• Controls bleeding and prevents infection. Allows visualization of site through transparent dressing.
• Secure tubing in loop fashion with tape.	• Prevents dislodgement of IV if tubing is pulled.
18. Remove gloves and dispose with all used materials.	**18.** Reduces transmission of microorganisms.
19. Place label with date and time of insertion and size and gauge of catheter on the dressing. Follow protocol for scheduled dressing change.	**19.** Provides information to schedule next dressing change.
20. Wash hands.	**20.** Reduces transmission of microorganisms.

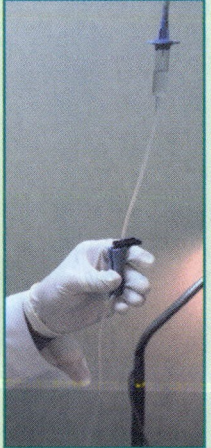

Figure 8-2-8 Begin the infusion at a slow rate to keep the vein open while you secure the catheter and dress the site.

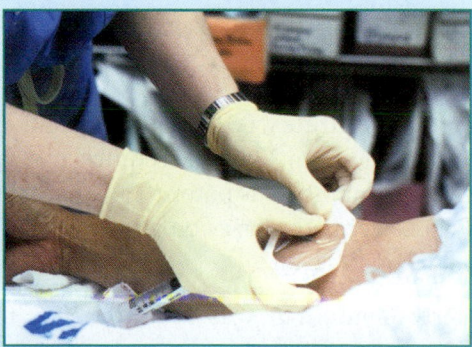

Figure 8-2-9 Cover the site with a transparent dressing.

▶ **REAL WORLD ANECDOTES**

Mrs. Kindzia was scheduled for surgery to have a medication pump replaced. The pump had been placed to provide Mrs. Kindzia with a steady dose of muscle relaxant medication to control severe muscle spasticity secondary to her multiple sclerosis. In the surgery preparation area the nurse attempted to start an IV for venous access during surgery. The nurse was unable to start the IV despite several attempts and reported this to the anesthesiologist. The anesthesiologist refused to participate in the surgery if Mrs. Kindzia did not have venous access. The nurse tried to start the IV multiple times, without success. Finally, in order to perform the surgery safely, the anesthesiologist placed an access catheter in Mrs. Kindzia's jugular vein. In all, the staff had attempted to start an IV 12 times before deciding on the jugular access. Because of her multiple sclerosis, Mrs. Kindzia was not able to protest the number of needle pokes she received. Long before she had been poked so many times her nurse should have stepped into the role of client advocate and discussed alternatives rather than continuing to traumatize the client. Most facilities recommend that after three attempts at an IV start, another more experienced person take over.

▶ EVALUATION

- The IV was inserted into the vein without complications and remains patent.
- Fluid and electrolyte balance were restored to the client.
- Nutrition was restored or maintained.
- The IV site remains free of swelling and inflammation.

▶ DOCUMENTATION

Nurses' Notes

- Note date and time the IV was inserted.
- Document type and gauge of catheter.
- Record date of dressing placement.
- Describe client's reaction to the procedure.
- Document fluid to be infused or if a saline or heparin lock.

Document on appropriate flow sheet or electronic medical record (EMR).

▶ CRITICAL THINKING SKILL

Introduction

When an IV infiltrates, it damages the vein and tissue surrounding it. Some clients require multiple venipunctures to maintain a patent IV. It is necessary to preserve the veins that are remaining for future use.

Possible Scenario

An elderly gentleman was admitted to the cardiac intensive care unit after complaining of chest pains. The nurse noted that the IV inserted in the emergency room was placed in the large vein in the antecubital space. A large-bore needle was used in case emergency medications were needed. However, the site appeared to be slightly swollen after the client had been moving his arm around during transport.

Possible Outcome

The nurse assessed the IV site and determined that the IV was still patent. As the site was already punctured and a large-bore needle was used, the nurse decided to place the client's arm on an arm board to prevent further trauma and continued to use this site. Shortly afterward, the client's blood pressure started to decrease, and his physician ordered dopamine to be started immediately. The nurse started to hang the dopamine and reassess the IV site and noted that the site was definitely swollen and infiltrated. This was the client's only venous access site, and with his low blood pressure, obtaining a new venous access site was difficult and time consuming. The nurse was able, finally, to secure a new IV site and the dopamine infusion was started. The client's blood pressure was stabilized but his life was unnecessarily jeopardized by the lack of patent venous access.

Prevention

The nurse looked for another vein more distal on the opposite arm after asking the client which was his dominant arm, and was successful in starting a large-bore IV that was in a much more comfortable site and preserved the proximal sites for later use if needed. The nurse then removed the IV that would soon be infiltrated.

In emergency situations, it is not always possible to select a comfortable site; however, planning for short-term IV therapy should be done whenever possible.

► VARIATIONS

Geriatric Variations:

- *The veins of elderly clients may be more fragile. Be aware of this when assessing IV sites for continued patency.*
- *Be careful to use only minimal pressure of the tourniquet because of fragile skin and veins.*
- *Use a 5- to 15-degree angle when inserting the needle as the elderly client's veins are more superficial.*
- *Elderly clients develop fluid imbalances more rapidly because of a larger extracellular fluid-volume.*
- *Some elderly clients may have cardiac or renal failure that requires specialized IV therapy because of increases in vascular volume or inability to eliminate extracellular fluid.*
- *Tourniquet should be left in place a minimal amount of time because of more fragile veins in the elderly.*

Pediatric Variations:

- *In neonates, veins of the scalp and feet can be used.*
- *Use the smallest gauge needle possible according to the IV therapy needed.*
- *Special precautions are needed to maintain an intact IV in very young clients.*
- *Allow older children to help in the selection of the IV site in order to increase cooperation and decrease anxiety.*
- *Teenagers and young adults often have thicker, tougher skin than a middle-aged client. The nurse should bear this in mind when starting an IV on someone this age.*

Home Care Variations:

- *A more secure dressing may be necessary if the client is active.*
- *Ensure that containers for proper disposal of equipment are in place.*
- *Arrange for delivery of IV supplies.*

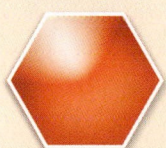

Long-Term Care Variations:

- *Clients in the long-term care setting may have more contact with nurses' aides than with nurses. The aides must be taught to recognize and report IV infiltrations or other problems.*
- *Be sure to assess the IV site often and to change the IV site every 3 days or according to the policies of the institution.*

► COMMON ERRORS

Possible Error:

The catheter is noted to be pulled out 1 inch at the time of the dressing change.

Prevention:

Be sure to secure the catheter with tape. Advise the client to be careful of the catheter during activity. If the catheter is pulled out, do not push catheter back into vein. Check for patency of the catheter. If it is patent, it may continue to be used when properly secured. If it is not patent, it will need to be replaced.

▶ **NURSING TIPS**

- Methods to promote venous dilation are:
  - Stroking the extremity from distal to proximal below the proposed venipuncture site

  - Opening and closing the fist

  - Light tapping with two or three fingers over the vein

  - Applying a warm washcloth or other heat to the extremity

- Be sensitive to the client's dominant arm and need for some movement.
- Use 18-gauge or larger needle if the infusion of blood products is anticipated.
- Always insert the IV needle/catheter in the direction of venous return (toward the heart) to avoid damaging the venous valve.

▶ **SPECIAL CONSIDERATIONS**

- *Approximately 14% of all hospital-acquired infections are catheter related and the result of bloodstream infections. Aseptic technique and adherence to handwashing are important measures in preventing catheter-associated infections.*
- *The most important extrinsic risk factors associated with infection caused by an intravascular catheter (bloodstream infection) are catheter location, duration of catheterization, type of catheter material, conditions of insertion, catheter-site care, and skill of the catheter inserter. Check institution policy regarding scheduled site changes as it is standard practice to decrease the potential for infection.*

Inserting a Butterfly Needle

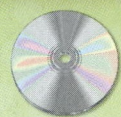

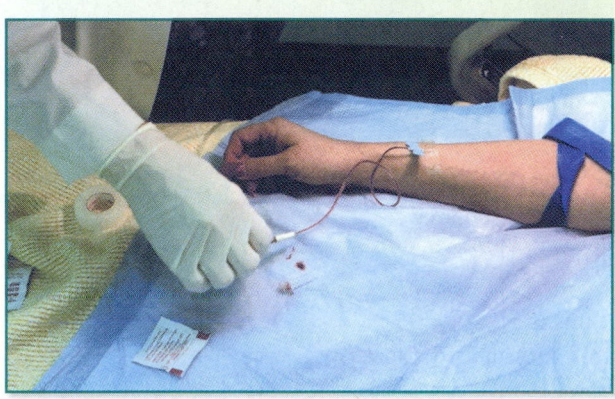

▶ OVERVIEW OF THE SKILL

Performing a venipuncture to establish a venous access is a priority for clients with fluid and electrolyte disturbances, clients who are critically ill, clients who are nothing per mouth (NPO) after surgery, or clients who for other reasons are not able to take fluids or food by mouth. Venous access can be used for infusions of intravenous (IV) fluids, emergency medications, parenteral nutrition, blood products, and routine IV medications.

A variety of IV needles and catheters exist, varying in gauge from small bore to large bore. A 20- to 22-gauge flexible catheter is used for adults, whereas a 22- to 24-gauge catheter is used for pediatric clients. If large volumes of fluid or blood products are expected to be given, a larger bore (18- or 19-gauge) is recommended.

A butterfly needle is commonly used for short-term venous access or for pediatric clients. It is called a butterfly because of the flexible wings on either side of a short needle and 2- to 3-inch tubing that ends with a hub. This design makes it easy for the nurse to guide the needle into a vein to draw blood or to infuse medication or fluid. Unlike the flexible catheters commonly used for IVs, the butterfly needle uses a rigid, sharp needle as the venous access port. Because the sharp tip remains in the vein during the IV infusion, infiltration of the IV is more common than with the flexible catheter. Butterfly needles are not commonly used for long-term IV therapy, although they may still be used in clients who have very small veins or in areas where a larger catheter cannot be advanced into the vein. Butterfly needles may be used when venous access is only required for short-term IV therapy. When a butterfly needle has been used for IV access, the nurse must check the IV site frequently for infiltration.

▶ ASSESSMENT

1. Assess the purpose of the IV. **Butterfly needles are more often used in short-term IV therapy.**
2. Assess the client's veins. **A butterfly needle may be necessary if the client's veins are small or the vein is in a difficult position to access.**
3. Check the client's fluid, electrolyte, and nutritional status **to provide baseline data for comparison with the client's response to IV therapy.**
4. Assess the client's understanding of the purpose of the procedure **so that client teaching can be used to decrease anxiety.**

▶ DIAGNOSIS

Deficient Knowledge

Excess Fluid Volume

Deficient Fluid Volume

Risk for Infection

Impaired Skin Integrity

Risk for Injury

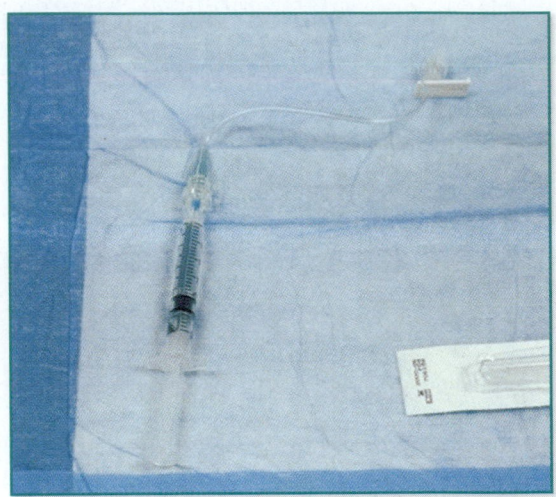

Figure 8-3-1A Needleless system, syringe, and extension tubing

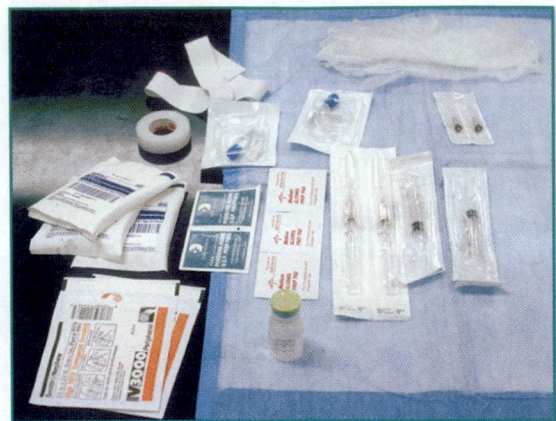

Figure 8-3-1B Transparent dressing, gauze, tape, extension tubing, povidone-iodine, alcohol pad, and sterile saline

▶ PLANNING

Expected Outcomes:

1. The IV will be inserted into the vein without complications and will remain patent.
2. The IV site will be without signs or symptoms of infiltration.
3. The IV will be started and will infuse with a minimum of trauma and discomfort to the client.

Equipment Needed (see Figures 8-3-1A and B):

- Appropriate gauge butterfly needle for venipuncture
- Tourniquet
- Povidone-iodine swabs (3) or chlorhexidine alcohol
- Alcohol swab sticks (3) (not needed if using chlorhexidine alcohol)
- Disposable gloves
- Arm board, if necessary
- Towel or absorbent drape
- Povidone-iodine ointment
- Gauze dressing or transparent dressing
- Tape
- Scissors
- IV tubing and solution

▶ CLIENT EDUCATION NEEDED:

1. Teach the client to report any signs of inflammation or swelling.
2. Teach the client how to bathe without getting the dressing wet.
3. Instruct the client how to prevent the IV from becoming dislodged.
4. Provide written and oral instructions about the care of an IV.
5. Instruct the client how to properly position the arm to maintain IV flow if the IV is positional.
6. Teach the client how to walk with an IV pole.
7. Discuss with the client what activities he or she engages in to be sure such activities are safe and will not cause damage to the IV.

Estimated time to complete the skill:
15 minutes

▶ DELEGATION TIPS

Initiating IV therapy via insertion of a butterfly needle device is a skill involving assessment and aseptic technique. It is an invasive procedure not delegated by the nurse unless other licensed personnel have been trained and certified to perform the procedure. Ancillary personnel who will be caring for the client need to be instructed to handle the extremity with the IV gently and to report any complaints about pain, numbness, or tingling to the nurse.

IMPLEMENTATION—Action/Rationale

Action	Rationale
1. Check health care provider's order for an IV, and identify client.	1. Ensures accurate insertion of IV needle in the correct client.
2. Wash hands; put on mask and gown, if needed.	2. Reduces the transmission of microorganisms.
3. Organize all equipment at bedside.	3. Ensures smooth procedure without accidents or contamination.
4. Explain procedure and reason the IV needle is being inserted.	4. Information decreases anxiety.
5. Assess the extremities for the presence of an arterio-venous shunt used for dialysis or history of mastectomy before selecting an appropriate site for the IV.	5. Extremities with a shunt or on the same side as the mastectomy should not be used for an IV site.
6. Inspect potential veins to be used (see Figure 8-3-2): • Place a tourniquet around the upper arm close to the axilla. • Examine the veins as they dilate. • Palpate the vein to test for firmness. • Release the tourniquet.	6. Promotes ease of placement of IV needle. • Distends vein to allow visual and tactile examination. • To assess blood return in veins. • To assess fragility of veins. • Prevents engorgement of blood.
7. Select vein for venipuncture: • Use most distal part of the vein first. • Avoid bony prominences. • Avoid client's wrist or hand. • Avoid client's dominant hand and arm. • Avoid an extremity with decreased sensation. • Avoid an area of skin affected by a rash or infection.	7. • If the vein is later damaged, the proximal part can be used. • Increases client comfort. • Bending of the wrist or hand increases the risk of infiltration or phlebitis. • Allows freedom of movement. • Promotes earlier detection of infiltration. • Decreases risk of infection.
8. Select appropriate gauge butterfly needle (see Figure 8-3-3).	8. Chooses needle necessary to puncture vein.

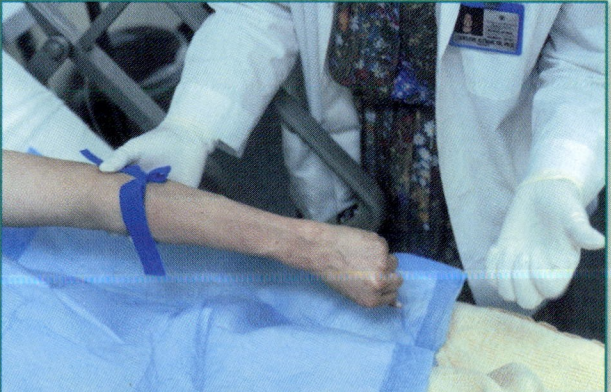

Figure 8-3-2 Inspect the veins and select the vein to be used.

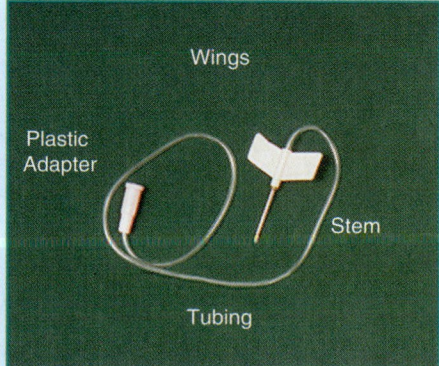

Figure 8-3-3 Butterfly IV catheter.

continues

Action	Rationale
9. Prepare supplies: • Place towel on table for supplies. • Place supplies on towel. • Open needle adapter end of IV tubing set.	9. Provides a clean working surface for an efficiently performed procedure.
10. Clip hair on skin at site, if necessary.	10. Ensures adherence of dressing and that removal is less painful. Shaving should be avoided as it causes microscopic abrasions that increase the risk of infection.
11. Ask client to rest arm in a dependent position, if possible.	11. Allows better venous dilation and visibility.
12. Put on disposable gloves.	12. Reduces transmission of microorganisms.
13. Prepare insertion site: • Place towel or absorbent drape under the arm. • Scrub the insertion site with 3 alcohol swabs then 3 povidone-iodine swabs or chlorhexidine alcohol antiseptic solution (see Figure 8-3-4). • Follow institution protocol for cleaning insertion site regarding use of iodine or chlorhexidine alcohol. • Allow the antiseptic solution to dry.	13. • Reduces transmission of microorganisms. • Alcohol removes fat on the skin and vigorous scrubbing in a circular motion with povidone-iodine removes bacteria. Using a separate swab and starting in the middle of the site working outward prevents bacteria from being reintroduced to the site. • Many institutions have switched to chlorhexidine alcohol swabs as clients may be sensitive to iodine. • Povidone-iodine or chlorhexidine alcohol must be dry to be effective.
14. Apply tourniquet 5–6 inches above the insertion site. • Secure it tightly enough to occlude venous flow, not arterial flow. • Check presence of distal pulse.	14. Tourniquet is needed to allow the vein to engorge for easier venipuncture. • Decreased arterial flow prevents venous filling. • Ensures arterial flow is present.
15. Perform the venipuncture: • Anchor the vein by placing thumb over vein and stretching the skin against the direction of insertion 2–3 inches distal to the site. • Grasp the wings of the butterfly needle and insert the butterfly needle at a 20- to 30-degree angle with the bevel up slightly distal to the venipuncture site (see Figure 8-3-5). • Watch for a blood return through the tubing of the butterfly needle. • Verify needle placement in a vein, not an artery. • Advance the butterfly needle into the vein until the hub rests at the venipuncture site (see Figures 8-3-6 and 8-3-7). • Release the tourniquet.	15. • Stabilizes the vein for ease of venipuncture. • Prevents puncture of posterior wall of vein. • Venous pressure from tourniquet causes backflow of blood into tubing. • Some veins are close to an artery. Arterial blood is bright red and pulses. • Ensures the IV needle is in the vein and proper placement of the IV needle. • Reestablishes venous blood flow.

continues

Action	Rationale

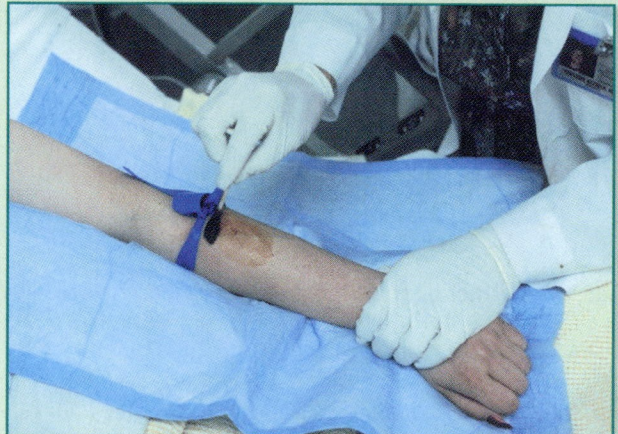

Figure 8-3-4   Scrub the insertion site with alcohol, then repeat with 3 povidone-iodine swabs or use chlorhexidine alcohol.

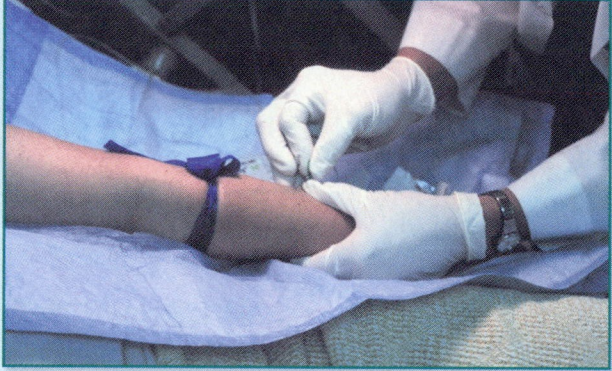

Figure 8-3-5   Insert the needle at a 20- to 30-degree angle with bevel up.

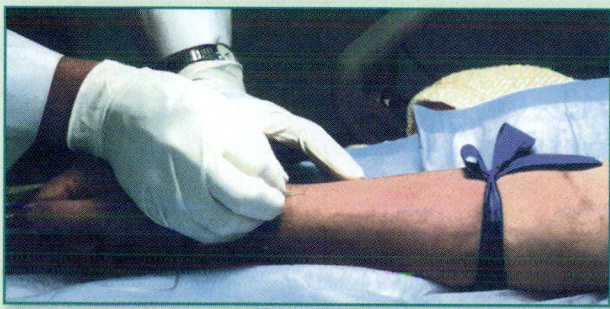

Figure 8-3-6   Still holding the butterfly wing, advance the needle into the arm.

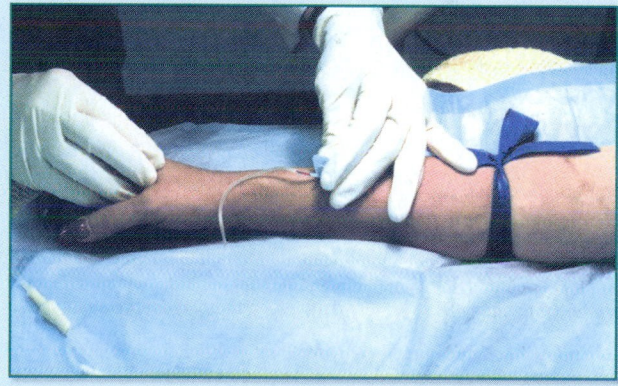

Figure 8-3-7   Stop when the hub rests at the venipuncture site. Note the blood return in the butterfly needle tubing.

16. Attach IV tubing to butterfly needle.
   - Stabilize the needle with one hand.
   - Connect needle adapter of IV set to hub of butterfly needle tubing.
   - Begin infusion at slow rate to keep vein open.

17. Secure needle in place (see Figure 8-3-8):
   - Place tape over the wings of the butterfly needle.
   - Place transparent dressing over insertion site and secure.

18. Remove gloves and dispose of all used materials.

16.
   - Maintains IV needle placement.
   - Reduces blood loss.

   - Prompt initiation of infusion maintains patency of IV.

17.
   - Ensures needle's safe position.
   - Controls bleeding and prevents infection. Allows visualization of site.

18. Reduces transmission of microorganisms.

continues

Action	Rationale
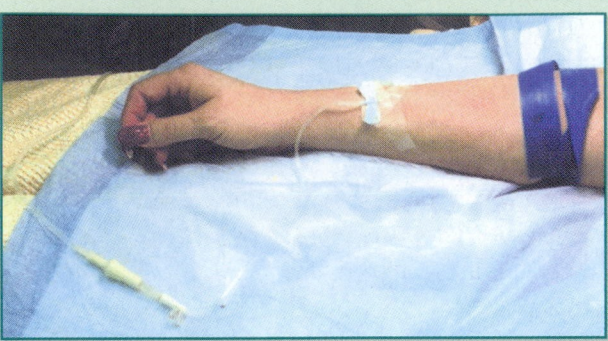	
	Figure 8-3-8 Attach the IV tubing to the needle and secure the needle in place.
19. Place label with date and time of insertion and size and gauge of needle on the dressing.	**19.** Provides information to schedule next dressing change.
20. Wash hands.	**20.** Reduces transmission of microorganisms.

► **REAL WORLD ANECDOTES**

Scenario 1

Jason, 2 years old, was admitted to the day surgery unit for placement of tubes in his ears after repeated ear infections. Because his need for an IV was short-term and his veins were small, the nurse selected a 23-gauge butterfly needle. As Jason's mother held him in her lap, the nurse explained what she was going to do and reassured him that when he woke up after his ears were fixed the needle would be taken out. The nurse demonstrated how she would put the needle into a vein using a teddy bear that Jason held. The demonstration with the teddy bear helped to reassure Jason, and with the help of his mother, Jason only whimpered when the needle was actually inserted. He chose a Band-Aid® with Mickey Mouse to put over the insertion site.

Scenario 2

Andrea, a 23-year-old with a history of IV drug use, was admitted to the emergency room with a suspected overdose. While trying to start an IV, the nurse noted that most of Andrea's veins were badly scarred. The nurse was unable to find a suitable IV site in either of Andrea's arms or the backs of her hands. The nurse was finally able to start an IV using a 21-gauge butterfly needle in the back of Andrea's right thumb. The nurse used a tongue blade as a splint to prevent movement of the site and carefully taped the site to prevent movement but allow inspection of the insertion point.

► **EVALUATION**

- The IV was inserted into the vein without complications and remains patent.
- The IV site is without signs or symptoms of infiltration.
- The IV was started and is infusing with a minimum of trauma and discomfort to the client.

► **DOCUMENTATION**

Nurses' Notes

Note the following:

- Date and time IV was started
- Type and gauge of needle used
- Insertion site
- Type of dressing placed over site
- Any unusual occurrences during the IV insertion
- Type and rate of fluid

Document on appropriate flow sheet or electronic medical record (EMR).

▶ CRITICAL THINKING SKILL

Introduction

Clients with small veins may require a small-gauge needle. Using a butterfly needle gives the nurse more control guiding it into a vein. The needle is also shorter so it may be less frightening to pediatric clients or people from another culture.

Possible Scenario

Mrs. Nguyen was admitted to the emergency room with complaints of abdominal pain. The emergency room physician ordered a complete blood count (CBC) and chemistry panel and then ordered an abdominal computerized tomography (CT) scan. The nurse noted that the woman's veins were quite small and delicate.

Possible Outcome

The nurse caring for Mrs. Nguyen felt that butterfly needles were never appropriate to use because of the frequency of venous trauma and infiltration. He attempted to gain IV access using a 21-gauge venous catheter. When he inserted the venous catheter, there was a blood flashback. However, when he attempted to advance the venous catheter, the vein tore and bled into the surrounding tissue. The nurse made three attempts at starting the IV using a 21-gauge venous catheter without success. Mrs. Nguyen became increasingly upset and agitated with each failure. Finally the nurse asked another staff member to try to start the IV.

The nurse chose a 21-gauge butterfly needle. She used it to draw the blood samples and then connected it to an IV solution of normal saline and set it at a rate to keep the vein open. When the client was sent for a CT scan, she had a vein open to be used for contrast dye.

Prevention

Keep in mind the reason for the IV when choosing an insertion site and infusion equipment. When the nurse realized that the client's veins were too fragile to sustain the passage of an over-the-needle catheter, he should have reevaluated the client's needs and his approach. Recognizing that the IV access was only required for a short time, the nurse could have saved the client undue trauma by changing to a butterfly needle sooner.

▶ VARIATIONS

Geriatric Variations:

- *The veins of elderly clients may be more fragile so care must be taken not to traumatize them with the tip of the needle.*
- *Be careful to use only minimal pressure of the tourniquet because of fragile skin and veins.*
- *Use a 5- to 15-degree angle when inserting the needle as the elderly client's veins are more superficial.*

Pediatric Variations:

- *In neonates, veins of the scalp and feet can be used.*
- *Use the smallest gauge needle possible according to the IV therapy needed.*
- *Special precautions are needed to maintain an IV intact in very young clients. Restraints may be required to immobilize the IV site.*
- *Allow older children to select the IV site in order to increase cooperation and control.*

Home Care Variations:

- *The butterfly needle can be inserted in the home by a nurse.*
- *A more secure dressing may be necessary if the client is active.*
- *Ensure that containers for proper disposal of equipment are in place.*

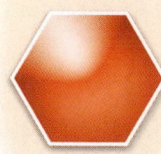

Long-Term Care Variations:

- *Butterfly needles are not generally used for long-term IV therapy.*
- *If a butterfly needle is placed for a long-term IV, the site should be inspected frequently for infiltration.*

▶ COMMON ERRORS

Possible Error:

Blood is noted in the tubing of the butterfly set after the venipuncture, but when the needle is advanced, a resistance is felt and no more blood flows into the tubing.

Prevention:

Be sure to advance the needle carefully at a 20- to 30-degree angle so it does not puncture through the vein. If this error does occur, pull back on the needle. If a brisk blood return in the tubing is seen, secure the needle to the skin. If no blood return is seen, the IV may need to be restarted in another site.

▶ NURSING TIPS

- Methods to promote venous dilatation are:
  - Stroking the extremity from distal to proximal below the proposed venipuncture site.
  - Opening and closing the fist.
  - Light tapping with two or three fingers over the vein.
  - Applying a warm washcloth or other heat to the extremity.
- Be sensitive to the client's dominant arm and need for some movement.
- Use the smallest gauge possible for pediatric and elderly clients with fragile veins.
- Always insert the IV needle in the direction of venous return (toward the heart) to avoid damaging the venous valves.

▶ SPECIAL CONSIDERATIONS

- Approximately 14% of all hospital-acquired infections are catheter related and associated with bloodstream infections. Aseptic technique and adherence to handwashing are important measures in preventing catheter-associated infections.
- The most important extrinsic risk factors associated with infection caused by an intravascular catheter (bloodstream infection) are: catheter location, duration of catheterization, type of catheter material, conditions of insertion, catheter-site care, and skill of the catheter inserter.
- Complications with peripheral intravascular catheters are more often associated with the following:
  - Lower extremities more than upper extremities
  - Wrist more than hand
  - Leaving the catheter in place for more than 3 days
- Catheter made from polyvinyl chloride and polyethylene-Teflon has been associated with fewer infections.

Preparing the IV Bag and Tubing

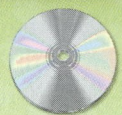

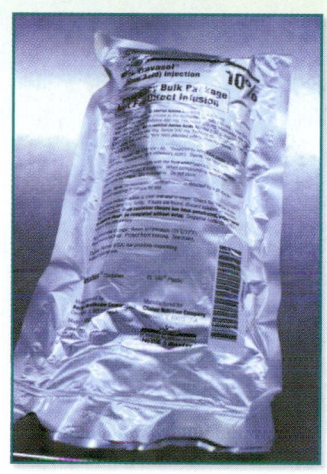

▶ OVERVIEW OF THE SKILL

An intravenous (IV) solution is a method of correcting or preventing a fluid and electrolyte disturbance. Clients who are acutely ill, are nothing per mouth (NPO) after surgery, or have severe burns are a few examples of those who require IV therapy.

The solution in an IV bag is ordered by the health care provider according to the client's needs and is changed at least every 24 hours. The tubing is used to connect the solution in the IV bag with the client's IV catheter or needle. The IV tubing should be changed every 72 hours and when the IV catheter is changed. These changes in solution and tubing are recommended to decrease the risk of infection.

There are many brands and types of IV tubing available. It is important to be familiar with the types you will be using most often. Tubing varies according to the number of ports required, for example, a primary tubing set may have no ports or multiple ports. Secondary tubing is used to add or "piggyback" another solution into a primary set. Blood transfusions require specific tubing with a filter. Tubing used in a controller is specific to the type of machine. Tubing size varies between brands and affects the drops (gtts) of solution for each cc, for example, macrodrops can vary from 10, 15, or 20 gtts per milliliter. Microdrops are 60 gtts per milliliter. The nurse must be aware of the drop size in order to accurately calculate the IV flow rate (see Skill 8-5).

▶ ASSESSMENT

1. Check the health care provider's order for the IV to be infused and rate of flow **to ensure accurate administration.**
2. Review information regarding the solution and nursing implications **in order to administer the solution safely.**
3. Check all additives in the solution and other medications **so that there will be no incompatibilities with the solution.**
4. Assess the patency of the IV **to ensure that the solution will enter the vein and not the surrounding tissue.**
5. Assess the skin at the IV site **so that the solution will not be administered into an inflamed or edematous site, which could cause injury to the tissue.**
6. Assess the client's understanding of the purpose of the IV infusion **so that teaching can be tailored to client's needs.**

▶ DIAGNOSIS

Impaired Skin Integrity

Risk for Infection

Deficient Knowledge

Deficient Fluid Volume

Excess Fluid Volume

▶ PLANNING

Expected Outcomes:

1. The IV tubing will be replaced without compromising the sterility of the system.
2. The new IV tubing will infuse the new solution without leaks or air bubbles.
3. The new IV solution will infuse at the prescribed rate.
4. The client will be able to discuss the purpose of the IV therapy.

Equipment Needed (see Figure 8-4-1):

- Disposable gloves
- IV solution in a bag
- IV tubing as ordered
- Sterile 2 × 2 gauze

▶ CLIENT EDUCATION NEEDED:

1. Teach the client the rationale for the IV therapy.
2. Teach the client the type of solution and additives he is receiving.
3. Instruct clients to report any swelling or pain at the IV site.

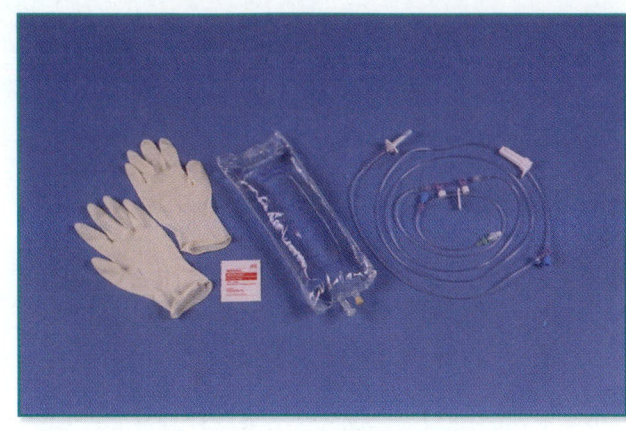

Figure 8-4-1   Gloves, alcohol pad, IV solution, and tubing

4. The client should know the rationale for changing the tubing.
5. Instruct the client to notify the nurse if any leaking from the tubing occurs.

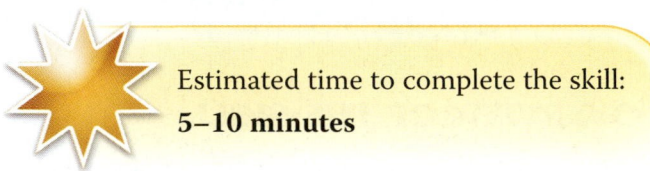

Estimated time to complete the skill:
5–10 minutes

▶ DELEGATION TIPS

Initiating IV therapy via IV bag and tubing preparation is a skill involving assessment and the use of medical asepsis. It is a procedure not delegated by the nurse unless other licensed personnel have been trained and certified to perform the procedure.

IMPLEMENTATION—Action/Rationale

Action	Rationale
1. Check health care provider's order for the IV solution.	1. Ensures accurate administration of the solution.
2. Wash hands.	2. Reduces transmission of microorganisms.
3. Check client's identification bracelet.	3. Ensures medication is given to the correct client.
4. Prepare new bag by removing protective cover. Check the expiration date on the bag and assess for cloudiness or leakage (see Figure 8-4-2).	4. Allows for quick, smooth preparation. Ensures that the solution is sterile.

continues

Action	Rationale
5. Open new infusion set. Unroll tubing and close roller clamp.	5. Prevents fluid from leaking after IV bag is spiked.
6. Spike bag with tip of new tubing and compress drip chamber to fill halfway (see Figures 8-4-3 to 8-4-6).	6. Promotes rapid flow of solution through new tubing without air bubbles.
7. Open roller clamp, remove protective cap from the end of the tubing, and slowly flush solution completely through tubing.	7. Removes air from tubing. Prevents entry of air into the venous system, a cause of air embolus. If fluid enters tubing too rapidly air bubbles occur.
8. Close roller clamp and replace cap protector.	8. Prevents fluid from leaking and maintains sterility of tubing.
9. Apply clean gloves.	9. Reduces the transmission of microorganisms.

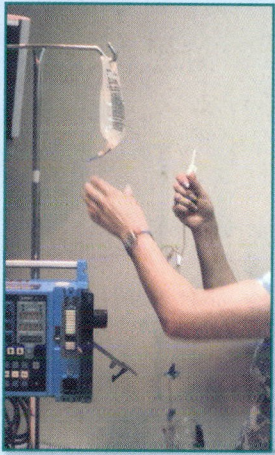

Figure 8-4-3   Remove the protective cap from the end of the IV tubing.

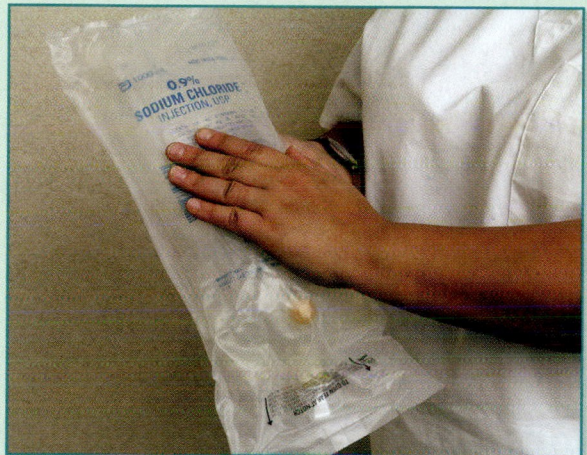

Figure 8-4-2   Check the expiration date on the bag and inspect for cloudiness and leakage.

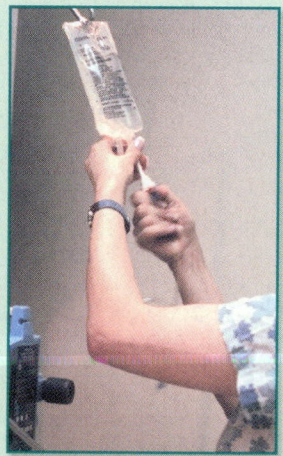

Figure 8-4-4   Spike the bag with the sharp tip of the new tubing.

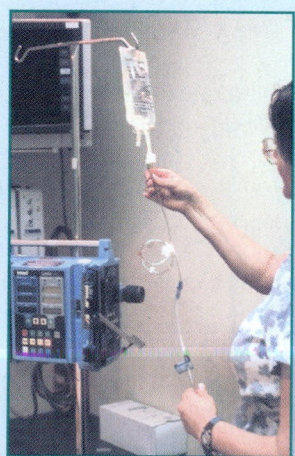

Figure 8-4-5   Compress the drip chamber and allow it to fill halfway with fluid.

continues

Action	Rationale

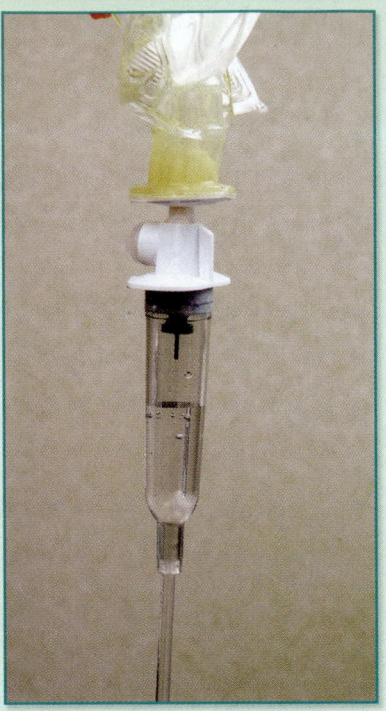

Figure 8-4-6   Make sure the drip chamber is at least half filled.

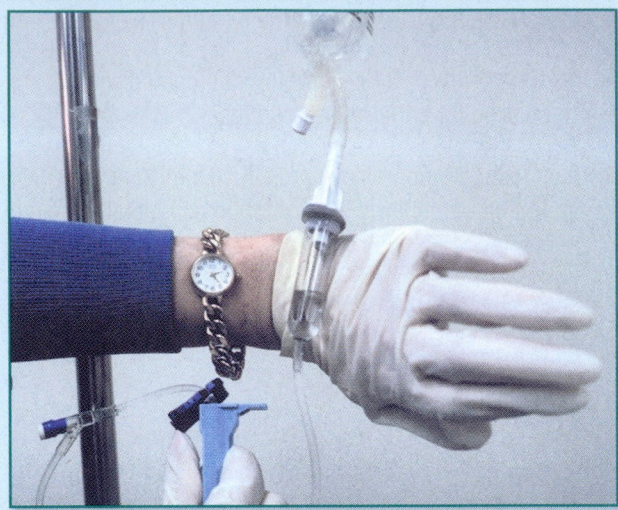

Figure 8-4-7   Establish the drip rate.

10. Remove old tubing and replace with new tubing:
  • Place sterile 2 × 2 gauze under IV catheter or heparin lock.
  • Stabilize hub of catheter or needle and gently pull out old tubing.
  • Quickly insert new tubing into hub of catheter or needle.
  • Open roller clamp to establish flow of IV solution.

  • Reestablish drip rate (see Figure 8-4-7).
  • Apply new dressing to IV site.

11. Discard old tubing and IV bag.

12. Remove gloves and dispose with all used materials.

13. Apply a label with date and time of change to tubing. Calculate intravenous drip rates and begin infusion at prescribed rate (see instruction on calculating drip rates).

14. Wash hands.

10.
  • Absorbs fluids that may drip during the procedure, preventing contamination of surrounding areas.
  • Prevents accidental dislodging of catheter or needle.
  • Prevents backflow of blood or the entrance of air into the vein.
  • Prevents catheter occlusion and maintains IV flow at prescribed rate.
  • Maintains IV flow at prescribed rate.
  • Provides protection from infection and accidental dislodgement.

11. Prevents accidental transmission of microorganisms.

12. Reduces transmission of microorganisms.

13. Allows for planning of next change.

14. Reduces transmission of microorganisms.

► **REAL WORLD ANECDOTES**

Mr. Hahn presented to the emergency room complaining of severe chest pain that radiated down his left arm. He was pale and clammy. His blood pressure was 108/64 and his ECG indicated that he was in the acute phase of a myocardial infarction. As the emergency room staff geared up to care for Mr. Hahn, his room quickly filled with people and equipment. Despite sublingual nitroglycerin, Mr. Hahn continued to have chest pain. The emergency room doctor ordered nitroglycerin IV to try to stop the chest pain. The emergency room nurse prepared the IV solution of nitroglycerin, spiked the bag, and primed the tubing. She put the tubing into an IV pump for accurate control of the infusion and, using a needle in one of the ports of the existing tubing, added the nitroglycerin into Mr. Hahn's IV. The emergency room doctor ordered the IV nitroglycerin rate to be increased until Mr. Hahn no longer had pain or until his blood pressure was too low to tolerate the nitroglycerin. The nurse started to increase the nitroglycerin infusion rate, slowly at first, but as the medication seemed to have no effect on Mr. Hahn, she increased it more aggressively. By the time the cardiologist arrived to see Mr. Hahn, the nurse had titrated the nitroglycerin drip beyond safe limits without any apparent effect on the client. She reported that she had checked the IV site and it was patent and she had checked the insertion site of the nitroglycerin tubing and it was intact. The nurse knew that something was wrong but did not know what it could be. In the meantime, Mr. Hahn continued to suffer with severe chest pain. The cardiologist took one look at the nitroglycerin bag and tubing and noted that the nurse had mixed the nitroglycerin in a plastic IV bag and had used standard IV tubing. She was not aware that nitroglycerin is absorbed by most plastics and must be mixed in a glass bottle and infused with special tubing. Mr. Hahn had not been receiving any medication at all. When the nurse mixed a new bottle of nitroglycerin using a glass bottle and special tubing, Mr. Hahn quickly received relief from his chest pain. Unfortunately, the delay in providing the appropriate treatment resulted in increased cardiac damage to Mr. Hahn and a longer hospital stay and home recovery period.

► **EVALUATION**

- The IV tubing was replaced without compromising the sterility of the system.
- The new IV tubing is infusing the new solution without leaks or air bubbles.
- The new IV solution is infusing at the prescribed rate.
- The client is able to discuss the purpose of the IV therapy.

► **DOCUMENTATION**

Flow Sheet

- Note date, time, and name of IV solution started.
- Note date and time IV tubing was changed.

Document on appropriate flow sheet or electronic medical record (EMR).

Intake and Output Record

- Note how much fluid was left in the IV bag to determine the amount of intake.

► **CRITICAL THINKING SKILL**

Introduction

The IV tubing should be changed every 72 hours in order to decrease the risk of infection. It should also be changed after infusion of blood products as it can become occluded with the viscous solutions.

Possible Scenario

A client has an IV of D_5W infusing at 75 mL/hr when the physician orders two units of packed red blood cells.

Possible Outcome

The nurse prepares the blood bag by spiking it with new tubing, filling the tubing, and piggybacking it into the current IV. She shuts the D_5W off and runs the blood in through the current IV tubing. Because the nurse was not aware that blood products are not compatible with dextrose solutions, the red cells are hemolyzed as they flow through the tubing which previously contained D_5W, the transfusion must be discontinued and discarded.

Prevention

The nurse prepares the blood with tubing designed for blood transfusions. She checks the hospital policy regarding blood transfusions and realizes that normal saline should be used to prime the blood tubing and to flush it following the transfusion. She carefully prepares the new tubing, double checks the blood bag with a second nurse, and changes from the D$_5$W tubing to the blood tubing. As the previous IV will resume after the transfusion of blood is completed, the nurse obtains a sterile cap to cover the end of the D$_5$W tubing to maintain its sterility when she attaches the blood tubing.

The nurse needs to know which solutions are compatible with other medications or blood products and if an IV solution will be used later in order to prevent contamination.

▶ VARIATIONS

Geriatric Variation:
- *Older clients and clients with heart failure or renal failure develop fluid imbalances more quickly. Accurate rates of infusion are crucial to prevent fluid overload or dehydration.*

Pediatric Variations:
- *Small children may develop fluid imbalances more quickly because of a larger extracellular fluid volume. Accurate infusion rates are essential in small children to prevent dehydration or fluid overload.*
- *Intravenous fluid rates are often prescribed for children based on their body weight. Most formulas used to calculate children's IV flow rates are based on the child's weight in kilograms. Most American institutions report weights in pounds. Be aware of the need to convert or report all weights in kilograms.*
- *The IV tubing connections should be very secure. Even sick children are active and may inadvertently disconnect tubing.*

Home Care Variations:
- *An approved receptacle needs to be provided for used IV tubing.*
- *Assess the home care setting. Teach the client or the caregiver to prepare the new IV bag and tubing in a clean area to reduce the risk of contamination.*

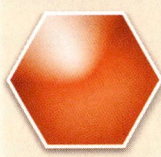

Long-Term Care Variation:
- *If the long-term care client will be cared for primarily by aides, the aides must be taught how to respond to incidents involving the IV site and infusion set. They need to know what to do if the IV tubing should come apart, if the solution bag becomes contaminated or is empty, and even what to look for to assess if something is not right with the IV infusion.*

▶ COMMON ERRORS

Possible Error:
The tubing is contaminated by a needle piercing through it during an IV piggyback injection.

Prevention:
Be sure to identify the port for the IV piggyback injection and carefully puncture only the port and not the tubing. If the error does occur, stop the IV piggyback administration of the medication. Remove the needle and replace the cap over the needle to maintain sterility. Stop the IV flow. Obtain new tubing for the IV solution and change it using sterile technique. Discard the contaminated tubing, place fresh IV solution and tubing, and proceed to administer the IV piggyback medication.

▶ **NURSING TIPS**

- Be sure the tape at the IV site is loosened so it is easier to change the tubing.
- Place a towel under the arm of the IV site where the tubing will be changed in order to keep the linen clean in case of blood leaking from the needle during IV tubing change.
- A special gown with snaps at the seams makes changing tubing easier.

▶ **SPECIAL CONSIDERATIONS**

- *In some areas, such as the operating room, IV fluids are warmed prior to use to help with thermoregulation. Always check that the temperature of the fluid is not too hot before administering it to the client.*
- *Encourage the alert client to become involved in his or her care. Advise the client that the fluid is not supposed to run out before being replaced and that the client can alert the nurse when he or she sees that it is due. This empowers the client in an environment where he or she often feels powerless.*

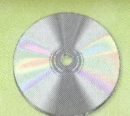

SKILL 8-5

Setting the IV Flow Rate

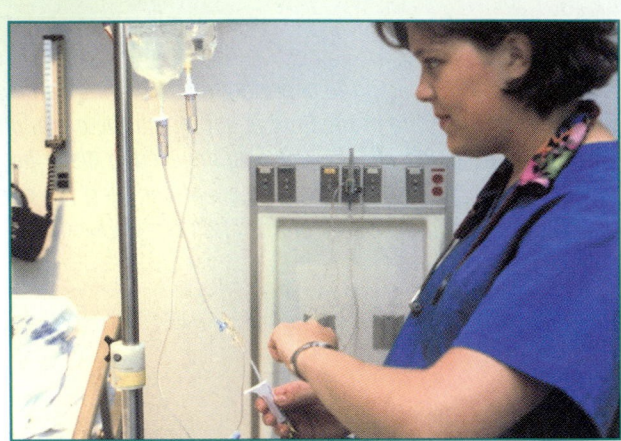

▶ OVERVIEW OF THE SKILL

Setting the rate of an intravenous (IV) infusion according to the health care provider's order is the responsibility of the nurse after he or she has established a patent IV. The flow rate can be controlled by the roller clamp on the IV tubing or by an infusion pump. It is important for the rate to be accurate to prevent complications in fluid balance. A rate that is too fast can result in fluid overload, which is potentially serious in clients with cardiovascular, renal, or neurologic impairment as well as in very young or very old clients. If an infusion is set too slow, the vein may clot or the more serious complication of circulatory collapse in a dehydrated or severely injured client who required large volumes of fluid could develop.

Sudden changes in the rate of infusion may be accidental or positional. A confused client may loosen the roller clamp or get tangled in the IV tubing. A client who gets up to walk may experience an increase in the IV rate. Changes in flow rate can occur with tubing and a roller clamp or infusion devices.

An infusion pump is an electronic device used to deliver a prescribed amount of fluid over a period of time in milliliters per hour. Pumps may have a drop sensor that counts each drop of fluid and sounds an alarm if the flow rate differs from what is programmed. An alarm sounds when the bag is empty or when pressure increases in the system, as in the case of an infiltrated IV.

An IV controller delivers fluid by gravity so the bag must be at least 36 inches above the IV site. The number of drops per minute as well as the IV tubing size and viscosity of the fluid are necessary to calculate the actual volume delivered per hour. The controller cannot force fluid into the vein like a pump so infiltrations are detected more quickly. However, the sensitivity of the pump system increases the number of alarms caused by client movement.

A volume control device is a calibrated chamber placed between the IV bag and the drip chamber so that a small volume of IV fluid (<200 mL) can flow into the chamber and then infuse without danger that the whole bag will be infused into the client.

▶ ASSESSMENT

1. Check the health care provider's order for the IV to be infused and rate of flow **to ensure accurate administration.**
2. Review information regarding the solution and nursing implications in order **to administer the solution safely.**
3. Assess the patency of the IV **to ensure that the solution will enter the vein and not the surrounding tissue.**
4. Assess the skin at the IV site **so that the solution will not be administered into an inflamed or edematous site, which could cause injury to the tissue.**

5. Assess the client's understanding of the purpose of the IV infusion **so that client teaching can be tailored to his needs.**

▶ DIAGNOSIS

Excess Fluid Volume

Risk for Deficient Fluid Volume

Deficient Knowledge

▶ PLANNING

Expected Outcomes:

1. The fluid will be infused into the vein without complications.
2. The IV catheter will remain patent.
3. The fluid and electrolyte balance will return to normal.
4. The client will be able to discuss the purpose of the IV therapy.

Equipment Needed:

- Watch with a second hand
- IV solution in a bag
- IV tubing
- IV infusion pump (optional) (see Figure 8-5-1A)
- Volume control device (optional) (see Figures 8-5-1B and 8-5-1C)
- Paper and pencil

▶ CLIENT EDUCATION NEEDED:

1. Teach the client the rationale for the IV therapy.
2. Teach the client the hourly flow rate of the fluid.
3. Teach the client the significance of the alarm if an infusion device is used.
4. Teach the client and caregiver to count the drops per minute.
5. Instruct clients to report any swelling or pain at the IV site.

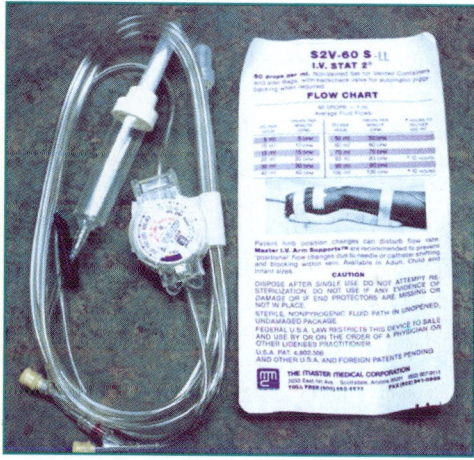

Figure 8-5-1B IV tubing and drip chamber with Dial-a-flo

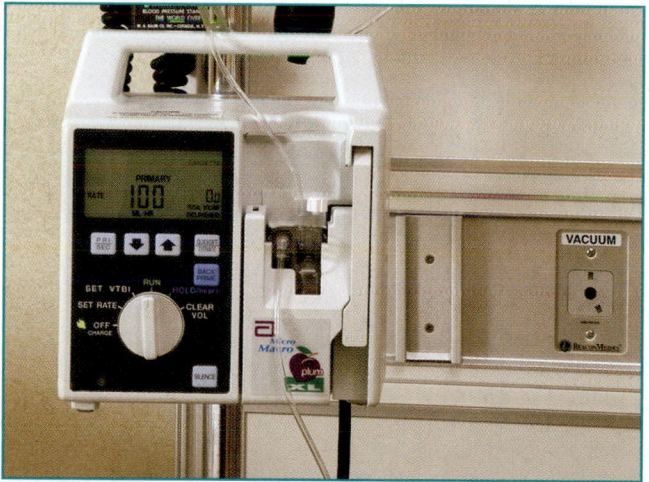

Figure 8-5-1A There are many types of IV pumps available.

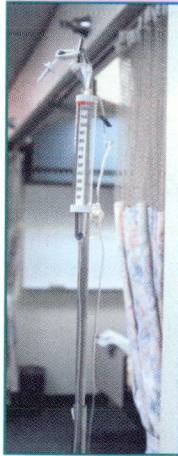

Figure 8-5-1C Volume control infusion chamber

▶ DELEGATION TIPS

Setting the rate of the IV after establishing the infusion is the responsibility of the nurse. It is a procedure not delegated unless other licensed personnel have been trained and certified to perform the procedure. Ancillary personnel may be instructed to report an infusion that is dripping too fast or an IV bag that is almost empty. It is the nurse's responsibility to monitor the infusion but ancillary personnel may also be instructed to report observations such as swelling, leaking, or client concerns about pain, numbness, or tingling at the site or in the extremity used for the infusion.

IMPLEMENTATION—Action/Rationale

Action	Rationale
1. Check health care provider's order for the IV solution and rate of infusion.	**1.** Ensures accurate administration of the solution.
2. Wash hands.	**2.** Reduces the transmission of microorganisms.
3. Check client's identification bracelet.	**3.** Ensures medication is given to the correct client.
4. Prepare to set flow rate: • Have paper and pencil ready to calculate flow rate. • Review calibration in drops per milliliter (gtt/mL) of each infusion set.	**4.** • A nurse unfamiliar with IV fluid rates should calculate the rate at first. • Drops per milliliter vary with manufacturer and tubing type. Macrodrip tubing varies from 10 to 15 gtt/mL. Microdrip tubing generally delivers 60 gtt/mL.
5. Determine hourly rate by dividing total volume by total hours. Example 1: The order reads 1000 mL D_5W with 20 mEq KCl over 8 hours: $$\frac{1000 \text{ mL}}{8 \text{ hr}} = 125 \text{ mL/hr}$$ Example 2: Three liters are ordered for 24 hours: $$\frac{3000 \text{ mL}}{24 \text{ hr}} = 125 \text{ mL/hr}$$	**5.** Provides a prescribed hourly rate with no sudden increases or decreases. The formula for calculation is: $$\frac{\text{mL/hr}}{60 \text{ min}} = \text{mL/min}$$
6. Mark a length of tape placed on the IV bag with the hourly time periods according to the rate (see Figure 8-5-2).	**6.** Provides a visual check of the fluid infused to be sure the rate is correct.
7. Calculate the minute rate based on the drop factor of the infusion set: $$\text{drop factor} \times \text{mL/min} = \text{gtt/min}$$ $$\frac{\text{mL/hr} \times \text{drop factor}}{60 \text{ min}} = \text{gtt/min}$$ $$\frac{\text{hourly rate} \times \text{drop factor}}{\text{infusion time in minutes}} = \text{gtt/min}$$	**7.** The nurse can use the formulas to calculate how many drops per minute will be infused, and can adjust the rate for a change in tubing (macrodrip, microdrip).

continues

Action	Rationale

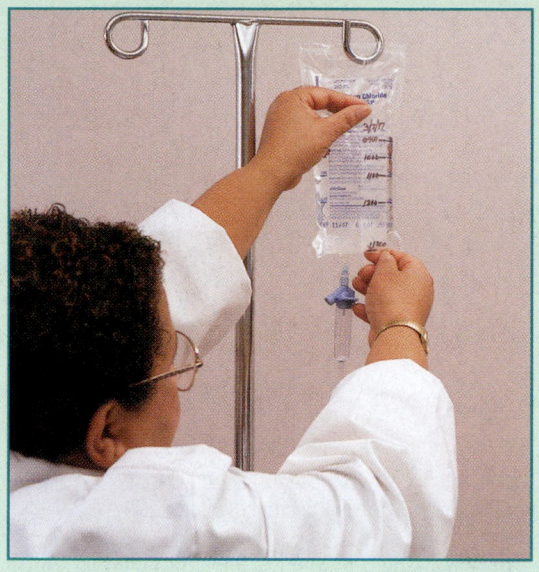

Figure 8-5-2   Apply time strip to IV bag.

- Microdrip example:

$$\frac{125\,\text{mL} \times 60\,\text{gtt/mL}}{60\,\text{min}} = \frac{7500\,\text{gtt}}{60\,\text{min}} = 125\,\text{gtt/min}$$

- Macrodrip example:

$$\frac{125\,\text{mL} \times 15\,\text{gtt/mL}}{60\,\text{min}} = 31\,\text{gtt/min}$$

8. Set flow rate:
   - For regular tubing without a device: Count drops in drip chamber for 1 minute while watching second hand of watch and adjust the roller clamp as necessary (see Figure 8-5-3).
   - For an infusion pump: Insert the tubing into the flow control chamber, select the desired rate (generally calibrated in milliliters per minute), open the roller clamp, and push start button.
   - For a controller: Place IV bag 36 inches above the IV site, select the desired drops per minute, open the roller clamp, and count drops for 1 minute to verify rate.
   - For volume control device: Place device between IV bag and insertion spike of IV tubing, fill with 1 to 2 hours, amount of IV fluid, and count drops for 1 minute (see Figure 8-5-4).

9. Monitor infusion rates and IV site for infiltration.

8.
   - Ensures that infusion is administered as ordered.

   - Pumps the solution through the tubing at the rate set.

   - The controller works by gravity.

   - The amount of fluid in the volume control chamber depends on the amount of fluid to be infused per hour:
     50 mL/hour = 50 to 100 mL of fluid
     100 mL/hour = 100 to 200 mL of fluid

9. Infusion devices may fail.

continues

Action	Rationale

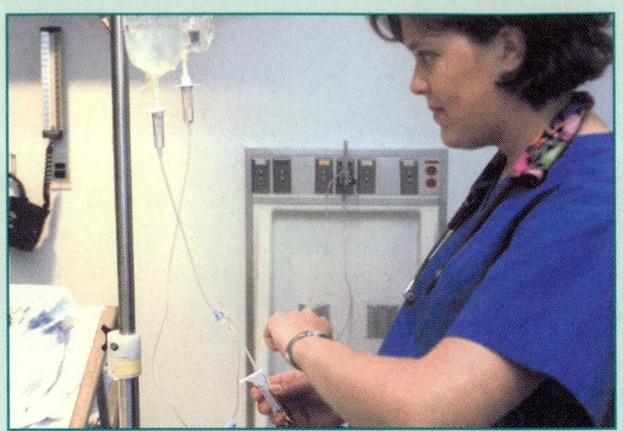

Figure 8-5-3 Count the drips in the drip chamber for 1 minute.

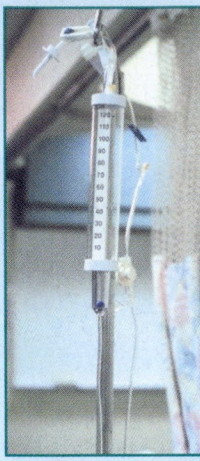

Figure 8-5-4 The controller is placed between the IV bag and the client. It is filled with 1 to 2 hours' worth of IV fluid.

10. Assess infusion when alarm sounds.

10. Alarms on infusion devices signal when a drip has not been sensed. It can be caused by an empty IV bag, a kink in the tubing, a clotted needle, an infiltrated IV, or another malfunction of the device.

11. Wash hands.

11. Reduces the transmission of microorganisms.

▶ REAL WORLD ANECDOTES

Anne, 3 years old, was hospitalized for meningitis. She was receiving IV antibiotics and fluids. She was usually somnolent but occasionally was restless. Her physician ordered IV fluids at 15 mL/hr and cautioned the nurse to be vigilant that she receive no more because of possible increased intracranial pressure. The nurse had already obtained a volume control set to attach to the IV tubing before spiking the IV bag. The nurse filled the chamber with 15 mL of the IV fluid, timed the drips, and checked the infusion frequently. When the level of the fluid reached 5 mL and it was 20 minutes before the hour, the nurse filled the chamber up to the 15-mL mark so that it would not run dry.

▶ EVALUATION

- The fluid is infusing into the vein without complications.
- The IV catheter remains patent.
- The fluid and electrolyte balance returned to normal.
- The client is able to discuss the purpose of IV therapy.
- The client receives the correct amount of IV fluid.

▶ DOCUMENTATION

Flow Sheet
- Date and time IV solution was started
- Rate of infusion in drops per minute and milliliters per hour
- Any changes in the IV rate

Nurses' Notes

- Client's response to the IV therapy
- Changes in condition caused by a complication in the IV infusion

Document on appropriate flow sheet or electronic medical record (EMR)

► CRITICAL THINKING SKILL

Introduction

Setting an IV infusion rate is part of delivering the prescribed fluid to the client. Knowledge of the size of tubing, the formulas used for calculating the number of drips per minute, and assessment of the client are all vital in successful administration of IV fluid.

Possible Scenario

A nurse reads the physician's order "$D_5$1/2NS 1000 mKL over 12 hours" and calculates a rate of 83 mL/hr and marks the tape on the IV bag accordingly.

The nurse selects an IV set and calculates the rate to be 13 to 14 gtt/min. After counting the drops while watching the second hand, the nurse sets the roller clamp to match the drops. However, upon returning an hour later, 120 mL has infused instead of 83 mL.

Possible Outcome

The difference of 40 mL has not made a difference in the client's assessment, but the nurse must explore the reason why more IV fluid has infused than wanted. The nurse looked more closely at the IV tubing and realized that the set delivered 15 gtt/mL instead of 10 gtt/mL. The calculation was correct for 10 gtt/mL instead of 15 gtt/mL.

Prevention

The nurse must look carefully at the product being used for an IV infusion in order to make the correct calculation.

► VARIATIONS

Geriatric Variation:
- *Older clients and clients with heart failure or renal failure are at greater risk for fluid overload.*

Pediatric Variations:
- *Small children may develop fluid imbalances more quickly because of a larger extracellular fluid volume.*
- *A volume control device is recommended for small children.*

Home Care Variations:
- *Clients and caregivers can be taught to control the rate of an IV infusion.*
- *The nurse should be in the home to teach the client and caregiver how to use an infusion device after checking the equipment.*
- *Be sure electronic equipment is properly grounded.*

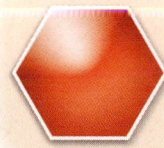

Long-Term Care Variation:
- *Infusion devices can be used in the long-term care facility. Be sure health care workers know how to use and care for the infusion pump.*

► COMMON ERRORS

Possible Error:

The infusion cassette is not snapped completely into place in the infusion pump. The alarm sounds whenever the pump is turned on and no fluid is infused.

Prevention:

Be sure the correct tubing for the infusion pump is placed according to the manufacturer's instructions. Infusion devices and tubing vary widely and, if the tubing is improperly loaded, the infusion device will not work correctly and will continue to sound the alarm.

► NURSING TIPS

- Anticipate the client's need for IV fluid so the next bag is ready to hang before the current one is finished.
- Watch for kinks in the IV tubing or other impediments to the infusion of the fluid.
- Remember not to depend entirely on an infusion pump or controller as they can fail.
- Always check IV infusions with a watch and monitor the tape on the IV bag to ensure the correct rate is being delivered.
- Do not write directly on the plastic IV bag. Some ink may migrate through the plastic and contaminate the IV fluid.

► SPECIAL CONSIDERATIONS

- *Encourage the alert client to become involved in his or her care. Advise the client that the fluid in the IV bag should not run out before being replaced and to alert the nurse when a replacement is due. This empowers the client in an environment where one often feels powerless.*
- *Some IV pumps work as a cassette where a predetermined quantity of solution is dispensed into the cassette at one time. With this system the nurse is not able to count the drip to ensure accuracy. The nurse must check that the cassette is programmed for the correct amount and periodically check the amount in the bag for accurate infusion.*
- *Shortcuts can be developed in calculating drip rates (mL per min). If the equipment's drip factor is 15 gtt per mL, cancellation of factors in the equation will leave 15/60, hence, 1/4 multiplied by the rate per hour or the rate per hour divided by 4* $\left(\dfrac{rate/hr}{4}\right)$.

  Example: Order of 1000 mL/10 hrs = 100 mL/hr

  $$\frac{100 \ mL/hr}{4} = 25 \ mL/min$$

  If the equipment is 10 gtt per mL, factors cancel so that the remainder is 10/60 or 1/6 multiplied by the rate per hour or the rate per hour divided by 6 $\left(\dfrac{rate/hr}{6}\right)$.

Assessing and Maintaining an IV Insertion Site

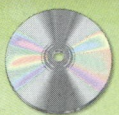

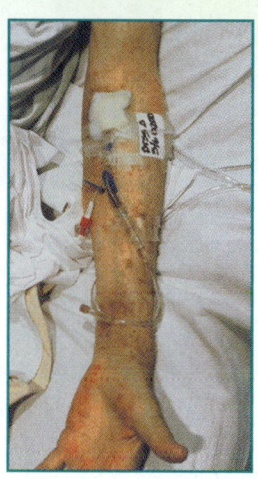

▶ OVERVIEW OF THE SKILL

Assessing a vein for an IV insertion requires knowledge of the anatomy of the veins of the upper extremities to determine the appropriate vein for the therapy ordered. It also requires the assessment knowledge of a healthy vein. A healthy vein is one that is round, firm, elastic, and engorged, without hardened, bumpy, or flattened areas. For most adults the first option for IV placement is in the hand or the large veins of the forearm, preferably in the nondominant hand. Appropriate veins would include the metacarpal, cephalic, basilic, and median veins using the most distal portion of the vein first. Areas to avoid when placing the IV include arms that have had previous mastectomy, edema, superior vena cava (SVC) syndrome, cerebrovascular accidents, infections, previous phlebitis, invading neoplasms, hematomas, sites distal to recent venipunctures, and areas of flexion and bony prominence, such as the wrist and antecubital fossa. Knowledge of both the IV solution and medications to be given and their potential side effects on the veins should be included in the assessment. Intravenous solutions with electrolytes and medications can have irritant properties that would require more frequent IV monitoring. Assessing an established IV site requires knowledge about the length of time since the insertion, the condition of the dressing, and the site itself. The site should be without redness, swelling,

pain, or discharge. When palpating the vein, it should have the characteristics of a healthy vein without signs of infection or phlebitis.

▶ ASSESSMENT

1. Review the order for IV therapy: Identify potential side effects from medication actions, and fluid rate. Consult drug reference books or pharmacists for information. **Decreases the risk of medication errors.**
2. Identify potential risk factors for your client's condition that might indicate fluid and electrolyte imbalances. **Allows targeted assessment and monitoring.**
3. Assess for dehydration: sunken eyes, dry skin, or mucous membranes, flattened neck veins, vital sign changes, inelastic skin turgor, decreased urine output, behavior changes, and confusion. **Allows intervention to increase fluids and reduce dehydration.**
4. Assess for fluid overload: periorbital edema, distended neck veins, auscultation of crackles or rhonchi in lungs, changes in vital signs, and level of consciousness. **Allows intervention to decrease fluids.**
5. Determine the client's risk for developing complications from IV therapy: very young or very old, heart or renal failure. **Allows the procedure to be**

modified if needed and promotes targeted assess-ment to look for signs of risk-related problems.

6. Observe IV site for complications, that is, signs of infection, phlebitis, or infiltration: redness, swelling, pallor, or warmth at the IV site and sur-rounding tissue, and bleeding or drainage. **Allows interventions to reduce further damage.**

7. Observe IV site for patency by briefly compress-ing the IV cannulated vein above the site. Note slowing or momentary cessation of IV rate with a positive blood return. **Provides ongoing assessment of current patency status. Allows early detection of changes.**

8. Assess the client's knowledge regarding the need for the IV therapy. **Allows for teaching, includ-ing information and education regarding medications, fluid needs, and signs of IV site irritation or phlebitis.**

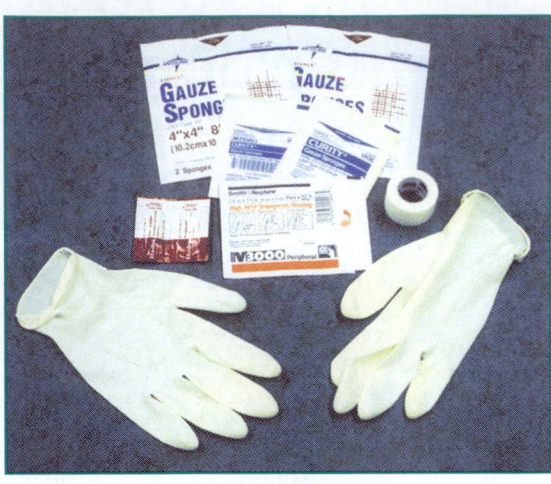

Figure 8-6-1 Transparent dressing, nonsterile gloves, tape, gauze sponges, and topical iodine ointment

▶ DIAGNOSIS

Impaired Tissue Integrity

Risk for Impaired Skin Integrity

Risk for Infection

Excess Fluid Volume

Deficient Fluid Volume

▶ PLANNING

Expected Outcomes:

1. The client will have a patent IV, without signs of infection or inflammation.
2. The client's fluid and electrolyte imbalances will return to normal and will be maintained.
3. The client will be able to report signs of inflammation or infiltration.
4. The client's IV rate will be administered and maintained per order.
5. The client's IV dressing will remain intact, clean, and dry.

Equipment Needed (see Figure 8-6-1):

* Clean gloves
* Gauze dressing
* Tape
* Nursing documentation record

▶ CLIENT EDUCATION NEEDED:

1. Explain to clients the reason they need IV fluids or medications.
2. Describe to the client the signs of inflammation or infiltration of IV.
3. Advise client to use nurse call light for assis-tance when getting out of bed.

Estimated time to complete the skill:

5–15 minutes, based on the nurse's knowledge of the IV therapy and the client's site assessment.

▶ DELEGATION TIPS

Assessing and maintaining the IV after establishing the infusion is the responsibility of the nurse. It is a procedure not del-egated unless other licensed personnel have been trained and certified to perform the procedure. Ancillary personnel may be instructed to report an infusion which is dripping too fast or an IV bag which is almost empty. It is the nurse's responsibility to monitor the infusion but ancillary personnel may also be instructed to report any observations such as swelling, leaking, client concerns about pain, numbness, or tingling at the site or in the extremity used for the infusion. Ancillary may also be involved in monitoring the client's daily weight, if ordered, along with intake and output. Ancillary personnel should be instructed not to obtain vital signs on an extremity with solutions infusing.

IMPLEMENTATION—Action/Rationale

Action	Rationale
1. Review health care provider's order for IV therapy.	1. Ensures accuracy in the administration of IV therapy.
2. Review client's history for medical conditions or allergies.	2. Decreases risk of fluid overload and allergic reactions.
3. Review client's IV site record and intake and output record.	3. Assesses for potential problems with fragile IV sites and fluid balance.
4. Wash hands.	4. Decreases transmission of microorganisms.
5. Obtain client's vital signs.	5. Assesses for changes in cardiovascular system.
6. Check IV fluid for correct fluid, additives, rate, and volume at the beginning of your shift (see Figure 8-6-2).	6. Ensures client is receiving correct therapy.
7. Check IV tubing for tight connections every 4 hours.	7. Ensures that no fluid leaks from tubing and connections.
8. Check gauze IV dressing hourly to be sure it is dry and intact (see Figure 8-6-3).	8. Ensures there is no sign of infiltration or infection at IV insertion site.
9. If the gauze is not dry and intact, remove the dressing and observe site for redness, swelling, or drainage.	9. Ensures there is no sign of inflammation or infection at IV site.
10. If an occlusive dressing is used, do not remove the dressing when assessing the site.	10. Ensures there is no sign of inflammation or infection at IV site.
11. Observe vein track for redness, swelling, warmth, or pain hourly.	11. These are early signs of phlebitis or infiltration.
12. Document IV site findings in the nursing record or flow sheet.	12. Provides documentation of frequent IV site observation.
13. Wash hands.	13. Decreases transmission of microorganisms.

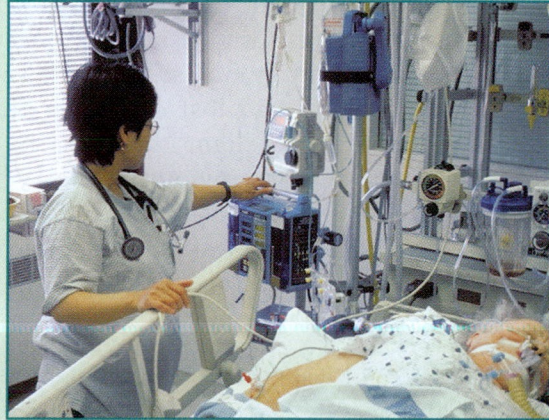

Figure 8-6-2 Check the IV fluid rate, volume, tubing, and additives at the beginning of the shift.

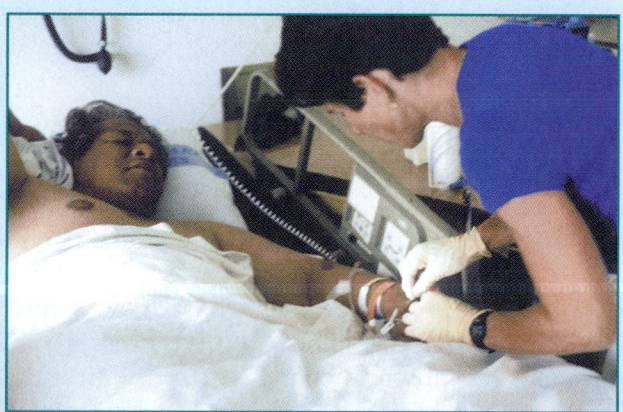

Figure 8-6-3 Check the IV dressing site every hour.

▶ **REAL WORLD ANECDOTES**

A nurse enters a client's room to assess the client at the beginning of her shift. The client is sleeping comfortably with the IV site hidden under the bed covers. The nurse hesitates and does not want to wake the client. The nurse uses all her observational skills: First she checks the IV solution, additives, and rate against the physician's order. Then the nurse reviews the previous nurse's documentation, noting when the IV site was last changed and checked, reviewing for any indication of problems. The previous nurse last checked the IV 2 hours previously and stated the site was clean, dry, and intact, without redness or swelling. The IV rate had slowed down from an hourly rate of 200 mL/hr to about 100 mL/hr over the past hour during shift change. The nurse tries to adjust the rate without success. The nurse gently follows the IV tubing to the client's arm and finds the tubing kinked. When the tubing is straightened, the IV flow returns to the normal rate of 200 mL/hr. The client begins to arouse, and the nurse introduces herself and finishes the IV site inspection, which is intact and unchanged. The client's vital signs are completed and the client is reminded to call for assistance when getting out of bed and to be careful of becoming tangled in the IV tubing when turning in bed.

▶ **EVALUATION**

- Nurse should observe the IV site on an hourly basis to avoid complications of phlebitis and infiltration.
- Have the client report signs and symptoms of redness, swelling, and pain to the nurse.

▶ **DOCUMENTATION**

Flow Sheet

- Name of IV solution with additives
- Hourly rate of fluids
- IV site condition
- Time checked
- Initials/signature of nurse

Document on appropriate flow sheet or electronic medical record (EMR).

▶ **CRITICAL THINKING SKILL**

Introduction

Look at the example of how a nurse prevents a large infiltration of an IV by thoroughly assessing the site and the surrounding tissue.

Possible Scenario

A dehydrated client came into an outpatient infusion setting to receive IV fluids for nausea and vomiting for the past 36 hours following a chemotherapy treatment. The physician ordered 1 liter of normal saline (NS) to be given over 2 hours and repeated if the client's blood pressure and pulse showed postural changes after the first liter. Compazine 10 mg IV was also ordered for nausea. An IV site was placed on the distal forearm of the client's nondominant left arm on the second

attempt. The nurse noted the client's veins to be flat and fragile from previous IV treatments and/or dehydration. The nurse initiated the NS IV drip at 500 mL/hr and went to obtain the Compazine injection to help the client's nausea. The nurse drew up the Compazine in a syringe and then diluted the medication with 10 mL of NS because she knew Compazine to be irritating to veins. The nurse administered the medication by slow IV push and asked the client to report any symptoms or burning or pain at the site. The nurse completed the administration of the medication and checked for a blood return in the IV. The blood return was present, but not as brisk as when the IV fluids were started. The nurse turned off the IV for a moment to see if a spontaneous blood return would appear after such rapid fluid rate. There was a blood-tinged solution present at the IV site. The nurse left the IV clamped and began to assess the tissue proximally from the site. The IV was in a small vein on the backside of the forearm where there tends to be more fleshy tissue surrounding the veins. The vein did not look swollen; however, the tissue felt cool and had lost color. On closer examination there was a slight thickness to the skin that was not present previously. The IV was discontinued and the nurse asked a colleague to assist her in starting a new IV site because she had already attempted 2 IVs on this client.

Possible Outcome

If the nurse had not persisted in the evaluation of the IV site and recognized the subtle changes in the client's IV rate and site, the client would likely have received a large infiltration caused by the rapid rate at which the fluids were infusing. This would have eliminated the left arm extremity for possible IV sites on a client who did not have many easily accessible IV sites.

Prevention

The nurse prevented the infiltration by closely monitoring the IV rate and site as well as diluting a medication known to be irritating to the veins.

▶ VARIATIONS

Geriatric Variations:

- Elderly clients have more fragile veins and need extra careful assessment for signs of infiltration.
- Veins in elderly clients tend to "blow" much more easily than those of younger clients.
- When you tape an IV on an elderly person, try not to use too much tape. Use the least abrasive tape available to reduce irritation to the skin.
- Be careful when removing tape as you may pull the skin off.

Pediatric Variation:

- Play therapy can be used with a child to help him or her understand the IV therapy. Play with the child as the child tapes and maintains an IV (without needles) on a doll or teddy bear. As you do, explain what is happening in simple terms appropriate for the child's age. Remind the child that this is one of the things nurses do to help sick people get better.

Home Care Variations:

- Educate the caregiver to recognize signs and symptoms of infiltration or phlebitis in any IV therapy. Make sure the caregiver knows who to call, day and night, for assistance and is comfortable calling as soon as symptoms appear.
- Make sure the caregiver can see well enough to recognize subtle skin changes. You may wish to enroll a second caregiver to specifically check the IV site.

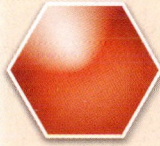

Long-Term Care Variations:

- A peripheral IV insertion site is not frequently chosen for long-term IV therapy.
- In clients who must have short-term IV infusions repeated over many months or years, assess for anticipatory anxiety, fear, or body image disturbances. Be especially aware of how these psychosocial factors develop over time secondary to pain, anxiety, and restricted mobility from IV therapy.

▶ COMMON ERRORS

Possible Error:

Not seeing the IV site clearly when assessing for irritation or infiltration.

Prevention:

Use enough light when assessing the IV site and vein path.

Possible Error:

Not catching an irritation or infiltration early.

Prevention:

If you question the IV site, increase the frequency of assessment.

► **NURSING TIPS**

• Be organized. Review the orders before examining the client's IV so you do not have to go back and check.
• Bring supplies with you for the assessment: gauze, tape, scissors, gloves.

• As you complete your assessment of the client's IV, incorporate teaching the client the signs and symptoms to report.
• Document every hour how the IV site looks and how the IV is functioning.

► **SPECIAL CONSIDERATIONS**

• *If the client complains of pain at the IV insertion site, thoroughly assess the area for edema, erythema, and patency of the IV. The catheter may be lodged against a valve and cause discomfort for the client and less than adequate flow capabilities. This may be relieved by simply repositioning the catheter.*
• *The transparent dressing does not need to be changed to assess the site. When it is necessary to change a transparent dressing, it is helpful to work your hand around the dressing as the edges are loosened. This prevents the dressing from sticking to itself or crimping at the edges. Difficulty in discerning the edge of the transparent dressing when it is on the client reflects a smooth application.*

Changing the IV Solution

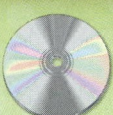

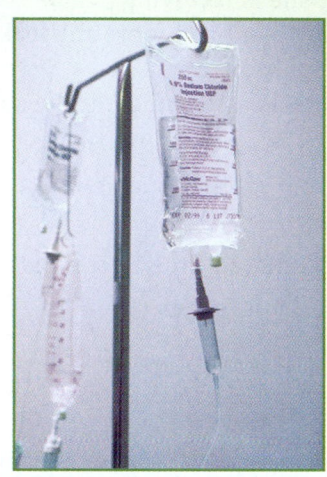

▶ OVERVIEW OF THE SKILL

An intravenous (IV) solution is a method of replacing fluids or correcting an electrolyte imbalance. Clients who are acutely ill, are nothing per mouth (NPO) after surgery, or have severe burns are examples of those who require IV therapy. Other clients require an IV solution infused slowly to keep the vein open (KVO) so that an IV medication can be administered every 4, 6, or 8 hours or venous access can be maintained.

The type of solution in an IV bag is ordered by a health care provider according to the client's needs. Changes in solution are ordered when the client's condition changes. To maintain sterility of the IV solution, the bag of solution is changed at least every 24 hours. Some solutions need to be changed more frequently because of the instability of some of the additives.

▶ ASSESSMENT

1. Check the health care provider's order for the IV to be infused, rate of flow, and any medications to be given **to ensure accurate administration.**
2. Review information regarding the solution and nursing implications **in order to administer the solution safely.**
3. Check all additives in the solution and other medications **so there will be no incompatibilities within the solution.**

4. Assess the patency of the IV **to ensure that the solution will enter the vein and not the surrounding tissue.**
5. Assess the skin at the IV site **so the solution will not be administered into an inflamed or edematous site, which could cause injury to the tissue.**
6. Assess the client's understanding of the purpose of the IV infusion **so client teaching can be tailored to his or her needs.**

▶ DIAGNOSIS

Impaired Skin Integrity

Risk for Infection

Deficient Knowledge

Excess Fluid Volume

Deficient Fluid Volume

▶ PLANNING

Expected Outcomes:

1. The ordered solution will be infused into the client's veins without complications.
2. The IV catheter will remain patent.
3. The client will be able to discuss the purpose of the IV therapy.
4. The solution infused will not harm the client because of additive incompatibilities or additive decomposition.

Equipment Needed (see Figure 8-7-1):
- Disposable gloves
- IV solution in a bag
- Additives as ordered
- IV tubing
- Alcohol swab (if needed)

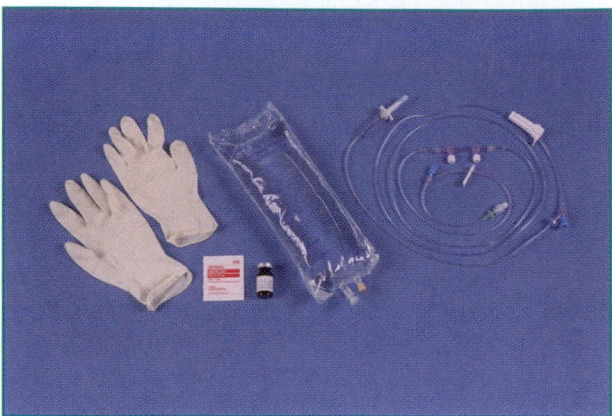

Figure 8-7-1 Gloves, alcohol pad, additive, IV solution, and tubing

▶ **CLIENT EDUCATION NEEDED:**

1. Teach the client the rationale for the IV therapy and need to change the solution.
2. Teach the client the type of solution and additives he or she is receiving.
3. Instruct the client to report any leakage of the bag of IV solution.
4. Instruct the client to report if the solution is at a low level.

Estimated time to complete the skill: **5–10 minutes**

▶ **DELEGATION TIPS**

Changing the IV solution after establishing the infusion is the responsibility of the nurse. It is a procedure not delegated unless other licensed personnel have been trained and certified to perform the procedure. Ancillary personnel may be instructed to report an infusion which is dripping too fast or an IV bag which is almost empty.

IMPLEMENTATION—Action/Rationale

Action	Rationale
1. Check health care provider's order for the IV solution.	1. Ensures accurate administration of the solution.
2. Wash hands and put on clean gloves.	2. Reduces the number of microorganisms.
3. Check client's identification bracelet.	3. Ensures IV solution is given to the correct client.
4. Prepare new bag with additives as ordered by health care provider. • Plan for new bag to be hung at least 1 hour before it is needed. • Change solution when an hour's infusion of solution remains in the IV bag (see Figure 8-7-2).	4. Laboratory tests may reveal a need for potassium, insulin, or magnesium. • Reduces clot formation in vein caused by empty IV bag. • Prevents air from entering tubing and vein from clotting from lack of flow of fluid.
5. Be sure drip chamber is at least half full (see Figure 8-7-3).	5. Prevents entry of air into IV tubing while bag is being changed.

continues

Action	Rationale

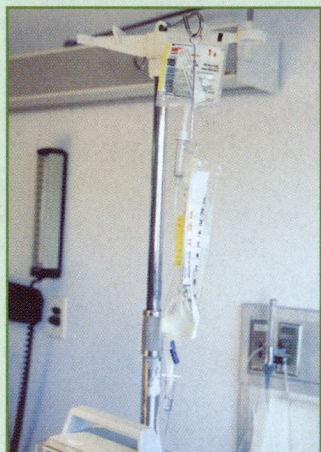

Figure 8-7-2 The IV bag needs to be replaced when an hour's infusion remains in the bag.

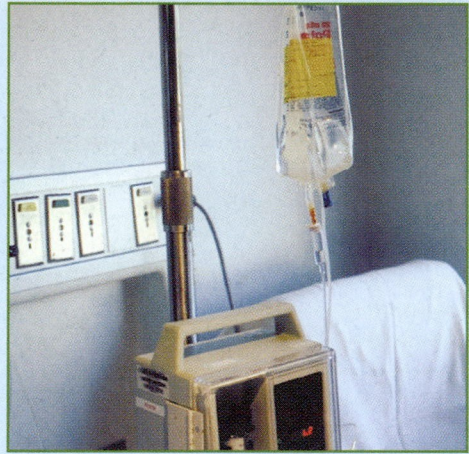

Figure 8-7-3 Make sure the drip chamber is at least half full of fluid.

6. Change IV solution:
- Move roller clamp to stop flow of fluid.

- Remove old IV bag from IV pole and hang new bag.
- Spike new bag with tubing (see Figure 8-7-4).
- Reestablish prescribed flow rate.

7. Check for air in tubing.
- If air bubbles are present, close the roller clamp. While stretching the tubing, flick the tubing with the finger and watch the bubbles rise to the drip chamber.
- If a large amount of air is in the tubing, insert a needle with an empty syringe into a port below the air (see Figure 8-7-5) and allow the air to enter the syringe as it flows to the client (see Figure 8-7-6).

6.
- Prevents fluid in drip chamber from emptying while changing solutions.
- Prepares equipment.
- Maintains sterility of solution.
- Prevents clotting of vein.

7. Reduces risk of air embolus.

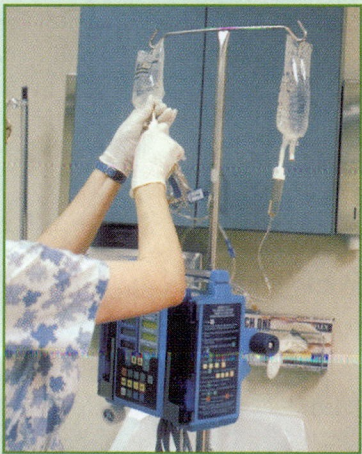

Figure 8-7-4 Spike the new bag with the sharp end of the tubing.

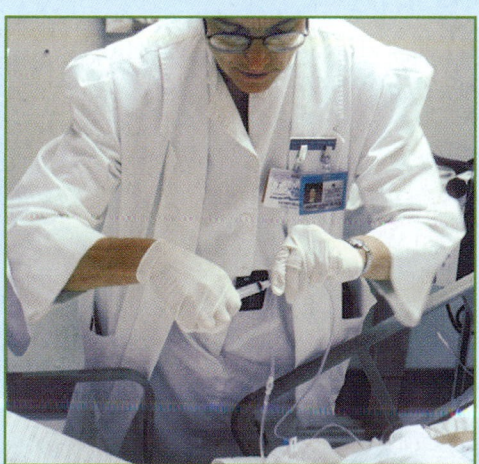

Figure 8-7-5 If there is a large amount of air in the tubing, insert a syringe into a port between the air and the client.

continues

Action	Rationale

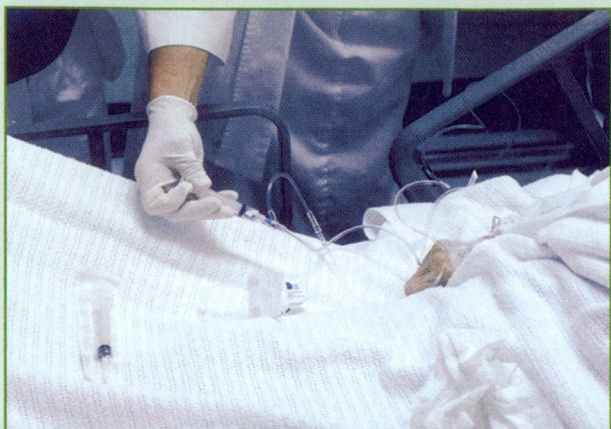

Figure 8-7-6   Allow the air to flow into the syringe.

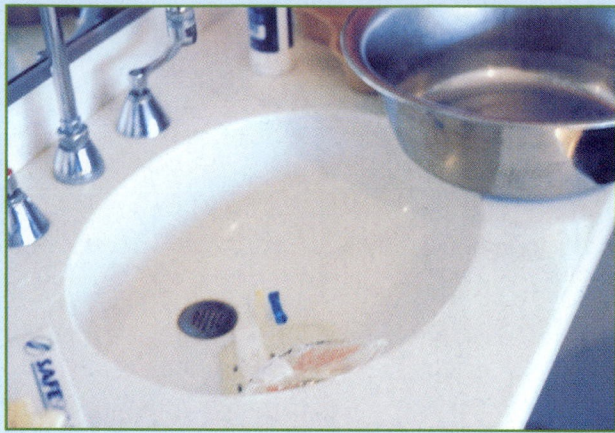

Figure 8-7-7   Drain the remaining fluid from the old IV bag.

8. Empty remaining fluid from old IV if needed (see Figure 8-7-7).

9. Remove gloves and dispose of all used materials.

10. Apply a label with date, time, and type of solution.

11. Wash hands.

8. Disposes of excess fluid. Reduces risk of spilling large amounts of fluid in waste can.

9. Reduces transmission of microorganisms.

10. Allows for planning of next change.

11. Reduces transmission of microorganisms.

▶ REAL WORLD ANECDOTES

Paul, a recently diagnosed diabetic, had been admitted to a medical unit with hyperglycemia. His blood glucose was very labile and his electrolytes were also out of control. His physician ordered IV insulin to control Paul's blood-glucose level. Paul's blood-glucose was checked hourly, and his IV insulin rate was adjusted according to the results. Because the first bottle of IV solution was being used quickly, the nurse decided to mix the next IV insulin solution in a 500-mL bag of fluid instead of a 250-mL bag of fluid to lengthen the time between IV bag changes. While mixing the new bag of solution, however, the nurse failed to double the amount of insulin as the amount of diluent was doubled. As a result, Paul's blood sugar once again soared out of control. Because the nurse did not recognize the error, Paul's physician was at a loss to explain why the insulin was no longer controlling Paul's blood-sugar levels. The head nurse, however, noted that Paul's blood-sugar levels had gone out of control at about the same time the new solution had been hung. The head nurse made up a new bag of solution and hung it herself. Paul's blood-glucose levels once again were controlled and the head nurse had a long discussion with Paul's nurse.

▶ EVALUATION

- The ordered solution infused into the client's vein without complications.
- The IV catheter remained patent.
- The client is able to discuss the purpose of the IV therapy.
- The solution infused did not harm the client because of additive incompatibilities or additive decomposition.

▶ DOCUMENTATION

Flow Sheet

- Date and time new IV solution was started
- Initials of nurse changing solution

Intake and Output Record

- Amount of fluid infused from old solution
- Amount of new solution hung

Nurses' Notes

- Any unusual findings or client teaching

Document on appropriate flow sheet or electronic medical record (EMR)

▶ CRITICAL THINKING SKILL

Introduction

Most IV solutions are commercially made or prepared by the pharmacist. It is the nurse's responsibility to hang them at the correct time.

Possible Scenario

On a busy surgical unit, the nurse had several postoperative clients to admit. One client, a young man who did not speak English, took longer than usual to assess and get settled. When the nurse returned to the first client, he noticed that the IV bag was empty and the fluid was halfway down the tubing. There was a small amount of blood at the hub of the IV needle.

Possible Outcome

As the nurse spiked the new bag he had previously brought into the room and hung it from the IV pole, he watched for the fluid to start to flow through the tubing. When this did not happen right away, he checked the client's IV insertion site. As he was inspecting the IV insertion site, he did not notice that the IV had started to infuse. The tubing was still half full of air. The nurse glanced up in time to see the air infusing into her client. Unsure of what to do, he removed the IV bag from the pole and held it below the level of the IV insertion site. Unfortunately, by the time he had accomplished this, the air had already infused into the client. Luckily there was not enough air in the tubing to cause an air embolism and the client was fine.

Prevention

As the nurse was inspecting the IV site, he noticed the air start to infuse through the venous catheter. He immediately pinched off the IV tubing and closed the roller clamp to prevent any further air from infusing into the client. He then used a syringe inserted into the lowest injection port to aspirate the air in the tubing. The nurse was reminded to always keep the roller clamp closed when the patency of an IV site is in question.

▶ VARIATIONS

Geriatric Variation:

- *Pay special attention to assessing the IV insertion site. A good time for that extra check is when you are changing the solution.*

Pediatric Variation:

- *Intravenous pump alarms can cause both anxiety and fear in younger and older children. Changing the IV solution is a good opportunity to teach children about the alarms. Remind children that the alarm going off is not an emergency and does not mean that they are in danger or becoming sicker.*

Home Care Variations:

- *An approved receptacle needs to be provided for used IV bags and tubing.*
- *The client or caregiver must be taught how to mix the IV solution if additives are required.*
- *The client or caregiver must be taught how to assess the new IV solution for breaks in sterility or contaminants.*

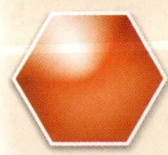

Long-Term Care Variation:

- *Monitor the client's laboratory results so that adjustments to the IV solution can be made if needed.*

▶ COMMON ERRORS

Possible Error:

The IV solution is not ready when the nurse needs it for a client.

Prevention:

The nurse should anticipate when the new IV solution will be needed and be sure it is ordered from the pharmacy. If this error does occur, slow the IV drip rate so that the IV bag will not run dry, following institution protocol. Obtain the new bag when it is ready and proceed to hang the IV solution.

▶ NURSING TIPS

- Anticipate the need for the next bag of IV solution to avoid the risk of an IV clotting because of the solution running out.

- Keep in mind the client's laboratory results and need for fluid to be sure the correct solution is given.

▶ SPECIAL CONSIDERATIONS

- *When using an infusion pump the nurse must not become reliant on the system's alarm device to diagnose site problems. The pump cannot replace nursing assessment and the critical thinking involved with assessing flow problems.*
- *IV systems should be regarded as closed systems and any break or entry should be accomplished through the injection ports after disinfection with an alcohol wipe.*

Discontinuing the IV and Changing to a Saline or Heparin Lock

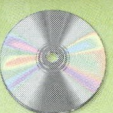

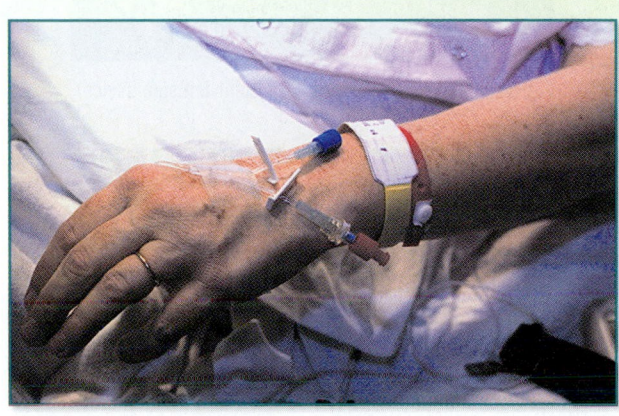

▶ OVERVIEW OF THE SKILL

A heparin or saline lock, also known as an intermittent infusion device, is a small plastic device with a resealing rubber entry that is screwed onto the hub of the existing IV catheter or butterfly needle tubing. It is used to "cap" the IV to maintain patent access to the vein without the necessity of running IV fluids into the body. Historically, heparin was used in these devices and, hence, became known as a "heparin lock." Research has shown that saline is adequate to keep IV lines patent, and that heparin may potentially interact with medications. Furthermore, in rare cases clients may be sensitive to heparin. In certain circumstances, such as with central lines, heparin may be indicated. For the purpose of this skill, "saline lock" will be used. "Saline flush" is another term used by some institutions. Heparin locks are regularly flushed with a heparin solution or normal saline to prevent clotting. They come in both needle and needleless styles, depending on the system used in the institution.

Saline locks are generally placed in two circumstances. First, when the client's need for continuous infusion of fluid or frequent medication changes, the IV line can be discontinued and plugged with a saline lock without losing access to the vein. Second, saline lock IV access sites are placed to provide access to the vein in situations where the client requires IV medications, but does not need continuous fluid infusions.

Saline locks are used to deliver IV medications into the vein. They can be quickly reattached to IV tubing in emergency situations when IV solutions or larger volumes of medication are required. Finally, saline locks are kept for emergency cases when quick administration of medications into the vein can be life saving. Changing to a saline lock, when possible, helps improve client mobility, as clients can walk and move without the IV stand, pump, and tubing.

▶ ASSESSMENT

1. Check the health care provider's order for the discontinuation of the IV or the insertion of the saline lock **to ensure appropriate placement of the saline lock.**
2. For existing IVs, assess the patency of the IV **to ensure that the saline will enter the vein.**
3. For existing IVs, assess the skin at the IV site **so the saline will not be administered into an inflamed or edematous site, which could cause injury to the tissue.**
4. Check the client's drug allergy history **as an allergic reaction could occur rapidly and be fatal.**
5. Assess the client's understanding of the purpose of the saline lock **so client's education can be tailored to his or her needs.**

▶ DIAGNOSIS

Risk for Infection

Impaired Skin Integrity

Deficient Knowledge

▶ PLANNING

Expected Outcomes:

1. The IV is discontinued and saline lock placed without complications.
2. The IV site remains patent and free of swelling and inflammation.
3. The IV will be changed to a saline lock with a minimum of trauma and discomfort to the client.
4. For new sites, the IV needle is inserted into the vein and the saline lock is attached with a minimum of trauma and discomfort to the client.

Equipment Needed:

• Disposable gloves
• Syringe, 3–5 mL
• Sterile needles, 25-gauge
• Antiseptic swab (usually alcohol unless control line)
• Syringe with saline flush solution
• Intermittent infusion device (see Figure 8-8-1)
• Transparent dressing, if required

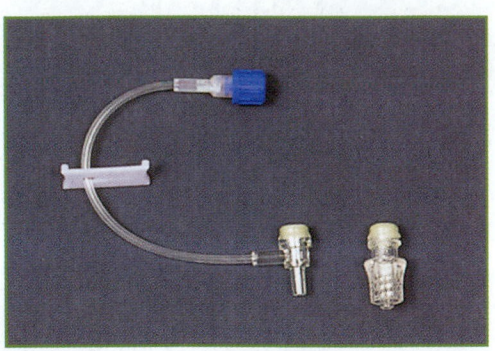

Figure 8-8-1   Saline lock (intermittent infusion device)

▶ CLIENT EDUCATION NEEDED:

1. Teach the client the rationale for maintaining the IV patent with a saline lock.
2. Teach the client to report any changes at the IV site, bleeding, or displacement of saline lock.

Estimated time to complete the skill:
3–5 minutes

▶ DELEGATION TIPS

Discontinuing or changing the IV to a saline lock is the responsibility of the nurse. It is a procedure not delegated unless other licensed personnel have been trained and certified to perform the procedure. Ancillary personnel may be instructed to report any bleeding, leaking, or client concerns after the procedure.

IMPLEMENTATION—Action/Rationale

Action	Rationale
1. Check health care provider's order to discontinue IV and to insert a saline lock.	1. Ensures accurate placement of saline lock.
2. Wash hands and put on clean gloves.	2. Reduces the number of microorganisms.
3. Check client's identification bracelet.	3. Ensures correct procedure is performed for the client.
4. Explain procedure and reason for discontinuing IV to client.	4. Information decreases anxiety.

continues

Action	Rationale
5. Prepare supplies at bedside: • Syringe with saline • Syringe with heparin • Saline lock	**5.** Ensures smooth procedure.
6. If inserting a new saline lock: Prime the extension tubing with saline and place the saline lock on it. Follow the procedures for starting an IV, including assessing and preparing the site, inserting the over-the-needle catheter (ONC) (see Figure 8-8-2) or butterfly needle, and obtaining a blood return. Do not attach the needle/ONC to the IV tubing. Instead, attach the ONC to the extension tubing. Dress the site (see Figure 8-8-3) per protocol. If inserting a new saline lock, prime extension tubing with solution and place connector in the hub of the angiocatheter. For needleless systems follow steps of manufacturer. In a spring-loaded, retractable needle system, press the button after a flashback of blood is observed. To ensure needle separation, turn angiocatheter 360 degrees at the hub before inserting the catheter into the vein. Advance the catheter and attach to extension tubing with the addition of a one-way needleless safety valve, which has been flushed with solution. Secure with dressing as per institution protocol.	**6.** Priming the extension tubing prevents air from being forced into the vein.
7. If discontinuing an IV and converting to a saline lock: Stop IV infusion. • For IV tubing, roll clamp to close IV tubing. • For infusion pump, turn switch to off.	**7.** Stops the flow of the fluid in the IV tubing.
8. Place saline lock: • Open sterile package with needleless adapter saline lock. • For existing IV, loosen IV tubing and remove.	**8.** Places the saline lock.

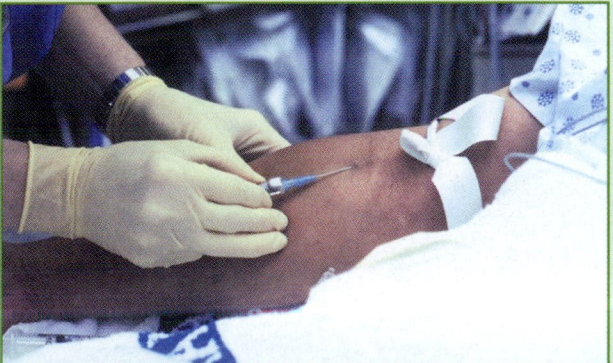

Figure 8-8-2 Insert an over-the-needle catheter.

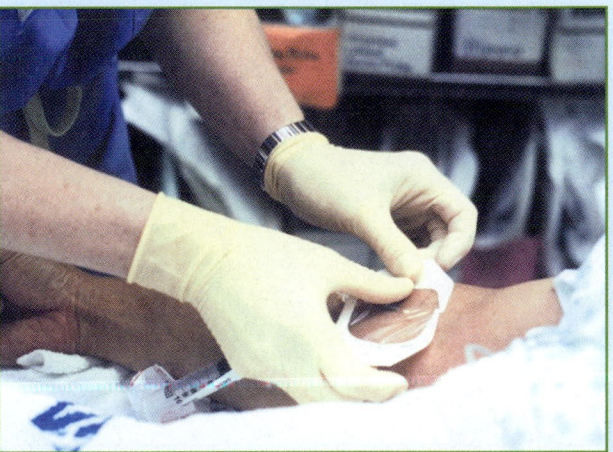

Figure 8-8-3 Cover the site with a transparent dressing.

continues

Action	Rationale
• Screw saline lock into hub of tubing (see Figure 8-8-4). • To check for patency remove cap from one-way valve following vigorous scrubbing with alcohol at the connection site. Connect needleless Leur-locking syringe to the valve. Inject solution into IV site per protocol, using gentle pulsating motions to create turbulence. Remove syringe and replace sterile cap at end of tubing.	
9. Check for patency of IV: • Clean saline lock with antiseptic solution (usually alcohol wipe). • Insert saline syringe with 25-gauge needle into center of diaphragm. (Needleless system will not require needle.) • Pull back gently on syringe and watch for blood return. • Inject saline slowly into lock (see Figure 8-8-5). • Assess client's pain at site.	9. Ensures the IV is patent so that the saline lock will function. Flushing with saline clears the lock. • Flushing should be done slowly. • Assess for pain to ensure site is patent.
10. Keep lock patent with heparin or normal saline. Every 8 hours: • Clean the rubber diaphragm with an antiseptic swab (not applicable if needleless system). • Insert the syringe or needleless adapter with heparin or saline into the diaphragm. • Inject heparin or saline slowly into lock (see Figure 8-8-6).	10. Ensures patency of saline lock. Only use heparin if prescribed as "flush with heparin" or if institutional policy requires it. Needleless system reduces risk of needle sticks.
11. Remove the syringe or needleless adapter from the diaphragm and swab it with an antiseptic swab. Discard needle or adapter in sharps container.	11. Reduces transmission of microorganisms. Reduces risk of needle sticks.

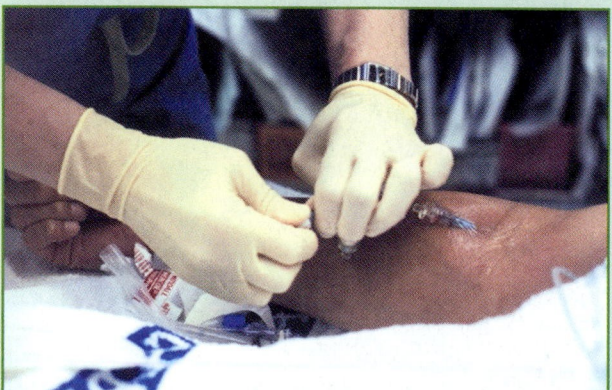

Figure 8-8-4 Screw the saline lock onto the hub of the extension tubing.

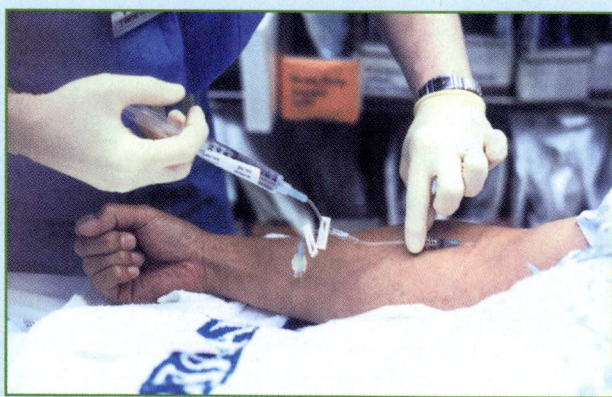

Figure 8-8-5 Inject saline slowly into the lock and extension tubing.

continues

Action	Rationale
12. Assess the site for any signs of leakage, irritation, or infiltration (see Figure 8-8-7).	**12.** Detects problems with the site that need additional assessment and intervention.
13. Remove gloves and dispose with all used materials.	**13.** Reduces transmission of microorganisms.
14. Wash hands.	**14.** Reduces transmission of microorganisms.

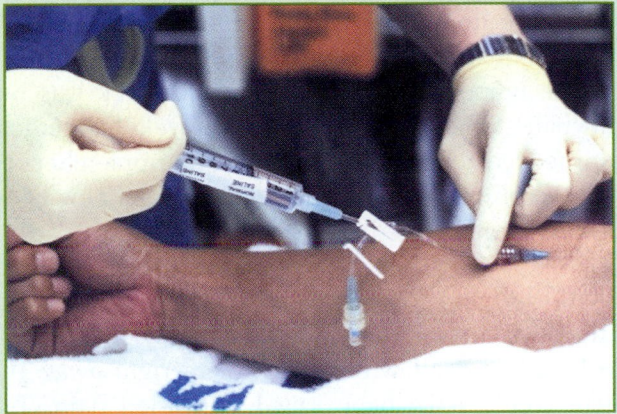

Figure 8-8-6   Maintain the saline lock by injecting saline slowly into the lock, every 8 hours.

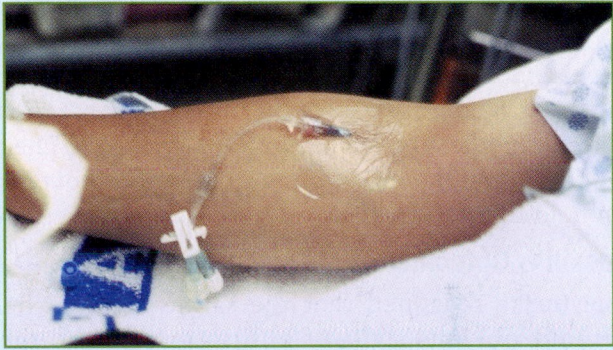

Figure 8-8-7   Assess the site for leakage, irritation, inflammation, or infection. Clean up and dispose of all materials.

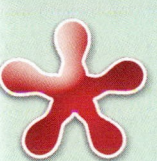

▶ REAL WORLD ANECDOTES

Paul was transferred from the coronary care unit to a medical floor with telemetry monitoring of his heart after having a myocardial infarction. He had recovered well and been off a lidocaine drip for cardiac arrhythmias for 48 hours. His doctor wrote in the chart that his IV fluids could be discontinued and a saline lock placed for emergency use. During the second night Paul was being monitored on telemetry and the monitor technician noted that Paul's rhythm was shifting between sinus rhythm and ventricular tachycardia. The monitor technician notified Paul's nurse and Paul was given a bolus of lidocaine via saline lock. Paul's doctor was notified and Paul was restarted on a lidocaine infusion and returned to coronary care. If Paul had not had the emergency venous access of the saline lock, precious minutes might have been lost trying to establish access while Paul's heart was throbbing in a life-threatening rhythm.

▶ EVALUATION

- The IV is discontinued and the saline lock placed without complications.
- The IV site remains patent and free of swelling and inflammation.
- The IV was changed to a saline lock with a minimum of trauma and discomfort to the client.

▶ DOCUMENTATION

Nurses' Notes

- Note date and time IV was discontinued and saline lock was placed.

- Note any unusual findings at insertion site.
- Document type of solution in lock (heparin or saline).

Document on appropriate flow sheet or electronic medical record (EMR).

Flow Sheet

- Note date and time IV was discontinued.

Medication Administration Record

- Chart solution infused every time lock is flushed.

Intake and Output Record

• Record the amount of IV solution left in the bag when the IV was changed.

► CRITICAL THINKING SKILL

Introduction

A saline lock needs to be checked for patency just as much as an IV catheter that has fluid infusing. If it is not patent, it has no value to the client.

Possible Scenario

A client has had a saline lock for 24 hours after his IV fluids were discontinued. The routine flushing of the saline lock has proven it to be patent; however, the last time it was flushed, the nurse felt some resistance. The nurse pulled back on the syringe to check for blood, and there was only a small amount of pinkish fluid that returned.

Possible Outcome

The nurse reasoned that the saline lock flushed without obvious signs of infiltration and the client was not getting any medication via the saline lock. The nurse decided to check the saline lock again later and perhaps restart it then. As the

shift ended the nurse was giving a report to the oncoming shift and remembered about the saline lock. The nurse reported these concerns to the oncoming nurse. The nurse who assumed this client's care assessed the saline lock prior to flushing it and noticed that the entire insertion site was red and swollen. The site was hot to the touch and the client was complaining of pain at the site. The nurse changed the saline lock site and placed a warm, moist compress on the reddened area. The nurse noted the inflamed area and reported it to the next shift for continued observation.

The nurse realized that the saline lock was not fully patent and would not function well if a medication needed to be administered. The nurse checked with the physician, who advised starting a new IV as the client still needed a patent venous access.

Prevention

If the nurse to first question the patency of the heparin lock had dealt with the problem right away, the client would have been saved unneeded pain. The nurse must always check the patency of IV access when a saline lock is used or it has no value for IV administration of medications or IV fluids.

► VARIATIONS

Geriatric Variations:

• Elderly clients may need special skin care and tape if a saline lock is used for an extended time.
• The veins of elderly clients may be more fragile and need more frequent changes of an IV with a saline lock.

Pediatric Variations:

• Giving a medication to a child through an established IV with a saline lock may be less traumatic than an IM or subcutaneous injection.
• Special precautions need to be taken to maintain a saline lock intact in very young clients.

Home Care Variations:

• The client or caregiver must be taught how to use and maintain a saline lock.
• Equipment for disposing of IV materials needs to be established.

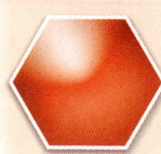

Long-Term Care Variation:

• Saline locks are not usually appropriate for long-term IV access. A permanent central line is often more appropriate in these circumstances.

▶ **COMMON ERRORS**

Possible Error:

When flushing a saline lock, there is swelling around the needle.

Prevention:

Be sure to assess the IV for patency before flushing the saline lock. If swelling does occur, stop pushing the saline lock. Pull back on the plunger to check for a blood return. If there is none, remove the needle and saline lock and start an IV in another site. When you are sure the needle is in the vein, attach a new saline lock and flush with saline.

▶ **NURSING TIPS**

- Sometimes no blood will return from a saline lock even though it is patent. Removing the screw-on cap, using sterile technique, may result in a blood return if the saline lock is patent. If in doubt, restart the saline lock at a new site.
- Be sure the IV site is visible and free of tape or dressing while checking for patency.
- Remember, a saline flush must inject enough saline to fill the entire set from the injection port to the needle tip.
- In some situations, such as with certain central lines, heparin may be used. Use heparin solution designated for flush and follow institution protocol.
- Replace the heparinized solution each time the heparin lock is used.
- If the drug to be administered through the saline lock is incompatible with heparin, flush the entire heparin lock set with normal saline before and after the medication is administered, then flush with heparin. Some institutions no longer flush heparin locks with a heparin solution. Some studies suggest that flushing with normal saline alone will maintain the patency of a heparin lock.

▶ **SPECIAL CONSIDERATIONS**

- *Most institutions are using the needleless system for all IV access to decrease nurses' risk of needle sticks. The nurse should be familiar with this system prior to entering the client's room to perform saline lock care.*
- *Prior procedures for heparin locks called for administration of saline, then administration of medication, followed by saline to flush the line, and heparin to keep the line patent. This was known as the SASH method. Research has indicated that heparin is not necessary to keep the vein open. Saline is sufficient to keep most veins accessible for medication administration.*
- *Heparin may be used in certain central lines or be ordered. Always check the strength of the heparin, usually 10 units per milliliter. Some heparin used for apheresis/wide-bore catheters is of strength up to 100 units per cc and should not be used in peripheral IV sites. Follow institution protocol. Furthermore, although a minimal risk, heparin may interact with medications or cause drug reactions in some clients and, therefore, drug interactions and allergy history must be assessed.*
- *Many institutions currently use the clave and one-way valve that is placed at the end of the extension tubing compatible with a heparin/saline lock device. The use of these devices eliminates the use of needles for administrations of medications and repeat flushes, thus preventing risk of needle sticks for the client and nurse.*

Administering a Blood Transfusion

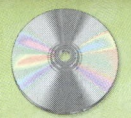

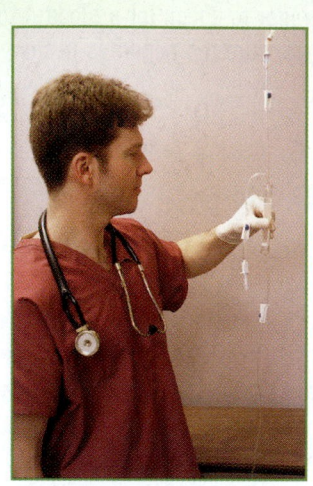

▶ OVERVIEW OF THE SKILL

A blood transfusion is the intravenous (IV) administration of a component of blood or whole blood. Red blood cells are given as whole blood or packed red blood cells; they may be modified by leukocyte reduction to prevent antibody formation or irradiation to prevent graft-versus-host disease in immunocompromised clients. Components used for clients with alterations in coagulation are fresh frozen plasma (FFP), cryoprecipitate, factors VIII and IX concentrates, and platelets. Components to enhance the immune system are granulocytes and immune serum globulin (IgG). Colloid components to treat hypoproteinemia or hypovolemia are plasma protein fraction and albumin. The most commonly used blood components are packed red blood cells, platelets, or FFP.

A client may require a transfusion for the following reasons: to increase blood volume after surgery, trauma, or hemorrhage; to increase the number of red blood cells in a client with severe anemia; to provide platelets to clients with low platelet counts caused by treatment with chemotherapy; to provide clotting factors in plasma; for clients with hemophilia, von Willebrand's disease, or disseminated intravascular coagulopathy (DIC); or to replace plasma proteins such as albumin.

The nurse should know why the health care provider has ordered a specific blood product to be given and the policies and procedures for giving that product. The nurse must know how to give the blood product and what adverse reactions to monitor in the client.

▶ ASSESSMENT

1. Assess the client for the indication of the blood product to be given, that is, low hematocrit or platelet count. **This will enable more specific evaluation of response to the transfusion.**
2. Verify the health care provider's order for the type of blood product to be given. **Only he or she may order blood products because of legal regulations.**
3. Review the client's transfusion history, especially any reactions or pretransfusion medications to be given. **If prior reaction has occurred, premedications can be given to prevent a subsequent reaction.**
4. Review the baseline vital signs in the client's medical record to **compare with vital signs during the transfusion. Changes in baseline may indicate a transfusion reaction.**
5. Assess the type, integrity, and patency of the venous access in place **so the transfusion will be completed without infiltration of the IV.**
6. Verify that a large-bore catheter (18- or 19-gauge) is to be used. **This prevents hemolysis as red blood cells are large and will not flow through a small-bore needle.**

7. Review institution policy and procedure for the administration of blood productions. Each institution has its own policies to ensure safe administration of blood products.

8. Ensure that the client has signed an informed consent release that includes potential risks and benefits.

▶ DIAGNOSIS

Risk for Infection

Potential for Excess Fluid Volume

Impaired Gas Exchange

Risk for Injury

Deficient Knowledge

Pain

▶ PLANNING

Expected Outcomes:

1. The client receives the blood component transfusion without any adverse reactions or has adverse reactions successfully managed.

2. The client demonstrates desired benefit from transfusion as evident by relief of symptoms or improvement in specific hematologic values.

3. The client describes the purpose and procedure for transfusion of a blood component.

4. The client describes the possible complications of a blood transfusion.

Equipment Needed (see Figure 8-9-1):

* Blood administration set and filter
* Intravenous solution of 0.9% sodium chloride (normal saline)
* Disposable gloves
* Infusion pump if compatible with the specific blood product
* Tape
* Leukocyte-depleting filter, if ordered
* Pressure bag, if needed
* Blood warmer, if needed

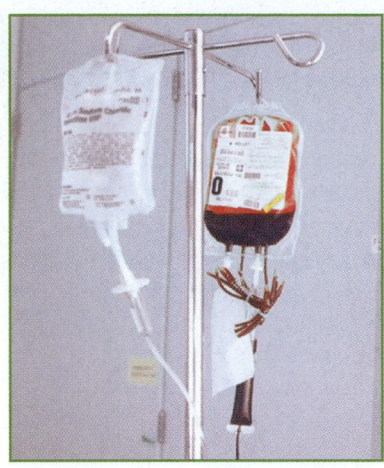

Figure 8-9-1 Blood and 0.9% sodium chloride

▶ CLIENT EDUCATION NEEDED:

1. Teach the client the rationale for the blood transfusion, the anticipated length of the transfusion, and the need for frequent vital sign monitoring while the transfusion is running.

2. Instruct the client to notify the nurse if he or she experiences any signs of reaction such as itching, swelling, dizziness, dyspnea, chest pain, or infiltration of the IV.

3. Teach the client and caregiver about the signs and symptoms of long-term reactions, such as delayed hemolysis and the need to report them to the health care provider immediately.

 Estimated time to complete the skill: **It will take approximately 15 minutes to initiate the infusion, 30 minutes to 2 hours to monitor the client during the infusion, and 10 minutes to discontinue the infusion and complete documentation. Infusion rates vary depending on the blood component to be transfused (see Table 8-9-1).**

Table 8-9-1	Blood Component Infusion Rates	
	PRODUCT	**INFUSION RATE**
	Red blood cells	1 unit over 2–3 hours (<4 hours)
	Platelets	30–60 min or more slowly (<4 hours)
	Fresh frozen plasma	200 mL/hr or more slowly
	Cryoprecipitate	1–2 mL/min

▶ DELEGATION TIPS

Initiating a blood transfusion is a skill involving assessment and knowledge regarding blood replacement techniques. It is an invasive procedure not delegated unless other licensed personnel have been trained and certified to perform the procedure. Ancillary personnel who will be caring for the client need to be instructed to handle the transfusion extremity gently and to take vital signs on another extremity. Vital signs should be recorded according to institution policy and the results reported promptly to the nurse. Any client complaints about chills, fever, itching or the appearance of hives, chest pain, dyspnea, or swelling at the IV site should be immediately reported to the nurse.

IMPLEMENTATION—Action/Rationale

Action	Rationale
1. Verify the health care provider's order for the transfusion.	1. Blood must be ordered by a health care provider.
2. If a venipuncture is necessary, refer to Skill 8-1.	2. Ensures a patent and adequate IV for infusion of blood.
3. Explain procedure to the client.	3. Ensures that client understands procedure and decreases anxiety.
4. Review side effects (dyspnea, chills, headache, chest pain, itching) with client and ask him or her to report these to the nurse.	4. Prompt reporting of a side effect will lead to earlier discontinuation of transfusion and minimize the reaction.
5. Have the client sign consent forms.	5. Most institutions require the client to sign a consent form.
6. Obtain baseline vital signs.	6. Allows detection of a reaction by any change in vital signs during the transfusion.
7. Obtain the blood product from the blood bank within 30 minutes of initiation.	7. Prevents bacterial growth and destruction of red blood cells.
8. Verify and record the blood product and identify the client with another nurse at the bedside (see Figure 8-9-2): • Client's name, blood group, Rh type • Cross-match compatibility • Donor blood group and Rh type • Unit and hospital number • Expiration date and time on blood bag • Type of blood product compared with health care provider's order • Presence of clots in blood	8. Strict verification procedures will reduce the risk of administering blood products to the wrong client. If there is an error during this procedure, notify the blood blank and do not administer the product.
9. Instruct client to empty the bladder.	9. A urine specimen after initiation of the transfusion will be needed if a transfusion reaction occurs.

continues

Action	Rationale

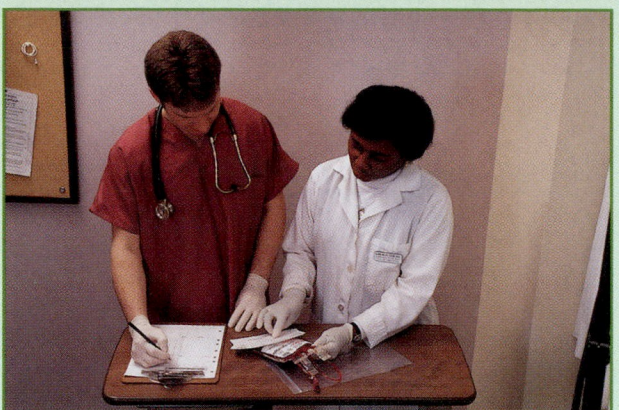

Figure 8-9-2   Verify the blood product with another nurse at the bedside.

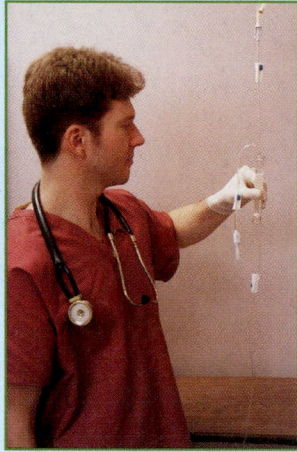

Figure 8-9-3   Close the roller clamp on the administration set and prime drip chamber.

10. Wash hands and put on gloves.

10. Reduces transmission of microorganisms and, therefore, risk of transmission of human immunodeficiency virus (HIV), hepatitis, or blood-borne bacteria.

11. Open blood administration kit and move roller clamps to "off" position.

11. Closed roller clamps prevents accidental spilling of blood.

12. For Y-tubing set:
- Spike the normal saline bag and open the roller clamp on the Y-tubing connected to the bag and the roller clamp on the unused inlet tube until tubing from the normal saline bag is filled. Close clamp on unused tubing.
- Squeeze sides of drip chamber and allow filter to partially fill (see Figure 8-9-3).
- Open lower roller clamp and allow tubing to fill with normal saline to the hub.
- Close lower clamp.
- Invert blood bag once or twice. Spike blood bag and open clamps on inlet tube to allow blood to cover the filter completely (see Figure 8-9-4).
- Close lower clamp.

12.
- The Y-tubing allows the nurse to switch from infusing normal saline to blood. This is especially helpful when multiple transfusions are given. Follow institutional guidelines for the number of units that can be given before tubing needs to be changed. Dextrose solutions are not used with blood transfusions as they can clot the donor blood.
- A correctly filled drip chamber enables an accurate drip count.
- Removes all air from tubing system.
- Prevents waste of IV fluid.
- Equal distribution of cells prevents clumping, which can lead to clotting of cells. Fragile blood cells may be damaged if they drop on an uncovered filter.
- Prevents blood from flowing until tubing is attached to venous catheter.

13. For single-tubing set:
- Spike blood unit.
- Squeeze drip chamber and allow the filter to fill with blood (see Figure 8-9-5).
- Open roller clamp and allow tubing to fill with blood to the hub.

13.
- Attaches tubing to blood unit.
- A correctly filled drip chamber enables an accurate drip count.
- Prevents air from being forced into the vein.

continues

Action	Rationale
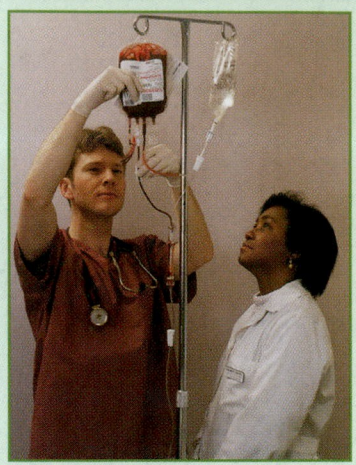 **Figure 8-9-4** Close the saline roller clamp and open the blood roller clamp.	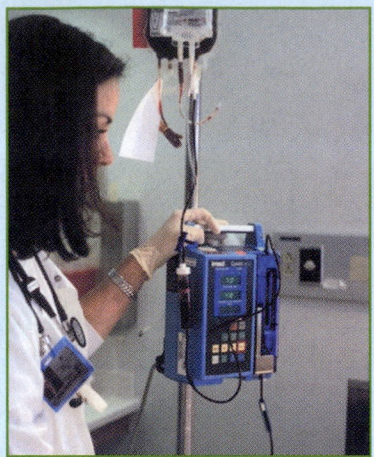 **Figure 8-9-5** Allow the filter to fill with blood.

Action	Rationale
• Prime another IV tubing with normal saline and piggyback it to the blood administration set with a needle and secure all connections with tape.	• The blood product should not be piggybacked into the normal saline line to avoid forcing blood cells through both a needle and a venous catheter.
14. Attach tubing to venous catheter using sterile precautions and open lower clamp.	14. Allows the blood product to be infused into the client's vein.
15. Infuse the blood at a rate of 2–5 mL/min according to the health care provider's order.	15. Packed red blood cells usually run over 1.5–2 hours; whole blood runs over 2–3 hours.
16. Remain with client for first 15–30 minutes, monitoring vital signs every 5 minutes for 15 minutes, then every 15 minutes for 1 hour, then hourly until 1 hour after the infusion is completed, or per institution policy.	16. If a reaction occurs, it generally happens during the first 15–30 minutes. Changes in vital signs can warn of a transfusion reaction.
17. After blood has infused, allow the tubing to clear with normal saline.	17. The client will receive all the blood that is left in the tubing.
18. Appropriately dispose of bag, tubing, and gloves. Wash hands.	18. Reduces transmission of microorganisms.
19. Document the procedure.	19. Ensures accurate records.

► REAL WORLD ANECDOTES

Scenario 1

One day after abdominal surgery, Marge's hematocrit was 26%, so her physician ordered two units of packed red blood cells (RBCs). The nurse noted the order and called the blood bank, but was told that only one unit was available of the type ordered because of a multivictim accident that had just occurred. The nurse knew that 26% was a low hematocrit but not life-threatening as the client showed no signs of active bleeding. The nurse started the unit and then called the physician to report that the second unit was not available.

continues

> ▶ **REAL WORLD ANECDOTES** *(continued)*

Scenario 2

Mr. Dobbs is a 70-year-old man currently receiving treatment for acute myelogenous leukemia. He also has a history of congestive heart failure (CHF). He has symptoms of anemia, such as fatigue and mild dyspnea on exertion. The nurse recently noticed the onset of bilateral pedal edema, although his exam was negative for other signs of CHF, such as pulmonary rales. Today, Mr. Dobbs's laboratory values showed a hematocrit of 27%, and he reported more shortness of breath after taking a shower. The physician prescribed a transfusion of two units of packed RBCs over a total of 4 hours.

The nurse was aware of the potential for fluid overload in this elderly gentleman with a history of CHF and contacted the physician to suggest a slower transfusion rate of 3 hours per unit. The nurse and physician also decided to administer furosemide 20 mg IV between the two units of packed RBCs to prevent fluid overload.

▶ EVALUATION

- Observe for signs of transfusion reaction.
- Observe client and laboratory values to determine response to transfusion.
- Monitor client for signs and symptoms of fluid overload.

▶ DOCUMENTATION

Nurses' Notes

- Record client name, ID number, blood component and component number, names of individuals verifying blood component, name of individual starting and ending transfusion, start and end times, volume transfused, and reaction, if any.
- Record date, time, type, and amount of the blood product administered.
- Document the condition of the venous access site and patency of the IV.
- Describe client's response to transfusion, including change in laboratory values and improvement of symptoms.

Document on appropriate flow sheet or electronic medical record (EMR).

Intake and Output Record

- Record volume of blood component transfused and urine output, if appropriate.

Medication Administration Record

- Record additional medications given to prevent or manage transfusion complications; for example, acetaminophen, diphenhydramine, furosemide.
- Document diagnosis and treatment of any transfusion reactions.

▶ CRITICAL THINKING SKILL

Introduction

Some clients require more than one unit of packed RBCs and more than one type of blood component.

Possible Scenario

Two units of packed RBCs, one unit of single donor platelets, and four units of FFP are ordered for an immunocompromised client who is actively bleeding. The client's hematocrit is 24%, and he is bleeding from his nose and upper gastrointestinal tract. Which blood product should be given first and in what order needs to be determined, as all of the products ordered need to be given so that the bleeding will slow down or stop and the laboratory values will return to normal.

Prevention

The nurse will need to plan the schedule of the blood products in order of importance and according to the physician's orders. As the platelets and the FFP take a shorter time to infuse and will help correct the coagulation problem, it may be beneficial to give them first. The packed RBCs each take 2 hours to infuse so they can be given later.

► VARIATIONS

Geriatric Variations:

- *Elderly clients may require longer infusion time because of decreased cardiac function in order to avoid fluid overload.*
- *Geriatric clients with a history of heart disease or hypertension may have an increased risk of fluid overload related to the transfusion.*
- *Elderly clients may have more fragile veins. Venous access may be more difficult, and these clients may be at a higher risk for IV infiltration.*

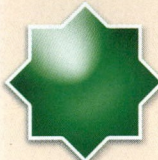

Pediatric Variations:

- *The first 50 mL of blood should be given slowly over 30 minutes. If no reaction occurs, the rate can be increased.*
- *A newborn's blood is cross-matched with the mother's serum which may have more antibodies than the newborn's. This will make an incompatibility more apparent.*
- *Pediatric infusion doses and rates are calculated by body weight. Volume of blood products may be divided into several units containing small volumes.*

Home Care Variations:

- *The blood component should be transported in an insulated container with ice according to the blood bank guidelines. The transfusion should be started as quickly as possible after leaving the blood bank.*
- *If the nurse is alone, she or he should be meticulous in cross-checking the unit of blood with the client to ensure correct administration of the product.*
- *The nurse must plan to have trained personnel available to monitor the client during the entire transfusion and for 1 hour after the transfusion in order to assess for a transfusion reaction.*
- *Assessing a client's eligibility to have a transfusion administered at home include no previous transfusion reactions, no angina or CHF, and being alert and oriented in order to report any symptoms of a reaction.*
- *Policies of the home health agency regarding administration of blood products in the home include preparation by the nurse, client eligibility, location of client in relation to the blood bank, blood transport and storage, disposal of biohazardous materials, and emergency procedures.*
- *Blood component transfusions may be carried out in a home setting. Nurses in this setting should be knowledgeable and prepared to treat acute transfusion reactions with standing orders to avoid the delay of contacting a health care provider or transporting the client for treatment.*

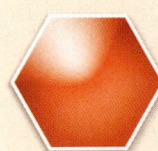

Long-Term Care Variation:

- *Personnel working in long-term care settings where blood is not frequently administered may need to review blood transfusion policies and procedures before the transfusion.*

► COMMON ERRORS

Possible Error:

The IV infiltrates halfway through the transfusion.

Prevention:

Assess the gauge of the IV and its patency before starting the transfusion. If this error does occur, stop the transfusion. Start a new IV in a different extremity, if possible. Restart the transfusion and observe the client for a transfusion reaction.

continues

► **COMMON ERRORS** *(continued)*

Possible Error:
Blood backs up into the bag of normal saline.

Prevention:
Clamp the normal saline bag before spiking the blood bag. If this error does occur, clamp the tubing to the normal saline bag and the blood bag. Obtain a new bag of normal saline. Remove the normal saline bag with the blood in it, and spike the new bag of normal saline. Open the clamp to allow the blood to flow out of the tubing and the normal saline to flow.

► **NURSING TIPS**

- Have all equipment prepared before ordering the blood from the blood bank.
- Use a pressure bag to increase the flow rate if the primary goal is volume replacement and a client is bleeding.
- Maintain another IV line if other fluids or medications are needed during the transfusion.
- Rotate the bag to prevent clumping of cells.
- A transfusion of packed RBCs requires planning and scheduling. A current type and cross-match specimen must be processed; the health care provider must obtain informed consent; IV access must be established; and premedication must be administered, if appropriate. Unless an emergency, a planning process of several hours should be anticipated.
- Medications should never be added to a blood product. If the client is receiving multiple IV medications on a strict schedule (e.g., antibiotics), consider starting a second IV line for a lengthy blood transfusion.
- Blood products should not be transfused simultaneously or immediately preceding or following medications also capable of causing allergic-type reactions. Distinguishing the etiology of the reaction could be difficult.
- Electromechanical infusion devices should be used for blood products only if they have been tested and approved for blood component infusion by the manufacturer.
- External pressure infusion cuffs may help speed a slow transfusion drip. However, do not exceed 300 torr when pressure transfusing an RBC product. Check with the manufacturer of specific venous access devices to determine how much pressure can be applied to a transfusion through the device.
- To avoid bacterial growth, do not leave a blood filter hanging for more than 4 hours.

► **SPECIAL CONSIDERATIONS**

- *Routine blood transfusions should not be warmed as hemolysis of blood occurs at temperatures above 104° F. However, in cases where massive transfusions are required (three or more units), such as a trauma or if hypothermia is present, a blood warmer may be used. The blood is warmed because rapid transfusion of multiple units of chilled blood may reduce the core temperature abruptly and lead to cardiac arrhythmias.*
- *Blood is sometimes administered perioperatively when the hemoglobin is less than 7 g/dL or when excessive loss of blood is anticipated.*
- *When the client receives a massive infusion of blood, a measurement of the prothrombin time (PT), partial thromboplastin time (PTT), and platelet count should be taken after the administration of every five to seven units of red cells. PT is an assessment of extrinsic coagulation blood factors (I, II, V, VII, X) that affect coagulation. PTT is an assessment of intrinsic coagulation factors (I, II, V, VII, IX, X, XI, XII) and is longer with heparin use. Some institutions use international normalization ratio (INR), which is a standardized system of reporting PT based on a calibration model comparing the client's PT with a control value.*

continues

► **SPECIAL CONSIDERATIONS** *(continued)*

- *A client with chronic anemia should be given red blood cell preparations containing minimal plasma, as volume replacement is not required.*
- *Autologous blood collecting devices should be used whenever possible. These devices allow rapid transfusion of autologous blood collected via chest tubes or aspirated from the pleural and peritoneal cavities. This technique may be particularly valuable when time does not allow for the process of a cross-match or compatible blood. It is also considered acceptable by some Jehovah's Witnesses, provided that the blood does not leave the bedside for processing. Nursing staff should check with the client or the client's family members to ensure that it is acceptable.*
- *Citrate is an anticoagulant used as a preservative in blood products and may bind with the calcium in the blood. Clients should be monitored for hypocalcemia.*

Assessing and Responding to Transfusion Reactions

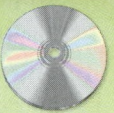

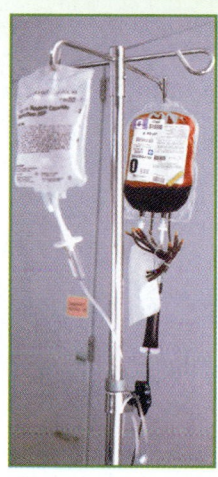

▶ OVERVIEW OF THE SKILL

A transfusion reaction can be caused by blood that is incompatible, blood that is contaminated, or a blood component that is infused too rapidly. It can also be caused by an allergic sensitivity to the leukocytes, the platelets, or the plasma protein components of the blood or the potassium or citrate preservative in the blood.

The types of reactions range from symptoms that appear within the first 15 minutes, such as fever, chills, and skin rash, that can progress to hypotension, shock, or a delayed reaction that can occur several days or weeks later.

The first type of transfusion reaction is an acute hemolytic reaction caused by an ABO incompatibility in which an antigen-antibody of the recipient responds to blood of the donor who has a different antigen. This may be related to the client's ABO blood type or the Rh factor. For example, people with type A blood cells produce anti-B antibodies in their plasma, so administering a unit of type B blood would cause the body to reject it with their anti-B antibodies. In the same manner, the Rh factor is an antigenic substance in the red blood cells (RBCs) of most people; they are Rh positive. If Rh-positive blood is given to an Rh-negative person, the Rh-negative antibodies will hemolyze or destroy the transfused RBCs. Intravascular hemolysis releases hemoglobin leading to hemoglobinemia or hemo-globinuria. The RBCs that are destroyed can damage the kidneys which may progress to renal failure. The coagulation system is also stimulated so the clotting cascade causes small clots to form in the circulating blood, which sets disseminated intravascular coagulation (DIC) in motion. A hemolytic reaction can be delayed for weeks or months but is still caused by antibodies reacting with their corresponding antigens other than the ABO system.

The second type of transfusion reaction is a febrile nonhemolytic reaction caused by the recipient's antibodies reacting with the transfused white blood cells, platelets, or plasma proteins.

The third type is an allergic reaction caused by a reaction to one or more donor plasma proteins.

The fourth type of reaction is a reaction to citrate. Citrate is an anticoagulant used as a preservative in blood products. When combined with serum calcium in the recipient, it produces hypocalcemia, which causes tingling in the mild reaction to muscle spasms in a severe reaction.

The fifth type is rare: an anaphylactic reaction. It may occur when immunoglobulin A (IgA) proteins are given to an IgA-deficient recipient who has developed IgA antibodies.

Other reactions can be septic shock caused by a blood product that is contaminated by bacteria or an endotoxin. The risk of acquiring a blood-borne infection is minimal as all blood products are tested by serology before being distributed for use. Infections that can be transmitted through blood products and not produce symptoms until weeks later are malaria, hepatitis, and human immunodeficiency virus (HIV). Hepatitis, for instance, has an incubation period of 1 to 6 months.

Graft-versus-host disease (GVHD) occurs in an immunocompromised recipient when donor lymphocytes recognize the recipient's cells as foreign and attack them. Blood products for these clients are usually irradiated to kill the lymphocytes and prevent this reaction.

▶ ASSESSMENT

1. Assess for symptoms of an acute hemolytic reaction, *including fever with or without chills, chest and lumbar pain, hypotension, dyspnea, oliguria or anuria, and abnormal bleeding.* **Early detection allows for implementation of appropriate treatments.**
2. Assess for a nonhemolytic reaction, *which includes symptoms of fever, chills, flushing, headache, muscle pain, anxiety.* **Early detection allows for implementation of appropriate treatments.**
3. Assess for an allergic reaction: flushing, hives, or itching or an anaphylactic reaction *in which symptoms of respiratory distress, chest pain, hypotension, abdominal cramps, vomiting and diarrhea, shock, loss of consciousness, or cardiopulmonary arrest will be present.* **Early detection allows for implementation of appropriate treatments.**
4. Assess for a citrate reaction, *including circumoral tingling, hypotension, nausea, vomiting, or cardiac dysrhythmias.* **Early detection allows for implementation of appropriate treatments.**
5. Assess for sepsis, *which includes symptoms of chills, fever, vomiting, diarrhea, hypotension, and shock.* **Early detection allows for implementation of appropriate treatments.**
6. Assess for circulatory overload, noting *dyspnea, cyanosis, severe headache, elevated systolic blood pressure, tachycardia, jugular vein distention, crackles, and elevated central venous pressure. Assess for hypothermia and cardiac dysrhythmias caused by cold blood cooling the right ventricle and affecting the conduction system.* **Early detection allows for implementation of appropriate treatments.**
7. Assess for GVHD in the immunocompromised client *who may present with fever, skin rash, diarrhea, bone marrow suppression, and liver dysfunction.* **Continued assessment**

is important to detect reactions and begin appropriate treatment.
8. Assess for a delayed hemolytic reaction: *continued anemia despite receiving a transfusion, or hepatitis that may present weeks after the transfusion with weakness, fatigue, nausea, and jaundice.* **Continued assessment is important to detect reactions and begin appropriate treatment.**

▶ DIAGNOSIS

Decreased Cardiac Output

Excess Fluid Volume

Risk for Infection

Hypothermia/Hyperthermia

Pain

Diarrhea

Impaired Gas Exchange

Impaired Skin Integrity

Risk for Allergic Response

▶ PLANNING

Expected Outcomes:

1. The client will have a normal temperature, no chills, and no signs of a transfusion reaction.
2. The client will have normal tissue perfusion and cardiac output.
3. The client will be calm and comfortable.
4. The client will show no signs of infection.

Equipment Needed (see Figure 8-10-1):

• Disposable gloves
• IV tubing
• Stethoscope
• Saline basal IV solution
• Sphygmomanometer
• Thermometer

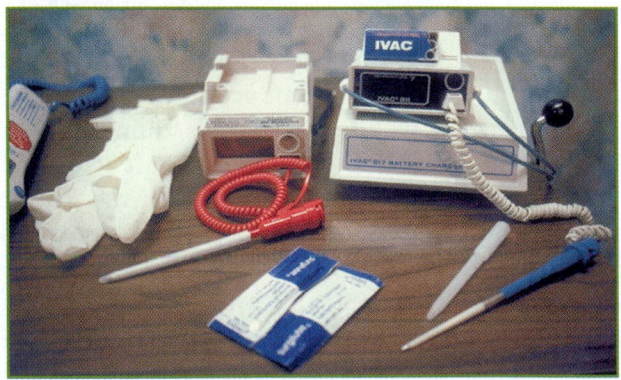

Figure 8-10-1 Thermometers

► **CLIENT EDUCATION NEEDED:**

1. Instruct the client on which symptoms should be reported to the nurse immediately.
2. Ask the client to verbalize previous experience with transfusions.
3. Assure the client of the measures taken to ensure safe blood products.
4. Assure the client that he or she is being carefully monitored for a possible reaction.

5. The client is given the call light and is able to verbalize potential adverse reaction symptoms.

Estimated time to complete the skill: **1 to several hours; until client is stable**

► **DELEGATION TIPS**

Responding to a blood transfusion reaction is a skill involving assessment and knowledge regarding blood replacement techniques and emergency responses. It is not delegated unless other licensed personnel have been trained and certified to respond.

IMPLEMENTATION—Action/Rationale

Action	Rationale
1. Immediately stop the transfusion.	1. Reduces risk of further reaction.
2. Using gloved hands, remove tubing with blood and replace with new tubing.	2. Prevents blood in the tubing from being infused.
3. Maintain a patent IV with normal saline. Do not use any solutions containing dextrose.	3. Ensures fluids or medications can be given in the event of anaphylaxis. Dextrose is incompatible with blood.
4. Obtain vital signs, including oxygen saturation.	4. Assesses client's hemodynamic stability.
5. Remove gloves and wash hands.	5. Maintains aseptic technique.
6. Notify health care provider of client's transfusion reaction, including vital signs and specific symptoms with severity of reaction and time frame. Know protocol to follow. Clients may need oxygen and to be placed in Trendelenburg position if shock occurs.	6. Transfusion reactions need prompt medical attention with efficient, accurate communication of the event.
7. Monitor client's vital signs at least every 15 minutes (see Figure 8-10-2).	7. Assesses client's cardiopulmonary status.
8. Read the blood component bag to ensure that the correct unit was given to the correct client.	8. Client may have received incompatible blood intended for another client.

continues

Action	Rationale

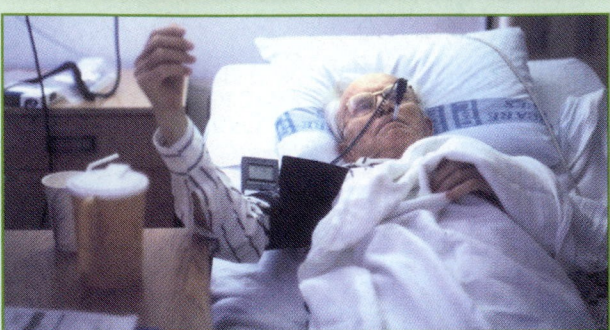

Figure 8-10-2   Monitor vital signs every 15 minutes.

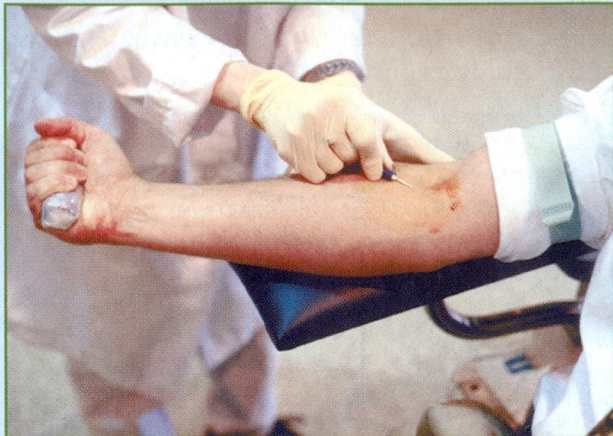

Figure 8-10-3   Obtain two blood samples from the arm opposite the transfusion.

9. Administer medications as prescribed:
   - Diphenhydramine

   - Epinephrine

   - Broad-spectrum antibiotics
   - Intravenous fluids

9.
   - Antihistamine given IV counteracts some allergic responses.
   - Stimulates alpha receptors and beta receptors in the sympathetic nervous system and decreases respiratory distress in anaphylactic reactions.
   - Given when bacterial sepsis is suspected.
   - Counteracts symptoms of septic shock.

10. Start cardiopulmonary resuscitation if indicated.

10. Prompt resuscitation may reverse cardiopulmonary arrest.

11. Obtain two blood samples from arm opposite transfusion (see Figure 8-10-3).

11. First sample is for cross-match to ensure that the correct ABO matched blood was given. In the second sample, the serum is tested for free hemoglobin, which indicates hemolysis.

12. Return the remaining blood and tubing to blood bank.

12. A sample of the blood will be cross-matched with the client's samples before and after the transfusion to check for any error in cross-matching.

13. Obtain first voided urine (within 1 hour of reaction).

13. Hemoglobinuria occurs with hemolysis so the urine may be red or black. Renal damage requires prompt treatment to promote diuresis and prevent renal tubular damage.

▶ REAL WORLD ANECDOTES

Scenario 1

Don was recovering from an abdominal aneurysm repair. His morning blood test showed a low hematocrit so his surgeon ordered two units of packed RBCs to be given. After checking the first bag of RBCs with another nurse, his nurse started the transfusion slowly to assess for a reaction. After taking his vital signs 5 minutes into the transfusion, he appeared to be tolerating it well. However, a few minutes later, Don felt some pain in his chest so

continues

► **REAL WORLD ANECDOTES** (continued)

he pushed his patient-controlled-analgesia (PCA) pump. When the nurse returned to take his vital signs, he said he was having difficulty breathing. The nurse immediately stopped the transfusion and then took his temperature, which was 38.8° C, and his blood pressure, which was 90/58, lower than his usual 124/78. The nurse called his surgeon and checked the unit of blood with the client's medical record again. The blood and urine tests sent to the laboratory showed an error in cross-matching the client with the donor blood.

Scenario 2

Trisha came to the outpatient department for her weekly platelet transfusion while she was recovering from her last cycle of chemotherapy for acute lymphocytic leukemia. She had a history of reacting to platelet transfusions so her nurse gave her medications to prevent a reaction before starting the transfusion. These medications included diphenhydramine, acetaminophen, and hydrocortisone. The volume of the platelet transfusion was also reduced as she weighed only 26 kilograms. The nurse started the transfusion slowly, and when Trisha appeared to tolerate it, the rate was increased. After 10 minutes, Trisha started feeling warm and restless. When her nurse took her temperature, it registered 38.4° C, and Trisha began shaking with chills. The nurse slowed the transfusion, called the physician, and gave her a dose of meperidine to calm the chills.

► **EVALUATION**

- Observe the client's response to discontinuing the transfusion and reaction to medications or other treatment administered.
- Observe for worsening of symptoms that could lead to a severe reaction and cardiopulmonary arrest.

► **DOCUMENTATION**

Nurses' Notes

Note:

- Date, time, and type of reaction that occurred
- Time the charge nurse and health care provider were notified
- Response of the client after discontinuing the transfusion
- Response to the treatment given for the reaction
- Time the blood and urine specimens were sent to the blood bank

Document on appropriate flow sheet or electronic medical record (EMR).

Medication Administration Record

- List medications and intravenous fluids given for the reaction.
- If client is being discharged, provide written instructions of symptoms to monitor along with follow-up health care provider appointment.
- Do not allow the client to drive if any medications were given that could cause sedation.

► **CRITICAL THINKING SKILL**

Introduction

The occurrence of a hemolytic reaction is life-threatening. Every precaution should be taken both in the laboratory where the type and cross-matching of the donor blood with the client's blood is done and while initiating the transfusion to ensure that the client and blood unit are identified correctly.

Possible Scenario

The client was scheduled to have two units of packed RBCs. The first one was completed without complications. The second unit was identified slightly differently from the first. Specifically, the last name was spelled "Smith" on the unit of blood and "Smythe" on the medical record and the client's wristband identification. The nurse started the transfusion as the other numbers and names were spelled correctly. Seven minutes after starting the second unit the client complained of pain in his back and feeling warm and weak.

Possible Outcome

The hemolytic reaction could progress and result in oliguria and renal failure. Hemolysis could lead to DIC and uncontrolled hemorrhage.

Prevention

If there is any variation in spelling of names, client identification numbers, or type of blood including Rh factor of blood, it must be returned to the blood bank. Only accurately identified cross-matched units of blood are safe to give a client. Check the blood components at the bedside and include the client in checking the name when applicable.

► VARIATIONS

Geriatric Variations:
- *Sodium citrate reactions can occur in clients with inadequate bone stores of calcium, clients with osteoporosis or bony tumors, or clients whose mobility is limited.*
- *In clients with poor cardiac function, the rate of a blood transfusion is critical in preventing cardiac overload.*

Pediatric Variations:
- *Children may react quickly to fluid overload unless the IV rate is carefully controlled.*
- *Citrate reactions can occur in infants receiving exchange transfusions.*

Home Care Variations:
- *Nurses working in the home setting must be meticulous in transporting, preparing, and verifying that the correct blood is on hand prior to administering it to the client.*
- *The nurse in the home setting must know the signs and symptoms of transfusion reactions, and closely watch for any symptoms that could signal the onset of a transfusion reaction. The nurse must know the proper steps to obtain help for the client, or transport, if necessary, should a transfusion reaction occur.*
- *Nurses working in the home setting must follow policies and procedures of the home health agency regarding administration of blood products.*

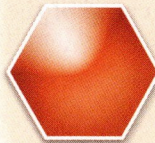

Long-Term Care Variation:
- *Personnel working in long-term care settings, where blood is not frequently administered, should review common symptoms of transfusion reactions prior to administering blood or blood products.*

► COMMON ERRORS

Possible Error:

The nurse did not give the client premedications because he or she did not look for a history of transfusion reactions in the medical record.

Prevention:

Assess the medical record and ask the client about his or her experience with transfusions before preparing the transfusion.

Possible Error:

The name on the blood bag is different from the medical record.

Prevention:

Assess the correct spelling of the client's name on the medical record. If this error does occur, do not give the blood. Call the blood bank to report the error in the spelling of the name and follow the hospital policy for returning the bag for correction.

▶ **NURSING TIPS**

- Organize your time so that you can remain with the client for the first 15 minutes of the transfusion.
- Have emergency medications at the bedside.
- Remember that anaphylactic reactions have two distinct features: the reaction occurs after only a few millimeters of blood or plasma has been infused and there is no fever.
- Review emergency measures such as cardiopulmonary resuscitation before starting a transfusion.

▶ **SPECIAL CONSIDERATIONS**

- *If the client in hepatic failure is to receive red blood cells, he or she may be at risk for ammonia toxicity. This can be avoided by selecting blood collected less than five days prior to transfusion. If the institution is unable to acquire these units, then whole blood, if available, can be packed immediately before infusion, or any unit of blood can be washed immediately before infusion. This washing removes the ammonia from the transfused unit(s).*
- *Routine blood transfusions should not be warmed as hemolysis of blood occurs at temperatures above 104° F.*

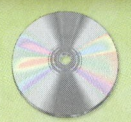

Assisting with the Insertion of a Central Venous Catheter

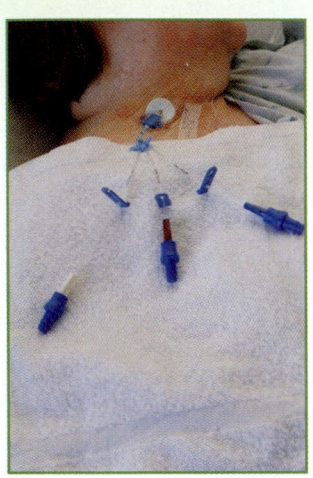

▶ OVERVIEW OF THE SKILL

A central venous catheter is an intravenous (IV) catheter designed to be inserted into a large central vein, with the catheter terminus usually in or near the right atrium. The reasons for central venous catheter insertion include long-term IV therapy, total parenteral nutrition administration, chemotherapy administration, dialysis, volume replacement, peripheral stem cell collections, and central venous pressure monitoring. Central venous catheter insertion can be performed on an outpatient basis with the client able to return home after insertion is complete. Discomfort may be experienced for a few days or for up to a week after this procedure. The length of time a central venous catheter can remain in place varies from a few months to years. Typically, it is necessary to cover the central venous catheter exit site with an air occlusive dressing to prevent potential bacterial contamination.

▶ ASSESSMENT

1. Verify policy regarding central venous catheter insertion. **This allows the nurse to ensure institutional policies are being followed.**
2. Review client's past medical history to see if central venous catheter insertion is contraindicated on one side of the client's body (e.g., on the same side as a mastectomy), if allergy exists to tubing, or if there is an optimal place to insert the catheter. **Identification of this information ensures that placement of central venous catheter will be in optimal position.**
3. Assess client's knowledge regarding central venous catheter insertion and care at home. **This determines need for further education and home care.**
4. Assess the client's ability to cooperate with the procedure, especially if the health care provider will want the client to hold his or her breath during insertion. **This allows any modifications to be made in technique that may be required if the client is confused or uncooperative.**
5. Assess whether or not signed consent is required by your institution and whether or not it has been obtained. **This allows the procedure to be performed in a timely manner without delays.**

▶ DIAGNOSIS

Risk for Infection

Impaired Skin Integrity

Disturbed Body Image Disturbance

Deficient Knowledge

Risk for Injury

▶ PLANNING

Expected Outcomes:

1. Central venous catheter will be placed in accordance with institution policy and in an optimal position for the client.
2. The client will not experience any adverse effects from the catheter insertion such as air embolus, infection, or pneumothorax.
3. The client will experience a minimum of anxiety and pain during the catheter insertion.

Equipment Needed (see Figure 8-11-1):

• Central venous catheter
• Central venous catheter insertion kit, if available (see Figure 8-11-2)
• Scalpel
• Suture kit
• Transparent occlusive dressing
• Gauze
• Sterile, latex-free gloves
• A 10-mL syringe with heparinized saline for each lumen
• Lidocaine
• Betadine
• Sterile gown
• Mask
• Sterile drape

▶ CLIENT EDUCATION NEEDED:

1. Explain sensation felt during central venous catheter insertion.
2. Explain with pictures what the central venous catheter will look like once it is inserted.
3. Explain care of the central venous catheter at home and troubleshooting (e.g., difficulty flushing, catheter leaking).
4. Describe signs of infection or thrombus formation involving the central venous catheter and how to handle these situations.

Estimated time to complete the skill: **20–30 minutes**

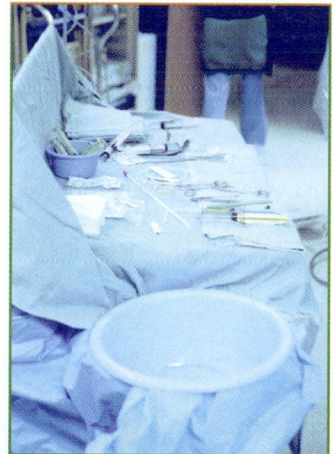

Figure 8-11-1 Central venous catheter and insertion equipment

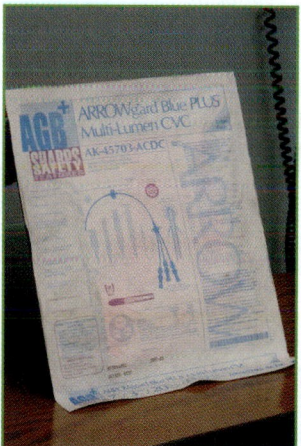

Figure 8-11-2 Central venous catheter kit.

▶ DELEGATION TIPS

Assisting with the insertion of a central venous catheter is a skill involving assessment and the use of sterile technique. It is an invasive procedure performed by the health care provider and assisting is not delegated by the nurse unless other licensed personnel have been trained and certified to assist with the procedure. Ancillary personnel who will be caring for the client need to be instructed to report any complaints of pain, redness, or swelling at the insertion site.

IMPLEMENTATION—Action/Rationale

Action	Rationale
1. Check the health care provider's written order for placement of a central venous catheter (see Figure 8-11-3).	1. Ensures accurate procedure is performed.
2. Obtain consent form from client.	2. Gives legal permission to perform the procedure and verifies client's understanding of the risks and benefits of the procedure.
3. Identify client and check for drug or iodine allergy.	3. Ensures proper client identification. Decreases risk of allergic reaction such as hives, urticaria, and anaphylactic reaction.
4. Position client in a supine position.	4. Allows for best visualization and access to appropriate vessel.
5. Apply mask to client and all other present in the room during the procedure.	5. Reduces spread of transmission of microorganisms.
6. Clean chest area with Betadine (see Figure 8-11-4) and drape appropriately (see Figure 8-11-5). (For more information on how to prepare a surgical site, see skill 4-21.)	6. Ensures minimal risk of contamination, which could cause infection.
7. Open package containing supplies for insertion and the catheter (see Figure 8-11-6).	7. Prepares a sterile field for the health care provider.
8. Assist health care provider with putting on a sterile gown (see Figure 8-11-7).	8. Reduces spread of microorganisms.
9. Open sterile gloves for health care provider.	9. Reduces spread of microorganisms.
10. Assist with administration of subcutaneous lidocaine by wiping off rubber top of vial and holding vial upside down for the health care provider to access.	10. Maintains a sterile field for the health care provider.

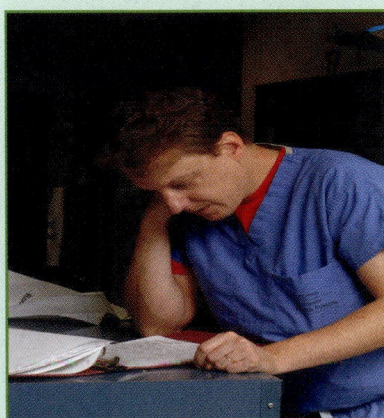

Figure 8-11-3   The order for the placement of the central venous catheter is verified.

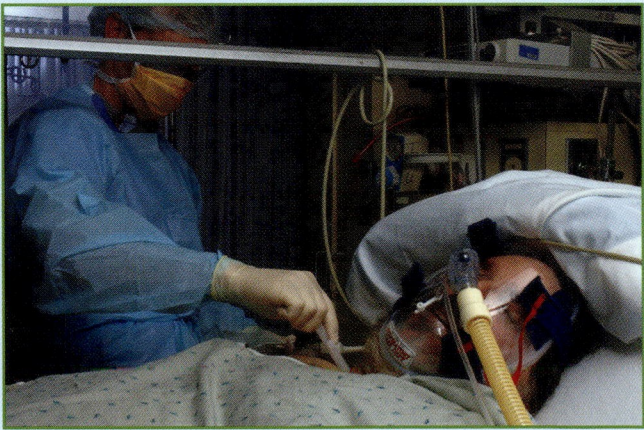

Figure 8-11-4   The area is cleansed with Betadine before the insertion of the central venous catheter.

continues

Action	Rationale

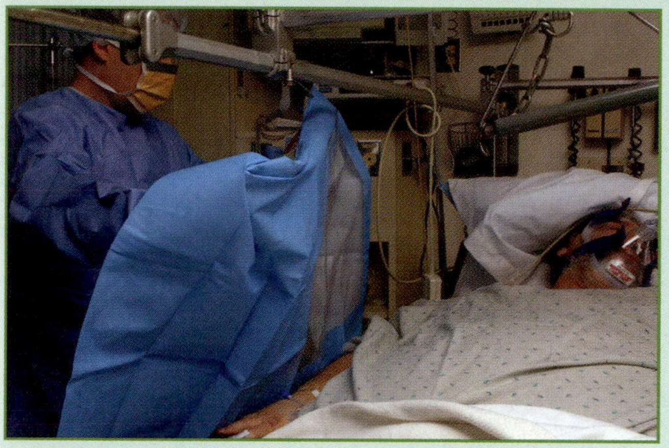

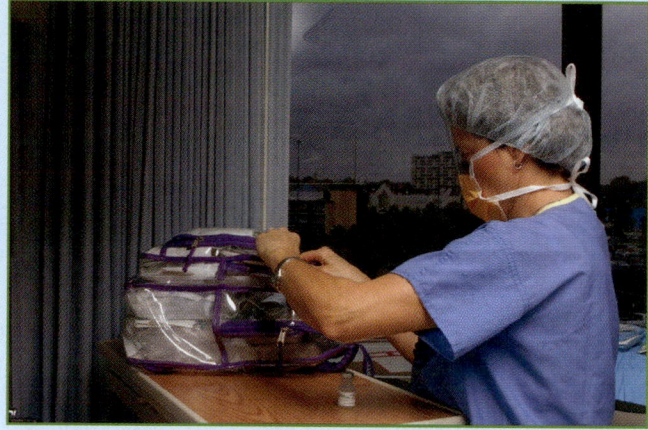

Figure 8-11-5   A sterile drape is applied around the central venous catheter insertion site.

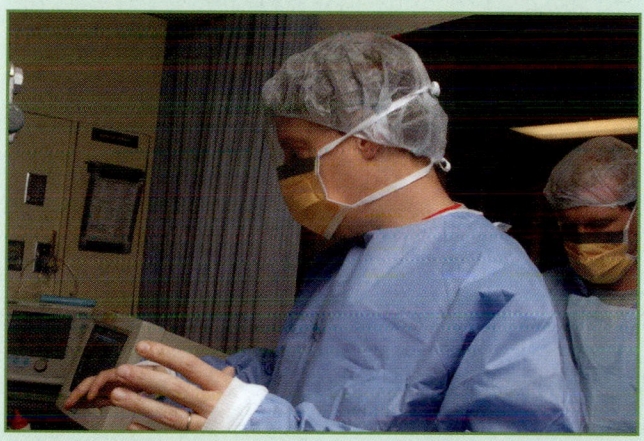

Figure 8-11-6   The package containing the necessary supplies for insertion of the central venous catheter is opened.

Figure 8-11-7   The nurse assists the health care provider with putting on a sterile gown.

11. Assist with priming the lumens of the central catheter by wiping off the top of the vial containing the sodium chloride and holding the vial upside down for the health care provider to access.

12. The procedure is only performed by a health care provider. The health care provider makes a small incision. The vein is percutaneously accessed by inserting a large bore needle attached to a syringe into the subclavian vein or jugular vein. When blood is aspirated the syringe is removed and a guidewire is threaded through the needle into the superior vena cava. After the guidewire is inserted the needle is removed. The catheter is threaded onto the guidewire and inserted into the superior vena cava. The lumens are aspirated and flushed with the saline or heparin (see Figures 8-11-8 through 8-11-11).

11. Maintains a sterile field for the health care provider.

12. There is a high volume of blood flow in the superior vena cava and the procedure requires specialized training to perform.

continues

Action	Rationale

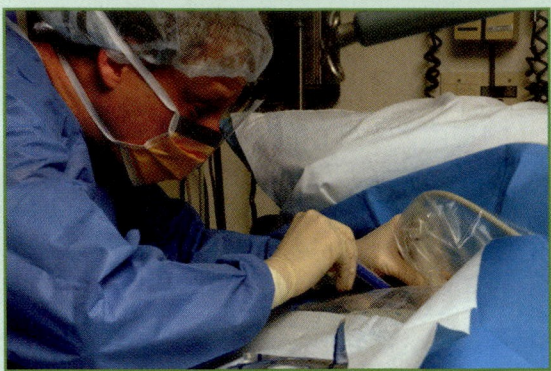

Figure 8-11-8   The health care provider accesses the subclavian with a needle attached to a syringe.

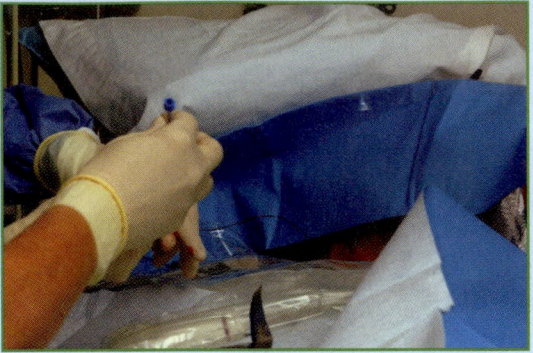

Figure 8-11-9   A guidewire is inserted through the needle and into the subclavian vein.

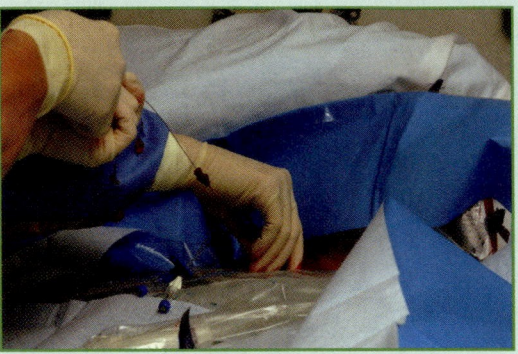

Figure 8-11-10   The catheter is threaded over the guidewire and inserted into the central vein.

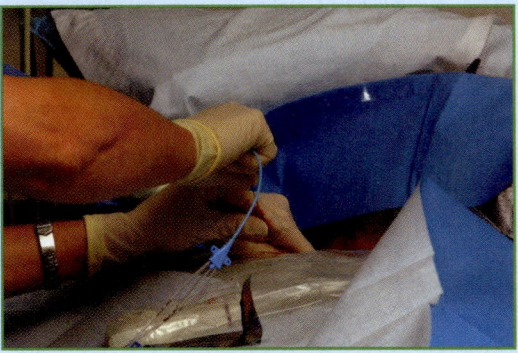

Figure 8-11-11   After the catheter is fully advanced into the central vein, the guidewire is removed.

13. The health care provider checks each lumen of the catheter for patency by flushing with normal saline or heparinized saline (depending on the type of catheter inserted) (see Figure 8-11-12).

13. Prevents clot formation in the lumens and keeps them patent. Helps to determine placement of the catheter.

14. The physician or qualified practitioner secures the central venous catheter with one suture (see Figure 8-11-13) and covers the wound with an air occlusive dressing.

14. Prevents bacterial contamination and the leakage of air into the insertion site.

15. Remove sterile drapes and dispose of sharps in the appropriate biohazard sharps container.

15. Prevents injury to health care providers.

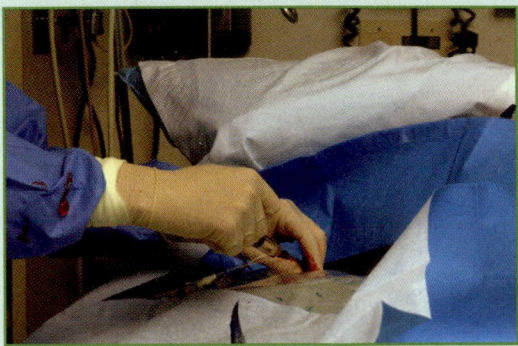

Figure 8-11-12   The lumens of the central venous catheter are each flushed with saline.

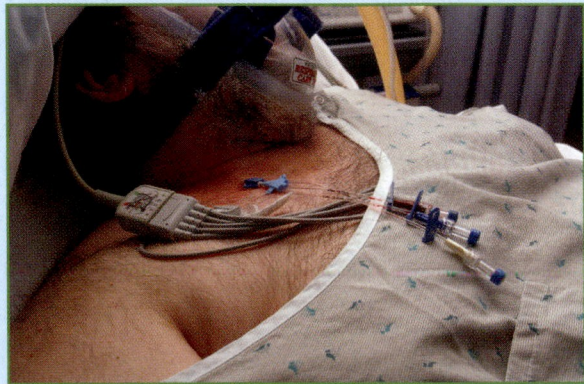

Figure 8-11-13   The central venous catheter after it is inserted. The catheter is then covered with a transparent dressing.

▶ **EVALUATION**

- Central venous catheter was placed in accordance with institution policy and in an optimal position for the client.
- The client did not experience any adverse effects from the catheter insertion such as air embolus, infection, or pneumothorax.
- The client experienced a minimum of anxiety and pain during the catheter insertion.

▶ **DOCUMENTATION**

Nurses' Notes:

- Document the date and time of catheter insertion.
- Note the type of catheter inserted, the insertion site, the chest X-ray results, and how the client tolerated the procedure.
- Note any unusual occurrences or observations.
- Chart if the client was started on IV therapy through the central line.

Document on appropriate flow sheet or electronic medical record (EMR).

▶ **CRITICAL THINKING SKILL**

Introduction

Central venous catheters are placed for a number of reasons, including long-term IV therapy, total parenteral nutrition administration, chemotherapy administration, dialysis, and peripheral stem cell collection. There are a number of different types and styles of catheters, and some are better for a specific purpose than others. Knowing the purpose for catheter placement is important so that the appropriate central venous catheter is placed.

Possible Scenario

Steven has lymphoma and is having a central venous catheter placed for peripheral stem cell collection in preparation for a stem cell transplant. The nurse reviews the physician's orders and gathers the required supplies. She notes that the orders state that Steven is to have a dual lumen 13.5-French catheter placed for phoresis of peripheral stem cells. She remembers that the last time she assisted with this procedure they needed to place a 12-French catheter to accommodate the phoresis machine. The nurse double-checks the order; it is in fact for a 13.5-French catheter. The last time she assisted with this procedure was quite a while ago, and she assumes that the physician must know what he is doing. Perhaps they have new phoresis equipment. She prepares a 13.5-French, double-lumen central catheter for insertion. The catheter insertion goes smoothly and Steven tolerates the procedure well.

Possible Outcome

When it is time for his first stem cell collection, the floor nurse receives a call regarding Steven's central line. The Bone Marrow Transplant Center is requesting information regarding the size of Steven's central line. When the nurse verifies that it is a 13.5-French catheter, the transplant center explains that their equipment will not work with anything smaller than a 12-French catheter. Steven has to return to the hospital for a replacement catheter of the correct size.

Prevention

If the nurse had been truly thinking like a client advocate, she would have questioned the original size of catheter ordered based on her previous experience. This would have saved Steven the additional trauma and expense of having a new catheter inserted. The nurse does not want to risk the possibility of the wrong central venous catheter being placed, so she decides to call the Bone Marrow Transplant Coordinator at the hospital to verify this order. The Bone Marrow Transplant Coordinator verifies that a 12-French catheter is needed and thanks her for catching this potential mistake. This lumen size is needed to ensure adequate volume can circulate through the phoresis machine. The nurse prevented an error in central venous catheter placement by verifying the correct catheter for the intended use.

► VARIATIONS

Geriatric Variation:
* *Elderly clients may not be able to tolerate lying supine while the central catheter is being inserted. A variation of client positioning may be necessary in order to place the central catheter.*

Pediatric Variations:
* *Children have smaller veins than adults. The central catheter will need to be shorter and smaller.*
* *Teenagers may have serious body image issues regarding long-term placement of a central line.*
* *The parents of a child receiving a central line need to be assessed for educational needs and anxiety about the placement.*

Home Care Variation:
* *If the nurse has a client who will receive a central line, the home care nurse can provide support and education to help the client prepare for the procedure.*

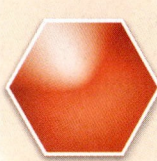

Long-Term Care Variation:
* *Central lines are not inserted in the long-term care setting.*

► COMMON ERRORS

Possible Error:

Assisting with insertion of a central line with catheter lumens full of air.

Prevention:

Remember that the lumens of the central line must be flushed as part of the equipment preparation. Remind the health care provider, if necessary.

► **NURSING TIPS**

- Become familiar with the central venous catheter insertion policy at the institution in which you work.
- Think through the steps and review written instructions if unsure about supplies needed for central venous catheter insertion.

- Ensure all supplies are available and ready for use before beginning this procedure. Be aware of any contraindications of catheter placement in the client. Be prepared to gently remind the health care provider of potential problems.

► **SPECIAL CONSIDERATIONS**

- *The surgeon may require hair to be removed from the insertion site. It is recommended that an electric razor or scissors be used for hair removal as shaving may cause micronicks and increase the potential for infection.*
- *When separating disposable from nondisposable items after the insertion of the catheter, make sure that all sharps are accounted for and disposed of properly. Those handling the trash may be stuck inadvertently with a contaminated needle if the nurse is not prudent about sharp object safety.*
- *Surgical conscience is imperative when working in the surgical arena. If a surgeon's glove should become contaminated, it is the nurse's responsibility to alert him or her to this and to change the glove without compromising the integrity of the sterile field.*

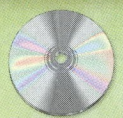

Changing the Central Venous Dressing

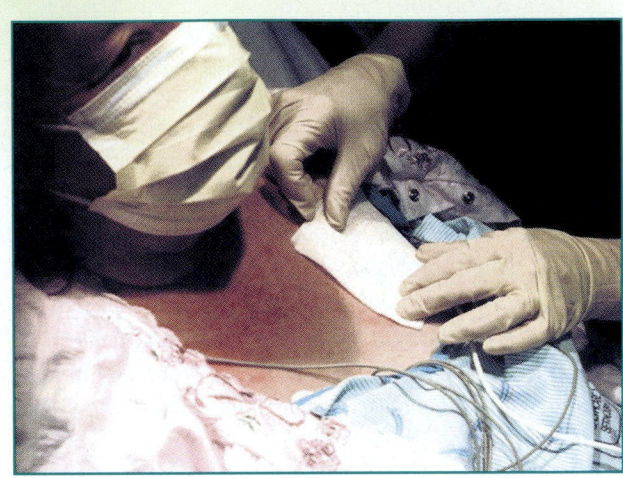

▶ OVERVIEW OF THE SKILL

Because the central venous catheter insertion site is a direct route to the circulatory system, care must be taken to keep the insertion site clean and infection-free. The insertion site must be inspected frequently for signs and symptoms of infection, such as inflammation, heat, or drainage. Regular, aseptic dressing changes can help decrease the possibility of infection at the insertion site and systemically. Policies vary from institution to institution regarding the type of dressing to apply as well as the frequency with which they are changed. Be aware of the policy at your institution and the rationale for it. Dressings that have become wet or are pulling loose from the insertion site must be changed immediately.

▶ ASSESSMENT

1. Assess the need for dressing change by noting the last dressing change documented in the medical record and standard of care recommended by the manufacturer and the institution. **This decreases the risk of infection by following the standard of care.**
2. Assess the timing of the dressing change as it relates to medication, IV fluid and transfusion schedules, as well as the time of the client's daily shower or bath. **This allows the nurse to avoid simultaneous administration of medication**

and the need for two dressing changes in one day.
3. Assess the type of central venous access in place **in order to obtain the appropriate supplies.**
4. Assess the integrity of the skin at the site **for signs of infection or bleeding.**
5. Assess the client and caregiver's knowledge of the purpose and care of the catheter **so a teaching plan can be developed.**

▶ DIAGNOSIS

Risk for Infection

Impaired Skin Integrity

Deficient Knowledge

▶ PLANNING

Expected Outcomes:

1. Skin is intact at catheter site, has normal color, is not edematous, and has no drainage.
2. Client has no signs of systemic infection such as fever, malaise, or chills.
3. Catheter and tubing are intact.
4. Client and caregiver are able to perform skin care and dressing change.

Equipment Needed (see Figure 8-12-1):

• Povidone-iodine swabs, chlorhexidine or agency-approved antiseptic solution

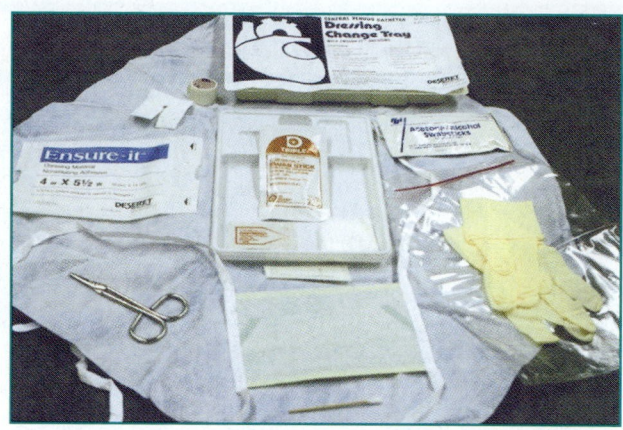

Figure 8-12-1   Central venous catheter dressing change tray, mask, clamp, and nonsterile gloves

- Mask
- Sterile gloves

- Povidone-iodine ointment
- Sterile gauze, tape, or moisture transparent dressing
- Label with date and time of dressing change
- Latex-free gloves

▶ CLIENT EDUCATION NEEDED:

1. Teach the client the rationale for the dressing change, the need for aseptic technique, and how to perform the dressing change if the catheter will be placed long term.
2. Provide written or illustrated instructions on how to change the dressing.
3. Ask the client or caregiver to demonstrate the skill.
4. Discuss the time of day the dressing change should be done.

Estimated time to complete the skill:
5–10 minutes

▶ DELEGATION TIPS

Changing the central venous catheter dressing is a skill involving assessment and the use of sterile technique. It is a procedure not delegated by the nurse unless other licensed personnel have been trained and certified to assist with the procedure. Ancillary personnel who will be caring for the client need to be instructed to report any disruption of the closed dressing, along with complaints of pain, redness, or swelling at the insertion site.

IMPLEMENTATION—Action/Rationale

Action	Rationale
1. Wash hands and put on clean gloves.	1. Reduces the number of microorganisms.
2. Put on mask.	2. Reduces the number of microorganisms.
3. Remove old dressing carefully (see Figures 8-12-2 and 8-12-3), being careful not to dislodge the central catheter.	3. Skin integrity may be impaired.
4. Note drainage on dressing.	4. Potential for bleeding or infectious material.
5. Inspect skin at insertion site for redness, tenderness, or swelling (see Figure 8-12-4).	5. Assesses for infection.
6. Palpate tunneled catheter for presence of Dacron cuff, using care not to palpate close to the exit site.	6. Documents proper placement of catheter.
7. Visually inspect catheter from hub to skin.	7. Checks whether catheter has a crack or is split or cut.

continues

Action	Rationale

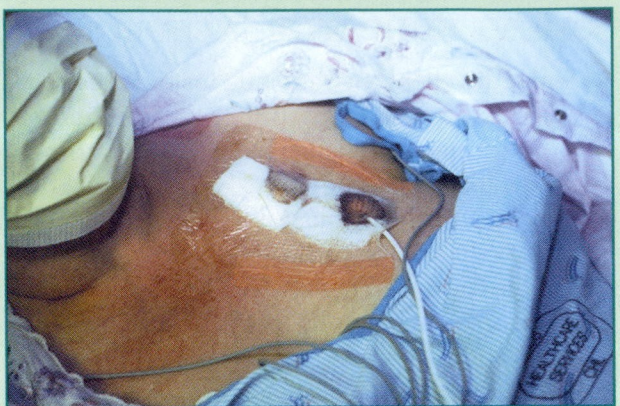

Figure 8-12-2 Inspect the dressing.

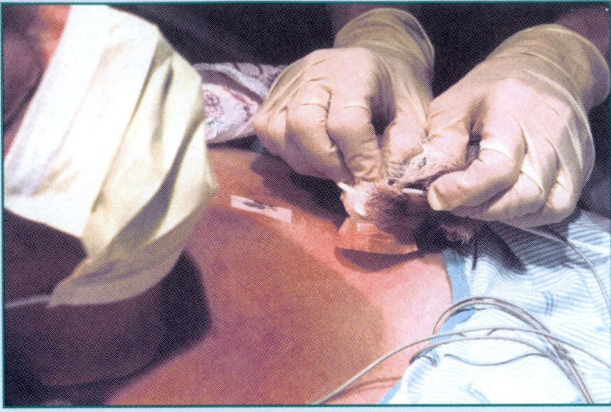

Figure 8-12-3 Remove the old dressing. Be careful not to dislodge the catheter.

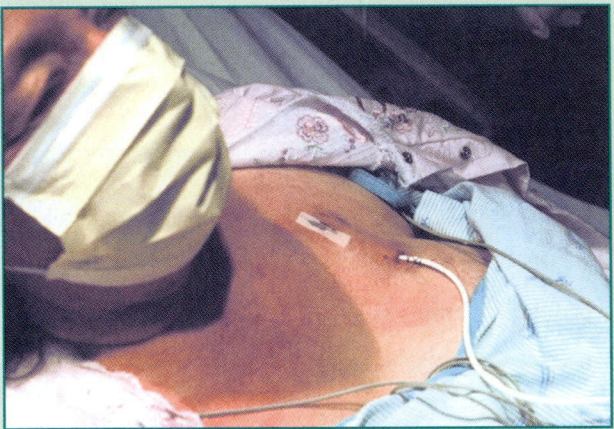

Figure 8-12-4 Inspect the site for redness, tenderness, and swelling.

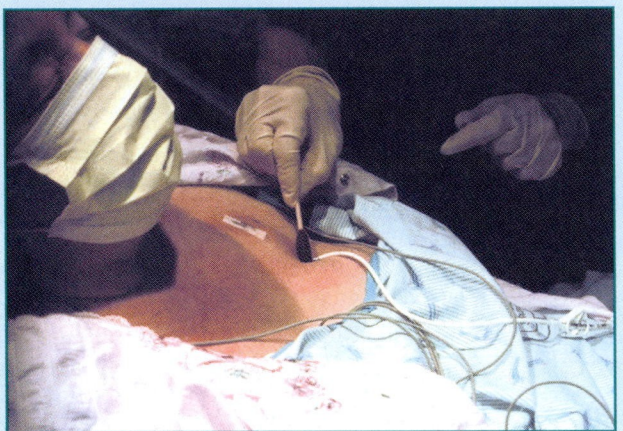

Figure 8-12-5 Clean the site with povidone-iodine swab.

8. Remove gloves and put on sterile gloves.

9. Clean exit site according to institution protocol. Most use alcohol wipes first, then povidone-iodine swab beginning at the catheter and moving out in a circular manner for 3 cm to maintain aseptic technique (see Figure 8-12-5).

10. Some institutions use povidone-iodine ointment to exit site (check agency policy).

11. Apply transparent dressing (see Figures 8-12-6, 8-12-7, and 8-12-8). Some institutions prefer to omit the gauze dressing to allow visualization of the site. In this case only the transparent dressing is applied.

12. Label with date and time of dressing change (see Figure 8-12-9).

13. Secure tubing to client's clothing.

8. Prevents transmission of microorganisms from skin to exit site.

9. Eliminates microorganisms by chemical and mechanical means.

10. Reduces growth of bacteria at exit site.

11. Prevents bacteria from entering exit site.

12. Documents time to plan for next change.

13. Prevents accidental displacement.

continues

Action	Rationale

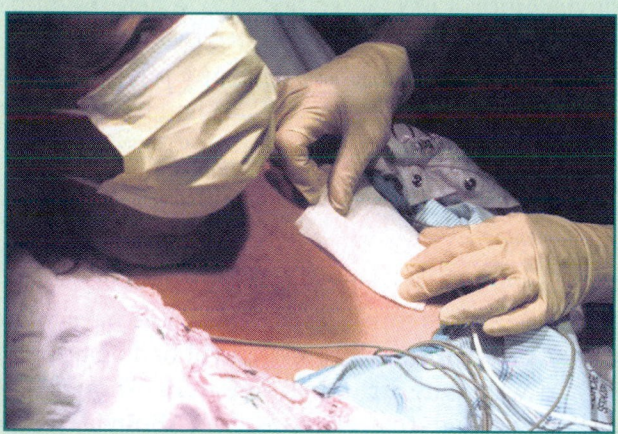

Figure 8-12-6 Slide the first piece of gauze directly over and under the catheter.

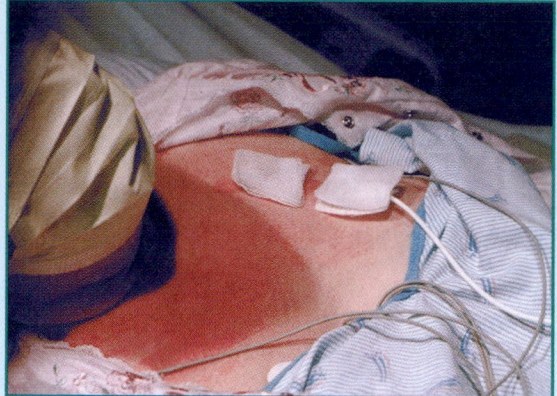

Figure 8-12-7 Place the next piece of gauze directly over the insertion site.

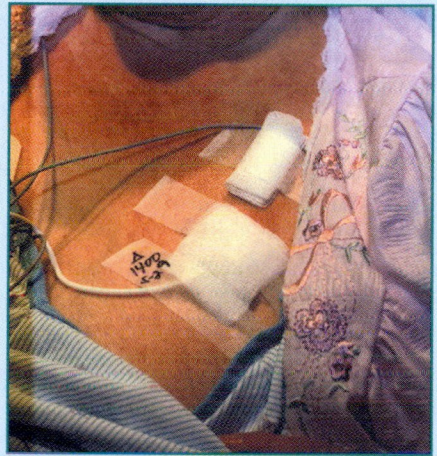

Figure 8-12-8 Place a larger piece of gauze over the area and secure with tape or transparent dressing.

Figure 8-12-9 Write the date and time of the dressing change on the dressing.

14. Remove gloves and dispose of all used materials.

14. Reduces transmission of microorganisms.

15. Wash hands.

15. Reduces transmission of microorganisms.

▶ REAL WORLD ANECDOTES

Mrs. Abukar was to be discharged to home with a central venous line in place. Mrs. Abukar was unable to change the dressing herself so the nurse planned to teach her caregiver how to change the dressing and care for the site. Mrs. Abukar's primary caregiver was her husband, Ali Abukar, who spoke no English. Mr. Abukar had seen the nurse change the central line dressing once but he had not participated, and the nurse was not sure he understood all the steps or the need for asepsis. Mr. Abukar was not able to come in during the day for teaching because he worked full time on the weekdays. Mrs. Abukar's nurse arranged for a translator to be present one evening when Mr. Abukar would be at his wife's bedside. She waited to change the central line dressing until Mr. Abukar and the translator were present. She then went through the procedure step by step as Mr. Abukar watched and the translator explained the rationale for

continues

▶ **REAL WORLD ANECDOTES** *(continued)*

each step. Mr. Abukar looked frightened and overwhelmed, but the nurse gently worked with him, showing him each step over again and having him help with each step until he felt somewhat at ease with the procedure. The nurse then arranged for Mrs. Abukar's next dressing change to be supervised by a home health nurse, and encouraged Mr. Abukar to have an English-speaking family member present to help with the translation of any questions he might have.

▶ EVALUATION

- The client's skin is intact at catheter site, has normal color, and is not edematous.
- The client has no signs of systemic infection such as fever or malaise.
- The central venous catheter and tubing are intact.
- Client and caregiver are able to perform skin care and dressing change.

▶ DOCUMENTATION

Nurses' Notes

Note:
- The date and time the dressing was changed
- The type of ointment and dressing applied
- The condition of the skin at the site
- The presence of any exudate or bleeding at the site
- The client or caregiver's ability to perform the dressing change

Document on appropriate flow sheet or electronic medical record (EMR).

▶ CRITICAL THINKING SKILL

Introduction

Mrs. Bouvier's tunneled central line exits in her upper chest right under her bra strap. The strap sometimes rubs the dressing at the site.

Possible Scenario

The skin around the exit site is red and, one day, she noticed a puslike drainage. She cleaned the area as instructed and reported the redness and drainage to her nurse by phone.

Possible Outcome

Mrs. Bouvier's nurse told her to continue to cleanse the area as instructed and apply an antibiotic ointment to the site. The nurse planned to come see Mrs. Bouvier within a day or two and would assess the site at that time. The nurse was unable to see Mrs. Bouvier until 3 days after her call. When the nurse did arrive, he noted that the central venous catheter insertion site was quite reddened and pus was visible around the catheter. The nurse notified the physician and received an order for IV antibiotics as well as more frequent dressing changes.

Prevention

The nurse should have talked to Mrs. Bouvier regarding the site and its care. This way, he would have found out that Mrs. Bouvier's bra strap rubbed against the site and was quite irritating. The nurse should then have mentioned that perhaps Mrs. Bouvier could obtain a bra that did not rub on the central line insertion site or she could discontinue wearing a bra until the insertion site was no longer inflamed. He should have then recommended that Mrs. Bouvier change the dressings more frequently to assess the site condition and then seen Mrs. Bouvier the next day to determine if there were any other steps that could be taken to reduce the irritation to the central line insertion site.

▶ **VARIATIONS**

Geriatric Variations:
- *The integrity of the skin of an elderly client may be impaired. Care should be taken when removing tape and the dressing, which may stick because of exudate.*
- *Teaching a geriatric client or caregiver about changing a dressing will need to be done after assessing his or her willingness and ability to perform this procedure.*

continues

▶ VARIATIONS *(continued)*

Pediatric Variations:
- *Children can be taught to help with the dressing change, such as opening and holding the sterile dressing or holding the tape.*
- *Children may need an extra means for securing the catheter, such as a vest to attach the catheter and tubing.*

Home Care Variations:
- *Supplies should be kept in a clean, dry space.*
- *The nurse can contact the client at home to see if he or she is having problems with the dressing change.*
- *Discharge planning should include referral for home health services.*
- *Client should be given a written list of providers of supplies and equipment.*

▶ COMMON ERRORS

Possible Error:

You accidentally pull the catheter while removing the dressing that is stuck to the catheter.

Prevention:

Assess the dressing for drainage that may have stuck to the catheter. Be sure gloves are the correct size so fingers are agile. If this error does occur, assess the area around the catheter for bleeding. Soak the dressing with sterile normal saline in order to remove the dressing without further trauma. Proceed with the dressing change.

Possible Error:

The sterile dressing falls on the floor before it is applied to the skin.

Prevention:

Have all supplies next to the client. Maintain sterile supplies on a sterile field. Be sure you do not have to reach over anything to use your equipment. If this does occur, discard the gauze, obtain another package, put on another pair of sterile gloves, and continue with the procedure.

▶ NURSING TIPS

- Gather extra supplies to have available in case you drop something.

- A cotton-tipped applicator dipped in normal saline may help loosen exudate on a catheter.

▶ SPECIAL CONSIDERATIONS

- *When using a transparent dressing, it is helpful to work your hand around the dressing as the tab is unraveled. This prevents the dressing from sticking to itself or crimping at the edges. Difficulty in discerning the edge of the transparent dressing when it is on the client reflects a smooth application.*
- *Asepsis is especially essential when changing a central line dressing because of the potential for infection and close proximity to the heart.*

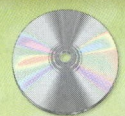

SKILL 8-13

Changing the Central Venous Tubing

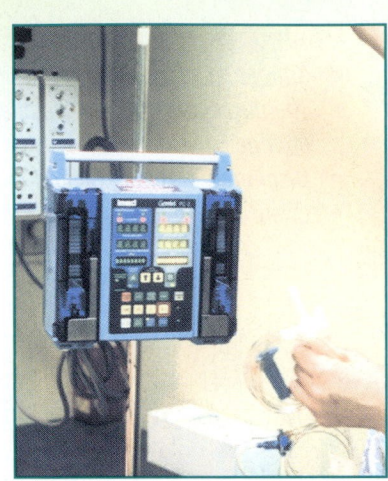

▶ OVERVIEW OF THE SKILL

Central venous catheter tubing is changed frequently to ensure minimal risk of infection. The frequency of change depends on institutional policy, the status of the client, and the type of fluid that is being infused. In clients receiving total parenteral nutrition or those with compromised immune systems, tubing may be changed daily. Clients who are neutropenic, such as cancer clients undergoing chemotherapy, also require more frequent central venous catheter tubing changes. However, if the client is receiving hydration such as normal saline and has an intact immune system, central venous catheter tubing may be changed just a few times a week. Central venous catheter tubing should be changed immediately if it is found to be damaged or contaminated.

▶ ASSESSMENT

1. Verify policy regarding frequency of central venous catheter tubing changes. **This allows the nurse to ensure institution policies are being followed.**
2. Check original fluid or medication orders regarding rate of infusion and duration. **Identification of this information ensures that fluid or medication is given at the correct rate for the intended amount of time.**
3. Assess client's knowledge regarding fluid or medications. **Determine need for fluid or drug education.**

4. Assess client's catheter site. **Determine need for dressing change and observe for signs of infection.**

▶ DIAGNOSIS

Impaired Skin Integrity

Risk for Infection

▶ PLANNING

Expected Outcomes:

1. Central venous catheter tubing will be changed in accordance with institutional policy.
2. The client will remain free of infection secondary to the central venous catheter tubing.
3. The client will remain free of infection secondary to the central venous catheter tubing change.

Equipment Needed (see Figure 8-13-1):

- Central venous catheter tubing
- Medication administration record (MAR) or original order containing documentation of the type and rate of medication or fluids to be administered
- Medication or fluids
- Tag or a piece of tape with the date tubing is due to be changed

▶ CLIENT EDUCATION NEEDED:

1. Explain type of medication or fluids.
2. Explain action of medication or fluids.

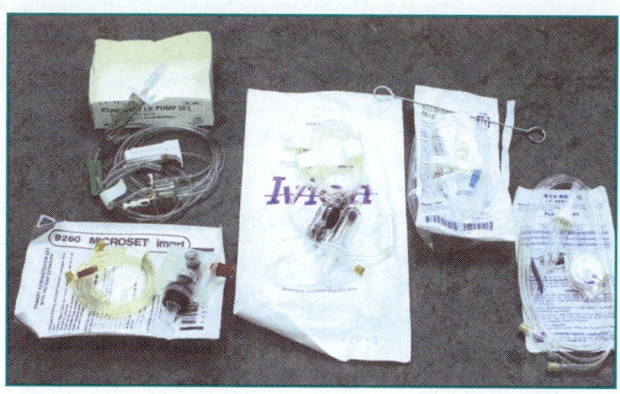

Figure 8-13-1 Types of IV tubing

3. Explain use of central venous catheter tubing and why it is changed on a schedule.

4. If the client is going to be administering medication or fluids at home using an infusion central venous catheter tubing, have client do a return-demonstration setting up the infusion set independently.
5. Make sure client knows whom to call with questions.
6. Reinforce verbal teaching with written instructions.

Estimated time to complete the skill:
5–10 minutes

▶ **DELEGATION TIPS**

Changing central venous line tubing is a skill involving assessment and the use of sterile technique. It is a procedure not delegated unless other license personnel have been trained and certified to perform the procedure.

IMPLEMENTATION—Action/Rationale

Action	Rationale
1. Wash hands.	1. Reduces the transmission of microorganisms.
2. Check MAR against health care provider's written orders.	2. Ensures accuracy in the administration of the fluid or medication.
3. Check for drug allergies.	3. Decreases risk of allergic reaction such as hives, urticaria, or anaphylactic shock.
4. Prepare the medication or fluids for one client at a time. Decide what type of central venous catheter tubing is needed and assemble equipment (see Figure 8-13-2).	4. Ensures that the right client receives the right medication using the right equipment.
5. Check the client's arm band before hanging the new central venous fluids (if appropriate).	5. Ensures right client.
6. Identify the fluids for the client and their therapeutic purpose.	6. Encourages client cooperation and increases client awareness of what to expect from the medication or fluids.
7. Clamp off new tubing. Spike bag of medication or fluids with new tubing. Squeeze drip chamber (if there is one) until it is about half full. Open clamp on new tubing until medication or fluids have filled tubing completely.	7. Prevents air from being infused through the central venous catheter and causing an air embolus.

continues

Action	Rationale

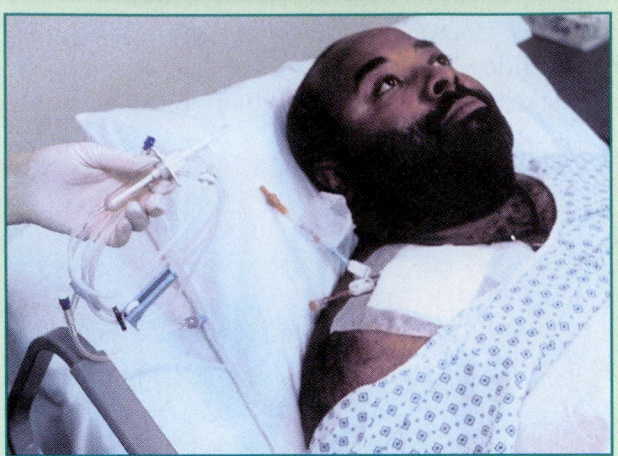

Figure 8-13-2 Select the correct tubing and take it with other equipment to the bedside.

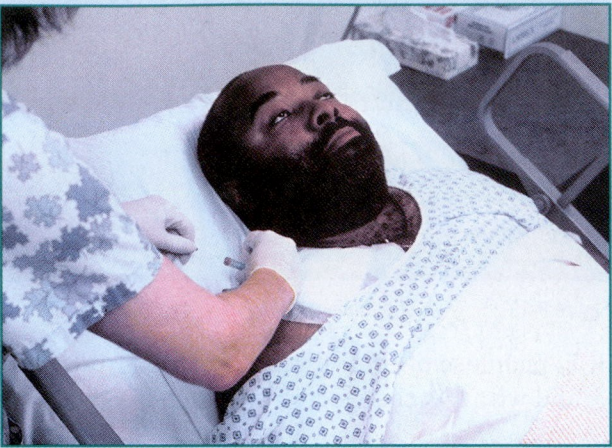

Figure 8-13-3 Disconnect old tubing.

8. Clamp off the central venous catheter and old tubing if it is currently hanging. Disconnect old tubing or cap from central venous catheter site. Cleanse the access port per institutional policy. Connect new tubing without letting the end of the catheter become contaminated (see Figures 8-13-3 and 8-13-4). Secure the connection (see Figure 8-13-5).

8. Sterile tips on catheter and tubing must be maintained to minimize risk of contamination and infection.

9. Insert tubing into pump if one is being used and unclamp new tubing. Set pump or adjust drip rate to infuse at ordered rate.

9. Necessary to ensure proper rate and to prevent fluid bolus.

10. Put tag on tubing with next date to be changed. Document tubing change in client's chart or on MAR if space is allotted.

10. Ensures that other nurses will be aware of date the tubing needs to be changed.

11. Wash hands.

11. Reduces the transmission of microorganisms.

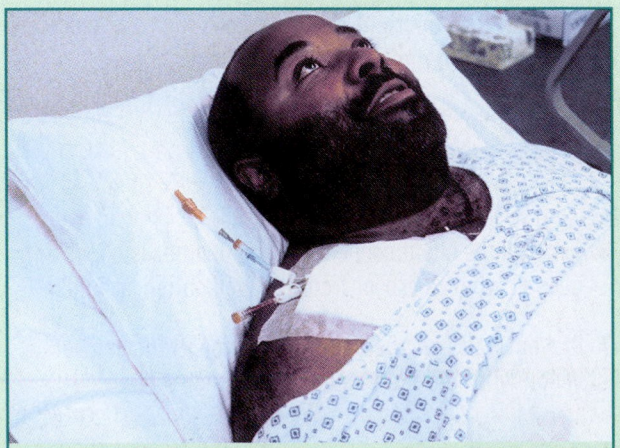

Figure 8-13-4 Connecting tubing using a needleless system.

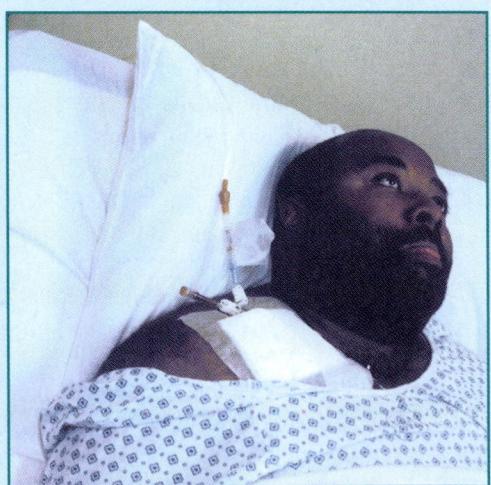

Figure 8-13-5 Secure the connection with tape.

▶ REAL WORLD ANECDOTES

Scenario 1

The nurse brought in the supplies to change the central venous tubing connected to Bill's central line. He clamped off the old tubing and disconnected it from the central line. He then uncapped the new central venous catheter tubing and connected it to the end of Bill's central venous catheter. The nurse then realized that he had forgotten to purge the tubing of air. He carefully disconnected the tubing from the central venous catheter and squeezed the drip chamber of the new tubing. He then opened the clamp to allow the fluid to replace the air in the tubing and reconnected the new tubing to the central venous catheter.

Scenario 2

The nurse notes that Jane's central venous catheter tubing and total parenteral nutrition (TPN) is due to be changed, so she gathers the supplies and heads into her room. She sets up the new IV solution and tubing, turns off the IV pump, carefully removes the old tubing, and replaces it with the new tubing. As she opens the IV pump to place the new tubing in it, she realizes that she has forgotten to close the clamp on the old tubing. She glances down to see a stream of yellow TPN draining onto her uniform and shoes. She quickly clamps the tubing and proceeds to place the new tubing into the IV pump. Unfortunately, the tubing she had so carefully primed and connected to the central catheter is not the type of tubing required by the IV pump in use. The nurse now finds herself, sticky with TPN, smelling of vitamins, having to redo the entire procedure. She is ruefully reminded to plan ahead and know what type of tubing will be required as well as to close all clamps prior to changing IV tubing.

▶ EVALUATION

- The central venous catheter tubing was changed in accordance with institutional policy.
- The client remains free of infection secondary to the central venous catheter tubing.
- The client remains free of infection secondary to the central venous catheter tubing change.

▶ DOCUMENTATION

Nurses' Notes

- Record any unusual findings.

Document on appropriate flow sheet or electronic medical record (EMR).

MAR Flow Sheet

- Record the time and date the tubing and fluids were changed. Sign and initial the entry.

▶ CRITICAL THINKING SKILL

Introduction

Take all precautions to ensure that the tubing is sterile.

Possible Scenario

The nurse is preparing to change the central venous fluids and infusion tubing for Mr. Xydis. She prepares the solution and tubing in the medication room, spiking the solution bottle, priming the tubing, and placing a sterile cover on the end of the tubing. Before she can take the prepared solution and tubing to Mr. Xydis's room, she is called away to care for another client. When she returns to the medication room, the end of the central venous infusion tubing is lying on the floor. The sterile cap is still in place.

Possible Outcome

Seeing that the sterile cap is still on the tubing, the nurse proceeds with the solution and tubing to Mr. Xydis's room and hangs them, replacing Mr. Xydis's old central line solution and tubing. Sixteen hours later Mr. Xydis spiked a temperature of 102° F. Blood cultures revealed staph sepsis. When she returned to duty the next day, the nurse wondered if Mr. Xydis's sepsis had been caused by the central venous tubing she had used.

Prevention

Upon seeing the end of the tubing lying on the floor, she should have started over with a new solution and tubing setup. The tubing was still capped, but contamination was possible. The best precaution is to take the tubing and solution to Mr. Xydis's room and prepare it at his bedside. The nurse can use the time to assess the old tubing and solution and to check his central line insertion site for infection or other complications. If there is any question in your mind regarding the sterility of an object, throw it away and start over. The cost and time savings are not worth endangering a client.

► VARIATIONS

Geriatric Variation:
- Elderly clients may have compromised immune systems and delicate, thin skin. Changing the tubing is a good time to assess for signs of infection and skin breakdown at the insertion site.

Pediatric Variations:
- Pediatric clients are very susceptible to small fluid balance changes. Be sure to use the correct tubing when changing the central line tubing. Some tubing sizes deliver large drops and some deliver small drops. You should use a volume control mechanism, such as a pump or Volutrol, on any pediatric IV.
- Remind the pediatric client that changing the tubing is not painful.

Home Care Variations:
- Make sure that you have supplies set up and a clear work field when changing tubing in the home setting. It can be difficult to replace contaminated tubing.
- Make sure the home caregiver knows how to work the IV pump and how to respond to alarms and emergencies.
- Make sure the home caregiver has the correct tubing and equipment for the pump.

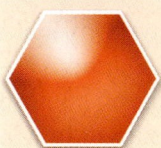

Long-Term Care Variations:
- Establish a regular schedule for changing tubing.
- Complications can occur in central lines that have been placed for long periods of time. Do not become complacent about assessment.
- People who care for the client daily should know what changes to look for, who to report them to, and how to respond to pump alarms.

► COMMON ERRORS

Possible Error:
One hour after changing the central venous catheter tubing, the nurse returns to the client's room to find that no fluid has infused during this time period.

Prevention:
Always check back within 20–30 minutes after setting up new central venous catheter tubing to see if it is infusing properly and to adjust the rate as needed. Consider using an infusion pump to ensure the desired rate of infusion is achieved.

Possible Error:
There is no tag with a date on the central venous catheter tubing.

Prevention:
Be sure to tag and chart the date and time of IV tubing changes. The potential for bacterial growth increases as the days pass without changing the central venous catheter tubing.

▶ **NURSING TIPS**

- Become familiar with the central venous catheter tubing policy at the facility in which you work.
- Think through the steps and review written instructions if unsure about how to change the central venous catheter tubing.

- If teaching a client this skill, use the same equipment he or she will be using at home.

▶ **SPECIAL CONSIDERATIONS**

- *Air bubbles trapped in the tubing are a potential risk for air embolus. Take the time to clear the line of bubbles or trapped air, especially when the fluid will enter the superior vena cava.*
- *Know institution protocol for the different types of central lines.*

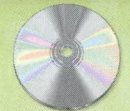

Flushing a Central Venous Catheter

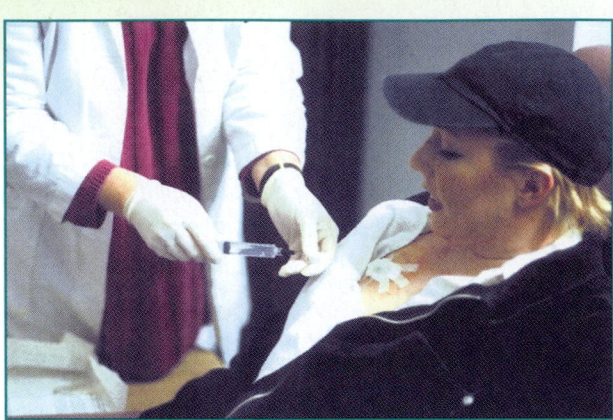

▶ OVERVIEW OF THE SKILL

A central venous line is a safe, convenient, and pain-less way to infuse fluid, medications, and blood products or obtain blood samples from clients who require specific therapy and monitoring. Frequent venipuncture and multiple intravenous (IV) lines increase the risk of infection and bleeding. Long-term therapy involving multiple treatments with corrosive medications can cause peripheral venous harden-ing or collapse. Central venous catheters, which are inserted through a large vein into the superior vena cava, can help avoid these problems.

There are several types of venous access devices. This skill deals with flushing peripherally inserted central catheters (PICCs), tunneled catheters, and nontunneled catheters.

- The PICC is inserted into a large vein in the ante-cubital fossa and advanced to the subclavian vein and finally into the superior vena cava.
- Tunneled central venous catheters are surgically inserted while the client is under general or local anesthetic in the operating room. They can have one to three lumens depending on the needs of the client. A tunnel is made through subcutane-ous tissue below the clavicle; then the catheter tip is inserted through one of the large veins, such as the internal or external jugular, and the distal end is threaded into the right atrium. The proximal end is pulled out through the tunnel where it can be anchored.

The patency of a central venous catheter depends on regular flushing with saline and possibly heparin solution to prevent clots from forming within the catheter or at the tip. Changing the dressing at the insertion site is detailed in Skill 8-12.

▶ ASSESSMENT

1. Assess the type of central venous line in place. **This allows the nurse to know how many lumens are available to access.**
2. Assess the function and patency of the catheter **to ensure minimal complications during a blood draw or infusion.**
3. Assess client's knowledge of the purpose of the central venous line **to determine the need for education.**

▶ DIAGNOSIS

Risk for Infection

Impaired Skin Integrity

Deficient Knowledge

▶ PLANNING

Expected Outcomes:

1. The nurse will be able to aspirate blood through the catheter.
2. The nurse will be able to infuse fluid through the catheter.
3. The client will not exhibit any signs or symptoms of systemic infection.

4. The visible portion of the catheter will be intact without leaks, holes, or tears.

Equipment Needed (see Figure 8-14-1):
- Povidone-iodine and alcohol swabs
- Syringes (10 mL)
- Vial or ampule of normal saline solution
- Vial of heparin solution (heparin flush or heparin 100 U/mL in saline) (check institution policy on heparin solution use)

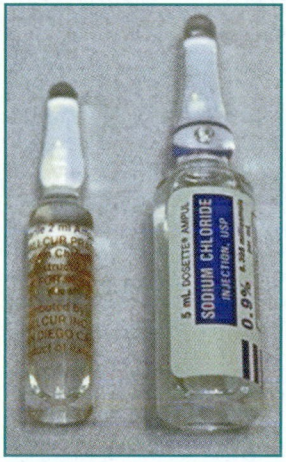

Figure 8-14-1 Ampules of sodium chloride

- Plastic clamp or metal bull-dog clamp
- Sterile needle (20- to 22-gauge)
- Sterile gloves, gown, and mask

▶ CLIENT EDUCATION NEEDED:

1. Teach the client the rationale for flushing the catheter with normal saline and/or heparin according to the institution's or manufacturer's guidelines.
2. Instruct the client about the need for aseptic technique.
3. Teach the client and caregiver how to flush the catheter.
4. Teach the client and caregiver what complications to look for and how to react to them.
5. Ask the client or caregiver to demonstrate their ability to flush the catheter after they have been taught.

Estimated time to complete the skill:
5 minutes

▶ DELEGATION TIPS

Flushing a central venous line is a complex skill requiring assessment and proper technique. It is a procedure not delegated unless other licensed personnel have been trained and certified to perform the procedure.

IMPLEMENTATION—Action/Rationale

Action	Rationale
1. Wash hands. Apply gloves, gown, and other protective equipment as needed.	1. Reduces transmission of microorganisms.
2. Prepare two syringes (see Figure 8-14-2): one with 10 mL of normal saline and one with 5 mL of heparin solution.	2. Preparing equipment in advance allows for a smooth procedure.
3. Swab injection cap or catheter hub with povidone-iodine and alcohol.	3. Prevents introduction of microorganisms into catheter.
4. Clamp catheter and remove cap.	4. Prevents entrance of air into catheter.
5. Check catheter for patency: • Attach syringe with normal saline. • Release clamp.	5. Ensures patency of catheter. • Connects syringe to catheter. • Opens catheter lumen.

continues

Action	Rationale

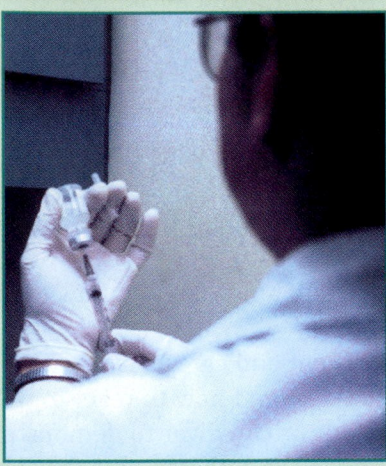

Figure 8-14-2 Prepare two syringes.

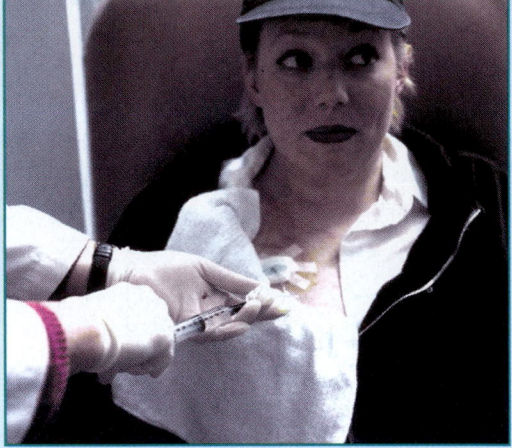

Figure 8-14-3 Aspirate heparin solution from the catheter and flush with saline.

- Aspirate heparin solution from catheter (see Figure 8-14-3).
- Observe blood return.
- Flush quickly with normal saline (see Figure 8-14-4).

- Reclamp.

- Remove empty syringe.
- Attach syringe filled with 5 mL heparin solution to catheter.
- Release clamp.
- Flush quickly.
- Reclamp.

6. Place new cap on end of catheter, tape all tubing connections, and attach tubing to client's clothing.

7. Dispose of soiled equipment and used supplies.

8. Wash hands.

- Removes old heparin solution.

- Verifies patency of catheter.
- Ensures that catheter will be cleared of any blood so it will not clot.
- Clamping catheter during changes of syringes prevents air from entering catheter.
- Continues procedure.
- Connects syringe to catheter.
- Opens catheter lumen.
- Injects heparin solution into catheter.
- Closes catheter lumen.

6. Maintains sterile seal to catheter.

7. Reduces transmission of microorganisms.

8. Reduces transmission of microorganisms.

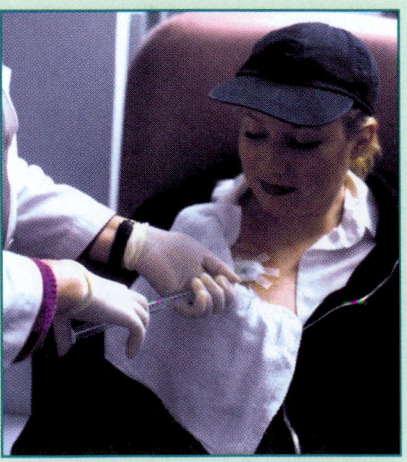

Figure 8-14-4 Flush with heparin solution.

► REAL WORLD ANECDOTES

Mr. Wilson had a central venous catheter placed for the infusion of total parenteral nutrition (TPN). He received 2 liters a day and liked to have a few hours away from the IV pump. His 13-year-old daughter had learned how to care for his central line in case his wife was not home. One day, she felt a slight resistance when she flushed the catheter after stopping the TPN. She had been taught to try to aspirate blood to check for patency. When she saw a small amount of blood appear in the syringe, she was relieved and assured that the catheter was patent, but as it still did not flow as easily as before, she notified the home health nurse who came later to evaluate the catheter for patency.

► EVALUATION

- The nurse was able to aspirate blood through the catheter.
- The nurse was able to infuse fluid through the catheter.
- The client does not exhibit any signs or symptoms of systemic infection.
- The visible portion of the catheter is intact, without leaks, holes, or tears.

► DOCUMENTATION

Nurses' Notes

- Report the condition of the catheter.
- Report the patency of the catheter, including the ability to draw blood and difficulty of infusing fluids.
- Report occlusions, damage to the catheter, or air embolus to the health care provider immediately.

Document on appropriate flow sheet or electronic medical record (EMR).

▪ CRITICAL THINKING SKILL

Introduction

There are several causes of difficulty in aspirating blood from a central venous catheter. It could be a thrombus, precipitation from incompatible medications, or malposition.

Possible Scenario

The client was lying on his side when the nurse came to check on his central line. He wanted to check on its patency before starting the IV infusion of antibiotics. When he tried to aspirate blood, nothing happened. He knew the catheter had been patent just 2 hours before.

Possible Outcome

He asked the client to turn on his other side, then raise his arms and cough. No blood returned into the syringe. Finally, he asked him to perform the Valsalva's (bear down and attempt to exhale while keeping the nose and mouth closed) maneuver and blood easily flowed into the syringe.

Prevention

The tip of the catheter can become lodged against the side of the blood vessel. Knowing how to cause the catheter to return to a good position will reestablish patency of the catheter.

► VARIATIONS

Geriatric Variation:
- *If the client is fluid compromised, adjust the volume of flushes.*

continues

> ▶ **VARIATIONS** *(continued)*

Pediatric Variation:
- *Be sure to reduce the volume of fluids used to aspirate and to flush the catheter.*

Home Care Variations:
- *A receptacle for disposing of soiled equipment is needed.*
- *Be sure the client or caregiver knows the signs and symptoms of complications and what steps to take if they occur.*

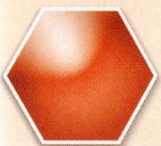

Long-Term Care Variation:
- *If the catheter has been indwelling for a long period, be sure to assess carefully for cracks, tears, or leaks.*

> ▶ **COMMON ERRORS**

Possible Error:

The catheter was not clamped between changing the saline syringe and the heparin syringe. When the client took a deep breath, an air embolus formed.

Prevention:

Keep one hand near the clamp in order to remember to clamp the catheter between changing syringes. If this error does occur, clamp the catheter. Attach an empty syringe and aspirate blood. Observe for air bubbles. Place client on left side with head slightly elevated. Assess for dyspnea, hypoxia, or tachycardia. Notify the health care provider immediately.

▶ **NURSING TIPS**

- Have all the equipment available for the procedure.
- Take advantage of this procedure to assess the client and provide emotional support.
- Different catheters require different amounts of heparin or no heparin at all.
- Some catheters do not require clamps.
- If maneuvers to aspirate blood are not successful, the health care provider should be notified so fibrinolytic therapy (urokinase) can be ordered and given according to institutional policy.

▶ **SPECIAL CONSIDERATIONS**

- Tunneled catheters have fewer infection complications than do nontunneled central venous catheters (CVCs). Examples of tunneled CVCs include Hickman, Broviac, Groshong, and Quinton catheters.
- PICCs are a popular alternative to the traditional CVC because they can be inserted with ease into the cephalic or basilar veins of the antecubital fossa, there is a low risk of complications, and the client seems to tolerate the PICC line well.
- The nurse may also find that the client has an antibiotic or antiseptic-impregnated catheter. These tend to demonstrate a decrease in bacterial colonization and infection. Some examples are: chlorhexidine/silver sulfadiazine and minocycline/rifampin-coated catheters.

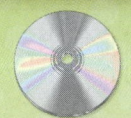

Measuring Central Venous Pressure (CVP)

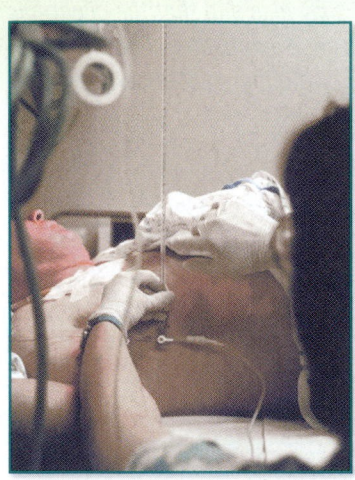

▶ OVERVIEW OF THE SKILL

Central venous pressure (CVP) is a measure of the pressure within the right atrium of the heart. Central venous pressure measures the ability of the right side of the heart to deal with the systemic fluid load. Central venous pressure changes reflect the client's overall fluid volume status. A low CVP is an indicator of hypovolemia, generally necessitating an increase in intravenous (IV) fluids. A high CVP can be caused by hypervolemia or poor cardiac function, which is usually treated by diuresing the client.

CVP is commonly measured by the use of a pressure transducer attached to a bedside monitor. The transducer must be leveled at the phlebostatic axis as well. Using a pressure transducer reduces the risk of air embolus while measuring the CVP.

CVP can be measured using a manometer attached to the intravenous fluid line. The CVP is measured in terms of fluid pressure in the column of the manometer. To ensure the accuracy of the CVP reading, the manometer must always be positioned in the same place, relative to the right atrium. This spot is called the phlebostatic axis. It is located on the midaxillary line in the fourth intercostal space. Once located, the phlebostatic axis should be marked with ink to ensure the accuracy of following measurements.

▶ ASSESSMENT

1. Assess the client's ability to lie in a supine position without a pillow. **This allows the nurse to take a more accurate reading of the CVP.**
2. Assess the client's vital signs and intake and output. **This information will aid the health care team in determining how best to manage the client.**

▶ DIAGNOSIS

Risk for Infection

Risk for Deficient Fluid Volume

Impaired Skin Integrity

▶ PLANNING

Expected Outcomes:

1. The client's CVP will be measured accurately.
2. Aseptic technique will be maintained.
3. The client will not suffer any complications as a result of the CVP measurement.

Equipment Needed (see Figure 8-15-1):

- Sterile gloves
- IV tubing
- Manometer set or pressure transducer setup
- Stopcock, if not included in manometer set

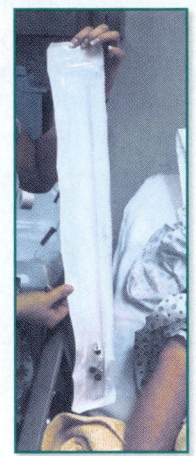

Figure 8-15-1 Manometer

- Indelible ink marking pen
- Tape
- Mask
- Normal saline

▶ **CLIENT EDUCATION NEEDED:**

1. Explain to the client why it is important to be placed in a supine position without a pillow for the measurement. Reassure the client that once the procedure is completed, the client can be placed in a more comfortable position.
2. Explain to the client the importance of leaving the "X" marking the right atrium in place. Reassure the client that once measurements are no longer needed, the mark can be washed off.

Estimated time to complete the skill:
5–10 minutes

▶ **DELEGATION TIPS**

The skill of measuring the CVP requires specific preparation, proper site assessment, and location for accurate results. It is a procedure not delegated by the nurse unless other licensed personnel have been prepared by the agency and certified to perform the procedure.

IMPLEMENTATION—Action/Rationale

Action	Rationale
Taking a CVP with a Manometer	
1. Wash hands and apply gloves.	1. Reduces transmission of microorganisms.
2. Explain procedure to client.	2. Reduces anxiety in client.
3. Gather equipment needed to bedside.	3. Maximizes efficiency and minimizes chance of breaking sterility once started.
4. Position the client in a supine or flat position. If this is not tolerated and the client is in a semi-Fowler position, take all measurements at the same angle. Mark the right atrium (at the midaxillary line about one-third of the distance from the anterior to the posterior chest wall, in the fourth intercostal space) with an "X" using indelible ink pen (see Figure 8-15-2). The term phlebostatic axis may be used to identify the level of the atrium (see Special Considerations).	4. The manometer should always be zeroed at the "X" to minimize variance in measurements.

continues

Action	Rationale

Taking a CVP with a Manometer *continued*

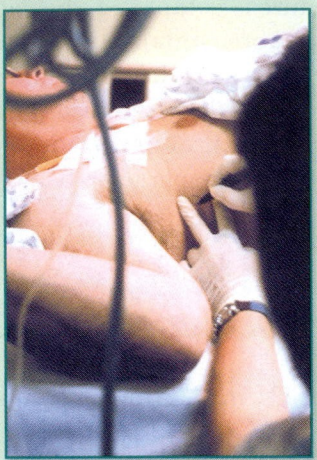

Figure 8-15-2   Mark the right atrium line directly on the skin using an indelible ink pen.

5. Connect the IV fluid (usually normal saline) to a three-way stopcock and flush the other two ports.

6. Apply sterile gloves and mask.

7. Connect the CVP manometer to the upper port of the stopcock (see Figure 8-15-3).

8. Connect the CVP tubing from the client to the second side port of the stopcock (see Figures 8-15-4 and 8-15-5).

9. Allow normal saline to drip rapidly into client for a few seconds, with stopcock closed to manometer.

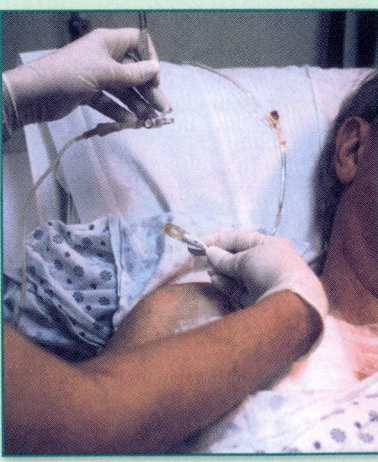

Figure 8-15-4   Connect the tubing from the client to the second port of the stopcock.

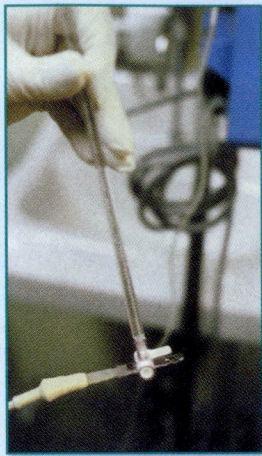

Figure 8-15-3   Connect the CVP manometer to the upper port of the stopcock.

5. Forces air out of the stopcock. Fluids with glucose are stickier than normal saline and may cause manometer to stick; thus, glucose should be avoided.

6. Aseptic technique should be used to minimize infection.

7. Inserts the CVP manometer into the central line system.

8. Establishes IV line from normal saline to CVP catheter.

9. Establishes that CVP line is patent. Fluids must flow freely for reading to be accurate.

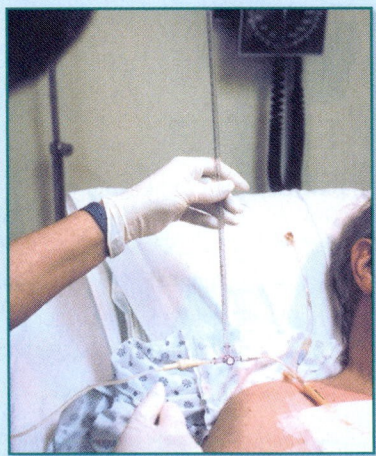

Figure 8-15-5   This is the correct setup. Note that the IV fluid, manometer, and the line to the client are all connected to the stopcock.

continues

Action	Rationale
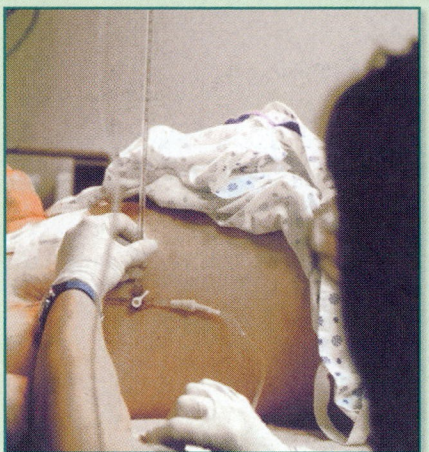 **Figure 8-15-6** Hold the manometer at the marking on the chest.	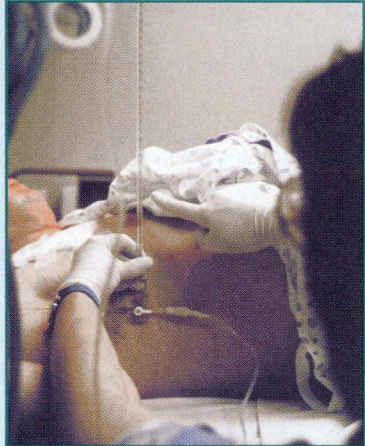 **Figure 8-15-7** Watch the fluid fall in the manometer. When the fluid level stabilizes, take a central venous pressure reading.
10. Turn stopcock off to client and fill manometer with normal saline to the 20-cm mark above the anticipated reading.	10. The normal CVP reading varies from 5 to 12 cm of water.
11. Hold manometer at the phlebostatic axis and turn the stopcock off to the normal saline (see Figure 8-15-6).	11. System is open from the manometer to the client.
12. Watch as the fluid falls in the manometer. Take the central venous pressure reading when the fluid stabilizes (see Figure 8-15-7).	12. The fluid will stabilize at a level equal to the pressure in the central veins or right atrium. If the fluid level fluctuates with the client's respirations, take the reading at the end of the client's expiration.
13. Turn the stopcock off to the manometer.	13. Reestablishes fluid flow from the IV to the client.
14. Store the manometer in an upright position (usually hanging from the IV pole) to prevent air bubbles from entering the fluid column or the client and to prevent contamination of the manometer.	14. The top of the manometer is open to the air. If the manometer is not properly stored, contaminants or air can enter the manometer and be flushed into the client.
15. Wash hands.	15. Prevents the spread of microorganisms.
16. Document reading.	16. Provides continuity of care.

Taking a CVP Using a Transducer

Action	Rationale
17. Wash hands.	17. Prevents the spread of microorganisms.
18. Prime the transducer and the IV lines that are attached to it using the ordered solution (usually heparinized normal saline).	18. The transducer provides a very low flow of IV fluids and the heparin helps to maintain the patency of the line.
19. Place the IV bag into a pressure bag and pressurize the IV solution.	19. The pressure prevents the backflow of blood into the central catheter and the IV line.
20. Attach the IV pressure tubing from the transducer to the central line.	20. Establishes a pathway for the pressure monitoring.

continues

Action	Rationale
Taking a CVP Using a Transducer *continued*	
21. Attach the transducer to the pressure-monitoring equipment.	21. Allows for the translation of the signal emitted by the transducer.
22. Place the client in the supine position with the bed flat, if tolerated.	22. Provides the most accurate measure of CVP.
23. Level the pressure transducer to the phlebostatic axis.	23. Obtains an accurate, consistent reading of the CVP.
24. Zero the monitor according to the manufacturer's instructions.	24. Obtains an accurate CVP reading.
25. The CVP will appear on the monitor. If the reading varies, use the reading obtained at the end of the client's expiration.	25. The end expiratory pressure is the most accurate measure of CVP.
26. Return the client to a position of comfort.	26. Increases client comfort and decreases client anxiety.
27. Wash hands.	27. Reduces transfer of microorganisms.
28. Document CVP reading.	28. Provides continuity of care.

► REAL WORLD ANECDOTES

Scenario 1

John was hospitalized after an automobile accident, in which he lost a large amount of blood. The physician inserted a catheter in the superior vena cava and ordered CVP readings to be performed every 4 hours. The first reading was 8. John's nurse was scheduled to be at lunch when the second reading was due, and she asked one of the other staff nurses to take the reading while she was gone. The staff nurse got a reading of 4 when she took it and reported this to John's nurse when she returned from lunch. John's nurse was concerned about the decrease in John's CVP. She was unsure if the decrease was caused by technique differences or an actual deterioration in John's condition. She reevaluated John, noting that his blood pressure was slightly lower than it had been 4 hours earlier, but his pulse had increased from a rate of 92 to 110. John's nurse took another CVP reading, being careful to hold the manometer at the same phlebostatic axis level she had used earlier. She obtained a reading of 5. When the nurse notified the physician of the CVP and John's vital signs, the physician ordered a stat complete blood count (CBC) to be drawn. The results of the CBC showed that John's hemoglobin had dropped 1.5 grams. John's physician ordered a stat computerized tomography (CT) scan, which revealed internal bleeding. John was taken directly to surgery.

Scenario 2

Ms. Robinson, a 70-year-old woman with a history of pneumonia, was transferred from the intensive care unit to the floor. Her physician was concerned about her fluid status and ordered CVP measurements every shift. She had multiple IV fluids infusing as well as total parenteral nutrition. Over the course of the shift Ms. Robinson's blood pressure increased from 110/76 to 140/90. The nurse was concerned about the increase but attributed it to Ms. Robinson's agitation caused by her noisy roommate. Following the shift change, the evening shift nurse measured Ms. Robinson's CVP. She noted that it had increased from the reported 10 cm to 14 cm. She releveled the transducer and recalibrated the monitor to be sure her reading was accurate. After confirming that Ms. Robinson's CVP was in fact 14 cm, she notified the physician, who asked for Ms. Robinson's intake and output totals for the last shift. Upon checking the totals, the nurse realized that Ms. Robinson's output had been significantly lower than her intake during the previous shift. The physician ordered 40 mg of furosemide IVP, and minimized her IV fluids. Over the next 8 hours, Ms. Robinson's output increased, her blood pressure dropped to 124/82, and her next CVP reading was 12. If the day shift nurse had reassessed Ms. Robinson's CVP after noting the increase in blood pressure, Ms. Robinson's treatment would have been initiated in a timelier manner.

▶ **EVALUATION**

- The client's CVP was measured accurately.
- Aseptic technique was maintained.
- The client did not suffer any complications as a result of the CVP measurement.

▶ **DOCUMENTATION**

Nurses' Notes

- Record CVP results on the graphic sheet, on a flow sheet, and/or in the narrative record.
- Actions based on the results should be documented (i.e., notifying health care provider, interventions performed based on results, and any results based on the interventions) in the narrative record.

Document on appropriate flow sheet or electronic medical record (EMR).

▶ **CRITICAL THINKING SKILL**

Introduction

The following is a scenario in which the nurse prevents an inaccurate measurement of CVP.

Possible Scenario

The nurse has just started her shift and is beginning to position Mr. Clark to measure his CVP. As he lowers the head of the bed and removes his pillow, the nurse notices that Mr. Clark immediately begins breathing more rapidly.

Possible Outcome

The nurse is aware that Mr. Clark's CVP has been taken the previous shift so he decides to simply take the reading quickly while Mr. Clark is lying flat. To compensate for Mr. Clark's respiratory distress, the nurse turns Mr. Clark's oxygen level up while he is taking the reading. As he is taking the reading, he can hear Mr. Clark's breathing become increasingly labored. Anxiously he waits for the fluid in the manometer to stop falling. As he is concentrating on the fluid level, he suddenly realizes that Mr. Clark's breathing is no longer labored and that, in fact, he cannot hear his breathing at all. As the nurse glances over at Mr. Clark, he realizes that he is no longer breathing and calls for emergency resuscitation.

Prevention

The nurse should have noticed a sign over the head of Mr. Clark's bed that was written by the nurse who cared for Mr. Clark on the previous shift. The sign stated that because of his history of chronic obstructive pulmonary disease (COPD), Mr. Clark had extreme difficulty lying flat, and thus all CVP readings were performed at a 45° angle. While this angle is not optimal for CVP monitoring, if all nurses were consistent in the positioning of the client, Mr. Clark's CVP measurement would be more consistent and a useful diagnostic tool.

▶ **VARIATIONS**

Geriatric Variations:

- *As a rule, geriatric clients are more sensitive to fluid shifts, and accurate CVP monitoring is even more important in this population.*
- *Geriatric clients may not be able to lie flat or even supine. The nurse may have to use a less-than-optimal position for measuring CVP to prevent injury to the client. Any unusual positioning or technique must be noted in the nurses' notes as well as both verbally and in the notes at change of shift.*

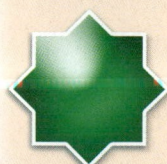

Pediatric Variations:

- *Children are sensitive to fluid imbalances, and a slight increase or decrease from the institution's norms for CVP monitoring may have serious implications for pediatric clients.*
- *It is important that the right atrium is clearly marked and that all readings are zeroed to ensure that all variations in the CVP measurements are hemodynamic changes, not technique variations.*

continues

► **VARIATIONS** *(continued)*

Home Care Variation:
- *Central venous pressure readings are not performed at home. A client may have a central venous catheter in place for IV fluids, frequent blood draws, or hyperalimentation. The client and family should be taught how to care for the catheter.*

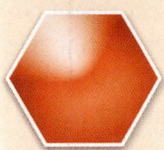

Long-Term Care Variation:
- *Central venous pressure measurements are rarely performed in long-term care facilities.*

► **COMMON ERRORS**

Possible Error:

Not using a consistent protocol when measuring CVP.

Prevention:

Make sure that the client is in the same position when CVP measurements are performed. The client should lie in a supine position without a pillow for CVP measurements. The position of the client should be standard in the institution and/or documented to ensure that all nurses caring for the client perform the measurement in the same manner.

► **NURSING TIPS**

- Consistency when positioning the client for CVP measurements will improve the accuracy of the measurements over time. Establish a standard client position for CVP measurements in the institution where you work so that all nurses will follow the same protocol to ensure accurate measurements.
- It is helpful to label the tubing that is used to measure the CVP. This makes it less likely that the nurse will flush the line with fluid other than normal saline, especially if the client is receiving multiple fluids.

- It is helpful to have extra sterile injection caps available at the bedside in case one drops during the manipulation of the stopcock. It is essential that the injection caps and stopcock be sterile and intact to minimize the risk of infection.
- Be careful to close the stopcock to the manometer after measuring the CVP to prevent air from entering the client's central venous catheter.
- When changing the heparin flush solution attached to a transducer for measuring CVP, mark the fluid loss from the old bag as intake on the intake and output record.

► **SPECIAL CONSIDERATIONS**

- *As a novice, it is suggested that another nurse confirm CVP readings until feeling confident and able to display competence with this procedure.*
- *The term phlebostatic axis may be used to determine the level of the atrium. This is an external measurement of the intersection of a plane drawn transversely from the fourth intercostal space at the sternum and a frontal plane drawn through the midchest that is halfway between the outermost anterior and posterior locations of the chest. If the client is elevated the axis remains at the same anatomic location, although progressively elevated from the floor. The zero reference point on the manometer must be repositioned with changes in the back rest of the bed to keep it at the phlebostatic level.*

Drawing Blood from a Central Venous Catheter

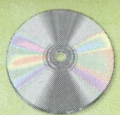

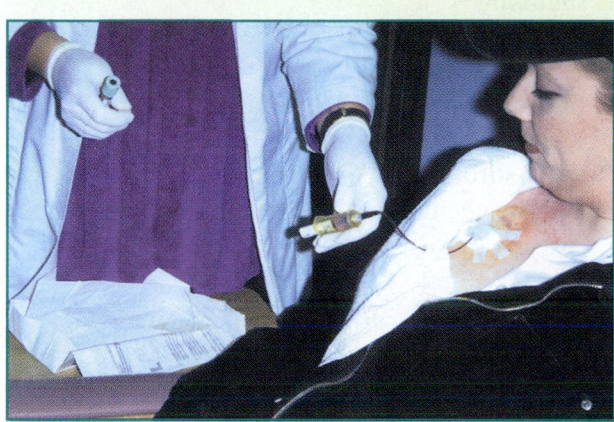

▶ OVERVIEW OF THE SKILL

A central venous line is a safe, convenient, and painless way to obtain frequent blood samples from clients with chronic disease or who require specific therapy and monitoring. Frequent venipuncture and multiple intravenous (IV) lines increase the risk of infection and bleeding. Clients receiving multiple doses of chemotherapy may have hardening of the veins so that it is difficult to find a vein to use for obtaining blood samples.

Central venous catheters are inserted into a large vein, usually the superior vena cava via the subclavian vein. This allows easy access to the right atrium of the heart.

▶ ASSESSMENT

1. Assess the type of central venous line in place. This allows the nurse to know how many lumens are available to access.
2. Assess the need to use the central venous line for blood samples. This ensures that a blood draw schedule can be established to minimize the number of times the catheter is accessed.
3. Assess the function and patency of the catheter. This ensures minimal complications during the blood draw such as the inability to infuse normal saline or aspirate blood.
4. Assess client's knowledge of the purpose of the central venous line in relation to obtaining blood

samples. Determines the need for education regarding the uses of a central venous line.
5. Check the health care provider's order for blood sampling. Ensures that only necessary testing is done for the client.

▶ DIAGNOSIS

Risk for Infection

Impaired Skin Integrity

Risk for Deficient Fluid Volume

▶ PLANNING

Expected Outcomes:

1. The blood sample obtained will be representative of the client's circulating blood, without undue dilution from fluids present in the central catheter.
2. The blood sample will not be contaminated by IV fluid or topical flora.
3. The blood will be collected in the appropriate containers for the ordered tests.
4. The client will not suffer any infection or complications as a result of the blood draw.
5. The client's central venous catheter will remain intact and patent during and after the blood draw.

Equipment Needed (see Figure 8-16-1):

- Antiseptic solutions
- Povidone-iodine and alcohol swabs
- Four to five syringes (10 to 20 mL)

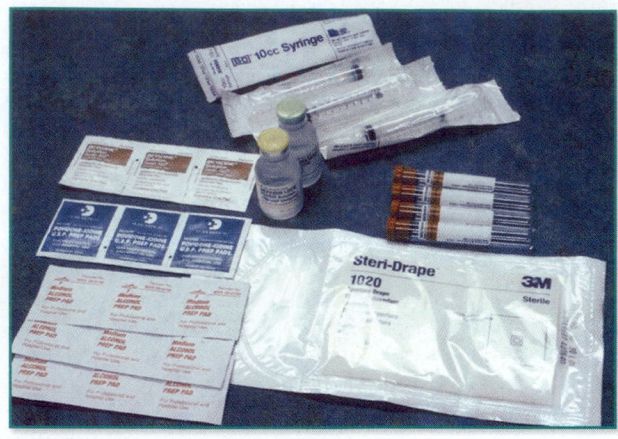

Figure 8-16-1 Povidone-iodine, alcohol pads, drape, blood collection tubes, syringes, sterile saline, and sterile heparinized saline.

- Sterile drape
- Vial of normal saline solution
- Vial of heparin or saline solution (heparin flush or heparin 100 U/mL in saline); solution determined by type of central line
- Plastic clamp or metal bull-dog clamp

- Sterile needle (20- to 22-gauge)
- Blood tubes with labels and requisitions
- Sterile gloves
- Gown, mask, and eye protection optional

▶ CLIENT EDUCATION NEEDED:

1. Teach the client the rationale for the blood sampling.
2. Instruct the client about the need for aseptic technique.
3. Explain to the client the reason for flushing with normal saline and/or heparin according to the institution's or manufacturer's guidelines.
4. Tell the client why the blood sample is needed.

Estimated time to complete the skill:
5–10 minutes

▶ DELEGATION TIPS

Blood drawing from central venous catheters is not delegated to ancillary personnel. The procedure requires sterile technique, and accessing the catheter improperly increases the client's risk for nosocomial infection, air emboli, and clotting of the line.

IMPLEMENTATION—Action/Rationale

Action	Rationale
1. Wash hands. Don gown and apply gloves, and identify client.	1. Reduces the transmission of microorganisms. Ensures proper client identification.
2. Prepare two syringes: one with 10 mL of normal saline and one with 5 mL of heparin solution.	2. Preparing equipment in advance allows for a smooth procedure.
3. Expose the venous access site. Swab injection cap, catheter hub, or catheter implantation site with povidone-iodine and alcohol.	3. Prevents introduction of microorganisms into catheter.
4. Shut off any IV solutions infusing through the other ports of the central line. This does not apply to life-sustaining fluids such as dopamine, nitroglycerin, nipride, or other medications that would adversely affect the client's condition if shut off even briefly.	4. Prevents dilution of the drawn blood by IV fluids infusing through nearby central line ports.

continues

Action	Rationale
5. Clamp catheter and remove cap if appropriate.	**5.** Prevents entrance of air into catheter.
6. Aspirate heparin solution in catheter: • Attach empty syringe or plastic vacutainer adapter and vacutainer tube to catheter. • Release clamp. • Aspirate 5 mL of blood. • Clamp catheter. • Remove syringe or vacutainer tube and discard.	**6.** Ensures patency of catheter. • Continues procedure. • Opens catheter lumen. • Aspirates heparin solution. • Prevents air from entering catheter. • Continues procedure.
7. Obtain blood samples: • Attach empty syringe (size according to the volume of blood to be obtained) or place appropriate vacutainer tube into the plastic adapter (see Figure 8-16-2). • Release clamp. • Collect blood (see Figure 8-16-3). • Clamp catheter. • Remove syringe or adapter and attach new needle with cap to it.	**7.** Clamping catheter during changes of syringes prevents air from entering catheter. • Allows all the blood to be obtained for laboratory analysis at one time. • Opens catheter lumen. • Obtains blood samples. • Prevents air from entering catheter. • Continues procedure.
8. Flush catheter: • Attach syringe filled with 10 mL of normal saline to catheter (see Figure 8-16-4). • Release clamp. • Flush quickly. • Reclamp. • Attach syringe filled with 5 mL of heparin solution to catheter. • Release clamp. • Flush quickly. • Reclamp.	**8.** Ensures that catheter will be cleared of any blood so it will not clot. • Connects syringe to catheter. • Opens catheter lumen. • Flushes blood from catheter. • Prevents air from entering catheter. • Connects syringe to catheter. • Opens catheter lumen. • Injects heparin solution into catheter. • Closes catheter lumen.

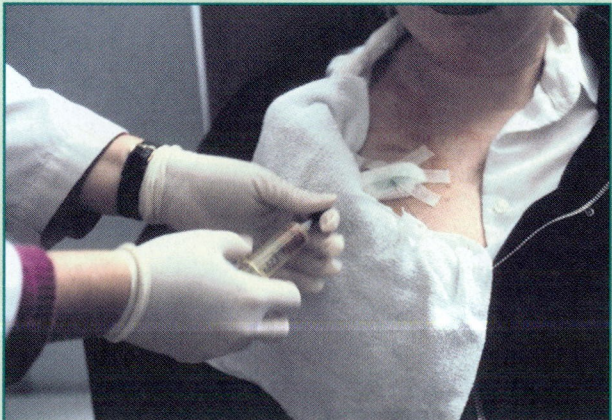

Figure 8-16-2 Attach vacutainer tube.

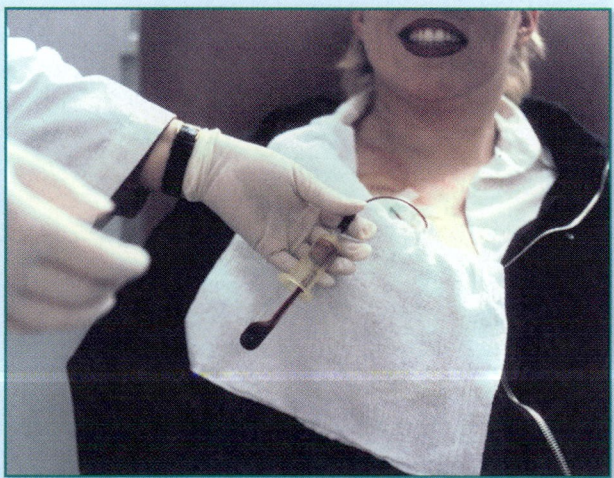

Figure 8-16-3 Collect blood.

continues

Action	Rationale

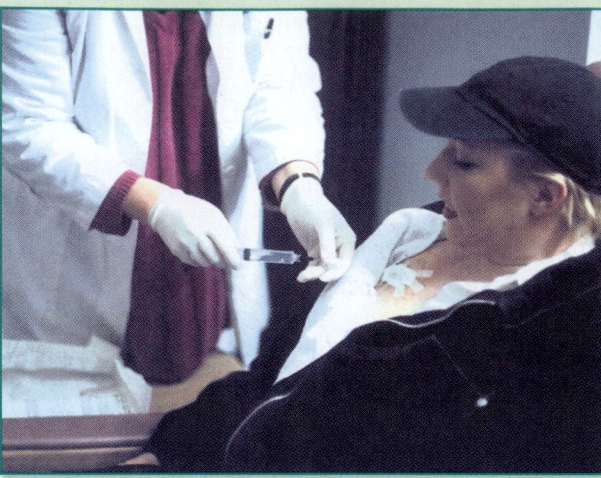

Figure 8-16-4   Flush with normal saline.

9. Place new cap on end of catheter, tape all tubing connections, and attach tubing to client's clothing.

10. Prepare blood samples:
    • Insert blood-filled syringe into blood tube if necessary and allow it to fill. Repeat for all tubes ordered.
    • Label blood tubes with client's identification (see Figures 8-16-5 and 8-16-6).
    • Fill out requisition forms and send to laboratory.

11. Dispose of soiled equipment and used supplies. Wash hands.

9. Maintains sterile seal to catheter.

10. Ensures the correct identification of the client for reporting correct laboratory results.

11. Reduces the transmission of microorganisms.

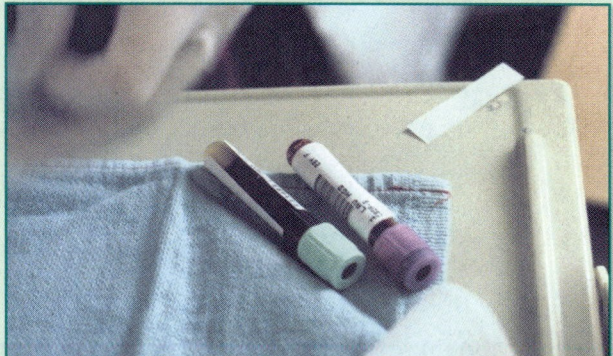

Figure 8-16-5   Label blood specimen tubes with client's identification.

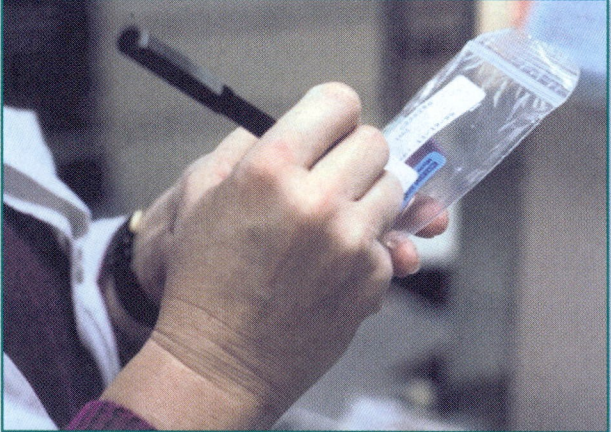

Figure 8-16-6   If blood specimen tubes are placed in a bag, label the bag with the client's identification.

▶ REAL WORLD ANECDOTES

Scenario 1

The doctor ordered a CBC and chemistries to be drawn on Mr. Ellison in the afternoon when he made rounds. The nurse checked the order and the previous laboratory reports and noticed that a CBC had already been ordered. The nurse reported to the physician that it had been ordered so another test was not duplicated.

Scenario 2

Mr. Arnold's central line had been functioning well for the 2 weeks since it had been inserted. One day, however, the nurse was unable to aspirate blood. She tried flushing the line with normal saline; it flushed easily, but she was still unable to aspirate blood. She then instructed Mr. Arnold to raise his arms and cough. There was no change. She suggested taking a deep breath and then performing Valsalva's maneuver. There was still no change. As Mr. Arnold was already sitting on the edge of the bed, he tried lying down on his side. Again no change. Finally, he turned to the other side and the nurse was able to aspirate the blood she needed for the test. The catheter must have been lodged against the vessel so that changing position freed it. Afterward, she flushed the line with saline and then heparin and recorded the event in the nurses' notes as well as reporting it to the physician.

▶ EVALUATION

- The blood sample obtained was representative of the client's circulating blood, without undue dilution from fluids present in the central catheter.
- The blood sample was not contaminated by IV fluid or topical flora.
- The blood was collected in the appropriate containers for the ordered tests.
- The client did not suffer any infection or complications as a result of the blood draw.
- The client's central venous catheter remained intact and patent during and after the blood draw.

▶ DOCUMENTATION

Nurses' Notes

- Record the date and time the blood was obtained.
- Report that the laboratory samples were sent.
- Note the condition of the catheter.
- Record the patency of the catheter, including the ability to draw blood and difficulty of infusing fluids.
- Report occlusions, damage to the catheter, or air embolus to the health care provider immediately. Note the condition of the client's skin at the insertion or implantation site.

Document on appropriate flow sheet or electronic medical record (EMR).

▶ CRITICAL THINKING SKILL

Introduction

There are several causes of difficulty in aspirating blood from a central venous catheter. It could be caused by a thrombus, precipitation from incompatible medications, or malpositioning.

Possible Scenario

The catheter was patent but sluggish after an incompatible drug was infused with total parenteral nutrition (TPN). Now, it is occluded. Attempts to change position, raise arms, cough, or perform Valsalva's maneuver have failed. It is unknown whether a precipitate or a clot is the cause.

Possible Outcome

A venogram shows a clot at the distal end of the catheter so the physician orders urokinase, a fibrinolytic agent, to be given to dissolve the clot.

Prevention

The nurse should carefully check each drug and IV fluid being given to the client to plan the administration so incompatible drugs do not result in a precipitate that can cause an occlusion in the central venous catheter.

▶ VARIATIONS

Geriatric Variation:
- *The volume of blood drawn should be assessed according to the client's hemoglobin and hematocrit.*

Pediatric Variations:
- *Children should have no more than 1 mL/kg of blood drawn per day.*
- *Children may not like the smell of normal saline or heparin flushes. Giving them a freshly cut lemon or peppermint candy to smell during the flushing process may help.*

Home Care Variation:
- *A receptacle for disposing of soiled equipment is needed.*

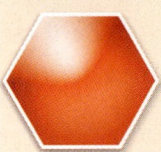

Long-Term Care Variations:
- *Be sure this procedure is performed by a person licensed to perform blood draws.*
- *Deposit the marked blood samples and laboratory requisition slips in the proper location for pickup by the laboratory.*
- *Note if the sample requires special handling so it can be properly stored until pickup.*

▶ COMMON ERRORS

Possible Error:

The catheter was not clamped after the blood sample was obtained and the syringe removed, so blood flowed out of the catheter and saturated the client's gown.

Prevention:

Keep one hand near the clamp to remember to clamp the catheter. If this error occurs, clamp the catheter. Attach the syringe with normal saline and flush. Then flush with heparin. Remove the blood-soiled clothing. Note the incident for follow-up regarding the amount of blood loss.

Possible Error:

The catheter was not clamped after the blood sample was obtained and the client took a deep breath, so an air embolus formed.

Prevention:

Keep one hand near the clamp to remember to clamp the catheter between changing syringes. If this error occurs, clamp the catheter. Attach an empty syringe and aspirate blood. Observe for air bubbles. Place client on left side with head slightly elevated. Assess for dyspnea, hypoxia, or tachycardia. Notify the health care provider immediately.

► **NURSING TIPS**

- Have all the equipment available for the procedure.
- Label the blood tubes before obtaining the sample.

- Check the label and requisition form and health care provider's order before obtaining the sample.
- Check for any special handling requirements for the blood sample, such as refrigeration, freezing, or specially prepared blood tubes.

► **SPECIAL CONSIDERATIONS**

- *As with any blood draw, make sure the tubes chosen are correct for the lab test requested. It is also imperative that the lab tubes are labeled correctly after the client's name is confirmed and all information, as per institution policy, is placed on the tube. Lab specimens should be transported in a bag with a biohazard label or in a receptacle designated by the facility.*
- *Aseptic technique must be maintained when drawing blood from a central line as blood infections may be the result of poor technique. Such an infection could increase the client's morbidity and/or mortality and increase the length of stay in the hospital.*

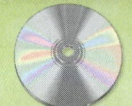

Infusing Total Parenteral Nutrition (TPN) and Fat Emulsion through a Central Venous Catheter

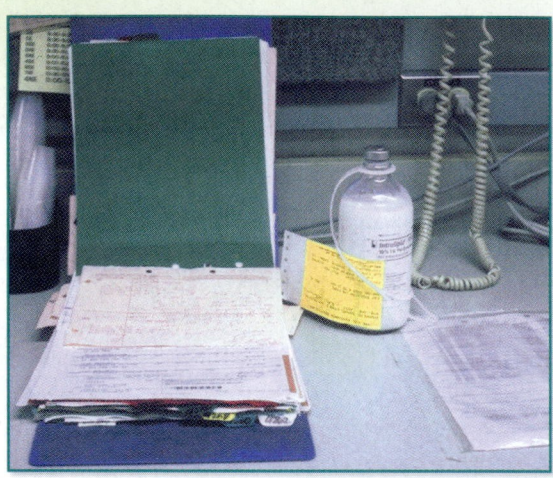

▶ OVERVIEW OF THE SKILL

Total parenteral nutrition (TPN) is the intravenous administration of varying combinations of hypertonic or isotonic glucose, lipids, amino acids, electrolytes, vitamins, and trace elements. Although the formulas vary for individual clients, they are designed to be nutritionally complete and meet the total nutrient needs of the client. The TPN formulas are used for clients who, because of their disease process or treatment, are unable to receive adequate nutrition through the gastrointestinal tract. The following are examples of disease states that require this type of nutritional intervention:

- Short bowel syndrome
- Inflammatory bowel disease
- Gastrointestinal fistula
- Hypermetabolic state (severe burns)
- Intractable diarrhea
- Serious acute alimentary disease (pseudomembranous colitis)
- Chronic idiopathic intestinal pseudo-obstruction

Total parenteral nutrition can be administered either through a peripheral (PPN) or central line (CPN). Determination of the type of venous access is based on a number of factors: the length of the therapy; concentration of the TPN solutions (more hypertonic solutions require a central line); and client contraindications for line placement. Table 8-17-1

outlines the comparison between peripheral and central line administration.

Another component of TPN is the addition of lipid emulsions. Lipid emulsions are a 10% or 20% combination of triglycerides, egg phospholipids, glycerol, and water. These solutions may be given as a separate infusion; however, more commonly they are incorporated into a total nutrient admixture or three-in-one emulsion. Fatty acids are an essential part of a normal diet. Clients at risk for fatty acid deficiency will exhibit signs and symptoms such as dry skin, sparse hair, impaired wound healing, liver abnormalities, and decrease in immune system function.

TPN is administered continuously over 24 hours or may be given intermittently (cyclic TPN). Cyclic TPN is given over 10–12 hours in a 24-hour period, which allows for easier integration of the therapy into the client's lifestyle and minimizes adverse effects of TPN. Intermittent therapy is desirable for those clients on long-term therapy at home.

Total parenteral nutrition may have both physiologic and psychological consequences for the client. Clients may feel socially isolated if they cannot eat and are unable to enjoy the usual atmosphere that centers on food. Client and family education and support become integral components of the treatment plan.

This skill focuses on the administration of TPN through a central line, also known as CPN.

Table 8-17-1	Comparison Between Peripheral and Central Line Administration	
PARAMETER	PERIPHERAL ADMINISTRATION	CENTRAL ADMINISTRATION
Osmolality	600–700 mOsm	1800–2000 mOsm
Usual daily caloric intake	700–2000	2000–4000
Fat emulsion	Major caloric source	Minor caloric source
Duration of therapy	3–7 days	>6 days
Objectives	Weight maintenance	Weight gain or maintenance

▶ ASSESSMENT

1. A nutritional assessment should be performed before initiating therapy. There should also be a plan of care for ongoing nutritional assessment as the client proceeds with this therapy. **CPN is indicated when a client has been or is expected to be unable to take adequate oral or enteral nutrition caused by the inability to ingest, digest, or absorb nutrients.**

2. Determine the type of venous access to be used for TPN. Anticipate placement of a central venous line if indicated. **Clients who require TPN short-term and have adequate peripheral assess may be candidates for PPN depending on the concentration of the solution ordered. If the client needs a central line for access, that procedure will be scheduled in advance and the nurse may be required to assist with the line placement.**

3. Review the health care provider's orders and the TPN formula. Compare the ordered solution with the venous access to be used. **Remember, the concentration of the TPN solution will determine the need for a central line. For example, a dextrose solution < 10% should be given via central versus peripheral line.**

4. Review the client's medical history and rationale for CPN. **The nurse should have an understanding of the disease process, treatment plan, or acute situation (burns, trauma) that has led to the need for CPN. This knowledge will help the nurse anticipate the length of time the client may expect to remain on CPN, and he or she will format the teaching plan for self-care accordingly.**

5. Review the client's normal range of vital signs, weight, electrolytes, liver function, triglyceride levels, glucose levels, and fluid balance. Also check blood counts in clients who may be at risk of neutropenia, either caused by their disease process or treatment. **CPN can produce serious complications such as metabolic changes, fluid and electrolyte imbalance, line maintenance, or sepsis. It is critical that the nurse understands the client's baseline data and monitor for complications.**

6. If the client is to receive a lipid emulsion, review the client's history of food allergies, particularly to egg, soybean, or safflower products. **Lipid emulsions may contain these products, and clients may experience adverse side effects such as fever, chills, or rash during administration.**

▶ DIAGNOSIS

Imbalanced Nutrition: Less Than Body Requirements

Risk for Infection

Anxiety

Ineffective Coping

Deficient Knowledge

▶ PLANNING

Expected Outcomes:

1. Client maintains ideal body weight (for those clients on preventative CPN).
2. Client gains 1 to 2 pounds per week to reach ideal body weight as appropriate.
3. Serum glucose levels are less than 120 mg/dL.
4. Venous access site remains patent and free of signs and symptoms of infection.
5. Client masters self-administration of CPN in those situations requiring long-term nutritional support.

Equipment Needed (see Figure 8-17-1):

- Disposable gloves
- IV infusion tubing
- IV infusion pump
- CPN solution
- IV filter (optional: 0.22 mm for dextrose/amino acids; 1.2 mm for three-in-one solutions)

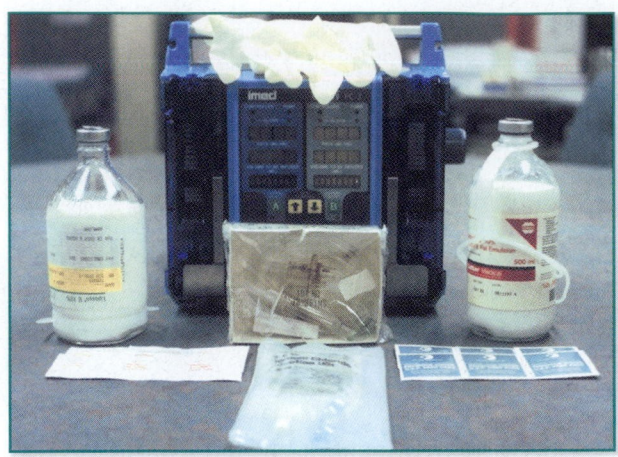

Figure 8-17-1   Gloves, IV pump, tubing, alcohol pads, povidone-iodine, and sodium chloride

▶ CLIENT EDUCATION NEEDED:

1. Explain the rationale for CPN as it relates to the client's disease state.
2. Instruct the client to report discomfort around the venous access site during infusion.
3. Teach the client and caregiver catheter care procedures for long-term administration as appropriate.
4. Instruct the client to report any symptoms of infection or sepsis, such as shaking, chills, malaise, fever (if not in a monitored setting), and redness or tenderness at catheter site.
5. Instruct the client to monitor glucose levels and to report any symptoms of hyperglycemia: thirst, malaise, flushed skin, nausea or vomiting, or polyuria, and symptoms of hypoglycemia: headache, drowsiness, diaphoresis, dizziness, tremor, tachycardia, muscle twitching, or seizure activity.
6. Review with the client symptoms related to venous thrombosis—a potential complication of CPN. These symptoms include edema and pain in neck or shoulder, leaking of infusate around catheter site, and inflammation or swelling at insertion site.
7. Instruct the client to report any symptoms associated with a potential allergic reaction such as rash, shortness of breath, headache, flushing, pain in chest or back, or chills.
8. Teach the client to report any adverse symptoms.
9. Teach the client emergency measures in the event of problems with the central line (breakage, disconnection from IV tubing). Include information regarding true emergencies (and calling 911) versus reporting minor problems to the health care provider or home care team.
10. In the home care setting, teach the client to call the home care provider with any questions related to the solution or the infusing device. The home care provider will usually work with the client over the phone to solve the problem and provide a nursing visit for those problems that the client cannot resolve by phone.
11. Teach the client to weigh self daily on the same scale and at the same time for more accurate results. The client may also need to know how to take his or her temperature.
12. Allow the client to observe the central line catheter site during routine care so he or she will have a baseline of what to expect when learning self-care.
13. Ask the client to tell you why he or she is receiving TPN and fat emulsion.
14. Tell the client how long to expect to receive TPN.
15. Discuss the need for setting aside a special place for IV fluids at home.

Estimated time to complete the skill:
15 minutes

▶ DELEGATION TIPS

Infusing total parenteral nutrition (TPN) is a skill involving assessment and knowledge regarding nutrition replacement techniques. It is an invasive procedure not delegated unless other licensed personnel have been trained and certified to perform the procedure. Vital signs should be recorded according to institution policy and any abnormal results reported promptly. Any client complaints about chills, fever, chest pain, dyspnea, or swelling at the IV insertion site should be immediately reported to the nurse.

IMPLEMENTATION—Action/Rationale

Action	Rationale
1. Remove TPN from refrigerator at least an hour before hanging, if appropriate (see Figure 8-17-2).	1. Some solutions must be refrigerated; this action decreases the risk of hypothermia or venous spasm.
2. Inspect fluid for presence of cracking or for precipitate or discoloration of solution. If the solution is a three-in-one solution, check for a cream layer of separation. Check label against order and check expiration date.	2. The CPN solution should be clear without clouding. The three-in-one solution should be uniform without areas of fat separation. If there is any problem with the solution, notify pharmacy and receive a new product.
3. Wash hands and identify client.	3. Reduces the transmission of microorganisms. Ensures proper client identification.
4. Using aseptic technique, attach tubing (with filter) (see Figure 8-17-3) to the CPN bag or bottle; prime tubing.	4. Reduces the transmission of microorganisms. Prevents air embolus.

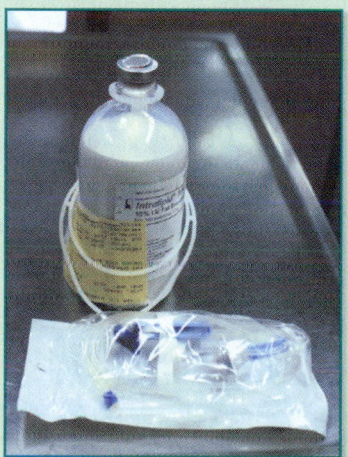

Figure 8-17-2 Remove lipid emulsion from the refrigerator at least an hour before hanging, if necessary. Inspect for cracking or discoloration.

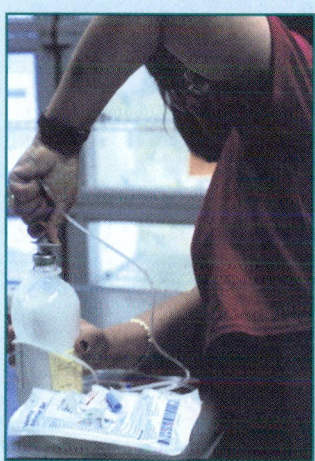

Figure 8-17-3 Attach the tubing to the lipid emulsion bottle.

5. Attach tubing into volume control infusion pump (see Figure 8-17-4). Connect the tubing to the catheter. With some infusion devices, you may connect the IV tubing first to the client's catheter and then to the infusion device.	5. Note that infusion pumps vary on tubing requirements, priming, and attachment to the central line. Review this information and be familiar with the equipment before beginning this step.
6. Regulate flow rate based on client's nutritional and metabolic needs.	6. Flow rate may begin at 40–60 mL/hr. The rate is increased each day toward a target goal. For example: Begin the infusion flow rate at one-half the end desired rate for 1 hour, then increase to the end desired rate. Institute more gradual tapering increments for pediatric clients.

continues

Action	Rationale

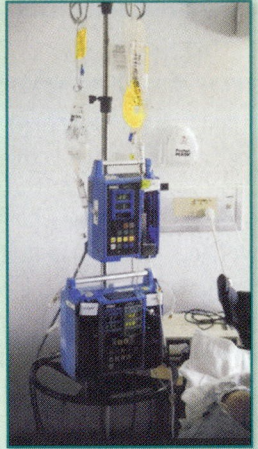

Figure 8-17-4   Connect the tubing to the volume control infusion pump.

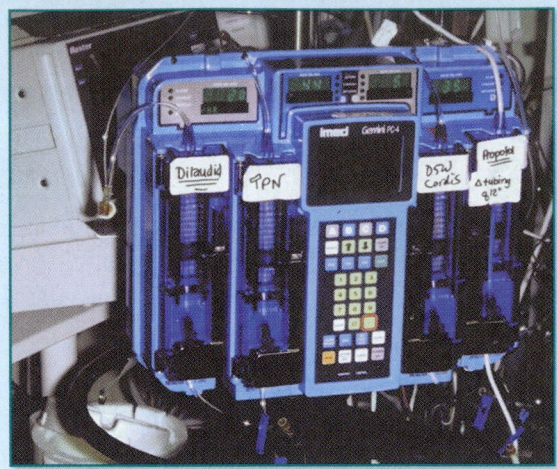

Figure 8-17-5   Check the infusion pump and the flow rate, and make sure the pump is on and operating correctly.

7. Check to see that all IV connections are secured.

8. Recheck flow rate on infusion pump; check to see that unit is plugged into wall or has adequate battery reserve (see Figure 8-17-5).

9. Wash hands.

7. Prevents disconnection of tubing. Many facilities tape the connections as an added measure of security.

8. Prevents flow rate errors.

9. Reduces the transmission of microorganisms.

▶ REAL WORLD ANECDOTES

Scenario 1

Mr. George was nearing hospital discharge and the staff were in the process of converting his CPN therapy from a 24-hour infusion to a 12-hour cyclic schedule. Upon routine assessment of Mr. George, the nurse found him to be very shaky, dizzy, and anxious. He called the physician, who suspected that the CPN had been stopped too rapidly and Mr. George was suffering from hypoglycemia. The nurse checked his blood glucose and provided him with $D_{10}W$ per the physician's order. The taper schedule was changed for the next cycle of TPN to a more gradual rate.

Scenario 2

Mike was a new nurse in the surgical unit. He knew how important it was to provide care to his clients in a timely fashion. Mike had three clients on CPN. One of them, Mr. Green, had an occlusion of his central line during the night and was 1½ hours behind in his CPN administration schedule. Mike felt it was important to keep Mr. Green on his schedule and increased the CPN infusion rate to "catch up" during his shift. Mr. Green reported symptoms of thirst and frequent urination. He was suffering from hyperglycemia from receiving the solution too quickly. Central parenteral nutrition therapy must be infused as ordered, without rate adjustments.

► **EVALUATION**

- If this is a new start of therapy, monitor the client's response hourly, assessing for complications such as allergic reactions, fluid overload, occlusion of the line, and electrolyte imbalance (mental status changes).
- Monitor blood glucose frequently with initiation of CPN; schedule will vary per facility routines.
- Monitor electrolytes daily, particularly liver function tests and triglyceride levels, and assess for the presence of jaundice. Clients on long-term CPN will require ongoing evaluation of liver function tests (at least monthly).
- Monitor client's weight daily and intake and output; assess for peripheral edema.
- Inspect venous access site for signs of infection and patency.
- Check breath sounds for crackles, indicating fluid overload.
- Table 8-17-2 outlines some of the more common complications of CPN therapy. The nurse should be familiar with these and incorporate the information into his or her ongoing assessment of the client.

► **DOCUMENTATION**

Nurses' Notes

- Document initiation of therapy; record client's preinfusion vital signs.
- On the medication record, document the components of the CPN solution (some facilities have pretyped labels that the nurse verifies and documents).
- Document client's response to initial flow rate and subsequent increase in rate.
- Document tubing changes and condition of venous access site. Review record for date that the venous access site dressing was last changed.
- Document client/caregiver education.
- Document results of the physical assessment (e.g., breath sounds) during the infusion.

Table 8-17-2 Complications of CPN Therapy		
TECHNICAL COMPLICATIONS	**SYMPTOMS**	**ACTION**
Pneumothorax	Sharp pain in chest, dyspnea after insertion of central line	Stop infusion; obtain chest X-ray as ordered by health care provider.
Air embolism	Chest pain, dyspnea, tachycardia, apprehension, shock	Clamp central line near insertion site; turn client to left side in Trendelenburg position; provide respiratory support.
Venous thrombosis	Edema and pain in neck, shoulder, and arm; leaking of infusate around site	Remove catheter as ordered; culture tip; administer anticoagulant therapy as ordered.
Clot or blockage in catheter	Infusion pump unable to deliver solution; occlusion	Check tubing for kinks; provide urokinase to dissolve blockage as ordered.
Difficulty aspirating blood from line	Catheter tip may be against atrium or vessel wall; fibrinous sheath around catheter tip	Have client change position; raise arms; take a deep breath; may need to declot.
METABOLIC COMPLICATIONS	**SYMPTOMS**	**ACTION**
Hyperglycemia	Thirst, malaise, polyuria, nausea and vomiting, flushed skin, dry mouth	Monitor blood glucose; insulin dose in solution may be adjusted; check urine for sugar and acetone.
Hypoglycemia	Headache, dizziness, drowsiness, diaphoresis, tachycardia, tremor, seizures	May administer $D_{10}W$ as ordered if CPN is stopped.

continues

Table 8-17-2 **Complications of CPN Therapy** *(continued)*

METABOLIC COMPLICATIONS	SYMPTOMS	ACTION
Protein intolerance	Nausea, vomiting, diarrhea, jaundice	Reduce rate of infusion as ordered. Reduce concentration of protein source in solution as ordered.
Electrolyte imbalance	Symptoms vary with specific disturbances; nausea, vomiting, muscle weakness, confusion, lethargy are common to many of these imbalances.	Treat imbalances as ordered; monitor electrolytes regularly; assess client behavior and associated symptoms.
Fatty acid deficiency	Dry, scaly skin; sparse hair; poor wound healing; thrombocytopenia; fatty degeneration of the liver	Monitor serum triglycerides; CPN solution should contain 4% to 10% of total caloric intake as lipids.
Trace element deficiencies	Dermatitis, hair loss, impaired wound healing, diarrhea (zinc); or anemia, neutropenia (copper)	Monitor serum copper and zinc levels; add trace elements to CPN.
Liver toxicity	Liver tenderness; elevated liver tests	Monitor liver function.
Allergic reaction to amino acids, peptides, or fats	Headache, fever, chills, nausea, vomiting, or rash	Check vital signs. Report symptoms; may result in discontinuation of CPN.
Excessive weight gain	Client gains more than 1/2 lb/day; signs of edema	Evaluate daily weights; monitor for fluid retention or overload.

INFECTION	SYMPTOMS	ACTION
Bacteremia/sepsis	Fever, chills, hypotension, tachycardia, tachypnea, change in level of consciousness	Discontinue CPN if ordered; obtain blood cultures; monitor vital signs; remove catheter as ordered; administer antibiotics as ordered.
Catheter site infection	Swelling; purulent drainage	Culture site; remove catheter as ordered; change dressing with aseptic technique; administer antibiotics as ordered.

PSYCHOLOGICAL COMPLICATIONS	SYMPTOMS	ACTION
Psychological complications	Anxiety, depression, oral cravings, feelings of isolation from social activities	Encourage verbalization of feelings; provide client education; encourage participation in self-care; provide diversional activities; provide support and encouragement for client and caregiver.

- Document glucose levels and pertinent electrolytes, such as the additives.

Document on flow sheet or electronic medical record (EMR).

▶ CRITICAL THINKING SKILL

Introduction

Caring for the client on CPN also means caring for the central line. Prevention of complications arising from the line placement or line maintenance is the key for clients receiving this therapy.

Possible Scenario

Mrs. Bauer had a subclavian catheter placed in anticipation of initiating CPN therapy. Currently she was only receiving normal saline to maintain the line until the compounding was completed for her CPN solution. Mrs. Bauer's call light went on. When the nurse entered the room, Mrs. Bauer was short of breath, very anxious, coughing, and reporting chest pain. The nurse quickly clamped the central line, placed the client on her left side, in Trendelenburg position, and immediately called the physician. Upon close inspection of the IV tubing, the nurse noticed that it was disconnected at the extension tubing site.

Possible Outcome

Most likely the client had received an air embolism from the disconnected central line.

Prevention

Carefully check all connections with each client assessment. Many settings require that the connection sites be taped together for added security. Teach the client to help monitor the connections as well; frequently it may be the client that reminds a nurse to tape a tubing connection.

► VARIATIONS

Geriatric Variations:

- *Older adults may have visual or mental impairment, which may interfere with their ability to perform self-care routines related to the central line dressing or administration of CPN. Precautions may be needed to protect the central line site, particularly if the client is disoriented.*
- *Elderly clients are also at risk for lipid intolerance and hyperglycemia.*
- *The geriatric client will need to be monitored for fluid overload and cardiac status when receiving these concentrated IV fluids.*

Pediatric Variations:

- *Central parenteral nutrition may be indicated for infants with gastroschisis, congenital anomalies of the gastrointestinal system, or short bowel syndrome. Infants are also more prone to complications such as hepatobiliary dysfunction.*
- *Care and protection of the central line for infants and young children are especially important. Young children should be carefully supervised at all times. Additional extension tubing may be required for children in order to allow them adequate room to play and move about.*
- *Glucose levels may be difficult to maintain in children.*
- *Children will need emotional support with frequent glucose monitoring if done by needle stick.*

Home Care Variations:

- *Extensive client and caregiver education is needed to successfully manage this therapy in the home setting. The therapy administration schedule will need to be integrated into the client's lifestyle; most of these clients will be on cyclic CPN.*
- *The client should have written information related to the storage, handling, preparation, and infusion instructions.*
- *Care should be taken to ensure that the client has a refrigerator, which can store the premixed solutions at 2° to 8° C (35.5° to 46.5° F).*
- *Client and caregiver should be taught aseptic technique for caring for central venous catheter, tubing, and IV fluids.*
- *Clients should be taught to record their weight, intake and output, and glucose levels.*

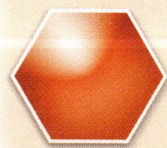

Long-Term Care Variation:

- *Long-term care facilities may not be equipped for the management of CPN. Some facilities will require pharmacy support from a qualified provider and extensive training of nursing personnel for the ongoing management of the client on this therapy.*

▶ COMMON ERRORS

Possible Error:

Upon removal from the refrigerator, the CPN solution (three-in-one) has a layer of separation, or "creaming," of the solution.

Prevention:

The nurse cannot actually "prevent" solution separation. However, the nurse's role is critical in inspecting the solution prior to administration for signs of discoloration, precipitation, or separation.

Possible Error:

The CPN solution is tapered too quickly.

Prevention:

Verify the health care provider's orders for the solution composition and for the rate ordered. Verify that the infusion pump is set for the correct rate and that it is operating properly. If this error does occur, call the health care provider. The client may exhibit symptoms of hypoglycemia. The health care provider may order $D_{10}W$ at the previous CPN rate and may also have the blood glucose checked.

▶ NURSING TIPS

- Prepare several syringes with normal saline to have available for flushing the catheter.
- Have a reference card for drug compatibility to refer to.
- Write a medication schedule to ensure safe administration.
- Have an extra cap and syringes at hand.
- Hyperglycemia is defined as a serum glucose of 160 mg/dl and causes thirst and increased urination because of a lack of insulin in the bag of TPN.
- Hypoglycemia is defined as a serum glucose of, 80 mg/dl and causes the client to be shaky, dizzy, nervous, and anxious because of an excess of insulin or TPN that is stopped abruptly.
- Be familiar with the infusion pump. Some pumps can be programmed for a tapering schedule. Other devices will require manual programming for each change.

- Allow adequate time for client teaching for those clients going home on this therapy. Always include a caregiver in the teaching session and allow for adequate opportunity for return demonstration. Provide written instructions and check client's insurance benefits for home care services.
- It is important that the home environment be reviewed with the client who is self-administering CPN. Does the client have, for example, adequate refrigeration, electricity, water supply, and access to 911?
- Check carefully the prepared CPN solution with the health care provider's orders. The solution is composed of many types of additives (i.e., trace elements) that are an important part of the therapy.
- Always use sterile technique when working with the central line because of the increased risk for septicemia.

▶ SPECIAL CONSIDERATIONS

- *Enteral nutrition is usually preferred over parenteral nutrition whenever possible. Enteral nutrition can be provided at lower cost, with less severe complications, greater wound healing, and lower rates of infection.*
- *Check that radiographic confirmation of central venous catheter placement is completed prior to starting TPN infusion.*
- *Clients currently receiving chemotherapy should not receive parenteral nutrition as it may increase the risk of complications and impair treatment response.*
- *Do not administer IV medications with the TPN.*

Removing the Central Venous Catheter

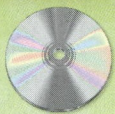

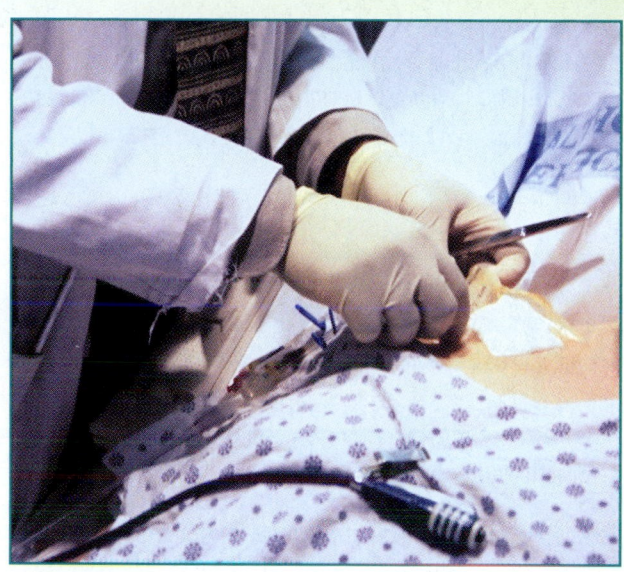

▶ OVERVIEW OF THE SKILL

Central venous catheters can remain patent and free from infection until treatment is no longer required. However, infections involving catheters do occur and often are indications for catheter removal. If the catheter is blocked, an effort should be made to attempt to aspirate the clot gently with a syringe. Any unusual sign or symptom (chills, fever) occurring immediately after a procedure may indicate septic thrombosis and is an indication for catheter removal. Removal of a central venous catheter can be performed in a clinic or in a client's hospital room. Catheter removal is performed by a qualified health care provider. Check your institution policies regarding specifics of whom this includes.

▶ ASSESSMENT

1. Verify policy regarding removal of central venous catheter. **This allows the nurse to ensure institution policies are being followed.**
2. Check original order regarding removal of central venous catheter. **Identification of this information assures the nurse that removal of the catheter is indicated at this time.**
3. Assess client's knowledge regarding central venous catheter removal. **Determines need for education about this procedure.**

▶ DIAGNOSIS

Risk for Infection

Risk for Ineffective Tissue Perfusion

▶ PLANNING

Expected Outcomes:

1. Central venous catheter will be removed in accordance with institution policy.
2. The client will experience minimal discomfort and no adverse effects from removal of the catheter.

Equipment Needed:

- Scalpel
- Gauze, 4 × 4s
- Tape
- Sterile container for culture of catheter tip (if ordered)
- Sterile scissors

▶ CLIENT EDUCATION NEEDED:

1. Explain sensation felt when central venous catheter is removed.
2. Explain what exit site will look like when central venous catheter is removed and care is needed.
3. Discuss how to care for exit site wound when the client is sent home.

4. Make sure client knows whom to call with questions.
5. Reinforce verbal teaching with written instructions.

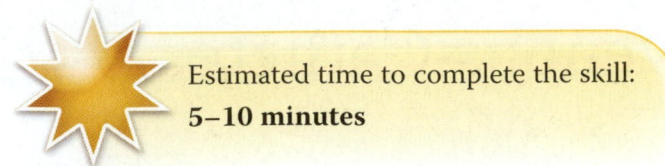

Estimated time to complete the skill: **5–10 minutes**

▶ **DELEGATION TIPS**

Removing the central venous line is a skill involving the use of sterile technique. It is a procedure not delegated unless other licensed personnel have been trained and certified to perform the procedure. It is frequently performed by the health care provider, and the nurse assists and then monitors the client following removal.

IMPLEMENTATION—Action/Rationale

Action	Rationale
1. Wash hands and apply gloves.	1. Practices sterile technique.
2. Check health care provider's written orders regarding removal of catheter.	2. Ensures that removal of catheter is indicated.
3. Check the client's arm band before removing catheter.	3. Ensures right client.
4. Set up equipment and supplies. Open sterile packages using sterile technique (see Figure 8-18-1).	4. Ensures a smooth procedure.
5. Remove tape and dressings from around catheter (see Figure 8-18-2). Cut the suture.	5. Allows visualization of the catheter.

Figure 8-18-1   Open sterile packages using sterile technique.

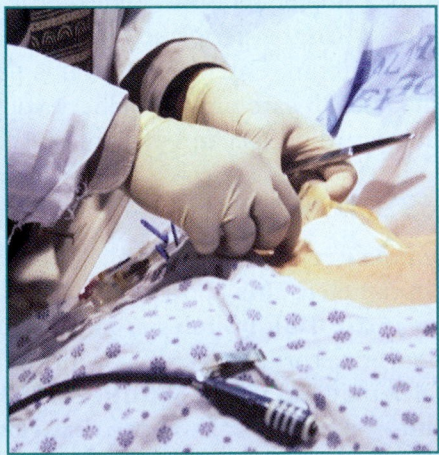

Figure 8-18-2   Remove the tape and dressing.

continues

Action	Rationale

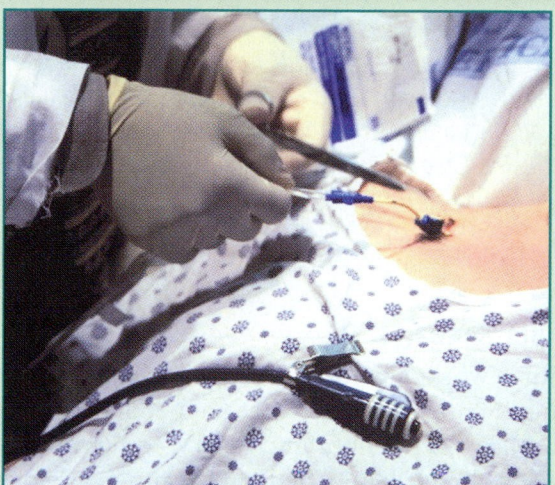

Figure 8-18-3   Free the cuff from the tissue.

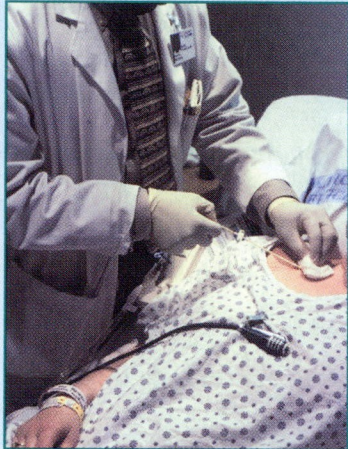

Figure 8-18-4   Remove the catheter by pulling in a gentle, smooth motion.

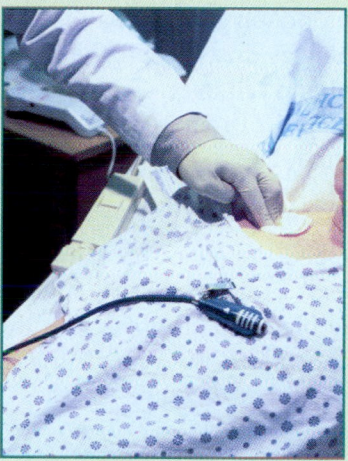

Figure 8-18-5   Apply pressure to the site.

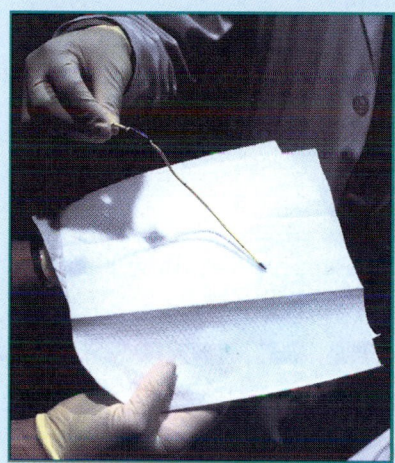

Figure 8-18-6   Make sure that the catheter tip is intact. Cut off the catheter tip into a sterile container if a culture has been ordered.

6. Place client in supine position. Instruct client to hold breath during removal. Remove the catheter by freeing the cuff from the tissue and pulling the catheter gently and smoothly (see Figures 8-18-3 and 8-18-4). Do not use a sharp, jerking motion or undue force.

6. Avoids breaking the catheter while removing and tearing tissue around the exit site.

7. Apply pressure to the site. Assess for bleeding (see Figure 8-18-5).

7. Prevents excess bleeding. Prevents air embolus.

8. Cut off tip of catheter into a sterile container if culture is ordered (see Figure 8-18-6).

8. Needed to diagnose infection of central venous catheter.

9. Place two or three 4 × 4s over exit site and hold pressure for a few minutes until bleeding stops. Apply a dressing using two 4 × 4s and tape.

9. Attempts to decrease bleeding.

10. Wash hands.

10. Decreases transmission of microorganisms.

► REAL WORLD ANECDOTES

The nurse gets an order from Jerry's physician to remove his central venous catheter. She gathers the supplies and enters his room. After preparing the client for this procedure, she frees the cuff from the tissue and gently pulls the catheter. The catheter offers resistance and will not give. The nurse decides to inject some subcutaneous lidocaine and performs a cutdown. She then removes all the sutures at the venotomy site and removes the catheter. The nurse was reminded of the importance of not using force or jerking movements when removing the catheter to prevent breakage.

► EVALUATION

- Return within appropriate time (10–20 minutes) to evaluate client's response to catheter removal and exit site.

► DOCUMENTATION

Nurses' Notes

Document:
- Date and time of central venous catheter removal
- Description of exit site
- Client's response
- Signature of nurse

Document on appropriate flow sheet or electronic medical record (EMR).

► CRITICAL THINKING SKILL

Introduction

Central venous catheter removal can be safely performed by a qualified health care provider in a clinic. However, occasionally catheters break, are accidentally cut, or fall out. It is important that the client and the nurse know how to handle these situations.

Possible Scenario

The nurse working with Mary heard a noise from her room and entered to see what happened. The nurse found Mary on the floor and her IV equipment with the central line still attached, on the other side of the room. Mary was holding her chest with her hands and the nurse noticed that there was a significant amount of blood on Mary's hands. Mary told her nurse that she was dizzy when she stood up to go to the bathroom and fell over. The nurse was reminded of the importance of making sure clients are helped out of bed when dizzy.

Possible Outcome

The nurse helped the client back to bed and covered the catheter exit site with three 4 × 4s, applying pressure until the bleeding stopped. She then contacted the client's physician to report the incident and inquire about new intravenous access.

Prevention

Remind clients to call for help when out of bed, especially if they are feeling dizzy. Warn them of the possibility of the catheter becoming dislodged.

► VARIATIONS

Geriatric Variation:
- *Older clients may have fragile skin. They may be more prone to bruising, tearing the skin, and hematoma development.*

Pediatric Variations:
- *Assess frequently for signs of infection. Small children are at greater risk for central line related bacteremia, which often requires removal and replacement of the catheter.*
- *Have another nurse or a parent assist with distracting or gently restraining the child during the procedure, if needed.*

continues

▶ **VARIATIONS** *(continued)*

Home Care Variation:
- *Central lines are generally removed in the hospital or clinic setting. Make a point to review the policy at the agency where you work. Have a contingency plan to arrange for this procedure if the home care client must have the catheter removed unexpectedly.*

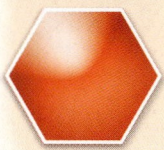

Long-Term Care Variation:
- *Watch for signs and symptoms of infection or bacteremia that may necessitate catheter removal in the long-term care client.*

▶ **COMMON ERRORS**

Possible Error:

One hour after removing the central venous catheter, the client calls the nurse into his room to find that the gauze dressing that was applied following central venous catheter removal was completely saturated with blood.

Prevention:

Always check back within 10–20 minutes after removing the central venous catheter to see if bleeding has stopped or if the dressing needs to be changed. If this error does occur, apply a new 4 × 4 gauze to catheter exit site. Apply pressure for a few minutes until bleeding has stopped.

▶ **NURSING TIPS**

- Become familiar with the central venous catheter removal policy at the institution in which you work.
- If the client is able to cooperate, have him or her perform Valsalva's maneuver (hold breath and bear down) during removal to prevent an accidental air embolism.
- Think through the steps and review written instructions if unsure about how to remove the central venous catheter.

▶ **SPECIAL CONSIDERATIONS**

- *With pediatric clients, most nosocomial bloodstream infections are related to the use of an intravascular device. Care should be taken to properly monitor clients with central venous catheters and also when removing the catheter to ensure it is removed in its entirety.*

Inserting a Peripherally Inserted Central Catheter (PICC)

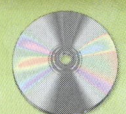

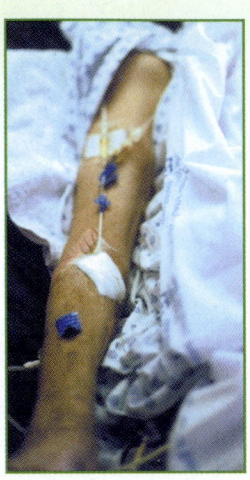

▶ OVERVIEW OF THE SKILL

A peripherally inserted central catheter (PICC) is used for clients who need a venous access for 1 week to 3 months. The advantages of a PICC compared to a central venous catheter include less risk of pneumothorax, hemothorax, or air embolism and less cost. A PICC is also preferred over a peripheral IV as it can remain in place longer and has less risk of infiltration and phlebitis.

A PICC can be used for infusions of IV fluids, parenteral nutrition, blood products, and medications. Some PICCs can be used to draw blood samples.

A client eligible for a PICC must have a palpable cephalic or basilic vein in the antecubital fossa.

The catheter is made of soft, nonirritating materials and may vary in size from 16 to 24 gauge with a length from 40 to 60 cm. The catheter can have a single, double, or triple lumen. It is inserted using a guidewire or stylet to make the catheter stiff and easier to advance into place. Complications of PICCs may include clotting, leaking, or breaking of the catheter.

▶ ASSESSMENT

1. Check the health care provider's order for the type of catheter **to ensure accurate placement of the PICC.**
2. Review information regarding the insertion of the catheter **in order to insert the catheter safely.**
3. Know the agency's policy regarding who may insert a PICC **as many institutions require special training for nurses before they can perform this procedure.**
4. Assess the pulse of the cephalic or basilic vein in the antecubital fossa **to ensure that the client is a good candidate for a PICC.**
5. Check the client's fluid, electrolyte, and nutritional status **to provide baseline data for comparison with the client's response to IV therapy.**
6. Assess the client's understanding of the purpose of the procedure **so client teaching can be used to decrease anxiety.**

▶ DIAGNOSIS

Risk for Infection

Impaired Skin Integrity

Risk for Peripheral Neurovascular Dysfunction

▶ PLANNING

Expected Outcomes:

1. The PICC will be inserted into the vein without complications and will remain patent.
2. The client will remain free of infection, thrombus, or other complications secondary to the insertion of a PICC.

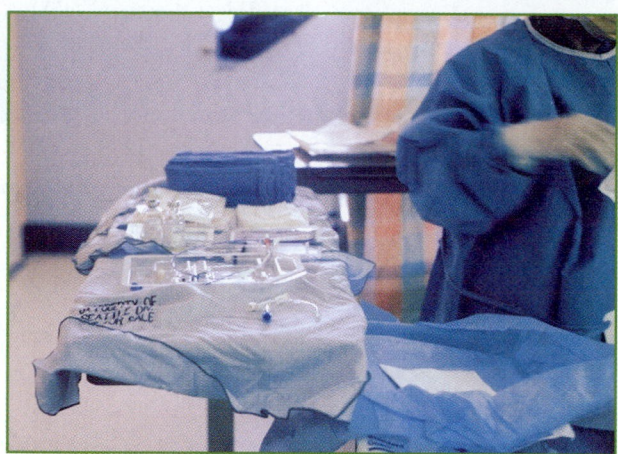

Figure 8-19-1 PICC catheter, catheter insertion kit, sterile drapes, lidocaine, and dressings

- Steri-Strips
- Six 10-mL syringes with 1-inch, 21-gauge needles
- Four-inch extension tubing (one for each lumen)
- Injection cap (one for each lumen)
- Two 10-mL vials of sterile normal saline for injection
- A 10-mL vial of heparin 10 to 100 U/mL (check institution policy for heparin solution use)
- Peripherally inserted central catheter (size and length determined by size of client's vein and type of infusion ordered)
- Two tape measures (one sterile and one nonsterile)
- Face mask, gown, goggles

3. The client will not suffer from neurovascular damage to the extremity secondary to the PICC insertion.
4. The client will be able to discuss the purpose of the PICC.

Equipment Needed (see Figure 8-19-1):
- Two pairs of sterile gloves
- Two drapes (one fenestrated and one non fenestrated)
- Sterile forceps without teeth
- Sterile scissors
- Tourniquet
- Three povidone-iodine swabs
- Three alcohol swab sticks
- Two sterile 2 × 2 gauze pads
- Two sterile 4 × 4 gauze pads
- Tuberculin syringe and 25-gauge needle
- Vial of 1% lidocaine
- Transparent dressing

▶ **CLIENT EDUCATION NEEDED**

1. Give the client oral and written instructions about the insertion of a PICC.
2. Teach the client to report any signs of inflammation, clotting, leaking, or breaking.
3. Teach the client how to bathe without getting the dressing wet.
4. Warn the client not to participate in activities that may dislodge the catheter such as weight-lifting or golf.
5. Assure the client that he or she can move the arm freely but may be restricted by the dressing on the antecubital fossa.

Estimated time to complete the skill: **30 minutes**

▶ **DELEGATION TIPS**

Assisting with the insertion of a PICC catheter is a skill involving assessment and the use of sterile technique. It is an invasive procedure performed by the health care provider and assisting is not delegated unless other licensed personnel have been trained and certified to assist with the procedure. Ancillary personnel who will be caring for the client need to be instructed to report any complaints of pain, redness, bleeding, or swelling at the insertion site. Vital signs should be obtained from another extremity.

IMPLEMENTATION—Action/Rationale

Action	Rationale
1. Check health care provider's order for PICC, and identify client.	1. Ensures accurate insertion of catheter.
2. Wash hands; apply mask and gown.	2. Reduces the number of microorganisms.
3. Organize all equipment at bedside.	3. Ensures smooth procedure without accidents or contamination.
4. Explain procedure and reason the catheter is being inserted. Obtain consent.	4. Information decreases anxiety. Consent gives permission for the procedures.
5. Assess the extremities for presence of an arteriovenous shunt used for dialysis or history of mastectomy prior to selecting an appropriate site for the PICC.	5. Extremities with a shunt or on the same side as the mastectomy should not be used for a PICC.
6. Identify vein to be used: • Place a tourniquet around the right upper arm close to the axilla. • Examine the veins in the antecubital fossa. • Release the tourniquet.	6. The cephalic or basilic vein may be used; however, the basilic vein is preferred because it is straighter. • Allows veins to fill with blood. • Determines the most appropriate vein. • Releases engorgement of vein.
7. Ask the client to lie flat in bed with arm extended at a 90-degree angle. Have client apply mask to cover mouth and nose (see Figure 8-19-2).	7. Ensures a straight course for the catheter to be advanced in the vein. Mask protects the sterile field.
8. Determine the length of catheter: • For subclavian placement, measure from the insertion site up the arm to the shoulder and across to the midclavicular line. • For superior vena cava placement, measure from the insertion site up the arm to the shoulder, across to the sternal notch, and down to the third intercostal space on the right of the sternum.	8. The health care provider's order will be carried out. • Anatomic landmarks correspond with the venous structures below. • Parenteral nutrition or any irritating solution should be infused into the superior vena cava with its high blood flow.

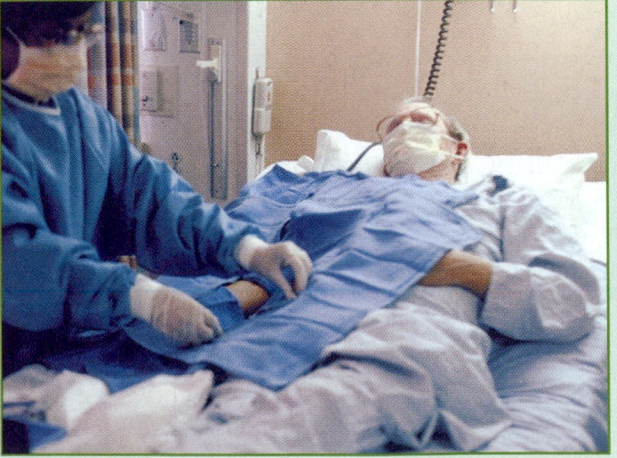

Figure 8-19-2 Have the client lie flat. Apply a mask to the client to cover the nose and mouth.

continues

Action	Rationale
9. Prepare supplies and sterile field: • Open sterile towel and place on table for the sterile field. • Open sterile supplies (gauze, extension tubing, and injection cap) and drop onto sterile field. • Place heparin and saline vials next to sterile field.	9. Provides a sterile working surface for an efficiently performed procedure.
10. Clip hair on skin at site if necessary.	10. Ensures adherence of dressing and that removal is less painful. Shaving should be avoided as it causes small abrasions that increase the risk of infection.
11. Put on sterile gloves.	11. Reduces transmission of microorganisms.
12. Prepare catheter and tubing: • Measure the catheter with the sterile tape to the length determined and add 1 inch. • Cut the catheter with sterile scissors at the appropriate length, or coil the excess catheter and tape to arm after insertion. • Attach the injection cap to the extension tubing. • Draw up 5 mL of normal saline into a syringe using a sterile gauze to hold the nonsterile vial. • Flush each cap, tubing, lumen with sterile saline, and leave the syringe in place. • Inspect the catheter for cracks or kinks. • Verify patency of introducer.	12. • Ensures the tip of catheter will be in desired position. • Cutting straight across may prevent the catheter tip from lying against the wall of the vein, causing an occlusion. • Continues procedure. • Prepares saline solution for flushing catheter. • Prevents air embolus. • Ensures proper function of catheter.
13. Prepare insertion site: • Place sterile drapes under the arm. • Scrub the insertion site with three alcohol swabs, then three povidone-iodine swabs (see Figure 8-19-3). • Allow the povidone-iodine to dry.	13. • Reduces transmission of microorganisms. • Alcohol removes fat on the skin and vigorous scrubbing in circular motion with povidone-iodine removes bacteria. Using a separate swab and starting in the middle of the site working outward prevent bacteria from being reintroduced to the site. • Povidone-iodine must be dry to be effective.

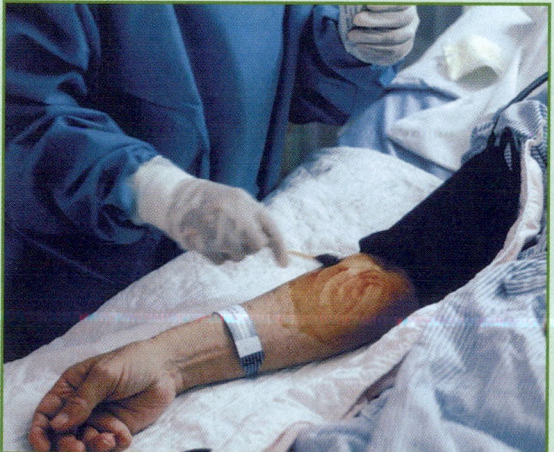

Figure 8-19-3 Swab the area with alcohol, then three povidone-iodine swabs.

continues

Action	Rationale

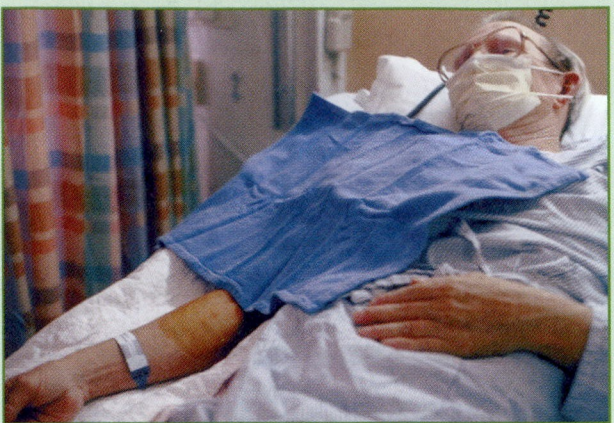

Figure 8-19-4 Place sterile drapes over the insertion site.

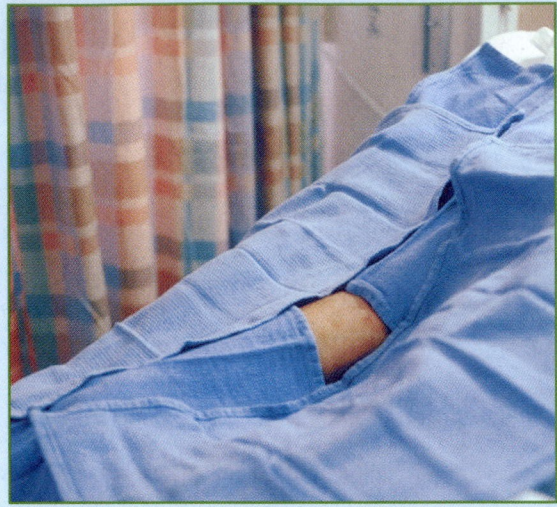

Figure 8-19-5 Sterile drapes should completely cover the area surrounding the insertion site.

14. Remove gloves and reapply tourniquet.

14. Nonsterile tourniquet should not be touched with sterile gloves. Tourniquet is needed to allow the vein to engorge for easier venipuncture.

- Place sterile 4 × 4 gauze over tourniquet.

- Allows release of tourniquet without contamination.

15. Put on new pair of sterile gloves without powder.

15. Reduces transmission of microorganisms during procedure. Powder could adhere to catheter.

16. Place sterile drapes over the insertion site (see Figures 8-19-4 and 8-19-5).

16. Provides a sterile field at the site.

17. Inject local anesthetic of 0.1–0.2 mL of 1% lidocaine at the insertion site (see Figure 8-19-6).

17. Reduces pain.

18. Insert the PICC:
- Insert the introducer needle at a 20- to 30-degree angle with the bevel up.
- Watch for a quick blood return through the introducer.
- Verify its placement in a vein, not artery.

- Advance the introducer 1/4 to 1/2 inch further into the vein while it is parallel to the skin.
- Insert the catheter through the introducer needle (see Figure 8-19-7).
- Advance the catheter slowly 2–3 inches using the non-toothed forceps, maintaining the end of the catheter on the sterile field.
- If a guidewire is used, be sure that it remains within the lumen of the PICC during insertion.

- Release the tourniquet using the sterile 4 × 4 gauze.
- Advance the catheter 6 more inches depending on the client's size until the tip of the catheter is at the shoulder.

18.
- Prevents puncture of posterior wall of vein.

- Indicates introducer has entered the vein.
- The brachial vein is close to the brachial artery. Arterial blood is bright red and pulses.
- Ensures the introducer is in the vein.

- Makes a path for the catheter to enter the vein.

- Prevents trauma to the vein when advanced slowly.

- Prevents contamination of catheter. Also, agency policy must be checked for use of guidewire or stylet to stiffen catheter during advancement.
- Prevents contamination of the sterile glove.
- Allows catheter to travel further up the vein.

continues

Action	Rationale

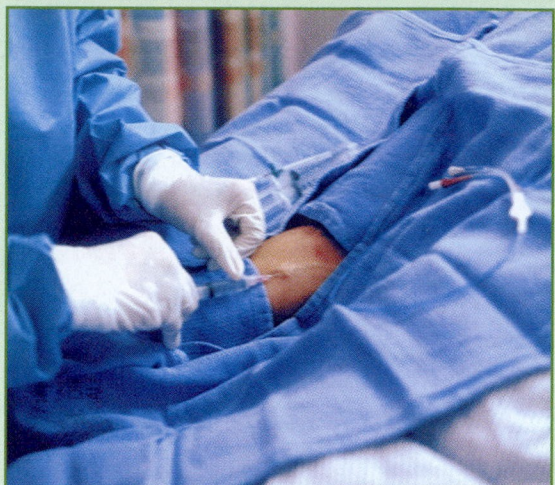

Figure 8-19-6   Numb the site by injecting local anesthetic.

- Instruct the client to turn head toward the venous access site and drop chin to chest (see Figure 8-19-8).
- Continue to advance the catheter to the predetermined length.
- Withdraw the introducer needle using the forceps. Apply pressure 2 inches above the insertion site to maintain the catheter in place (see Figure 8-19-9).

- Tell the client he or she will hear a snapping sound when the needle is removed.
- Press the wings together until they snap, then peel the needle from around the catheter.
- If a guidewire has been used, remove it with a gentle twisting motion.

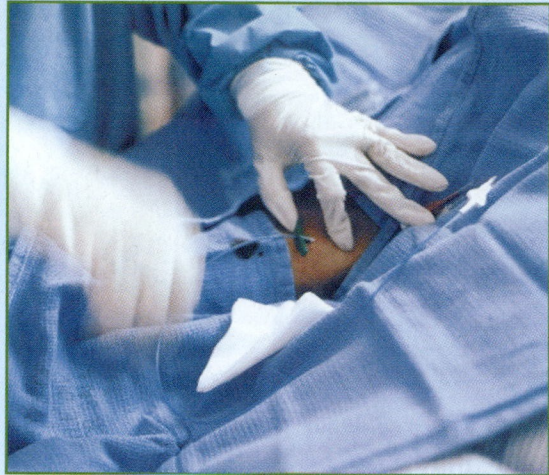

Figure 8-19-7   After inserting the introducer, insert the catheter through the introducer needle and advance 2–3 inches.

- Facilitates the catheter to enter the subclavian vein.

- Ensures proper placement of the catheter.

- Prevents accidental puncture of the vein with the introducer. Ensures that the catheter will not be withdrawn with the introducer as it could cut off the catheter and cause a catheter embolism.
- Prevents anxiety during procedure.

- Prevents the catheter from being punctured by the needle.
- Opens lumen for use. Prevents injury to catheter and vein.

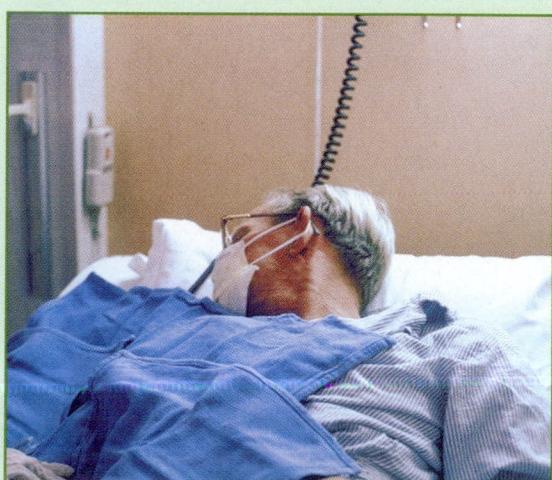

Figure 8-19-8   Have the client turn his head and drop his chin to help the catheter enter the subclavian vein.

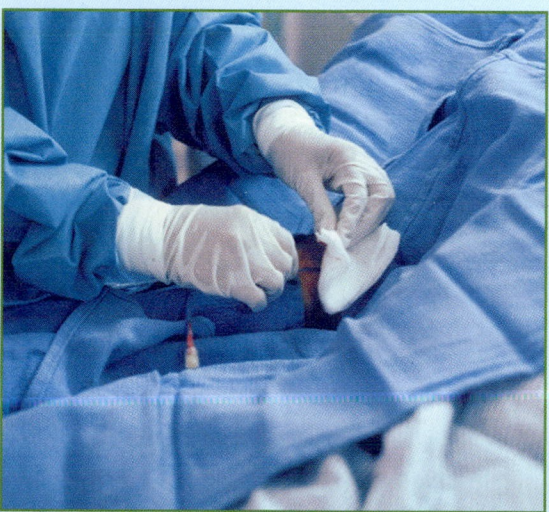

Figure 8-19-9   Withdraw the introducer while applying pressure 2 inches above the site to keep the catheter in place.

continues

Action	Rationale

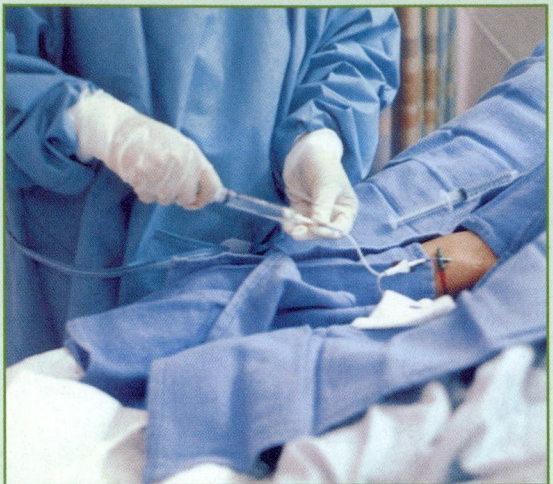

Figure 8-19-10 Attach a syringe with 3 mL of normal saline to the catheter lumen and flush the catheter.

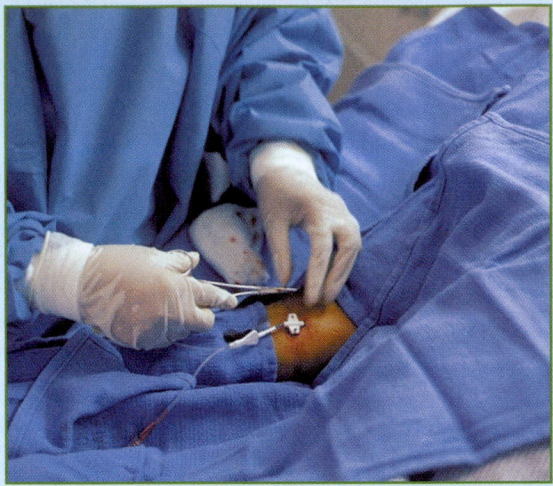

Figure 8-19-11 Suture the catheter in place.

19. Check catheter placement:
    - Attach a syringe filled with 3 mL of normal saline to the lumen (see Figure 8-19-10).
    - Aspirate blood.
    - Flush the catheter with normal saline.
    - Repeat if there is more than one lumen.

20. Secure catheter in place:
    - Remove the syringe and attach the extension tubing and cap to the lumen.
    - Place Steri-Strips over the hub of the catheter or suture in place (see Figure 8-19-11).
    - Place 2 × 2 gauze pads over insertion site and cover with transparent dressing (see Figure 8-19-12).
    - Coil the extension tubing and tape to client's arm.

19. Verifies patency of the catheter.
    - Prepares saline for injection.

    - Verifies patency of the catheter
    - Prevents blood from clotting in the catheter.
    - Ensures all lumens are patent.

20.
    - Maintains sterile, closed system.

    - Ensures catheter's safe position.

    - Controls bleeding by pressure for first 24 hours after insertion.
    - Prevents accidental dislodgment.

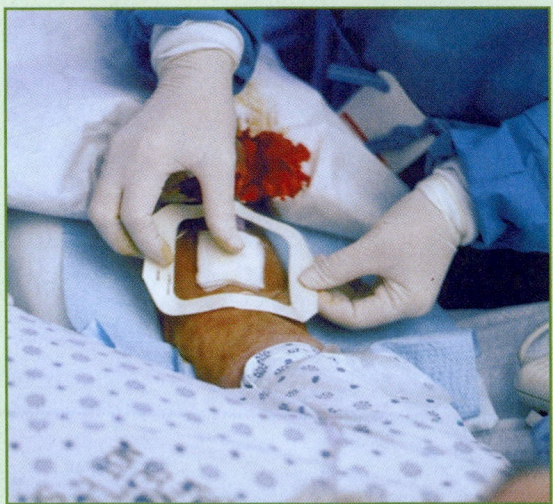

Figure 8-19-12 Dress the site with gauze and transparent dressing.

continues

Action	Rationale
21. Fill syringe with 3 mL of heparin and flush each lumen (please note, not all PICCs require heparin).	21. Maintains patency of lumen.
22. Remove gloves and dispose with all used materials.	22. Reduces transmission of microorganisms.
23. Place label with date and time of insertion and size and gauge of catheter on the dressing (see Figure 8-19-13).	23. Provides information to schedule next dressing change.
24. Wash hands.	24. Reduces transmission of microorganisms.
25. Order chest X-ray to document correct placement of PICC.	25. Ensures solution will be infused into the subclavian vein or superior vena cava.
26. Postinsertion care of the PICC: • Replace 2 × 2 gauze with sterile, transparent occlusive dressing 24 hours after insertion. • Change dressing every 3–7 days. • Check length of external tubing with each dressing change. • Flush the catheter with normal saline, then heparin (if necessary, per institution policy) after any infusion.	26. • Allows visual inspection of the site and prevents the entrance of microorganisms. • A clean, intact dressing reduces the transmission of microorganisms and protects the wound. • Ensures the catheter has not become dislodged. • Maintains patency.

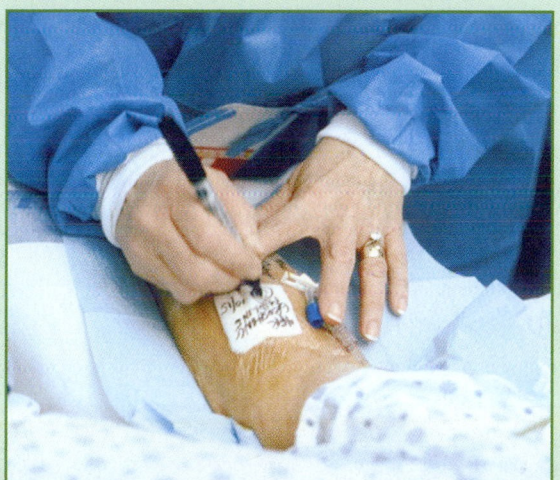

Figure 8-19-13 Label the dressing with the date and time of the insertion.

▶ REAL WORLD ANECDOTES

When Jennifer was ready to be discharged from the hospital after several weeks in the intensive care unit after a septic shock episode, she still required parenteral nutrition. She had had many peripheral venipunctures for IV fluids and medications; however, her basilic veins were still intact. Her nurse prepared her for the last venipuncture in order to send her home with a PICC and total parenteral nutrition. The nurse assured her that when she could eat and drink normally and maintain her weight she would no longer need IV fluids. Jennifer was glad to have only one line left after her serious illness and felt she could care for it with her mother's help and a daily visit from a home health nurse.

▶ EVALUATION

- The PICC was inserted into the vein without complications and remains patent.
- The client remains free of infection, thrombus, or other complications secondary to the insertion of a PICC.
- The client does not suffer from neurovascular damage to the extremity secondary to the PICC insertion.
- The client is able to discuss the purpose of the PICC.

▶ DOCUMENTATION

Nurses' Notes

Document:

- Date and time the PICC was inserted
- Length and gauge of catheter
- Results of chest X-ray checking for placement of catheter
- External length of catheter for comparison with each dressing change
- Serious side effects and report to the health care provider immediately

Document on appropriate flow sheet or electronic medical record (EMR).

▶ CRITICAL THINKING SKILL

Introduction

When the catheter is inserted through the introducer needle and is advanced up the basilic vein to the subclavian vein, it should never be withdrawn as the catheter could be pulled against the sharp edge of the needle and cut off.

Possible Scenario

After a successful insertion of the introducer needle and advancement of the catheter, the nurse asked the client to turn his head toward the insertion site and then drop his head. The nurse thought this should help advance the catheter into the subclavian vein; instead, she was not able to advance the catheter at all. She pulled back on the catheter to try again, but met resistance. She could not advance or withdraw.

Possible Outcome

The resistance the nurse felt could mean that the catheter was against the edge of the needle. There was a risk of cutting off the catheter and causing an embolism, a life-threatening event.

Perhaps the nurse realized that is was wrong to pull the catheter out through the introducer needle. If she was sure she could not advance it, she could either have asked for assistance from a coworker or removed the introducer needle, then the catheter, and start again with new supplies.

Prevention

When resistance is met while advancing the catheter, the nurse needs to know what other methods may help, such as a change in the client's position of arm or head. The nurse should be especially alert to the danger of removing a catheter through the introducer needle.

▶ VARIATIONS

Geriatric Variations:
- *Elderly clients may have greater risk of dependent edema in the arm where a PICC is placed because of decreased circulation.*
- *The veins of elderly clients may be more fragile.*

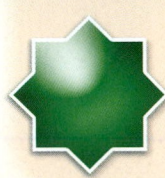

Pediatric Variations:
- *In neonates, other veins can be used such as the antecubital, saphenous, superficial temporal, external jugular, popliteal, ankle, and axillary veins.*
- *Special precautions are needed to maintain a PICC intact in very young clients.*

continues

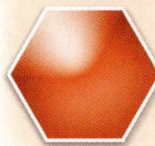

► **VARIATIONS** *(continued)*

Home Care Variations:
- *The PICCs are easily adaptable to the home care setting.*
- *The catheter can be inserted in the home by a nurse.*
- *Clients may receive antibiotics, pain medication, or parenteral nutrition at home.*
- *A more secure dressing may be necessary if the client is active.*

Long-Term Care Variation:
- *The PICCs can be useful in the long-term care setting in older clients as well as younger clients requiring rehabilitation.*

► **COMMON ERRORS**

Possible Error:

The catheter is noted to be pulled out 1 inch at the time of the dressing change.

Prevention:

Make sure the catheter is secure. Advise the client to be careful of the catheter during activity. If this error does occur, do not push catheter back into vein. Check for patency of the catheter. Report the dislodgment to the health care provider. A chest X-ray may be ordered to check placement if it was in the superior vena cava.

► **NURSING TIPS**

- Use the dominant arm when placing a PICC intended to be placed in the superior vena as movement enhances blood flow and reduces the risk of edema.
- Use only 10-mL syringes with a PICC.
- The catheter has marks at regular intervals to aid in advancing it to the correct length.
- Be sensitive to the client's restriction of flexing the elbow of the arm with a PICC.
- Use an 18-gauge or larger catheter if the infusion of blood products is anticipated.

► **SPECIAL CONSIDERATIONS**

- *One drawback of the PICC line is that the catheter tip displaces with arm movement. The catheter should be well secured and the client should be advised to use care when moving.*
- *Peripherally inserted central catheters (PICCs) appear to be associated with a lower rate of bloodstream infection than centrally inserted CVCs. With this concept in mind, inform the health care provider of this option as needed.*

Administering Peripheral Vein Total Parenteral Nutrition

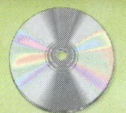

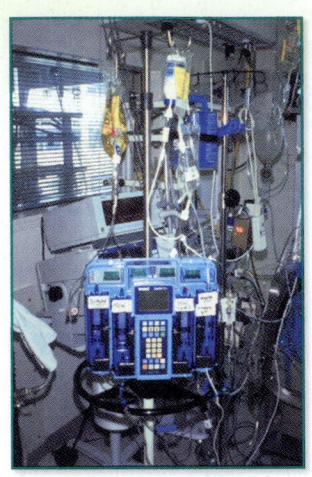

▶ OVERVIEW OF THE SKILL

Peripheral parenteral nutrition (PPN) is the intravenous (IV) administration of a nutritionally balanced solution via a peripheral vessel. Peripheral parenteral nutrition tends to be used as short-term therapy (3 weeks or less) for clients who are unable to eat secondary to surgery or illness and who require supplemental nutritional support. Approximately 1,400–2,000 calories per day are provided from a solution containing protein, carbohydrates, electrolytes, vitamins, trace elements, and water. Carbohydrates are provided from a 5% to 10% dextrose solution. Crystalline amino acids, 2.75–4.25%, provide protein. (In some facilities, dextrose 20% and crystalline amino acids 8.5% are approved to be administered in PPN.) Lipid emulsion, 10–20%, is administered daily to provide calories and essential fatty acids.

Before a client is started on PPN, a baseline nutritional assessment is completed that includes the client's weight and the following laboratory work: electrolytes, blood-urea-nitrogen (BUN), creatine, prealbumin, glucose, albumin, transthyretin, triglycerides, and liver enzymes. While on PPN, daily blood work should include electrolytes, BUN, prealbumin, creatine, and glucose. Initiation of PPN begins slowly. The first bag, approximately 1 liter, is administered over 24 hours. Daily lipid emulsion is administered at the same time and runs concurrently with PPN to minimize vein irritation. As the client tolerates, the volume, rate, and concentrations of dextrose and protein in PPN are increased over several days until the client's caloric needs are met. If a client is unable to tolerate a relatively high volume of fluid, PPN is not an effective means of caloric support. At the conclusion of the PPN therapy, the rate of administration of PPN should be decreased to half the original rate for the last 30–60 minutes to minimize hypoglycemia.

It is important to assess the nutritional status of the client. This can be done by looking at weight, laboratory values, client's ability to eat, and extent of NPO status. Dietitians are excellent resources to verify that clients are at risk for healing because of poor caloric intake. In some institutions, dietitians are often actively involved in overseeing PPN orders and ensuring the proper solution is ordered.

▶ ASSESSMENT

1. Before starting a client on PPN, assess the client's knowledge of the therapy, including what to expect before, during, and after PPN administration **to determine the client's need for education and provide information as indicated.**
2. Check for an allergy to eggs. **Clients who are allergic to egg protein may have an acute or allergic reaction to lipid emulsion.**
3. Assess the client's veins, selecting the largest peripheral vein available for the venipuncture. Also, consider the proposed length of treatment

and begin with the most appropriate distal vein. A large vein will minimize the irritation from PPN by better hemodilution. **By using distal sites first, the nurse will have access to proximal sites later on in therapy (see Figure 8-20-1).**

4. Assess the client's IV site several times daily for phlebitis or infiltration. Peripheral parenteral nutrition is irritating to the veins because of its high osmolarity. Administration of the lipid emulsion over 24 hours or the duration of the PPN will diminish the irritation from the PPN solution by directly protecting the endothelium. **Sometimes low-dose heparin or hydrocortisone may be added to PPN to decrease vein irritation.** Changing the IV site is indicated if erythema, edema, hardness of the vein, or pain is identified. Also, designate that the IV site be solely used for PPN and lipids.

5. Assess for signs of sepsis. **Elevated temperature, leukocytosis, chills, or malaise may indicate sepsis.**

6. Monitor blood sugars according to the health care provider's guidelines. This can be as often as every 6 hours for the first 48 hours. Peripheral parenteral nutrition is often more concentrated in sugars than the IV solution and can cause hyperglycemia. **For diabetic clients, glucose monitoring can be more extensive and require adjustments to insulin.**

7. Check daily for the health care provider's order of PPN in advance of the finish time of the present bag. **Verifying the order will ensure that the next bag of PPN is available and ready to be used, thus avoiding an interruption in administration.**

8. Check the client's laboratory results daily, reporting abnormal values to the health care provider when indicated. If electrolyte replacement is indicated, the health care provider often will include the replacement orders in the next bag of PPN. **If the blood-glucose level is elevated, the health care provider may wish to include insulin in the PPN or orders may include a sliding scale for glucose administration. Serum triglyceride levels are monitored to assess client's response to the lipid infusion.**

9. Check that the label on the bag of PPN exactly matches the order prior to hanging the bag. **This verifies that the correct solution will be administered.**

10. Check identification band when hanging a new bottle of PPN. **Peripheral parenteral nutrition is administered via IV and should be managed as though it were an IV medication because complications can occur quickly.**

11. Daily weight assessment is needed **to help assess nutritional status.**

▶ DIAGNOSIS

Imbalanced Nutrition: Less Than Body Requirements

Risk for Infection

▶ PLANNING

Expected Outcomes:

1. Client will receive adequate nutritional support via PPN during the course of administration.
2. Client will maintain weight.
3. There are no complications at peripheral site.

Equipment Needed (see Figure 8-20-2):

- Health care provider's order
- PPN and lipid solution, verified with the order
- Two IV controllers or pumps (lipid emulsion should be administered over 24 hours or the duration of

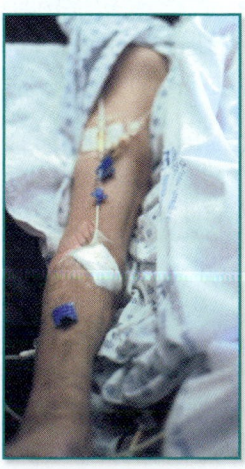

Figure 8-20-1 PPN may be administered through a PICC line.

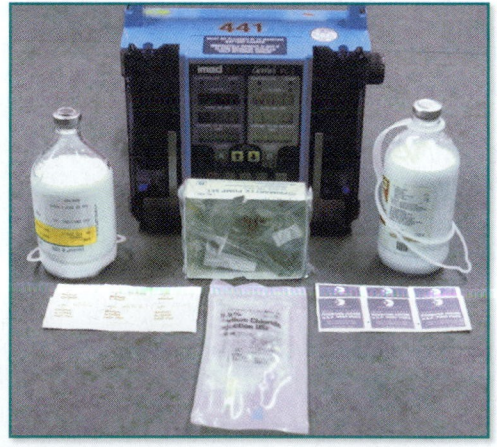

Figure 8-20-2 Gloves, IV pump, lipid emulsion, tubing, alcohol pads, povidone-iodine, and sodium chloride

the PPN and should also be on an IV controller or pump)
- Appropriate IV tubing with filter for the PPN line. Vented tubing for the lipids. Include a Y-type administration or connector in order that PPN and lipids can be administered together.
- Alcohol pads
- IV pole
- Gloves

► CLIENT EDUCATION NEEDED:

1. Explain the procedure involved with PPN, including venipuncture, monitoring of daily laboratory values, and the use of the IV controllers.
2. Instruct the client to notify the nurse if pain or swelling develops at the IV insertion site.
3. Explain associated procedures (blood glucose monitoring, frequent blood draws, daily weights, etc.).

► EVALUATION

- Check the IV site several times during each shift for signs of infiltration or phlebitis.
- Discontinue the PPN and lipid administration if erythema, edema, hardness of the vein, or pain is detected and start a new IV site.
- Monitor the client's laboratory values daily, including blood sugars, reporting abnormal results to the health care provider.
- Check insulin requirements for diabetic clients.

Estimated time to complete the skill:
10–20 minutes

► DELEGATION TIPS

Infusing total parenteral nutrition is a skill involving assessment and knowledge regarding nutrition replacement techniques. It is an invasive procedure not delegated unless other licensed personnel have been trained and certified to perform the procedure. Ancillary personnel who will be caring for the client need to be instructed to handle the infusion extremity gently and to take vital signs on another extremity. Vital signs should be recorded according to institution policy and abnormal results reported promptly. Any client complaints about chills, fever, chest pain, dyspnea, or swelling at the IV site should be immediately reported to the nurse.

IMPLEMENTATION—Action/Rationale

Action	Rationale
1. Check the label on the PPN bag against the health care provider's order. Check expiration date.	1. Ensures that the correct solution will be administered within the proper time frame.
2. Inspect the PPN bag for precipitates, cloudiness, or leakage.	2. Prevents the inadvertent administration of precipitates into the client. If the bag is leaking, inform pharmacy so a new bag can be prepared.
3. Inspect the lipid solution for separation, oiliness, or particles (see Figure 8-20-3).	3. Prevents administration of possibly contaminated solution.
4. Check that the client does not have an allergy to eggs.	4. Client's who have an allergy to eggs may develop an allergic reaction to the lipid infusion.

continues

Action	Rationale

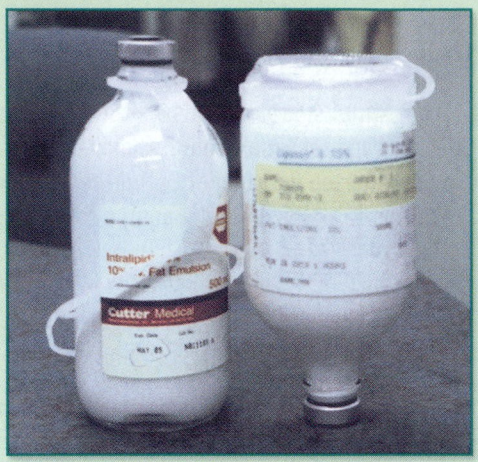

Figure 8-20-3 Inspect the solution for separation, oiliness, or particles. Check the bottle for cracks.

Action	Rationale
5. Gather IV controller tubing and a filter (0.22 mm) for the PPN. If the lipids come in a bottle, vented tubing is essential for administration. If a lipid filter is used, 1.2 mm is recommended.	**5.** PPN is filtered to remove unseen precipitates from reaching the client. A filter may not be used with lipids, but vented tubing is essential to ensure that the tubing does not develop an air lock.
6. Wash hands.	**6.** Decreases the transmission of microorganisms.
7. Attach the filter to the IV controller tubing and close the roll clamp. Remove the protective cap from the PPN bag and insert the tubing spike into the bag using aseptic technique.	**7.** Assures that the PPN bag is correctly attached to the tubing.
8. Hang the PPN and squeeze the drip chamber until the fluid reaches desired level. Prime the tubing according to the manufacturer's directions. Date the tubing.	**8.** Prevents air embolism by correctly priming tubing. Dating the tubing will ensure that tubing is changed according to institution policy.
9. Remove the protective cap from the lipid container and cleanse the rubber stopper with alcohol.	**9.** Decreases the transmission of microorganisms.
10. Close the roll clamp on the vented tubing and insert the tubing spike into the bottle using aseptic technique.	**10.** Ensures that the lipid bottle is correctly attached to the tubing.
11. Hang the lipids and squeeze the drip chamber until the fluid reaches the desired level. Prime tubing according to the manufacturer's directions. Date the tubing.	**11.** Prevents air embolism. Dating the tubing will ensure that tubing is changed according to the hospital policy.
12. Attach the lipid tubing to the PPN tubing via the Y-connector.	**12.** Ensures that PPN and lipids will be administered together.
13. Attach IV pumps to IV pole and insert tubing for PPN and lipids into the machines according to the manufacturer's directions.	**13.** An IV pump or controller is necessary for the administration of PPN. Because the lipids (usually 500 cc) will be administered throughout the duration of the PPN (usually 24 hours), an IV controller is used to ensure accuracy of the drip rate.
14. Check client's armband before beginning infusion.	**14.** Ensures identity of client.
15. Verify patency of IV site or perform venipuncture, if necessary.	**15.** Ensures proper administration of PPN and lipids and avoids infiltration.

continues

Action	Rationale
16. Wear gloves to connect the IV administration set to the IV catheter using aseptic technique.	16. Decreases the transmission of microorganisms and prevents body fluids from contacting the nurse's skin.
17. Turn on the IV controllers and set them to the prescribed rate. The initial infusion of PPN should start slowly, at half the prescribed rate for the first 30 to 60 minutes (see Figure 8-20-4).	17. An initial slower rate allows the client's body to adjust to the hypertonic solution. If the client tolerates the slower rate for the first bag of PPN or has been on a continuous infusion of PPN, set the pumps to the prescribed rate.
18. Monitor client for an allergic reaction during the initial lipid administration.	18. An adverse reaction to lipids occurs in less than 1% of clients and can include fever, diaphoresis, flushing, dyspnea, syncope, and chest and back pain.
19. Record the PPN and lipid administration on the appropriate flow sheets.	19. Provides documentation of administration.
20. Check the IV site several times during the day for signs of infiltration or phlebitis.	20. The major side effect of PPN, phlebitis, can be avoided or minimized by careful IV site monitoring.
21. Wash hands.	21. Reduces transmission of microorganisms.

Figure 8-20-4 Set the IV controller at the prescribed rate.

▶ REAL WORLD ANECDOTES

Scenario 1
Earlier in the day, Barbara was started on PPN and lipids via a new IV site. Upon awakening from a nap, she noticed that her bed was wet and smelled like vitamins. She called the nurse to check on her IV site. The nurse noted that the IV tubing was not connected tightly to the IV catheter and had been leaking onto the bed. Applying gloves, the nurse cleaned the IV connection site with alcohol before tightening the connection and applied spiral taping to the connection site. The nurse then changed the linens and assisted Barbara with the changing of her gown.

Scenario 2
While checking the PPN label with the physician's orders, the nurse noted that the percentage of dextrose listed did not match the physician's order. The nurse called the pharmacy to clarify the discrepancy. After checking the orders, the pharmacist stated that an error had been made in the percentage of dextrose. The nurse was asked to return the incorrect bag to the pharmacy and wait for the new bag of PPN to be made. Accurate checking by the nurse prevented an error from occurring.

▶ DOCUMENTATION

Medication Administration Record

Document:

- Client's response to initiation of PPN
- Percentage and amount of solution
- Any unusual reactions
- Route
- Signature of nurse
- Site
- Time hung
- Initials of nurse
- Signature of nurse identifying initials

Intake and Output Record Flow Sheet

Record:

- Time and date
- Site
- Amount of fluid infused/hung
- Initials of nurse hanging PPN and lipids
- Signature of nurse identifying initials

Document on appropriate flow sheet or electronic medical record (EMR).

▶ CRITICAL THINKING SKILL

Introduction

Three days ago, 86-year-old Charlie Black had an extensive bowel resection for cancer resulting in a colostomy and large midline abdominal incision. His bowel function is slow to return, evident by his lack of bowel tones and no flatus or stool via his colostomy bag. Mr. Black also has been reporting generalized weakness with his daily activities. His doctor has decided to start Mr. Black on PPN and lipids until he is able to eat.

Possible Scenario

The nurse decided to use Mr. Black's existing IV site, started 3 days ago, for the PPN and lipid infusions. Shortly after beginning the infusion, Mr. Black began complaining of pain at the site. On inspection, the nurse noticed that the IV site was cold, hard, and edematous.

Possible Outcome

Infiltration: The nurse stopped the PPN and lipid infusion and discontinued the IV site. A new IV site was started on the opposite arm using one of the larger vessels of the forearm. Then, the PPN and lipid infusion was restarted. A warm pack was applied to the old IV site.

Prevention

This situation could have been prevented by carefully checking out the existing IV site prior to starting the PPN and lipids. The IV site should have been flushed with saline to verify patency and inspected for redness and edema. By palpating, the nurse could detect hardness or a firm cord if the vein was inflamed. Also, asking the client if the site was tender to the touch would have provided additional information. Usually, when IV sites are 72 hours old, they should be changed to minimize problems with phlebitis.

▶ VARIATIONS

Geriatric Variation:
- *If PPN is ordered for a frail, malnourished older adult, it will take longer to achieve an adequate caloric intake parenterally.*

Pediatric Variations:
- *Strength of the nutritional solution and rate of administration are less than that of the adult.*
- *Check your drug guide book.*

Home Care Variations:
- *Peripheral parenteral nutrition can be given at home and family members can be trained to hang the IV bags.*
- *Follow-up with a home infusion company is essential to ensure that the client has adequate supplies and IV access.*

continues

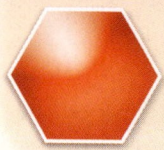

► **VARIATIONS** *(continued)*

Long-Term Care Variation:
- *PPN is not generally given in the long-term care setting. If parenteral nutrition is needed in this setting, it is generally given through a central line.*

► **COMMON ERRORS**

Possible Error:

The wrong PPN solution was administered.

Prevention:

Carefully check the label on the PPN bag against the health care provider's orders. If there are any discrepancies, verify with the pharmacist who prepared the PPN solution. If this error does occur, inform the health care provider of the error and complete a hospital incident report. Replace the wrong solution with a mixture of dextrose 10% until the new bag of PPN is available.

Possible Error:

Using the PPN-designated IV line for other IV medication administration resulting in precipitation.

Prevention:

Only administer PPN and lipids through the IV site designated for that purpose. If it is absolutely essential to give additional IV medication through the designated IV line, generously flush the IV line with normal saline before and after IV medication administration. If this error does occur, wearing gloves, disconnect the IV tubing from the IV site. Aspirate back at the IV site to remove any precipitate and ensure blood supply. If unable to verify the patency of the IV site, discontinue the IV site and start a new IV. Change the IV tubing for the PPN and lipids before reconnecting the tubing.

► **NURSING TIPS**

- Administer lipid emulsion over 24 hours concurrently with PPN to protect the endothelial lining and minimize phlebitis.
- Designate one IV site only for PPN and lipids, thus preventing medication incompatibilities. It is hard to see precipitate forming when the lipids are also infusing.
- Use vented tubing on the IV lipid line to prevent an air lock.

- Check the IV site frequently for phlebitis and infiltration; restart the IV site when indicated.
- Check the client's laboratory values, and report abnormal values to the health care provider before the new bag of PPN is mixed. It is possible that the health care provider may want to change the composition of the PPN based on the current laboratory values.

► **SPECIAL CONSIDERATIONS**

- *Total parenteral nutrition is a great expense for the client. If the next parenteral feeding will not be required because of a change in the client's status, alert the pharmacy to prevent mixing costly ingredients and adding additional cost to the client.*

Hemodialysis Site Care

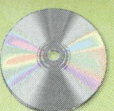

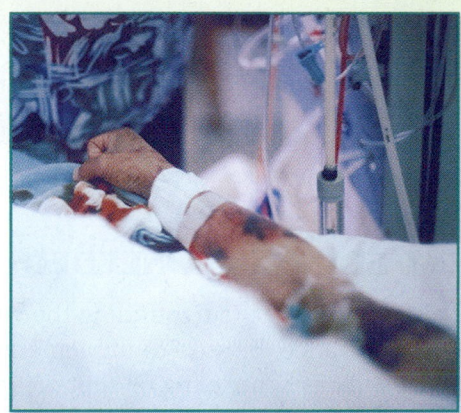

► OVERVIEW OF THE SKILL

Hemodialysis is a renal replacement therapy for clients with end-stage renal disease (ESRD). It uses the principles of osmosis, diffusion, and ultrafiltration to replace some of the kidney's major functions. Waste products, fluid, and excess electrolytes are removed to help maintain a more stable weight, acid-base balance, and blood pressure in the ESRD client. To accomplish this, the blood must be taken from the client by the use of some type of vascular access device. This can be an internal shunt or graft or an external double-lumen catheter. The arteriovenous fistula, shunt, or graft (bovine or Gore-Tex) is surgically created in a client's extremity (most frequently the arms) to enlarge the veins for easy venipuncture and attachment to the hemodialysis machine. The fistula takes 2–6 weeks to mature so that blood flow is adequate to support hemodialysis. Over the maturation process the vein distends as a result of the high-pressure arterial flow. This causes the wall of the vein to become thicker and tougher and allows for frequent puncture of the fistula for hemodialysis. The fistula/graft will only have a dressing in the immediate postoperative period, and dressing changes are usually not required.

Catheters may be permanent or temporary. The temporary double-lumen catheter is a large lumen catheter inserted into the subclavian or jugular vein and threaded to the superior vena cava or right atrium. It is used until the permanent one is ready or for longer periods in the client with venous access problems related to circulation or infection. This catheter is also used for the client in acute renal failure to facilitate dialysis until the kidneys recover. There are also permanent double-lumen catheters that are usually made of a flexible and less reactive plastic such as silastic. They have a cuff similar to other long-term venous access devices to decrease infection.

There are various manufacturers of these catheters so they may appear differently from client to client. Most will be kept patent by a predetermined amount of heparin and saline and have a transparent dressing that needs to be changed every 48 to 72 hours depending on institution policy and frequency of hemodialysis.

► ASSESSMENT

1. Identify the cause of the client's renal failure and other chronic diseases **to determine risk for other complications related to the access device.**
2. Assess the venous access site for redness or swelling and dressing for bleeding or other drainage **to detect infection or bleeding complications at an early stage.**
3. Assess vital signs **for signs of infection.**
4. Check for the presence of pain or numbness in the extremity where the access is located **to determine whether the change in blood flow is taking blood supply from the tissue distal to the fistula. Clients may develop a problem known as steal syndrome as the fistula changes blood patterns and "steals" oxygen from parts of the extremity.**

5. Check for the presence of audible bruit and palpable thrill in the fistula/graft **to determine patency and monitor flow through the access.**
6. Assess client's knowledge of access care and hemodialysis **to determine need for education.**

▶ DIAGNOSIS

Risk for Infection

Impaired Skin Integrity

Risk for Deficient Fluid Volume

Ineffective Tissue Perfusion

Deficient Knowledge

▶ PLANNING

Expected Outcomes:

1. Access is patent for dialysis without evidence of any redness, drainage, or swelling.
2. Client is able to state rationale for access and self-care principles and practices.
3. The client is able to verbalize care of fistula or catheter.

Equipment Needed (see Figure 8-21-1):

- Povidone-iodine swabs or antiseptic solution as determined by institution protocol
- Sterile and nonsterile gloves
- Mask
- Alcohol swabs
- Transparent dressing or gauze dressing supplies
- Heparin (concentration depends on hospital policy for flushing)

Note: Many institutions package the first five items in a sterile pack with sterile drapes and a plastic tray.

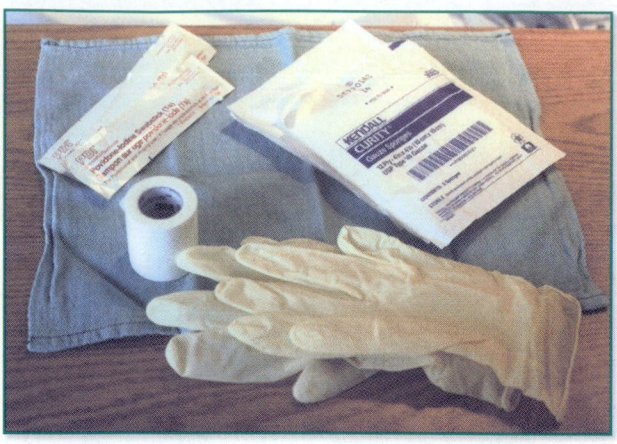

Figure 8-21-1 Gloves, tape, gauze, and povidone-iodine swabs

▶ CLIENT EDUCATION NEEDED:

1. There is much anxiety surrounding the whole dialysis experience. Be sure to implement interventions, such as counseling or support groups, to deal with this anxiety or very little will be heard by the client and family.
2. Demonstrate proper techniques for assessment of sites and determination of fistula patency. Models are very helpful to reinforce the teaching and evaluate the client's abilities to provide safe self-care.
3. Communicate teaching plan with home health care providers so that learning can continue to be evaluated.
4. Teach the client not to wear constrictive clothing on the extremity with the permanent shunt.

Estimated time to complete the skill: **10–15 minutes**

▶ DELEGATION TIPS

Caring for a hemodialysis access line is a skill involving the use of sterile technique. It is a procedure not delegated unless other licensed personnel have been trained and certified to perform the procedure. Ancillary personnel need to know to avoid the extremity for vital signs and to report any client concerns about the integrity of the site to the nurse.

IMPLEMENTATION—Action/Rationale

Action	Rationale
Arteriovenous Fistula: Shunt or Graft	
1. Wash hands.	1. Prevents the spread of microorganisms.
2. Position extremity so that you can easily palpate the fistula.	2. Prevents trauma to fistula.
3. Palpate gently over the area with fingertips or palm of your hand to feel for thrill (vibration).	3. Tests for adequate blood flow through the fistula.
4. Auscultate over the area with a stethoscope to detect a bruit (swishing noise).	4. Tests for adequate blood flow through the fistula. Notify the health care provider if bruit and thrill are absent. Surgical interventions may be necessary to restore flow.
5. Palpate pulses distal to the fistula and observe capillary refill in the extremity.	5. Checks for adequate blood flow and perfusion to the fistula extremity.
6. Assess for symptoms of infection, bleeding, or sensation impairment in the area around the fistula and the entire extremity.	6. Monitors for potential complications.
7. Post signs in the client's room to let all caregivers know to avoid venipuncture and blood pressure in the fistula extremity.	7. Prevents restriction of flow and possible clotting or rupture of fistula. Reduces chances for infection.
8. Inform client to avoid any activities that will restrict flow or cause injury to the affected extremity.	8. Prevents unnecessary loss of access site because of occlusion or infection.
9. Once the surgical incision is healed, the skin over the fistula or graft requires only routine care with soap and water.	9. Prevents infection at the puncture sites.
Double-Lumen Catheter	
10. Wash hands.	10. Prevents the spread of microorganisms.
11. Fill two 5-mL syringes with heparin and saline per institution protocol.	11. Used to fill both lumens of catheter at end of site care. Actual volume used may vary, but most catheters hold <3 mL.
12. If changing caps, prime with heparin and saline.	12. Prevents air from entering the system.
13. Open central line care kit or assemble needed supplies and place on sterile field.	13. Maintains sterile technique.
14. Put on mask and nonsterile gloves.	14. Protects site from expired pathogens and used in removal of dressing as part of Standard Precautions.
15. Remove old transparent dressing and discard with gloves in appropriate receptacle.	15. Complies with Standard Precautions.

continues

Action	Rationale
Double-Lumen Catheter *continued*	
16. Put on sterile gloves.	16. Maintains sterile technique.
17. Cleanse site with alcohol and assess site for any redness, swelling, or drainage.	17. Removes any remaining iodine, skin oils, and drainage to allow clear visualization of site.
18. Cleanse area surrounding the catheter site with povidone-iodine swabs beginning at insertion site and going out in a circular motion. Repeat for a total of three times.	18. Removes pathogens from the skin and prepares the skin for a new dressing.
19. Let air dry and apply transparent dressing.	19. Allows the iodine solution to complete the disinfectant process and ensures that the dressing will adhere tightly to the skin.
20. Close clamp to both lumens and remove and discard old male adapters (caps).	20. Clamping prevents air from entering the system when the client inspires and creates a negative pressure.
21. Cleanse ends of catheter with alcohol pads and then attach new primed male adapters.	21. Removes any old blood or drainage.
22. Unclamp lumens and flush with heparin and saline per agency protocol. Close clamp as the last 0.5 cc is being injected.	22. Creates a positive pressure within the catheter, thereby preventing backup of blood into the catheter.
23. Note: Some institutional policies will include aspirating the heparin solution in the catheter before flushing. The permanent catheters may also require flushing with normal saline before the heparin depending on the frequency of dialysis. • Normal saline is never used without heparin unless the client has an allergy to heparin.	23. Aspirating the heparin solution before flushing prevents over-anticoagulating the client, who may already have bleeding tendencies. • Heparin maintains patency of dialysis catheters.

▶ REAL WORLD ANECDOTES

Mike was a middle-aged client in chronic renal failure. He was scheduled for dialysis three times a week at the clinic but often missed appointments. He was not compliant with dietary restrictions or fistula care. When he came in after two missed appointments, the clinic nurse assessed the fistula. He noted that Mike's fistula did not have a thrill or a bruit. He also noted what appeared to be fresh puncture wounds over the fistula. When questioned, Mike became defensive and hostile. He accused the nurse of not knowing how to properly assess a fistula. When it became clear that the fistula was actually clotted, he accused the clinic staff of not flushing the fistula properly the last time he had dialysis. When confronted by his doctor, Mike admitted that he had been injecting IV drugs using his fistula. He did not have any heparin and so was unable to flush the fistula after the injections. The doctor ordered a lytic agent to attempt to reopen the fistula. This was unsuccessful and Mike had to have a new fistula created surgically. His doctor counseled Mike regarding fistula care and IV drug abuse. Mike promised to keep appointments at the clinic and to take better care of his fistula.

▶ EVALUATION

- Assess catheter site for signs of infection or bleeding.
- Determine if catheter or fistula is patent and provides adequate blood flow for dialysis.
- Determine client's understanding of rationale for fistula/catheter and related care.

▶ DOCUMENTATION

Medical Administration Record

- Document heparin/saline concentration used and when flushed.

Nurses' Notes

Record:
- Location of access, status of site, and dressing
- Vital signs
- Dressing changes
- Result of assessment of bruit and thrill; pulses and sensation distal to access as applicable

Document on appropriate flow sheet or electronic medical record (EMR).

▶ CRITICAL THINKING SKILL

Introduction

The nurse must be astute in the assessment of the client returning from dialysis. They are prone to many complications. The site is in particular need of assessment to determine if appropriate hemostasis has been achieved and patency of the access has been maintained.

Possible Scenario

Jim just returned from dialysis. He complained of being cold, so the nurse placed several blankets over him, tucking them in close to his body to help him warm up. Shortly after getting warm, Jim fell asleep.

Possible Outcome

Since Jim had been so miserable earlier, the nurse was reluctant to wake him and check his fistula site. She waited as long as she could before returning to his room to check the site. When she pulled back all the blankets, she saw that the site had been actively bleeding and there was a large pool of blood beneath Jim's arm at the fistula site. She immediately placed pressure on the site of the bleeding and called for help. The dialysis nurse arrived to assess the situation and noted that the floor nurse was applying quite a bit of pressure in an attempt to stop the bleeding.

Prevention

The nurse was reluctant to wake Jim to assess his fistula site, but she wanted to be sure the site was not bleeding or clotted. She washed her hands with warm water to try to have them warm when she assessed Jim's fistula site. She pulled the blankets back just enough to expose Jim's arm and fistula site. As she did this, she noted some blood on the sheets and discovered that Jim's fistula had been bleeding. Because she had not waited too long before checking the graft site, the bleeding was minimal. The nurse applied moderate pressure to the site and called for the dialysis nurse. She was careful to feel for the thrill of blood through the fistula even when she was holding pressure on the site. It is critical to apply only enough pressure to stop bleeding but still be able to detect flow through the fistula.

▶ VARIATIONS

Geriatric Variations:
- *Frail skin may necessitate use of different dressings if tears are noted when the dressing is removed.*
- *The elderly have less total body water and more sclerotic vessels and so respond slower to changes in blood volume with initiation of treatment. They may also have more cardiac abnormalities and poor tolerance of dialysis.*

Pediatric Variations:
- *Children have more total body water and may respond differently to dialysis. Peritoneal dialysis is the preferable method to dialyze children.*
- *The catheter will need to be covered well to prevent dislodgment. Supervise play to make sure the catheter or access is not pulled on or damaged in any way.*

continues

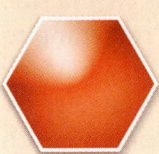

▶ VARIATIONS (continued)

Home Care Variation:
- *The family will need to be taught to perform the site care.*

Long-Term Care Variation:
- *The client may need transportation to dialysis.*

▶ COMMON ERRORS

Possible Error:

Cutting off blood flow while taking blood pressures or applying a tourniquet to the extremity with the shunt.

Prevention:

Do not perform any procedure that will cut off any blood flow in the shunt extremity. Post signs in the client's room reminding that no blood pressures or venipunctures are to be performed on the shunt extremity.

▶ NURSING TIPS

- Dialysis catheter can be used for medications and fluids if there is no other venous access. Generally a health care provider's order is required. Strict aseptic technique must be used to ensure patency and sterility of this lifeline. A pump should be used to control flow as clients with renal failure cannot tolerate any excess fluids.
- Dialysis staff may provide care to catheters in some institutions and may ask that no other staff work with the catheter except in emergencies.

- If the dialysis double-lumen catheter is clotted, the health care provider may order a urokinase injection to lyse the clot and restore patency. Follow institutional protocol to administer.
- If the fistula or graft is suspected of being clotted, Doppler and/or angiography studies are done to determine if surgical intervention is needed to restore patency or if an alternate site will need to be created. If no thrill is felt or no bruit heard, suspect that the graft is clotted.

▶ SPECIAL CONSIDERATIONS

- *The leading cause of morbidity and mortality in dialysis clients is infectious complications. This is why nurses must be trained and observed carefully when learning to access dialysis sites.*
- *Experienced dialysis nurses may be required to cannulate new fistulas. Fistulas are often more difficult to insert a needle into than are grafts, so dialysis staff usually prefer grafts to fistulas for ease of care.*

Using an Implantable Venous Access Device

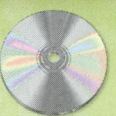

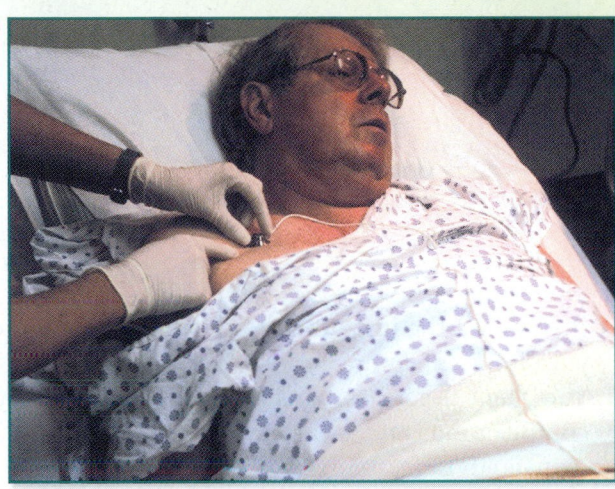

▶ OVERVIEW OF THE SKILL

Venous access devices (VADs) are inserted in clients who require long-term IV therapy and/or frequent blood sampling. The VADs promote client comfort by minimizing repeated venipunctures and offer reliable venous access to maximize safe medication delivery. Implanted venous access ports are one type of VAD. It is used for administering blood or blood products, chemotherapy, fluid replacement therapy, medication, and for blood sampling.

The port is a self-sealing, silicone domed reservoir connected to a silicone or polyurethane catheter. The system remains under the skin for months to years. Implantable VADs may have a Groshong tip, with a slit-valve that opens with negative pressure to allow blood aspiration and opens with positive pressure to permit infusion of fluids. When not is use, the valve remains closed and heparin instillation is not necessary.

The port is inserted using local anesthesia (see Figure 8-22-1). The catheter is threaded into a large vein, most commonly the subclavian vein, with the distal tip positioned in the superior vena cava close to the entrance to the right atrium (see Figure 8-22-2). The port is sutured into a subcutaneous pocket near the vessel where the catheter is inserted, generally around the third rib, lateral to the sternum.

An implanted port is accessed aseptically through the skin with a noncoring needle, called a Huber needle, after skin preparation. Port access is usually completed with minimal client discomfort, and, once accessed, the needle can be left in place for up to 7 days. When the port is not accessed, the catheter should be flushed with a saline or heparin solution at least once a month.

Complications associated with implantable ports include infection, malposition, and occlusion. Ports are removed as a minor surgical procedure using a cut-down method to remove the port and catheter.

▶ ASSESSMENT

1. The client should be assessed for criteria that favor the placement of an implantable port.

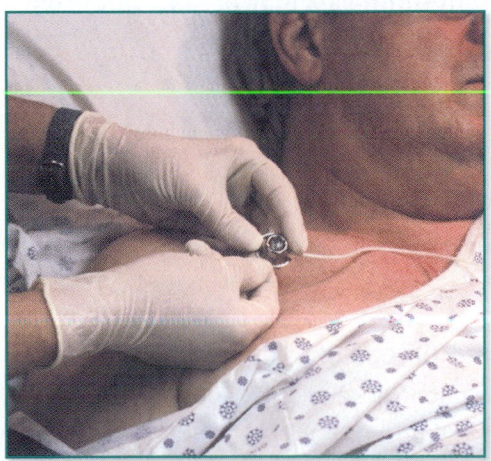

Figure 8-22-1   Implantable venous access device

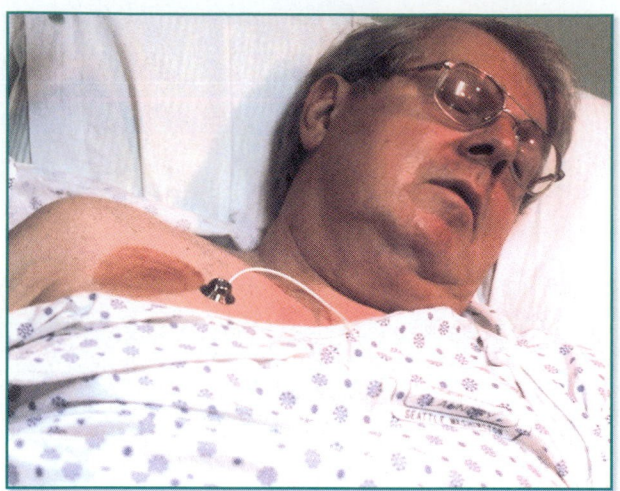

Figure 8-22-2 The port is sutured into a subcutaneous pocket and the catheter is threaded into the subclavian vein.

Physical factors such as obesity, chest wall disease, or superior vena cava abnormalities usually contraindicate placement of an implantable port.

2. The client's treatment plan should be considered for suitability of delivery via an implantable port. **Clients requiring continuous long-term infusions, such as bone marrow transplants, are not good candidates for a port.**

3. The client's knowledge of VAD insertion, procedures for use, and removal should be examined before a VAD is placed. **Client education promotes client comfort and compliance and decreases anxiety.**

4. The function of the catheter should be verified before each use by assessing the condition of the skin over the port site, presence of a blood return via the catheter, and infusion without resistance. **The presence of complications requires interventions to restore catheter patency and vascular or skin integrity.**

► DIAGNOSIS

Potential for Infection

Acute Pain

Deficient Knowledge

Disturbed Body Image

► PLANNING

Expected Outcomes:

1. The client describes the purpose, benefits, and risks of an implantable venous access device.

2. The client reports minimal discomfort when the implantable venous access device is accessed.

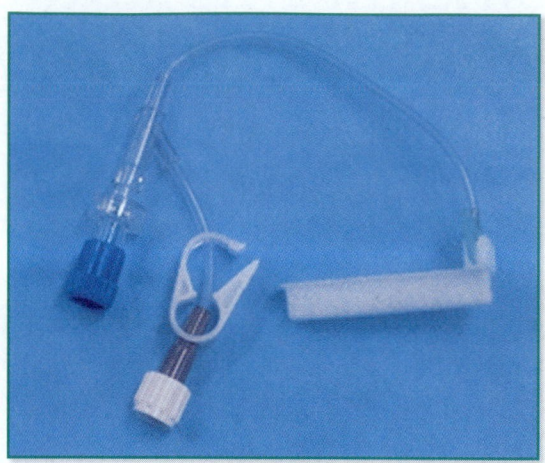

Figure 8-22-3 Noncoring port needle

3. The client completes blood sampling and IV therapy via the implantable venous access device with minimal complications.

4. The client describes signs and symptoms of port complications and measures to prevent and manage these complications.

Equipment Needed (see Figure 8-22-3):

- Extension set/noncoring port needle (e.g., Huber needle)
- Sterile gloves
- Sterile barrier
- Three alcohol swabsticks
- Three povidone-iodine swabsticks
- Dressing material of choice (e.g., transparent, gauze)
- Normal saline solution
- Heparin solution (100 U/mL) if establishing an intermittent access (check institution policy for heparin solution use)
- Local anesthetic of choice (EMLA® cream or lidocaine), if necessary

► CLIENT EDUCATION NEEDED:

1. The client and family should receive the following information about the implantable VAD:
   - Purpose
   - Benefits and risks
   - Insertion procedure
   - Procedures for use for blood sampling and medication administration
   - Management of complications

Estimated time to complete the skill: **15 minutes**

► **DELEGATION TIPS**

Use of implanted venous devices is not delegated to ancillary personnel. The procedure requires sterile technique, and accessing the catheter improperly increases the client's risk for nosocomial infection, air emboli, and clotting of the line.

IMPLEMENTATION—Action/Rationale

Action	Rationale
1. Review the prescribed order for blood sampling and/or medication administration.	1. Prevents laboratory and medication errors.
2. Identify client and explain the procedure to the client.	2. Ensures proper client identification and promotes client comfort and compliance.
3. Gather supplies.	3. Organization promotes efficiency.
4. Wash hands.	4. Prevents infection.
5. Expose skin and palpate port septum.	5. Identifies exact location for needle insertion and assesses for infection at port site. Deeper ports should be accessed with a longer needle (1 1/2 inches). Superficial ports can be accessed with shorter needles (3/4 or 1 inch).
6. Although most needle insertions can be performed with minimal discomfort, administer local anesthetic if necessary. EMLA® cream may be applied 1 hour before the insertion. Lidocaine may be injected subcutaneously just before insertion.	6. Local anesthetics reduce client discomfort.
7. Put on sterile gloves.	7. Prevents infection.
8. Clean area with alcohol and povidone-iodine swabsticks (see Figure 8-22-4).	8. Prevents infection.
9. Prime needle and extension set with normal saline solution.	9. Prevents air embolism.
10. Stabilize port and firmly insert needle, at a right angle to the skin, through the skin and septum until needle touches the back of the port.	10. Stabilization is essential for correct entry and to minimize discomfort. Twisting or inserting needle at the wrong angle may result in incorrect needle placement.
11. Aspirate blood to verify needle placement and function of port.	11. No blood return may indicate incorrect needle placement, presence of fibrin sheath at the tip of catheter, or clot in the catheter. The presence of a blood return is critical before administering medications, especially irritant or vesicant drugs.
12. Obtain blood samples as prescribed.	12. A small amount (4–5 mL) of blood must be discarded prior to obtaining blood samples to remove heparin from sample.

continues

Action	Rationale
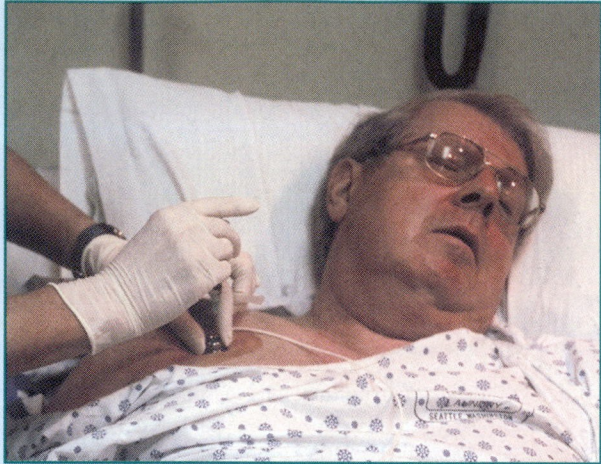	

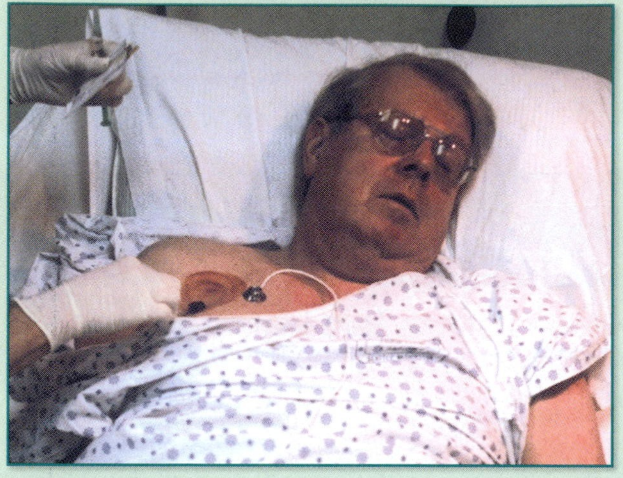

Figure 8-22-4   Clean the area with povidone-iodine swabsticks.

Figure 8-22-5   Flush the line with normal saline, using a noncoring needle.

13. Flush the line with normal saline solution to clear blood and establish patency of the line (see Figure 8-22-5).

14. Proceed with medication administration as indicated.

15. If needle will be left in place, secure needle with a sterile dressing. If left in place for continuous use, the needle should be changed every 7 days. The dressing should be changed every 2–3 days or whenever it is not clean and intact.

16. If needle will be removed, flush needle with heparin solution to establish heparin lock, maintaining positive pressure at the end of the heparin instillation. Positive pressure may be created by clamping the tubing while instilling the last ½ mL of heparin solution.

17. Remove needle by stabilizing port and pulling with a firm and straight motion.

18. Apply pressure and dressing to needle insertion site.

19. Document interventions with implantable VAD in client record. Documentation should include function of VAD, blood samples drawn, medications administered, and client response.

13. Inability to flush the line or client discomfort during flush may indicate incorrect needle placement or clot in the catheter. Recommended for use are 10-mL syringes.

14. Provides client with ordered medication regimen.

15. Stabilizes needle and prevents site infection.

16. Heparin prevents blood clots in the line. Positive pressure prevents blood reflux into the catheter.

17. Minimizes discomfort.

18. Minimizes bleeding and prevents infection.

19. Accurate documentation provides a record of the procedure.

▶ **EVALUATION**

- Correct catheter placement and patency is confirmed before the catheter is used for medication administration.
- If blood return is absent or sluggish or when there is resistance to infusion, the catheter should be evaluated for possible occlusion, damage, or displacement.
- If fluids infuse freely but blood return is absent or sluggish, possible causes include fibrin sheath formation, a kinked catheter, or "pinch-off" syndrome.

- Patency resolution solutions have been tried including changing client position, alternately flushing and aspirating the catheter, and performing a dye study and/or X-ray to verify catheter position.
- A trial of urokinase to dissolve a thrombotic occlusion or other solutions to dissolve occlusions from precipitates is indicated. A follow-up dye study may illustrate the site of an occlusion, if indicated.
- Catheter has been removed if the occlusion is not able to be dissolved.

▶ **DOCUMENTATION**

Nurses' Notes

- Record function of VAD.
- Indicate blood samples drawn.
- Report client response.

Document on appropriate flow sheet or electronic medical record (EMR).

Medical Administration Record

- Record medications administered.

▶ **REAL WORLD ANECDOTES**

Scenario 1

Mrs. Rogers had an implantable VAD placed 3 months ago to facilitate monthly chemotherapy infusions. She relates that during each visit nurses have had difficulty placing the needle because the port "moves." Even when the needle is successfully placed, the catheter has to be flushed several times and her position changed numerous times before a blood return can be obtained. She reports that repeated needle punctures of the VAD are uncomfortable and the VAD site stays sore during the month it is not used. Her port is palpable deeper than usual and closer than usual to the axillary line, and it is tender to palpation. She elects to have a local anesthetic used for access, and lidocaine is injected subcutaneously before access, which makes the access less painful. The needle is inserted into the port, with metal contact confirming correct needle placement. However, despite numerous flushing and aspirating techniques and client repositioning, a blood return is absent. In addition, when the catheter is flushed, the client reports a tingling sensation close to her axilla. Heparin is instilled into the catheter and a dressing is applied. The physician is notified, and a chest X-ray is ordered to check correct placement of the needle as well as placement of the catheter. The X-ray reveals that the catheter is kinked close to the axilla and the end of the catheter is in the axillary vein rather than in the superior vena cava. As the client was near the completion of her therapy, she elected to have the catheter removed and to complete her treatments using peripheral veins.

Scenario 2

Mr. Minifield was at home and self-administering intermittent antibiotic therapy via an implanted VAD. When an antibiotic is not infusing, the needle is left intact in the port and flushed with heparin to create a heparin lock. At a scheduled time one afternoon, Mr. Minifield assembled his supplies to begin an antibiotic infusion. With a 10-mL syringe of normal saline, he attempted to check for a blood return to verify catheter patency. When he did not obtain a blood return, he changed positions, ambulated, and tried again with no success. He gently tried to flush the catheter and met resistance. When he checked under the dressing, he noted that the needle was pulled halfway out of the port. He replaced the dressing and contacted his home care nurse. The nurse visited the client, reinserted the needle, and verified catheter patency before antibiotic therapy was resumed.

▶ **CRITICAL THINKING SKILL**

Introduction:

Too little knowledge can be a dangerous thing.

Possible Scenario:

The nurse on the previous shift was new. He had never worked with an implantable port and did not know that he needed special training prior to accessing the port to administer chemotherapy. He placed the Huber needle into the edge of the port at a 15-degree angle and started the medication. The client complained of burning pain at the site. The nurse stopped the medication immediately and notified the nurse practitioner.

Possible Outcome:

Extravasation, or leaking of the fluid into the surrounding subcutaneous tissue, had occurred because of improper needle placement. The nurse practitioner looked up the specific agent to determine if an antidote was available and to determine if hot or cold compresses should be used at the site. She ordered cold compresses placed every 2 hours for 3 days. As less than 0.5 mL of the chemotherapeutic agent leaked into the skin, the damage was painful but did not require grafting or other interventions.

Prevention:

The nurse needed to ask for help when faced with a new procedure.

▶ **VARIATIONS**

Geriatric Variations:
- *The elderly have fragile skin and the site should be monitored closely after needle removal.*
- *A confused elderly individual might push or rub a device enough to displace it. Monitor closely for signs the site has been disturbed.*

Pediatric Variations:
- *Pediatric clients may require consistent and/or additional measures to minimize the discomfort associated with needle placement.*
- *Children may need to be distracted or watched closely to make sure they do not dislodge the needle placed in the port.*

Home Care Variations:
- *The home caregiver can be taught to use the Huber needle. Stress the need for proper technique.*
- *Stress the need to report any signs or symptoms of extravasation around the port site early, so further damage can be prevented and treatment can be started.*

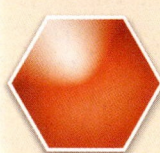

Long-Term Care Variation:
- *As the port can remain in place for months or years, displacement or leakage of the catheter may occur well after the site has healed.*

▶ **COMMON ERRORS**

Possible Error:

Trying to access the port with a needle that is too short.

Prevention:

A short needle may be inadequate when the port is deeper than usual. Always palpate the port first before preparing supplies. Choose a longer needle when the port feels deeper in the subcutaneous tissue.

Possible Error:

Tissue infiltration or extravasation around the port.

Prevention:

Catheters should have a free blood return and allow rapid infusions before being used for medications. Any complications should be addressed prior to using the catheter for access.

▶ **NURSING TIPS**

- Place the client in a comfortable position to access an implantable VAD. Be sure to assess the location of the port before use and determine any previous complications with the VAD that have occurred.
- Be patient when problem solving with an implantable VAD that has a sluggish blood return.

Try flushing and aspirating using different pressures with the syringe and reposition the client to change intrathoracic pressures, which affect catheter function.

- Clients may be placed on low-dose systemic anti-coagulants (Coumadin 1 mg PO daily) in an attempt to prevent fibrin sheath formation.

▶ **SPECIAL CONSIDERATIONS**

- *Accessing the implanted port may cause the client to experience some discomfort. A helpful technique is to have the client take a big breath and then exhale, as the needle is inserted.*
- *Implantable devices are not likely to become dislodged during activity. Examples of implantable devices include Mediports, Infus-a-ports, and Port-a-caths.*

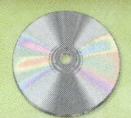

SKILL 8-23

Caring for an Implanted Venous Access Device

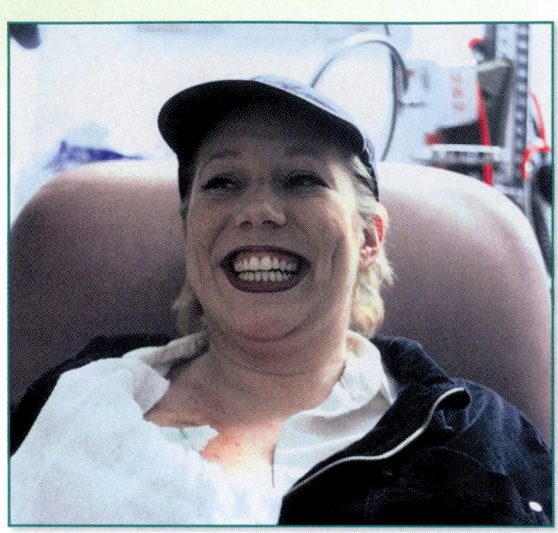

▶ OVERVIEW OF THE SKILL

An implanted venous access device (VAD) is a safe and convenient method of accessing the right atrium of the heart. VADs are used to administer intravenous (IV) fluids, antibiotics, chemotherapy, parenteral nutrition, other medications, and blood products or to obtain blood samples for clients who require specific therapy and monitoring. An implanted VAD differs from other central VADs in that the entire device, including the injection port, is internal. The implanted VAD consists of a self-sealing injection port in a plastic or metal case connected to a silicone venous catheter. The injection port may have one or two lumens. The injection port is implanted in a subcutaneous pocket at the infraclavicular fossa under sterile conditions. The catheter is inserted into a large vein and threaded into the right atrium. The procedure is performed in the operating room after the client has been given local anesthesia.

Caring for an implanted VAD differs somewhat from caring for other central VADs. As well as preventing infection or clotting, the self-sealing integrity of the injection port must be maintained. The plastic of the injection port is preserved by using a noncoring needle, such as a Huber needle.

▶ ASSESSMENT

1. Assess the type of VAD in place **in order to know how to care for the device.**
2. Assess the function and patency of the catheter **to ensure minimal complications during a blood draw or infusion such as the inability to infuse normal saline or aspirate blood.**
3. Assess client's knowledge of the purpose of the central venous line **to determine the need for education.**
4. Check the manufacturer's and institution's policies regarding maintaining patency of an implanted VAD **to ensure the proper care of the catheter.**

▶ DIAGNOSIS

Risk for Infection

Impaired Skin Integrity

Deficient Knowledge

▶ PLANNING

Expected Outcomes:

1. The nurse will be able to aspirate blood through the catheter without difficulty.
2. The nurse will be able to infuse fluid through the catheter without difficulty.

3. The skin at the catheter insertion site and the puncture site will remain intact and without redness or swelling.
4. The client will have no signs or symptoms of localized or systemic infection.
5. The catheter injection port will remain intact and without leaks.
6. The client and caregiver will be able to explain the purpose of the VAD and the proper method of maintaining the VAD.
7. The client and caregiver will be able to perform dressing changes and skin care.
8. The access site will be free of signs or symptoms of infiltration of blood or IV fluids.

Equipment Needed:

- Povidone-iodine and alcohol swabs
- Four to five syringes (10 mL)
- Vial of normal saline solution
- Vial of heparin solution (heparin flush or heparin 100 U/mL in saline)
- Sterile needle (20- to 22-gauge)
- Sterile Huber needle (20- to 22-gauge) (see Figure 8-23-1)
- Sterile drape
- Sterile gloves, gown, and mask, as needed

► CLIENT EDUCATION NEEDED:

1. Teach the client the rationale for flushing the VAD with normal saline and/or heparin

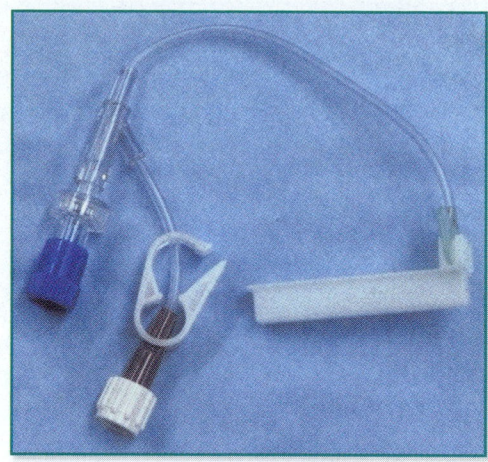

Figure 8-23-1 Noncoring port needle

according to the institution's or manufacturer's guidelines.
2. Instruct the client about the need for aseptic technique.
3. Teach the client and caregiver how to change the dressing at the insertion/access site of the VAD.
4. Discuss with the client how to care for the VAD.
5. Ask the client or caregiver to demonstrate ability to care for the VAD after having been taught.

Estimated time to complete the skill: **10–15 minutes**

► DELEGATION TIPS

Use of implanted venous devices is not delegated to ancillary personnel. The procedure(s) require sterile technique, and accessing the catheter improperly increases the client's risk for nosocomial infection, air emboli, and clotting of the line.

IMPLEMENTATION—Action/Rationale

Action	Rationale
1. Wash hands. Apply gown and mask, if required by institutional policy.	1. Reduces the transmission of microorganisms.
2. Prepare sterile field and lay out supplies (see Figure 8-23-2).	2. Protects sterile supplies from contamination.

continues

Action	Rationale

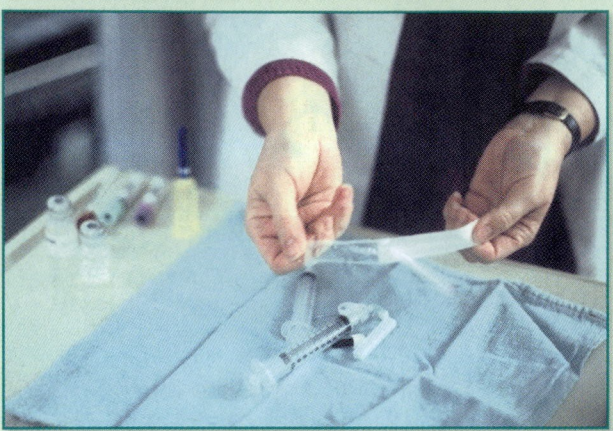

Figure 8-23-2 Lay out supplies on a sterile field.

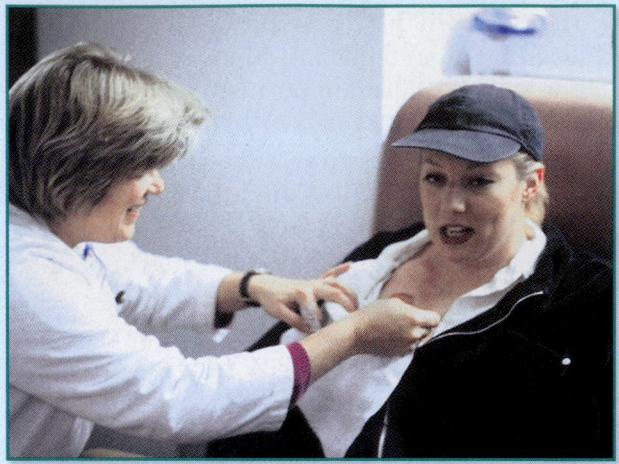

Figure 8-23-3 Swab skin over injection port.

3. Swab skin over injection port with alcohol and then povi-done-iodine using a circular motion and moving from the center outward (see Figure 8-23-3).

3. Prevents introduction of microorganisms into system.

4. Apply sterile gloves.

4. Reduces transmission of microorganisms.

5. Prepare sterile syringe with 20 mL of normal saline.

5. Flushing solution is ready for procedures.

6. Prepare Huber needle:
   • Attach sterile extension tubing between saline-filled syringe and Huber needle (see Figure 8-23-4).
   • Fill tubing with saline solution.

6. Removes air from tubing to reduce the risk of air embolus.

7. Apply sterile drape to port site.

7. Provides sterile work area.

8. Access port:
   • Palpate port septum using aseptic technique (see Figure 8-23-5).
   • Insert Huber needle through skin.
   • Push down until needle penetrates the septum and rests against needle stop.

8.
   • Ensures proper needle entry of port.
   • Huber needle is bent at a 90-degree angle.

9. Flush port with 20 mL normal saline.

9. Ensures patency of device.

10. Obtain blood sample, if ordered:
    • Aspirate 5 mL of fluid and discard.
    • Aspirate blood with syringe size equal to desired amount.
    • Flush port with 20 mL normal saline.
    • Flush port with 5 mL heparin solution if no IV infusion is started.

10.
    • Ensures undiluted sample.
    • Avoids repeated puncture of port.
    • Clears blood from port.
    • Prevents clot formation.

continues

Action	Rationale

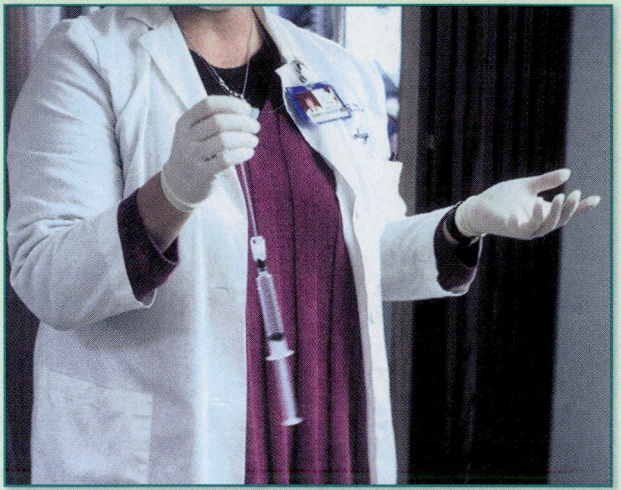

Figure 8-23-4   Attach syringe to extension tubing.

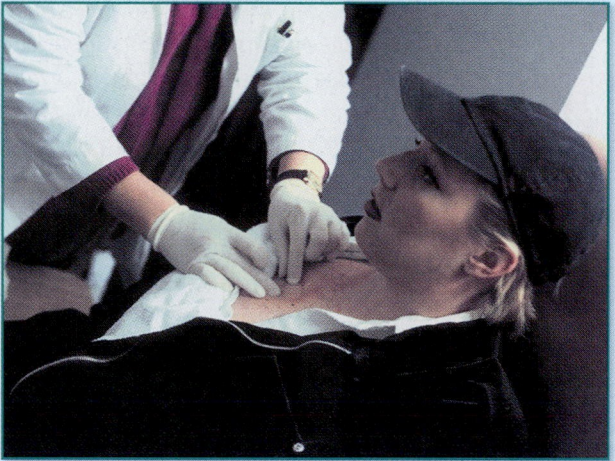

Figure 8-23-5   Using aseptic technique, palpate to find the port.

11. Set up IV infusion:
   • Secure Huber needle with sterile gauze or transparent dressing.
   • Connect IV tubing to tubing from Huber needle.
   • Set flow rate of infusion as ordered.
      When the infusion is finished:
   • Flush port with 20 mL normal saline.
   • Flush port with 5 mL heparin solution if no further therapy is ordered (see Figure 8-23-6).

12. Dispose of soiled equipment and used supplies. Remove gloves and wash hands.

11.
   • Prevents accidental dislodging of needle and maintains aseptic technique.
   • Maintains sterile system.
   • Ensures correct administration of fluid.

   • Clears blood from port.
   • Prevents clot formation.

12. Reduces the transmission of microorganisms.

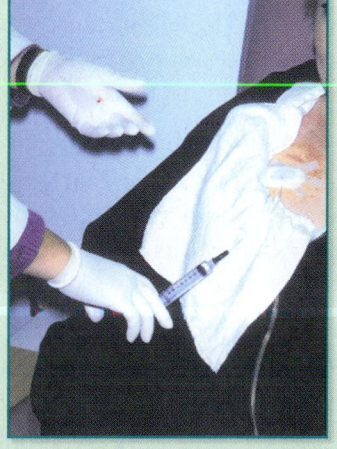

Figure 8-23-6   Flush with heparin solution.

► REAL WORLD ANECDOTES

Ms. Chen had an implanted VAD placed for blood draws and chemotherapy infusions. Several weeks later, she reported to the outpatient clinic for blood work and chemotherapy. The nurse caring for Ms. Chen was not familiar with implanted VADs and was not aware of the need to use a Huber needle to access the implanted port. He prepared the tubing and the saline and heparin flushes. The nurse then attached a 2-inch, 18-gauge needle to the tubing for the blood draw to allow a quicker draw without damaging the red blood cells. As he was getting ready to insert the needle into the VAD access port, Ms. Chen pointed out that the needle looked very different from the one that was normally used. She told the nurse that the needle she was supposed to use should be bent. The nurse stopped and sought out the nurse practitioner in the clinic for advice and prevented a potentially dangerous mistake. He had learned to listen to his clients when they pointed out discrepancies in technique.

► EVALUATION

- The nurse was able to aspirate blood through the catheter without difficulty.
- The nurse was able to infuse fluid through the catheter without difficulty.
- The skin at the catheter insertion site and the puncture site is intact and without redness or swelling.
- The client does not have signs or symptoms of localized or systemic infection.
- The catheter injection port remained intact and without leaks.
- The client and caregiver were able to explain the purpose of the VAD and the proper method of maintaining the VAD.
- The client and caregiver were able to perform dressing changes and skin care.
- The access site is free of signs or symptoms of infiltration of blood or IV fluids.

► DOCUMENTATION

Nurses' Notes

- Record the condition of the skin at the site of the VAD.
- Document the client's response to therapy.
- Record the patency of the catheter, including the ability to draw blood and difficulty of infusing fluids.
- Immediately report occlusions, damage to the catheter, or air embolus to the health care provider.
- Report signs or symptoms of infection or infiltration.
- Report client teaching or concerns voiced by the client or caregiver.
- Report laboratory specimens drawn and their disposition.

- Record date, time, type, and volume of fluids given.

Document on appropriate flow sheet or electronic medical record (EMR).

Medication Administration Record

- Record medications and dose infused via the venous access device.
- Report the heparin flush.

► CRITICAL THINKING SKILL

Introduction

One of the most common complications in clients with an implanted VAD is infection. Aseptic technique must be maintained when accessing the device to obtain blood samples or infuse fluids. Assessment of the site and systemic symptoms is necessary for early detection and treatment.

Possible Scenario

The client with an infusion port was feeling tired at home the day after his clinic visit when he had blood drawn. He felt slightly warm, and when he took his temperature, it was 38.3° C. He called the clinic and reported it to the nurse.

Possible Outcome

The nurse knew that he had an infusion port and asked about the skin above the port. When he told her that it was pink and warm, she instructed him to come to the clinic to be assessed.

Prevention

The infusion port may not have been properly prepared before the blood draw the previous day. Scrubbing the skin over the port is the only way to prevent transmission of microorganisms from entering the circulation.

▶ VARIATIONS

Geriatric Variation:
- *Elderly clients often have thin skin. Be careful not to tear their skin when inserting the Huber needle or when removing tape.*

Pediatric Variation:
- *Have the child's caregiver distract the child while inserting the Huber needle and during the therapy to prevent the child from dislodging the needle.*

Home Care Variations:
- *An infusion port needs to be flushed only every 4 weeks if not in use.*
- *A receptacle for disposing of soiled equipment is needed.*

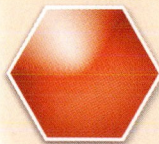

Long-Term Care Variation:
- *If an implanted VAD is being used for long-term therapy, be sure the access port is not damaged during use. Multiple sticks can break down the plastic of the access port leading to infiltration of blood or IV fluids.*

▶ COMMON ERRORS

Possible Error:
When flushing the infusion port, too much force is used and a small clot is pushed into the muscular tissue around the port.

Prevention:
If resistance is felt when flushing the port, do not irrigate with force. If this error occurs, stop flushing the port. Aspirate into the syringe to observe for clots. Use another syringe to flush more gently.

▶ NURSING TIPS

- Have all the equipment available for the procedure.
- Take advantage of this procedure to assess the client and provide emotional support.

▶ SPECIAL CONSIDERATIONS

- *The Huber needle is unlike other injection needles; it is thicker, may be curved, and is noncoring. The nurse should become familiar with the needle and the process prior to accessing the port.*
- *When accessing the implanted port, the client may experience some discomfort. A helpful technique is to have the client take a big breath and then exhale while the needle is easily inserted.*
- *Implantable devices are not likely to become dislodged during activity. Examples of implantable devices include Mediports, Infus-a-ports, and Port-a-caths.*

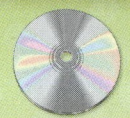

Obtaining an Arterial Blood Gas Specimen

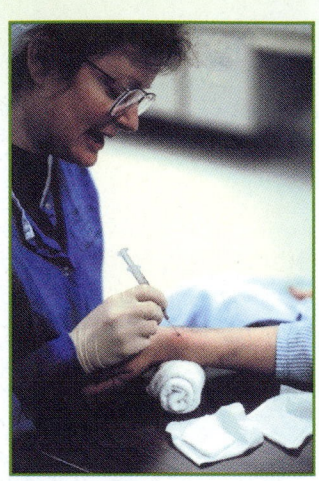

▶ OVERVIEW OF THE SKILL

Arterial blood gases are measured to assess a client's oxygenation, ventilation, and acid-base balance. The blood sample is easily, although often painfully, obtained from an artery and is analyzed for arterial blood pH, partial pressure of oxygen (PaO_2), partial pressure of carbon dioxide ($PaCO_2$), and arterial oxygen saturation (SaO_2). The analysis can quickly provide information on the client's respiratory or metabolic status and response to a disease process. Clients who require mechanical ventilation or have sudden respiratory distress or change in level of consciousness may benefit from this test for diagnosis and treatment.

▶ ASSESSMENT

1. Assess the type of symptom and lung sounds that require an arterial blood gas (ABG) sample. Signs and symptoms may include dyspnea, sudden change in respiratory rate or pattern, unequal breath sounds, unequal chest expansion, cyanosis, change in level of consciousness, self-extubation, and increased work of breathing. **Determines when an ABG is needed.**
2. Assess if the client has just awakened, just been suctioned, or had a change in oxygen or ventilator settings within the last half hour. **Identifies factors that may affect an ABG measurement.**
3. Assess collateral blood flow by performing Allen's test **to choose a site for ABG sample.**

4. Assess tissue surrounding artery **to avoid sites of previous punctures and proximity to veins.**
5. Assess baseline or most recent ABG for client **to compare with current status.**
6. Assess client's knowledge about the procedure of obtaining an ABG sample **to ensure cooperation and reduce anxiety.**

▶ DIAGNOSIS

Risk for Injury

Impaired Gas Exchange

Pain

▶ PLANNING

Expected Outcomes:

1. The client will have normal ABG results.
2. The pulse, color, and temperature of the client's extremity distal to the puncture will be unchanged.
3. The client will be calm and free of pain.
4. The client will have minimal bleeding from the site following the puncture.

Equipment Needed (see Figure 8-24-1):

- Heparinized syringe with cap, 3 mL (check institution policy for heparin solution use)
- A 23- or 25-gauge needle
- Povidone-iodine and alcohol swabs
- Gauze pad, 2 × 2
- Heparin 1:1000 solution

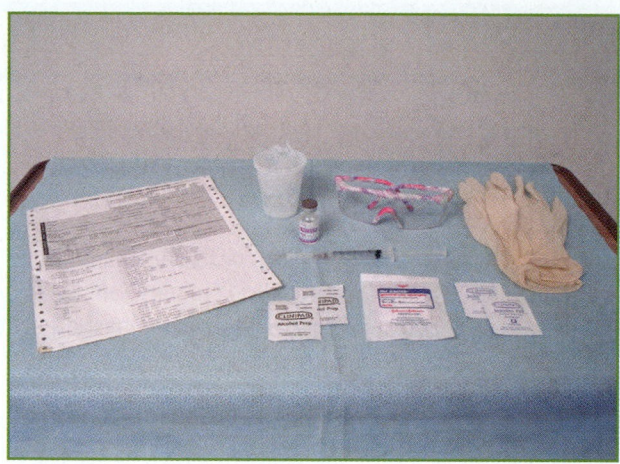

Figure 8-24-1 Alcohol, syringes, gauze, heparinized solution, and a cup of ice

- Cup with crushed ice
- Label with date, time, and client's name
- Laboratory requisition

- Disposable gloves
- Protective eye wear

▶ **CLIENT EDUCATION NEEDED:**

1. The client should be taught the rationale for the ABG sample.
2. Prepare clients by telling them that the needle stick will be painful so they do not reflexively pull their arm away.
3. Client should be instructed to breathe slowly and deeply.
4. The client should be taught to report these symptoms immediately: numbness, burning, tingling, or bleeding in the hand that was punctured.

Estimated time to complete the skill: **15–20 minutes**

▶ **DELEGATION TIPS**

Obtaining a blood gas specimen is not delegated to ancillary personnel. The procedure(s) require sterile technique, and accessing the artery improperly increases the client's risk for nosocomial infection, air emboli, and neurovascular damage. Ancillary personnel should report any client concerns regarding numbness, tingling, coolness, cyanosis, or paleness of the extremity to the nurse.

IMPLEMENTATION—Action/Rationale

Action	Rationale
1. Identify client and explain procedure to client in calm tone of voice.	1. Ensures proper client identification and reduces anxiety and promotes cooperation.
2. Prepare syringe with heparin: • Aspirate 0.5 mL of sodium heparin (1000 U/mL) into syringe from vial. • Withdraw plunger entire length of syringe and eject all heparin out of syringe.	2. Needed if a heparinized syringe is not available. • Prevents blood from clotting before analysis is performed. • Coats the barrel of syringe with heparin. More than 0.25 mL of sodium heparin in 3 mL of blood may affect the pH level.
3. Select safest and most accessible site for ABG sample: • Perform Allen's test. Have client make tight fist and apply direct pressure to both radial and ulnar arteries. When client opens hand, release pressure over ulnar artery and observe color of fingers, thumbs, and hand. Fingers should flush within 15 seconds—a positive Allen's test.	3. Arterial puncture may result in spasm, clotting, or hematoma, which could reduce blood flow, so collateral flow is essential. • Determines adequate blood flow to the hand by removing blood from hand, obstructing blood flow, then allowing blood to flow into hand through the ulnar artery. Indicates collateral flow is positive.

continues

Action	Rationale
• If Allen's test is positive, use the radial artery.	• The radial artery is the safest and most accessible site.
• Brachial artery should be used if radial artery is inaccessible or Allen's test is negative.	• Has collateral blood flow but is less superficial and more difficult to palpate and stabilize and has risk of damage to adjacent structures such as brachial nerve or vein.
• Femoral artery should be used only by specially trained nurses or health care providers.	• Has no collateral blood flow if obstructed below the inguinal ligament, is difficult to stabilize, and is adjacent to femoral vein. However, this is the best artery to use in an emergency such as cardiac arrest or shock.
4. Wash hands and put on gloves.	4. Reduces number of microorganisms.
5. Palpate selected radial site with fingertips and stabilize artery by slightly hyperextending wrist.	5. Determines area of maximal impulse for puncture site and facilitates successful insertion of needle.
6. Use alcohol swab to clean in a circular motion the area above the pulse (see Figure 8-24-2).	6. Reduces number of bacteria on surface of skin.
7. Hold alcohol swab in fingers of one hand while keeping a fingertip from the other hand on the artery.	7. Keeps swab accessible during procedure.
8. Insert needle with bevel up into artery at a 45-degree angle (see Figure 8-24-3).	8. Allows for better arterial flow into needle. Oblique hole in artery seals more easily.
9. Hold the needle and syringe still when blood appears in the syringe.	9. Prevents traversing needle through artery.
10. Allow arterial pulsing to slowly pump 2–3 mL of blood into heparinized syringe.	10. Prevents air bubbles from entering sample, which can alter results.
11. When sample is collected, hold alcohol swab over the puncture site and withdraw needle.	11. Swab minimizes pulling of skin as needle is withdrawn.
12. Apply pressure with the alcohol swab over the puncture site for 5 minutes, or 10 minutes if the client is on anticoagulant therapy or has a bleeding disorder.	12. Ensures adequate coagulation at puncture site.

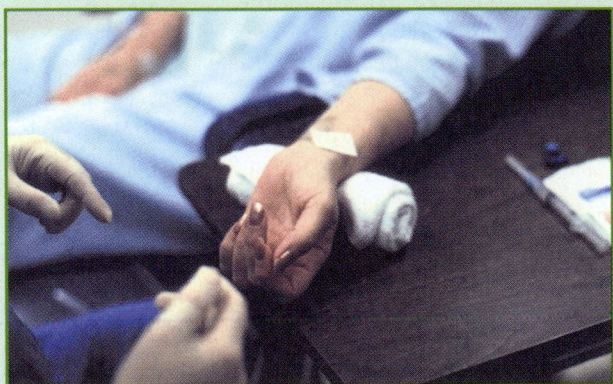

Figure 8-24-2   Clean the area with an alcohol swab.

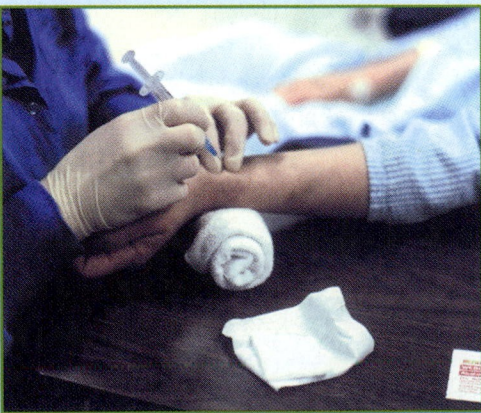

Figure 8-24-3   Insert the needle with the bevel up at a 45-degree angle.

continues

Action	Rationale
13. Inspect site for signs of complications: • Bleeding • Change or disappearance of pulse • Color of hand	13. Determines need for further treatment. • Indicates need to exert pressure. • Shows change in blood flow to hand. • Paleness may indicate obstruction of blood flow.
14. Remove gloves and wash hands.	14. Reduces transmission of organisms.
15. Prepare sample for laboratory and send it: • Expel air bubbles from syringe. • Label syringe with client identification. • Place syringe in cup of crushed ice. • Fill out requisition form, including amount of oxygen the client is receiving (e.g., 2 liters O_2 by nasal cannula, room air, 70% on ventilator) Note: Some laboratories also require a recent body temperature.	15. • Prevents false ABG results. • Ensures results are correct for client. • Reduces blood cell metabolism. • Ensures proper identification of sample.
16. Review results of ABG sample and compare with normal values: • pH 7.35 to 7.45, $PaCO_2$ 35 to 45 • PaO_2 80 to 100 • SaO_2 94% to 98%	16. Identifies abnormality: • pH and decreased $PaCO_2$—respiratory alkalosis; pH and increased $PaCO_2$—respiratory acidosis • PaO_2—inadequate oxygenation • SaO_2—contamination of sample
17. Report ABG results to health care provider and perform nursing measures accordingly: • Respiratory acidosis • Respiratory alkalosis	17. Ensures proper treatment of client: • Encourage coughing and deep breathing; perform tracheal suctioning, elevate head of bed, administer or increase oxygen therapy, hold pain medication if possible. • Encourage slow, deep breaths; have client breathe into a paper bag, administer pain medication, help client alleviate anxiety.

▶ REAL WORLD ANECDOTES

Mrs. Anderson was admitted to the hospital with pneumonia. She was started on IV antibiotics and IV fluids. Her daily chest X-ray was stable and she had a low-grade fever. One afternoon, the nurse noticed that her temperature was 38.9° C and her respirations were 36 and shallow. She seemed less alert than earlier and restless. The nurse reported her symptoms to the physician, who ordered oxygen to be given at 40% by mask and that ABGs and a chest X-ray be done immediately. The nurse obtained a blood gas sample while waiting for the portable chest X-ray to arrive. The blood gas results showed a reduced PaO_2 level, indicating inadequate oxygenation. The nurse notified Mrs. Anderson's physician of the ABG results immediately. The physician ordered Mrs. Anderson's oxygen to be increased, and she informed the nurse that she would be right in to see the client. Because the nurse had noted and correctly assessed Mrs. Anderson's symptoms in a timely manner, the appropriate care was administered before Mrs. Anderson's condition could deteriorate to a life or death situation.

▶ EVALUATION

- The client has normal ABG results.
- The pulse, color, and temperature of the client's extremity distal to the puncture is unchanged.
- The client was calm and free of pain.
- The client had minimal bleeding from the site following the puncture.

▶ DOCUMENTATION

Note: When the blood gas results are delivered to the nurse, they should be reported to the client's physician.

Nurses' Notes

- The date and time of the ABG sampling should be recorded in the narrative notes.
- Also record the reason for the test, the results of Allen's test, the client's response to the blood sampling, and any unusual observations.
- Note the route and amount of oxygen the client is receiving and any respiratory assessment observations.
- Record the condition of the puncture site prior to the blood draw and after the blood draw.
- Be sure to note the follow-up check on the condition of the site.
- For the laboratory requisition slip, record the date and time of the sample, the client's name and room number, the site the sample was drawn from, and the amount and route of oxygen delivery.

Document on appropriate flow sheet or electronic medical record (EMR).

▶ CRITICAL THINKING SKILL

Introduction

The rate and depth of respirations can affect the results of an ABG sample. It is necessary to assess the client's respirations before obtaining the sample.

Possible Scenario

A 19-year-old client presents to the emergency department complaining of difficulty breathing. Her lungs are clear and her physical assessment does not seem to indicate poor oxygenation. The emergency room doctor orders ABGs to be sure the teenager's blood oxygen level is normal. As the nurse explains the test to the client and prepares the needle and syringe, the client becomes increasingly anxious. Her respiratory rate increases to 36 breaths per minute.

Possible Outcome

The test results show respiratory acidosis. While examining the results, the nurse remembers that the client had been very anxious about the procedure and that her respiratory rate had increased dramatically. As the nurse gives the doctor the blood gas results, she reports this observation. The doctor recognizes that the blood gas results are probably not indicative of the client's actual blood gas levels. As the client's other symptoms do not indicate respiratory acidosis, the physician pursues other possible causes for the client's shortness of breath. The eventual cause is found to be a sinus infection that has caused swelling of the nasopharyngeal mucosa.

Prevention

Assess the client for deficient knowledge of the procedure as well as fear and anxiety. Take time to explain the procedure to allay the client's fears. Instruct the client to breathe normally. Note and record the client's respiratory rate and depth at the time of the ABG test. If the test is not consistent with the client's observable condition, treat the client, not the test results.

▶ VARIATIONS

Geriatric Variations:
- *Blood vessels can be fragile in elderly clients.*
- *Capillary refill can be slow in older clients.*
- *If Allen's test is failed in hands, it may be necessary to use the brachial or femoral artery.*

Pediatric Variations:
- *A heel stick for obtaining a capillary blood gas may be used in neonatal or pediatric clients.*
- *Values for neonatal clients may be different from adult values.*

continues

► VARIATIONS *(continued)*

Home Care Variations:

- *Arterial blood gas samples are less stable than venous blood samples and should be tested as soon as possible. When drawing this sample in the home care situation, take the blood to the laboratory as soon as possible.*
- *Between the time the arterial blood is drawn and the time it is tested, it should be stored in ice. Be sure to have ice in a cup or plastic bag available prior to drawing the sample. If the weather is hot or the drive to the laboratory is long, the nurse might want to have a small, portable ice chest available for transporting the sample.*

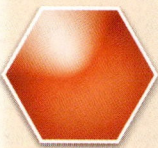

Long-Term Care Variations:

- *Clients with chronic obstructive pulmonary disease may have peripheral vascular insufficiency and may require a brachial or femoral sample.*
- *Clients with chronic obstructive pulmonary disease often have abnormally high $PaCO_2$ levels. The nurse should be aware of this when assessing blood gas results.*
- *The high $PaCO_2$ levels should not be treated with increased oxygen as this could cause the client to stop breathing.*

► COMMON ERRORS

Possible Error:

Air bubbles enter the syringe while obtaining the ABG.

Prevention:

Do not pull back on the plunger of the syringe while obtaining arterial blood. Be sure the needle is attached securely to the syringe before inserting the needle into the artery. If a sufficient amount of blood has been obtained, remove the needle and expel the air bubbles from the syringe. If not, remove the needle, apply pressure to the site, wait 5 minutes, and obtain the sample at another site with a new needle and syringe.

► NURSING TIPS

- Prepare the heparinized syringe before going into the client's room.
- Remember that superficial arteries are at the distal ends of extremities.
- Be sure to calmly warn the client before you insert the needle so he or she does not pull back the hand.
- A rolled towel placed under the client's wrist helps to relax the hand and allows easier access to the artery.
- Never pull back on the plunger of the syringe while sampling arterial blood.
- Bring a cup of ice into the room to have available to transport the sample.

► SPECIAL CONSIDERATIONS

- *Local anesthetic, such as 2% lidocaine, may be injected preprocedure to reduce the client's discomfort.*
- *If air bubbles are left in the syringe and occupy more than 1% to 2% of the blood volume, then the client may exhibit artificially high arterial PaO_2. This can be prevented by gently removing the bubbles, taking care not to agitate the sample. Air bubbles in the tip of the syringe can be removed by pushing the plunger to expel bubbles into a container designed for biohazard waste.*

Assisting with the Insertion and Maintenance of an Epidural Catheter

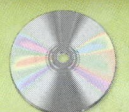

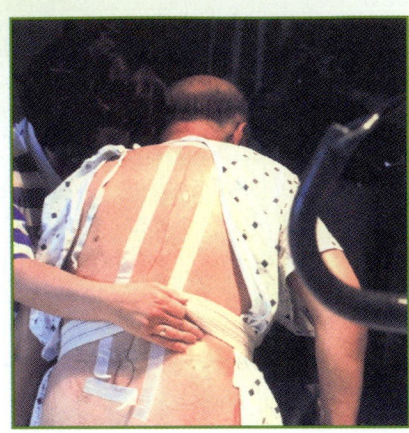

▶ OVERVIEW OF THE SKILL

Epidural catheter placement is an effective method used to administer regional anesthesia and/or analgesia. Epidural placement is performed by qualified personnel. Qualification guidelines are determined by law and institutional policy. Persons assisting with placement must be knowledgeable about the routine, possible complications, desired outcomes, and client support.

▶ ASSESSMENT

1. Perform a thorough history and physical before epidural placement. Report positive findings to the anesthetist/anesthesiologist. **Prior experiences with anesthesia, medical problems, and current medical status are vital information and must be assessed prior to therapy.**
2. Assess baseline vital signs. **Alterations in blood pressure and pulse will indicate reactions to medications used in epidural dosing.**
3. Assess client's ability to follow direction and communicate. **Client must be able to maintain a steady position and convey any symptoms to the practitioner.**

▶ DIAGNOSIS

Anxiety

Pain

Risk for Infection

1174

▶ PLANNING

Expected Outcomes:

1. Client will experience relief of pain or lack of sensation in accordance with the reason for the epidural.
2. Client will experience no untoward effects of epidural anesthesia.
3. Client will perform self-medication as appropriate (e.g., client-controlled analgesia).
4. Client will experience desired effect of anesthesia/analgesia until it is appropriate to discontinue treatment.

Equipment Needed (see Figure 8-25-1):

- Oxygen
- Suction

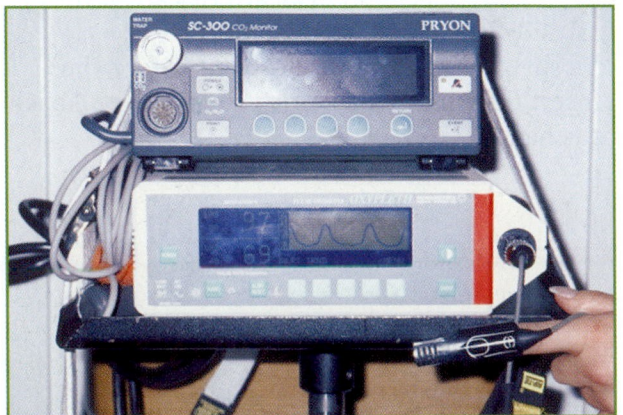

Figure 8-25-1 Pulse oximeter

- Anesthesia equipment
- Emergency medication
- Automated blood pressure recorder
- Oximeter
- ECG monitor
- Drugs as requested by anesthesia personnel
- Positioning aids, e.g., pillows, sandbags

▶ CLIENT EDUCATION NEEDED:

1. Describe the procedure to the client in easy-to-understand terms. Clients experiencing anxiety may require calm reassurance throughout the procedure and benefit by knowing ahead of time sensations they may feel.
2. Remind client to maintain position during the procedure.
3. The most uncomfortable part of the procedure for most people is numbing the skin. After the skin is numb, most people feel pressure as the anesthetist places the catheter.
4. Ask the client to report any sudden shooting pain or back pain, which might indicate that the skin is not numb. Some practitioners prefer to teach this themselves, and it is important to check before the client is present if the anesthesiologist/anesthetist has a preference.
5. If anesthesia is desired, client will not be able to ambulate and may not have sensation below the level of anesthesia effect.

6. If analgesia is provided on a client-controlled analgesia device, ensure that the client understands that medication is available on demand and is able to demonstrate the technique for medication delivery.
7. If client is to have intermittent bolusing: Teach client to report when he or she begins to feel pain. Notify anesthesia practitioner immediately for bolus (or follow institution protocol) as feeling often returns rapidly.
8. If client is to receive client-controlled analgesia: Ensure that the client understands medication principles associated with his or her dosing scheme.
9. Reinforce that if the epidural is not providing adequate relief there are changes that can be made to dosage and administration. Often, clients may think that there are no alternatives to the current treatment.
10. If therapy is to be long-term, ensure that the client understands mobility limitations and learns to identify sensations that indicate, for example, full bladder and pressure over bony prominences.

Estimated time to complete the skill: **10–30 minutes. Time requirements will vary with anesthesia practitioners, difficulty of the procedure, and institution policy for monitoring.**

▶ DELEGATION TIPS

Assisting with the insertion and maintenance of an epidural catheter is a skill involving assessment and the use of sterile technique. It is an invasive procedure performed by the health care provider, and assisting is not delegated unless other licensed personnel have been trained and certified to assist with the procedure. Ancillary personnel who will be caring for the client need to be instructed to report any complaints of pain, numbness, tingling, or alteration in movement of the extremities to the nurse.

IMPLEMENTATION—Action/Rationale

Action	Rationale
1. Identify client and review preanesthesia orders.	1. Ensures proper client identification and that the client has received medications and fluids before start of the procedure. Some practitioners will ask that fluid boluses be given within an hour of epidural starts.
2. Obtain consent from client.	2. Client gives permission for procedure.

continues

Action	Rationale
3. Assemble equipment. Label tubing, provide appropriate filters, and ensure that tubing is correct for designated purpose and has no injection ports. Use solutions without preservatives.	**3.** Ensures functionality of emergency equipment. Extra and alternative supplies are brought to the room in case of contamination or client needs.
4. Apply client monitors in accordance with institutional policy.	**4.** Ensures correct monitors will be utilized during surgery or evaluates oxygenation and cardiac function following epidural insertion. Alerts to sudden changes in the client's status that will require immediate attention.
5. Assist client to lying or sitting position.	**5.** Positioning will depend on practitioner preference, client condition, and environmental constraints.
6. Assess that the client can maintain a stable position (see Figure 8-25-2). Assist if necessary.	**6.** If the client is unable to maintain a stable position, alternative anesthesia/analgesia methods must be used.
7. Maintain calm milieu; encourage client to follow anesthesia practitioner's directions. Instruct client to report symptoms to the anesthesia practitioner throughout the procedure.	**7.** Provides clues as to the progress of insertion, especially in difficult cases.
8. Monitor for: • Untoward effects of intravenous administration of medication or anesthesia. • Untoward effects associated with a dural puncture.	**8.** Detects adverse signs including ringing in the ears, sudden tachycardia, and metal taste in the mouth. • Some medications used in epidurals will cause seizure. This is the reason test dose is used before initial dosing. • If a dural puncture occurs, the client will be immediately and profoundly numb as soon as medication is administered. Respiratory assistance may be required in this instance as dosages for epidural therapy are much higher than those required for intrathecal (spinal) therapy.
9. Assist anesthesia practitioner to stabilize catheter. Often the catheter will be taped along the client's back, then over the shoulder for easy access. Take care to prevent kinks in the soft material.	**9.** Prevents catheter from becoming dislodged.
10. Follow anesthesia practitioner's direction for client positioning after anesthesia is administered.	**10.** Positioning may be used to "even out" the drug and therefore the effect. Epidural anesthesia does not provide instantaneous relief; rather it requires several minutes to set up depending on which drugs are used, the client's anatomy, and position of the catheter.

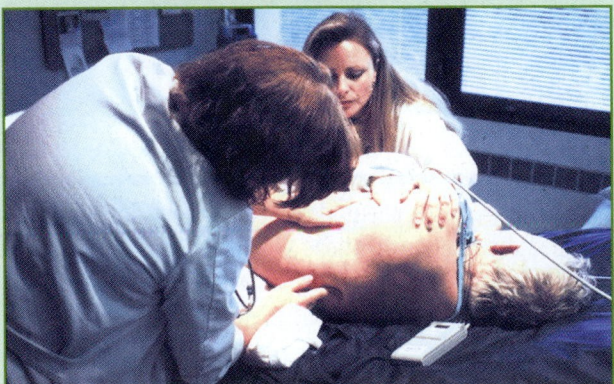

Figure 8-25-2 Help the client maintain a position lying on side.

continues

Action	Rationale
11. Initiate automatic drug delivery system (if appropriate to institutional policy). Some state laws require that automatic drug delivery be started by anesthesia personnel. Know your practice act (see Figure 8-25-3).	**11.** Provides drug administration as ordered.
12. Perform frequent blood pressure and neurologic exams in compliance with institutional policy.	**12.** Regional anesthesia may cause motor blockade and lead to vasodilation.
13. Monitor client at frequent intervals for ability to void, pressure and positioning, analgesic and/or anesthetic effects, and compliance with mobility limitations, if appropriate.	**13.** Basic assessment ensures effectiveness and reduces risk of complications from the intervention.

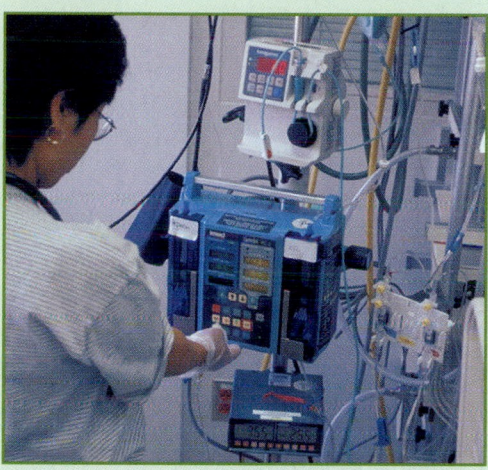

Figure 8-25-3   Initiate drug delivery system.

▶ **EVALUATION**

- The client experiences relief from pain or lack of unpleasant sensation.
- The client does not experience the untoward effects of epidural anesthesia.
- The client understands the purpose and action of the epidural anesthesia, and performs self-medication if appropriate.

▶ **DOCUMENTATION**

Nurses' Notes

Following epidural placement:
- Use a pain scale for evaluation and document client's response on a 1- to 10-point scale. Sensation absent at T_{10}. (Describe client positioning and any supportive intervention used to prevent injury.)
- Document sensation or absence of sensation at the T_{10} dermatome.

Document on appropriate flow sheet or electronic medical record (EMR).

Medical Administration Record

- Personnel from the anesthesia department will document medications on the anesthesia record. Ensure that all partial narcotics doses are documented according to institution and state and federal regulations.

Vital Signs Flow Sheet

- Vital signs are recorded at greater frequency during surgery, during recovery, and anytime a client's condition may change unexpectedly because of continuously infusing medication or other reasons. Check your institution's policy for recording parameters for the anesthetized client.

▶ **REAL WORLD ANECDOTES**

Scenario 1

Often in surgery, it seems that everything happens at once. For the circulating nurse, many tasks must be accomplished in a short time before the procedure begins. Be aware that when clients are brought to the surgical suite they may have had antianxiety medication and may not be able to protect themselves.

The nurse received a report on Adeline, who was scheduled for an abdominal hysterectomy. In the operating room, the nurse was almost ready for the case. The anesthetist was ready to perform the epidural but the scrub technician was a little late getting started. As the anesthetist helped Adeline to lie on her side, the nurse stood in front of her to protect her from falling off the edge. Just as the anesthetist began looking for a good place for insertion, the scrub technician asked the nurse to tie her gown. The nurse moved away from the table "just for a second." Adeline began to fall, but the quick action of the anesthetist prevented her from falling to the floor. The nurse learned the hard way that clients must never be left unattended, even for a moment.

Scenario 2

Don, a 68-year-old client, had an epidural catheter placed for client-controlled analgesia following an exploratory laparotomy. Over the evening, he kept complaining of pain, even though he was using the client-controlled analgesia correctly. His nurse checked the equipment several times and was considering requesting an increased dosage rate of pain medication. When the family came to visit, the daughter noticed that the catheter had pulled out of her father and was lying in the bedclothes. The sweat from his skin and the friction of the bedsheets had caused the tape to roll and the catheter became dislodged. He had been medicating the bed all afternoon. The nurse needed to check the epidural catheter as well as the pump and the client (see Figures 8-25-4 and 8-25-5).

▶ **CRITICAL THINKING SKILL**

Introduction

Positioning is important during epidural catheter placement. The anesthesia practitioner must navigate the structures of the spine by the feel of the needle. Recall that the spaces in the spine open up as the client bends.

Possible Scenario

Mario is a large man. He is scheduled for hernia surgery and has elected to have an epidural for surgery and postoperative pain control. Mario has a protruding abdomen and cannot seem to bend in the middle when instructed to do so.

Possible Outcome

If Mario is still unable to bend sufficiently, the anesthetist may elect to have Mario sit up for catheter insertion.

Prevention

Try to help Mario understand the need to bend. It may help to demonstrate "bending in the middle" for Mario. Try to think of analogies for an arched back.

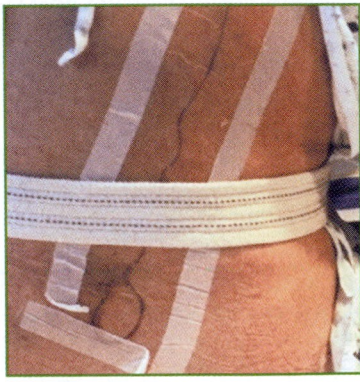

Figure 8-25-4 Check the epidural catheter to make sure it has not become dislodged.

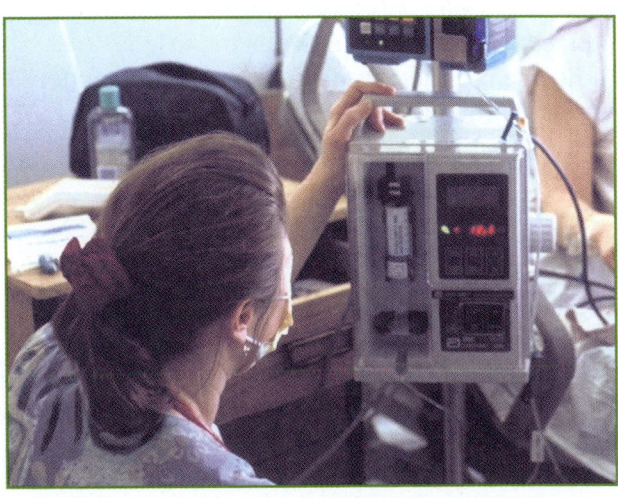

Figure 8-25-5 Check the pump to make sure it is functioning correctly.

▶ VARIATIONS

Geriatric Variations:
- Older clients may overestimate their ability to tolerate pain, or have expectations that they can "bear up."
- Visual, hearing, and cognitive impairments might interfere with accurate assessment of side effects and pain control.
- Older clients may have more complex medication regimens, and may have greater responses to medications, including opioids. Careful assessment of potential medication interactions is important.

Pediatric Variations:
- Educate parents about the epidural catheter and the type and effects of medications being delivered.
- Educate parents about the child's mobility. Tell them that the child can be out of bed, if the medical condition permits. Assist the parent to position and hold the child without accidentally dislodging the epidural catheter.

Home Care Variations:
- Home care clients with long-term epidural catheters for pain control or medication administration must be monitored on a continuous basis to adjust dosages and assess for potential complications.
- Home care clients should have telephone access to health care providers for consultation and know what to do in case complications arise.

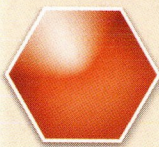

Long-Term Care Variations:
- Long-term assessment of the epidural catheter should include regular monitoring for signs of infection, the need for dosage adjustment for pain control, or signs of fibrotic encapsulation, which may reduce the therapeutic effect of drugs.
- Know what alternatives for pain control are available to the client if the catheter must be removed. Discuss with the client.

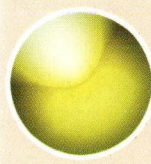

Pregnancy Variations:
- When assisting during the placement of an epidural for labor or cesarean section, it is imperative the assistant be competent in FHR monitoring. Appropriate response is critical if the FHR displays signs of distress (i.e., bradycardia, late decelerations) or if labor unexpectedly progresses to birth. The anesthesia personnel should be prepared to abandon the procedure in the instances cited. It is imperative for the assistant to be mindful of the effect of regional anesthesia on the progress of labor in addition to the physical effects on the mother and fetus.
- Never place the mother in a supine position, regardless of desirability for anesthesia efficacy.

▶ COMMON ERRORS

Possible Error:
The client requires oxygen because of profound hypotension. You cannot find a face mask anywhere.

Prevention:
Make sure that all emergency equipment is available and functional.

▶ **NURSING TIPS**

- Do not attempt to do other duties while assisting with epidural placement. If there are competing demands, insist on extra personnel. (For example, in surgery do not count sponges or pour liquids when client is positioned.) Client safety must be your first concern.

- Maintain proper body mechanics during the procedure as you may need to hold your position for a prolonged time.
- If anesthesia personnel ask the client to bend, it is sometimes helpful to ask the client to arch like a "Halloween cat."

▶ **SPECIAL CONSIDERATIONS**

- *After the epidural catheter is in place, it is important to monitor the client for signs of infection. Some initial signs may be fever, malaise, and back pain. If the client has severe, localized back pain that increases upon percussion, coupled by the presence of an elevated temperature, then infection should be suspected and the health care provider notified. If untreated, epidural site infection could progress to irreversible paralysis.*

Skin Integrity and Wound Care

Bandaging

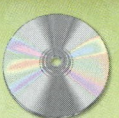

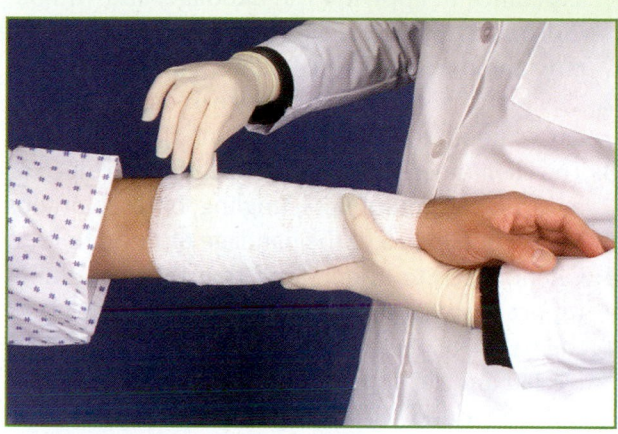

▶ OVERVIEW OF THE SKILL

Bandages are narrow strips of fabric, gauze, or elastic material used on wounds to aid and promote the healing process. Bandages are used to cover wounded areas, hold dressings in place, and reduce edema. Bandages may also be used to apply pressure or support to a specific area without compromising circulation, alignment, or mobility. Gauze bandages are readily available in a variety of widths, so the size of the bandage can be chosen to correspond to the size of the wound and body part involved. Another advantage of gauze is that it is porous, which promotes healing by allowing circulation of air to the wound.

Elastic bandages are also available in a variety of widths and have the added advantage of applying more pressure/compression because of their elastic quality. Therefore, they are used more often to prevent edema on lower extremities (see Skill 10-1 on applying elastic bandages). Fabric bandages are not routinely used. Fabric bandages can be made from many available sources and can be used in emergency situations.

▶ ASSESSMENT

1. Assess the wound to be covered if a wound is involved. **If there is active bleeding, the bleeding must be controlled to prevent hemorrhage and possible hypovolemia. A pressure dressing can be applied using a bandage to hold the pressure compress in place if necessary. A bandage should not be applied to a** wound that does not have a dressing over the bleeding area. Immobilizing a joint or broken bone is one of the most important factors in controlling blood loss, and a properly applied bandage can aid in immobilization.

2. Assess the client's level of consciousness. **This is important so that the client can report if the bandage is too tight and is possibly restricting circulation.** If the client has a decreased level of consciousness, use extra caution to ascertain that the dressing is not too constricting.

3. Assess the client's skin integrity, paying special attention to the presence of edema, ecchymosis, urticaria, lacerations, abrasions, any bony prominence, and the condition of the skin (dry, cracked, infected, thin). **These factors will help determine what bandage products and techniques to use.**

4. Assess neurovascular status. Check capillary refill, temperature, and color of the skin in the area surrounding and distal to the bandage. Check motion, sensation, and pulses. **These factors will help determine a baseline for future assessments as well as what type of bandaging product or technique to use.**

5. Assess that client is not allergic to latex products. **Elastic bandages often contain latex and may cause local irritation or anaphylaxis in the presence of severe latex allergy.**

▶ DIAGNOSIS

Acute Pain

Impaired Skin Integrity

Impaired Physical Mobility

Ineffective Tissue Perfusion

Risk for Fluid Volume Deficit

Risk for Infection

Risk for Peripheral Neurovascular Dysfunction

▶ PLANNING

Expected Outcomes:

1. The client does not become hypovolemic, and bleeding is controlled.
2. The wound is supported and in alignment.
3. The bandage is applied properly, with adequate anchoring and no loose or dangling ends.
4. The client does not experience pain or discomfort from the bandaging.
5. There is adequate circulation to the wound and distal body parts before, during, and after application of the bandage.
6. The client does not report any numbness or tingling.
7. The wound heals, without breakdown of skin or neurovascular status.

Equipment Needed (see Figures 9-1-1 and 9-1-2):

- Dressing for wound, if present
- Bandage, either gauze, elastic, or fabric (emergency situation)
- Gloves to maintain body fluid precautions if there is the potential for body fluids
- Tape or clips to secure bandage

▶ CLIENT EDUCATION NEEDED:

1. It is important that clients understand what the nurse is doing and why the bandage is being applied (to control the bleeding, support the wound/limb, hold a dressing in place, reduce edema). If clients are part of the process, they will experience less discomfort, will be of more assistance in applying the bandage, and will be more compliant in keeping the bandage in place after the nurse has finished applying it.
2. Teach the client the importance of having the bandage smooth to avoid any unwanted constriction.
3. The client needs to understand the importance of reporting any numbness, tingling, or discoloration of skin in the area of the bandage or distal to it.
4. Clients need to understand that they should report any drainage that has soaked through the bandage. Active bleeding needs to be controlled and reported. It is important to maintain a clean wound with less potential for secondary infection.

Estimated time to complete the skill:
5–15 minutes depending on whether a wound is involved and the complexity of the bandage, which is dependent on the body part involved.

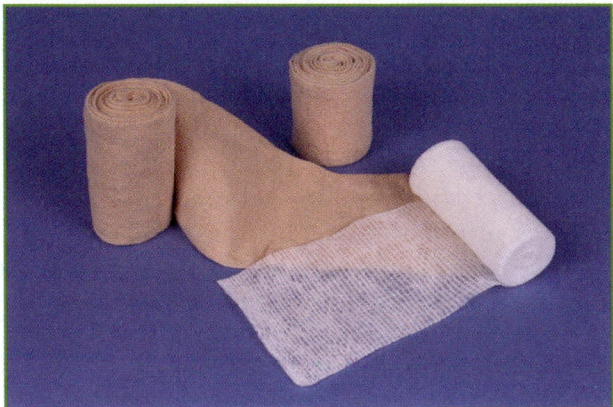

Figure 9-1-1 Select the appropriate size bandage for the body part.

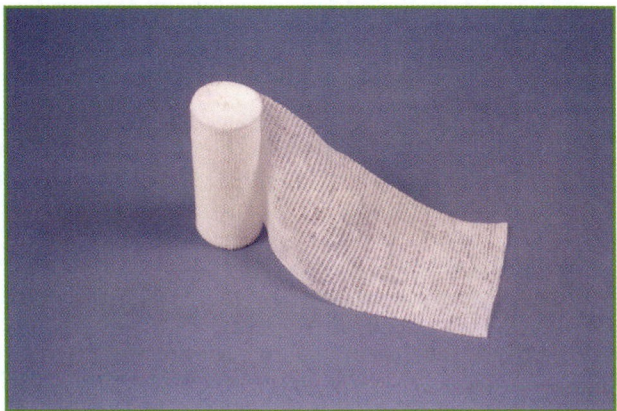

Figure 9-1-2 Kling gauze bandage

The application of bandages to the client is not delegated to ancillary personnel. Family members may be taught this skill before the client's discharge. Occasionally, ancillary personnel will be delegated the task of applying a clean dry gauze as skin protection, but the nurse is responsible for the assessment of the integrity of the client's skin.

IMPLEMENTATION—Action/Rationale

Action	Rationale
1. Provide privacy for the client, then wash hands and apply gloves.	1. Reduces the transmission of microorganisms and ensures client comfort.
2. Provide wound care as ordered or required. Determine the need for the bandage. Will it be used to: • Cover a wound? • Hold a dressing in place? • Apply pressure? • Support a wound/limb? • Maintain circulation? • Decrease edema?	2. If the need is to control bleeding and the risk of hemorrhage exists, the nurse must apply a pressure dressing immediately. A clean bandage can be used to control the bleeding in emergency situations, but use a sterile dressing when available.
3. Assess the neurovascular status. Check pulse, capillary refill, skin color, and warmth. Check sensation. Neurovascular status needs to be assessed at the wound or area to be bandaged and the body part distal to the area.	3. If the neurovascular status is compromised, it will be necessary for the nurse to fully assess and document this prior to applying the bandage and to correct the compromised status, if possible.
4. Assess skin integrity. Check for dryness, fragility of the skin, any apparent breakdown, and signs of bleeding or infection.	4. If there is excessive dryness or fragility, extra care will be needed to prevent breakdown of the skin. If the skin around the existing wound is already impaired as evident by swelling, bleeding, or infection, this breakdown must be dealt with before applying the bandage.
5. Assess need for immobilization.	5. Proper immobilization is essential for controlling bleeding, supporting the area, protecting the wound from further damage, and maintaining client comfort.
6. Assess client's comfort and level of consciousness. Explain procedure to client.	6. Makes client more comfortable and determines how aware the client is and able to understand and cooperate with the nurse during the process of bandaging.
7. Gather supplies needed, based on above assessment.	7. If the nurse knows what will be needed, the process will be more effective and time efficient.

continues

Action	Rationale
8. Apply the bandage. The technique will vary depending on the area of body to be bandaged.	8. If the bandage is properly applied, it will be more effective in doing what it was applied for: controlling bleeding, covering the wound, applying necessary pressure or compression, reducing edema, supporting wound/limb to maintain circulation and immobilization, if needed.
• Hold roll of bandage in dominant hand, with the loose end on the distal portion of the area to be bandaged (see Figure 9-1-3). The end is held with nondominant hand.	• Wrap with the dominant hand for dexterity.
• The roll of bandage is applied by starting at the distal and moving toward the proximal part of the body. Apply slight tension as the bandage is unrolled around the body part.	• Proper application promotes venous return and maintains consistent bandage tension.
• The first two or three turns of the bandage should overlap to secure the loose end.	• Prevents the bandage from unwrapping.
• The roll of bandage can be transferred from hand to hand and should be applied evenly and firmly, but caution should be taken to avoid the bandage being too tight (see Figure 9-1-4).	• A bandage that is uneven or too tight can create a tourniquet effect, reducing circulation, with the possibility of causing skin breakdown and nerve damage.
9. Common bandaging methods:	9.
• **Figure eight:** Anchor bandage at center of joint. Ascend obliquely in circular fashion around extremity above and below joint, in a figure-eight fashion, overlapping until necessary immobilization is obtained. Secure end of bandage (see Figure 9-1-6D).	• Used for bandaging joints and providing immobilization.
• **Spiral:** Anchor bandage at distal aspect with two or three circular turns. Then proceed upward, overlapping one-half to two-thirds the width of the bandage with each turn (see Figure 9-1-6B). Secure end of bandage (see Figure 9-1-5).	• Used to cover cylindric body parts.

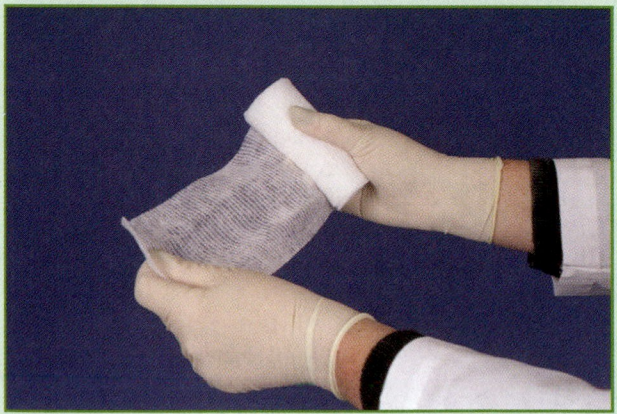

Figure 9-1-3 Hold the bandage in the dominant hand and loosen the end of the bandage.

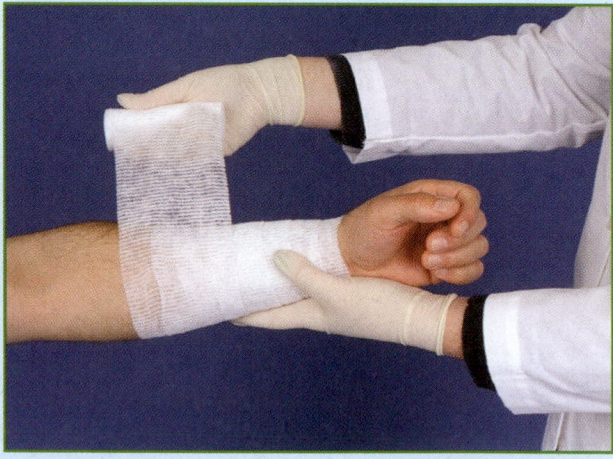

Figure 9-1-4 Wrap the bandage from distal to proximal. Do not wrap the bandage too tightly.

continues

Action	Rationale
• **Recurrent turns (also known as the stump method):** Anchor bandage with two circular turns around proximal end of area to be bandaged. Then make a reverse turn at center front, taking roll of bandage over the distal end of the area to the center back. Then make another reverse turn and take roll of bandage over the distal end to the center front. Continue front to back with reverse turns in this fashion until the wound is covered. Then anchor with two more circular turns and secure end of bandage (see Figure 9-1-6E).	• Used to cover top of head or stump wounds.
• **Reverse spiral:** Anchor bandage at distal border with 2 to 3 turns. Advance roll of bandage proximally at about a 30-degree angle. Halfway through each turn, fold bandage toward the nurse and continue in a downward fashion. Continue bandaging proximally in this manner until the area to be bandaged is covered. Secure the end of the bandage (see Figure 9-1-5).	• Used to cover cone-shaped body parts, such as the forearm and lower leg.
10. Remove and appropriately dispose of gloves and wash hands.	**10.** Reduces the transmission of microorganisms.

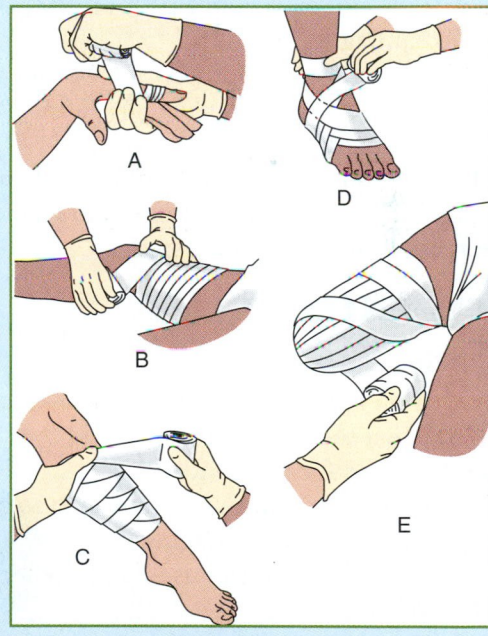

Figure 9-1-6 Common bandaging methods. **A.** *Circular turns* are wrapped around a body part several times to anchor a bandage or supply support. **B.** *Spiral turns* begin with one or two circular turns, then proceed up the body part, with each turn covering two-thirds the width of the previous turn. **C.** *Reverse spiral turns* begin with a circular turn. Then the bandage is reversed or twisted once each turn to accommodate a limb that gets larger as the bandaging progresses. **D.** *Figure-eight turns* criss-cross in the shape of a figure eight and are used on a joint that requires movement. **E.** *Recurrent turns* are anchored with circular turns and follow a back-and-forth motion, and are completed with circular turns; used to cover a fingertip, head, or amputated stump.

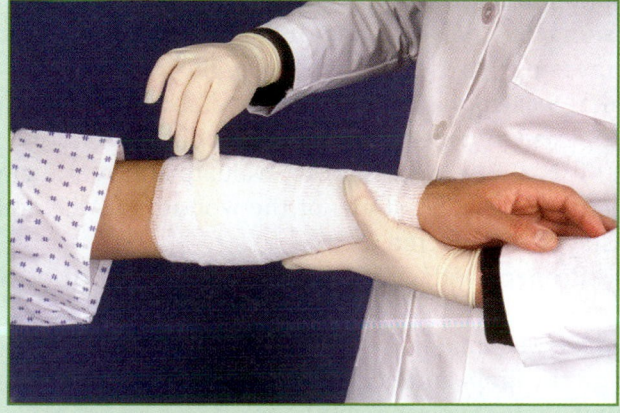

Figure 9-1-5 Anchor bandage at the center of joint.

▶ REAL WORLD ANECDOTES

Joe is a 36-year-old painter who fell off his painting platform 2 hours before arriving in the emergency department. He is complaining of left elbow pain and bleeding. He is holding a towel on the wound, which is not actively bleeding at the time of arrival. Joe is alert and oriented, and his vital signs are stable. He has decreased range of motion of his left elbow and arm. It is determined that he needs an X-ray. The nurse checks the wound and determines that with a proper bandage, it will be safe for Joe to go to X-ray prior to having the laceration sutured. A light-pressure, sterile dressing is applied over the wound. The nurse then proceeds to bandage the wound and limb to keep the dressing in place, which will control bleeding and immobilize the elbow. The nurse applies a figure-eight bandage with 2.5 cm gauze over the dressing, checking neurovascular status before applying the bandage. After she is done she asks Joe if he has any numbness or tingling in the arm and fingers distal to the wound. Capillary refill is checked and appears to be brisk. His radial and ulnar pulses are full and intact. When Joe returns from X-ray, the bandage is reassessed. The bandage is now wrinkled and has been reapplied tightly, causing some intermittent tingling in Joe's left fingers. The bandage is removed to improve circulation and so the wound can be further assessed and sutured as necessary.

▶ EVALUATION

- The client did not become hypovolemic, and bleeding was controlled.
- The wound was supported and in alignment.
- The bandage was applied properly, with adequate anchoring and no loose or dangling ends.
- The client did not experience pain or discomfort from the bandaging
- There is adequate circulation to the wound and distal body parts before, during, and after application of the bandage.
- The client did not report any numbness or tingling.
- The wound is healing without breakdown of skin or decrease in neurovascular status.

▶ DOCUMENTATION

Nurses' Notes

- Document on appropriate flow sheet or electronic medical record (EMR).
- Record the need for the bandage.
- Record the condition of the wound/area to be bandaged prior to the bandaging.
- Record the type of material used and the technique used.
- Record the neurovascular status of the wound before, immediately after, and 20 minutes after the bandage was applied.
- Record the client's comfort level.

▶ CRITICAL THINKING SKILL

Introduction

A nurse's timely assessment prevented well-intentioned first aid interventions from increasing the victim's injuries.

Possible Scenario

You are out hiking on your day off. A climber has fallen from a rock ledge and is unconscious with a head injury and an obviously fractured left arm. A fellow climber has taken appropriate first aid measures, which include splinting the arm very tightly.

Possible Outcome

Because this climber is unconscious, he cannot report the tingling and numbness in his fingers. His neurovascular status could become compromised. You assess his neurovascular status, adjust the splint, and return your attention to his head injury while awaiting the search-and-rescue team.

Prevention

If the bone was broken and the joint had not been immobilized, the climber could have had further trauma to the area and increased bleeding, thus increasing his risk of hypovolemia. In this case, a splint was applied along with the bandage to ensure proper alignment as well as immobilization.

It is always necessary to evaluate and reevaluate the neurovascular status of the wound and the area distal to the affected area.

Proper bandaging in this scenario applied pressure to a bleeding wound; kept the dressing in place; reduced edema; helped to support, immobilize, and align the limb; and helped to reduce the pain that the climber was experiencing.

▶ VARIATIONS

Geriatric Variations:
- *Normal increased fragility of the skin in elderly clients can make the skin more likely to break down. Apply dressing with less pressure.*
- *Less resilient cardiovascular status may increase the risk of hypovolemia, so the bleeding must be closely watched.*

Pediatric Variations:
- *Be aware of increased movement and the fact that a child may take off the bandage. A child's bandage needs to be more secure (but not tighter) than an adult's.*
- *Explaining what you are doing is very helpful and helps to decrease the child's anxiety.*

Home Care Variations:
- *Make sure the care provider knows where to purchase supplies, if needed. Research available options for cost and location prior to the home care visit.*
- *A plastic storage bin with a lid will help keep bandage supplies together, clean, and dry in the home setting.*
- *Store liquids in a different container to reduce the chance of spillage and contamination of the sterile dressings.*
- *Teach the client or home caregiver to frequently launder reusable bandages, such as Ace wraps or stockinette, to keep them clean.*

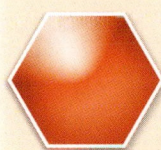

Long-Term Care Variations:
- *Discuss alternatives to taping and removing tape several times a day if the bandage will be in place for the long term. Mesh net, ties, or a light Ace wrap may be solutions that will be easier on the skin surrounding the bandage.*
- *Choose the lightest tape that will do the job. Check for allergies to the tape, which do not necessarily show up immediately but may appear over the long term.*
- *Teach the client the proper techniques and allow as much bandaging self-care as possible to promote a sense of independence and control.*

▶ COMMON ERRORS

Possible Error:
The bandage slips out of place.

Prevention:
Select the proper bandage for the area. Make sure the bandage is not too loose.

Possible Error:
The bandage impairs circulation distal to the site.

Prevention:
Do not apply the bandage too tightly. Select a bandage large enough to cover the area without applying too much pressure. If a circular or spiral wrap is used, make sure it is applied from distal to proximal and has not been wrapped too tightly.

▶ **NURSING TIPS**

• Assess need for a bandage, the wound, and the area involved before attempting to bandage to determine the technique that will be best suited to the situation.

• When applying a bandage, hold the rolled bandage so that it unrolls from the bottom of the roll (see Figure 9-1-3), thus making application easier.

• Gather all needed supplies before starting.

• Explain what you are doing and why to the client.

▶ **SPECIAL CONSIDERATIONS**

• *At times topical skin products may be used as a protectant for the lower limbs. These products are called Dome paste bandage, Unna's boot, or Zinc gelatin boot. The dressing comes as a 3 inch × 10 yards or 4 inch × 10 yards bandage and is applied as an occlusive boot. It provides support to varicosities or lesions on the legs. The dressing remains on for approximately 2 weeks, after which it is removed by soaking the boot in warm water.*

• *Elastic and stretchable bandages generally contain natural rubber latex. Avoid use if client has history of latex allergy, urticaria, or rash.*

Applying a Dry Dressing

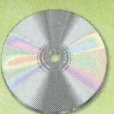

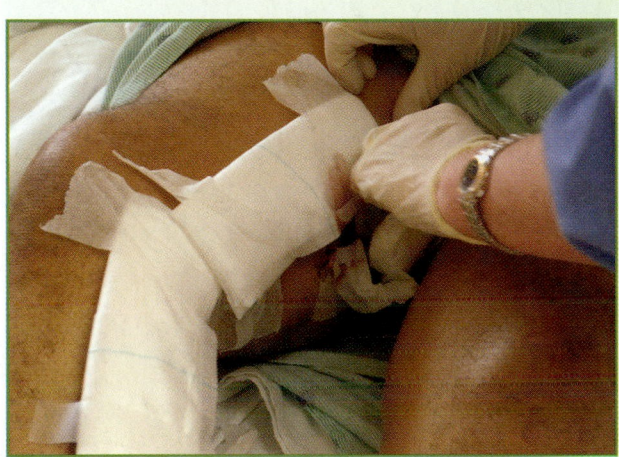

▶ OVERVIEW OF THE SKILL

A closed surgical wound can be described as a wound that was caused, revised, or debrided by a surgical intervention. Closed wounds are generally categorized as clean. They may be closed with sutures, staples, or tapes. The general purpose of the closed wound dressing is to cover and protect as well as absorb the minimal drainage that may occur with this type of wound. Dressing care may vary according to the surgeon's preference and institutional policy. General guidelines for the closed surgical wound dressing will be covered in this skill.

As there are different types of wounds, there are different approaches to wound care. Wound care agents, including povidone-iodine, hydrogen peroxide, Dakin's solution, or other cleaning solutions may need to be avoided, diluted, or used sparingly according to institutional policy. Cleaning solutions can dry the wound and interfere with wound healing at the cellular level. Furthermore, clients may be allergic or sensitive to these solutions. Although they reduce the risk of infection, frequent application may not be necessary. In many cases, sterile normal saline, sterile water, or pH neutral solutions will be adequate to cleanse the wound. It is important for nurses practicing in the profession to follow agency guidelines, observe the preferences of the health care provider, and to review recent research and published information on the optimal care for the type of wound being treated.

▶ ASSESSMENT

1. Assess the client's comfort level postoperatively upon arrival from the operating room, before wound care, and as needed throughout the postoperative course. **Surgical wounds are painful. If the client is made comfortable with appropriate pain medications and positioning, there will be better tissue gas exchange from deep breathing, coughing, and early ambulation, thereby promoting healing of tissues. The clients will be more cooperative and less anxious during dressing changes if they are comfortable.**

2. Assess the external appearance of the initial postoperative dressing and subsequent dressings. **The initial dressing may need to be reinforced. Excess saturation with drainage, blood, or other bodily fluids, dislodgement, or anything unusual about the dressing should be brought to the attention of the health care provider. The appearance of the external portion of the dressing provides information about needed supplies.**

3. Assess the appearance of the wound and drains once the dressing is removed. **Inspection of the wound is important for assessment of the skin and tissues and for determining dressing supply needs. Assessment includes noting signs of infection as evident by redness,**

swelling, foul odor, amount of drainage, color of wound exudate (yellow and viscous would indicate purulent) or unusual pain or tenderness; signs of tissue trauma as evident by swelling or ecchymosis; evidence of bleeding or leakage of tissue fluids from the site; and the position of indwelling catheters, drainage tubes, and the sutures or stabilizing devices closing the wound and supporting the drains.

4. Assess the client's understanding about the postoperative care of the surgical wound site. **It is important to take into consideration the client's ability to understand verbal and written instructions and the cultural and social variations that may affect the delivery of health care and client/family education.**

5. If solutions are to be used on the wound, assess the client's allergy status and test a drop of solution on the skin. **This prevents an adverse reaction.**

▶ DIAGNOSIS

Impaired Skin Integrity

Impaired Tissue Integrity

Risk for Infection

▶ PLANNING

Expected Outcomes:

1. The initial postoperative dressing will be reinforced until changed by the health care provider.
2. The site will be inspected for signs of infection, tissue trauma, position of stabilizing devices (sutures or staples), and drainage tubes.
3. The site will have the appropriate dressing applied.
4. The client/family will verbalize and/or demonstrate understanding and the ability, if indicated, to perform the dressing change and associated wound care of the surgical wound site.

Equipment Needed (see Figure 9-2-1):

- Clean exam gloves
- Container for proper disposal of soiled dressing

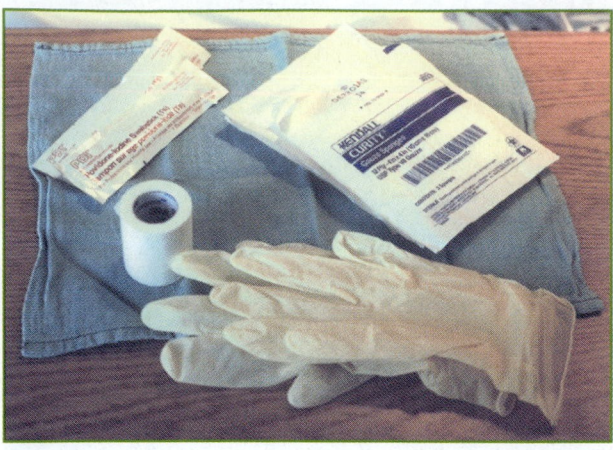

Figure 9-2-1 Gauze sponges, clean gloves, tape, and antiseptic solution are used to change a dry dressing.

- Sterile 4 × 4 gauze pads
- Washcloth (optional)
- ABD pads (optional)
- 2-inch tape (foam or paper)
- Cleaning solution (if ordered)

▶ CLIENT EDUCATION NEEDED:

1. Review where and how to obtain additional supplies.
2. Review how to properly dispose of contaminated dressings.
3. Review discharge instructions which should include how to care for the dressing at home, and when and who to call if the client experiences problems with the dressing change or wound care.
4. Review problems that might occur during dressing changes, including fever, bleeding, infected wound, and pain management.

Estimated time to complete the skill: **5–10 minutes**

▶ DELEGATION TIPS

The application of bandages to the client is not delegated to ancillary personnel. Family members may be taught this skill before the client's discharge. Occasionally, ancillary personnel will be delegated the task of applying a clean dry gauze as skin protection, but the nurse is responsible for the assessment of the integrity of the client's skin.

IMPLEMENTATION—Action/Rationale

Action	Rationale
1. Gather supplies.	1. Promotes a smooth workflow.
2. Provide privacy; draw curtains; close door.	2. Maintains client comfort and privacy while body is exposed during procedure.
3. Explain procedure to client.	3. Provides information about the procedure.
4. Wash hands.	4. Reduces the transmission of microorganisms.
5. Apply clean exam gloves.	5. Promotes infection control and protection from body fluids.
6. Remove dressing and place in appropriate receptacle. Remove soiled gloves with contaminated surfaces inward and discard in appropriate receptacle; apply clean gloves.	6. Dressings and gloves soiled with body fluids are considered contaminated and subject to biohazard disposal in the correct manner per institution protocol. It is standard for the surgeon to do the first postoperative dressing change. The initial dressing is maintained for 24–48 hours postoperatively, unless conditions of the dressing call for contacting the health care provider for a dressing change order. Until the removal of the initial dressing, the nurse will reinforce the dressing as needed. The frequency of the dressing change is dependent upon the needs of the wound and the preference of the health care provider. This will usually be specified in the orders.
7. Assess the appearance of the undressed wound bed for healing.	7. Assess for signs of redness, foul odor, swelling, irritation, drainage, dehiscence, bleeding, or skin breakdown.
8. Remove used exam gloves.	8. Exam gloves that are used to remove the old dressing are considered dirty and should be removed and discarded appropriately.
9. Wash hands.	9. Hands should be washed prior to setting up dressing supplies to reduce the transmission of microorganisms.
10. Set up supplies. Open 4 x 4 gauze packages • If incision requires cleaning (consult orders of health care provider and/or institution policy regarding cleaning incisions), pour cleaning solution on 4 × 4 gauze pads.	10. Following the removal of the dressing, you will have a better idea of what supplies are needed and in what amount. • Remove microorganisms.
11. Apply a new pair of clean exam gloves.	11. This is considered to be a clean procedure after the initial dressing is removed if the skin margins are approximated with the skin closures.

continues

Action	Rationale
12. Cleanse wound if indicated. Grasp the edges of gauze that contains cleaning solution. • **Incision:** Moving from top to bottom, clean incision line first (see Figure 9-2-2). Clean each side of incision, using a new gauze for each swipe. • **Drain:** Using a circular motion, begin at the drain site and clean outward. If additional cleaning is required, obtain a new gauze and clean from drain site outward.	12. Wounds are cleansed from least contaminated to most contaminated.
13. Apply a new dressing: Fold a 4 × 4 gauze pad in half to make a 2 × 4 size. Place the folded gauze pad lengthwise on the wound and tape lightly (see Figure 9-2-3). **Optional:** An ABD pad may be applied on top of the dressing for added protection or for client comfort.	13. Reduces the transmission of microorganisms and protects the incision.
14. Initial the dressing, citing date and time it was changed.	14. Maintains a record of the dressing change for the next nurse.
15. Dispose of dressings appropriately, remove gloves, and then wash hands.	15. Reduces the transmission of microorganisms.
16. Conduct client/family education about the dressing, which may include teaching the dressing technique to the client/family.	16. Educates the client/family and prepares for discharge.

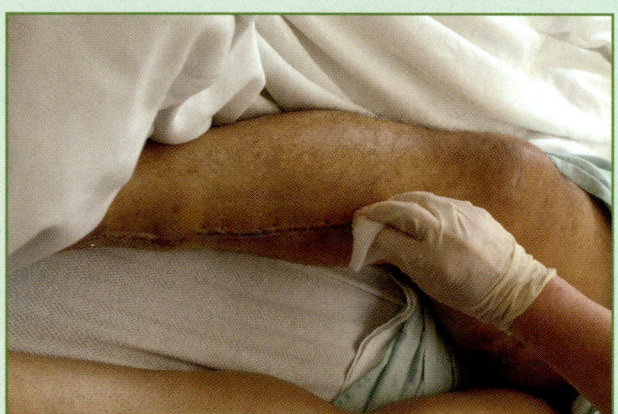

Figure 9-2-2   Clean the suture lines gently, if necessary.

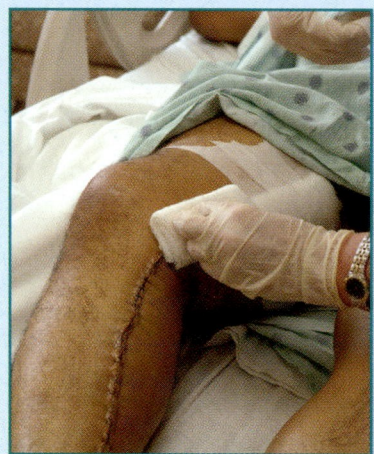

Figure 9-2-3   Apply 4×4 gauze pads, folded in half. Tape the gauze in place.

▶ REAL WORLD ANECDOTES

Josh is a 13-year-old who had an emergency appendectomy. He has stayed overnight on the short stay unit. On rounds, the surgery resident removes the postoperative dressing and inspects the wound, which measures about 3 inches in the right lower quadrant. The wound is stapled and appears clean with no redness present. The resident tells Josh and his mom that the wound can be left open. A postoperative appointment is made to have the staples removed the following week. Josh gets dressed and notices that the staples are being irritated by his clothing. You suggest a light dressing of a folded 4 × 4 gauze and paper tape. You wash your hands, apply clean gloves, and place the dressing to the incision. In addition to their basic postoperative discharge teaching, you review with Josh and his mom the dressing care for the closed wound. They are provided with enough supplies for one dressing a day until the follow-up appointment.

► EVALUATION

1. The initial postoperative dressing was reinforced until changed by the health care provider.
2. The site was inspected for signs of infection, tissue trauma, position of stabilizing devices (sutures or staples), and drainage tubes.
3. The site had the appropriate dressing applied.
4. The client/family verbalized and/or demonstrated understanding and the ability, if indicated, to perform the dressing change and associated wound care of the surgical wound site.

► DOCUMENTATION

Nurses' Notes

Documentation should include the following:

- Date and time dressing done
- Brief description of the wound site
- Brief description of the site care done and dressing applied
- Client comfort before and after dressing change
- Client/family education done and evaluation of the teaching

Document on appropriate flow sheet or electronic medical record (EMR).

► CRITICAL THINKING SKILL

Introduction

It is appropriate to intervene when you observe a potentially risky situation.

Possible Scenario

You are on morning rounds with the surgery team on your unit. You observe the first-year resident forget to wash hands or apply exam gloves before removing the initial wound dressing.

Possible Outcome

The result could be transmission of bacteria to the wound from the resident's unwashed hands, transmission of bacteria from the wound or dressing to the resident's hands, or potential exposure of the resident to body fluids.

Prevention

Refer the resident to the institutional policy for body substance precautions.

Remind the resident to wash his or her hands before the next client contact and offer exam gloves.

► VARIATIONS

Geriatric Variations:

- *Elderly people have thin skin, which can be sensitive to tape and solutions. Special attention should be given to the skin when removing the dressing.*
- *Elderly clients often live alone and may need home health care to assist with dressings.*

Pediatric Variations:

- *Remind all children who are old enough to understand not to touch the dressing site or play with the drainage tubes. Make sure that the dressing is secure and the small child cannot easily pull or dislodge a drain.*
- *Demonstration of wound care on a doll or stuffed animal may be appropriate for younger children.*
- *Young children will require explanation that their wound will heal and that having a wound does not mean that their body part is missing or that their insides will leak out.*
- *Older children can be taught to participate in self-care of dressings. Special bright stickers, bright Band-Aids®, or brightly colored wrap (Coban) are options for securing and decorating children's wound dressings.*

continues

▶ VARIATIONS *(continued)*

Home Care Variations:

- *Where and how to obtain additional supplies should be reviewed with the client/family.*
- *Review proper disposal of contaminated dressings.*
- *Discharge instructions need to include how to care for the dressing at home and when and whom to call if the client experiences problems with the dressing change or wound care.*
- *Problems that might occur should be reviewed with the client/family and include fever, bleeding, infected wound, and pain management during dressing changes.*

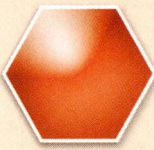

Long-Term Care Variations:

- *Special supplies are most likely not going to be needed for the clean, closed surgical wound other than 4 × 4 or 2 × 2 gauze pads and tape.*
- *Review with the long-term care facility the physician's or qualified practitioner's preference for wound care, as the facility may have to special order or replace with equivalent supplies. If necessary, provide the client with a 3-day supply until supplies can be obtained by the facility.*

▶ COMMON ERRORS

Possible Error:

You apply a dressing to a clean, closed abdominal surgical wound on a young man with quite a bit of abdominal hair. The next day you inspect the wound and find it very difficult to remove the dressing without causing pain to the client because the hair is stuck to the tape.

Prevention:

Instead of tape, consider using Montgomery straps, tubular mesh, or other nonadhesive methods to secure the dressing. If tape is used, first remove the hair from the area to be taped.

▶ NURSING TIPS

- Dressing changes to clean, closed wounds are very simple and require minimal supplies.
- Do not overdress the wound.
- Check the room for supplies before bringing more into the room.
- Order specially needed supplies in advance of the procedure; do not wait until the last minute.
- Client/family education and preparation for discharge begins upon admission.

▶ SPECIAL CONSIDERATIONS

- *Surgical glue or Dermabond has been approved by the Food and Drug Administration for simple wound closure. The glue is applied to an incision or wound that normally would have required stitches. It is applied in at least three thin layers and goes on with a bluish-purple color. It takes about 50 seconds to set and the approximated wound must be held in place to ensure that skin edges line up correctly. Removal is unnecessary as the glue sloughs off in 5–10 days. It cannot be used at joints (elbows, knees), or for hands, feet, mouth, groin, or any moist area.*
- *A surgical zipper is another option being used to close a surgical wound. A surgeon actually zippers the wound closed. This is possible on surgical incisions and lacerations up to 47 cm long. It can be used in orthopedic, neurovascular, heart, abdominal, and gynecologic surgeries. It is applied by two multilayered adhesive support strips attached to the zipper. The strips are lined up on both sides of the surgical incision and the zipper closes, thereby drawing the edges of the wound together. This provides atraumatic closure of the wound.*

Applying a Wet to Damp Dressing (Wet to Moist Dressing)

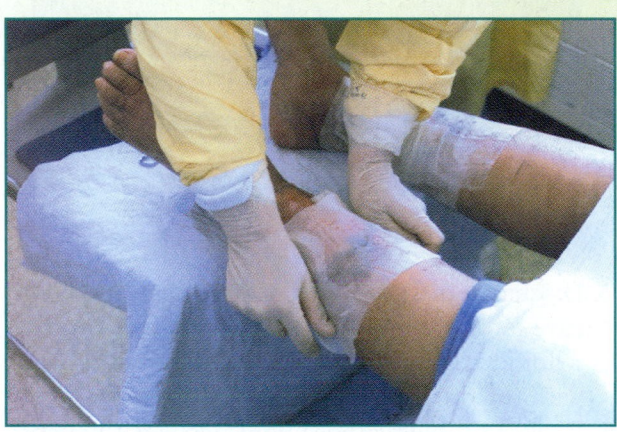

▶ OVERVIEW OF THE SKILL

The purpose of a wet to damp dressing (also known as wet to moist dressing) is to cover and protect the wound, collect exudate, promote healing, and promote light surface debridement. The decision to apply a wet to damp dressing will depend on the wound bed, type of tissue and presence of eschar, amount of exudate, stage of wound healing, state of surrounding tissue, and the presence of infection.

Wound healing is promoted by a warm, moist environment; however, it is imperative to avoid moisture on the surface of the dressing. A wet external dressing can act as a wick with the external environment and draw contamination into the wound. Gentle debridement of a red wound is accomplished with a wet to damp dressing. One must be careful not to apply a dressing so wet that it ends up macerating the surrounding good tissue. Wet dressings are contraindicated in black eschar wounds, where the eschar represents full-thickness tissue destruction, as bacteria will multiply under such a dressing.

The wet to damp or moist dressing consists of gauze, applied wet and allowed to become "near dry" before the next dressing change. Specifics of the wet to damp dressings vary according to the preferences of the surgeon and wound specialist, institutional policy, and outcome measurement standards used to evaluate the effectiveness of the dressing. Current research regarding dressing types and tracking wound outcomes should be reviewed periodically to help make the best dressing treatment choices in the clinical setting. General guidelines for a simple wet to damp or wet to moist dressing are covered in this skill.

▶ ASSESSMENT

1. Assess the client's comfort level **to assess the need for medication before the dressing change. Clients will be more cooperative and less anxious during dressing changes if they are comfortable.**
2. Assess the external appearance of the dressing **to evaluate dressing adequacy as well as needed supplies.**
3. Assess the appearance of the wound and drains once the dressing is removed, noting redness, swelling, purulent drainage, or ecchymosis **to determine the condition of the wound and the effectiveness of the wet to damp dressing.**
4. Assess the client's understanding regarding the dressing changes and wound care **to determine any client teaching needed.**
5. Assess the client's healing response to previous treatments. The effectiveness of the wet to moist application should be routinely reassessed and the treatment modified if healing is not occurring.

▶ DIAGNOSIS

Impaired Skin Integrity

Impaired Tissue Integrity

Risk for Infection

Acute Pain

▶ PLANNING

Expected Outcomes:

1. The site will be inspected for healing (granulation tissue and approximation of edges) and signs of infection and drainage.
2. The site will have the appropriate dressing applied.
3. The procedure will be performed will minimal discomfort to the client.

Equipment Needed (see Figure 9-3-1):

- Clean exam gloves
- Container for proper disposal of soiled dressing
- Sterile gloves
- Moisture-proof gown (optional)
- Sterile towel
- Normal saline or ordered solution
- Sterile bowl
- Sterile 4 × 4 gauze pads, multiple
- Cover sponges or fluffs (optional)
- ABD dressing pads
- 2-inch tape (foam or paper)
- Tubular mesh (optional)
- Montgomery straps (optional)

▶ CLIENT EDUCATION NEEDED:

1. Review where and how to obtain additional supplies with the client/family.
2. Review proper disposal of contaminated dressings.

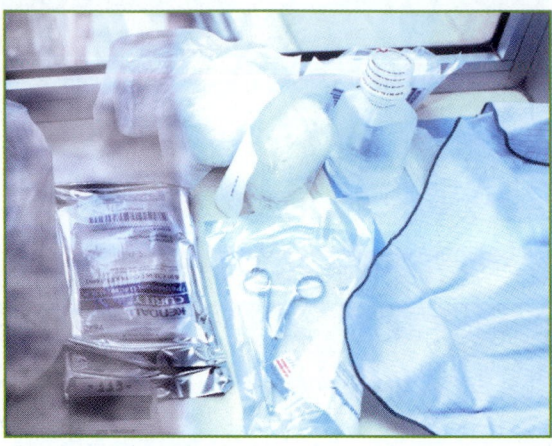

Figure 9-3-1   Sterile bandages, sterile saline, sterile field, and sterile scissors are used to create a wet to damp or moist dressing.

3. Discharge instructions need to include how to care for the dressing at home and when and whom to call if the client experiences problems with the dressing change or wound care.
4. Review problems that might occur with client/family including fever, bleeding, infected wound, and pain management during dressing changes.
5. Encourage handwashing before and after dressing changes, site care, or emptying of drainage collection devices.

Estimated time to complete the skill: **15–20 minutes**

▶ DELEGATION TIPS

Applying a wet to dry dressing requires sterile technique and professional assessment skills and cannot be delegated to ancillary personnel.

IMPLEMENTATION—Action/Rationale

Action	Rationale
1. Review order of health care provider for wound care and gather supplies.	1. Promotes a smooth work flow.
2. Provide privacy; draw curtains; close door.	2. Maintains client comfort and privacy while body is exposed during procedure.

continues

Action	Rationale
3. Explain procedure to client.	**3.** Provides information about the procedure.
4. Wash hands.	**4.** Reduces the transmission of microorganisms.
5. Apply clean exam gloves, a moisture-proof gown, mask, and eye protection, if needed.	**5.** Provides infection control and protection from body fluids. If there is copious drainage or the wound is infected, a gown, a mask, and eye protection should be worn. A mask will also help the nurse when the drainage is foul-smelling.
6. Assess need for pain medication. Pain is rated on a scale from 0 (lowest) to 10 (greatest). Assess need based on quality, pain pattern, location, and last pain medication received. Medicate with analgesic 60 minutes before procedure if medication is to be given orally (PO) or intramuscularly (IM).	**6.** Removal of a wet to damp or moist dressing may be painful to the client, so careful assessment of his or her pain medication needs before the dressing change is important. Allows time for the medication to be absorbed to increase the analgesic effect.
7. Inform client that the dressing is going to be removed.	**7.** This helps prepare client and alleviates anxiety.
8. Remove wet to damp dressing noting number of gauze pads used and place in appropriate receptacle (see Figure 9-3-2).	**8.** The dressing should be removed slowly yet deliberately. It is not recommended to moisten the dressing with saline because this defeats the purpose of the debriding and cleaning action. If it is found that the dressing is extremely dry and removal will result in injury, a small amount of saline to loosen that portion of the dressing is indicated (see Figure 9-3-3). To counteract the problem of an extremely dry dressing, increase the wetness of the dressing or increase the frequency of dressing changes. Count the number of gauze pads so you know how many to use when replacing the dressing.
9. Observe the undressed wound for healing (granulation and approximation of edges), signs of infection (inflammation, edema, warmth, pain), and drainage.	**9.** Allows for evaluation of effectiveness of treatment.
10. Cleanse the skin around the incision if necessary with a clean, warm, wet washcloth.	**10.** Dried blood or drainage on the surrounding skin can be an irritant and a medium for microbes.

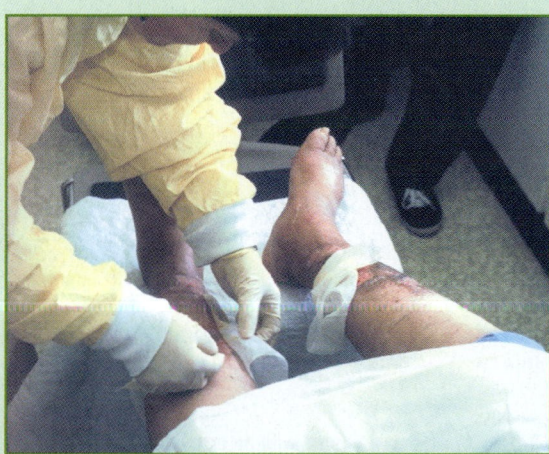

Figure 9-3-2   Carefully remove the old dressing, allowing the old dressing to debride the wound as you pull it away.

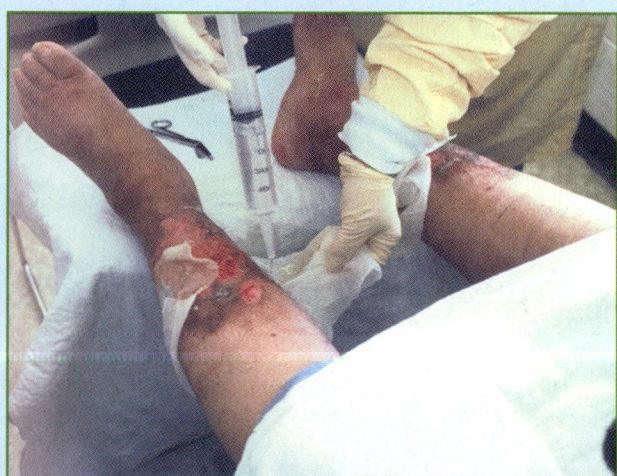

Figure 9-3-3   If the dressing is too dry and removing it will cause injury, use a small amount of saline to loosen the portion of the dressing that adheres too tightly to the wound.

continues

Action	Rationale
11. Remove used exam gloves.	11. Exam gloves used to remove the old dressing are considered dirty and should be removed and discarded appropriately.
12. Wash hands.	12. Reduces the transmission of microorganisms.
13. Set up supplies in a sterile field, including pouring ordered solutions into appropriate containers if indicated for the dressing change.	13. Following the removal of the dressing, you will have a better idea of what supplies are needed and in what amount.
14. Apply sterile gloves.	14. This is a sterile dressing change.
15. Place gauze or packing material to be moistened in the bowl with the normal saline or other solution. • Wring gauze or packing of saline until damp. • Unfold the moist gauze sponge into a single layer. Place gauze loosely to entire wound surface. Do not allow moist gauze to touch the surrounding skin. • Use a cotton swab to place the gauze into tunnels or deep spaces.	15. If a solution is not specified, then normal saline is used. Wounds that are considered dirty or contaminated may have special solutions ordered by the health care provider to moisten the wound packing. Follow institutional guidelines. • Avoid overwringing of the dressing to prevent excessive drying. The dressing should be wet to damp depending upon the depth and size of the wound and the interval of the dressing change. • Overpacking can cause trauma to the wound. Moist gauze to the surrounding skin can cause maceration of the skin. • All wound surfaces need to be covered for debridement.
16. Apply external dressing of dry 4 × 4 gauze pads, cover sponges, fluffs, or ABD pads. • Secure dressing in place with tape, Montgomery straps, or tubular mesh (see Figure 9-3-4).	16. The external dressing is determined by the size and shape of the wound. • Tape for short-term dressings in clients who are not sensitive to adhesives is the method of choice for securing dressings. For long-term dressings or for those who are sensitive to tape, use Montgomery straps or tubular mesh. Tubular mesh is a nice alternative to hold the dressing in place because tape is not involved—the mesh is simply pulled up or down to accommodate the dressing change.
17. Remove gloves and wash hands.	17. Reduces the transmission of microorganisms. Be sure to discard gloves in appropriate receptacle.

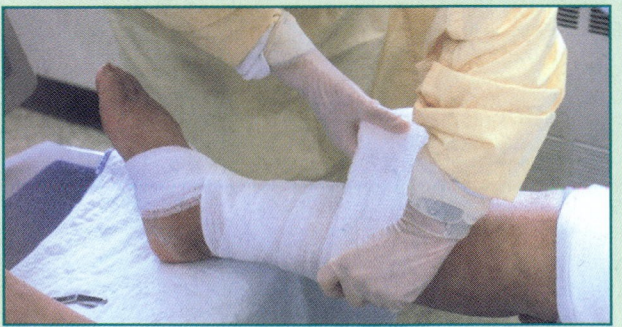

Figure 9-3-4 Wrap the wet gauze with an external dressing of dry gauze bandages.

continues

Action	Rationale
18. Mark the dressing with the date and time it was changed. Initial the dressing.	18. This maintains a record of the dressing change for the next nurse and provides for continuity of care.
19. Conduct client/family education about the dressing, which may include teaching the dressing technique to the client/family.	19. Educates the client/family and prepares for discharge.

▶ REAL WORLD ANECDOTES

Mrs. Gold is a 63-year-old woman who was admitted to the emergency department with a temperature of 103° F, chills, and abdominal pain not adequately controlled with her postoperative pain medication. She is 7 days post a total abdominal hysterectomy and bilateral salpingo-oophorectomy (TAH/BSO) for uterine carcinoma. She was discharged from the hospital 48 hours previously. Her physical exam reveals an elderly woman in pain; she is guarding her abdomen, which is tender to the touch. Her incision is red, with the erythema extending beyond the incision line by 1.5 cm along the length of the wound. Beneath the Steri-Strips, there is evidence of wound dehiscence and purulent drainage at the lower 2 cm of the wound. An IV is started; blood, urine, and wound cultures are taken; and a chest X-ray is obtained. Mrs. Gold is started on a broad spectrum antibiotic intravenously. She is taken to the operating room where her wound is opened and irrigated. Postoperatively, Mrs. Gold's dressing change order reads: "wet to damp dressing changes q 8h, teach client to do dressing."

The plan in the chart is for Mrs. Gold to be discharged home in 48 hours with an open wound and do dressing changes b.i.d., with a follow-up appointment in 1 week with the surgeon. Mrs. Gold has a stated allergy to tape. Montgomery straps are applied over hydrocolloid patches (DuoDerm) to avoid using tape to secure the dressing. Mr. Gold was identified as the one who will be doing the dressing. He is instructed to use sterile technique. The dressing consists of three packages of sterile 4 × 4 gauze pads, which are moistened with sterile normal saline; these are then packed into the wound. The wet gauze pads are then covered with two packages of dry 4 × 4 pads and two ABD pads. The dressing is held securely by the Montgomery straps using safety pins and rubber bands. Mr. Gold demonstrates competence in performing the sterile dressing change. He is given 48 hours of dressing supplies and instructed where to obtain additional dressing supplies in the community. A visiting nurse referral is completed to assess wound healing and to offer support for Mr. Gold in his role as caregiver.

▶ EVALUATION

1. The site was inspected for healing (granulation tissue and approximation of edges) and signs of infection and drainage.
2. The appropriate dressing was applied to the site.
3. The procedure was performed with minimal discomfort to the client
4. The client/family verbalized or demonstrated understanding and the ability, if necessary, to perform the dressing change and associated wound care of the surgical wound site.

▶ DOCUMENTATION

Nurses' Notes

Document:

- Administration of pain medication before dressing change
- Date and time dressing done
- Brief description of the wound site
- Brief description of the site care done and dressing applied
- Client comfort before and after dressing change
- Client/family education done and evaluation of the teaching

Document on appropriate flow sheet or electronic medical record (EMR)

▶ CRITICAL THINKING SKILL

Introduction

Planning ahead can save anxiety and frustration during the dressing change.

Possible Scenario

You have arrived to do a wet to damp dressing change on a client who has a large abdominal wound. You apply your sterile gloves and proceed with the dressing change and suddenly realize that you have not opened the bottle of sterile normal saline.

Possible Outcome

The dressing change is delayed as you remove your sterile gloves, pour the normal saline into the bowl, and go to the supply area to get another pair of sterile gloves. The client becomes more anxious.

Prevention

There are many steps to most dressing changes and reviewing the steps ahead of time will minimize the chance of interruptions due to missed steps. You could also ask a visitor to open the saline and pour it into the container for you.

▶ VARIATIONS

Geriatric Variations:

- *Elderly people have thin skin, which can be sensitive to tape and solutions.*
- *Special attention should be given to the skin when removing the dressing.*
- *Elderly clients often live alone and may require home health care to assist with dressings changes that need to be done in the home setting.*

Pediatric Variations:

- *Remind all children who are old enough to understand not to touch the dressing site. Make sure that the dressing is secure and the small child cannot easily pull or dislodge the dressing.*
- *Demonstration of the wound care on a doll or stuffed animal may be appropriate for younger children.*
- *Young children will require explanation that their wound will heal and that having a wound does not mean that their body part is missing or that their insides will leak out.*
- *Older children can be taught to participate in self-care of dressings.*
- *Special bright stickers, bright Band-Aids®, or brightly colored wrap (Coban) are options for securing and decorating children's wound dressings.*

Home Care Variations:

- *Where and how to obtain additional supplies should be reviewed with the client/family.*
- *Review proper disposal of contaminated dressings.*
- *Discharge instructions need to include how to care for the dressing at home and when and whom to call if the client experiences problems with the dressing change or wound care.*
- *Problems that might occur should be reviewed with client/family and include fever, bleeding, infected wound, and pain management during dressing changes.*

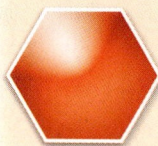

Long-Term Care Variations:

- *Special supplies may need to be ordered. A dressing change order may need to be written by the attending health care provider at the facility.*
- *A review of the specific dressing change procedure may need to be presented to the staff caring for the client at the long-term care facility along with aspects of the home care and geriatric variations mentioned previously.*

▶ **COMMON ERRORS**

Possible Error:

You have just applied a dressing and taped it in place when the client gets up out of bed to ambulate and the dressing falls out onto the floor.

Prevention:

Before placing the bandage, consider how to hold it in place. Assess for skin condition, size of wound area, location, and types of wrap available.

Possible Error:

You have applied your sterile gloves, grab the container of normal saline, and pour the solution into the sterile bowl when you suddenly realize that you have contaminated your sterile gloves by touching the unsterile exterior of the normal saline container.

Prevention:

Mentally review the sequence. If you are concerned about remembering the proper sequence of steps, write notes to remind yourself.

▶ **NURSING TIPS**

- Dressing changes require organization to be done efficiently. Gather data about the dressing change from the following:
  - Shift report
  - Nurses who have cared for client
  - The client/family
  - Chart notes
  - Orders
  - Care map, care plan
  - Observation of the dressed wound
  - Supplies already in room
- Make a list, if necessary, of needed supplies to take into the room.

- If you are going to be in a client's room for some time, let others know so that they can cover your call lights and you can devote your attention to the dressing change.
- When doing very small wet to damp dressing changes, the normal saline can be carefully poured on open packets of sterile 4 × 4 pads, thus by-passing the need for a sterile bowl.
- Order specially needed supplies in advance of the procedure; do not wait until the last minute.
- Client/family education and preparation for discharge begins upon admission.
- Carefully evaluate and communicate client's wound healing response to dressing treatments.
- Consult wound specialist and change treatment as recommended or as ordered.

▶ **SPECIAL CONSIDERATIONS**

- *At times when a small dressing change is performed, a container of sterile water or normal saline with a spout or nozzle may be used to moisten the gauze.*
- *Wet to moist dressings are contraindicated in the presence of eschar as moisture encourages bacterial growth with such wounds.*
- *Wet to moist dressings must be changed frequently enough to avoid drying out, as dried tissue will adhere to the gauze. Wet to moist dressings may not be useful with small wounds since they may require too frequent of changes to maintain moisture.*

Applying a Transparent Dressing

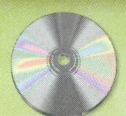

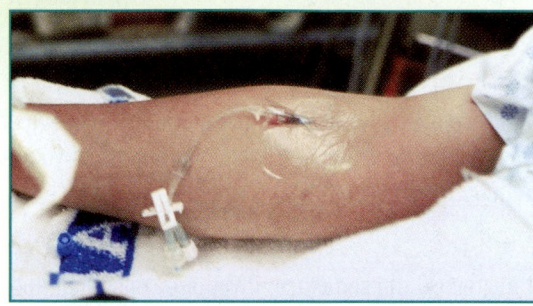

▶ OVERVIEW OF THE SKILL

A transparent dressing may be used on various intravenous, surgical, or wound sites. This type of dressing allows easy visibility of the wound and serves like other dressings in preventing infection and promoting healing by retention of serous products to enhance epithelial growth. These dressings also allow for a tight seal in preventing microorganisms from entering the wound site. Transparent dressings are particularly useful over intravenous (IV) sites in that direct visualization of the IV site is possible, which allows for immediate observation of changes, such as infiltration around the IV sites or inflammation. Transparent dressings generally do not require changes as frequently as other dressings and do not adhere to the wound. Because of their elasticity, transparent dressings mold more easily over body parts, such as joints, and allow clients to use the shower without removal. As with adhesive products, allergic reactions can occur.

▶ ASSESSMENT

1. Question the client regarding any previous reactions to adhesive products (such as latex allergy). **Helps determine allergies or sensitivities that may contribute to discomfort and skin breakdown.**
2. Assess the client's skin and wound site carefully before applying dressing. **Affects which dressings may be used and how the procedure is performed. Establishes a baseline for future comparison.**
3. Assess the client for skin reaction to transparent dressing products (such as latex allergy). **Detecting allergies or sensitivities early will**

alert the nurse to change dressing type and monitor closely.

▶ DIAGNOSIS

Impaired Skin Integrity

Impaired Tissue Integrity

Risk for Infection

▶ PLANNING

Expected Outcomes:

1. The wound site will have promotion of the healing process, such as granulation tissue and adherence of edges.
2. The wound site will be free of signs and symptoms of infection.
3. The client will have no adverse reaction to adhesive material.

Equipment Needed (see Figure 9-4-1):

- Transparent dressing

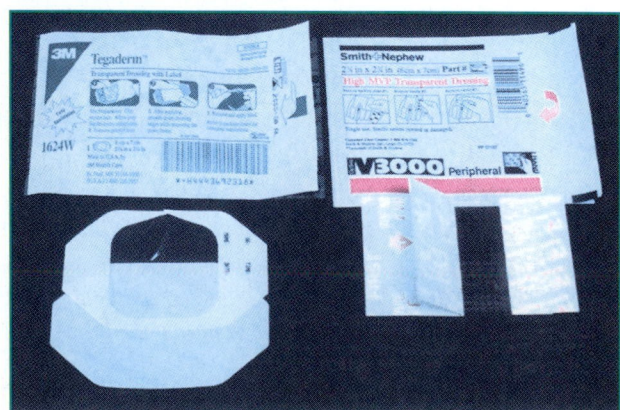

Figure 9-4-1 Transparent dressings

- Examination gloves
- Disposable bag

▶ **CLIENT EDUCATION NEEDED:**

1. Teach the client to report any allergic reactions, such as itching, hives, or inflammation.
2. Teach the client to report whether dressing edges are loose.

3. Teach the client to report any signs of infection, such as redness, pain, or increased swelling.

Estimated time to complete the skill:
5–10 minutes

▶ **DELEGATION TIPS**

Applying a transparent dressing requires the problem-solving and assessment skills of a nurse and cannot be delegated.

IMPLEMENTATION—Action/Rationale

Action	Rationale
1. Review the order of the institutional policy and procedure or standing order for applying a transparency dressing. Provide wound care as ordered.	1. Promotes wound healing and prevention of infection.
2. Check the client's medical record for previous reactions to adhesives and date of last dressing change.	2. Avoids allergic reaction and assesses the need for dressing change.
3. Wash hands.	3. Reduces the transmission of microorganisms.
4. Remove any clothes or coverings from area of dressing change and put on examination gloves.	4. Allows easy access to area needing dressing. Gloves reduce the transmission of microorganisms.
5. Remove old dressing. Hold the client's skin taught, lift the edges of the dressing and, if possible, remove the dressing in the direction of hair growth. If removing the dressing from an IV, stabilize the IV site and remove dressing in the direction of the insertion site.	5. If the skin is held taut, the old dressing will pull off more easily. Following the direction of hair growth will cause less pain for the client. Removing dressing in the direction of insertion site decreases catheter dislodgement.
6. Discard the used dressing in disposable bag.	6. Reduces the transmission of microorganisms.
7. Assess the area of the wound bed for healing (granulation and approximation of edges), signs of infection (inflammation, edema, warmth, pain), and drainage.	7. Allows for evaluation of effectiveness of treatment.
8. Remove the gloves with contaminated surfaces inward and discard in a disposable bag.	8. Reduces the transmission of microorganisms.
9. Open the package with transparent dressing.	9. Allows easy access to dressing.
10. Reglove in clean or sterile gloves per institutional policy and dressing change requirements.	10. Reduces the transmission of microorganisms.

continues

Action	Rationale

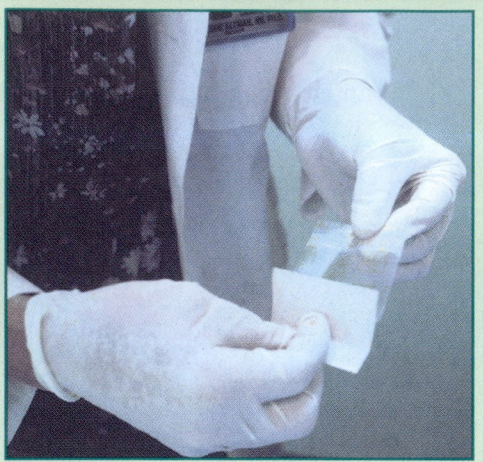

Figure 9-4-2   Remove part of the backing from the transparent dressing.

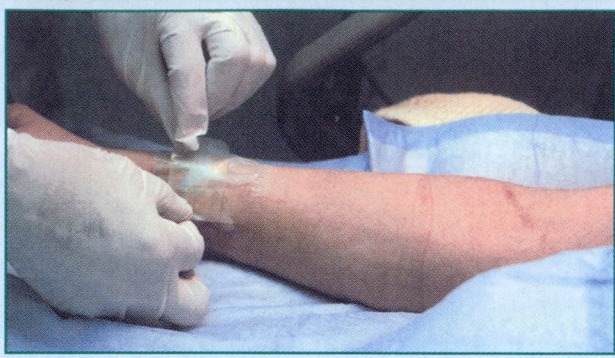

Figure 9-4-3   Place the adhesive side over the area to be covered, sliding smoothly from one side to the other.

11. Grasp the tab on the back and underside of the transparent dressing and separate about 1 inch of the backing from the dressing (see Figure 9-4-2).

11. Applying a small portion of the dressing first allows for better control of dressing and smoother application.

12. Place the adhesive side over the area to be covered; while holding the dressing in place with one hand, with the other hand peel the backing off from the dressing and slowly smooth out the dressing as it is moved over the site (see Figure 9-4-3).

12. If the process of placing the dressing is done in a smooth fashion and small portions at a time, fewer wrinkles and better adherence will occur.

13. Press gently and smooth out any wrinkles.

13. Allows for better adherence and less risk of microorganisms entering under dressing.

14. Reinforce any edges with tape as needed (see Figure 9-4-4).

14. If large dressings are used or are used over movable parts, such as joints, reinforcement may be necessary.

15. Date and initial the dressing.

15. Provides easier communication regarding need for dressing changes. Generally, standards exist requiring routine dressing changes of transparent dressing, such as every third day. Initials provide accountability and maintain a record of the dressing change for the next nurse.

16. Discard old dressing, remove gloves, and wash hand.

16. Reduces the transmission of microorganisms.

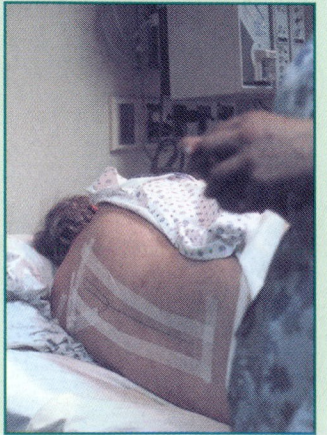

Figure 9-4-4   Reinforce the edges of the transparent dressing with tape, if necessary, to prevent the edges from rolling up or becoming dislodged.

▶ REAL WORLD ANECDOTES

Deon had a transparent dressing over a wound site. The nurse told Deon that he could have a shower with the transparent dressing in place. The nurse did not anticipate how hard Deon would scrub around the sensitive surgical site. The edges of the dressing peeled loose and soapy water entered the site. The site had to be cleaned and the dressing changed immediately after the shower. The wound site was monitored for infection. For subsequent showers, the nurse advised Deon to wrap the area with plastic wrap and reminded him to keep it as dry as possible.

▶ EVALUATION

1. The wound site has the promotion of the healing process, such as granulation tissue and adherence of edges.
2. The wound site was free of signs and symptoms of infection.
3. The client had no adverse reaction to adhesive material.

▶ DOCUMENTATION

Nurses' Notes

- Document on appropriate flow sheet or electronic medical record (EMR).
- Document date and time of dressing change in chart and on dressing.
- Document any signs of allergic reaction or infection, such as inflammation, urticaria, pain, increased warmth, or purulent drainage.

▶ CRITICAL THINKING SKILL

Introduction

You are checking IV sites on the evening shift. You note moisture under a transparent dressing over an IV site.

Possible Scenario

The IV may be leaking around the entry site.

Possible Outcome

First check the IV connection to see whether it is secure. If the IV is in a movable area, such as the anticubital site, reinforcement of the dressing and an arm board may be needed or the IV may need to be moved to another site.

Prevention

Place IVs in stable areas. If a client has veins that are difficult to find and the need exists to use certain IV sites, use an arm board as needed.

▶ VARIATIONS

Geriatric Variations:

- *Older clients have skin that wrinkles easily; therefore, transparent dressings are useful. However, in application it is necessary to keep the skin taut.*
- *Older clients may have skin sensitivity to adhesive products and require paper tape or hypoallergenic tapes.*
- *Because elderly clients have thin, sensitive skin, as adhesives are removed skin may tear. In clients with very sensitive skin, the nurse may need to have alternative choices of dressings.*

Pediatric Variation:

- *Children may experience anxiety at being able to see the wound or IV. If the nurse chooses to use a transparent dressing for increased protection of the wound site, loose gauze, mesh, or other air-permeable external cover can be placed over the transparent dressing to obscure view of the wound.*

continues

▶ VARIATIONS (continued)

Home Care Variations:
- *Transparent dressings are useful in home care settings. They are generally more expensive than other dressings, and, therefore, clients may request to use a different type of dressing.*
- *Teach the caregiver what the wound site should look like, what is normal, and what is not normal.*
- *Outline signs of infection, irritation, or skin breakdown.*
- *Make sure the caregiver knows whom to contact with concerns or questions.*

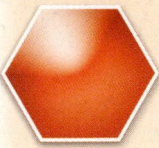

Long-Term Care Variations:
- *Caregivers in long-term settings may not be as familiar with dressing care as those in acute care settings. Assess and teach care providers as needed.*
- *Outline signs of infection, irritation, or skin breakdown.*
- *A dressing order will need to be written by the attending health care provider of the facility.*

▶ COMMON ERRORS

Possible Error:
Skin is not held taut and wrinkles occur under the dressing. This allows for entry of microorganisms, and the dressing does not stay in place.

Prevention:
Plan ahead how you will hold the skin and apply the dressing. Get help if you need extra hands.

Possible Error:
The dressing sticks to itself while it is being opened or placed.

Prevention:
Open dressing carefully. Plan ahead and visualize how the dressing will go on the site prior to opening the dressing. For technique, observe nurses with more experience using the dressings, and practice when possible.

▶ NURSING TIPS

- Use a smooth, slow application to avoid wrinkles.
- Apply a small portion of the dressing first and create firm adhesion with the client's skin before applying the rest of the dressing.

▶ SPECIAL CONSIDERATIONS

- *Be aware that the use of topical medication under an occlusive dressing, such as a transparent dressing, will enhance drug absorption.*
- *It is helpful to work your hand around the dressing as the tab is unraveled. This prevents the dressing from sticking to itself or crimping at the edges. Difficulty in discerning the edge of the transparent dressing when it is on the client reflects a smooth application.*
- *If a transparent dressing is used over an IV site, label the date and time the new dressing was applied.*

Applying a Pressure Bandage

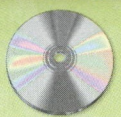

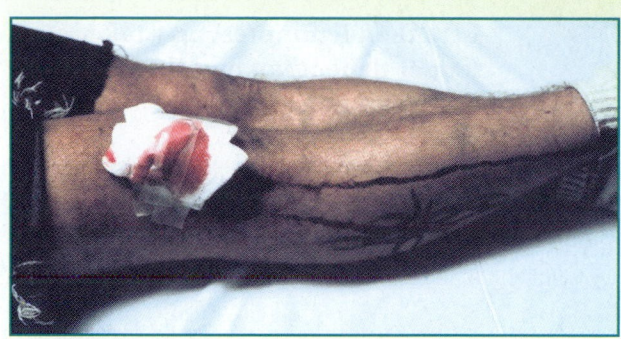

▶ OVERVIEW OF THE SKILL

Pressure dressings are used to prevent or control bleeding. Examples of wounds that require pressure dressings are those from trauma, suicide attempts, arterial puncture sites, or after debridement. The pressure applied with a sterile dressing is used at the puncture site to halt bleeding. Rapid assessment and action is required. Clients with bleeding disorders are especially at risk for uncontrolled bleeding.

▶ ASSESSMENT

1. Observation, rapid assessment of bleeding site, and immediate action are required **to minimize blood loss.**
2. Identification of the origin of bleeding is necessary **to determine the next steps of intervention.**
3. Assessment of vital signs and general client condition is necessary **to detect early signs of shock.** If the client is bleeding profusely, hypovolemic shock may occur. Tachycardia, change in blood pressure (initially elevated, then decreased), and change in color, anxiety/restlessness, and change in level of consciousness may all be indicators of shock. Although a decrease in blood pressure is associated with shock, initially the blood pressure may be increased as a compensatory mechanism. If the client has an underlying medical anticoagulation disorder, adjunct treatment may be necessary.

▶ DIAGNOSIS

Decreased Cardiac Output

Risk for Peripheral Neurovascular Dysfunction

Ineffective Tissue Perfusion

Risk for Deficient Fluid Volume

Impaired Skin Integrity

Risk for Infection

▶ PLANNING

Expected Outcomes:

1. Bleeding is stopped.
2. Circulating blood volume is maintained and the client has no adverse systemic consequences, such as shock.
3. Underlying causes are identified and treated.
4. If there is debridement, sterile technique is used and infection is prevented.
5. If there was a suicide attempt, the client is referred for appropriate treatment.

Equipment Needed:

- Gauze compresses (usually 4 × 4) depending on amount of bleeding
- Sterile gloves
- Roll of gauze or elastic or Ace bandages
- Stethoscope
- Sphygmomanometer
- Scissors
- Tape

▶ **CLIENT EDUCATION NEEDED:**

1. The client should understand the need for pressure.
2. The client should understand the importance of rapid response to minimize blood loss and reduce the possibility of hypovolemic shock in addition to knowing the symptoms of hypovolemic shock.
3. Educating the client will depend on what condition precipitated the need for the pressure dressing, underlying condition of the client, and potential complications associated with the wound, surgery, or trauma.

4. The client and caregivers should know the emergency response and treatment, especially if the client is in an at-risk occupation, or has a bleeding tendency.

Estimated time to complete the skill:
Less than 5 minutes; may take longer depending on other trauma and other sites involved

---

▶ **DELEGATION TIPS**

Applying a pressure dressing requires assessment and intervention by a nurse and cannot be delegated to ancillary personnel.

IMPLEMENTATION—Action/Rationale

Action	Rationale
1. Wash hands (time may not permit this in emergency situations). Immediately put on gloves. Apply additional protective gear including mask, eyewear, and gown, if available, if there is a risk of contact with bodily fluids.	1. Reduces the transmission of microorganisms. In emergency situations gloves will suffice because the priority is to stop the bleeding and prevent complications.
2. Rapidly assess the wound and determine origin of bleeding—either arterial, which is seen as pulsating or spurting bright red blood, or venous, which is seen as oozing or flowing darker blood (see Figure 9-5-1).	2. Arterial bleeds can occur rapidly and cause hemorrhage. Venous bleeds also require quick response but do not lead to life-threatening complications as rapidly.
3. Call for assistance as needed. Notify health care provider of hemorrhage.	3. If large areas of profuse bleeding occur, assistance will be needed and medical orders will be required. If bleeding is life-threatening, the client should never be left alone.

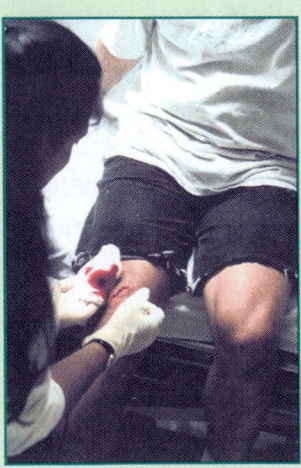

Figure 9-5-1 Assess the wound and determine whether the bleeding is arterial or venous.

continues

Action	Rationale
	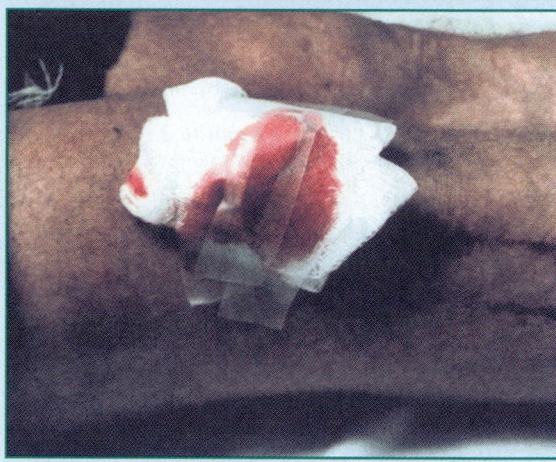

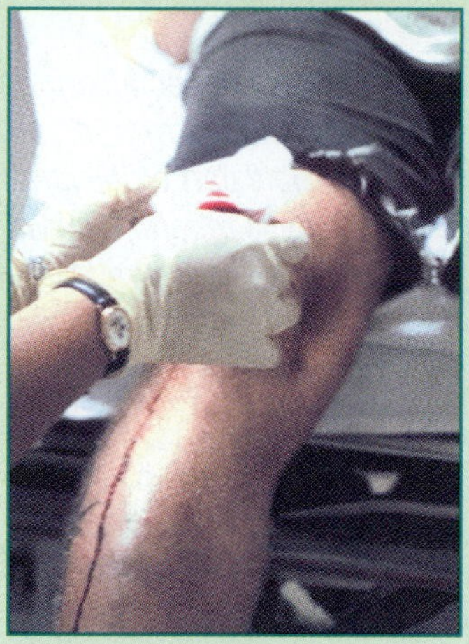

Figure 9-5-2   Completely cover the wound and apply pressure.

Figure 9-5-3   This bandage has become saturated with blood.

Action	Rationale
4. Apply firm pressure with sterile gauze.	4. Pressure will help control bleeding and decrease blood loss.
5. If an extremity is involved, completely cover the wound (see Figure 9-5-2) and if gauze becomes soaked with blood, do not remove but add additional layers and maintain pressure (see Figure 9-5-3). Elevate the extremity.	5. Constant pressure is needed until bleeding has stopped. Elevating the extremity reduces blood flow to the area.
6. Apply tape firmly over site, maintaining pressure.	6. Constant pressure is required until the bleeding stops.
7. Apply an Ace bandage or elastic wrap over the sterile dressings; snugly wrap the elastic bandage and completely cover the wound. Use a figure-eight configuration if wrapping a joint.	7. Elastic wraps allow for more pressure to remain in place for long periods of time.
8. Remove gloves and wash hands.	8. Reduces the transmission of microorganisms.
9. Check the client's pulse distal to the wound.	9. Indicates blood flow to the distal area of an extremity.
10. Assess the client and obtain a complete set of vital signs. Assessing the client's mental status, color, warmth, and capillary refill.	10. Provides an indication of early signs of hypovolemic shock or decreased tissue perfusion.
11. If hemorrhage was large or unexpected, initiate intravenous fluids. Select a site and a needle size that will accommodate blood administration if it becomes necessary.	11. Required for replacement if large volume loss.
12. Monitor vital signs and signs and symptoms associated with blood loss every 15 minutes or more often if necessary.	12. Provides indication of ongoing cardiovascular status.
13. Wash hands.	13. Reduces the transmission of microorganisms.

► REAL WORLD ANECDOTES

Scenario 1

A client with severe rheumatoid arthritis was noted to have had a significant drop in hematocrit and hemoglobin in the 24-hour period following total hip surgery. Because the client was difficult to turn, dressings had been checked with the client in a recumbent position. No blood was noted on the visible part of the sheet. Because the hematocrit and hemoglobin were decreased, a more careful assessment was made regarding blood loss. With the help of another nurse, the client was fully turned, at which point the nurse noted the pressure dressing was soaked with a bloody, serous drainage. The pressure dressing was removed and another one applied, placing a firm surface under the client. This client had probably been oozing all night without notice. This is why it is important to turn clients in positions to assess all the area of dressings and edges.

Scenario 2

A nurse was working alone in a small emergency room. A client came in at about 2:00 a.m. complaining of diarrhea. He stopped at the admission desk and was filling out forms when he suddenly asked to use the bathroom. When he did not come out after 5 minutes, the nurse knocked on the door and went in. The client was sitting on the edge of the toilet. He was pale, diaphoretic, and complained of dizziness and nausea. There was blood in the toilet bowl, on the floor, and soaking the client's trousers. What the client had not had time to mention was that he had undergone an outpatient surgical procedure for hemorrhoids that afternoon. He was bleeding profusely from the anus. The nurse hit the emergency help button and, with the help of the doctor, was able to hold pressure on the bleeding, using gauze pads. She held pressure until suction could be set up and the incisions resutured. The man required several units of blood, but recovered.

► EVALUATION

- The bleeding was stopped.
- Circulating blood volume was maintained and the client had no adverse systemic consequences, such as shock.
- Underlying causes were identified and treated.
- If there was debridement, sterile technique was used and infection was prevented.
- If there was a suicide attempt, the client was referred for appropriate treatment.

► DOCUMENTATION

Nurses' Notes

- Document amount of blood loss, site of blood loss, vital signs, and assessment of client during and following treatment for blood loss.
- Document type of pressure dressings used and amount of time required to stop bleeding.
- Document follow-up treatment.
- Document any education to client and family member.

Document on appropriate flow sheet or electronic medical record (EMR).

► CRITICAL THINKING SKILL

Introduction

Mrs. Foster had a total hip replacement 2 days ago. She is receiving a blood transfusion. When the nurse walks in to check the IV, she notes that the client appears lethargic, can barely speak, and is pale. Ten minutes after a blood transfusion was initiated, Mrs. Foster's blood pressure was 76/54. Three hours earlier it had been 106/70.

Possible Scenario

Initially, the nurse stopped the blood and assessed the client for a blood transfusion reaction. The client was in a recumbent position. Her dressing, a pressure dressing with elastic tape holding it in place, was on the lateral side of her hip and leg. The dressing had been checked a half hour prior and no bleeding was noted. The nurse turned the client to the opposite side and noted a pool of blood under the client, with no evidence on the dressing. Because of the client's position and the thick elastic dressing, nothing was visible until the client was turned to the side. The nurse quickly pulled off the dressing and assessed the site, and noted a small arterial spurt. Rapidly the nurse replaced the dressing, placed pressure on the wound, and called for help. In obtaining more information, it was learned that the client's HemoVac had been pulled out 45 minutes before this episode.

Possible Outcome

The client was placed on oxygen, the hanging blood was sped up, and the physician was notified. A new pressure dressing was applied and a sandbag placed for added pressure. The client was evaluated for return to surgery or cauterization of the small arterial bleed; however, the client was able to be treated with pressure dressings, appropriate intravenous fluids, and additional blood transfusions.

Prevention

Check dressings carefully after any line or drains are pulled that approximate blood vessels. Apply new pressure dressings after drains are pulled. Turn clients in positions to assess all areas of dressings and edges. Use care when nonabsorbent materials are used that do not allow blood seepage to be recognized. In this situation, the blood accumulated under the dressing and under the client.

▶ VARIATIONS

Geriatric Variations:

- *Elderly clients are not able to tolerate large blood losses and may experience complications more readily than younger clients.*
- *The vascular system in elderly clients is not as readily able to compensate with constriction as it is in younger clients.*
- *Bruising may occur more readily after bleeding.*
- *A Medic-Alert bracelet or necklace should be worn if the client has hemophilia, bleeding tendencies, or is receiving anticoagulation therapy.*

Pediatric Variations:

- *It may be difficult to hold a pressure dressing in place with a crying and active child. You may require assistance.*
- *If the child is frightened, you may require the assistance of the child's parents.*
- *If a child has hemophilia or may have bleeding tendencies, it is crucial that the child always wear a Medic-Alert bracelet and understand medical needs.*

Home Care Variations:

- *Teach emergency treatment of bleeding.*
- *If the client has bleeding tendencies or is on anticoagulant therapy, a Medic-Alert bracelet should be worn and significant others taught emergency procedures for acute bleeding.*
- *Encourage the caregiver and other family members to take the basic Red Cross first aid course in their area.*

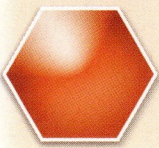

Long-Term Care Variations:

- *Teach emergency treatment of bleeding.*
- *If the client has bleeding tendencies or is on anticoagulant therapy, a Medic-Alert bracelet should be worn and significant others taught emergency procedures for acute bleeding.*
- *Make sure staff members know where first aid supplies are kept and exactly what to do in a bleeding emergency.*

> ▶ **COMMON ERRORS**

Possible Error:

A client's bleeding is undetected.

Prevention:

Be alert to changes in client vital signs, color, or complaints. Look for undetected bleeding sites.

Possible Error:

There is an undetected foreign object in wound.

Prevention:

Determine the cause of the wound. Was glass or other debris involved? Prior to applying pressure, quickly assess the wound for presence of foreign objects. Request an X-ray if needed.

▶ **NURSING TIPS**

- Check all dressings sites, carefully observing all edges of the dressing for signs of bleeding.
- If a pressure dressing is in place, be sure to palpate the dressing with gloves on. Assess for any spongy or watery feel, which may indicate trapped bleeding under the dressing.
- Assess the area distal to the bleed for inadequate perfusion.
- Clients may require pressure dressings for non-emergency situations, such as following the access of the radial artery to obtain an arterial blood sample. In this situation pressure should be applied over the site for 5 minutes with sterile gauze and using gloves. Pulses and capillary refill distal to the artery should be assessed after the procedure and periodically.
- If the bleeding was unexpected and a large amount of blood was lost, the client should be monitored carefully for hypovolemic shock, and appropriate protocol followed for hypovolemic shock.
- If bleeding occurred following debridement, pressure dressings should be applied and any seepage of blood should be outlined on the dressing to track any continued bleeding. If the dressing is in an area not readily observed, the client should be moved to enable the nurse to note any drainage leaking under the client.
- Avoid use of elastic bandages if client has a history of latex allergy, rash, or urticaria.

▶ **SPECIAL CONSIDERATIONS**

- *It is important to assess if the client is on anticoagulation therapy or has any systemic disease (hemophilia, sickle cell anemia) that would further complicate the bleeding wound.*

Changing Dressings Around Therapeutic Puncture Sites

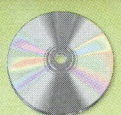

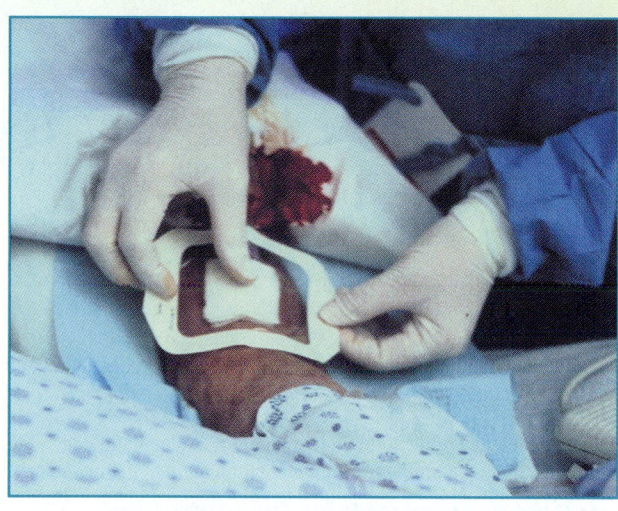

▶ OVERVIEW OF THE SKILL

Therapeutic puncture is a term applied to any procedure in which the client's skin is punctured for diagnostic or therapeutic purposes. As a result of the procedure, there may exist one or more puncture wound sites or an indwelling device remaining in place such as an IV catheter, percutaneous indwelling central catheter (PICC) line, triple lumen catheter (TLC), external long-term venous access device (Hickman, Broviac, Groshong catheters), or percutaneously inserted drainage tubes (biliary or nephrostomy). The puncture site(s) will need dressings for one or more of the following reasons: to apply temporary pressure, protect the site, contain drainage, and/or secure, support, and stabilize any indwelling device. The dressing may be short term (24–48 hours) for those sites that do not have an indwelling device, or the dressing may be a long-term, recurring process as with dressings around indwelling devices. Agency or institutional policy will dictate the frequency of the dressing change.

▶ ASSESSMENT

1. Assess the client's comfort level **to determine whether any premedication will be needed.**
2. Assess the appearance of the therapeutic puncture site **to evaluate for signs of infection, tissue trauma, or ecchymosis.**

3. Assess the position and condition of any indwelling catheters, drainage tubes, and the sutures or stabilizing devices supporting the indwelling items **to evaluate the patency and stability of the indwelling device.**
4. Assess the client's understanding about the care of the therapeutic puncture site **to determine client teaching needed.**

▶ DIAGNOSIS

Impaired Skin Integrity

Impaired Tissue Integrity

Risk for Infection

▶ PLANNING

Expected Outcomes:

1. The therapeutic puncture site will be free from infection, redness, swelling, or ecchymosis.
2. The therapeutic puncture site will be cleaned and dressed appropriately.
3. The client will verbalize or demonstrate understanding about the therapeutic puncture site.

Equipment Needed:
Dressing Removal and Site Inspection (all therapeutic puncture sites)

- Clean exam gloves

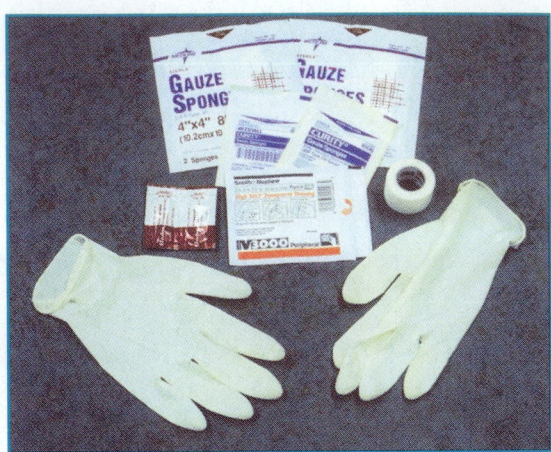

Figure 9-6-1 Transparent dressing, gauze sponges, gloves, tape, and povidone-iodine ointment

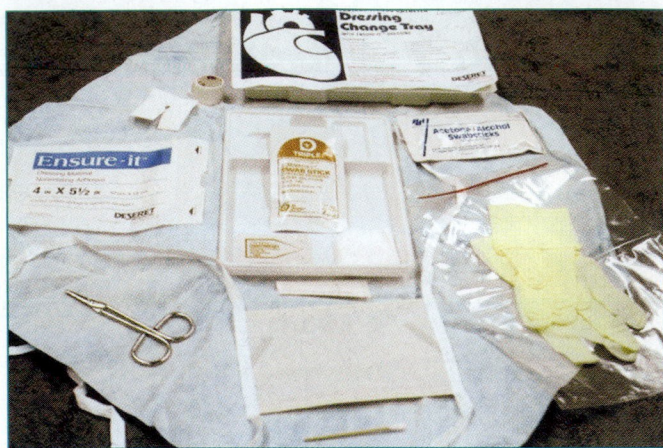

Figure 9-6-2 Central venous catheter dressing change kit

- Container for proper disposal of soiled dressing
- Masks for nurse and client for central line care

Dressing Applications for Peripheral IV Cannulas Newly Inserted (see Figure 9-6-1)

- Clean exam gloves
- Transparent semipermeable dressing (TSM) or sterile 2 × 2 gauze pad
- Tape

Dressing Applications for PICC Line, TLC or Single Subclavian Line, and Central Venous Access Devices Needing Redressing (see Figure 9-6-2)

- Clean exam gloves
- Sterile gloves
- Masks for nurse and client
- Central venous catheter dressing change kit

Dressing Applications for Peripherally Inserted Drainage Tubes (nephrostomy tubes, biliary tract tubes)

- Clean exam gloves
- Povidine-iodine swabs or other wound-cleaning solution and sterile swabs (as per agency protocol)
- Alcohol swabs

- Small sterile container
- Sterile saline
- Sterile cotton-tip applicators
- Steri-Strips
- 4 × 4 gauze pads
- Tape

Dressing Applications for Puncture Sites Following Diagnostic Procedures (angiogram, thoracentesis, paracentesis, lumbar puncture)

- Clean exam gloves
- Band-Aids® (latex-free, if necessary)
- 4 × 4 gauze pads
- 2 × 2 gauze pads
- Latex-free tape
- Sandbag (optional)

▶ CLIENT EDUCATION NEEDED:

1. Teach the client or caregiver to monitor the site for pain, redness, swelling, or purulent drainage. This is especially important if the client will go home with a therapeutic device in the puncture site.

Estimated time to complete the skill:
2–15 minutes, depending on procedure being performed

▶ DELEGATION TIPS

Dressing changes around therapeutic puncture sites require assessment and the use of aseptic technique by a nurse. This skill is not delegated to ancillary personnel.

IMPLEMENTATION—Action/Rationale

Action	Rationale

Dressing Removal and Site Inspection (all therapeutic puncture sites)

1. Review order of health care provider, institutional policy/ procedures, or standing orders and gather supplies.

2. Provide privacy; draw curtains; close door.

3. Explain procedure to client.

4. Wash hands and set up supplies.

5. Apply clean exam gloves; nurse and client apply mask for central line dressing removal.

6. Remove dressing and place dressing in appropriate receptacle (see Figure 9-6-3).

Dressing Applications for Peripheral IV Cannulas Newly Inserted

7. Place a TSM dressing (Op-site or Tegaderm) over the newly placed cannula (see Figure 9-6-4).

---

1. Institutional policy/procedures dictate the frequency of changing and supplies needed. Having all supplies in the room increases consistency of client care.

2. Maintains client comfort and privacy while body is exposed during procedure.

3. Providing information about the procedure can help reduce client anxiety.

4. Reduces the transmission of microorganisms and promotes organization.

5. Provides infection control and protection from body fluids.

6. Dressings and gloves soiled with body fluids are considered contaminated and subject to biohazard disposal in the correct manner per institution protocol.

7. Reduces the transmission of microorganisms. TSM dressings anchor the cannula with their adhesive properties as well as provide for visualization of the site. The dressing is left intact until a new cannula is placed, usually every 48–72 hours or as needed for signs of phlebitis or infiltration. The dressing must be changed if it becomes wet, soiled, or loose. Check institutional policy.

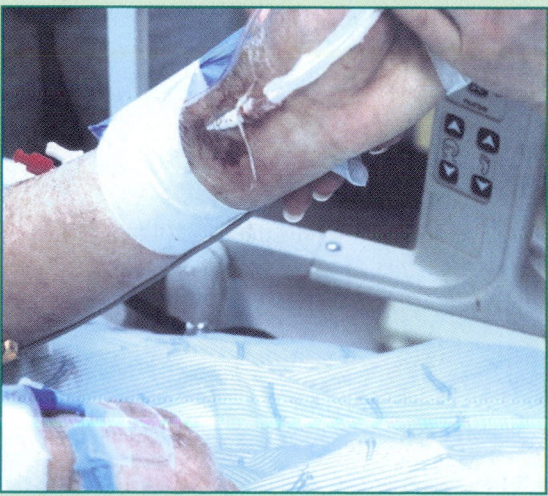

Figure 9-6-3 This is an example of a transparent dressing that should be removed and replaced. Note the soiled transparent dressing holding the cannula in place. Note how the edges have rolled, exposing the cannula.

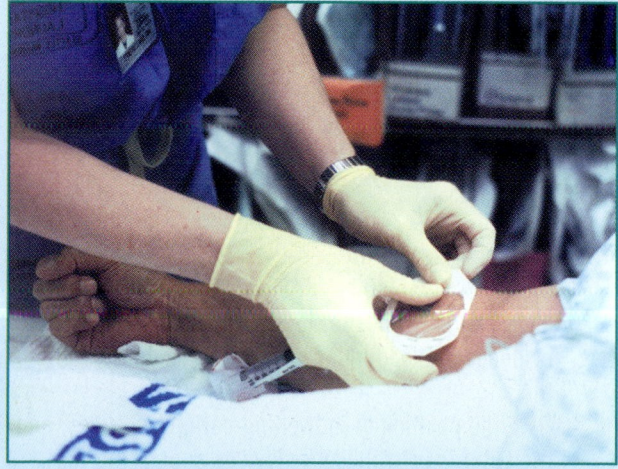

Figure 9-6-4 Place a new transparent dressing over the cannula.

continues

Action	Rationale

Dressing Applications for Peripheral IV Cannulas Newly Inserted *continued*

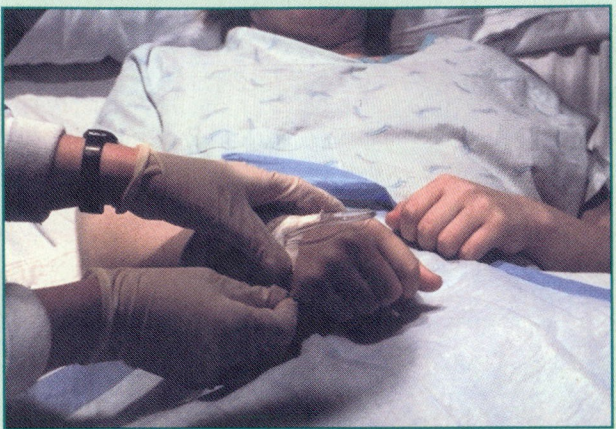

Figure 9-6-5 Tape the hub of the cannula and tubing in place.

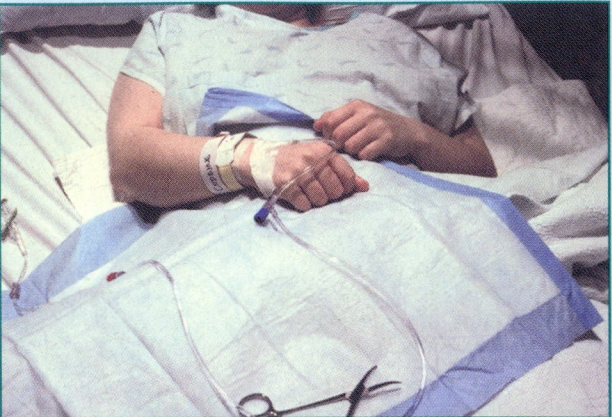

Figure 9-6-6 Tape is not considered to be sterile so it must be placed over the transparent dressing.

8. Tape the hub of the cannula and connected tubing in place externally over the TSM dressing (see Figures 9-6-5, 9-6-6, and 9-6-7).

8. Taping should be on top of the TSM dressing because tape is not considered sterile next to the newly placed IV cannula. Taping anchors the hub and tubing so as to avoid pulling that might lead to dislodging or phlebitis.

9. Discard dressings, remove gloves, and wash hands.

9. Reduces the transmission of microorganisms.

10. Document the time and date of the dressing.

10. Provides information related to when the dressing was done. This can be written on the label provided with the TSM dressing and applied to the dressing site, or it can be written on the treatment sheet or progress notes.

Dressing Applications for PICC Line, TLC or Single Subclavian Line, and Central Venous Access Devices Needing Redressing

11. Review institutional policy for dressing change procedure.

11. Ensures protocol is followed.

12. Repeat Actions 1 to 5.

12. See Rationales 1 to 5.

13. Hold tubing and remove dressing in the direction of the insertion site. Be careful not to dislodge the catheter (see Figure 9-6-8).

13. Removing dressing in the direction of the insertion site decreases chance of catheter dislodgement.

14. Observe site (see Figure 9-6-9).
   • Check for complaints of pain, redness, swelling, purulent drainage, unusual tenderness, ecchymosis, or evidence of bleeding or leakage of tissue fluids from the site.
   • Note the position of indwelling catheters, tubes, and the sutures or stabilizing devices supporting the indwelling items.

14.
   • To evaluate for signs and symptoms of infection or tissue trauma.

   • To evaluate the patency and stability of indwelling devices.

continues

Action	Rationale

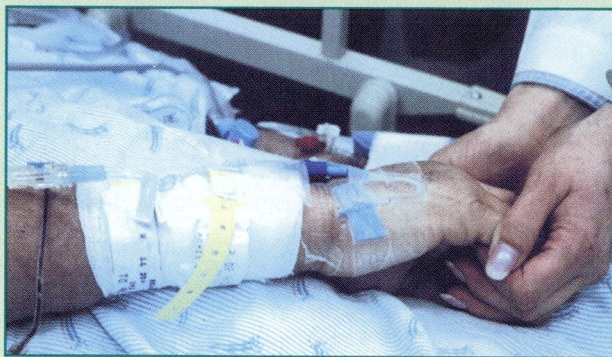

Figure 9-6-7 This cannula has been covered with a transparent dressing. The tubing has been securely taped so it will not become dislodged.

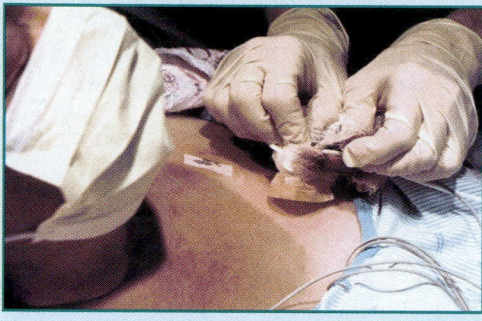

Figure 9-6-8 Removal of a central venous dressing.

15. Discard dressing and remove gloves.

16. Open dressing tray and apply sterile gloves.

17. Clean exit site according to institution policy. Most use povidone-iodine. Clean from insertion site to the periphery using a circular motion. Cleanse a 2.5- to 5.0-cm (1- to 2-inch) area. (see Figure 9-6-10). Cleanse two more times if needed. Allow for a 2-minute contact with site.

18. If povidone-iodine was used, remove dried povidone-iodine with alcohol swabs, using same circular motion as described previously. Allow alcohol to dry.

15. Reduces the transmission of microorganisms.

16. Dressing changes on central lines are sterile procedures.

17. Cleansing from insertion site out to periphery decreases microorganism entering insertion site. Povidone-iodine decreases skin microbes. Chlorhexidine gluconate may be used to cleanse site if client is sensitive to povidone-iodine solution. The chlorhexidine gluconate is removed with sterile saline.

18. Povidone-iodine solution may be irritating to the skin. (Avoid use if clients have history of iodine allergy.)

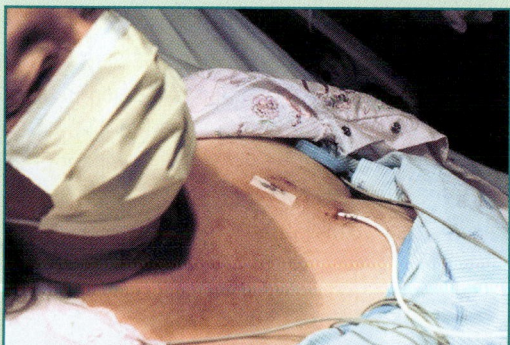

Figure 9-6-9 Inspect insertion site for redness, drainage, and swelling.

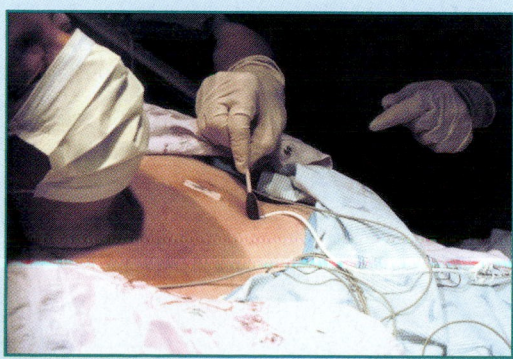

Figure 9-6-10 Cleanse the site with povidone-iodine.

continues

Action	Rationale
Dressing Applications for PICC Line, TLC or Single Subclavian Line, and Central Venous Access Devices Needing Redressing *continued*	
19. Apply dressing to site. **PICC Line:** • Apply a TSM dressing. The site may also be over-wrapped with a continuous gauze wrap such as Kling or Kerlix for client comfort and protection. **Triple Lumen Catheter:** • Apply a TSM dressing. **External Long-Term Venous Access Device, Tunneled with Cuff:** • Apply a TSM dressing.	19. • TSM dressing allows for visualization of site. • TSM dressing allows for visualization of site. • TSM dressing allows for visualization of site.
20. Apply necessary tape to indwelling line or tubing.	20. Ensures stability and prevents tugging on line.
21. Remove mask from client. Dispose of equipment. Remove gloves and mask. Wash hands.	21. Reduces the transmission of microorganisms.
22. Conduct client/family education about the dressing, which may include teaching care of the long-term venous access device.	22. Educates the client/family and prepares for discharge.
Dressing Applications for Peripherally Inserted Drainage Tubes (nephrostomy tubes, biliary tract tubes, and similar tubes)	
23. Repeat Actions 11 to 18.	23. See Rationales 11 to 18.
24. Apply dressing. Apply folded gauze under tube. Apply one or two layers of flat gauze pads on top of tube. Tape dressing securely. Variation: If body fluids from the cavity being drained are leaking from around tubing site, a protective barrier such as Duoderm may be applied around the tube to protect the skin from the drainage.	24. Size of gauze to use when a dressing is applied around a tube is determined by the size, location, and position of the tube. Some tubes are flat against the body and need minimal support; other tubes protrude and are stiff and need support of the dressing for client comfort and tube support.
25. Apply necessary tape to tube.	25. Ensures stability and prevents tugging on tube.
26. If indicated, empty or change the drainage collection container and record the amount in the appropriate location.	26. Emptying of drainage collection containers is often done along with the dressing change. Documentation of the amount and nature of the drainage is an important aspect of the care of a client with indwelling drains. Removal of the drain often depends upon documentation of decreasing amount of drainage.
27. Dispose of equipment. Remove gloves and mask. Wash hands.	27. Reduces the transmission of microorganisms.
28. Conduct client/family education about the dressing, which may include teaching care of the drain site to the client/family.	28. Educates the client/family and prepares for discharge.

continues

Action	Rationale
Dressing Applications for Puncture Sites Following Diagnostic Procedures (angiogram, thoracentesis, paracentesis, lumbar puncture, needle biopsy sites)	
29. Review agency/institutional policy for dressing change procedure.	29. The basic technique is described; however, there may be an agency/institutional policy that deviates from this one.
30. Repeat Actions 1 to 4.	30. See Rationales 1 to 4.
31. Apply clean gloves unless sterile gloves are specifically indicated.	31. Sterile gloves may be indicated for some clients.
32. Observe site.	32. Assessment includes noting signs of infection as evident by redness, swelling, purulent drainage, or unusual tenderness; signs of tissue trauma as evident by swelling or ecchymosis; and evidence of bleeding or leakage of tissue fluids from the site.
33. Apply dressing to site. **Lumbar Puncture:** • Band-Aid® is applied following pressure to the site for a brief period. **Thoracentesis:** • Apply sterile petrolatum gauze, 4 × 4, and 2-inch tape. **Paracentesis:** • Apply several thicknesses of 4 × 4 gauze as a bulky dressing and tape to secure. **Angiography:** • A Band-Aid® or 4 × 4 gauze pad is placed on the site following a period of pressure being applied to achieve homeostasis of the site. Variation: A sandbag may be ordered to be applied directly to the site. **Needle Biopsy Sites:** • Tape a Band-Aid® or 2 × 2 gauze in place.	33. • The puncture wound is small, and a Band-Aid® is sufficient. • The dressing needs to be occlusive to air to avoid a potential pneumothorax. Two-inch foam tape works well. • A bulky dressing is needed because often the ascitic fluid leaks from the puncture site, especially if paracentesis is done routinely. • Involves a puncture to large vessels, usually the femoral artery or vein or the brachial artery or vein. A Band-Aid is sufficient once the artery or vein is stabilized after a period of compression. • A 5-lb. sandbag may be applied for added pressure for a brief period. This is optional and determined by the institutional policy. • A Band-Aid® or 2 × 2 gauze taped in place is sufficient because the puncture sites are small.
34. Dispose of equipment, remove gloves, and wash hands.	34. Reduces the transmission of microorganisms.
35. Conduct client/family education about the dressing and any procedure-specific activity limitations or positioning requirements.	35. Educates the client/family.

► REAL WORLD ANECDOTES

Mrs. Jones presented to the laboratory for routine lab work, including a prothrombin time. The nurse drew her blood and placed a cotton ball and tape dressing over the puncture site. As Mrs. Jones was putting on her coat, she noticed blood soaking through her shirt sleeve. Mrs. Jones sat down while the nurse applied pressure over the puncture site for 5 full minutes. The nurse then redressed the site with a pressure dressing and advised Mrs. Jones to monitor the dressing for bleeding and not to remove the dressing until that evening. Mrs. Jones's prothrombin was later found to be quite elevated.

► EVALUATION

- The therapeutic puncture site remains free from infection, redness, swelling, or ecchymosis.
- The therapeutic puncture site is clean and dressed appropriately.
- The client can verbalize or demonstrate understanding about the therapeutic puncture site.

► DOCUMENTATION

Nurses' Notes

Document on appropriate flow sheet or electronic medical record (EMR):
- Date and time dressing was done
- Brief description of the puncture site including any unusual findings
- Brief description of the site care done and dressing applied
- Client/family education done and evaluation

► CRITICAL THINKING SKILL

Introduction

Be aware of all potential sources of contamination in the environment.

Possible Scenario

You are doing the dressing change on a double lumen Hickman catheter placed in Mr. Beeson for chemotherapy. He had his chemotherapy 7 days ago and today his absolute neutrophil count is 450. You have applied your mask and gloves and have removed the old dressing. Mr. Beeson is happy to have you attending to him because his family lives 200 miles away and he gets lonely. He is quite talkative. You proceed to cleanse the site and suddenly realize that the client has his head turned in your direction, is not wearing a mask, and is talking over the site as you clean.

Possible Outcome

You ask the client to turn his head in the other direction and, realizing that you have an extra sterile towel opened on your sterile field, you carefully drape the client's head as you explain to him what you are doing and the rationale. With his neutrophil counts down, he is at risk for developing an infection and should not be breathing on his Hickman site.

Prevention

It is important to assess the surrounding conditions during dressing changes. Clients, families, and support staff may not understand the rationale behind your actions and may inadvertently compromise the dressing change. In the preceding situation, either covering Mr. Beeson's face with a towel or having him don a mask would prevent further contamination of the site. A thorough cleaning would then be required to protect Mr. Beeson from infection.

► VARIATIONS

Geriatric Variations:
- *Elderly people have thin skin, which can be sensitive to tape and solutions.*
- *Special attention should be given to the surrounding skin when removing the dressing around the exit site.*
- *If the skin appears to be sensitive to the iodine, this should be reported to the health care provider and this step eliminated.*
- *Elderly clients often live alone and may require home health care to assist with dressings and management of drainage tubes that need to be done in the home setting.*

continues

▶ VARIATIONS *(continued)*

Pediatric Variations:
- *Remind all children who are old enough to understand not to touch the therapeutic puncture site or play with the drainage tubes.*
- *Make sure that any tubing is secure and the small child cannot easily pull or dislodge the drain.*
- *Older children can be taught to care for the drainage tubes.*
- *Young children will require explanation that their puncture wound will heal and that their insides will not leak out of the wound.*
- *Special bright Band-Aids® are an option to cover the puncture sites of children.*

Home Care Variations:
- *Where and how to obtain additional supplies should be reviewed with the client/family.*
- *Review proper disposal of contaminated dressings.*
- *If the therapeutic puncture was performed as an outpatient or short-stay procedure, discharge instructions need to include how to care for the puncture site at home and when and whom to call if the client experiences problems with site management at home.*
- *Problems that might occur should be reviewed with the client/family and include the following:*
  —Fever
  —Bleeding, internally or externally from an angiography site
  —Leakage from paracentesis or around biliary and nephrostomy tubes
  —Leakage and possible headache from lumbar puncture
  —Difficulty breathing from thoracentesis

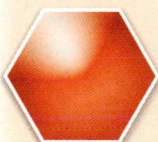

Long-Term Care Variations:
- *Special supplies may need to be ordered.*
- *A dressing change order may need to be written by the attending health care provider at the facility.*

▶ COMMON ERRORS

Possible Error:
While dressing a newly placed IV cannula, you first secure the hub with tape that you had in your pocket, then apply the TSM dressing over the tape, thereby compromising the sterility of the site.

Prevention:
Tape the hub after placing the TSM dressing. The TSM dressing will preserve the sterility of the puncture site and prevent contamination by the tape.

▶ NURSING TIPS

- When dressing a newly placed IV, have all the supplies for the dressing ready to apply. Lack of planning at this phase can lead to an easily dislodged IV.

- If the health care provider is performing a therapeutic puncture at the bedside or in the clinic, anticipate the dressing needs so the correct dressing can be applied postprocedure.
- Familiarize yourself with the institution's policy and procedure for care of the specific puncture site.

- Before doing a dressing change for the first time around a drainage tube, review the progress notes, treatment sheet, or care map for care tips. Ask colleagues because they are a good source of information if they have cared for the client in the past; ask the client what has been comfortable with regard to the dressing. Then view the dressing, assess room for leftover unopened supplies, and gather needed supplies.

- If home care of the therapeutic puncture site is necessary, identify who is going to do the dressing or site care. If an agency referral is needed to provide for the client's dressing care needs, start this process as early as possible.
- Check aging protocol for use of antiseptic solutions.

> ► **SPECIAL CONSIDERATIONS**

- The use of topical medication under an occlusive dressing, such as a transparent dressing, will enhance drug absorption.
- A larger dressing may be required if the client is confused and there is risk of contamination to the puncture site.
- When venipuncture is performed in the field, sterile technique may be compromised because of field conditions. As soon as possible, cleanse the area and apply a sterile dressing. Check institution policy regarding site change.

Irrigating a Wound

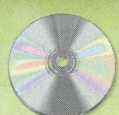

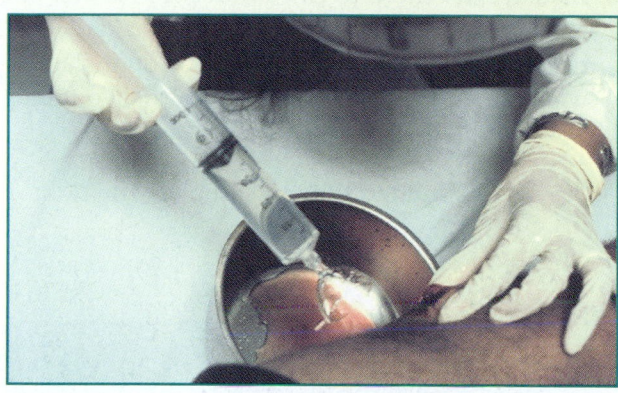

▶ OVERVIEW OF THE SKILL

Wound irrigation is the process of washing debris, drainage, or exudate out of the wound to promote healing. The fluid used to irrigate a wound varies depending on the health care provider's orders. Fluids commonly used include normal saline and specially prepared antibiotic solutions. Wounds that require irrigation also vary. They may be simple open lacerations; tunneled pressure ulcers; or complex, open abdominal wounds extending down to the abdominal fascia. Wound irrigation is a sterile procedure because the skin's integrity, the body's primary defense against infection, has been breached. The nurse must take care not to contaminate the wound, but must also take care not to become contaminated with wound drainage.

▶ ASSESSMENT

1. Assess the current dressing **to determine what equipment will be needed to replace it with a clean dressing and whether the dressing has been adequate to protect the wound and contain any drainage or exudate.**
2. Assess the client to determine whether he or she is able **to understand the need for the wound irrigation and cooperate with the procedure.**
3. Assess whether the client has concerns about pain or body image regarding this wound and the irrigation **to determine what client teaching and support will be most effective.**
4. Assess the client's environment **to ensure whether the necessary equipment and**

supplies are available, including irrigant, hand-washing facilities, and an adequate work area to lay out supplies and establish a sterile field.

▶ DIAGNOSIS

Impaired Skin Integrity

Risk for Infection

Acute Pain

▶ PLANNING

Expected Outcomes:

1. The wound will be free of exudate, drainage, and debris.
2. The wound will be free of signs and symptoms of infection.
3. The procedure will be performed with a minimum of trauma and pain to the client.

Equipment Needed (see Figure 9-7-1):

- Sterile gloves
- Disposable gloves
- Gown
- Mask with protective eye gear
- Sterile irrigation kit (basin, piston irrigation syringe, solution container)
- Irrigation solution (per health care provider's order)
- Waterproof pad
- Sterile dressing material to redress the wound
- Moisture-proof container or bag for use after the irrigation procedure

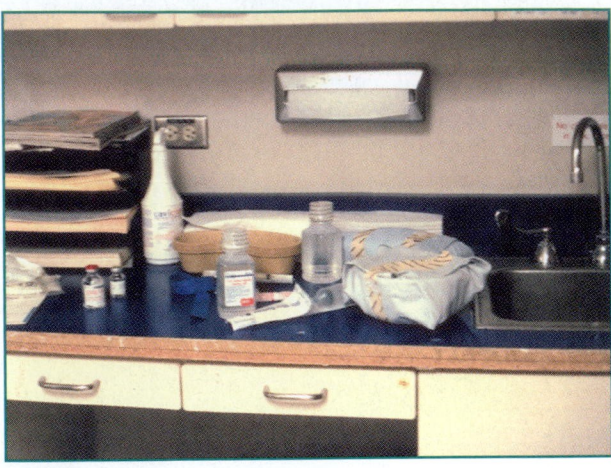

Figure 9-7-1 Sterile basin, sterile irrigating solution, and sterile syringes are used to irrigate a wound.

▶ **CLIENT EDUCATION NEEDED:**

1. Instruct the client about the reason for the wound irrigation and answer any questions the client may have.
2. Explain to the client the reason for the sterile procedure and ways the client can assist in maintaining the sterile field.
3. Instruct the client to call a nurse for further assistance if the dressing becomes soaked with drainage. A dressing that is wet through can wick infectious agents through to the wound.

Estimated time to complete the skill:
20–30 minutes

▶ **DELEGATION TIPS**

Wound irrigation requires nursing assessment, aseptic technique, and monitoring of wound healing. This procedure is not delegated to ancillary personnel.

IMPLEMENTATION—Action/Rationale

Action	Rationale
1. Confirm the health care provider's order for wound irrigation and note the type and strength of the ordered irrigation solution.	1. Wound irrigation is a dependent nursing action that requires a medical order stating the type of solution to be used.
2. Assess the client's pain level and medicate if needed with analgesic 60 minutes before the procedure if the medication is to be given orally (PO) or intramuscularly (IM).	2. Allows time for medication to be absorbed to increase the analgesic effect.
3. Explain the procedure to the client.	3. Helps to decrease the client's anxiety and increase the client's cooperation.
4. Place a waterproof pad on the bed. Assist the client onto the pad. Then assist the client into a position that will allow the irrigant to flow through the wound and into the basin from the cleanest to dirtiest area of the wound.	4. Positioning of the client and placement of a waterproof pad will decrease contamination of bed linen.
5. Wash hands and put on clean gloves. Apply gown, and mask with protective eye gear if splashes from wound fluid or blood are anticipated. Remove and discard old dressing.	5. Gloves reduce the transmission of microorganisms. Gown and mask with protective eye gear protects the nurse from splashes of wound fluid or blood.
6. Assess the wound: measure length and depth, appearance, and note quality, quantity, color, and odor of drainage.	6. Provides assessment of the status of the wound.

continues

Action	Rationale

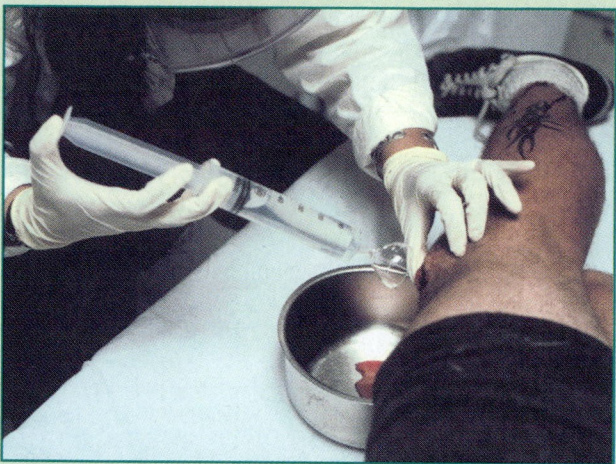

Figure 9-7-2   Gently flush the wound.

7. Remove and discard the disposable gloves and wash hands.

8. Prepare the sterile irrigation tray and dressing supplies. Pour the room-temperature irrigation solution into the solution container.

9. Apply sterile gloves.

10. Position the sterile basin below the wound so the irrigant will flow from the cleanest area to the dirtiest area and into the basin.

11. Fill the piston syringe with irrigant. Attach a 19-gauge needle hub if pressure irrigation is required. Hold the syringe tip approximately 1 inch above the wound bed to irrigate. Refill the syringe and continue to flush the wound until the solution returns clear and no exudate is noted or until the prescribed amount of fluid has been used (see Figures 9-7-2 and 9-7-3).

12. Dry the edges of the wound with sterile gauze (see Figure 9-7-4).

7. Reduces the transmission of microorganisms.

8. Aseptic technique is used to prevent introduction of microorganisms into the wound. Room-temperature solution reduces client discomfort.

9. Promotes sterile environment.

10. Decreases possibility of wound contamination.

11. Irrigating the wound removes debris. Pressure irrigation loosens and removed devitalized tissue.

12. Drying the edges of the wound prevents maceration of tissues caused by excess moisture.

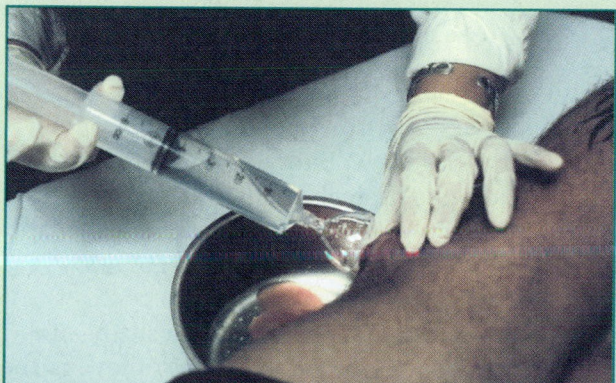

Figure 9-7-3   Hold the syringe close to the wound, but be careful not to touch the wound with the syringe.

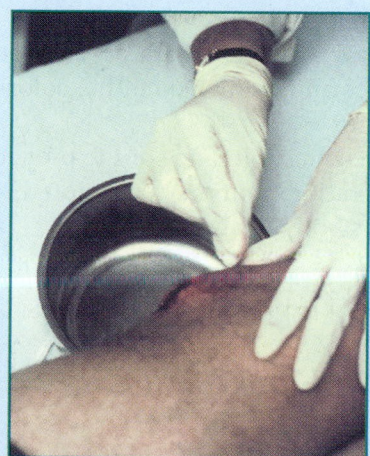

Figure 9-7-4   Dry the edges of the wound with sterile gauze.

continues

Action	Rationale
13. Assess the wound's appearance and drainage.	13. Provides indication of change in wound status.
14. Apply a sterile dressing.	14. Application of a sterile dressing protects the wound from microorganisms.
15. Dispose of old dressings and equipment. Remove gloves, mask with protective eye gear and gown. Wash hands.	15. Reduces the transmission of microorganisms.
16. Document all assessment findings and actions taken.	16. Records information for evaluation.

▶ REAL WORLD ANECDOTES

Mrs. Korpinen is an elderly client in a long-term care facility. She has a pressure ulcer on her right hip that extends into the muscle. The wound has started to tunnel and now extends under the skin in a 2-inch pocket. Mrs. Korpinen's doctor has ordered irrigation of the wound with normal saline every shift. Nurse Ung is the charge nurse on the night shift at this facility, and 5 nights a week she irrigates Mrs. Korpinen's wound. She uses a large amount of normal saline and makes sure the pocketed area is completely irrigated with the solution. She has noted that when she returns from her days off that the pocketed area of Mrs. Korpinen's wound is filled with pus and the irrigation takes much longer to return clear of exudate. Upon investigation Nurse Ung discovers that the other nurses performing this procedure "irrigate" the wound by pouring normal saline over the exposed open area. She carefully and tactfully explains the need to take the time to irrigate the pocketed area underneath the skin in order to heal Mrs. Korpinen's wound.

▶ EVALUATION

1. The wound was free of exudate, drainage, and debris.
2. The wound was free of signs and symptoms of infection.
3. The procedure was performed with a minimum of trauma and pain to the client.

▶ DOCUMENTATION

Nurses' Notes

- Record your findings regarding the wound's appearance and quality, quantity, color, and odor of drainage.
- Note the client's tolerance of the procedure and any observations you may have noted regarding the client's body image.

Document on appropriate flow sheet or electronic medical record (EMR).

▶ CRITICAL THINKING SKILL

Introduction

Thoughtful client assessment and careful procedure planning can prevent serious complications.

Possible Scenario

Mrs. Abelson has a large midline abdominal surgical incision. The upper end of the incision is draining purulent fluid. Her doctor has ordered irrigation of the area and a dressing change every 8 hours. As you prepare to perform the procedure, you note that Mrs. Abelson is sitting propped up in bed with several pillows. Upon checking her chart you find that she has emphysema and cannot lie flat in bed. The area to be irrigated is at the top of the incision, nearest Mrs. Abelson's xiphoid process.

Possible Outcome

- If you lay Mrs. Abelson flat and turn her on her side so the irrigant will not drain into the rest of the incision, the drainage will not contaminate the incision; however, Mrs. Abelson will probably not tolerate this position and could go into respiratory distress.
- If you allow Mrs. Abelson to remain sitting and place the bowl for irrigant in her lap, allowing the irrigant to bathe the entire incision, Mrs. Abelson will be able to breathe, but her entire surgical

incision will be contaminated with whatever is causing the purulent drainage. Because the incision goes through to the abdomen, contaminating the entire length of the incision increases the chance of the infection traveling to the peritoneal cavity.

Prevention

Have another staff member apply sterile gloves and hold the bowl to catch the irrigant directly under the area to be irrigated. This allows Mrs. Abelson to continue to sit up and prevents contamination of the rest of the incision.

► VARIATIONS

Geriatric Variation:
- Be aware that an elderly client may not be able to hear your instructions, see what you are doing, or remember the education you have provided. Be ready to explain the procedure step by step, answer questions, and encourage the client to participate in the care.

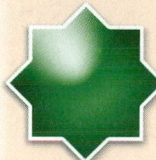

Pediatric Variation:
- A child's skin is tender and may react to solutions that are used routinely on adults. Be aware of any potential allergic-type reactions or topical allergies.

Home Care Variation:
- Clients with slow-healing wounds are often sent home to be cared for. The nurse is often in the position of teaching the client or a caregiver how to perform the irrigation and dressing change. The nurse should periodically assess the irrigation and dressing change to ensure it is still being done correctly.

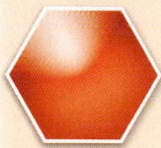

Long-Term Care Variations:
- Clients with long-term wounds need to plan a regular schedule of wound care and a clear method to document the progress of healing and signs of infection.
- An irrigation order and dressing change order will need to be written by the attending health care provider of the facility.

► COMMON ERRORS

Possible Error:

Being too aggressive or not aggressive enough with the irrigation.

Prevention:

Aggressively irrigating the wound in an effort to remove all tissue debris risks damaging fresh tissue that is just starting to granulate on the walls of the wound. Irrigating the wound too gently risks not removing infected debris, thus prolonging the client's recovery and risking infection. Before irrigating the wound, assess the amount of drainage, the condition of the wound, and the stage of healing. With inflammation present, granulation cannot take place, and therefore a more aggressive approach would be appropriate. If the wound contains mostly pink tissue with small amounts of tissue debris, granulation and healing are progressing, and a more gentle irrigation is needed.

▶ **NURSING TIPS**

- Always ask the client for a preferred way of doing the irrigation that has worked in the past without difficulties. Many clients have developed their own shortcuts and in turn educate the nurse on an easier way to irrigate.

- Be sure the irrigant is at room temperature or ideally body temperature to avoid traumatizing the granulating tissues and avoid client discomfort.
- A small wound can be irrigated with a syringe and solution poured into a sterile specimen cup.

▶ **SPECIAL CONSIDERATIONS**

- *Ideal pressure for irrigation can be achieved with a 19-gauge syringe or a catheter on a 60-cc syringe. An IV bag pressurized with 400 mm Hg from a blood pressure cuff is also effective. If lower pressures are indicated, then a bulb syringe can be used.*
- *Very high-pressure irrigation is reserved for highly contaminated wounds or debridement of devitalized tissue. It is effective in removing bacteria from the surface of the wound and decreasing infection rates.*

Packing a Wound

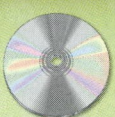

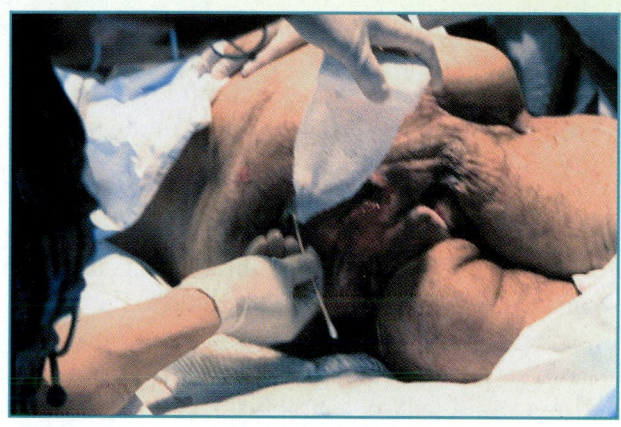

▶ OVERVIEW OF THE SKILL

Dressings are placed on wounds to accomplish a number of goals ranging from aesthetic comfort for the client to immobilizing and protecting the wound area. Wounds such as ulcers and open surgical incisions are generally left open to heal by tissue granulation from the edges of the wound. This is known as healing by secondary intention. Wounds that heal by secondary intention may have copious exudate, necrotic or infected tissue on the surface, tunneling, or may be in high pressure or low circulation sites. These types of wounds are often "packed" as part of the dressing process. Dressing a wound using packing material is done primarily to protect an open wound from contamination, absorb drainage, protect from mechanical injury, fill dead space, and debride the wound.

There are many new dressings on the market specifically designed for packing and caring for wounds that are healing by secondary intention. Traditionally, gauze has been used to pack wounds.

Gauze

Gauze has a number of advantages as a packing material. It is inexpensive as well as versatile. It can be used to fill dead space, protect the wound from contamination and injury, absorb drainage, and debride necrotic and infected debris. It is easily applied and easily removed. It is readily available in most settings and requires no special handling.

While gauze is versatile and multifunctional, it often does not perform any one specific function well. In addition, although gauze will debride necrotic tissue, it also removes newly granulated tissue. Gauze can provide some protection from contamination, but studies have shown that bacteria can penetrate 64 thicknesses of gauze. Gauze does absorb drainage, but it can absorb so much drainage that the wound surface becomes desiccated, slowing healing. Gauze will fill dead space but if packed too tightly can restrict blood flow and oxygenation at the wound surface.

Hydrocolloids

Hydrocolloids are a synthetic material available as a powder or paste. This type of dressing material can be used to fill dead space in a wound and to maintain a moist healing environment. Although hydrocolloids are absorptive, they can be overwhelmed with drainage in wounds with large amounts of exudate. Hydrocolloid pastes or powders may be inappropriate packing for tunneled areas or areas that may be difficult to cleanse of packing material during dressing changes.

Alginates

Alginates are derived from brown seaweed and are highly absorptive. This type of material is available as a pad or in the form of a rope. Alginates can be used to fill dead space and to absorb wound drainage.

Hydrophilic Polyurethane

Hydrophilic polyurethane foams are available in sheets or as a filler. Foam can be used to fill dead space, absorb drainage, and maintain a moist wound environment. Foam may require a secondary gauze dressing.

The primary goals in packing a wound are to protect, absorb, fill, or debride the wound. The wound packing material used should be chosen based on the reasons for packing the wound, the availability of the packing material, and the skill level of the caregiver.

Wound VAC

A vacuum assisted closure (VAC) device can be used to facilitate healing and closure of an open wound. An evacuation tube is embedded in a polyurethane foam dressing which is placed in the wound and sealed with an occlusive dressing. The tube is attached to a vacuum. The negative pressure causes the foam to collapse and removes excess fluid. As a result blood flow is increased and bacterial growth decreased, which promotes granulation tissue and wound closure. The vacuum may be indicated for clients with venous or arterial insufficiency ulcers, neuropathic ulcers, chronic pressure ulcers, dehisced wounds, wounds around exposed orthopedic hardware, and certain acute wounds such as poststernotomy mediastinitis. VAC generally should not be used with cancerous wounds, where fistulas open to organs or body cavities, or with necrotic tissue in the presence of eschar.

▶ ASSESSMENT

1. Assess the dressing currently in place **to determine effectiveness of the current regimen.**
2. Assess the client's comfort level **to determine whether the client will need medication prior to the dressing change.**
3. Assess the client's understanding regarding the wound, the healing process, and the reason for the particular type of dressing **to determine whether any client teaching is needed.**
4. Assess the wound for infection, necrotic tissue, exudate, tunneling, circulation, and tissue **granulation to determine the effectiveness of the current care regimen.**
5. Assess the wound size and depth **to determine wound healing and effectiveness of the current care regimen.**

▶ DIAGNOSIS

Risk for Infection

Impaired Skin Integrity

Impaired Tissue Integrity

Body Image Disturbance

Deficient Knowledge

Acute Pain

▶ PLANNING

Expected Outcomes:

1. The wound will not exhibit signs or symptoms of infection.
2. The client will experience a minimum of pain and trauma related to the wound and wound care.
3. The client will understand the reason for the current wound care regimen.
4. If the wound is to be cared for at home, the client or the client's caregiver will be able to demonstrate appropriate wound care and explain the reasons for the wound care regimen.
5. The wound will measurably heal.
6. Wound drainage will be adequately absorbed.

Equipment Needed:

- Gloves (gown, goggles, and mask prn)
- Sterile gloves
- Tape (Montgomery straps or stockinette)
- Gauze or other wound packing material (see Figure 9-8-1)
- Biohazard waste receptacle
- Dressing material to cover the packing
- Cotton-tip applicators, sterile
- Tweezers or forceps, sterile
- Normal saline
- Sterile 4 × 4 gauze pads
- ABD dressing

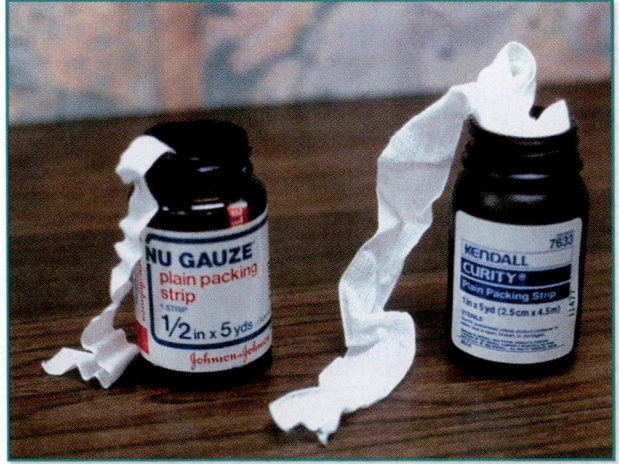

Figure 9-8-1 Wound packing gauze

► **CLIENT EDUCATION NEEDED:**

1. Explain the reasons for packing the wound and for the use of the chosen packing material.
2. Explain the need to avoid pressure at the wound site.
3. Explain the need to keep the exterior of the dressings dry.
4. Emphasize to the client not to lie on the wounded area, even if it is the client's preference.
5. Have clients rate their pain on a 0 to 10 scale during the wound-packing procedure.
6. Encourage clients to tell you when they are experiencing pain so you can provide appropriate pain relief prior to the procedure.
7. Encourage the client or family members to watch and assist with the dressing change, especially if they will be performing the dressing change at home.
8. Some clients may be uncomfortable with knowing that dressings and gauze are being placed inside of them. Encourage the client to talk about feelings and concerns, and provide emotional and educational support.

Estimated time to complete the skill: **15–30 minutes**

► **DELEGATION TIPS**

Wound packing requires nursing assessment, aseptic technique, and skilled insertion. This procedure should never be delegated to ancillary personnel.

IMPLEMENTATION—Action/Rationale

Action	Rationale
1. Wash hands.	1. Reduces the transmission of microorganisms.
2. Provide for client privacy.	2. Promotes client comfort and cooperation.
3. Assemble dressing change material at bedside (see Figure 9-8-2).	3. Prevents a break in technique during the dressing change.
4. Apply gloves.	4. Reduces the transmission of microorganisms.
5. Remove the old dressing, noting the integrity of the old dressing and the way it was applied (see Figures 9-8-3 and 9-8-4).	5. If the old dressing adequately contained wound drainage, debrided the wound, or performed the necessary function, use it as a template for applying the new dressing. If it was not adequate, evaluate and implement ways to improve the dressing.
6. Dispose of the old dressing in the appropriate receptacle.	6. Reduces the transmission of microorganisms.
7. Remove gloves with contaminated surfaces inward and dispose of them appropriately.	7. Prevents contamination of the new dressing material.

continues

Action	Rationale

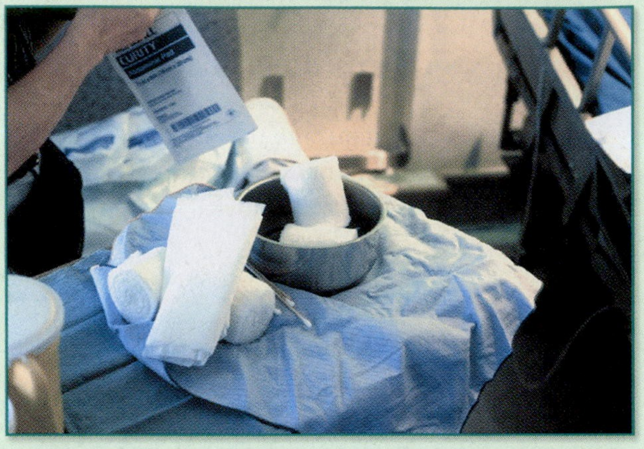

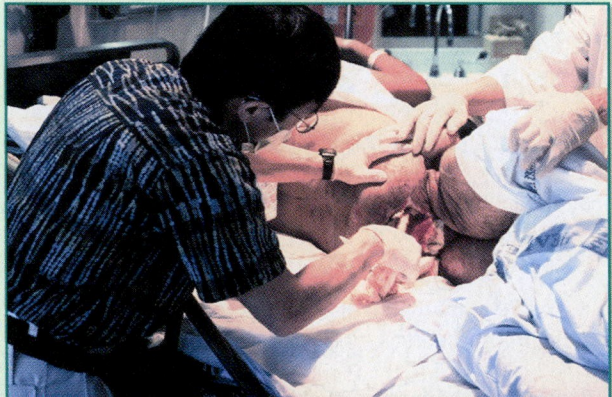

Figure 9-8-2   Assemble dressing change material.

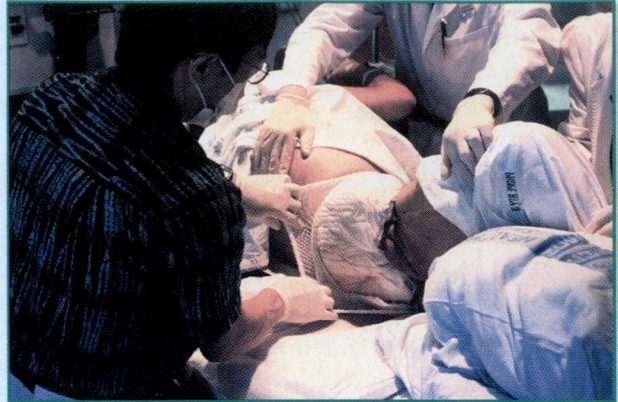

Figure 9-8-3   Carefully remove the old dressing.

8. Open and prepare the dressing materials. If this is a sterile dressing change, establish a sterile field for the dressing materials.

9. Apply sterile gloves (see Figure 9-8-5).

10. Inspect the wound (see Figure 9-8-6). Using the cotton-tip applicator as a measuring tool, gently measure the depth, width, length, depth of undermining, and depth of tunneling of the wound.
    • Carefully assess that no packing material has been left in the wound from prior wound packing.

11. Cleanse, irrigate, or treat the wound according to the prescribed wound regimen as stated by institutional policy, active orders, or as recommended by a wound specialist. For irrigation, see Skill 9-7.

8. Prevents breaks in technique during the dressing change.

9. Reduces the transmission of microorganisms.

10. Documents progress in healing. Gentle measurement will prevent damage to any new tissue granulation.

    • Old packing material can lead to infection and delay healing.

11. Promotes wound healing.

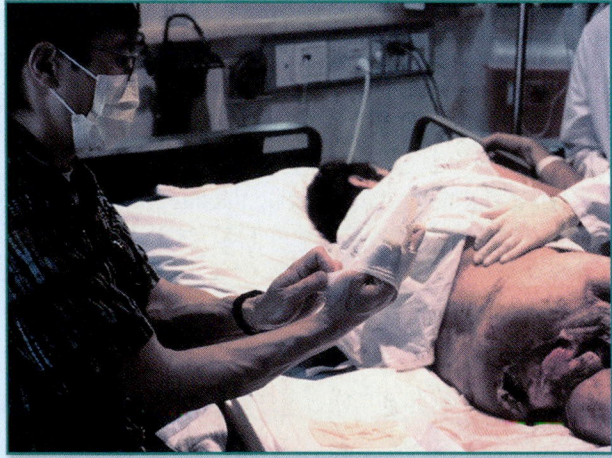

Figure 9-8-4   Examine the old dressing as it is removed. Note what dressings were applied, in what order, and assess the effectiveness of the old dressing.

Figure 9-8-5   Apply gloves.

continues

Action	Rationale

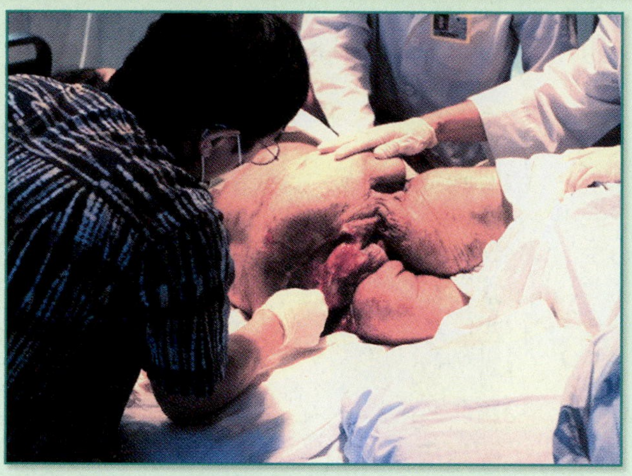

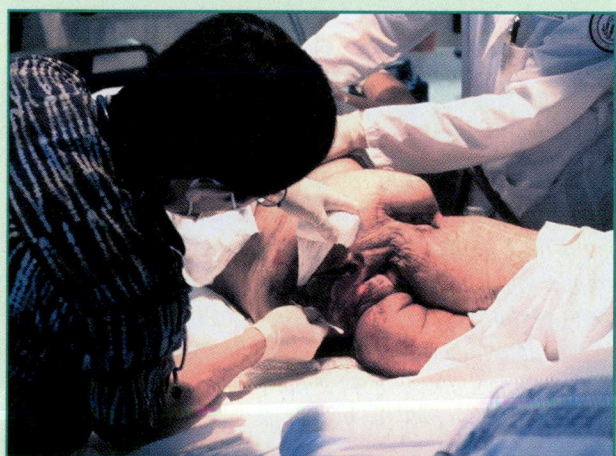

Figure 9-8-6 Inspect the wound. Gently probe the length and depth, and assess for tunneling and undermining in the wound.

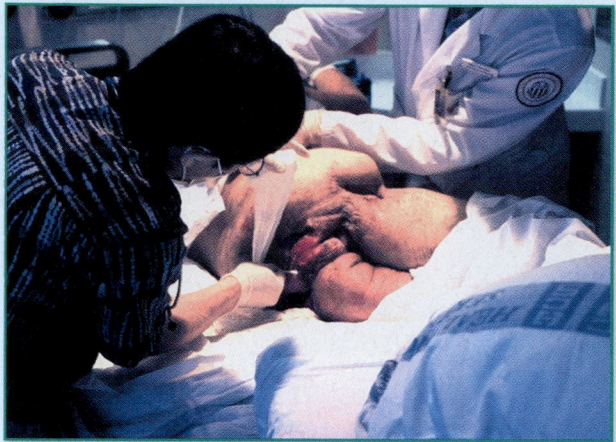

Figure 9-8-7 Gently pack the wound.

12. Using the information you obtained while removing the old dressing, gently place the prescribed packing material into the wound (see Figure 9-8-7).

13. If the wound packing is for debridement, be sure the packing material contacts all the surfaces to be debrided (see Figure 9-8-8).
  • If wound requires a wet to dry dressing, wring out excess moisture on gauze prior to packing.

14. If gauze is being used to absorb drainage, fluff the gauze before packing.

15. Pack all tunneled areas, being sure not to pack too tightly (see Figure 9-8-9).

12. Gentle packing will prevent damage to any new tissue.

13. Contacting all surfaces to be debrided will increase effectiveness of the wound packing.

  • A moist gauze absorbs wound drainage and aids in debridement of wound.

14. Fluffing increases moisture absorption and helps the gauze conform to the ulcer surface.

15. Packing tunneled areas helps to prevent mechanical injury to the newly granulated tissue. Packing too tightly impairs circulation to the area and slows healing.

Figure 9-8-8 Make sure the packing reaches all the surfaces that need to be debrided.

Figure 9-8-9 Place packing into all tunneled areas.

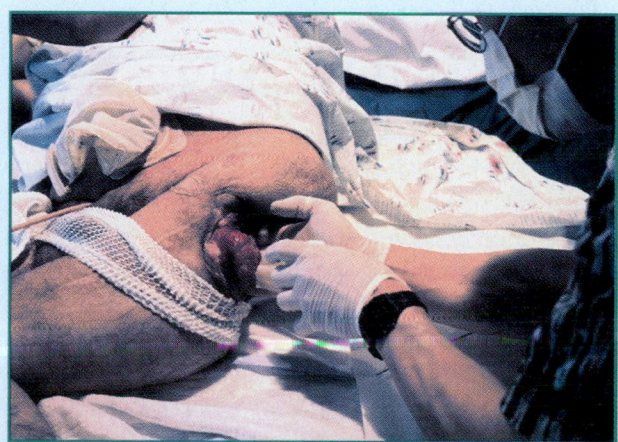

continues

Action	Rationale

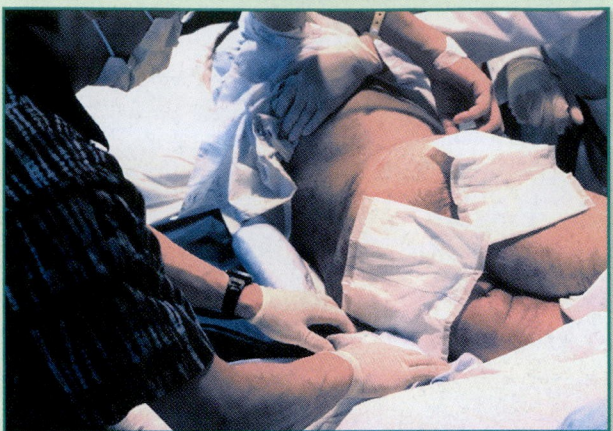

Figure 9-8-10   Apply an external dressing over the packing, if needed, to hold the packing in place.

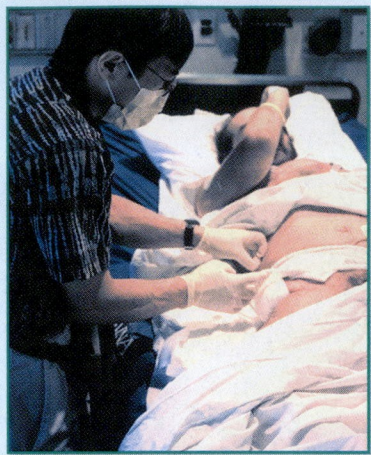

Figure 9-8-11   Stockinette is used to secure the dressing in place.

Action	Rationale
16. If the packing material requires a secondary dressing to hold it in place, apply that now (see Figure 9-8-10).	16. Protects the dressing from external contamination and holds the packing material in place.
17. Using tape, Montgomery straps, or stockinette, secure the dressing in place (see Figure 9-8-11).	17. Secures the dressings in place. If the dressing is being changed frequently, Montgomery straps or stockinette may be a preferable method of securing the dressing to prevent skin damage from tape.
18. Dispose of any waste appropriately.	18. Reduces the transmission of microorganisms.
19. Remove any bedding soiled by drainage, remove any foul-smelling dressing material, and freshen the air, if necessary.	19. Promotes client comfort.
20. Remove gloves and dispose of them properly.	20. Standard Precautions.
21. Wash hands.	21. Reduces the transmission of microorganisms.

▶ **REAL WORLD ANECDOTES**

Mrs. Harmston was a bedridden client in a long-term care facility. She had an undermined pressure ulcer on her right hip, which was to be irrigated and packed three times per day. Every night, when the night shift nurse changed Mrs. Harmston's dressing, she noted that the previous shift packed only the visible open area of the pressure ulcer with a small amount of gauze. The undermined area was not packed and contained a large amount of purulent drainage. The night shift nurse routinely took the time to irrigate all portions of the pressure ulcer, especially the undermined area, and she gently packed the undermined area with gauze moistened with sterile saline. During morning report she noted the way she had treated Mrs. Harmston's pressure ulcer but refrained from criticizing the previous nurse. She later discovered that the day shift also packed and irrigated only the visible portion of Mrs. Harmston's wound. Despite only one careful dressing change a day, Mrs. Harmston's wound drainage and general appearance would improve for a few days and the night shift nurse was happy to see the progress. However, when she would return from her two days off, she would be discouraged to note that Mrs. Harmston's ulcer was once again filled with purulent drainage and only barely packed. Unwilling to compromise her client's care, the night shift nurse reported the inadequate dressing changes being performed during the day shift. The problem was addressed, and as time went on, Mrs. Harmston's wound improved.

▶ EVALUATION

- The wound does not exhibit signs or symptoms of infection.
- The client experienced a minimum of pain and trauma related to the wound and wound care.
- The client understands the reason for the current wound care regimen.
- If the wound is to be cared for at home, the client or the client's caregiver was able to demonstrate appropriate wound care and explain the reasons for the wound care regimen.
- The wound has measurably healed.
- The wound drainage was adequately absorbed.

▶ DOCUMENTATION

Nurses' Notes

- Document the time and date of the dressing change.
- Note the size and depth measurements you made during the dressing change.
- Indicate any changes in the wound condition you observed, including an increase or decrease in drainage or purulence, changes in the size or shape of the wound, odor, or necrosis.
- Note the condition of the client's skin surrounding the wound, including any tape blisters or tissue maceration.
- Record any questions or concerns the client expressed regarding the wound or the dressing change.

Document on appropriate flow sheet or electronic medical record (EMR).

▶ CRITICAL THINKING SKILL

Introduction

Investigate the unusual to avoid the unexpected.

Possible Scenario

You are changing the dressing on a pressure sore with undermining and tunneling. You have cared for this client in the past and are familiar with this wound. While removing the old gauze packing, you realize that you cannot find any gauze tail at the opening to the tunneled area.

Possible Outcome

After poking around at the entrance to the tunneled area, you decide that the previous nurse did not pack this area. You pack the tunneled area with gauze, making sure to leave a tail for easy removal later. Over the course of the next few days, the tunneled area of this wound becomes increasingly purulent and starts to drain foul-smelling exudate. Determined to find the cause of this new drainage, you probe the tunneled area with cotton-tip applicators and tweezers. Using a flashlight and tweezers to hold the tunnel open, you see what appears to be matted gauze deep in the tunneled wound. Further exploration with the tweezers and flashlight reveals an old 4 × 4 gauze that had been pushed deep into the tunneled area and had provided a breeding ground for infection. Removing the gauze resulted in some excoriation of the wound surface, providing an excellent entry point for the infection. The client developed a septic infection and had to be placed on a course of intravenous antibiotics. The wound healing was severely delayed because of the infection and the damage from removing the gauze.

Prevention

When packing a wound, especially in tunneled and undermined areas that are difficult to see, be sure to leave a means of removing the packing. Think ahead to the next nurse who will be caring for this client and place the packing the way you would want to find it for ease of removal.

▶ VARIATIONS

Geriatric Variations:
- *Do not pack the wound too tightly. Elderly clients may already have compromised circulation, and packing the wound tightly will impair it even further.*
- *Be aware of the condition of the client's skin surrounding the wound. Elderly clients are at high risk of skin breakdown, and tape, frequent handling, and drainage or antiseptic solutions from the wound care can cause further breakdown.*

continues

▶ VARIATIONS *(continued)*

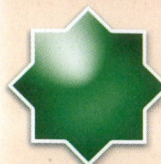

Pediatric Variation:
- *Children may need to be restrained to prevent them from interfering with the dressing change.*

Home Care Variations:
- *Be sure to dispose of soiled dressings appropriately.*
- *Monitor the client's or caregiver's dressing change technique periodically. If caregivers do not completely understand the reasons for each step, they might become careless in performing the dressing change.*
- *Educate the caregiver and the client regarding the need to avoid pressure on the wound site.*
- *Even if it does not hurt to lie on the site, pressure can compromise wound healing.*
- *Ensure that the client understands the need to monitor for infection by monitoring systemic temperature and color and healing of wound.*

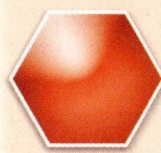

Long-Term Care Variations:
- *The client's primary caregiver in a long-term setting may not be a licensed person. Be sure that the primary caregiver is aware of how to care for the dressing and the signs and symptoms to report to the licensed staff.*
- *Teach the caregivers not to turn a client onto the wounded area.*
- *Emphasize to the client not to lie on the wounded area, even if it is the client's preferred way to lie.*
- *A dressing change order will need to be written by the attending health care provider of the facility.*

▶ COMMON ERRORS

Possible Error:
The wound is packed too tightly.

Prevention:
Packing the wound tightly will allow for more drainage absorption and does reduce dead space more completely. However, packing the wound tightly also compromises circulation to the wound surface, which slows new tissue growth and healing. If gauze is used to tightly pack the wound, it can cause mechanical injury to the wound surface as well. Be sure to pack the wound well enough to fill the dead space and absorb drainage but not so tightly that circulation is compromised. If wound drainage is overwhelming the dressings, change the dressing more often or change the packing to a more absorbent material rather than trying to pack in more dressings.

▶ NURSING TIPS

- If the old packing material is adhered to the wound surface, moisten the packing with sterile saline. This allows easier removal and helps prevent damage to any new tissue.

- Be sure to assess whether the client will require premedication for the dressing change. Client cooperation and understanding improves greatly if the client is not focused on the pain.

- If the wound is large, odoriferous, or otherwise unpleasant, do not indicate disgust or displeasure during the procedure. The client is already painfully aware of the wound and may interpret your expression of disgust personally. The wound is a part of the client and the client is always treated with respect.
- When packing tunneled areas, be sure to leave a piece of gauze or other packing material visible and easy to reach with forceps or tweezers to facilitate removal of the packing material.
- Assess that all old packing material is removed with each treatment.
- Use cotton-tip applicators to gently push the packing material into tunneled or undermined areas of the wound.
- Do not perform complex, painful, or odoriferous dressing changes around mealtimes.

▶ SPECIAL CONSIDERATIONS

- *A transparent dressing may be placed over a packed wound. This provides an occlusive dressing and allows the client to shower while the healing process continues.*
- *Often clients are sent home with open wounds and need clear instructions on the packing procedure and prevention of infections. Ensure that the client understands the need for aseptic technique. Ensure that the client has good eyesight and lighting and is able to avoid mistakenly leaving old packing material in the wound, especially when tunneled cavities are present.*

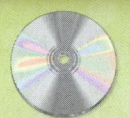

SKILL 9-9

Cleaning and Dressing a Wound with an Open Drain

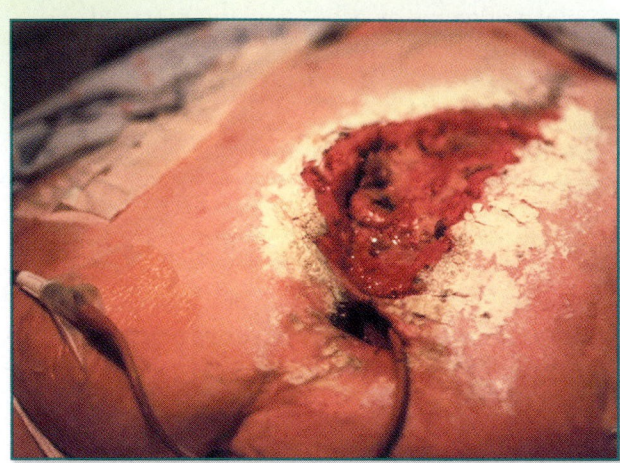

▶ OVERVIEW OF THE SKILL

Wounds may have drains placed in them during surgery or during the healing process. The purpose of the drain is to drain sanguineous, serosanguineous, purulent, biliary drainage, or other body fluids from the surgical site or cavity. The drain may exit through a stab wound near the main incision or may exit through the incision line or open wound. Common types of drains consist of a collection device that can be emptied (see Skill 9-13) and is connected to a catheter inserted in the wound. Examples of this type of drain are the Jackson-Pratt or HemoVac. Other types of drains, such as the Penrose, are a hollow tube or rubber catheter drain that is not connected to a collection device and simply drains into a dressing.

Dressings and drain care vary according to the surgeon's preference and agency or institutional policy. This skill presents a general guideline for a wound dressing with an open drain either exiting from the incision line or exiting from a nearby stab wound and terminating in a dressing. This skill may also be used when providing care around an open drain that may be present with open wounds requiring wet to dry dressing or deep packing or wounds with retention sutures.

▶ ASSESSMENT

1. Assess the client's comfort level **to determine whether pain medications are needed.**

2. Assess the external appearance of the dressing. Reinforce the dressing if necessary. **Documents the initial condition of the dressing and places additional dressing if needed to absorb drainage.**

3. Assess the appearance of the wound for bleeding, intactness, drainage and the presence of drains, sutures, or other devices. **Helps plan care needed and establishes a baseline for later assessments.**

4. Assess the client's understanding about the postoperative care of the surgical wound site. **It is important to take into consideration the client's ability to understand verbal and written instructions and the cultural and social variations that may affect the delivery of health care and client/family education.**

▶ DIAGNOSIS

Acute Pain

Impaired Skin Integrity

Impaired Tissue Integrity

Risk for Infection

▶ PLANNING

Expected Outcomes:

1. The dressing change will be performed with minimal discomfort to the client.

2. The wound site and drains will be assessed for signs of healing and infection.

3. The site will have the appropriate dressing applied over the wound and around the drains.

4. The surgically placed drains will be monitored for proper functioning and placement.

5. The client/family will verbalize and/or demonstrate the purpose of the drains, and, if required, care of the wound site.

Equipment Needed (see Figure 9-9-1):

- Clean exam gloves
- Moisture-proof gown (optional)
- Mask (optional)
- Eye protection (optional)
- Container for proper disposal of soiled dressing
- Washcloths (optional)

- Sterile gloves
- Normal saline
- Small sterile bowl (optional)
- Sterile cotton-tip applicators (optional)
- Sterile towel
- Sterile 4 × 4 gauze pads, multiple
- Precut 4 × 4 drain sponges, multiple
- ABD dressing (optional)
- Tubular mesh (optional)
- 2-inch tape (foam or paper)

▶ CLIENT EDUCATION NEEDED

1. Instruct the client how frequently the dressing should be inspected and changed.

2. Discuss how the site will heal, when drains might be removed, and how long sutures or staples will remain in place.

3. Instruct the client not to reach onto the sterile field to help with the dressing change.

4. Instruct the client to report any symptoms of pain or discomfort associated with the incision or dressing.

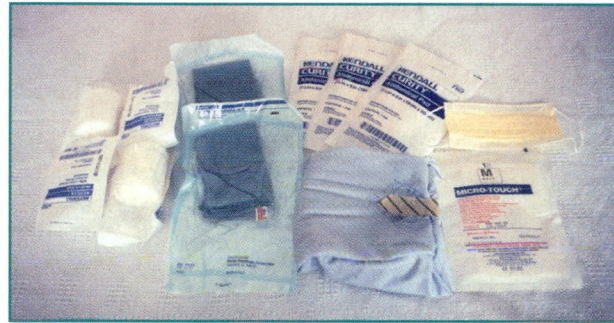

Figure 9-9-1   Sterile gloves, dressings, basin, and towels are used to dress a closed wound with an open drain.

Estimated time to complete the skill:
15 minutes

▶ DELEGATION TIPS

Cleaning and dressing a wound with an open drain requires nursing assessment, aseptic technique, and skilled insertion and removal. This procedure should never be delegated to ancillary personnel.

IMPLEMENTATION—Action/Rationale

Action	Rationale
1. Gather supplies.	1. Having all supplies in the room increases the consistency of client care.
2. Provide privacy; draw curtains; close door.	2. Maintains client comfort and privacy while body is exposed during procedure.
3. Explain procedure to client.	3. Provides information about the procedure.

continues

Action	Rationale

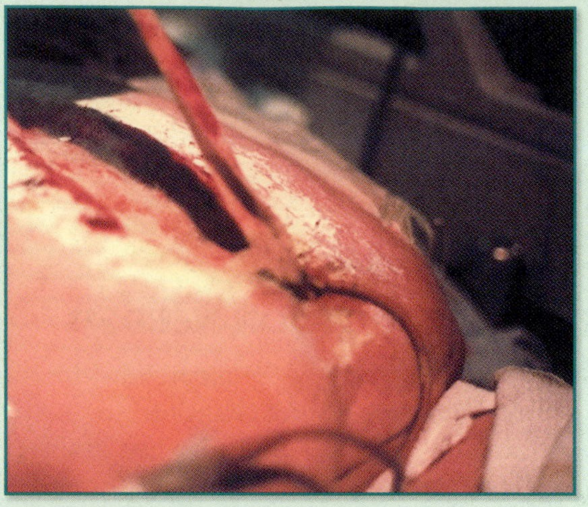

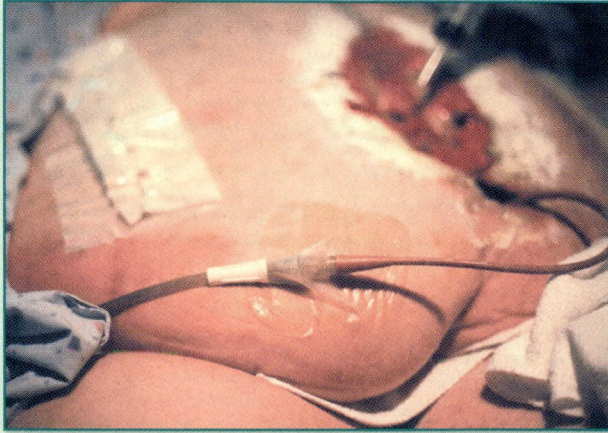

Figure 9-9-2 Remove the old dressing.

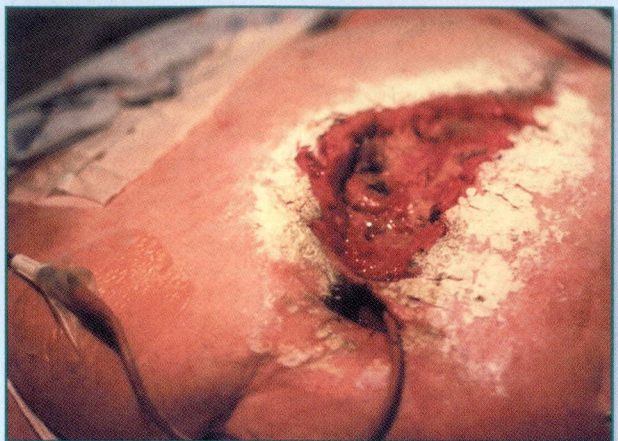

Figure 9-9-3 Observe the undressed wound and the drain.

4. Wash hands.

5. Apply clean exam gloves, a moisture-proof gown, mask, and eye protection, if needed.

6. Remove dressing and place in appropriate receptacle (see Figure 9-9-2).

7. Assess the undressed wound for signs of healing and infection. The drain may be observed to exit directly from the incision line or from a separate stab wound near the incision (see Figure 9-9-3). Ensure that the drain is securely attached to the skin to prevent it from being accidentally dislodged (see Figure 9-9-4).

4. Reduces the transmission of microorganisms.

5. Provides infection control and protection from body fluids. If there is copious drainage or the wound is infected, a gown, a mask, and eye protection should be worn.

6. Dressings soiled with body fluids are considered contaminated and subject to biohazard disposal in the correct manner per institution protocol.

7. Allows for evaluation of effectiveness of treatment.

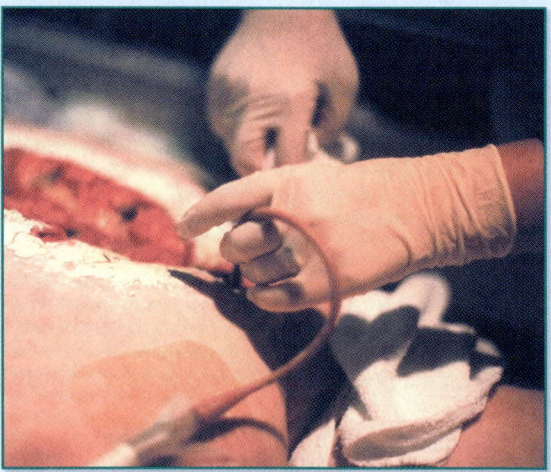

Figure 9-9-4 Make sure the drain is secured to the skin so it will not be accidentally dislodged from the wound.

Figure 9-9-5 The drain is gently elevated to facilitate cleaning.

continues

Action	Rationale
8. Cleanse the skin around the incision if necessary with a clean, warm, wet washcloth. Do not disturb the drain or the area under the drain at this point.	8. Dried blood or drainage on the surrounding skin can be an irritant and a medium for microbes. Move the drain as little as possible to avoid dislodging or shifting the drain, and to minimize trauma to the tissues.
9. Remove used exam gloves.	9. Exam gloves used to remove the old dressing are considered dirty and should be removed.
10. Wash hands.	10. Reduces the transmission of microorganism.
11. Set up supplies.	11. Following the removal of the dressing, you will have a better idea of what supplies are needed and in what amount.
12. Set up a sterile field, including pouring ordered solutions into appropriate containers, if indicated for the dressing change. Apply sterile gloves.	12. This is a sterile dressing change.
13. • If necessary, cleanse the suture line using sterile normal saline or other approved cleaning solution applied with sterile cotton-tip applications or 4 ×4 gauze pads. • Clean the incision, using a separate cotton-tip applicator or gauze pad for each swipe. Moving from top to bottom, clean the incision line first, then clean each side of the incision. • Remove excess moisture after cleaning with dry cotton-tip applicators or gauze pads. If the wound is open and requires wet-to-dry dressings, deep packing, or retention suture wound care, perform this care at this time.	13. • If the suture line is grossly bloody, it should be cleaned first. In absence of a stated preference, normal saline will not interfere with healing of the suture line and is routinely used. • Cleansing should be from clean to contaminated to avoid introduction of microorganisms into the wound. • Excessive moisture from the cleansing may cause excoriation if left on the skin and suture line.
14. Cleanse the area under the drain. The open drain should be handled minimally. The drain may be elevated with a sterile finger or a cotton-tip applicator to facilitate cleansing (see Figure 9-9-5). • Cleanse the drain site using sterile normal saline or other approved cleaning solution applied with sterile cotton-tip applicators or gauze pads. Using a circular motion, begin at the drain site and clean outward. Use a new cotton-tip applicator or gauze for each cleaning, and clean from drain site out.	14. If the drainage is excessive or not adequately absorbed by the dressing, the skin beneath the drain will need to be cleaned. Drainage on skin can be an irritant and a medium for microbes. The open drain is a portal of entry into the surgical site. It may or may not be sutured in place and requires care in handling to avoid spreading contaminants or dislodging. Drains are cleansed from least to most contaminated.
15. Apply needed layers of precut drain sponges around the drain. Top with one to two layers of uncut drain sponges.	15. Precut drain sponges allow a close fit of the dressing around the drain while allowing the drainage to exit onto a maximum absorbent

continues

Action	Rationale

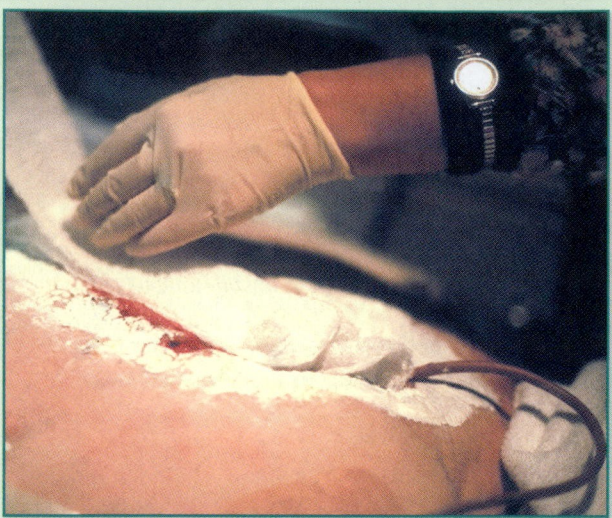

Figure 9-9-6   Apply dressing.

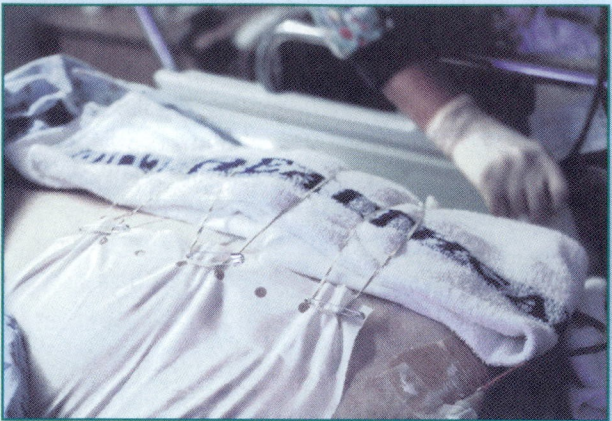

Figure 9-9-7   Secure dressing in place with Montgomery straps.

16.
- Apply external dressing of dry 4 × 4 gauze pads, cover sponges, fluffs, or ABD pads (see Figure 9-9-6).
- Secure dressing in place with tape, Montgomery straps, or tubular mesh (see Figure 9-9-7).

16.
- The external dressing is determined by the size and shape of the wound.
- Tape for short-term dressings in clients who are not sensitive to adhesives is the method of choice for securing dressings. For long-term dressings or for clients who are sensitive to tape, use Montgomery straps or tubular mesh. Tubular mesh is a nice alternative to hold the dressing in place because tape is not involved—the mesh is simply pulled up or down to accommodate the dressing change.

17. Conduct client/family education about the dressing, which may include teaching the dressing technique to the client/family.

17. Educates the client/family and prepares for discharge.

18. Dispose of old dressings appropriately. Remove gloves and wash hands.

18. Reduces the transmission of microorganisms.

► REAL WORLD ANECDOTES

Ms. Stacy is a 25-year-old woman who is recovering from a ruptured appendix and resulting peritonitis. She has a midline wound, which is closed with staples, and a 3/4-inch latex Penrose drain exiting from a stab wound in her right lower quadrant. She is having her dressing changed around the Penrose every 8 hours because of moderate amounts of purulent drainage. Upon removing the dressing, you find that the drain has slipped out of the wound. There was no suture holding the drain in place. You notify the surgical resident on call who arrives to assess the client. Because the drainage is still a moderate amount, the resident obtains a new sterile Penrose and using sterile technique replaces the drain in the tract in the stab wound and places a suture to hold the new drain in place. The client is instructed that the drain will be slowly advanced and removed once the drainage is minimal. The drain site is dressed with drain sponges and cover sponges, and tubular mesh secures the dressing in place.

▶ EVALUATION

- The dressing change was performed with minimal discomfort to the client.
- The wound site and drains were inspected for signs of healing and infection.
- The site had the appropriate dressing applied over the wound and around the drains.
- The surgically placed drains were monitored for proper functioning and placement.
- The client/family verbalized and/or demonstrated the purpose of the drains, and, if required, care of the wound site.

▶ DOCUMENTATION

Nurses' Notes

- Record date and time the dressing was changed.
- Write a brief description of the wound and drain site.
- Note the position, length, and condition of drains, and description of drainage.
- Write a brief description of the site care provided and dressing applied.
- Document client comfort before and after dressing change.

Document on appropriate flow sheet or electronic medical record (EMR).

- Document client family education provided and evaluation of the teaching.

▶ CRITICAL THINKING SKILL

Introduction

Skin in elderly or compromised clients may be very thin. A split or a tear can put the client at greater risk of infection.

Possible Scenario

Mr. Goff has a closed midline abdominal wound and two red, rubber catheter drains sutured in place in his right upper quadrant and left upper quadrant to drain his subphrenic abscess. He has rheumatoid arthritis and is on prednisone daily. His skin is thin and friable. The last nurse taped the wound dressing on with paper tape. You pull off the tape quickly, thinking it will cause less pain to the client, and a 1 cm circle of skin pulls off with the tape and the tissue begins to bleed.

Possible Outcome

Potential skin ulceration and infection from exposed tissue near a drain site could result.

Prevention

Remove the tape slowly. Think of using an alternate method of securing the dressing rather than tape.

▶ VARIATIONS

Geriatric Variations:

- *Elderly people have thin skin. Special protective barriers such as special creams or hydrocolloid (Duoderm) pads may need to be applied to the areas under the drains if the drainage is causing excoriation.*
- *Protect the elderly client's skin from pressure, or friction, by the drain on the skin around the wound.*
- *Elderly clients may need help with dressings and management of drainage tubes in the home setting.*

Pediatric Variations:

- *Remind all children who are old enough to understand not to touch the dressing site or play with the drainage tubes.*
- *Make sure the dressing is secure and the small child cannot easily pull or dislodge a drain.*
- *Placing a drain in a stuffed animal and allowing the child to change the dressing may be appropriate play therapy for younger children.*
- *Young children will require explanation that their wound will heal and the drain does not mean that their insides will leak out of the wound.*
- *Older children can be taught to participate in self-care of dressings.*

continues

► VARIATIONS *(continued)*

Home Care Variations:
- *Where and how to obtain additional supplies should be reviewed with the client/family.*
- *Review proper disposal of contaminated dressings.*
- *Discharge instructions need to include how to care for the dressing at home, and when and whom to call if the client experiences problems with the dressing change or wound care. Specific instructions need to be given on what to do if the drain becomes dislodged or pulls out.*

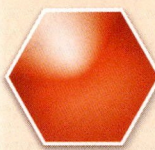

Long-Term Care Variations:
- *Special supplies will need to be ordered.*
- *A dressing change order will need to be written by the attending health care provider of the facility.*

► COMMON ERRORS

Possible Error:

The drain care is done in advance of the dry dressing to the closed wound. You have drainage on your sterile gloves. You pick up a sterile 4 × 4 gauze from your sterile field and apply it on top of the closed wound. You do not change your soiled sterile gloves before applying the closed wound dressing.

Prevention:

Change gloves before completing the care of the closed wound. Be aware of what is clean and what has been contaminated as you proceed through the dressing change.

Possible Error:

The dressing change is ordered t.i.d., 6:00 a.m., 2:00 p.m., and 10:00 p.m. It is 1:45 p.m. and you are about to do a dressing change around a Penrose drain. Four packages of drain sponges have been used for each dressing. You go to gather your supplies and there are no drain sponges. Quickly you order some from the central supply department. They arrive at 2:30 p.m.

Prevention:

As you acquire dressings for a dressing change, note how many dressings remain in the supply. Order supplies in advance.

► NURSING TIPS

- Dressing changes require organization to be done efficiently. Gather data about the dressing change from the following:

    –Shift report

    –Nurses who have cared for client

    –The client/family

    –Chart notes

    –Orders

    –Care map, care plan

    –Observation of the dressed wound

    –Supplies already in room

- Make a list, if necessary, of needed supplies to take into the room.
- If you are going to be in a client's room for some time, let others know so that they can cover your call lights and you can devote your attention to the dressing change.
- Order special needed supplies in advance of the procedure; do not wait until the last minute.
- Client/family education and preparation for discharge begins upon admission.
- Make sure the container for proper disposal of the removed dressing is nearby so that you have something to drop the dressing into immediately upon removal.
- Avoid elastic dressings if history of latex allergy.

▶ **SPECIAL CONSIDERATIONS**

- *The Penrose drain uses wicking action to drain the wound. This may resemble a wet noodle to the inexperienced care giver and proper instruction must be given so it is not inadvertently pulled out.*
- *When a drain is placed in a contaminated wound it may potentially increase the risk of wound infection. Careful monitoring of the site and frequent monitoring of vital signs are necessary.*

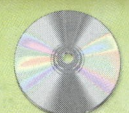

Dressing a Wound with Retention Sutures

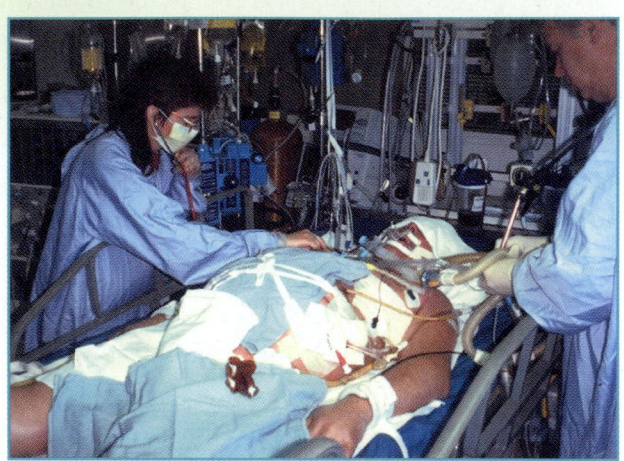

▶ OVERVIEW OF THE SKILL

Large wounds that are at risk for dehiscence may be closed with wires or heavy nylon or silk suture material known as retention sutures. The suture material or wires may be additionally stabilized by commercially available plastic guide devices commonly referred to as "spoons." These devices look like bridges across the suture line. The plastic guides also protect the client's skin from the wires or heavy suture material. Surgical wounds at risk for dehiscence are those that occur in obese individuals, in individuals who have had repeat abdominal surgeries in the same site, and clients whose wounds are at risk for delayed healing; such as diabetics and those who are immunosuppressed or are on steroids. Wounds with retention sutures may also have drains. Drains may be of the Jackson-Pratt or HemoVac type, exiting in a collection device that can be emptied (see Skills 9-12 and 9-13), or the drain may be a hollow-type drain such as a Penrose drain or rubber catheter drain that is not connected to a collection device and simply drains into the dressing (see Skill 9-9). Dressings and drain care vary according to the surgeon's preference and agency or institutional policy. A general guideline for care of the wound with retention sutures is covered in this skill.

▶ ASSESSMENT

1. Assess the client's comfort level postoperatively upon arrival from the operating room.

Determines the need for pain medications and other comfort measures. Good pain control promotes compliance with other postoperative care regimes.

2. Assess the external appearance of the initial postoperative dressing and compare with subsequent dressings. **The initial dressing may need to be reinforced if it becomes saturated with drainage. A disrupted or saturated dressing should be brought to the attention of the health care provider. Inspecting the dressing helps determine what supplies will be needed.**

3. Assess the appearance of the wound and drains once the dressing is removed. Assess for signs of infection, tissue trauma, evidence of bleeding or leakage of tissue fluids. Note the position of indwelling catheters, drainage tubes, and the presence of sutures or stabilizing devices closing the wound and supporting the drains. **Establishes a baseline for later comparisons.**

4. Assess the client's understanding about the postoperative care of the surgical wound site. **Determines what education and support is needed.**

▶ DIAGNOSIS

Impaired Skin Integrity

Impaired Tissue Integrity

Risk for Infection

▶ PLANNING

Expected Outcomes:

1. The wound and retention sutures will be assessed for signs of healing, infection and skin irritation.
2. The appropriate dressing will be applied to the site.
3. The surgically placed drains will be monitored for proper functioning.
4. The client/family will verbalize and/or demonstrate the ability, if indicated, to perform the dressing change and associated wound care of the surgical wound site.

Equipment Needed (see Figures 9-10-1 and 9-10-2):

- Clean exam gloves
- Container for proper disposal of soiled dressing
- Moisture-proof gown (optional)
- Protective eyewear (optional)
- Sterile gloves
- Approved cleaning solution
- Normal saline
- Small sterile container
- Small sterile bowl (optional)
- Sterile cotton-tip applicators
- Sterile 4 × 4 gauze pads, multiple
- ABD dressing (optional)
- Montgomery straps (optional)

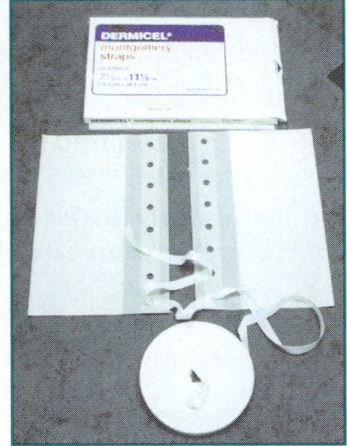

Figure 9-10-2 Montgomery straps

- Tubular mesh (optional)
- 2 rolls of tape (foam or paper)

▶ CLIENT EDUCATION NEEDED:

1. Educate the client about the need for the retention sutures, the signs and symptoms of infection, the anticipated course of healing, and how the wound will be managed.
2. Teach the client to wash hands before and after dressing changes, site care, or emptying of drainage collection devices.
3. Make sure the client's pain is controlled before beginning a teaching session.
4. If family is to be involved in care, plan teaching when they are present, if possible.
5. Employ the aid of a translator if there is a language barrier.
6. Take into consideration the client/family's cultural and social background when deciding what to teach and when eliciting feedback.
7. Use visual aids such as flip charts, models, and videos, if available.

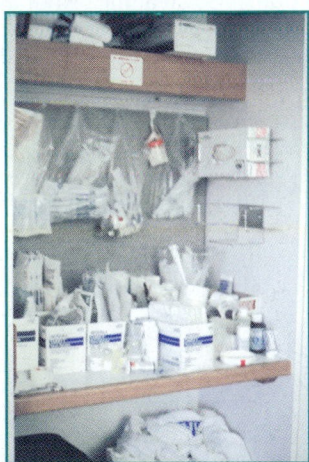

Figure 9-10-1 Dressing supplies are kept in the client's room.

Estimated time to complete the skill:
15–20 minutes

▶ DELEGATION TIPS

Wound dressing with retention sutures requires nursing assessment of wound edge proximity and tissue integrity and cannot be delegated to ancillary personnel.

IMPLEMENTATION—Action/Rationale

Action	Rationale

Dressing Application for Closed Surgical Wounds with Wire Retention Sutures

1. Gather supplies.

2. Provide privacy; draw curtains; close door.

3. Explain procedure to client.

4. Wash hands.

5. Apply clean exam gloves.

6. Remove dressing and place in appropriate receptacle (see Figure 9-10-3).

7. Assess the wound, retention sutures, and drains for signs of healing, infection and skin irritation.

8. Remove used exam gloves with contaminated surfaces inward and discard in appropriate container.

9. Wash hands.

10. Set up supplies.

1. Avoids having to break aseptic technique.

2. Maintains client comfort and privacy while body is exposed during procedure.

3. Provides information about the procedure.

4. Reduces the transmission of microorganisms.

5. Provides infection control and protection from body fluids.

6. Dressings soiled with body fluids are considered contaminated and subject to biohazard disposal in the correct manner per institution protocol.

7. Allows for evaluation of effectiveness of treatment.

8. Exam gloves used to remove the old dressing are considered dirty and should be removed.

9. Reduces the transmission of microorganisms.

10. Following removal of the dressing, you will have a better idea of what supplies are needed and in what amount.

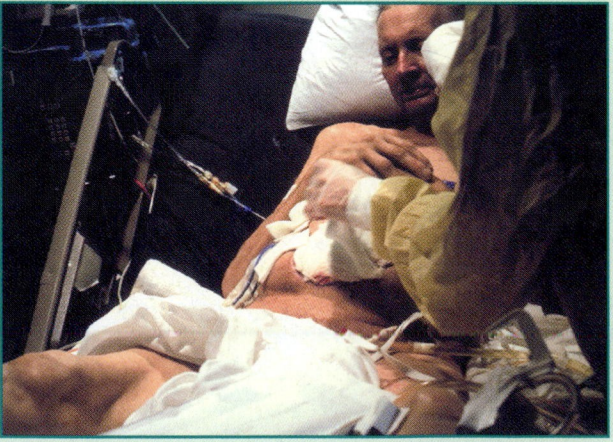

Figure 9-10-3 Remove the old dressing.

continues

Action	Rationale
11. Set up a sterile field, including pouring ordered solutions into appropriate containers, if indicated for the dressing change. Apply sterile gloves.	**11.** This is a sterile dressing change.
12. Cleanse the suture line, areas around the retention sutures and plastic guard devices using sterile normal saline or other approved cleaning solution applied to cotton-tip applicators or 4 × 4 gauze pads. Cleanse the incision, using a separate cotton-tip applicator or gauze for each swipe. Moving from top to bottom, clean the incision line first, then clean each side of the incision. Use cotton-tip applicators to clean under retention sutures.	**12.** Blood and drainage can be an irritant and a medium for microbes and should be removed from the incision line, exit sites of the retention sutures, and plastic guard devices supporting the retention sutures. Normal saline will not interfere with healing of the suture line and may be used. Cleansing should be from clean to contaminated to avoid introduction of microbes into the clean wound.
13. Apply external dressing of dry 4 × 4 gauze pads, cover sponges, fluffs, or ABD pads (see Figure 9-10-4). Secure dressing in place with tape, Montgomery straps, or tubular mesh (see Figure 9-10-5).	**13.** The external dressing is determined by the size and shape of the wound. Tape may be an option; however, because of the size of most wounds requiring retention sutures, Montgomery straps, tubular mesh, or an abdominal binder with Velcro closures are the best alternatives to securing large dressings over retention sutures. Tubular mesh and abdominal binders are a nice alternative to hold the dressing in place because adhesive application is not involved.
14. Conduct client/family education about the dressing, which may include teaching the dressing technique to the client/family.	**14.** Educates the client/family and prepares for discharge.
15. Dispose of old dressing appropriately. Remove gloves and wash hands.	**15.** Reduces the transmission of microorganisms.

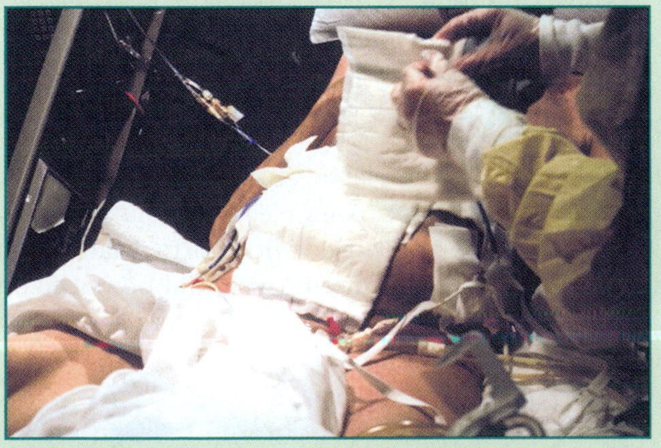

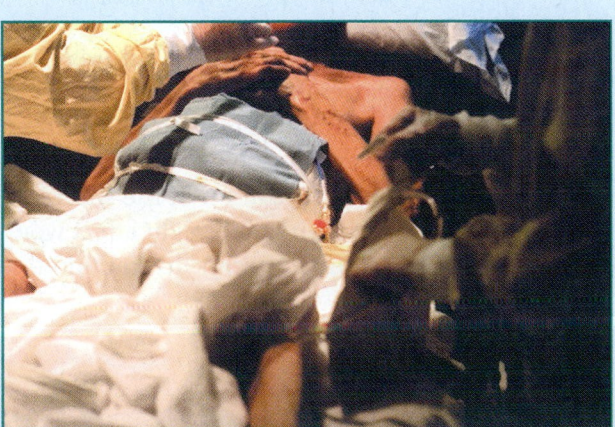

Figure 9-10-4 Apply ABD pads as external dressing.

Figure 9-10-5 Secure dressings in place.

▶ REAL WORLD ANECDOTES

Mr. Russell is a 39-year-old man who is 5 days postoperative for an exploratory laparotomy for a recurring intra-abdominal abscess. The client had gastric bypass surgery 3 years ago which did not reduce his obesity. Because of the client's large size of 152 kg and history of diabetes and recurrent abdominal surgeries, the surgeon has placed retention sutures for wound closure intermittently spaced with nylon sutures. During the first 72 hours after surgery, Mr. Russell experienced fluid retention and abdominal distention. The plastic guards supporting the retention sutures were pressed tightly against the abdominal skin. With the ensuing postoperative diureses and a nasogastric tube connected to low continuous suction, his distention resolved. A wound and skin assessment revealed skin ulcerations beneath the plastic guard devices and crusting around the retention wire exit sites.

The skin under each plastic guard and around each exiting retention suture is cleansed with normal saline and dried. Hydrocolloid patches (Duoderm) are applied to the ulcerated areas under the plastic guards, and 2 × 2 gauze pads are applied to the areas under the plastic guards that are not ulcerated. Below the last retention suture, the inferior portion of the wound was left open and a wet to dry dressing is applied every 8 hours. The remaining suture line is cleansed of crusts using approved cleaning solution as needed. Dry 4 × 4 gauze pads are folded lengthwise along the suture line. Two ABD pads are applied on top and the dressing is secured with Montgomery straps.

▶ EVALUATION

- The wound and retention sutures were assessed for signs of healing, infection, and skin irritation.
- The appropriate dressing was applied to the site.
- The surgically placed drains were monitored for proper functioning.
- The client/family verbalized and/or demonstrated the ability, if indicated to perform the dressing change and associated wound care of the surgical wound site.

▶ DOCUMENTATION

Nurses' Notes

- Record date and time the retention sutures were inspected and the dressing changed.
- Write a brief description of the wound, sutures, and retention sutures.
- Note the condition and position of the sutures.
- Document any risk factors that might affect wound healing, such as obesity or poor skin condition.

Document on appropriate flow sheet or electronic medical record (EMR).

▶ CRITICAL THINKING SKILL

Introduction

Assessing, but not intervening to reduce pressure from a retention suture guard, allowed a pressure ulcer to develop.

Possible Scenario

You observe that the skin is pressed tightly against the plastic guards of the retention sutures. The rest of the suture line is clean and dry and approximated. After a visual inspection of the wound, you apply a dry gauze dressing on top of the wound. The next shift finds an ulceration under one of the plastic guards.

Possible Outcome

Plastic guards pressing tightly against the skin can cause ulceration of the skin.

Prevention

The skin beneath the plastic guards should always be cleansed using an approved cleaning solution and a cotton-tip applicator, rinsed with normal saline, and dried. The health care provider should be notified if the plastic guards appear to be pressing too tightly against the client's skin.

► VARIATIONS

Geriatric Variations:
- *Elderly people have thin skin, which can tear. Do not tug at the skin when removing the dressing. Assess the skin carefully after removing the dressing.*
- *Elderly clients may require assistance with wound management in the home setting.*

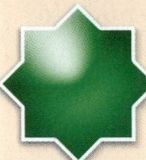

Pediatric Variations:
- *Make sure that the dressing is secure and the small child does not have access to the retention sutures.*
- *Demonstrate retention sutures on a doll or stuffed animal.*
- *Teach older children how to participate in placing dressings over retention sutures.*

Home Care Variations:
- *Advise the client/family on how to obtain additional dressing supplies.*
- *Make sure the client/family follows proper disposal of contaminated dressings. Make sure they have appropriate disposal materials available.*
- *Wounds with retention sutures can be complex and difficult to heal. Make sure the client knows whom to contact for questions and assistance with wound care. Make sure the client understands the symptoms of infection and what to do if bleeding or dehiscence occurs. Make sure the client can obtain adequate pain control during dressing changes.*

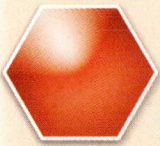

Long-Term Care Variations:
- *Special supplies necessary to dress large wounds may not be available in the long-term care setting. A review of the specific dressing change procedure may need to be presented to the staff caring for the client at the long-term care facility.*
- *A dressing change order will need to be written by the attending health care provider of the facility.*

► COMMON ERRORS

Possible Error:
You have applied your sterile gloves and are ready to proceed with the dressing change when you notice that you did not bring enough 4 × 4 gauze pads into the client's room, necessitating removal of sterile gloves, leaving the room, and obtaining more supplies.

Prevention:
Perfect your organizational skills. Assess what will be needed and bring the proper supplies to the client. Open all wound care supplies prior to applying sterile gloves.

Possible Error:
You are teaching a dressing change to a young Hispanic woman who will be caring for her husband at home. She demonstrates basic conversational English skills. You proceed to explain the dressing change using medical terms. You assume she understands. Her return demonstration the next day indicates she did not understand.

Prevention:
You may need to employ the aid of a translator when giving care or instructions to a client or family member whose first language is not English.

▶ **NURSING TIPS**

- Dressing changes require organization to be done efficiently. Gather data about the dressing change from the following:

  –Shift report

  –Nurses who have cared for the client

  –The client/family

  –Chart notes

  –Orders

  –Care map, care plan

  –Observation of the dressed wound

  –Supplies already in room

- Make a list, if necessary, of needed supplies to take into the room.
- If you are going to be in a client's room for some time, let others know so that they can cover your call lights and you can devote your attention to the dressing change.
- Avoid elastic dressings and tubes if history of latex allergy.

▶ **SPECIAL CONSIDERATIONS**

- *Retention sutures with large gauge wire provide a good choice of support for the obese client. These bridges help support deep tissues while more superficial fascia and skin tissues heal.*
- *Retention sutures are also used when clients have undergone preoperative radiation. These clients often have an increased risk of dehiscence, which delays healing and increases risk of infection.*

Obtaining a Wound Drainage Specimen for Culturing

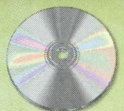

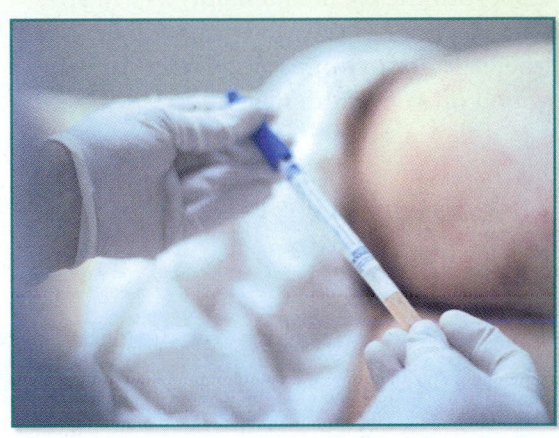

▶ OVERVIEW OF THE SKILL

Bacterial wound contamination is one of the most common causes of altered wound healing. A surgical wound can become infected with microorganisms preoperatively, intraoperatively, or postoperatively. During the preoperative period, the wound may become exposed to pathogens because of the manner in which the wound was infected, such as in traumatic injuries. Nicks or abrasions created during preoperative shaving may also be a source of pathogens. The risk for intraoperative exposure to pathogens increases when the respiratory, gastrointestinal, genitourinary, and oropharyngeal tracts are opened. Nonsurgical wounds from trauma, pressure ulcers, or disease can become infected as well.

If the amount of bacteria in the wound is sufficient or the client's immune defenses are compromised, clinical infection may result and become apparent 2 to 11 days postoperatively. Infection slows healing by prolonging the inflammatory phase of healing, competing for nutrients, and producing chemicals and enzymes that are damaging to the tissues. Identifying when a wound is contaminated and the infectious agent is an important step in wound healing.

▶ ASSESSMENT

1. Assess the wound and the surrounding tissues for signs of infection. Check for heat, redness, inflammation, and drainage. Check the color and consistency of the drainage. Check the smell and color of the wound. **Allows for intervention to detect and treat infection.**
2. Assess the client's overall status, including vital signs, for signs of infection such as fever, chills, or elevated white blood cell count (WBC). **Allows for intervention to detect and treat infection.**

▶ DIAGNOSIS

Risk for Infection

Impaired Tissue Integrity

Impaired Skin Integrity

Disturbed Body Image

▶ PLANNING

Expected Outcomes:

1. The wound culture will be collected with a minimum of pain and trauma to the client.
2. The wound culture will be representative of the flora present in the wound, without contamination by flora outside the wound.

Equipment Needed (see Figure 9-11-1):

- Disposable gloves
- Sterile gloves and dressing supplies
- Normal saline and irrigation tray

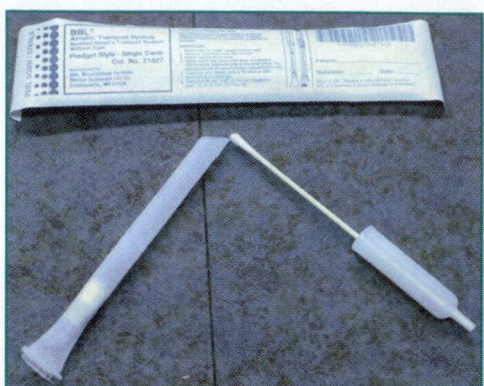

Figure 9-11-1   Sterile culture tube and swab

- Culture tube and swab
- Moisture-proof container or bag

▶ **CLIENT EDUCATION NEEDED:**

1. Explain to the client the reason the wound culture is being collected and how the procedure will be done.
2. Be aware of verbal and nonverbal communication indicating the client is concerned about being dirty or contaminated. Provide teaching and support to the client and family as needed.
3. Teach the client to wash hands frequently, especially after coming in contact with the wound or wound drainage.

Estimated time to complete the skill: **15 minutes**

▶ **DELEGATION TIPS**

Obtaining a wound culture requires nursing assessment and aseptic technique, and is potentially an invasive procedure; therefore, delegation to ancillary personnel is not appropriate.

IMPLEMENTATION—Action/Rationale

Action	Rationale
1. Wash hands, apply disposable gloves, and remove old dressing. Place old dressing in moisture-proof container and remove and discard gloves. Wash hands again.	1. Reduces the transmission of microorganisms. Makes the wound accessible for obtaining the culture.
2. Open the dressing supplies using sterile technique and apply gloves.	2. Maintains sterile environment.
3. Assess the wound's appearance; note quality, quantity, color, and odor of discharge.	3. Provides assessment of the amount and character of the wound's drainage prior to irrigation. Reddened areas and heavy drainage suggest infection.
4. Irrigate the wound with normal saline prior to culturing the wound; do not irrigate with antiseptic.	4. Irrigation decreases the risk of culturing normal flora and other exudates such as protein; irrigating with an antiseptic prior to culturing may destroy the bacteria.
5. Using a sterile gauze pad, absorb the excess saline, then discard the pad.	5. Removal of excess irrigant prevents maceration of tissue caused by excess moisture.
6. Remove the culture tube from the packaging (see Figure 9-11-2). Remove the culture swab from the culture tube and gently roll the swab over the granulation tissue. Avoid eschar and wound edges (see Figure 9-11-3).	6. Decreases the chance of collecting superficial skin microorganisms.

continues

Action	Rationale

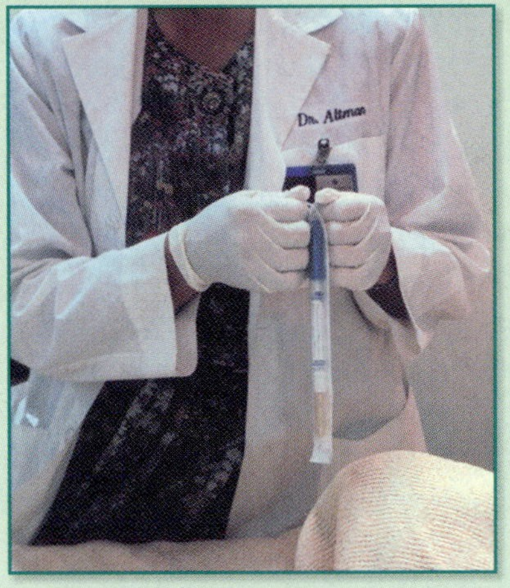

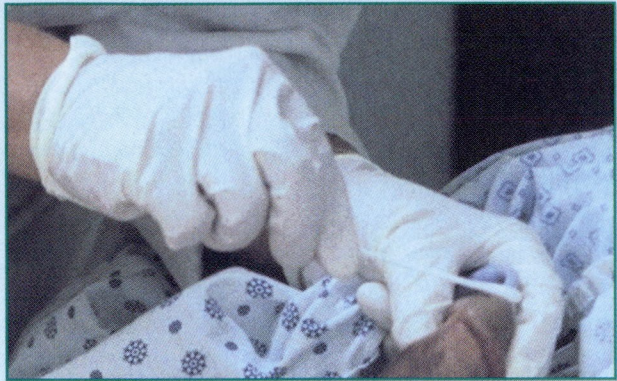

Figure 9-11-3 Roll the swab over the area to be cultured.

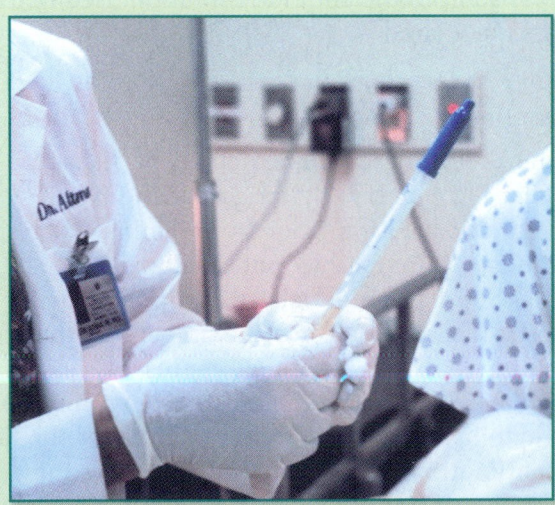

Figure 9-11-2 Remove the culture tube from the packaging.

7. Replace the swab into the culture tube, being careful not to touch the swab to the outside of the tube. Recap the tube. Crush the ampule of medium located in the bottom or cap of the tube (see Figure 9-11-4).

8. Remove gloves, wash hands, and apply sterile gloves. Dress the wound with sterile dressing.

9. Label the specimen, place in biohazard transport bag, and arrange to transport the specimen to the laboratory according to institutional policy.

10. Remove gloves and wash hands.

11. Document all assessment findings and actions taken. Document that a specimen was obtained.

7. Avoids contamination with microorganisms. Releases the medium to surround the swab.

8. Prevents contamination of the wound.

9. Ensures proper handling of specimen.

10. Reduces the transmission of microorganisms.

11. Records information for evaluation and promotes continuity of care.

Figure 9-11-4 Crush the ampule to release the medium inside the culture tube.

▶ REAL WORLD ANECDOTES

Mrs. Smith has advanced stage ovarian cancer. She was admitted to the hospital for wound care for an ulceration on her coccyx. The ulceration required frequent dressing changes, and while a client in the hospital, Mrs. Smith developed an infection in the wound. Cultures revealed that the infection was a particularly resistant strain of Staph. This same strain had been found in a wound in another part of the hospital. Her physicians determined that Mrs. Smith was suffering from a nosocomial infection, probably caused by poor handwashing on the part of a caregiver. A barrage of multiple antibiotics failed to destroy the infection. Mrs. Smith's doctors wanted to send her home with home care nurses and instructions regarding her wound care. Unfortunately, Mrs. Smith's daughter suffered from a congenital heart defect and Mrs. Smith's doctors felt that the infection was a hazard to the daughter's health. Mrs. Smith was told that while she could return home she would not be able to see her daughter because of the danger of infection. Citing exhaustion and discouragement with this latest setback as well as her poor prognosis, Mrs. Smith arranged for a guardian for her daughter and then refused any further antibiotic therapy. Shortly thereafter she developed a systemic infection from this same resistant bacteria and within weeks died without ever having the chance to see her daughter one last time.

▶ EVALUATION

- The wound culture was collected with a minimum of pain and trauma to the client.
- Determined whether the wound culture was representative of the flora present in the wound, without contamination by other bacteria.

▶ DOCUMENTATION

Nurses' Notes

- Document the time and method of collection of the culture, and what was done with the specimen.
- The lab requisition form must be filled out with the client's information as well as the time and date the specimen was collected, location of the culture, and the requested tests. Often there are duplicate numbered or coded labels on the lab slips. One copy is placed in the chart.

Document on appropriate flow sheet or electronic medical record (EMR).

▶ CRITICAL THINKING SKILL

Introduction

Know the proper technique for culturing a wound to get accurate results.

Possible Scenario

You are assisting another nurse in changing a dressing. You note that she has the equipment present to collect a wound specimen for a sensitivity analysis. The nurse removes the dressing and starts to cleanse the wound according to the physician's orders for this client. Part of the cleansing routine is to irrigate the wound with an antibiotic solution. After she has finished cleaning the wound, just before placing a clean dry dressing over the wound, the nurse uses the culture swab sticks to obtain a specimen to send to the lab.

Possible Outcome

- The specimen returns no growth despite clinical observations that indicate an infection.
- The specimen returns with growth of one type of bacteria. Even after being treated for that type of bacteria, the wound continues to appear infected.
- The specimen returns with bacterial growth that is resistant to the antibiotic solution used to irrigate the wound.

Prevention

All the preceding outcomes could be hazardous to the client's recovery. By irrigating the wound with an antibiotic solution prior to obtaining the culture specimen, the nurse has potentially altered the lab results. She has potentially destroyed many of the bacteria that are causing the infection; therefore, the culture will not accurately represent the flora of the wound. The culture should be taken prior to placing anything in the wound that might alter the flora. Any antibiotics used in the wound or that the client is receiving systemically should be noted on the lab slip.

▶ VARIATIONS

Geriatric Variations:
- *Explain the procedure step-by-step to clients who cannot hear or see well so they know what you are doing.*
- *Enlist help if needed to hold an older or debilitated client in position so you can obtain a proper culture.*

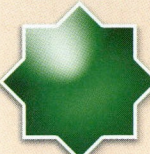

Pediatric Variations:
- *Explain to the child in age-appropriate terms what the culture procedure is for.*
- *Allow older children to assist in positioning and watch the procedure if they wish.*
- *Answer questions and reassure the child that the procedure will not hurt any more than the normal dressing change.*

Home Care Variations:
- *When conducting a home care visit, make sure you know where to send the culture after you have collected it. Will it be picked up by the lab? Will you or a caregiver be responsible for delivery to a location? Will the lab be open, or do you need to make special arrangements?*
- *Make sure you bring the correct equipment to the visit. A cotton-tip applicator and a sandwich bag will not provide the appropriate sterile culture receptacle.*
- *Make sure that the culture can be sent without excessive delay.*

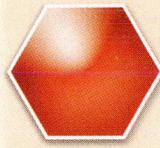

Long-Term Care Variations:
- *If the long-term facility does not stock the necessary equipment, make sure you know where to obtain the culture tubes and where to deliver the specimen before you initiate obtaining a wound drainage specimen.*
- *A culture order must be written by the attending health care provider of the facility.*

▶ COMMON ERRORS

Possible Error:

The swab is contaminated either before or after obtaining the specimen.

Prevention:

Be sure the swab touches only sterile items and the area to be cultured. Touching anything else will cause the test to be invalid and require a fresh specimen to be obtained. This increases cost to the client and wastes nursing time.

▶ NURSING TIPS

- Do not irrigate the wound with anything except sterile saline or sterile water prior to obtaining the specimen.
- Be aware of what you are doing while holding the culture swab. Touching the swab to anything but the area to be cultured and sterile surfaces contaminates the swab and invalidates the test.
- In anaerobic cultures be sure the specimen is immersed in the medium at the bottom of the tube.

► SPECIAL CONSIDERATIONS

- *Labeling the specimen with the right label for the right client is essential when culturing a wound. If mislabeled, client A could receive antibiotics needed by client B. Client A is put at risk to develop a resistance to the antibiotic while client B's infection is left untreated.*

Maintaining a Closed Wound Drainage System

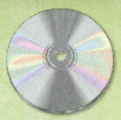

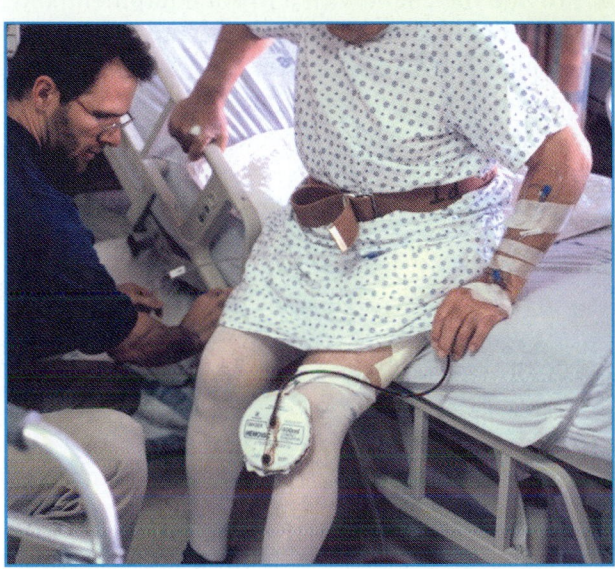

▶ OVERVIEW OF THE SKILL

Closed wound drainage systems are used whenever the drainage from a wound is greater than 100 mL in 24 hours. Closed wound drainage systems create a vacuum environment providing suction to remove the drainage from the wound environment. Small amounts of drainage are often contained using a Jackson-Pratt system (see Skill 9-13). Larger amounts of drainage are contained by using a HemoVac system (see Figure 9-12-1).

▶ ASSESSMENT

1. Identify the type and amount of drainage coming from the wound. **This will allow the nurse to determine which type of system (i.e., ostomy appliance versus a suction system) is required.**
2. Inspect the condition of the skin surrounding the wound. **Alterations in skin integrity will prohibit a closed drainage system from adhering to the skin.**
3. Measure the dimensions of the wound or determine the type of drainage system previously used prior to obtaining a closed drainage system from central supply. **This will alleviate the problem of obtaining the wrong equipment.**

▶ DIAGNOSIS

Risk for Impaired Skin Integrity

Risk for Deficient Fluid Volume

Risk for Infection

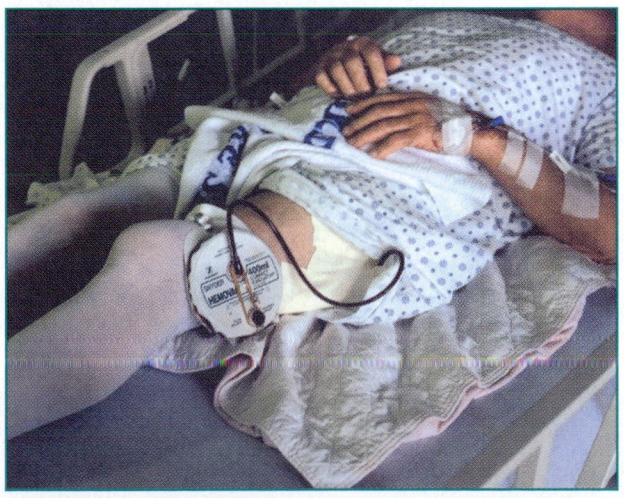

Figure 9-12-1   Wound drainage reservoir

1261

▶ PLANNING

Expected Outcomes:

1. Drainage will be contained within the system. There will be no leakage to the surrounding skin.
2. Wound drainage will be accurately measured and documented.
3. The wound drainage system will not decrease the client's mobility.
4. Odor from the wound will be controlled

Equipment Needed (see Figures 9-12-2 and 9-12-3):

- Gauze pads, 4 × 4
- Normal saline
- Gloves, clean and sterile
- Suction equipment
- Protective eyewear
- Red rubber catheter, HemoVac or Jackson-Pratt drainage system
- Transparent film or Steri-drape
- Scissors
- Pen or pencil
- Measuring guide

▶ CLIENT EDUCATION NEEDED:

1. Teach the client how to disconnect from the suction apparatus to ambulate.
2. Instruct the client to inform the nurse whenever there appears to be drainage from the closed wound drainage system. This is an indication that the system needs to be removed and reapplied.
3. Provide the client with a list of equipment and product numbers and a list of retailers where supplies can be purchased.
4. Educate the client regarding reasons and situations when to call the health care provider and/or wound care nurse expert. If necessary, provide the client with a written list.

Estimated time to complete the skill: **15–30 minutes**

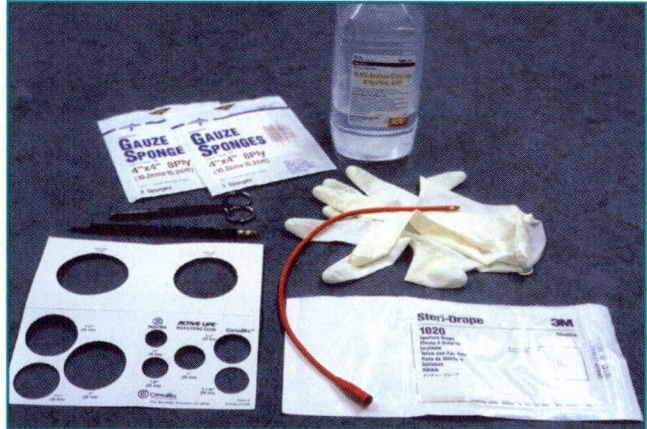

Figure 9-12-2 Gauze, gloves, catheter, measuring guide, pencil, scissors, and cleaning solution

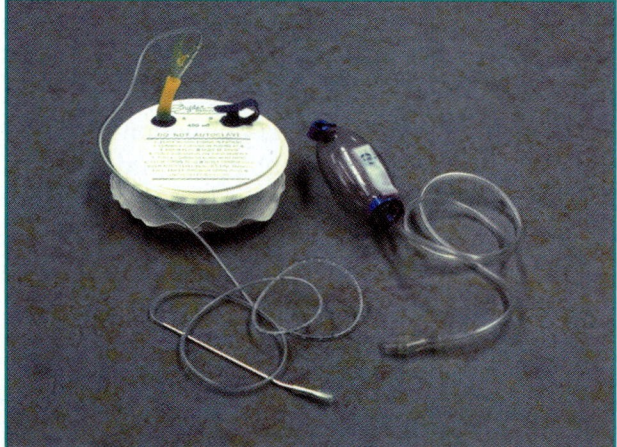

Figure 9-12-3 Jackson-Pratt and HemoVac drainage systems

▶ DELEGATION TIPS

The nurse is responsible for assessment of the wound, any drainage, and maintenance of drainage devices. Ancillary personnel may be delegated to empty and measure drainage device output. Ancillary personnel need proper training in handling drainage devices and in preventing transmission of microorganisms.

IMPLEMENTATION—Action/Rationale

Action	Rationale
1. Assess client's level of comfort and/or pain prior to beginning procedure.	1. Performing a dressing change may increase client's current pain level.
2. Medicate client for pain, if needed.	2. Promotes client comfort.
3. Assemble equipment.	3. Ensures that all equipment is ready to use.
4. Wash hands.	4. Reduces the transmission of microorganisms.
5. Apply clean gloves and remove old dressing, placing it in an appropriate receptacle.	5. Clean technique is appropriate for removing old dressings.
6. Assess site.	6. Check for signs of infection, drainage, and skin irritation.
7. Remove gloves and wash hands.	7. Reduces the transmission of microorganisms.
8. Open sterile packages of gauze, suction catheter, and transparent film or Steri-drape.	8. Ensures that all equipment is ready to use.
9. Moisten several packages of gauze with normal saline (NS).	9. Preparing work materials decreases exposure time of wound to environment.
10. Apply sterile gloves	10. Practices aseptic technique.
11. Cleanse wound bed with moistened normal saline gauze pads (see Figure 9-12-4).	11. Removes wound debris, which could impede wound healing.
12. Lay drain/catheter over the wound site.	12. Provides for adequate removal of wound drainage.
13. Open moistened gauze pad and lay them in the wound bed over the drain/catheter.	13. Maintains moist wound environment.

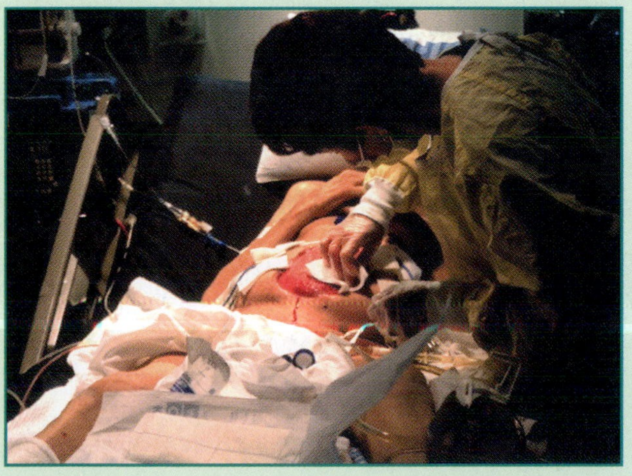

Figure 9-12-4 Clean the wound bed with moistened gauze.

continues

Action	Rationale

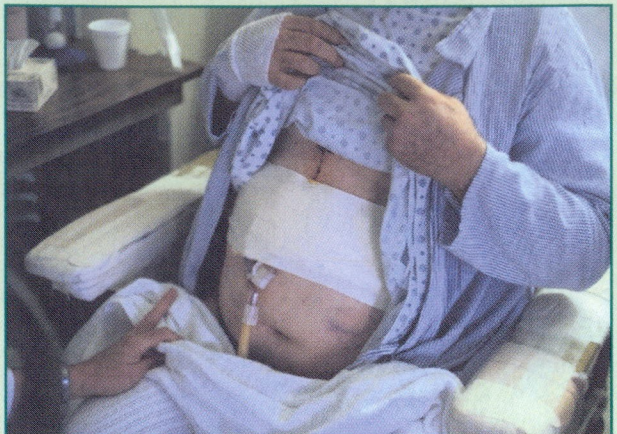

Figure 9-12-5   Cover the wound with an occlusive dressing to seal the wound environment.

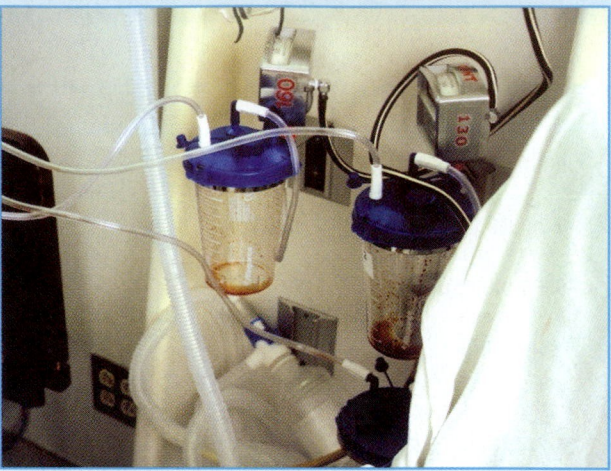

Figrue 9-12-6   Empty the collection container and record the amount of drainage.

14. Cover the entire wound with the transparent film, Steri-drape, or other occlusive dressing (see Figure 9-12-5).

14. Provides a sealed wound environment.

15. Attach drain/catheter to intermittent low wall suction, or compress HemoVac system, Jackson-Pratt, or Blake reservoir.

15. Provides suction removal of drainage from wound.

16. Dispose of contaminated supplies, remove gloves, and wash hands.

16. Reduces the transmission of microorganisms.

17. Change dressing system as needed depending on the intactness of the seal.

17. Maintains an adequate seal for suctioning of wound drainage.

Empty Drainage

18. Wash hands and apply clean gloves.

18. Reduces the transmission of microorganisms.

19. If attached to suction, empty and record drainage from suction apparatus every 8 hours (see Figure 9-12-6)

19. Maintains accurate output record.

20. If attached to Hemovac system, Jackson-Pratt, or Blake reservoir, empty and record drainage every 8 hours.
   a. Assess the drainage container for contents and compression.
   b. Open the drainage spout being careful not to touch the tip of the spout cap or spout to anything.

   c. Turn drainage collection container upside down and pour contents into measuring container.
   d. Press the container flat and replace the plug.

20. Maintains accurate output record.

   a. The drainage container needs to be compressed in order to work properly.
   b. Decreases microorganisms on the spout, thereby minimizing introduction of microorganisms into the closed system.
   c. Measures the drainage output.

   d. Drainage container needs to be compressed in order to work properly.

21. Dispose of drainage, remove gloves, and wash hands.

21. Reduces the transmission of microorganisms.

► REAL WORLD ANECDOTES

A client developed a fistula at the site of a previous drain following exploratory surgery for intestinal obstruction, which resulted in an ileostomy. The client had a history of bladder cancer with a continent urinary diversion. As the fistula output increased, the ileostomy output decreased. Skin irritation was prevented by immediately applying a drainable ostomy appliance when drainage began to occur from the drain stab wound. As the drainage from this enteric fistula increased beyond 100 mL in 24 hours, the pouching system was changed to a urinary appliance attached to a bedside drainage bag.

► EVALUATION

1. Drainage was contained within the system. There was no leakage to the surrounding skin.
2. Wound drainage was accurately measured and documented
3. Odor from the wound was controlled.
4. The wound drainage system did not decrease the client's mobility.

► DOCUMENTATION

Nurses' Notes

- Document assessment of periwound skin.
- Record wound dimensions (length, width, depth).
- Note color and amount of drainage.
- Document periwound skin care if alteration in skin integrity was noted.
- Describe type of closed wound system applied.

Document on appropriate flow sheet or electronic medical record (EMR).

► CRITICAL THINKING SKILL

Introduction

The client is experiencing a postoperative complication secondary to an enterocutaneous fistula.

Possible Scenario

A 65-year-old woman with a history of abdominal pain following lysis of adhesions and removal of a benign ovarian mass develops drainage from the midline incision. Within 7 days after surgery, the midline incision dehisces and large amounts of dark green drainage appear on the incisional dressing.

Dressing changes are initially done using gauze and changed every 30–90 minutes. The client's periwound skin is beginning to become excoriated.

Possible Outcome

The wound was not healing well. The nature and amount of wound drainage from the surgical wound should have alerted the nurse to the immediate need for further assessment. This client was at risk for wound infection, further dehiscence or evisceration of the wound, and further skin breakdown around the wound.

Prevention

The nurse consults with the wound care nurse expert for assistance in managing this complex wound. The nurse expert proceeds to apply a closed wound drainage system using suction after completing a thorough assessment of the client's wound environment.

The nurse should immediately notify the health care provider of the change in the client's status. The second nursing action is to apply a closed wound drainage system to quantify the amount of drainage. This action will allow for continued monitoring of the client's fluid status.

► VARIATIONS

Geriatric Variations:

- If elderly clients are confused, they may pull at dressings or tubes. Watch for signs that this is occurring.
- Increased monitoring of the client, and changes in the dressing may be indicated.
- The elderly may have thinner, more delicate skin, which may be more prone to breakdown and more sensitive to tapes and adhesives.

continues

▶ VARIATIONS *(continued)*

Pediatric Variation:
* *Have a parent in the room to support and distract the child while drainage system care is being performed.*

Home Care Variations:
* *When discharging a client with a newly healed fistula or wound, teach the client how to continue to care for the wound at home, if additional care is needed.*
* *Teach the client the signs and symptoms of infection.*
* *Teach the client how to tell what is normal redness and tenderness and what needs further evaluation.*

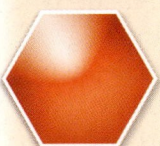

Long-Term Care Variations:
* *Some wounds are very slow to heal. Be especially watchful for signs of infection if the wound remains open for many weeks.*
* *Consider the long-term effects of constant dressings on the surrounding skin.*
* *Consider the long-term effects of restrictions in position or prolonged immobility that may develop as the wound fails to heal normally.*
* *Watch for signs of further skin breakdown caused by immobility.*
* *A client with a slow-healing wound may feel an increased sense of helplessness and depression.*
* *A dressing change order will need to be written by the attending health care provider of the facility.*

▶ COMMON ERRORS

Possible Error:
The closed wound drainage system is too small for the wound's dimensions

Prevention:
Measure the dimensions of the wound prior to the application of the drainage system. If this error occurs, remove the leaking appliance and remeasure the wound dimensions before reapplying the closed wound drainage system.

▶ NURSING TIPS

* Recognize that all draining wounds are not the same. Each wound must be treated individually, which requires that the nurse assess the dimensions, type, and amount of drainage, and the periwound skin's condition.
* Client teaching is easily incorporated into the care of the draining wound by encouraging the client to be your assistant during the application process.
* Use of a closed drainage system on a draining wound will increase the client's comfort level and thereby the client's participation in self-care activities.
* Costs to the client and the health care institution are reduced when draining wounds are maintained in a closed wound system. The cost reduction is realized in a decreased use of sterile dressings, linen changes, pain medication used by the client, and nursing time.

▶ SPECIAL CONSIDERATIONS

* *Closed drainage systems are often used in conjunction with IV antibiotics.*
* *Some complications associated with drains are infection, hemorrhage, kinking, and hernia. The closed system usually requires small incisions and herniation is rarely seen.*

Care of the Jackson-Pratt (JP) Drain Site and Emptying the Drain Bulb

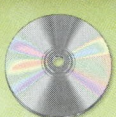

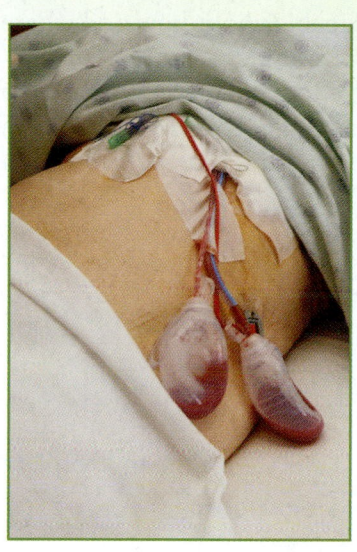

▶ OVERVIEW OF THE SKILL

Jackson-Pratt (JP) or similar drains are placed surgically to allow for draining of body fluids postoperatively. The drain ends in a bulb that compresses to allow for creation of gentle suction, thereby enhancing the flow of the fluid from the operative site. The drains may be in place for 24 hours to several weeks.

▶ ASSESSMENT

1. Assess the client's understanding about the drain care procedure. **It is important to take into consideration the client's ability to understand verbal and written instructions and the client's cultural and social background.**
2. Assess the external appearance of the dressed drain exit site, drain, and bulb. **Assessment of the external appearance of the dressing is important for determining dressing supply needs and for noting effectiveness of the closed drainage system.**
3. Assess the drain exit site once the dressing is removed. **Assessment should include noting any signs of infection, excessive drainage from around the drain, normal position of the drain, or sutures that are loose or not intact.**

4. Assess the client/family response to the drain care procedure. **Assessment of the client's response is necessary for determining client/family readiness for involvement with the drain care procedure.**

▶ DIAGNOSIS

Risk for Infection

Impaired Tissue Integrity

Impaired Skin Integrity

Deficient Knowledge

▶ PLANNING

Expected Outcomes:

1. The JP drain site will be free of drainage and signs of infection.
2. The JP drain site will be cleansed and redressed.
3. The external JP drainage bulb will be intact and functioning properly.
4. The JP drainage bulb will be emptied, and the amount measured and documented.
5. The JP drain will be secured to the client's gown or clothing.
6. The client/family will verbalize and/or demonstrate understanding about the drain care procedure.

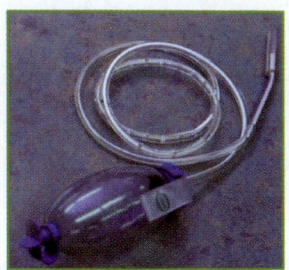

Figure 9-13-1 Jackson-Pratt drainage system

Equipment Needed (see Figure 9-13-1):

- Clean exam gloves
- Container for collecting and measuring the drain output
- Iodine swabs
- Approved cleaning solution
- Normal saline
- Sterile 4 × 4 gauze pads or split drain dressings
- Sterile cotton-tip applicators
- Tape

▶ **CLIENT EDUCATION NEEDED:**

1. Make sure the client is comfortable before teaching.

2. If family members are to be involved, plan to teach when they are present if possible.
3. Encourage handwashing before and after dressing change and bulb emptying.
4. Clients need to have a written set of instructions to take home with them.
5. Make sure the client has supplies to get started doing the dressing change at home and is knowledgeable about how and where to obtain additional supplies.
6. Make sure the client knows whom to contact for the postoperative visit, signs of infection, a dislodged drain, or a malfunctioning system.
7. Have the client record all drainage output and give totals to the health care provider during the postoperative visit.

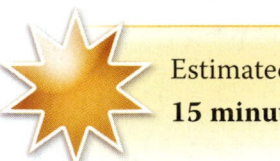

Estimated time to complete the skill:
15 minutes

▶ **DELEGATION TIPS**

The nurse is responsible for assessment of the wound and any drainage, and maintenance of drainage devices. Ancillary personnel may be delegated to empty and measure drainage device output. Ancillary personnel need proper training in handling drainage devices and preventing transmission of microorganisms.

IMPLEMENTATION—Action/Rationale

Action	Rationale
1. Review order of health care provider, institutional policy and procedure, or standing order for drain care.	1. The basic technique is described here. Remember to check for an institutional policy or specific orders.
2. Gather supplies.	2. Ensures that all supplies are ready and prevents interruption during the procedure.
3. Provide privacy; draw curtains; close door.	3. Maintains client comfort and privacy while body is exposed during procedure.

continues

Action	Rationale
4. Explain procedure to client/family.	**4.** Provides information about the procedure, allows for feedback, helps alleviate client anxiety, and promotes cooperation.
5. Wash hands and set up supplies.	**5.** Reduces the transmission of microorganisms and promotes organization.
6. Apply clean exam gloves.	**6.** Provides infection control and protection from body fluids.
7. Unpin drain tube from gown or clothing. Remove old dressing and dispose in appropriate waste location.	**7.** Unpinning allows for ease of removal of the old dressing. Dressings soiled with body fluids are considered contaminated and subject to biohazard disposal in the correct manner per institutional protocol.
8. Assess site (see Figure 9-13-2).	**8.** Checks for signs of infection; ascertains that the sutures that secure tube to skin are intact; checks the placement of the drain and that tubing is not kinked.
9. Remove gloves and wash hands.	**9.** Reduces the transmission of microorganisms.
10. Apply clean gloves. • Cleanse around drain with approved cleaning solution using sterile cotton-tip applicator, using gentle rolling motion of the applicator around the wound edge. • Cleanse away from the drain exit site. Do not roll one applicator more than halfway around the exit site. Use as many applicators as needed to clean the site. Dry with dry applicators.	**10.** • If there are crusts, this is an effective removal technique. This step may be omitted if crusts are not present. • Reduces the transmission of microorganisms.
11. Avoid contamination of the swabs and solutions. Do not dip the swabs into the solution container. Pour a small amount of the solution into a sterile bowl. Do not redip a used swab in the solution.	**11.** Reduces the transmission of microorganisms.
12. Apply a single folded 4 × 4 gauze pad under the drain and another folded 4 × 4 on top and tape in place. A drain sponge may be used if available as it has a slit opening for the drain.	**12.** Collects potential drainage and protects site.
13. Secure drain tube to dressing. To do this, tape a loop of the drain on the dressing. Then secure to gown/clothing by creating a tape tab on the drain and pinning to gown/clothing.	**13.** Minimizes the potential for dislodging the drain.

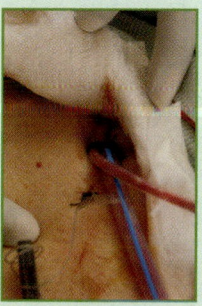

Figure 9-13-2   Assess insertion site for signs of infection.

continues

Action	Rationale
14. Dispose of dressings, remove gloves, and wash hands.	**14.** Reduces the transmission of microorganisms.
15. Assess the bulb for contents and compression.	**15.** The bulb should be emptied when it is one-half to two-thirds full. The bulb needs to be compressed to maintain suction in the closed system. The fluid in the JP drain system is red immediately post-op up to about 24 hours, then changes to light red 1–3 days postoperatively, then changes to straw-colored.
16. Wash hands, set up supplies, and apply gloves, if the bulb was not emptied in conjunction with the dressing change.	**16.** Reduces the transmission of microorganisms and promotes organization.
17. Remove the cap to the spout, being careful not to touch the tip of the spout cap or the spout to anything (see Figure 9-13-3).	**17.** Prevents contamination of the spout by microorganisms.
18. Pour the drainage collected in the drain bulb into the measuring container. Use a small calibrated cup, such as a urine specimen cup (see Figure 9-13-4).	**18.** Measures the drainage for intake and output.
19. Once emptied, while the cap is still off and the system is open, squeeze the bulb and while compressed reapply the cap to the spout (see Figure 9-13-5).	**19.** Functioning of the system is dependent upon a compressed bulb. If the bulb is compressed with the cap in place, the drainage contents in the tubing will be forced retrograde into the wound and could potentially introduce microbes into the wound. Also, the bulb will not maintain its compression if squeezed when closed.

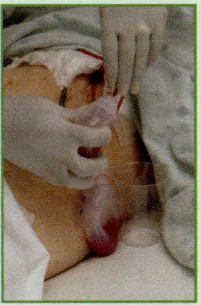

Figure 9-13-3   Remove the cap to the collection bulb spout.

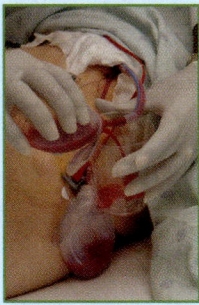

Figure 9-13-4   Pour the drainage into a measuring container.

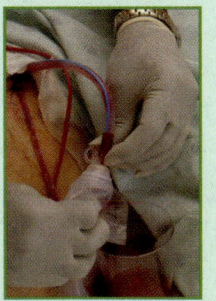

Figure 9-13-5   Squeeze the bulb and reapply the cap to the spout while the bulb is compressed.

continues

Action	Rationale
20. Secure drainage tube to client gown or clothing (see Step 13).	**20.** Minimizes the potential for dislodging the drain.
21. Dispose of the drainage.	**21.** Reduces the transmission of microorganisms.
22. Remove and properly dispose of equipment and gloves and wash hands.	**22.** Reduces the transmission of microorganisms.
23. Record the drainage on the intake and output record.	**23.** Maintain a record of output.

▶ REAL WORLD ANECDOTES

Mrs. Johnson is a 63-year-old woman who had a left axillary node dissection and lumpectomy of her left breast the previous day. While reaching for the phone, her JP drain becomes caught on the bed rail. She experiences a sharp pain in her left axillary region and puts on her call light. The nurse caring for Mrs. Johnson finds her holding her right hand over her left axillary area. She says, "I think something is wrong here; I felt a sharp pain as I reached for the phone." The nurse looks at the drain exit site to find that the sutures have torn from the skin and the JP drain tubing appears to have advanced about 2 cm. The system remains intact with a compressed bulb. There is a small amount of blood oozing from where the sutures were torn loose. The drain was temporarily secured with Steri-Strips, a new dressing was applied, and Mrs. Johnson was reassured that the system was intact. Pain medication was offered and the health care provider was notified of the incident.

▶ EVALUATION

- The JP drain site was free of drainage and signs of infection.
- The JP drain site was cleansed and redressed.
- The external JP drainage bulb was intact and functioning properly.
- The JP drainage bulb was emptied, and the amount measured and documented.
- The JP drain was secured to the client's gown or clothing.
- The client/family verbalized and/or demonstrated JP drain care.

▶ DOCUMENTATION

Nurses' Notes

- Date and time the exit site dressing change and emptying of the bulb occurred
- Appearance of the exit site
- Amount and character of the drainage

- Client/family education that took place, their level of understanding, and nursing observations of the return demonstration of the exit site care and emptying of the bulb
- Any contacts with the health care provider and the reason for the contact

Document on appropriate flow sheet or electronic medical record (EMR).

▶ CRITICAL THINKING SKILL

Introduction

Caring for the heart and mind as well as the body is a critical nursing challenge.

Possible Scenario

While working as a student nurse on a medical-surgical floor, you are assigned to care for a 30-year-old woman who has just had a right mastectomy for breast cancer. She needs to learn about her JP drainage system. You approach her to teach her the technical care of the JP drain and she bursts into tears. Feeling uncomfortable and not sure what to say, you excuse yourself and promise to return later.

Possible Outcome

The client's emotional needs are neglected. She remains upset and does not want to even speak about, or look at, her JP drainage system.

Prevention

It is usual for breast surgery clients to have JP drains in place postoperatively up to 1 week. It is not uncommon for women to have an emotional episode related to the loss of a breast while they are in the hospital. The nurse has the responsibility to recognize the loss and offer the client the chance to verbalize her feelings and concerns about the loss and changes in body image. Once the client has had a chance to verbalize her feelings, the nurse can begin to review the care of the JP drainage system with the client.

▶ VARIATIONS

Geriatric Variations:
- *Elderly people have thin skin, which can be sensitive to tape and solutions.*
- *Special attention should be given to the surrounding skin when removing the dressing around the exit site. If the skin appears to be sensitive to the iodine, it should be reported to the health care provider and this step eliminated.*
- *Elderly clients often live alone and may need home health care to assist with the care of the JP drainage system.*

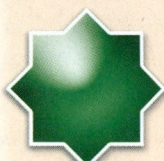

Pediatric Variations:
- *Remind all children not to touch the exit site or play with the bulb.*
- *Make sure the tubing is secure and the small child cannot pull or dislodge the drain.*
- *Older children can be taught to care for the JP drainage system.*
- *Elbow restraints may be necessary for younger children to prevent them from pulling on the drain site.*

Home Care Variations:
- *Where and how to obtain additional supplies should be reviewed with the client/family.*
- *Review proper disposal of contaminated dressings.*

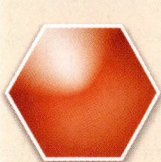

Long-Term Care Variations:
- *Special supplies may need to be ordered.*
- *A dressing change order may need to be written by the attending health care provider at the facility.*
- *A review of the above procedure may need to be presented to the staff caring for the client because they may not know how to care for a JP drainage system.*

▶ COMMON ERRORS

Possible Error:

While you are removing the client's gown, she feels a tug at her skin and you realize you did not unpin the tubing from the gown.

Prevention:

Remember to unpin the tube. Assess the client carefully before attempting any procedure that might dislodge tubes or drains.

continues

► **COMMON ERRORS** *(continued)*

Possible Error:

You complete your care and place a clean gown on the client, but you forget to pin the drainage tube to the gown.

Prevention:

Remember to pin the tube. If the client were to ambulate with the drainage bulb filled with fluid, the drain would become dislodged. Assess all tubes and drains on a regular basis to make sure they are properly secured.

Possible Error:

You forget to compress the bulb after emptying.

Prevention:

Review the basics of the JP tube, including the need to compress the bulb for a suction source. Ask for assistance if necessary.

► **NURSING TIPS**

- Assess the room for supplies before gathering additional supplies.
- Make sure to record all drainage because drain removal is based upon declining amount of drainage.
- If the client is going home with a drain in place, encourage the client to wear older blouses or shirts because of the iodine and potential soiling from the drainage. If the bulb does not retain its compression, there is most likely an air leak in the system or the bulb may need to be replaced.
- Empty the bulb any time it is half full because the suction created is better with an empty bulb. This may be every 2–3 hours postoperatively if there is a lot of drainage.

► **SPECIAL CONSIDERATIONS**

- *If the client is experiencing a leak in the JP system, the nurse must assess for location of the leak prior to informing the health care provider. If the leak is in the tubing proximal to the bulb, it may be necessary to cut the tubing and reapply the bulb further up. Provide an accurate description including the client's vital signs, antibiotic schedule (if applicable), last amount drained from bulb (whether amount is decreasing), where the leak appears to be located, and client's tolerance of the drain when you call the health care provider.*

Removing Skin Sutures and Staples

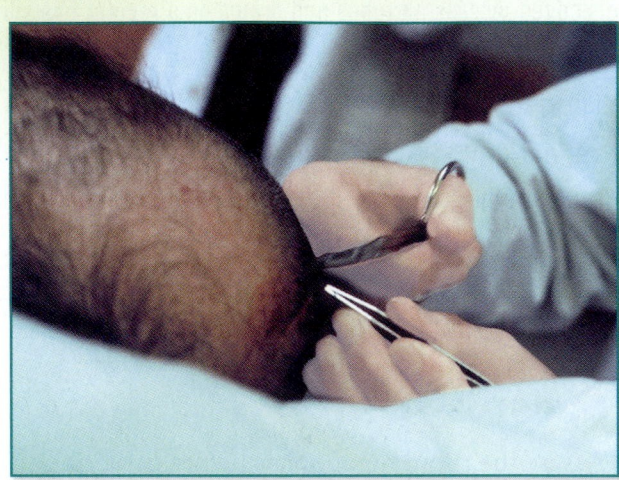

▶ OVERVIEW OF THE SKILL

Sutures and staples are a surgical means of closing a wound by sewing, wiring, or stapling the edges of the wound together. Most wounds are sutured in layers to maintain alignment of the tissues and reduce scarring. Sutures are generally removed 7–10 days after surgery, depending on where the wound is located and how well it is healing. Suture removal requires a health care provider's orders. Timing is important because sutures left in too long can increase the risk of infection and irritation from a foreign substance.

Sutures placed deep within the tissue layers are made of absorbable materials. Surface sutures are made of wire, nylon, or cotton. Continuous sutures are made with one thread, tied at the beginning and end of the suture line. Interrupted sutures are tied individually. Staples are used for large incision areas where the risk of dehiscence is greater, such as in sternotomies, in clients with increased adipose tissue, abdominal areas, and wounds that fail to heal or adhere.

▶ ASSESSMENT

1. Assess the wound **to determine whether the edges are approximate and healing. In deep wounds, palpate around the suture site for edema or any evidence of failure of tissue to adhere below the skin's surface.**

2. Assess **for any signs of infection, such as increased warmth, redness, exudate or drainage, and pain.**

3. Assess for any conditions **that impede the healing process**, such as age, immunosuppression, diabetes, obesity, smoking, radiation, poor cellular nutrition, infection, and deep wounds.

▶ DIAGNOSIS

Impaired Skin Integrity

Risk for Infection

Acute Pain

Impaired Physical Mobility

▶ PLANNING

Expected Outcomes:

1. The wound is intact, with the edges of the wound well-approximated.
2. There is no redness or signs of infection.
3. The procedure is performed with a minimum of pain and trauma to the client.

Equipment Needed (see Figure 9-14-1):

- Suture removal kit or sterile forceps with sterile suture removal scissors
- Gauze size as appropriate for wound area to be covered
- Biohazard bag or appropriate waterproof disposable bag

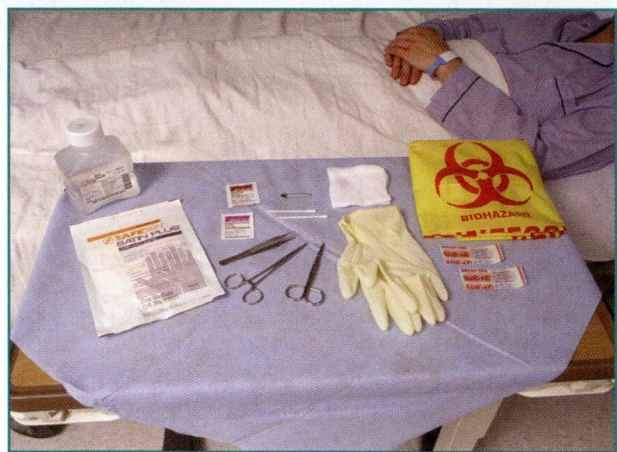

Figure 9-14-1 Suture removal supplies, including sterile saline, gloves, tweezers, scissors, gauze, and swabs

- Sterile saline, prepackaged antiseptic swabs, or gauze for cleaning, if appropriate
- Examination gloves
- Sterile gloves if dressings are to be applied
- Adhesive strips or butterfly adhesive tape as needed
- Sterile gauze to wipe stitches or sutures from forceps and scissors
- Tincture of benzoin as indicated

▶ **CLIENT EDUCATION NEEDED:**

1. Teach client to check for signs of infection, such as redness, pain, and increased warmth.
2. Teach client to assess body temperature daily at home for appropriate period of time depending on wound.
3. Teach client if deep wound with internal sutures, to observe for swelling or increased pain over the incision area.
4. If staples have been used, instruct the client to protect the area with a pillow when coughing.
5. If sutures or staples were used in abdominal wounds, instruct the client to avoid any lifting for up to 6 weeks.
6. If the client is sent home with sutures, teach how to assess for infection and set up appointment for suture removal. Let the client know that timing is important.

Estimated time to complete the skill: **Varies with type of wound, location, and need for cleaning and dressing—anywhere from 10–20 minutes**

▶ **DELEGATION TIPS**

Suture removal is a skill requiring aseptic technique and wound assessment by a nurse and, therefore, is not delegated to ancillary personnel.

IMPLEMENTATION—Action/Rationale

Action	Rationale
1. Wash hands.	1. Reduces the transmission of microorganisms.
2. Assess the wound to determine whether the edges of the wound are well-approximated and healing has occurred (see Figure 9-14-2).	2. Health care providers often have standing orders for sutures to be removed at a specified date. If the wound is not well-healed, sutures should be left in place longer and the health care provider notified.
3. Ascertain whether the client has had sutures removed before. If not, explain the procedure.	3. Explanation can help reduce anxiety.
4. Close the door and curtains around the client's bed.	4. Provides for privacy.

continues

Action	Rationale

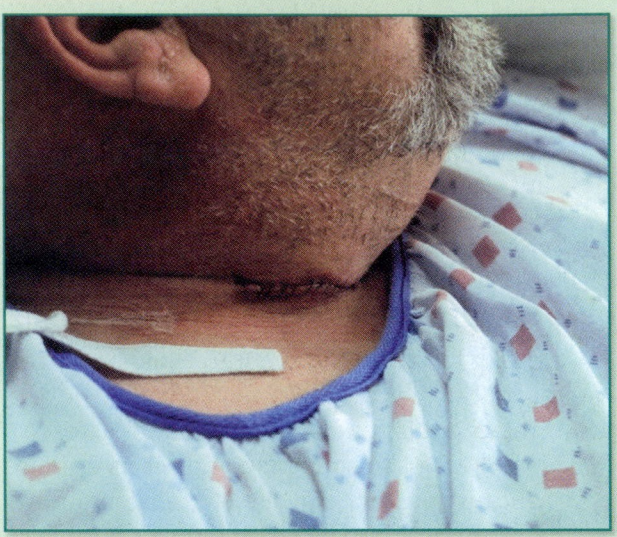

Figure 9-14-2 Inspect the wound to determine whether the edges are well-approximated and healing.

5. Raise the bed to a comfortable level.

5. Facilitates the procedure and provides for proper body mechanics for the nurse.

6. Position the client for comfort with easy access and visibility of the suture line.

6. Facilitates removal of the sutures and allows for careful observation of suture line.

7. Drape the client so that only the suture area is exposed.

7. Provides for privacy.

8. Open the suture removal kit, and assemble any supplies needed within easy access on a clean surface.

8. Facilitates removal of sutures.

9. Apply clean gloves to remove the old dressing and place it in a disposable bag.

9. Protects the client from transmission of microorganisms and protects the staff. Standard Precautions protocol.

10. Remove gloves and rewash hands.

10. Reduces the transmission of microorganisms.

11. If dressings are to be used, assemble equipment and supplies on sterile field.

11. Protects client from microorganisms.

12.
- Apply sterile gloves according to institutional policy.

- Clean the incision with saline-soaked gauze pads, antiseptic swabs, or per institutional policy (see Figure 9-14-3).

12.
- Protects the incision from microorganisms on the nurse's hands. Protects the nurse from possible contact with bodily fluids. Glove application policies vary for specific procedures. Nurses need to keep up-to-date with wound research and follow the guidelines of the institution where they practice.
- Various opinions exist regarding use of cleansing solutions for wound care.

13. When removing an interrupted suture, hold forceps in your nondominant hand and grasp the suture near the knot (see Figure 9-14-4).

13. Pulls the suture up and away from the client's skin.

14. Place the curved edge of the scissors under the suture or near the knot (see Figure 9-14-5).

14. Facilitates clipping of the suture.

continues

Action	Rationale

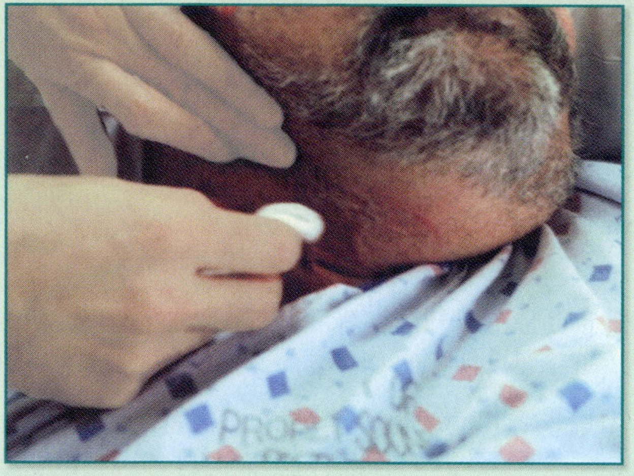

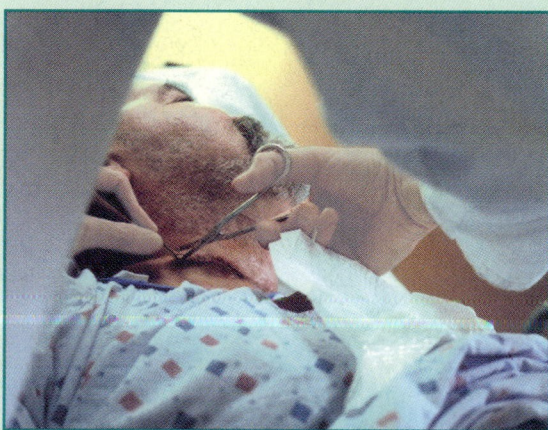

Figure 9-14-3 Clean the incision.

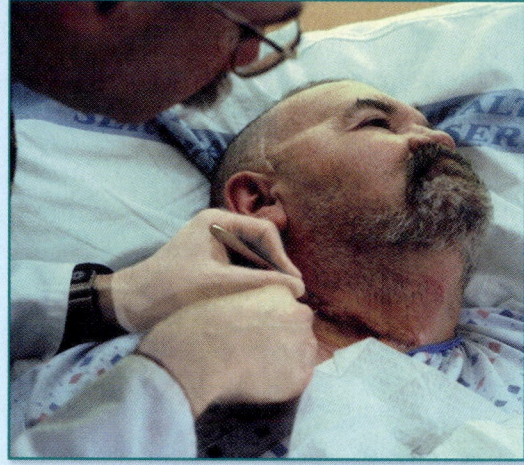

Figure 9-14-4 Hold forceps in your nondominant hand and grasp the suture near the knot.

15. Cut the suture close to the skin where the suture emerges from the skin (not in the middle). Pull the long end and remove it in one piece.

15. Facilitates suture removal. Cutting close to the skin avoids pulling large amounts of contaminated suture through tissue.

16. If the client has a continuous suture, cut both the first and second suture before removing them.

16. Facilitates suture removal without traumatizing the incision line.

17. Some policies require the removal of every other suture, with the remaining sutures removed at a later time. Assess the suture line to ensure that the edges remain approximated.

17. Any dehiscence should be detected early, and every other suture can be left in place.

18. Discard the sutures onto the gauze squares as they are removed and then place the gauze squares in the disposable bag when all the sutures have been removed.

18. Decreases the transmission of microorganisms.

19. Assess the suture line to ensure that the edges remain approximated and that all sutures have been removed (see Figure 9-14-6).

19. Detects early signs of dehiscence. Ensures that sutures do not remain in the skin when they are no longer needed.

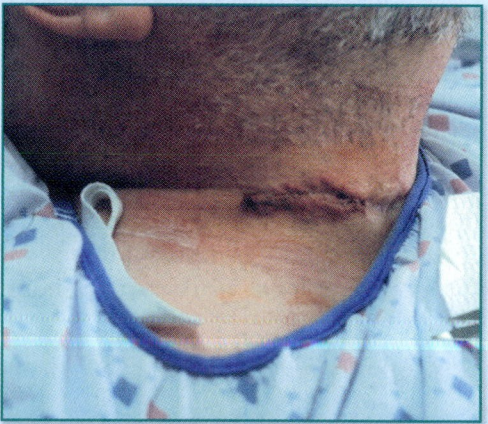

Figure 9-14-6 Reassess the suture line. Make sure the skin is still approximated and all sutures have been removed.

Figure 9-14-5 Hold the scissors in your dominant hand. Place the curved edge of the scissors under the suture.

continues

Action	Rationale
20. • Apply adhesive strips or butterfly tape adhesive strips across the suture line to secure the edges. The amount of reinforcement varies depending on the adherence of the suture line and the length of the suture line. Adhesive skin closures may be placed 1 inch apart or closer together. • Tincture of benzoin may be applied to the skin adjacent to the incision.	**20.** • If the suture line pulls apart a little after the sutures are removed, adhesive skin closures can be used to reinforce the suture line. • Helps adhesive strips adhere to skin.
21. Dispose of the soiled equipment.	**21.** Reduces odors in the client's room and reduces the transmission of microorganisms.
22. Remove gloves and wash hands.	**22.** Reduces the transmission of microorganisms.
23. If removing staples: • Repeat Actions 2 to 12. • Use a staple extractor to remove every other staple. Place the lower tip of staple remover under the staple and squeeze the handles together. The ends of the staple will extract from the skin. Move the staple away from the skin surface and release the staple into a disposal container. Assess the wound for adherence. Move on to the next staple if the skin has adhered well. • Repeat Actions 20–22.	**23.** • Prepares for staple removal. • When removing staples, it is best to remove every other staple and assess wound adherence before removing all staples. A staple extractor is designed to remove the staple with a minimum of discomfort and trauma to the surrounding skin and tissue. • See Rationales 20–22.

▶ REAL WORLD ANECDOTES

A client came back to the nurse after having his stitches removed because the suture line was reddened. The nurse explained that he might have slight redness around sutures because of irritation and not infection. He noted that the suture line was in an area where the client's waistband was irritating the skin.

▶ EVALUATION

• The wound is intact, edges are adhered, and there are no signs of infection or drainage.
• There was no redness or signs of infection
• The procedure was performed with a minimum of pain and trauma to the client.

▶ DOCUMENTATION

Nurses' Notes

• Document procedure and findings at wound site, such as redness, pain, or drainage.

• Document the time sutures were removed.
• Document that follow-up instructions and client teaching were provided.

Document on appropriate flow sheet or electronic medical record (EMR).

▶ CRITICAL THINKING SKILL

Introduction

Follow a procedure only when it is safe and correct to do so.

Possible Scenario

An obese client had an abdominal surgery 7 days previously. Her suture line looks clean; however, she is complaining of abdominal pain around the incision site.

Possible Outcome

Rather than remove any stitches, the nurse palpates the wound site for edema and possible poor internal healing and reports the findings. The client is diagnosed with both dehiscence and peritonitis related to surgery.

Prevention

Assess clients carefully who may be at risk for failure to heal. Carefully inspect the site for healing before removing sutures or staples. Internal wound healing may not have occurred.

▶ VARIATIONS

Geriatric Variations:
- *Elderly clients heal more slowly and sutures may need to remain in place for a longer period of time.*
- *Elderly clients may have increased risk of failure to heal or infection because of other medical diagnoses, such as diabetes or cancer.*
- *Poor nutrition in an elderly client may slow wound healing.*

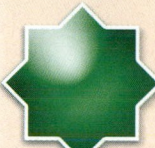

Pediatric Variation:
- *Children may need a covering over stitches so they do not pick at sutures.*

Home Care Variations:
- *Teach the client to assess the wound site, and set up an appointment for suture removal.*
- *Teach the client how to assess the site after suture removal.*
- *Remind the client and home caregiver not to remove the stitches early or at home, even if the wound appears healed. Plan and facilitate their return to the appropriate care provider as needed.*

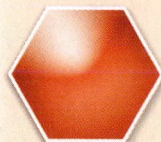

Long-Term Care Variations:
- *Staff in long-term care facilities may not encounter many opportunities for suture removal and may need to review the procedure. Make sure the proper equipment is available and the person who will receive the order to remove the sutures is comfortable with the procedure.*
- *Identify an alternate provider for suture removal, if necessary.*
- *Review the procedure with the appropriate staff, if necessary.*

▶ COMMON ERRORS

Possible Error:

Sutures are removed too early.

Prevention:

To avoid early removal, review when the sutures were placed. Consider factors that may slow healing. Examine the wound to determine whether healing has occurred. Instruct the client not to remove sutures independently. If the wound edges gape or separate when a suture is removed, do not continue. Place a Steri-Strip over the suture site holding the wound edges together, document your findings, and notify the appropriate health care provider.

To avoid late removal, actively follow up with clients who do not return for appointments. Stress the need to return for suture removal and identify with the client where to go (e.g., urgent care clinic, nurse practitioner, health center) to get sutures removed.

▶ NURSING TIPS

- Avoid pulling sutures back through the skin. Sutures beneath the skin surface are sterile, while those that are visible are contaminated. Pulling sutures through tissue introduces a risk of infection. Cut the suture as close to the skin as possible on one side and pull it through the skin from the other side
- Obese clients may not heal as well because adipose tissue has decreased circulation.
- Clients with compromised circulation will not heal as well and may require butterfly strips after sutures are removed. Check carefully that adherence has occurred before removing sutures. If staples are used, the health care provider may request that every other staple be left in place until adherence is present.
- Many clean surgical sites may not require cleaning with antiseptic solutions or dressings.
- Know policies of facilities and health care provider preference. Keep up-to-date with current research regarding wound care.
- Dressing, fabric, or bedsheets over the incision area may cause irritation.

▶ SPECIAL CONSIDERATIONS

- *When removing staples, it is important to go slowly to avoid pain for the client. When the lever is squeezed it allows the curled staple edges to release; the staple can now be raised painlessly. If the nurse fails to pause and pulls up before the edges are completely released, they may get caught on tissue and cause discomfort for the client.*

Preventing and Managing the Pressure Ulcer

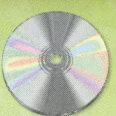

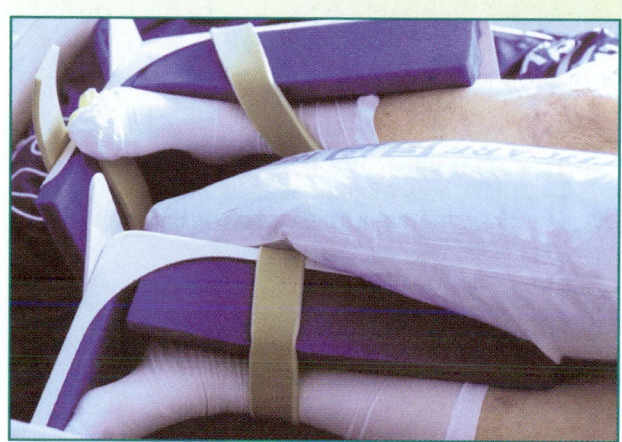

▶ OVERVIEW OF THE SKILL

A pressure ulcer is a localized injury to the skin and/or underlying tissue as a result of pressure, or pressure in combination with shear and/or friction. Pressure ulcers have also been called bedsores, decubitus ulcers, and dermal ulcers. Pressure ulcers are due to ischemia, or decreased blood supply, and commonly occur in areas subject to high pressure from body weight on bony prominences. The reduction of blood flow causes blanching (white color) of the skin when pressure is applied. When pressure is relieved, the skin takes on a brighter color (reactive hyperemia) due to vasodilation, the body's normal compensatory response to the absence of blood flow. If the area blanches with fingertip pressure or if the redness disappears within an hour, no tissue damage is anticipated. If, however, the redness persists, then tissue damage is present.

Other factors, such as shearing and/or friction, in conjunction with pressure contribute to pressure ulcer formation. Shearing is the force exerted against the skin when a client is moved or repositioned in bed by being pulled or allowed to slide down in bed. The skin and subcutaneous tissue tend to adhere to the bed surface and remain stationary, while deeper tissue pull away and slice in the direction of movement. This action results in the stretching and tearing of blood vessels, reduced blood flow, and necrosis. Shearing force accounts for a high incidence of sacral ulcers.

Friction is the force of two surfaces moving across one another. When a client moves or is pulled up in bed, rubbing of the skin against the sheets creates friction. Friction can remove the superficial layers of the skin, making it more prone to breakdown.

Pressure ulcers are staged according to the degree of tissue damage. The National Pressure Ulcer Advisory Panel (NPUAP, 2007) has developed definitions for the staging of pressure ulcers (See Table 9-15-1). The recommendations from the NPUAP may or may not be followed at your facility. It is always important to know agency policy and follow the guidelines that are required for compliance.

Pressure ulcers can be prevented if at-risk clients and the specific factors placing them at risk can be identified. Many risk factors have been associated with pressure ulcer formation including immobility and inactivity, incontinence, malnutrition, decreased mental status, diminished sensation, and age-related changes. A pressure ulcer risk assessment should be performed on each client upon admission to acute health care and long-term care facilities. The Braden Scale is a tool that may be used to predict a client's risk of developing a pressure ulcer.

Interventions to prevent the development of pressure ulcers include monitoring nutritional status, hygiene and skin care, repositioning and the use of supportive devices (pillows, heel protectors, and specialty beds). The wound care dressings for

TABLE 9-15-1   National Pressure Ulcer Association Staging System (2007)

Suspected Deep Tissue Injury:

Suspected deep tissue injury is a purple or maroon localized area of discolored intact skin or blood-filled blister due to damage of underlying soft tissue from pressure and/or shear. The area may be preceded by tissue that is painful, firm, mushy, boggy, warmer, or cooler as compared to adjacent tissue.

Stage I

Stage I is characterized by intact skin with nonblanchable redness of a localized area usually over a bony prominence. The area may be painful, firm, soft, warmer, or cooler as compared to adjacent tissue. Darkly pigmented skin may not have visible blanching, but the color may differ from the surrounding area.

Stage II

Stage II is a partial-thickness loss of dermis presenting as a shallow open ulcer with a reddish pink wound bed, without slough or bruising. The ulcer may be shiny or dry. The ulcer may also present as an intact or open/ruptured serum-filled blister. This stage should not be used to describe skin tears, tape burns, perineal dermatitis, maceration, or excoriation. Bruising indicates suspected deep tissue injury.

Stage III

Stage III is characterized by full thickness tissue loss. Subcutaneous fat may be visible but bone, tendon or muscle are not exposed. Slough may be present but does not obscure the depth of tissue loss. May include undermining and tunneling.

Stage IV

Stage IV is characterized by full thickness tissue loss with exposed bone, tendon, or muscle. Slough or eschar may be present on some parts of the wound bed. Often includes undermining and tunneling.

Unstageable

Full-thickness tissue loss in which the base of the ulcer is covered by slough (yellow, tan, gray, green, or brown) and eschar (tan, brown, or black) in the wound bed. Until enough slough and/or eschar is removed to expose the base of the wound, the true depth, and therefore stage, cannot be determined. Stable (dry, adherent, intact, without erythema or fluctuance) eschar on the heels serves as "the body's natural (biological) cover" and should not be removed.) See Figure 9-15-1.

pressure ulcers depends on the stage of the ulcer, the type and amount of drainage, the location of the ulcer, presence of infection and the condition of the surrounding skin. The primary functions of a pressure ulcer dressing are to provide protection from infection, improve client comfort, and optimized wound healing by providing a clean moist environment protected from both chemical and mechanical trauma. Table 9-15-2 identifies wound dressing guidelines and includes the category of the dressing, indications, advantages, disadvantages, and tips for using. It is essential that the nurse is knowledgeable in the assessment of pressure ulcers and the indications for the various wound care products. The nurse should consult available resources such as

wound care nurse specialists and physical therapists in the care of pressure ulcers.

Vacuum-assisted wound closure therapy may be used for the treatment of Stage III and Stage IV pressure ulcers. Vacuum-assisted closure therapy uses negative pressure to evacuate wound fluid, improve circulation, and promote the formation of granulation tissue and accelerates wound healing. The application of vacuum-assisted wound closure therapy may be done by a nurse but is often performed by a wound care specialist or physical therapist.

This skill will describe the interventions for preventing the development of pressure ulcers and the procedure for vacuum-assisted wound closure therapy.

TABLE 9-15-2	Wound Dressing Guidelines			
DRESSING TYPE AND EXAMPLES*	**INDICATIONS**	**ADVANTAGES**	**DISADVANTAGES**	**TIPS FOR USING**
Transparent adhesive films (ACU-Derm, Bioclusive OpSite, Tegaderm, Transeal, UniFlex, Polyskin	• Minor burns, lacerations • Skin donor sites • Pressure ulcers: stage I and some stage II (partial thickness, lightly exuding) • Secondary dressing in certain situations • Dry necrotic wounds that need autolytic debridement	• Impermeable to external fluids and bacteria • Transparent • Conformable • Don't require secondary dressing • Promote autolytic debridement • Reduce surface friction	• Nonabsorptive • Application can be difficult • Can't be used on wounds with fragile surrounding skin, infected wounds, or draining wounds	• Defat surrounding skin with acetone or alcohol as needed • Shave surrounding hair • Allow 1- to 2-inch margin around wound bed
Hydrocolloids (Comfeel, Cutinova hydro, DuoDERM, IntraSite Restore, Tegasorb, Hydrocol, Ultec)	• Partial-thickness wounds • Pressure ulcers: superficial stage III and some approved clean stage IV • Wounds with necrosis or slough • Wounds with mild to moderate exudate	• Conformable • Impermeable to external bacteria and contaminants • Support autolytic debridement • Minimally to moderately absorptive • Can be used with compression (treatment of venous stasis ulcers) • "Thin" forms diminish friction • Reduces pain	• Not recommended for wounds with heavy exudates, sinus tracts, infections; wounds that expose bone or tendon; or wounds with fragile surrounding skin • Not transparent • May curl or "seep" under edge	• Characteristic odor as well as yellow exudate that looks similar to pus is normal when dressing is removed from wound • Allow 1- to 1 1/2-inch margin of healthy tissue around wound edges • Taping edges will help prevent curling • Contour dressing to area to increase adhesion • Change every 3 to 7 days and as needed with leakage
Collagens (Fibracol Medifill particles/gel/pads, skin temp sheets, OASIS)	• Partial- and full-thickness wounds • Pressure ulcers • Stage III and some IV • Dermal ulcers • Donor sites • Surgical wounds	• Comfortable • Absorbent, nonadheren • May be used in combination with topical agents	• Contraindicated: sensitive to bovine and porcine products and third degree burns • May require rehydration • Not recommended for necrotic wounds	• Requires secondary dressing to secure

continues

TABLE 9-15-2 **Wound Dressing Guidelines** *(continued)*

DRESSING TYPE AND EXAMPLES*	INDICATIONS	ADVANTAGES	DISADVANTAGES	TIPS FOR USING
Hydrogels (Aquasorb, Carrasyn Hydrogel Wound Dressing ClearSite, ElastoGel, IntraSite Gel, Normigel, Transorb, Vigilon)	• Partial- and full-thickness wounds • Wounds with necrosis or slough • Burns and tissue damaged by radiation • Dermal ulcers • Painful wounds	• Soothing, cooling • Fill dead space • Rehydrate dry wound beds • Promote autolytic debridement • Provide minimal to moderate absorption • Conform to wound bed • Transparent to translucent • Many are nonadherent • Can be used when infection is present	• Most require secondary dressing • Not used for heavily exuding wounds • May dry out, then adhere to wound bed (sheet form in particular) • May macerate surrounding skin	• Sheet forms work best on superficial wounds • Dressing change schedule varies from every 8 to 48 hours • Use skin barrier wipe on surrounding intact skin to decrease risk of maceration
Exudate absorbers (AlgIDERM, Bard Absorption Dressing, Debrisan DermaSORB Spiral Dressing, Mesalt, Kaitostat Sorbsan)	• Wounds with moderate to large amounts of exudate • Wounds with combination exudate and necrosis • Wounds that require packing and absorption • Easy to apply • Infected, exuding wounds	• Absorb up to 20 times their weight in drainage • Fill dead space • Support debridement in presence of exudate	• Require secondary dressing • Not recommended for dry or lightly excuding wounds • Can dry wound bed	• Can use gauze pad or transparent film as secondary dressing • Change schedule varies (with type of product used and amount of exudates) from every 8 hours to every 3 to 4 days
Polyurethane foams (Allewn, Epi-Lock, Hydrosorb, Lyofoam, Mitraflex)	• Partial- and full-thickness wounds with minimal to moderate exudate • Secondary dressing for wounds with packing to provide additional absorption • Around draining tubes	• Nonadherent; easy to apply and remove • Conformable; may be used under compression • Manage light to moderate amounts of exudate • Can be used on wounds that have surrounding body hair • Can be used on infected wounds	• Require secondary dressing, tape, or net to hold in place • Not for use with day eschar, wounds with no exudate, or wounds with sinus tracts unless packed	• Protect intact surrounding skin with skin sealant to prevent maceration • Change schedule varies from 1 to 5 days
Lubricating sprays of emollients (Dermagran, Granulex, Proderm)	• Partial-thickness wounds • Saturate gauze packing for use in full-thickness wounds • Moisturize wound and stimulate local circulation	• Easy to use • Inexpensive • Nonadhesive	• Apply two to three times daily to maintain moist wound environment • May require secondary dressing	• May stain clothing or sheets

continues

TABLE 9-15-2	Wound Dressing Guidelines *(continued)*			
DRESSING TYPE AND EXAMPLES*	**INDICATIONS**	**ADVANTAGES**	**DISADVANTAGES**	**TIPS FOR USING**
Enzymatic debriders (Accuzyme, Panafil, Collagenase/ Santyl, Gladase)	• Debride full thickness necrotic wounds, pressure ulcers, dermal ulcers, post-op wounds, Infected wounds	• Nonsurgical debridement	• Inactivated by soaps, detergents, acidic solutions, metallic ions • Must be covered by secondary dressing • Can damage healthy tissue	• Requires daily or twice daily dressing changes
Nonadherent dressings (Adaptic, ExuDry, Sofsorb, Telta, Vaseline Gauze, Xeroform)	• Skin donor sites • Abrasions, skin tears • Lacertions • Infected wounds, partial- and full-thickness wounds that require packing	• Readily available • Don't adhere • Cover partial- and full-thickness wounds without exudates • Can be used with topical antimicrobials, ointments, or creams	• Limited moisture retention • Require secondary dressing to retain moisture, protect from outside contaminants, and keep in place • May stick to wound if dressing dries out, causing wound damage with removal	• Change schedule varies from 8- to 24-hour intervals
Gauze dressings (numerous products available)	• Exudative wounds • Wounds with dead space, tunneling, or sinus tracts • Wounds with combination exudate or necrotic debris	• Readily available • Can be used with appropriate solutions such as gels, normal saline, or topical antimicrobials to keep wounds moist • Can be used on infected wounds	• Will disrupt wound healing if allowed to dry • Require secondary dressing	• Change schedule varies with amount of exudate • Pack loosely into wound; tight packing compromises blood flow and delays wound closure • If too wet, dressing will macerate surrounding skin; protect surrounding skin with moisture barrier ointment or skin sealant as needed

Source: Adapted from Thompson, J. (2000). A practical guide to wound care. RN 83 (1), 48–53; Ayello, E., & Cuddigan, J. (2004). Conquer chronic wounds with wound bed preparation. The Nurse Practitioner 29 (3), 8–25.
*The products listed are representatives of type; this list is not meant to be all-inclusive. Refer to manufactures' directions for product usage.

▶ ASSESSMENT

1. Assess client's level of mobility. **Clients who are paralyzed or have their mobility restricted (either physically or chemically) are not able to reposition themselves independently. Therefore, they are at risk for prolonged pressure against their bony prominences.**
2. Assess client's control over bowel and bladder. **Clients who are incontinent would be at risk for experiencing a moist, bacteria-saturated environment against their skin, thus making them prone to skin breakdowns and infection.**
3. Assess client's sensation. **Clients with peripheral neuropathy or loss of sensation are unable to feel discomfort from prolonged pressure.**
4. Assess client's nutritional status by monitoring serum albumin levels and glucose levels. **Clients with low serum albumin levels are experiencing malnutrition by a lack of protein. A low protein level is not conducive to wound healing. Likewise, clients with high glucose levels will experience poor wound healing.**
5. Assess client's hemoglobin and hematocrit levels. **Clients with low hemoglobin and hematocrit levels lack tissue oxygenation and perfusion of nutrients required for wound healing.**
6. Assess client's temperature. **Clients with elevated temperatures have increased metabolic needs and absorb nutrients at an increased rate.**
7. Assess client's weight. **Clients who lack nutrition will experience weight, muscle, and tissue loss. This loss decreases the amount of padding between skin and bone, causing an increase in pressure on the skin from the bony prominence.**
8. Assess client's hydration level. **Clients with dehydration have a decrease in tissue elasticity and skin turgor, causing them to be more at risk for pressure ulcers.**
9. Assess client for edema. **Clients with edema do not tolerate pressure and friction and are more prone to skin breakdown.**
10. Assess whether the client has equipment or material that is in prolonged contact with skin. **Equipment such as endotracheal tube, nasogastric (NG) tubes, and Foley catheters that are in con- tact with skin can be a source of pressure. Material such as tape can also be a source of constant pressure (i.e., if tape was too tight on tip of nose for NG tube).**
11. Assess client's skin for early signs of breakdown/ progression of tissue healing. **Clients need to have their skin monitored for prevention of and healing of pressure ulcers.**

▶ DIAGNOSIS

Impaired Tissue Integrity

Acute Pain

Deficient Knowledge

Imbalanced Nutrition: Less Than Body Requirements

Risk for Infection

Risk for Impaired Skin Integrity

Impaired Physical Mobility

Disturbed Body Image

▶ PLANNING

Expected Outcomes:

1. The client will not experience a disruption of skin integrity.
2. The client will benefit from wound care and pressure-reducing supportive measures to begin tissue healing.
3. The client will experience regular turning and passive range of motion (ROM).
4. The client will have an increase in nutrition to meet metabolic demands.
5. The client will not experience an increase in white blood count (WBC) or other signs or symptoms of infection.
6. The client will be pain-free.
7. The client will develop positive coping mechanisms in dealing with the pressure ulcer.
8. The client will verbalize and return-demonstrate the proper techniques in preventing pressure ulcers.

Equipment Needed (see Figures 9-15-1):
For Prevention of the Pressure Ulcer

*   Pillows
*   Rolled-up blankets or towels
*   Egg-crate mattress
*   Specialty beds, if ordered by physician or qualified practitioner
*   Heel and elbow protectors
*   Lotion or powder as needed
*   Soap and water

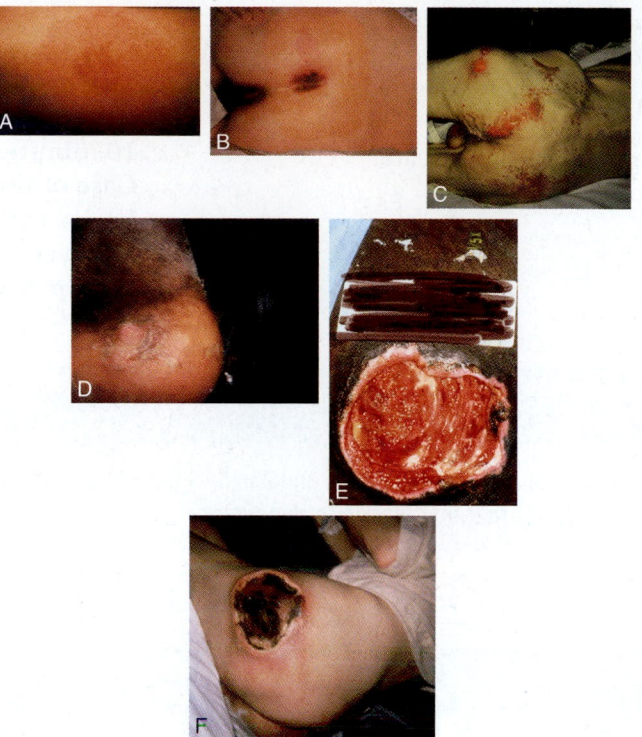

Figure 9-15-1   A. Suspected deep tissue injury (bruising under intact skin typically progresses to full-thickness ulceration). B. Stage I pressure ulcer (persistent erythema). C. Stage II pressure ulcer (loss of epidermis and possible penetration into dermis; superficial with pink-red wound base). D. Stage III pressure ulcer (extension into subcutaneous tissue). E. Stage IV pressure ulcer (note extension iinto muscle). F. Unstageable ulcer; cannot be staged because entire wound bed is obscured by necrotic tissue. (With permission from Emorgy University Wound Ostomy Continence Nursing Education Center.)

For Care of the Pressure Ulcer

- Dressings as ordered by health care provider
- Wound care solutions as ordered by health care provider (Dakin's, normal saline, Betadine, half-strength hydrogen peroxide, or other approved cleansing solution)

For Wound Vacuum-Assisted Closure

- Computerized vacuum therapy unit (see Figure 9-15-2)
- Foam Dressing
- Tubing for computerized vacuum unit

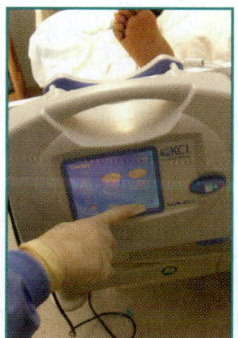

Figure 9-15-2   Computerized vacuum therapy unit

- Transparent Dressing
- Skin adhesive
- Gloves, clean and sterile
- Gown, and mask with protective eye gear, if splashing of wound drainage anticipated.
- Sterile irrigation tray (basin, piston irrigation syringe)
- Irrigation solution (normal saline or solution ordered by physician)
- Waterproof pad
- Moisture-proof container or bag for use after the irrigation procedure

► CLIENT EDUCATION NEEDED:

1. Teach clients to change position as often as they can and use supportive devices between their bones (e.g., put a pillow or towel between their knees when lying on their side). This will keep pressure off of bony prominences.
2. Teach client to increase nutrition and fluids as tolerated if not contraindicated by the client's health care provider. This will increase healing to the body.

3. Teach the client to follow health care provider's directions for the care of the pressure ulcer if applicable. Request assistance with dressing changes, if needed.
4. If client is diabetic, inform client that a greater need to provide good foot care exists.

Estimated time to complete the skill:
Prevention of the Pressure Ulcer: 10 minutes
Care of the Pressure Ulcer: Varies with the degree of skin involvement and specific health care provider's orders

---

▶ DELEGATION TIPS

Assessment of pressure ulcers is the role of the nurse. Licensed and ancillary personnel may observe the wound for improvement or deterioration during daily care and report that information to the nurse.

IMPLEMENTATION—Action/Rationale

Action	Rationale
Prevention of Pressure Ulcers	
1. Check the health care provider's order for specific positioning of client and dressing change instructions.	1. Because of the client's medical condition, the health care provider may want the client in a specific position and/or may have ordered dressing changes for a pressure ulcer.
2. Gather all the equipment you will need.	2. Having all your equipment in the room will increase the consistency of client care.
3. Identify the client and explain the procedure to the client.	3. Providing explanations to the client will employ his or her cooperation and provide time for client education.
4. Wash hands.	4. Reduces the transmission of microorganisms.
5. Provide for client privacy and apply gloves.	5. Shows respect for client's privacy. Gloves protect both client and nurse from potential body fluid contact.
6. Adjust the bed to your level and lower the side rail nearest you without leaving client unattended.	6. Adjusting the bed to your level will make the procedure easier on your back. Lowering the side rails will allow you closer contact with your client to provide care.
7. Assess client's risk for developing pressure ulcers by using the Braden Scale or similar risk chart.	7. Informs you as to the extent of client education of risk factors and what preventive care needs to be instituted immediately.
8. Assess client's skin over all pressure points, such as sacrum (see Figure 9-15-3), ischial tuberosities, feet, heels (see Figure 9-15-4), elbows, back of head.	8. A reddened area in light-skinned clients and a bluish or purple area in dark-skinned clients indicates that the tissue was under pressure.

continues

IMPLEMENTATION—Action/Rationale

Action	Rationale

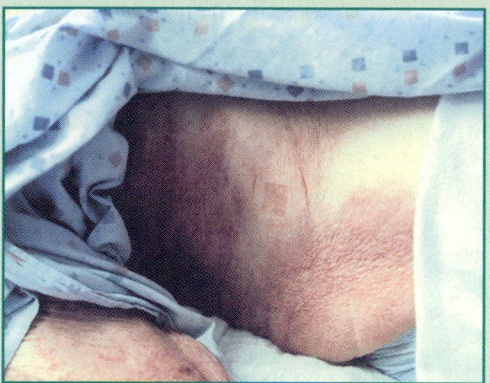

Figure 9-15-3 Assess the sacrum.

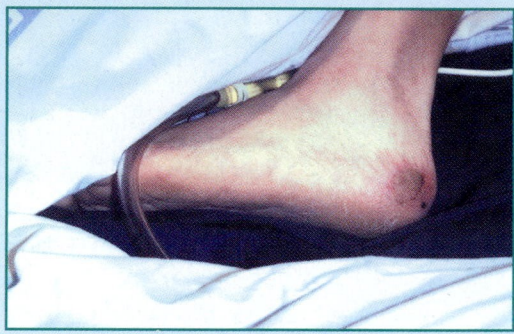

Figure 9-15-4 Assess the feet and heels.

Action	Rationale
9. Assess other sites for potential areas of pressure points.	**9.** Other potential sites and causes of pressure include the nasogastric (NG) tube and tape on tip of nose, IV dressing tape, a Foley catheter touching labia or taped area of skin, endotracheal tube and tape, and side rails touching the skin.
10. Change client's position (refer to Skills 4-3 and 4-4).	**10.** Refer to Skills 4-3 and 4-4.
11. Keep client's position at 30 degrees or less.	**11.** A position of 30 degrees or lower will limit the pressure on the sacrum.
12. Provide skin care if area is soiled or sweaty, but do not massage pressure points.	**12.** Skin care keeps skin clean and dry, and new preliminary evidence documents that massaging bony prominences may actually cause deep tissue trauma.
13. Use support devices such as special beds (see Figure 9-15-5), eggcrate mattresses, pillows (see Figure 9-15-6), towels, blankets, and heel protectors to support the body.	**13.** Lifting the heels and elbows off of the bed will limit the pressure to these areas. Also providing support between the legs will limit the pressure.
14. Perform dressing change to a pressure ulcer as ordered or per agency policy, remembering aseptic or sterile technique.	**14.** Providing wound care to existing pressure ulcers will facilitate wound healing and begin to protect the client from a potential infection.
15. Return side rail to the upright position and lower the bed.	**15.** Provides for client safety.
16. Remove gloves and wash hands.	**16.** Reduces the transmission of microorganisms.
17. Document appearance of pressure points and/or ulcers, including skin care and wound care provided and position changes.	**17.** Provides a picture of skin surface and interventions instituted to prevent pressure points and/or provide for tissue healing.

continues

Action	Rationale

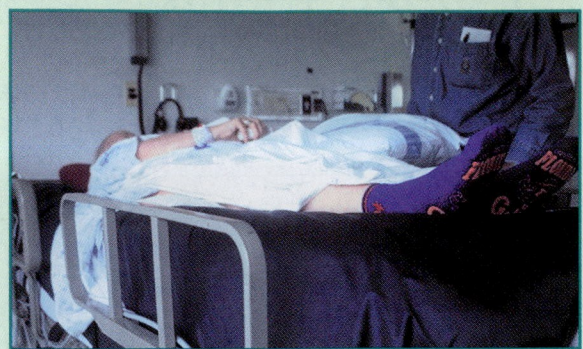

Figure 9-15-5 Special beds have air- or fluid-filled mattresses and are used to reduce the pressure on bony prominences.

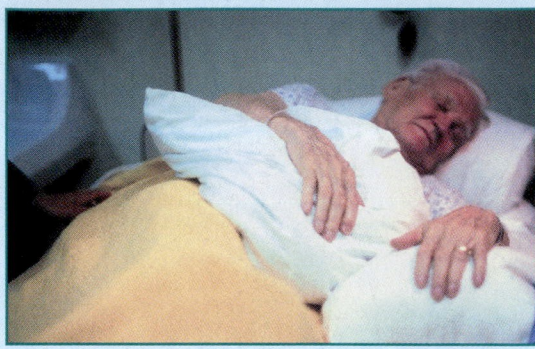

Figure 9-15-6 Pillows are used to support the hands and elbows.

18. Create an every-2-hours turning schedule if one is not available.

18. A turning schedule helps to promote more compliance with preventive measures for providing care.

Wound Vacuum-Assisted Closure

19. Follow Steps 1-6.

19. See Rationale Steps 1-6.

20. Place waterproof pad under pressure ulcer.

20. Protects linens.

21. Prepare supplies and equipment.

21. Facilitates the procedure.

22. Apply clean gloves, gown, mask, and face shield (if splashing is anticipated)

22. Protects against microorganisms.

23. Remove old dressing and place in appropriate receptacle.

23. Prevents the transmission of microorganisms.

24. Measure the wound and assess location, drainage, and appearance (see Figure 9-15-7).

24. Provides baseline data of wound.

25. Remove gloves and wash hands.

25. Reduces the transmission of microorganisms.

26. Apply sterile gloves.

26. Promotes sterile environment.

27. Irrigate the wound with normal saline or solution ordered by physician (see Skill 9-7).

27. Removes debris from the wound.

28. Using sterile scissors, cut the foam to the shape and size of the wound including tunneling.

28. This is a sterile procedure. Negative pressure must be applied to the entire wound. Choose the appropriate foam based upon the assessment of the wound. The foam may be polyurethane (black foam) or polyvinyl alcohol (white foam). Polyurethane foam has larger pores and is more effective for stimulating granulation tissue and wound contraction. Polyvinyl alcohol has small pores and is recommended when granulation tissue needs to be somewhat restricted.

continues

Action	Rationale

Wound Vacuum-Assisted Closure *continued*

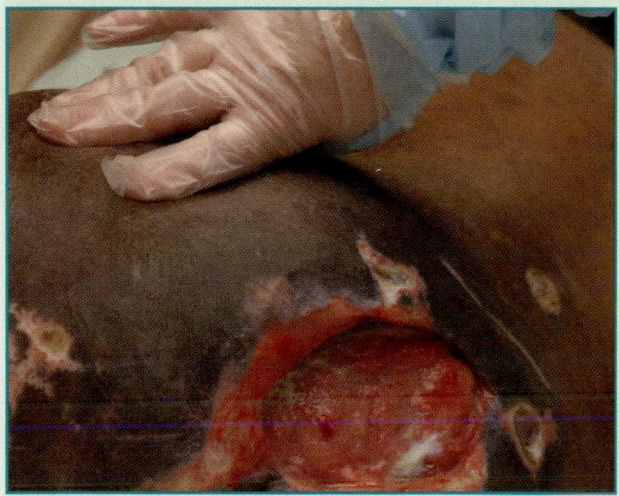

Figure 9-15-7   Assess pressure ulcer wound.

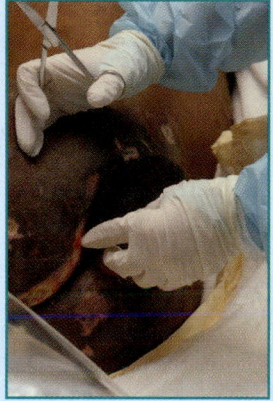

Figure 9-15-8   Place foam in wound.

29. Place foam gently in wound covering wound base, tunneling, and undermining (see Figure 9-15-8). If using polyurethane foam, protect exposed tendons, nerves and blood vessels by moving available muscle or fascia over the exposed structures and then place foam.

29. Negative pressure must be applied to entire wound; however, tendons, nerves, and muscles must not be injured from the negative pressure.

30. Apply tubing to the foam.

30. Connects to canister which provides the negative pressure.

31. Shave surrounding skin, if needed. Apply skin adhesive.

31. Transparent dressing will adhere to skin.

32. Apply transparent dressing to cover wound and 1–2 inches of surrounding skin (see Figure 9-15-9).

32. Creates an airtight seal.

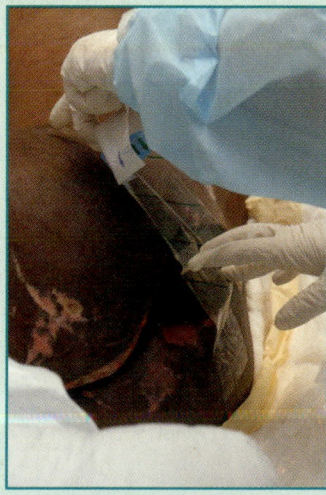

Figure 9-15-9   Apply transparent dressing to cover wound and 1–2 inches of surrounding skin.

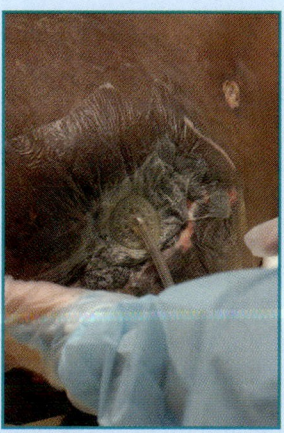

Figure 9-15-10   Vacuum-assisted closure applied to wound.

continues

Action	Rationale
33. Connect tubing to computerized vacuum therapy unit making sure tubing clamps are open.	33. Ensures that negative pressure will be applied to wound.
34. Turn on vacuum therapy unit and program the appropriate pressure and cycle (see Figure 9-15-10).	34. Provides the negative pressure.
35. Remove and discard supplies in appropriate receptacle.	35. Prevents the transmission of microorganisms.
36. Remove gloves, gown, and face shield, and wash hands.	36. Reduces the transmission of microorganisms.

► REAL WORLD ANECDOTES

Mr. Grecco was a thin, elderly man. He lived independently in his home, shopped for himself, and worked in the garden during the day. Every evening, he sat and watched television in his favorite chair. Upon a routine clinic visit, the nurse noticed the skin on his elbows was reddened and starting to break down. Mr. Grecco's favorite chair had wooden armrests. When he sat for 4 to 6 hours at a time, the skin on his elbow was compressing against the armrest. The nurse realized that even a mobile, active person is susceptible to skin breakdown.

► EVALUATION

- The client did not experience a disruption of skin integrity.
- The client benefited from wound healing care and pressure-reducing supportive measures to begin tissue healing.
- The client experienced regular turning and passive range of motion.
- The client's nutrition met the metabolic demands of the body.
- The client did not experience an increase in white blood count (WBC) or other signs and symptoms of infections.
- The client was pain free.
- The client developed positive coping mechanisms for dealing with the pressure ulcer.
- The client verbalized and demonstrated the proper techniques for preventing pressure ulcers.

► DOCUMENTATION

Nurses' Notes

- Describe in detail what the pressure area/ulcer looked like, noting its location, color, size, shape, and drainage, and the depth of tissue involved.

- Describe what procedure was done (wound care), what solutions or skin care were used, and how it was done, noting either aseptic or sterile techniques per orders.
- Describe the client's response to the procedure and how the client tolerated it.
- Document what interventions are being done to decrease/limit pressure to bony prominences.
- Document client education about risk factors and prevention of pressure ulcers and client's understanding of this education.

Document on appropriate flow sheet or electronic medical record (EMR).

Medication Administration Record

- Document wound care medications or solutions.
- Document whether any preprocedural pain medications were given for the client's comfort.

► CRITICAL THINKING SKILL

Introduction

Pressure sores can develop in unexpected places. Assess the whole client when determining pressure sore risk.

Possible Scenario

Mrs. McFaraday is an obese client in your nursing care facility. When she is awake, she is very active and agitated much of the time. This keeps her sweaty. She waves her arms around and lifts herself off of the wheelchair several times an hour. You do not consider her at risk for pressure sores.

Possible Outcome

One day the nursing assistant bathing Mrs. McFaraday reports that she had developed an open sore in the folds of her abdomen. You realize that, although Mrs. McFaraday is active, she is always leaning forward in her chair. This is a pressure sore.

Prevention

Although pressure sores frequently develop over bony prominences, they can also develop where obesity, poor skin condition, friction, and moisture come together, such as the folds of Mrs. McFaraday's abdomen. Keeping the skin clean and dry, allowing air circulation, relieving pressure, and dusting with cornstarch were are all interventions that could have helped Mrs. McFaraday avoid this complication.

► VARIATIONS

Geriatric Variations:

The elderly experience the following effects of aging, making them more prone to develop pressure ulcers:
- *Less tissue between skin and bone*
- *Dehydration*
- *Malnutrition*
- *Loss of bowel and bladder control*
- *Limited mobility*
- *Limited vision and/or fine motor skills to treat skin conditions*
- *Slower wound healing*
- *An increased risk for injuries*

Pediatric Variations:

- *Young children are dependent upon others for nutrition and skin care, and may be more vulnerable to skin breakdown when these areas have been neglected.*
- *Children are very mobile and do not stay in one position for very long. A child with a medical or psychiatric condition which restricts mobility must be assessed for the risk of developing pressure ulcers.*
- *Active children may need extra measures to keep wound care dressings or protective padding in place.*
- *Young children may not be able to communicate discomfort or pain. Careful assessment of skin condition, and identification of risks for skin breakdown, is very important.*

Home Care Variations:

- *Be creative in finding ways to devise homemade padding for bony prominences.*
- *Make sure the caregiver understands the need to assess for skin breakdown.*
- *Teach the caregiver proper skin care techniques.*
- *Remind the caregiver that pressure sores or bedsores can often develop when the client is not in bed.*
- *Remind the caregiver not to "scrub" skin areas susceptible to breakdown. The added friction can contribute to skin breakdown.*

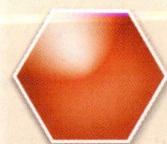

Long-Term Care Variation:

- *Teach clients to self-manage prevention of bedsores as much as possible.*
- *Repositioning themselves, massaging the skin around (not over) bony prominences, keeping their skin clean and dry, and reporting pressure areas that they need assistance in relieving will all help protect skin from breakdown.*

▶ COMMON ERRORS

Possible Error:

Not following specific positioning orders.

Prevention:

Because of the client's medical condition, the health care provider may want the client in a certain position (e.g., "head of bed up 30 degrees at all times," "elevate right arm continuously," "flat on back for 24 hours"). The nurse must tailor positioning changes, provide padding, and relieve pressure points so that positioning guidelines can be followed without increasing the risk for skin breakdown.

Possible Error:

The client does not change position enough to relieve pressure over bony prominences. The skin over several bony prominences starts to break down.

Prevention:

If the client is unable to, or is just not changing positions frequently enough, the nurse would need to assess the client's knowledge about changing positions and provide client education and movement as needed (e.g., a postoperative client may be afraid to move or may need pain medication to help move more frequently). Also, the client may need to be educated about risk factors for developing pressure ulcers and ways to decrease risks.

▶ NURSING TIPS

- Look at the client's skin, especially the pressure areas, at least every 2 hours and reposition the client as often as you can.
- Use towels, washcloths, pillows, and blankets to keep pressure off bony prominences.
- Do not massage the skin over the site. Recent research has discouraged massaging the area because of the potential to cause deep tissue trauma.

- Look for pressure ulcers in unexpected places such as under any area that has tape on it, including the nasogastric tube, IV dressing, and wound dressing. Also inspect the back of the head, ears, and elbows.
- When taking dressings off a pressure ulcer, note the sequence and size/type of dressings used so you can repeat the sequence when reapplying the dressings. Be familiar with the health care provider's order.
- Avoid elastic bandages if history of latex allergy.

▶ SPECIAL CONSIDERATIONS

- *The probe-to-bone test is a simple bedside technique used to detect osteomyelitis in infected diabetic foot ulcers and may be useful for pressure ulcers as well. A sterile probe is used to examine the pressure ulcer, and if bone is directly palpated it is seen as a positive test.*
- *Nutritional status is always relevant in the prevention and treatment of pressure ulcers. Studies have proven that increased dietary protein intake promotes healing of pressure ulcers.*
- *Specialized air-fluidized or air-loss beds may be ordered for the care of the client with large ulcers at multiple sites on the body. These beds can be very costly to the client but most pressure ulcers can be managed successfully without them.*

Managing Irritated Peristomal Skin

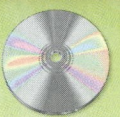

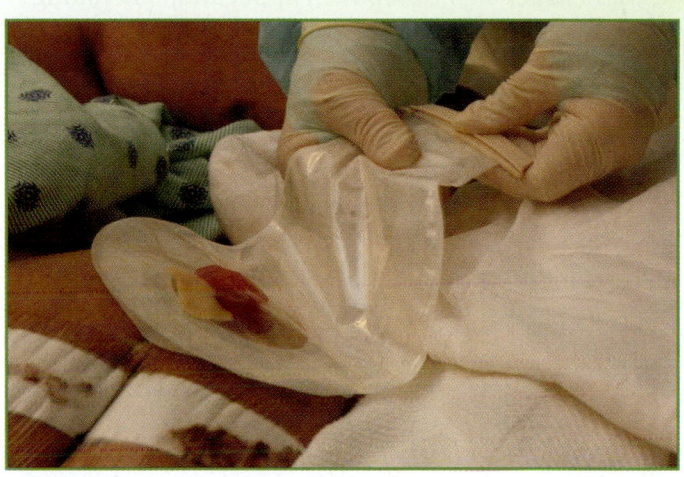

▶ OVERVIEW OF THE SKILL

This skill covers the management of irritated, denuded, or macerated peristomal skin for those clients with either a bowel or urinary diversion.

Skin irritation can have several causes. The most common cause of skin irritation for someone with an ostomy is leakage of urine/stool onto the skin when the stoma pattern is cut too large. Clients with ostomies can develop fungal infections underneath the wafer of their ostomy system. Exposure to digestive enzymes, stool, chemicals, or urine can cause irritation. Mechanical trauma from tape, adhesives, improper removal of protective barriers, friction, pressure, or shearing can cause irritation.

Moisture and heat can promote irritation. Finally, allergic reactions may develop to products used to clean, protect, or adhere appliances to the skin surrounding the stoma.

Irritated peristomal skin can make caring for the stoma more difficult and cause pain at the site. Irritated skin may increase the sense of frustration, depression, or anxiety about the stoma and increase the difficulty of adjusting to a changed body image. Finally, irritated skin increases the negative impact that the stoma and its care has on an individual's daily life.

▶ ASSESSMENT

1. Inspect the stoma for color and appearance. **This will allow the nurse to determine the viability and direction (retracted, orifice pointing downward toward skin) of the stoma.**
2. Inspect the condition of the skin surrounding the stoma. **Alterations in skin integrity will prohibit an ostomy appliance system from adhering to the skin.**
3. Measure the dimensions of the stoma prior to obtaining an ostomy appliance system from central supply. **This will alleviate the problem of obtaining equipment that is the wrong size.**

▶ DIAGNOSIS

Risk for Infection

Risk for Impaired Skin Integrity

Disturbed Body Image

Deficient Knowledge

▶ PLANNING

Expected Outcomes:

1. Client exhibits improved or healed areas of affected peristomal skin.
2. Client reports increased comfort.
3. Client is able to identify and report factors which lead to skin breakdown and discuss ways to prevent skin breakdown from recurring.
4. Client is able to demonstrate skin care regime.
5. Client voices feelings about change in body image.

Equipment Needed (see Figure 9-16-1):

- Clean washcloth or 4 × 4 gauze pads
- Warm tap water
- Appropriate urinary or drainable ostomy appliance
- Scissors
- Pen or pencil
- Clean gloves
- Pectin powder (i.e., Stomahesive Powder, Premium Powder)

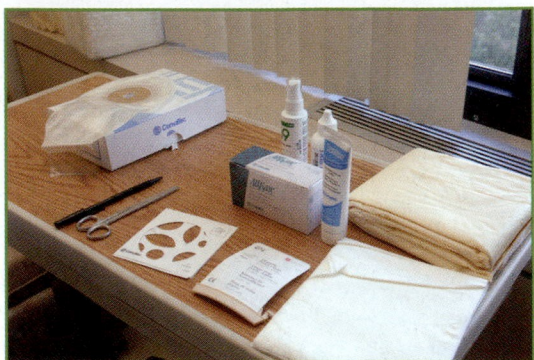

Figure 9-16-1   Ostomy appliance, scissors, measuring guide, ostomy bag closure clamp, skin sealant, pectin powder, pectin paste, and absorbent pads

- Pectin paste (i.e., Stomahesive Paste, Premium Paste)
- Skin sealant (i.e., Skin Prep, 3M No Sting™)

▶ **CLIENT EDUCATION NEEDED:**

1. Instruct the client on the use of skin care products to heal irritated or denuded peristomal skin.
2. Instruct client on pouch application, including frequency of change. Most pouching systems can be maintained for a minimum of 3 days to a maximum of 7 days.
3. Instruct client to report on changes in skin condition to wound/ostomy care nurse.
4. Provide client with a list of equipment and product numbers and a list of retailers where supplies can be purchased.

Estimated time to complete the skill: **15–20 minutes**

▶ **DELEGATION TIPS**

Assessment and treatment of peristomal skin is the role of the nurse. Ancillary personnel may observe the area around the stoma for improvement or deterioration during daily care and report that information to the nurse.

IMPLEMENTATION—Action/Rationale

Action	Rationale
1. Wash hands.	1. Reduces the transmission of microorganisms.
2. Assemble appropriate ostomy pouch and wafer, pectin paste, pectin powder, and skin sealant.	2. Ensures that all equipment is ready to use.
3. Apply clean gloves.	3. Practices clean technique.
4. Empty pouch of stool/urine, if present. Remove current ostomy appliance (see Figure 6-16-2).	4. Prevents contamination of surrounding environment if stool/urine accidentally leaks from appliance when it is removed from the client's skin.
5. Dispose of appliance in appropriate waste container.	5. Practices infection control principles.
6. Remove gloves and wash hands.	6. Reduces the transmission of microorganisms.

continues

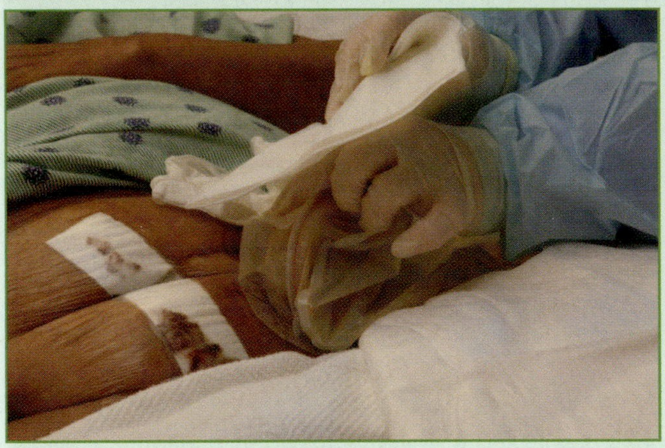

Action	Rationale

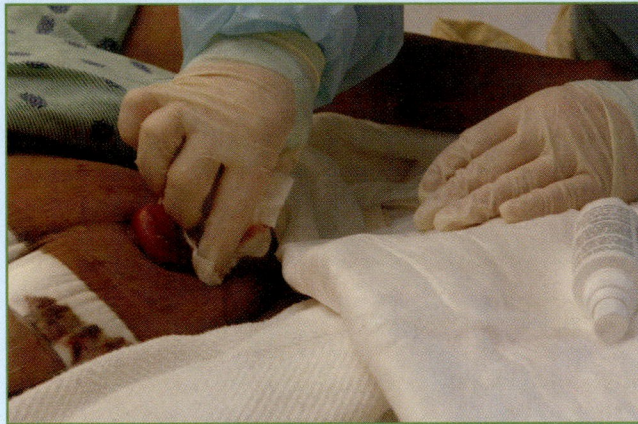

Figure 9-16-2 Remove ostomy appliance.

Figure 9-16-3 Cleanse stoma and skin with tap water.

7. Apply clean gloves.

8. Cleanse stoma and skin with warm tap water (see Figure 9-16-3). Pat dry.

9. Measure stoma using a measuring guide for appropriate length and width of stoma at base (where skin meets stoma) (see Figure 9-16-4).

10. Place gauze pad over orifice of stoma to wick stool/urine while you are preparing the wafer and pouch for application.

11. Trace pattern onto paper backing of wafer (see Figure 9-16-5).

7. Practices clean technique.

8. Gentle care of the stoma prevents injury to the mucosa, which has no nerve endings and is very friable.

9. Correct measurement of the stoma's dimensions will ensure a good fit of the ostomy appliance without excess skin at the base of the stoma exposed to stool/urine.

10. Using something to wick stool/urine away from the skin will ensure a good seal of the wafer to the client's skin.

11. It is important to trace the measurements of the stoma and not "eyeball" the stoma measurements. Inaccurate pattern size will result in either laceration of the stoma by the wafer or maceration of peristomal skin from constant contact with stool/urine.

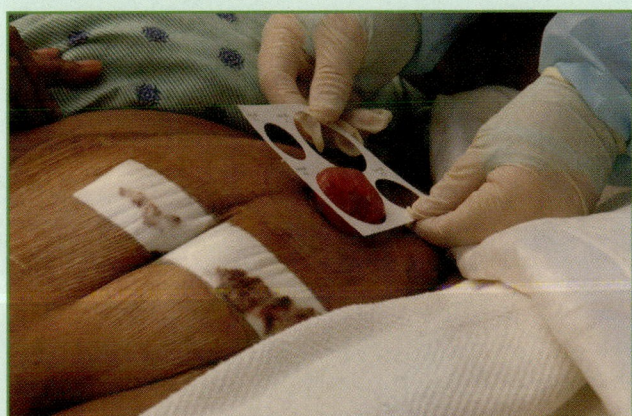

Figure 9-16-4 Measure stoma using measuring guide.

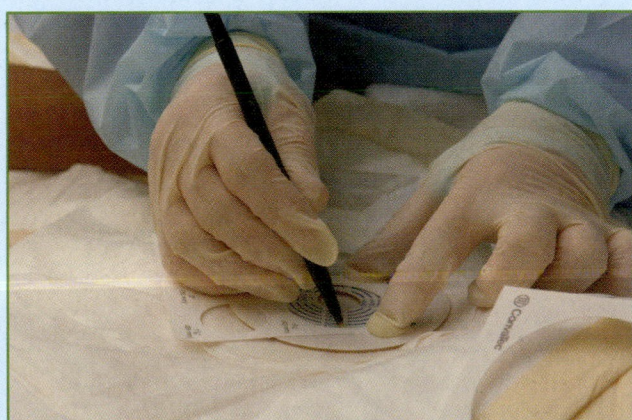

Figure 9-16-5 Trace pattern onto paper backing of wafer.

continues

Action	Rationale
12. Cut wafer as traced.	**12.** Accurately cutting the traced pattern will ensure a snug fit.
13. Attach clean pouch to wafer.	**13.** Preattaching the pouch to the wafer will save time and prevent stool from leaking underneath the wafer during the application process.
14. Remove gauze pad from orifice of stoma.	**14.** It is easier to see the stoma.
15. Sprinkle a light coating of pectin powder onto the irritated, weepy peristomal skin (see Figure 9-16-6).	**15.** The powder will absorb the peristomal drainage.
16. Brush off any excess pectin powder using a gauze pad.	**16.** Prevents caking of any excess pectin powder.
17. Dab the skin sealant over the pectin powder (see Figure 9-16-7). Allow to dry.	**17.** Dabbing the skin sealant will allow the pectin powder to remain where it was originally applied. The skin sealant creates an invisible bandage.
18. Remove paper backing from wafer. Apply a ring of pectin paste onto the sticky side of wafer at the edge of opening cut for the stoma (see Figure 9-16-8).	**18.** Paper backing needs to be removed from wafer for it to adhere to the skin. The paste will caulk between the base of stoma and wafer, creating a tighter seal.
19. Apply stoma appliance to skin with stoma centered in cutout opening of wafer (see Figure 9-16-9).	**19.** Intestinal contents will drain into pouch.
20. Apply closure clamp to pouch (see Figure 9-16-10)	**20.** Keeps intestinal contents in pouch.
21. Cover edges of wafer with hypoallergenic tape (optional).	**21.** This ensures that the edges of the wafer will not adhere to the client's clothing.

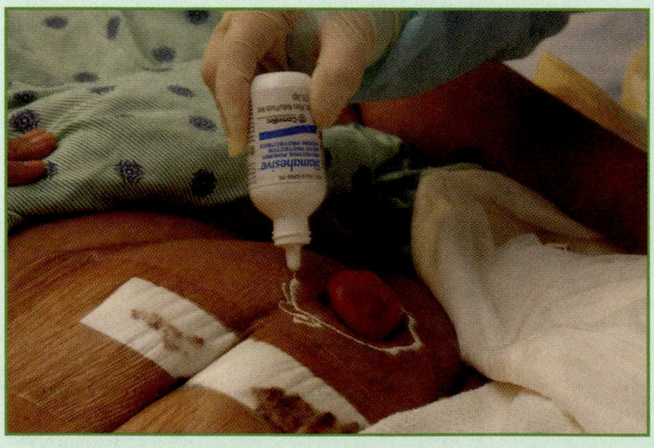

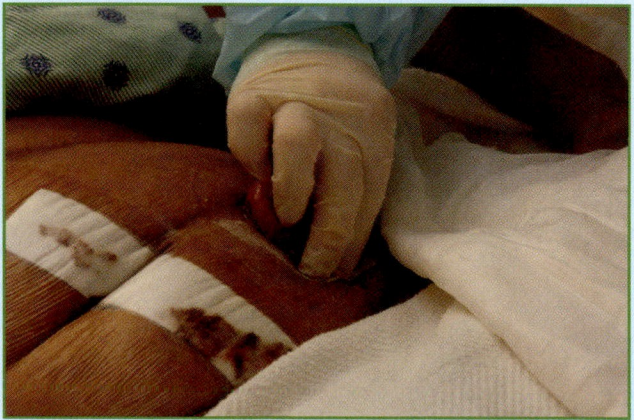

Figure 9-16-6 Sprinkle pectin powder onto irritated peristomal skin.

Figure 9-16-7 Dab skin sealant over pectin powder.

continues

Action	Rationale
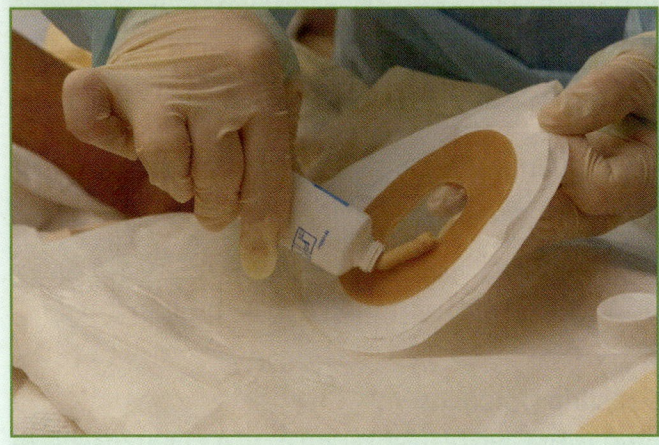	
	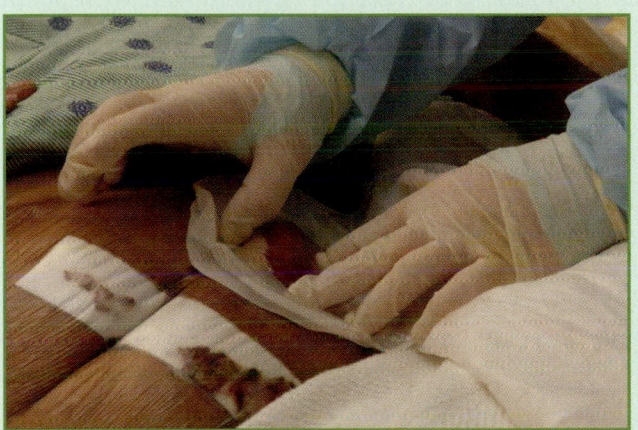... wait

Action	Rationale

Figure 9-16-8 Apply a ring of pectin paste onto sticky side of wafer.

Figure 9-16-9 Apply stoma appliance to skin.

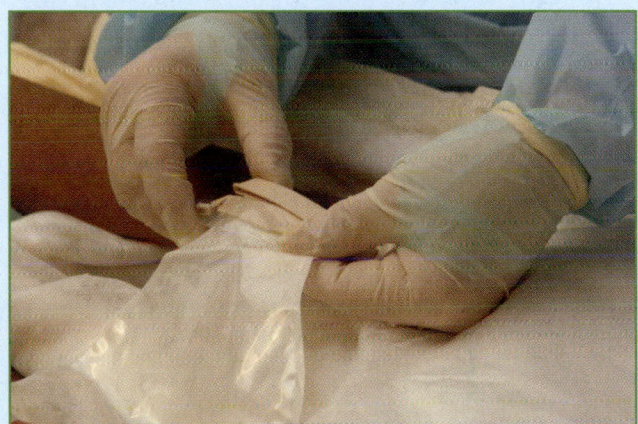

Figure 9-16-10 Apply closure clamp to pouch.

Action	Rationale
22. Dispose of used materials, remove gloves, and wash hands.	**22.** Reduces the transmission of microorganisms.

▶ REAL WORLD ANECDOTES

A 45-year-old woman has recently had a temporary loop ileostomy and ileoanal anastomosis for familial polyposis. Two weeks postoperatively, she is complaining of frequent appliance changes caused by leakage of stool beneath the wafer. Examination of peristomal skin reveals dimpling of the stoma at 3 o'clock and a deep skin crease when she sits. The peristomal skin is severely irritated from 2 o'clock to 6 o'clock without loss of epithelium. A consultation is arranged with the enterostomal therapy/ostomy nurse for evaluation of the current pouching system.

► EVALUATION

- Client exhibited improved or healed areas of affected peristomal skin.
- Client reported increased comfort.
- Client was able to identify and report factors which lead to skin breakdown and discuss ways to prevent skin breakdown from recurring.
- Client was able to demonstrate skin care regime.
- Client verbalized feelings about change in body image.

► DOCUMENTATION

Nurses' Notes

- Describe and document assessment of peristomal skin.
- Describe and document assessment of stoma.
- Record stoma measurements (length, width, height).
- Note color and amount of drainage.
- Describe what was done for peristomal skin care.
- Note type of ostomy pouch applied.

Document on appropriate flow sheet or electronic medical record (EMR).

► CRITICAL THINKING SKILL

Introduction

The client is 3 weeks postop from creation of a temporary loop ileostomy and ileoanal anastomosis with J pouch.

Possible Scenario

The client is a 23-year-old man with a history of ulcerative colitis who elected to have removal of the colon with creation of a temporary loop ileostomy and ileoanal anastomosis with J pouch. He is now complaining of severe burning of the skin around the stoma, and the appliance needs to be changed every 12 to 24 hours.

Removal of the appliance reveals severely denuded peristomal skin from 3:00 to 10:00 that extends for 1 inch from the base of the stoma outward. The lower portion of the stoma is noted to be flush to the skin.

Possible Outcome

The astute nurse realizes that this client needs to have the fitting of his appliance reassessed by the enterostomal therapy/ostomy nurse and arranges an immediate consult. The second action to be taken by the nurse is to treat the irritated skin with pectin powder and dab over it a nonsting skin sealant before reapplying the client's ostomy pouch.

Prevention

This problem can be prevented by encouraging and arranging for the client to be seen by the enterostomal therapy/ostomy nurse, who is well-versed in the various methods of managing complicated ostomies and skin care needs.

► VARIATIONS

Geriatric Variations:
- *Elderly clients often have vision difficulties. Make sure the person caring for the stoma can see the stoma and can see well enough to assess and apply the appropriate-size wafer to the stoma.*
- *Elderly skin can be very fragile. Tearing or shearing forces, reactions to tape, or reactions to the contents of the bowel remaining on the skin can cause increased irritation.*

Pediatric Variations:
- *If the child is participating in the care of the stoma and the changing of the appliance, remind the child it is best not to "rush" the job. Remind the child to remove any adhesives carefully, rinse any soap from the site, and report any signs of irritation early.*
- *Adolescence is a time of increased needs for privacy and concerns about body image. It may be difficult for an adolescent to ask for help or education about caring for the stoma. It may be tempting for the adolescent to ignore signs of growing irritation for fear of losing a sense of control over stoma care.*

continues

▶ **VARIATIONS** *(continued)*

Home Care Variations:

• *Teach the client and other care providers in the home how to detect and remedy peristomal skin irritations, including those caused by improper wafer size, tape allergies, or skin trauma.*
• *Make sure the home care setting has the facilities and equipment to adequately clean and manage the stoma. Interventions may include helping the client seek sources of supplies, arranging to have plumbing fixed, and verifying adequate laundry facilities.*

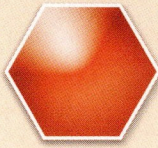

Long-Term Care Variations:

• *Encourage the client to manage stoma care as much as possible.*
• *Long-term care facilities may not have the staffing levels for prolonged or intensive wound care procedures. This can both contribute to peristomal skin irritation and delay healing. A clear, comprehensive assessment of wound care needs, including time involved, supplies needed, and knowledge of the appropriate care procedure, can help the facility plan the needed care.*

▶ **COMMON ERRORS**

Possible Error:

The appliance chosen is appropriate in size for the ostomy, but the peristomal skin has deep creases, causing effluent to leak beneath the wafer.

Prevention:

Consult with the enterostomal therapy/ostomy nurse as soon as there is evidence of atypical appearance to skin surrounding the stoma. Obtain an appliance with convexity or use pectin paste to caulk between stoma and wafer. Remove the leaking appliance and caulk the area between the stoma and wafer with pectin paste.

▶ **NURSING TIPS**

• Recognize that all stomas are not the same. Each stoma must be treated individually, which requires that the nurse assess the dimensions and location in relation to the client's body movements (i.e., sitting, bending) and the peristomal skin's condition.
• Client teaching is easily incorporated into the care of the ostomy by encouraging the client to be your assistant during the application process.

• Use of an ostomy appliance that is intact, comfortable, and easy to use will increase the client's comfort level and thereby the client's participation in self-care activities.
• Costs to the client and the health care institution are reduced when simplistic ostomy care is provided and an intact seal can be maintained for a minimum of 3 days.

> ► **SPECIAL CONSIDERATIONS**

- *Clients may need added support when they leave the hospital setting. One source of support available is the United Ostomy Association. It is prudent for the health care team to provide this information to the client before he or she leaves the hospital.*
- *An added resource for nurses is the Wound Ostomy Continence Society in Chicago, Illinois or www.wocn.org*
- *Fungal infections may develop and present as a rash with distinct satellite lesions. Assure the client that this can be treated with antifungal powder that is lightly blotted with a skin sealant.*
- *Clients may have an allergic reaction to the adhesives or the products used to protect the skin. The treatment usually involves eliminating the allergen and changing to a less caustic product. Steroids may be required if the reaction is severe.*
- *Odor or gas may be a concern for the client with an ostomy. Encourage the client to keep the tail of the pouch clean and give assurance that the pouch is odor-proof. When the pouch is emptied, odors are normal and should be anticipated by making room deodorant sprays/wicks available. If the client has a continued concern, the health care provider may recommend bismuth subgallate or chlorophyllin copper complex to reduce stool odor. Possible side effects should be reviewed with the client (thickened stool/diarrhea) before discharge.*

Applying a Pouch to a Draining Wound

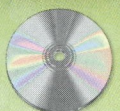

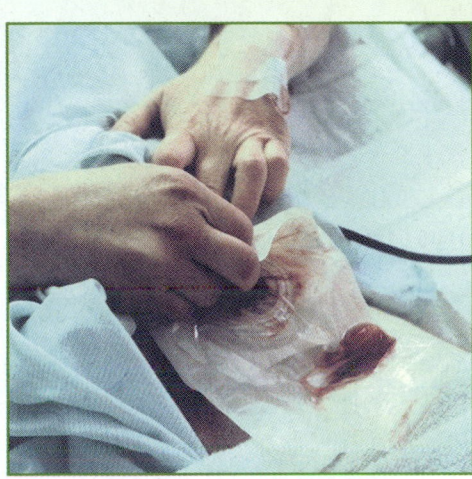

▶ OVERVIEW OF THE SKILL

A draining wound is pouched whenever the drainage from a wound is greater than 100 mL in 24 hours. It is an alternative to gauze dressings. Applying a pouch to a draining wound results in fewer dressing changes, allows more accurate measurement of drainage, and protects the surrounding skin from the drainage and irritation. It reduces the odor, mess, and contamination from saturated dressings. The most common method to pouch a draining wound is to use an ostomy appliance or a pouching system designed specifically to accommodate various sizes of draining wounds.

▶ ASSESSMENT

1. Identity the type and amount of drainage coming from the wound. **This will allow the nurse to determine which type of appliance (i.e., urinary or bowel pouch) or wound collector is required.**
2. Inspect the condition of the skin surrounding the wound. **Alterations in skin integrity will prohibit a closed drainage system from adhering to the skin.**
3. Measure the dimensions of the wound prior to obtaining a closed drainage system from central supply. **This will alleviate the problem of obtaining equipment that is the wrong size.**

▶ DIAGNOSIS

Risk for Impaired Skin Integrity

Disturbed Body Image

Deficient Fluid Volume

Risk for Infection

Social Isolation

▶ PLANNING

Expected Outcomes:

1. The skin around the wound will be protected from contact with the drainage and will not break down or become infected.
2. The drainage from the wound will be contained in the pouch and will facilitate accurate measurement of wound drainage.
3. Odor from the wound will be minimized.
4. The pouch will not decrease the client's mobility.

Equipment Needed (see Figures 9-17-1A–D):

- Clean washcloth or 4 × 4 gauze pads
- Normal saline
- Appropriate ostomy appliance (fecal or urinary) or wound drainage collector and wafer
- Scissors
- Pen or pencil
- Measuring guide

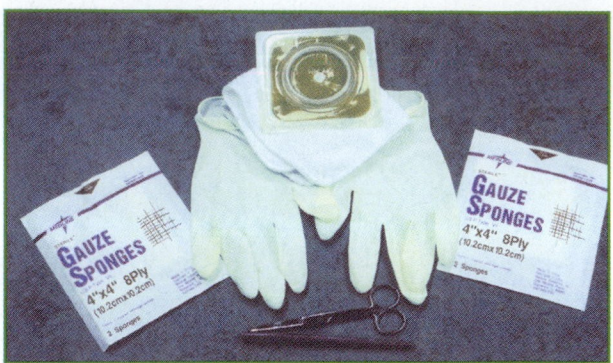

Figure 9-17-1A Gloves, wash cloth, wafer, gauze, scissors, and marking pen

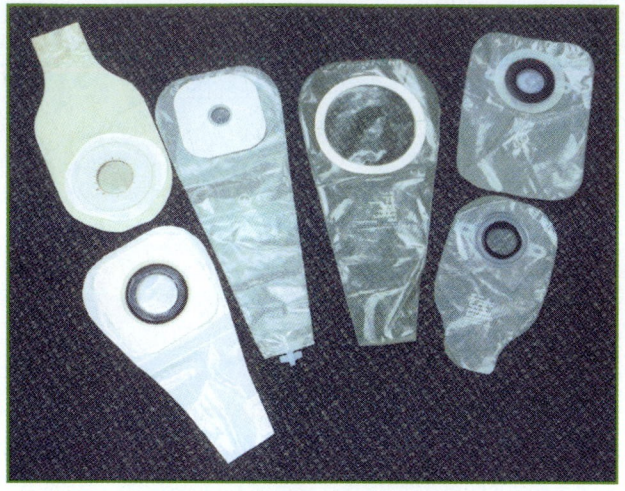

Figure 9-17-1B Ostomy appliances

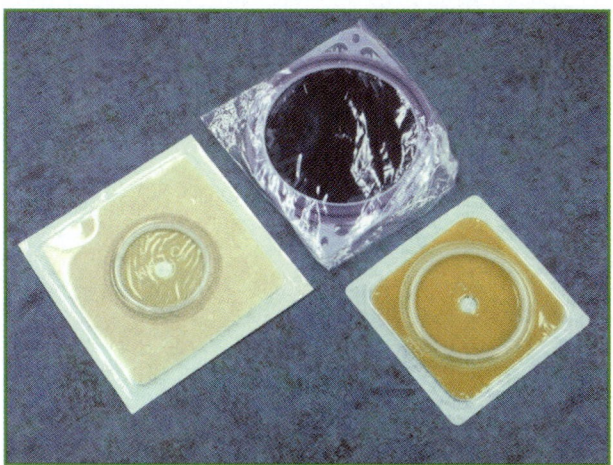

Figure 9-17-1C Wafers

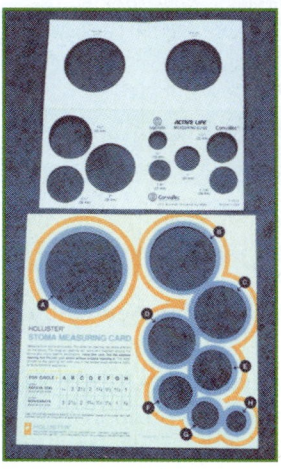

Figure 9-17-1D Measuring guides used to determine the length and width of the wound

▶ CLIENT EDUCATION NEEDED:

1. Teach the client about pouch application, including frequency of change. Most enterostomies are able to be maintained with a pouching system for a minimum of 24 hours to a maximum of 5 days.
2. Instruct the client to report changes in drainage or skin condition to health care provider or wound/ostomy care nurse.
3. Client should be provided with a list of equipment and product numbers and a list of retailers where supplies can be purchased.

Estimated time to complete the skill:

This is dependent on the type of draining wound being pouched and its location. A simple draining wound can be pouched in 15 minutes. A more complex wound requiring the expertise of a wound care nurse expert may take up to 60 minutes to pouch.

▶ DELEGATION TIPS

The assessment and treatment involved in pouching a draining wound is the responsibility of the nurse. Ancillary personnel may observe the site for improvement or deterioration during daily care and report those observations to the nurse.

IMPLEMENTATION—Action/Rationale

Action	Rationale
1. Wash hands.	1. Reduces the transmission of microorganisms.
2. Assemble appropriate pouch and wafer.	2. Ensures that all equipment is ready to use.
3. Apply clean gloves.	3. Practices clean technique.
4. Remove current appliance, after emptying pouch of drainage, if present (see Figures 9-17-2 and 9-17-3). Remember to measure drainage for intake and output record (see Figure 9-17-4).	4. This prevents contamination of surrounding environment if contents of pouch accidentally leak from appliance when it is removed from the client's skin.
5. Dispose of appliance in appropriate waste container.	5. Practices infection control.
6. Wash hands.	6. Reduces the transmission of microorganisms.
7. Apply clean gloves.	7. Practices clean technique.
8. Cleanse periwound area with normal saline on 4 × 4 gauze. Pat dry (see Figure 9-17-5).	8. Gentle care of the periwound area prevents injury to skin.
9. Measure fistula/wound opening using a measuring guide for appropriate length and width of fistula, adding an additional 1/8 inch clearance from edge of fistula.	9. Correct measurement of the fistula's dimensions ensures a good fit of the ostomy appliance without excess skin being exposed to drainage.
10. Place gauze pad over orifice of fistula to wick drainage while you are preparing the wafer and pouch for application.	10. Using something to wick drainage away from the skin ensures a good seal of the wafer to the client's skin.

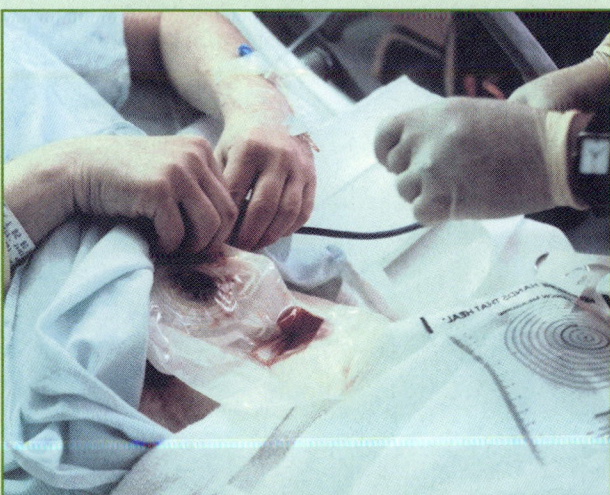

Figure 9-17-2 Remove the current appliance, gently peeling back the wafer.

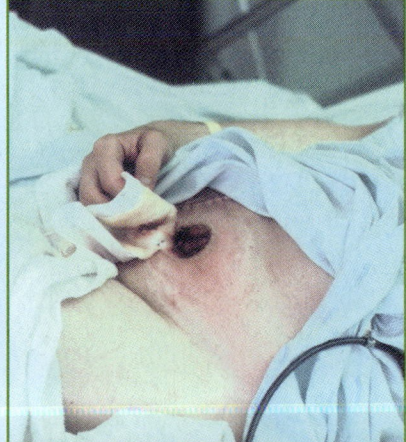

Figure 9-17-3 The appliance is almost completely removed. Note the wafer and appliance peeled away from the skin.

continues

Action	Rationale

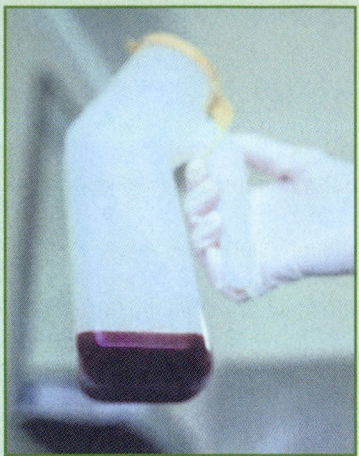

Figure 9-17-4   Measure the drainage for the intake and output record.

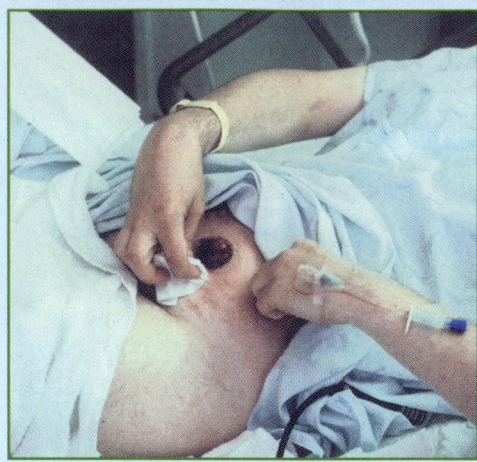

Figure 9-17-5   Clean the stoma area and pat dry.

11. Trace pattern onto paper backing of wafer.

11. It is important to trace the measurements of the fistula and not "eyeball" the fistula measurements. Inaccurate pattern size results in either leakage of drainage beneath the wafer or maceration of periwound skin from constant contact with the drainage.

12. Cut wafer as traced.

12. Accurately cutting the traced pattern ensures a snug fit.

13. Remove gauze pad from orifice of fistula. Dry the skin surrounding the fistula with a gauze.

13. It is easier to see the fistula opening for accurate placing of the wafer. Wafer does not adhere to wet skin.

14. Attach clean pouch to wafer, then wafer to skin. Alternatively, attach wafer to skin then pouch to wafer depending on institutional policy.

14. Preattaching the pouch to the wafer will save time and prevent drainage from leaking underneath the wafer during application process. Attaching the wafer first allows better visualization of the placement of the wafer.

15. To attach wafer to skin, remove paper backing from wafer and place on skin (see Figure 9-17-6). Center the cutout hole of the wafer over the fistula opening.

15. Paper backing needs to be removed from wafer for it to adhere to the skin.

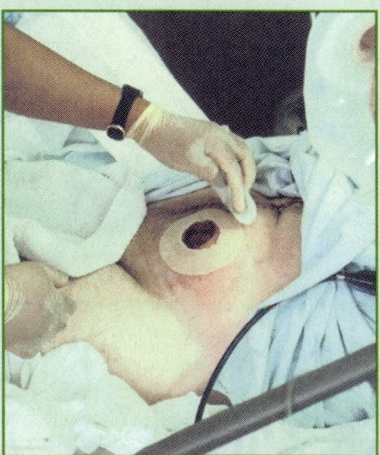

Figure 9-17-6   Place the wafer on the skin, centering the cutout hole over the fistula opening.

continues

Action	Rationale
16. To attach pouch to wafer, make sure port closure of pouch is closed or tail closure is attached, remove adhesive backing, and place on wafer (see Figures 9-17-7 and 9-17-8).	**16.** Prevents leakage of pouch contents onto client's skin and/or clothing.
17. Cover exposed areas of the wafer with hypo-allergenic tape.	**17.** Ensures that the edges of the wafer will not adhere to client's clothing.
18. Remove gloves and wash hands.	**18.** Reduces the transmission of microorganisms.

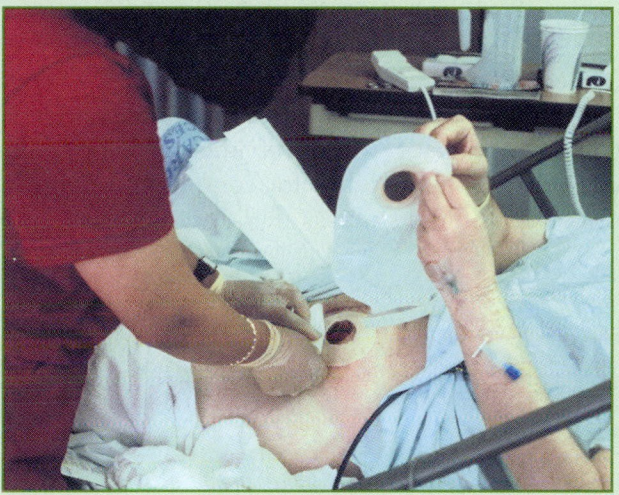

Figure 9-17-7   Remove the adhesive backing from the pouch.

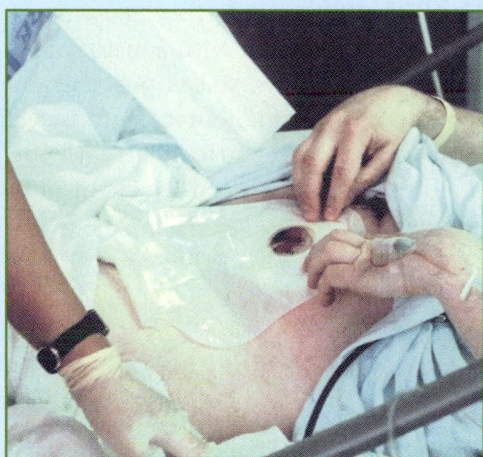

Figure 9-17-8   Place the pouch on the wafer.

► REAL WORLD ANECDOTES

A home health care nurse learned a valuable lesson when she "precut" half a dozen wafers to save steps during later visits. The size of the fistula changed over time, and the nurse had to throw out the precut supplies and order new wafers.

► EVALUATION

- The skin around the wound was protected from contact with the drainage and did not break down or become infected.
- The drainage from the wound was contained in the pouch and facilitated accurate measurement of wound drainage.
- Odor from the wound was maintained.
- The pouch did not decrease the client's mobility.

► DOCUMENTATION

Nurses' Notes

- Assessment of periwound skin
- Wound dimensions (length, width, depth)

- Color and amount of drainage
- Periwound skin care if alteration in skin integrity was noted
- Type of pouch applied

Document on appropriate flow sheet or electronic medical record (EMR).

► CRITICAL THINKING SKILL

Introduction

The client is experiencing a postoperative complication secondary to cancer therapy for recurrent rectal cancer.

Possible Scenario

A 65-year-old female client with a history of previous pelvic radiation is 3 days status post an abdominal perineal resection (permanent colostomy) and ileal conduit for recurrent rectal cancer with metastasis to cervix. The nurse caring for the client notices that there is increased drainage on the surgical dressing. The urinary output from the ileal conduit has decreased within the past 12 hours. The nurse should immediately notify the health care provider of the change in the client's status.

Possible Outcome

If the nurse is not astute enough to pick up the correlation between decreased urinary output and increased drainage from the surgical wound, the client is at potential risk for wound infection and alteration in the periwound environment.

Prevention

The second nursing action is to apply a closed wound drainage system (i.e., urinary ostomy pouch attached to bedside drainage) to quantify the amount of drainage. This action will allow for continued monitoring of the client's fluid status.

► VARIATIONS

Geriatric Variations:
- *If a client has arthritic hands, it is best to use either a one-piece appliance that is precut or a two-piece appliance that is adaptive to decreases in hand dexterity.*
- *Make sure the client can see and hear your teaching instructions. Ask for feedback to assess whether the client heard and understood the procedure.*
- *If the client needs assistance, instruct a willing family member or caregiver on the procedure.*

Pediatric Variation:
- *A pouch located near a child's groin will need an appliance that is very flexible and can bend with the client's movement and play without becoming nonadherent.*

Home Care Variations:
- *Make sure the client has the necessary supplies and facilities to clean and change the pouch.*
- *Changes in body image from a draining wound could cause the client to withdraw from social situations or even become isolated in the home. As the home care nurse entering the home, you are in a unique position to assess psychosocial needs and changes resulting from the changes in body image.*

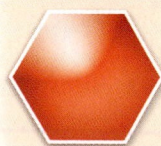

Long-Term Care Variations:
- *Consider the ongoing stress of a slowly healing or draining wound, and the potential changes to body image that large scars and marks will cause even after they have healed.*
- *Connect the client with support groups or further assessment if needed.*

► **COMMON ERRORS**

Possible Error:

Part of the wafer sticks to the client's gown or bed linen and dislodges the pouch.

Prevention:

Check the application for comfort before leaving the client's bedside. Make sure sticky areas are covered with hypoallergenic tape, if necessary.

► **NURSING TIPS**

- Recognize that all draining wounds are not the same. Each wound must be treated individually, which requires that the nurse assess the dimensions, type and amount of drainage, and the peri-wound skin's condition.
- Client teaching is easily incorporated into the care of the draining wound by encouraging the client to be your assistant during the application process.

- Use of a closed drainage system on a draining wound will increase the client's comfort level and thereby the client's participation in self-care activities.
- Costs to the client and the health care institution are reduced when draining wounds are maintained in a closed wound system. The cost reduction is realized in a decrease in the use of sterile dressings, linen changes, pain medication used by the client, and nursing time.

► **SPECIAL CONSIDERATIONS**

- *The drainage pouch should be emptied when it is one-third full to prevent spillage and inaccurate measurement of wound drainage.*
- *Changing the pouch may produce an odor in the client's room. Make sure that a room deodorant spray or deodorant wick is available.*

Immobilization and Support

Applying an Elastic Bandage

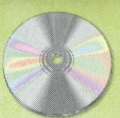

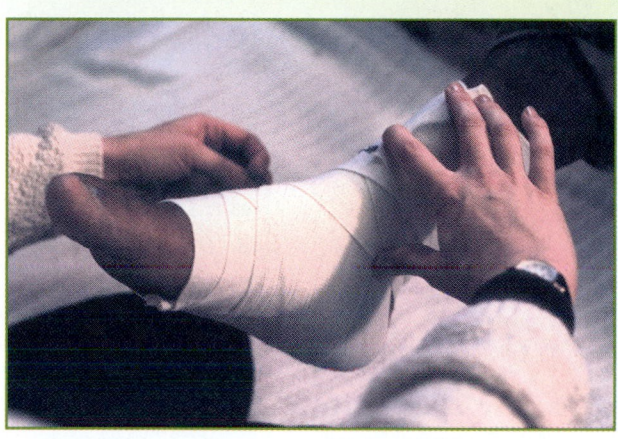

▶ OVERVIEW OF THE SKILL

Elastic bandages or wraps are used to secure dressings in place, immobilize joints, decrease swelling, maintain circulation, support or immobilize a body part, stabilize an extremity, or secure equipment, such as traction, to a body part. Elastic bandages can be used on any body part and to apply compression to any area, with the exception of the neck. The type and size will vary with the body part or area to be covered. Elastic bandages are often used on the lower extremities to prevent edema and to support varicose veins. Elastic bandages can also be used to support the knee, ankle, elbow, and wrist for conditions such as strains and sprains.

▶ ASSESSMENT

1. Check the client's skin integrity and previous reactions to bandages to establish a baseline and avoid allergic reactions to bandages. Inspect the site to be bandaged. Indications of edema, abrasions, discoloration, or bony prominences need to be noted before bandaging. **These assessments will affect the type of bandage used and how the bandage is placed (see Figure 10-1-1).**

2. Assess circulation. Inspect skin temperature, color, pulses, and sensation of body parts to be covered **to determine a baseline neurovascular status.**

3. Assess for the presence of a wound. If a dressing is to be applied under an elastic bandage, assess that wound prior to application of the elastic

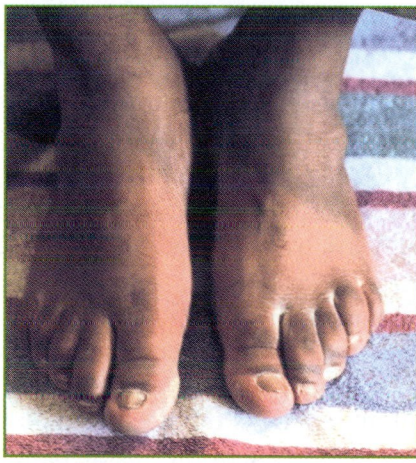

Figure 10-1-1 Examine the site to assess the condition of the skin and to determine the size and type of bandage needed.

bandage. **Determines whether the bandage will put pressure on the wound, or compromise the sterile wound dressing.** Make sure there is a sterile bandage between the elastic bandage and an open wound.

▶ DIAGNOSIS

Acute Pain

Impaired Physical Mobility

Ineffective Tissue Perfusion: Peripheral

Risk for Impaired Peripheral Neurovascular Dysfunction

▶ PLANNING

Expected Outcomes:

1. The client will have decreased edema.
2. The client will have decreased pain.
3. The client's body will be supported and in proper alignment.
4. The client will not experience tingling or numbness distal to the elastic bandage.
5. The client will have good perfusion in parts distal to the elastic bandage.
6. The bandage will be properly anchored and the ends secured with no looseness or stricture.
7. The client will not experience skin irritation or decreased skin integrity related to the bandage.

Equipment Needed (see Figure 10-1-2):

- Elastic bandage (latex-free elastic bandage if client allergic to latex)
- Gloves, if body fluids or wounds are involved
- Dressings, as appropriate, if covering open wounds
- Clips or tape to secure bandage in place

▶ CLIENT EDUCATION NEEDED:

1. Client understands the purpose of the elastic bandage (e.g., for support, to decrease edema, or to secure dressing in place).
2. Client understands the need to keep bandage smooth and wrinkle-free, and to avoid constriction.
3. Client understands the need to report any tingling, numbness, discoloration, or any increased pain.
4. Client understands the need to report any oozing of blood through the elastic bandage.

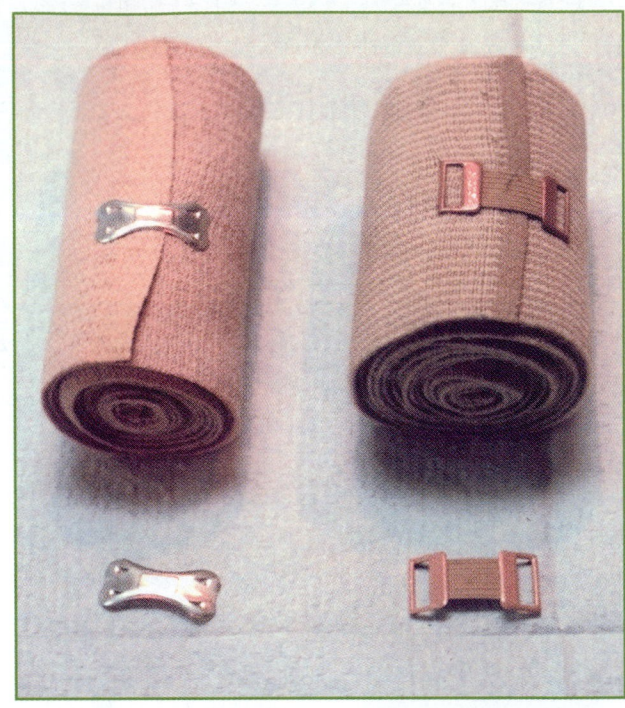

Figure 10-1-2 Elastic bandages

5. Client understands the need to report cool extremity, blanching, or mottling.

 Estimated time to complete the skill: **10 minutes for elastic wrap; if dressing change is involved, more time will be needed depending on the type of wound**

▶ DELEGATION TIPS

Application of bandages over wounds is not delegated to ancillary personnel but may be taught to family members/caregivers for the provision of long-term or home care. Ancillary personnel should be aware of the purpose of the elastic bandage and any reportable conditions such as complaints of pain, tingling, rubbing, pressure, edema, changes in skin condition, or any indications of neurovascular compromise.

IMPLEMENTATION—Action/Rationale

Action	Rationale
1. Assess size of material needed and gather materials (see Figure 10-1-3). Elastic bandages are available in 2-, 2½-, 3-, 4-, 6-, and 8-inch widths. Lengths are usually available in 3 yards. Assess client's reaction to elastic products, and use latex-free wraps if indicated.	1. Provides appropriate support, which will depend on the purpose, injury, or stabilization required. Elastic products may contain latex and are contraindicated if client has a history of latex allergy or contact dermatitis to latex products. Too small a bandage constricts circulation. Too large a bandage will not properly support the body part.
2. Wash hands.	2. Reduces the transmission of microorganisms.
3. Explain purpose and need for bandages to client.	3. Understanding the need to keep a bandage in place can facilitate cooperation. The purpose can be for support, alignment, decreasing edema, or securing dressings.
4. Assess the skin to be covered for redness, swelling, or open lesions. Assess that the client is in a correct position for application; for example, if supporting a fracture, arm, or other body part, it must be anatomically aligned. If elastic wrap is for edema of the lower extremity or for varicose veins, the client's leg must be elevated.	4. Avoids increased injury, infection, or improper alignment. Promotes healing, decreased edema, and proper support for varicosities.
5. Apply the bandage. Technique may vary depending on the body part to be covered and the purpose of the bandage.	5. Proper application maintains consistent bandage tension, conforms to body part, promotes stabilization of body part, and promotes venous return.

5. (continued)
- Hold roll of elastic bandage in dominant hand while using the other hand to lightly grasp the start of the bandage (see Figure 10-1-4). Starting at the distal point, begin by wrapping around body part twice to stabilize start of bandage, then begin working toward the proximal point by transferring hand-to-hand, making sure to overlap at least one-third of bandage on each pass. Bandage should be stretched slightly as it is wrapped; however, two fingers should still fit between bandage and skin to ensure it is not too tight (see Figure 10-1-5). Toes or fingertips must be visible to allow follow-up assessment (see Figure 10-1-6). Secure first bandage before applying additional rolls. Apply additional rolls without exposing any skin surface.
- If the feet and legs are to be covered, wrap twice around the foot, leaving the toes exposed. Use a figure-eight pattern to wrap the ankle. Continue wrapping the leg, using a circular pattern until all bandage is used (see Figure 10-1-7).
- A figure-eight pattern is also useful to cover and immobilize joints (see Figure 10-1-8).
- Use a circular pattern to bandage digits or wrists.
- Use spiral turns to apply a bandage to cover areas such as slender wrists or the forearms.

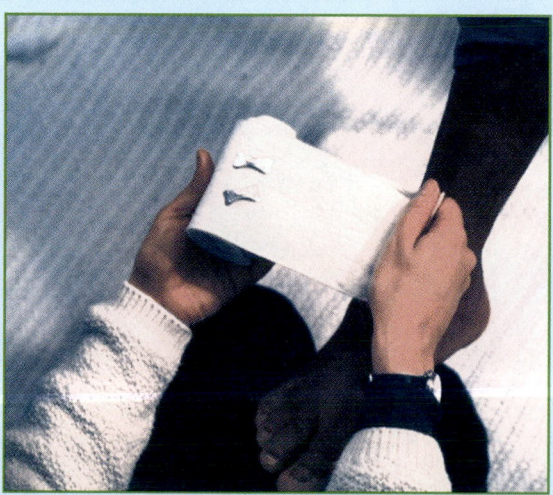

Figure 10-1-3 Remove material from packaging and set the clips aside where they may be easily reached.

continues

Action	Rationale

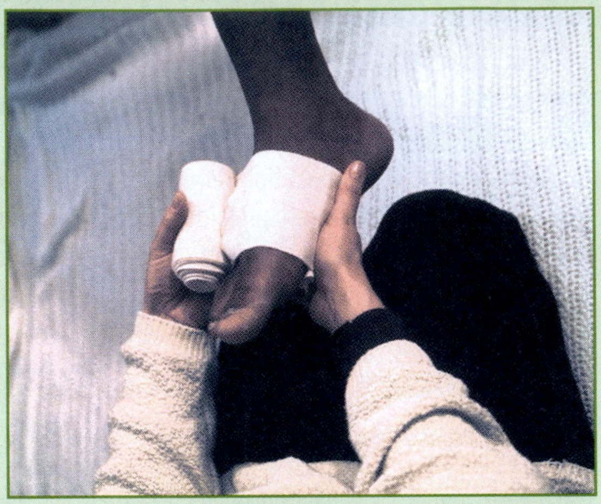

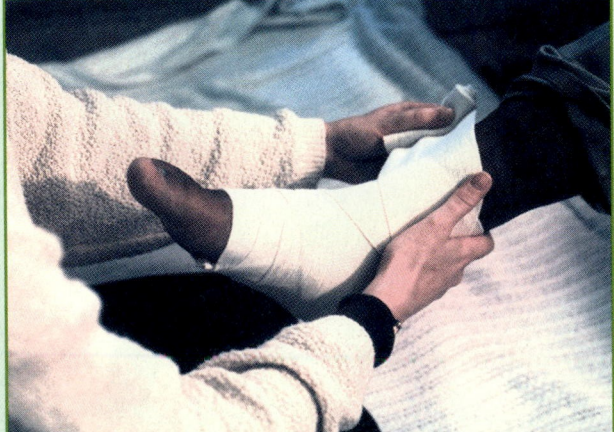

Figure 10-1-4 Hold the bandage in the dominant hand and anchor the end of the bandage against the skin with the nondominant hand.

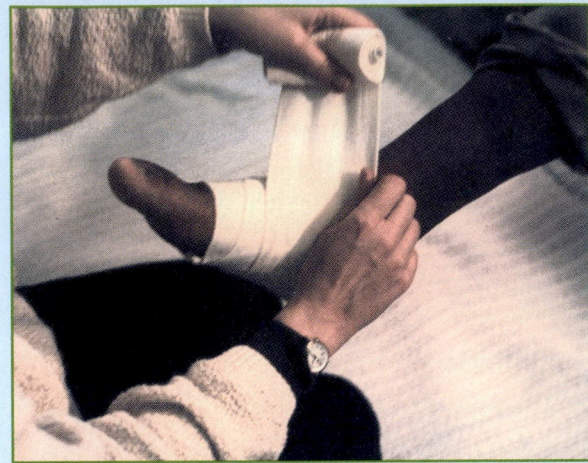

Figure 10-1-5 Apply the bandage from the distal to proximal area. You may transfer the bandage from hand to hand as you wrap.

- If securing equipment in place, such as Buck's traction, use a circular pattern around the leg and traction.
- Spiral reverse turns are used to cover parts of the body that are the shape of an inverted cone (begin small and get larger), such as the thigh or forearm.
- Recurrent turns are used to bandage the head or the stump of an amputated limb.

6. Secure in place with the tape, pins, or hooks provided with bandage (see Figure 10-1-9).

7. Check whether wrinkles are present; if so, smooth out.
   - Check that no constrictive areas are present
   - Check color, movement, sensation (CMS), and warmth distal to wrap.
   - If elastic wrap is used for traction, see Skill 10-7.

6. Prevents loose ends and unraveling of dressing.

7. Prevents skin breakdown and decreased circulation.

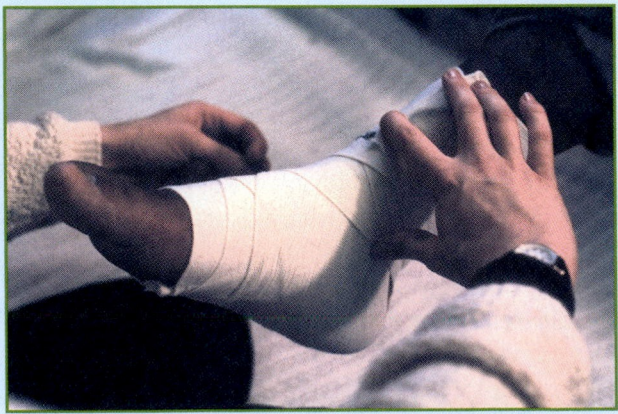

Figure 10-1-6 Wrap the bandage up the limb. Keep the toes visible to allow assessment of circulation.

Figure 10-1-7 Continue until the entire elastic bandage is used.

continues

Action	Rationale
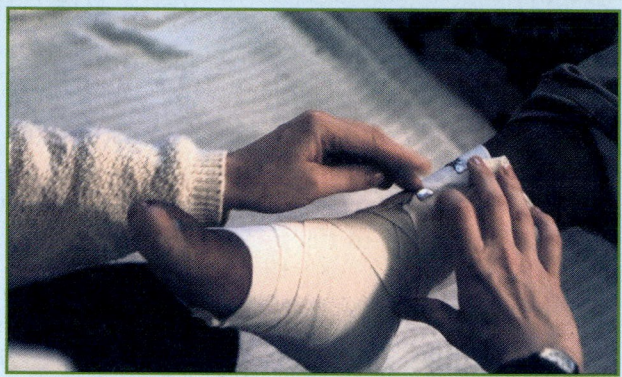	

Figure 10-1-8 The bandage is wrapped using the figure-eight method.

Figure 10-1-9 Secure the bandage with clips. When applying clips be careful they do not scratch the skin.

Action	Rationale
8. Wash hands.	**8.** Reduces the transmission of microorganisms.

▶ **REAL WORLD ANECDOTES**

Chai recently attended an in-service seminar given by a nurse with 20 years of experience in an orthopedic clinic. Chai learned about several problems with elastic bandages, or Ace wraps, commonly seen in both inpatient and outpatient settings. The most serious problem is when a client develops tingling in the fingers or toes if the bandage is wrapped too tightly. This can also occur if swelling continues after the bandage is placed. It is often seen when clients rewrap their own bandages at home. Younger clients especially will move around extensively and disrupt the smoothness of the bandage, which can lead to variations in pressure. The friction of the bedsheets can also disrupt the smoothness of elastic bandages. If the elastic bandage becomes wrinkled, skin tissue injury can occur at the points of compression. Sometimes a client will have a wound and dressing under the elastic wrap. If the dressing is inadequate or not changed often enough, oozing is noted through the elastic wrap. The wrap becomes contaminated with wound exudate and must be cleaned. The wound is not protected against infection, because bacteria can enter the wound.

▶ **EVALUATION**

- The client has decreased edema.
- The client has decreased pain.
- The client's body is supported and in good alignment.
- The client does not experience tingling or numbness distal to the elastic bandage.
- The client has good perfusion in parts distal to the elastic bandage.
- The bandage is properly anchored and the ends secured with no looseness or stricture.

▶ **DOCUMENTATION**

Nurses' Notes

Document:

- Procedure, type of wrap, and reason for wrapping
- Assessment of color, movement, warmth, and sensation initially and 20 minutes later
- Distal pulses, if applicable
- Vital signs, if needed, in acute injury situation

Document on appropriate flow sheet or electronic medical record (EMR).

► CRITICAL THINKING SKILL

Introduction

Assessment after the bandage is applied must include all possible complications of the injury.

Possible Scenario

A client is admitted to the unit after a motor vehicle accident. He fractured his leg, which is now wrapped in an elastic bandage. He rings his call light and complains of deep throbbing pain in his calf.

Possible Outcome

The nurse rewraps the leg, explains to the client that fractures can be painful, and offers medications. The client continues to develop a deep venous thrombosis as a result of the injury.

Prevention

The nurse needed to listen to the client's complaints of pain and should have done a thorough assessment, including assessing the leg for deep venous thrombosis by checking for pain, warmth, redness, discoloration, or pain in calf.

► VARIATIONS

Geriatric Variations:
- *Elderly clients have very frail skin and may find elastic bandages useful in enabling the healing process.*
- *Elderly clients may find more comfort and added support from elastic bandages than from an elastic stocking for varicose veins because elastic stockings may roll at the top and are difficult to put on.*
- *Elderly clients usually require assistance with elastic bandages.*
- *Elastic bandages may be useful in securing dressings in elderly clients with skin that is frail or tears easily.*

Pediatric Variations:
- *Children often do not like feeling constricted; therefore, assess frequently if the child plays with the bandage.*
- *A younger child can assist with the procedure by holding the clips used to secure the bandage, by counting and feeling the toes or fingers, or by counting the number of "wraps" taken.*
- *If the bandage does not stay on during active play, extra tape or clips can be used.*
- *If the parents will be rewrapping the bandage, teach them how to assess neurovascular status, the basics of handwashing, and keeping the bandage clean.*
- *Remind parents not to wrap the bandage "extra tight" in an effort to keep it in place.*
- *Younger clients may not be able to complain of pain or tingling. These clients need extra careful assessment.*
- *An older child or adolescent can be taught how to rewrap the bandage. This teaching must include how to assess neurovascular status, the basics of handwashing, and keeping the bandage clean.*

Home Care Variations:
- *Some clients find elastic bandages more useful than stockings and less expensive.*
- *Put bandages in a mesh "delicates" laundry bag before putting them in the washing machine. This keeps them from getting twisted and tangled in the laundry. Also, bandages may be hand-washed in the sink and rolled between towels to dry.*
- *Make sure client is not using a bandage that is too large or too small for the limb being treated. Bandages that are too small will constrict circulation and will not stay in place. Bandages that are too large will not properly support the injured limb.*

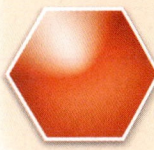

Long-Term Care Variations:
- *Elastic bandages lose their elasticity over time. Replace as needed.*
- *Same as home care variations.*

► COMMON ERRORS

Possible Error:

The bandage is wrapped too tightly or too loosely.

Prevention:

Use a steady, gentle stretch as you wrap the bandage. Do not tug at a bandage that is too short to cover an area. Add a second bandage if needed. Keep pins and clips within reach so you can anchor the bandage when you finish the wrap.

Possible Error:

Edges are not overlapped properly.

Prevention:

Pay attention to the wrapping process. Visualize ahead where the next wrap will go. If you run out of bandage before you run out of limb to cover, add a second bandage.

► NURSING TIPS

- Gently stretch the bandage as you apply it to make sure it is secure.

- If wounds are involved, check under bandages periodically.

► SPECIAL CONSIDERATIONS

- If the bandage is placed soon after injury, swelling is likely to occur and bandage may need to be rewrapped.
- Bandages lose elasticity after a time; be sure to replace them periodically.
- When wrapping the tip of a digit or a stump, be sure there is enough pressure at the end, but not too much around the circumference; this can act as a tourniquet instead of an anchor for the rest of the bandage.
- In the past, Homans' sign was used to rule out deep vein thrombosis. However, positive Homans' sign alone is no longer considered a diagnostic tool. Considering the entire clinical picture Homans' sign can be used as a guide for the need for further assessment, addition of diagnostic tools, or treatment.
- Latex-free bandages are available and should be used if the client has a history of latex allergy or contact dermatitis related to previous bandage use.

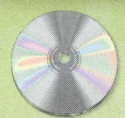

Applying a Splint

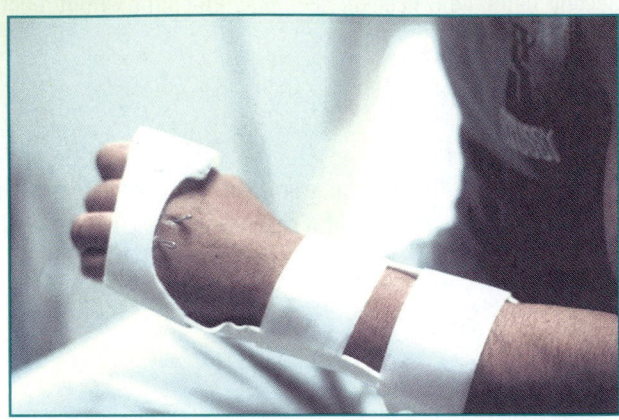

▶ OVERVIEW OF THE SKILL

Splinting is the process of applying a rigid device to a limb, joint, or wound to prevent movement of displaced or injured areas (see Figure 10-2-1). Splinting is used primarily for immobilization of broken bones or dislocated joints in emergency situations and to prevent movement in the injured area after the extent of the injury is known in nonemergency situations. When a fractured or dislocated area has been correctly immobilized, the splint allows complete rest of the injured area in the anatomically correct position (see Figure 10-2-2). This facilitates proper and complete healing. A properly applied splint is also important in controlling blood loss and pain. If a fracture with sharp bone ends is not immobilized, further tissue trauma, blood loss, and pain will occur. See Table 10-2-1 for types of splints and their indications.

A splint can be made from any rigid material, from a stick to plaster or fiberglass, or a premade aluminum padded splint can be used. Ideally the material should be light and rigid enough not to change shape if the client moves. It is very important that the splint be long enough to extend beyond the joint distal to the involved area. If the injury is close to the proximal joint, that joint should also be immobilized to avoid movement in the injured area. The splint should be as wide as the area being immobilized. For client comfort, and to avoid further trauma, padding is recommended on the side next to the client's skin. This is also of benefit if the area swells, as the padding will reduce interference with circulation. Splints are held in place with bandages (see Skill 10-1, Applying an Elastic Bandage), Velcro straps, or tape.

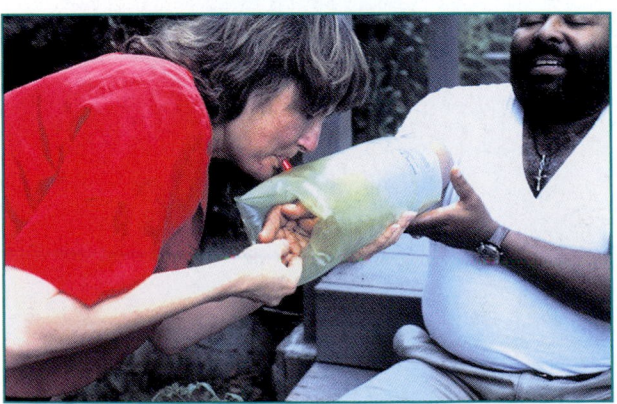

Figure 10-2-1 Applying an air splint to immobilize an injured wrist.

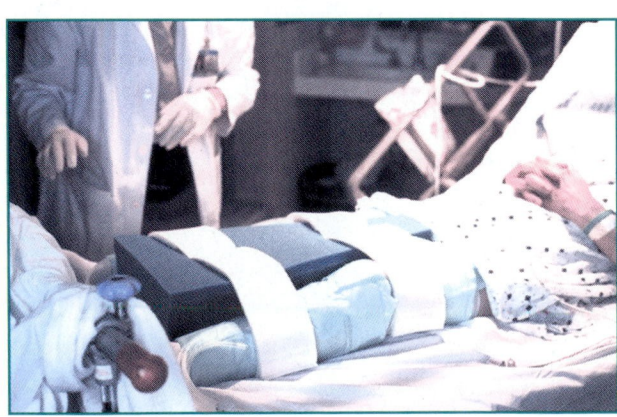

Figure 10-2-2 After surgery, a splint is applied to maintain the position of the limb.

Table 10-2-1 Types of Splints and Their Indications	
TYPE OF SPLINT	**INDICATION**
• *Volar splint*	Sprains of the wrist or soft tissue injuries
• *Dorsal splint*	Sprains of the wrist or soft tissue injuries
• *Radial gutter splint*	Immobilization of the second or third finger
• *Thumb spica splint*	Immobilization of the thumb
• *Ulnar gutter splint*	Immobilization of the third or fourth finger
• *Sugar tong splint*	Immobilization of the wrist and the elbow, for fractures of the proximal forearm and elbow
• *Anteroposterior splint*	Fracture of the distal forearm
• *Posterior long arm splint*	Injuries around the elbow and the forearm
• *Posterior short leg*	Ankle injuries
• *Sugar tong or stirrup short leg*	Ankle injuries (either sprains or fractures)
• *Posterior gutter—long leg*	Knee and upper tibia or fibula injuries

▶ ASSESSMENT

1. Assess the area where the splint is to be applied. Check for bleeding, raw bone ends, or debris. Note if the site is in correct alignment. Do not attempt to align a suspected fracture when splinting. **Affects how the splint will be applied, or if the procedure is contraindicated.**

2. Assess the client's skin integrity, paying special attention to the presence of an open fracture, edema, ecchymosis, lacerations, abrasions, and the condition of the skin (dry, cracked, infected, thin). **Alerts to possible complications such as skin breakdown and infection.**

3. Assess the neurovascular status. Circulation can be assessed by checking capillary refill and pulses in the distal area, and by checking the skin temperature and color. The nerve status can be assessed by asking the client, if conscious, if there is any numbness or tingling in the involved area or distal to it, and by actually checking sensation. **Provides baseline for future assessments.**

4. Assess the client's level of pain and how client is dealing with it. **Pain may cause the client to thrash, which could cause increased injury.**

▶ DIAGNOSIS

Acute Pain

Chronic Pain

Impaired Physical Mobility

Risk for Disuse Syndrome

Risk for Peripheral Neurovascular Dysfunction

Risk for Trauma

▶ PLANNING

Expected Outcomes:
1. The client will not experience unnecessary pain.
2. The client will not sustain further tissue damage and blood loss.
3. The injury will be well supported and immobilized in correct anatomic alignment.
4. There will be adequate circulation to the wound and distal body part.
5. The client will not experience any skin breakdown as a result of the splinting.
6. The client will verbalize an understanding regarding care of the injured area and use of the splint.

Equipment Needed:
- Dressing for wound, if present
- Gloves
- Padding for under splint (Webril or gauze)
- Appropriate splint (see Figure 10-2-3)

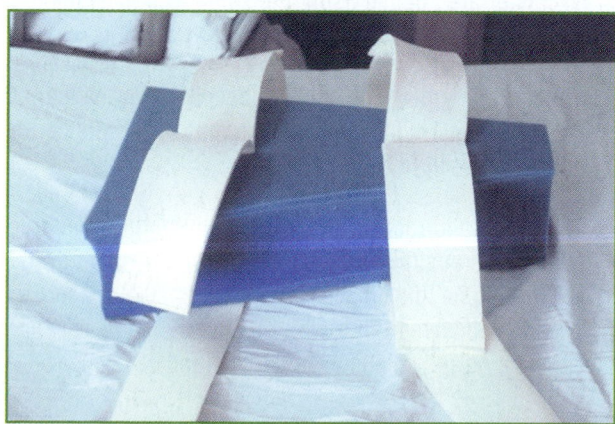

Figure 10-2-3 Abduction splint

- Elastic bandage, Ace wrap, Velcro straps, or tape to hold splint in place

▶ **CLIENT EDUCATION NEEDED:**

1. Explain to the client that the splint will impair mobility.
2. Reinforce the need to report any numbness, tingling, or cool skin distal to the splint.
3. Explain to the client that the splint needs to remain dry and in place until a health care provider has removed it.

Estimated time to complete the skill:
15–30 minutes depending on whether there is a wound involved and the complexity of the splint, which is dependent on the body part involved

---

▶ **DELEGATION TIPS**

Splinting is used primarily to immobilize broken bones or dislocated joints in emergency situations and may be applied by any properly trained emergency personnel. In nonemergency situations, a nurse would assess the extremity and apply a splint. Instruct ancillary personnel to report any evidence of decreased limb mobility, increased pain, numbness, tingling, coolness, bleeding, or cyanosis of the extremity. For routine application of a splint ordered by a physician, orthotist, physical therapist, or occupational therapist, the skill may be delegated to ancillary personnel or family members. They should be aware of the purpose of the splint, the proper application of the appliance, the schedule of application, and any reportable conditions such as complaints of pain, rubbing, pressure, changes in skin condition, or any indications of neurovascular compromise.

IMPLEMENTATION—Action/Rationale

Action	Rationale
1. Wash hands.	1. Reduces the transmission of microorganisms.
2. Assess the need for a dressing if there is an open wound.	2. Decreases the risk of blood loss or infection.
3. Check the health care provider's orders to see what kind of splint was ordered. This skill will concentrate on removable, preformed splints. Splints made of fiberglass or plaster are applied using the same technique found in Skill 10-10 and Skill 10-12.	3. The splint will vary depending on the area to be splinted and the type of injury.
4. Measure the area to be splinted according to the manufacturer's instructions. Be aware that some splints are made for the right or left side.	4. The correct size splint will aid healing and help prevent skin damage and ulceration.
5. Apply the splint according to the manufacturer's instructions. Generally this will involve sliding the splint over the area to be immobilized (see Figures 10-2-4 and 10-2-5), and securing it with an elastic bandage, tape, or Velcro straps (see Figures 10-2-6 and 10-2-7).	5. Correct application is important to avoid further damage to the area as well as to promote healing.

continues

Action	Rationale

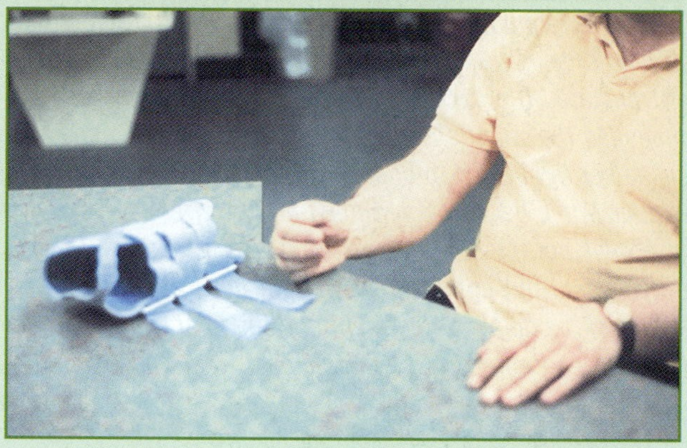

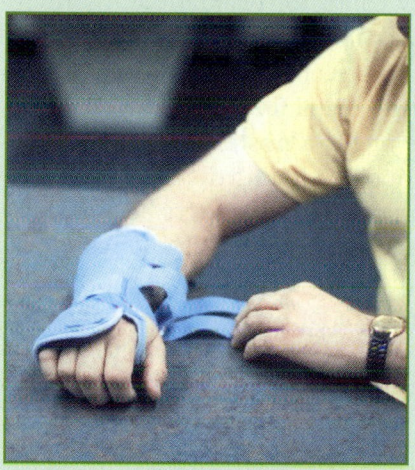

Figure 10-2-4 Align the splint with the limb to be immobilized.

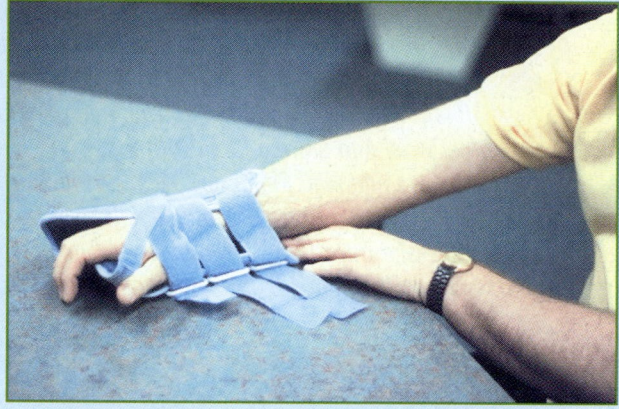

Figure 10-2-5 Slide the splint onto the area to be immobilized.

Figure 10-2-6 Secure the splint with attached fasteners, tape, or Velcro.

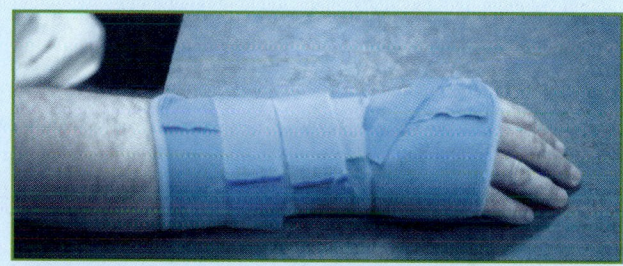

Figure 10-2-7 Assess the neurovascular status of the area distal to the splint. Make sure the splint provides adequate support for the injured area.

6. Check neurovascular status of the area distal to the splint as indicated by color, warmth, and CMS (circulation, movement, and sensation).

7. If the client will be taking the splint off and reapplying it at home, instruct regarding the use and care of the splint. Be sure client can perform the skill alone prior to discharge.

8. Check the neurovascular status of the area distal to the splint prior to discharging the client. Teach proper assessment.

9. Wash hands.

6. Establishes baseline assessment. Splints can compromise the neurovascular status of extremities that are distal to them. This should be checked often and taught to the client.

7. Client education is important to promote compliance and healing.

8. Neurovascular compromise is not always immediately apparent and must be checked often.

9. Reduces the transmission of microorganisms.

► REAL WORLD ANECDOTES

Mrs. Phum presented to the emergency room complaining of severe pain in her right wrist. The doctor noted that she was wearing a splint on her wrist. He noticed that it was designed for clients with carpal tunnel syndrome. Mrs. Phum spoke very little English and her daughter translated the doctor's questions. The doctor asked Mrs. Phum when her wrist pain started and who had recommended the splint she was wearing. Mrs. Phum noted that her wrist had started to hurt after she had fallen and used her right hand to break her fall. Her daughter was out of town and Mrs. Phum had been unable to see a physician. When her wrist continued to hurt after several days, she purchased a splint at a garage sale. She had been wearing it for a week but the pain had not improved. When Mrs. Phum's daughter returned she questioned her mother about the splint and her wrist, and immediately brought her to the emergency room. X-rays showed that Mrs. Phum's wrist had been fractured. Because of the delay in treatment and the improper splint, her wrist had started to heal in misalignment. The fracture that might have been treated with a simple cast would now require a much more complex procedure to align and set the bones.

► EVALUATION

- The client did not experience unnecessary pain.
- The client did not sustain further tissue damage and blood loss.
- The injury is well-supported and immobilized in correct anatomic alignment.
- There is adequate circulation to the wound and distal body part.
- The client did not experience any skin breakdown as a result of the splinting.
- The client has verbalized understanding regarding care of the injured area and use of the splint.

► DOCUMENTATION

Nurses' Notes

- Record the reason the splint was applied and the area the splint was applied to as well as the type of splint that was placed.
- Note the condition of the client's skin prior to placing the splint.
- Note the neurovascular status of the area distal to the splint both before and after placement.
- Record any client teaching.

Document on appropriate flow sheet or electronic medical record (EMR).

► CRITICAL THINKING SKILL

Introduction

Client education is an essential part of nursing care.

Possible Scenario

Betty is a 34-year-old lab technician who fell and hurt her left ankle while jogging. She presents to the emergency room for evaluation. There are no obvious fractures or dislocations and she is stable so she is sent in a wheelchair for an X-ray. The X-ray reveals that she has a distal fibular fracture with no misalignment. She needs a posterior splint and to follow up with orthopedics for further evaluation. During the application of the splint, Betty becomes very agitated and moves around a great deal, making it difficult to size and properly apply the splint. After the posterior leg splint is put on and she is being discharged, she complains of numbness and tingling of her toes below the splint that you just applied.

Possible Outcome

You reassure Betty that she should put her leg up and ice it when she gets home. This will reduce the swelling and the splint will feel much better. Betty stays home for 2 days, with her leg elevated and iced, taking her prescribed pain pills. Her foot is still numb and her toes are white, but she assumes that is the way it should be. When she sees her orthopedic doctor 2 days after the incident he notes that Betty seems to have nerve damage in her left foot.

Prevention

Betty needed to be educated and included in the process of the splint application to ensure that she would remain cooperative. Her pain status and how she was managing the pain needed to be assessed before and during the process. The importance of a good fit to avoid interference with blood flow to the area and the neurovascular status cannot be overstressed. The neurovascular status needs to be evaluated before, during, and after the process.

► VARIATIONS

Geriatric Variations:
- Pay special attention to the condition of the skin and the neurovascular status because these areas can be compromised in the elderly. Their skin is more easily broken down, so they need to be checked more often when in a splint.
- If a client has a compromised mental status, it is important to have someone check on the client and ascertain that he or she get follow-up care.
- It is often difficult for the elderly to walk with crutches, so a wheelchair or walker may be needed.

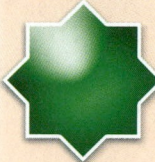

Pediatric Variations:
- Children tend to move a great deal more when anxious, so it is important to include them in the process as much as possible to get the best splint application possible.
- Children need someone to check the splint often to ensure there is no compromise to the neurovascular system.
- Children will need help with mobility while in a splint.

Home Care Variations:
- Clients who will be wearing a splint at home must be taught to watch for signs and symptoms of neurovascular compromise.
- Be sure to explain follow-up care and weight-bearing movement.

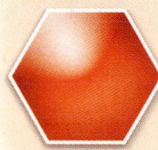

Long-Term Care Variations:
- Clients who wear a splint regularly must be sure to check for ongoing fit and wear and tear on the appliance.
- Fit and appliance wear should be checked by a professional at regular intervals.

► COMMON ERRORS

Possible Error:
Using a splint designed for the opposite extremity.

Prevention:
There are differences in splints made for a right hand or foot and ones made for a left hand or foot, so it is crucial that you are familiar with the splints and orthopedic appliances used in your facility. Health care providers have preferences, so familiarizing yourself with those appliances can increase your efficiency and decrease the number of errors and problems.

► NURSING TIPS

- Be sure the distal portion of the extremity is exposed for neurovascular assessment, if possible.
- Check and document the client's neurovascular status before, during, and after applying the splint.
- Familiarize yourself with the splints and appliances available in your facility. Know what they are supposed to look like and how they work both on and off the client.

> **SPECIAL CONSIDERATIONS**

- *Watch for clues in the splint that guide proper alignment and positioning. These may be things such as a bend in the splint where the knee or wrist can flex.*
- *Some splints are not used during all hours of the day; rather, some time is spent in and some time is spent out of the splint. Be sure you know what the orders are for its usage.*
- *In most facilities resting splints (usually made of white hard plastic material) are made and adjusted by occupational therapists. If there is a problem, or a question about a splint, call the occupational therapist on staff.*
- *"CMS" may be used at some agencies to refer to color, movement, and sensation.*

Applying an Arm Sling

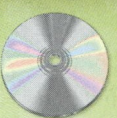

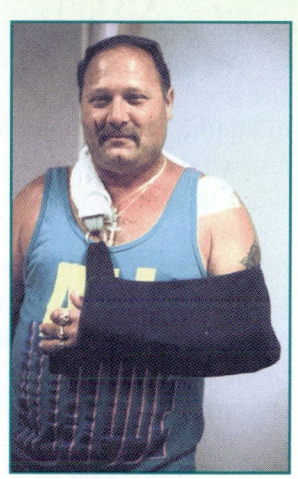

▶ OVERVIEW OF THE SKILL

Slings are used to immobilize an injured arm or shoulder caused by sprain, strain, dislocation, or fracture. Slings are used to prevent dependent edema, control pain, promote rest to aide healing, and, if a fracture is present, support the upper extremity. Slings are often used after an arm has been casted to avoid unnecessary pull on the neck and shoulders from the weight of the cast. In an emergency situation slings are used as first aid to prevent further tissue damage, bleeding, and to control pain. Slings are also used to hold dressings in place.

Slings can be made of various materials. In the emergency situation any large triangular piece of fabric can be used. In the nonemergency situation commercially made slings are generally used. These are usually made from sturdy canvas, which forms a sleeve that fits around the client's injured limb, with a supporting strap that is padded and fits around the neck. Some slings also have a strap that fits around the client's waist to further immobilize the upper arm, especially the shoulder.

▶ ASSESSMENT

1. Assess the arm, shoulder, and clavicle that is to have the sling applied. In an emergency situation, any possibility of a neck injury would preclude the use of a sling. **In a nonemergency situation,** **assess for any other deformities or injuries that might preclude the use of an arm sling.**

2. Assess the client's skin integrity on the entire upper extremity and the neck. The sling is supported by the neck strap. **If a triangular bandage is used as the sling, extra padding in the neck area will make the sling more comfortable and may prevent skin breakdown. Extra padding on a manufactured sling may be used as well for client comfort (see Figure 10-3-1).**

3. Assess the client's level of consciousness to determine how he or she will tolerate the process of applying the sling and deal with it after it is applied. **If the client is noncompliant, the**

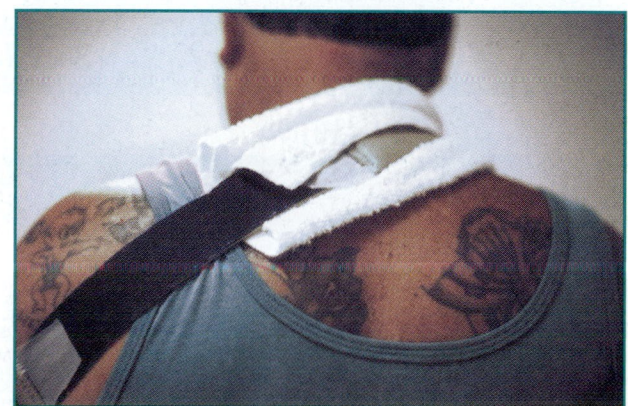

Figure 10-3-1 Extra padding around the neck area will make the sling more comfortable for the client.

1327

waist strap may be necessary to establish the needed immobilization.

4. Assess the client's level of pain. **If the client is having a great deal of pain, he or she may move around more, which could cause further tissue damage, bleeding, and improper immobilization.**

▶ DIAGNOSIS

Acute Pain

Impaired Physical Mobility

Risk for Disuse Syndrome

Risk for Impaired Skin Integrity

Risk for Peripheral Vascular Dysfunction

▶ PLANNING

Expected Outcomes:

1. The client will not experience any unnecessary pain.
2. The procedure will be performed with a minimum of trauma to the client.
3. The injured area is adequately supported to allow healing in proper alignment.
4. The client will not experience any skin breakdown or neurovascular damage as a result of the arm sling.

Equipment Needed:

- Dressing for wound(s), if needed
- Sling: either large triangular piece of cloth or pre-made sling
- Padding, if needed

▶ CLIENT EDUCATION NEEDED:

1. Teach the client how to put on and remove the sling if he or she will be wearing it at home.
2. Be sure the client understands to keep the hand just above the level of the elbow to prevent swelling and edema in the hand, as well as prevent unnecessary strain on the shoulder.
3. Teach the client to remove the sling once or twice a day to perform range of motion exercises as ordered by the health care provider.
4. Have the client or the caregiver perform a return demonstration of applying and removing the sling.
5. Teach the client how to check the neurovascular status of the fingers and hand. Instruct client to notify his health care provider if he or she notes any impairment.

Estimated time to complete the skill: **5 minutes**

▶ DELEGATION TIPS

Application of a sling may be delegated to ancillary personnel. For routine application of a sling ordered by the health care provider, physical therapist, or occupational therapist, the skill may be delegated to ancillary personnel or family members. Proper instruction dictates that they should be aware of the purpose of the sling, the proper application of the appliance, the schedule of application, and any reportable conditions such as complaints of pain, rubbing, pressure, changes in skin conditions, or any indications of neurovascular compromise.

IMPLEMENTATION—Action/Rationale

Action	Rationale
1. Wash hands.	1. Reduces the transmission of microorganisms.
Applying the Triangular Sling Used in Emergency Situations and for Brief Periods of Time	
2. Place the affected arm across the client's chest with the fingers higher than the hand and the hand higher than the elbow.	2. Keeping the hand above the elbow will prevent edema, which could compromise the client's neurovascular status.

continues

Action	Rationale
3. Place the base of the triangle under the client's wrist with the apex of the triangle under the client's elbow. The endpoints at the base of the triangle should be pointing up and down, one on the client's unaffected shoulder and the other on the knee.	**3.** Allows for proper positioning of the sling.
4. Pull the point at the client's knee up over the affected arm to meet with the point on the unaffected shoulder. Tie the two points together with a square knot at the client's unaffected shoulder.	**4.** Avoids pressure from the knot on the neck.
5. Fold the apex of the triangle neatly around the affected elbow and secure it with a safety pin.	**5.** Provides elbow support and holds the arm in alignment.
6. Pad any areas where the sling presses against soft tissues, such as the neck, axilla, or around a cast.	**6.** Helps prevent skin breakdown in pressure areas.
7. Have the client sit up or stand, if indicated, and check the alignment of the arm. The elbow should be enclosed, the fingers exposed, and the knot at the side of the neck, not in back. The client's hand should be above the level of the elbow. Be sure to check alignment and positioning when the arm is in the position it will be in most often.	**7.** Prevents further injury caused by misalignment or undue strain from improper fit.

Applying a Manufactured Sling Most Commonly Used When Immobilization Will Be Needed for a Long-Term Treatment

Action	Rationale
8. Position the sling next to the arm. Read the manufacturer's directions if you are unclear how to lay out the sling in the proper position (see Figure 10-3-2).	**8.** Allows for a smooth procedure.
9. Support the arm as you guide it into the sleeve (see Figure 10-3-3).	**9.** Places sling with a minimum of discomfort.

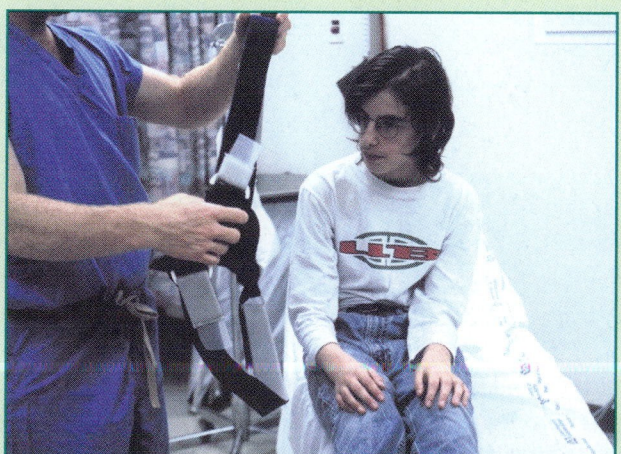

Figure 10-3-2   Align the sling next to the arm in the correct position.

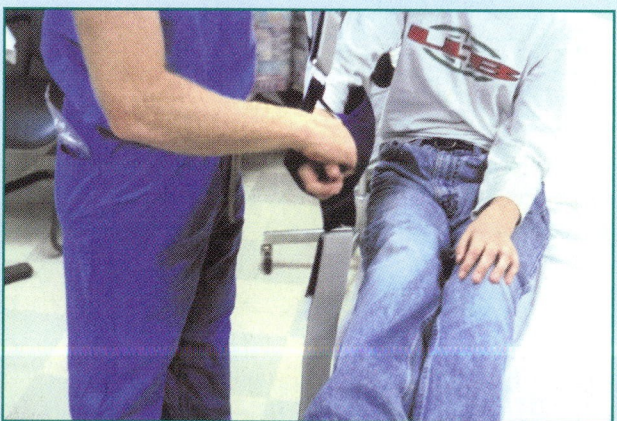

Figure 10-3-3   Support the arm and gently guide the arm into the sleeve of the sling.

continues

Action	Rationale
Applying a Manufactured Sling Most Commonly Used When Immobilization Will Be Needed for a Long-Term Treatment *continued*	
10. Adjust the shoulder strap. The straps should be snug but not tight; the hand should be held above the level of the elbow. Be sure fingers can be viewed with minimal movement of the sling (see Figure 10-3-4). Assess circulatory and neurovascular status of extremity.	**10.** Ensures proper alignment of the arm as well as client comfort. Establishes baseline assessment.
11. Adjust the waist strap. If the client has a shoulder injury the waist strap will be needed to provide further immobilization.	**11.** Allows for client comfort.
12. If the client will be wearing the sling while at home, teach client or caregiver to apply and remove the sling.	**12.** Education promotes compliance and faster healing.
13. Wash hands.	**13.** Reduces the transmission of microorganisms.

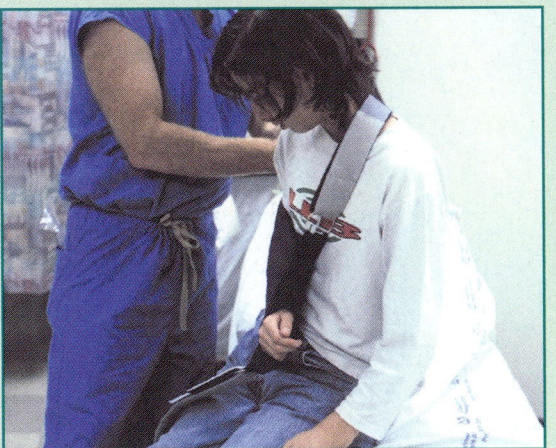

Figure 10-3-4 Adjust the shoulder strap. Make sure the hand is positioned higher than the elbow when the sling is resting comfortably on the shoulder.

► **REAL WORLD ANECDOTES**

While working nights in a long-term care facility, a confused client fell, striking her upper arm on the toilet. The charge nurse was called to the scene. The client was trying to get up despite two assistants trying to keep her still. She was holding her upper arm, which was obviously dislocated. The charge nurse sent one of the assistants to call for an ambulance. The client continued to struggle to return to bed. Rather than cause more damage to the client's arm, the second assistant helped the client back to bed while the nurse supported the client's arm in alignment. When the client was safely in bed, the nurse sent the second assistant for a triangle bandage. As they waited for the ambulance, the nurse applied a sling to the client's arm and attempted to calm and reassure the client.

▶ **EVALUATION**

- The client did not experience any unnecessary pain.
- The procedure was performed with a minimum of trauma to the client.
- The affected arm is adequately supported to allow healing in proper alignment.
- The client is not experiencing any skin breakdown or neurovascular damage as a result of the arm sling.

▶ **DOCUMENTATION**

Nurses' Notes

- Record the reason a sling was required and the type of sling applied. Note the condition of the client's arm, including neurovascular status, prior to placement of the sling.
- Note the neurovascular status of the client's arm after placement of the sling.
- Record the client's comfort level and understanding of the instructions received regarding care of the arm and placement of the sling.

Document on appropriate flow sheet or electronic medical record (EMR).

▶ **CRITICAL THINKING SKILL**

Introduction

The proper equipment in the correct size is essential to good care.

Possible Scenario

You are working in the infirmary at a summer camp. During the initial check-in you notice one of the campers is wearing an arm sling. His left forearm is in a cast and the cast is in the sling. Upon questioning the child he gives you a note from his doctor.

The note indicates that the boy had recently sustained a hairline fracture of the wrist but that he would be able to participate in most camp activities as long as he wears his sling. Upon closer examination you note that the boy's fingers have good capillary return but they are a little cool. You also note that the sling the boy is wearing extends well past the end of his fingers. When you ask about the sling, you are told that the clinic did not have a small sling so they used a larger one instead. You can see that the sling is so large it is not holding the boy's hand above his elbow. Additionally his fingers are hidden from view for neurovascular assessment. Because the boy had not been wearing the cast very long and the possibility of bumping and injuring his arm is increased at camp, you are concerned that you cannot tell at a glance if the boy's fingers are pale or swollen. You are reluctant to allow the boy to stay at camp with the oversized sling, but his parents have already left and he is obviously looking forward to camping.

Potential Outcome

You resolve the dilemma by replacing the oversized sling with a triangle bandage sling. You carefully adjust the size of the triangle bandage so it will support the boy's arm in proper alignment and will allow the boy's fingers to be visible for inspection. When the boy's fingers started to swell after a particularly vigorous day, you had the boy elevate his hand and arm and put ice on it. The swelling went down in his fingers and the boy was able to finish out the week at camp.

Prevention

In areas that serve a specialized population, equipment of the proper size and variety should be on hand.

▶ **VARIATIONS**

Geriatric Variation:
- *Older people often have thin, fragile skin. Extra care must be taken to pad the pressure points to prevent skin breakdown.*

Pediatric Variation:
- *Young children may need a strap around the waist to ensure immobilization because young children tend to thrash around when in pain.*

continues

▶ VARIATIONS *(continued)*

Home Care Variation:
- *Home care clients need to be assessed regularly for compliance. Check that they are wearing their sling and be sure they are wearing the sling in a manner that actually provides support.*

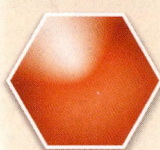

Long-Term Care Variation:
- *Long-term care clients need to be reassessed regularly regarding their ongoing need for a sling. They also need to be reevaluated for fit because people can gain and lose weight over time, perhaps requiring a different size sling.*

▶ COMMON ERRORS

Possible Error:

Allowing the hand to fall below the level of the elbow.

Prevention:

Be sure that the sling fits properly and keep the hand elevated above the level of the elbow. Teach the client about the need to keep the hand elevated to prevent venous pooling and edema.

▶ NURSING TIPS

- Have the client demonstrate applying and removing the sling if he or she will be doing it at home.
- Assess the client's ability to perform the skill prior to discharge.
- Check neurovascular status before and after applying the sling. Assess circulation, movement, and sensation (CMS).

▶ SPECIAL CONSIDERATIONS

- *With an arm sling it is best to have the tips of the fingers exposed; however, not all facilities have adjustable slings. Be sure the fingers are easily accessible for inspection.*
- *Be sure the sling always supports the wrist joint as well as the elbow. If a wrist is limp in a downward position, there may be injury to the wrist joint.*
- *Slings are not a reliable way to immobilize or maintain a joint in an anatomically correct position; they are used mostly for support and to decrease use of that extremity. If immobilization is needed, there are special types of slings or equipment for this purpose.*

Applying Antiembolic Stockings

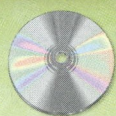

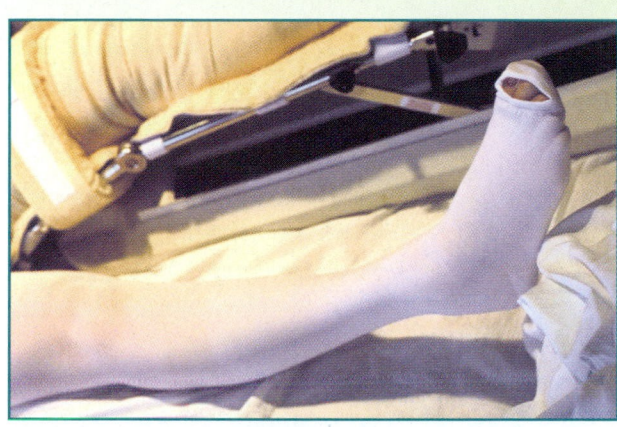

▶ OVERVIEW OF THE SKILL

Antiembolic hose, also called TED® hose or elastic stockings, are used to promote circulation by compression and are useful to prevent thrombophlebitis. They are used on the legs of a client after surgery, on clients who are immobile, and on clients who have vascular disorders such as thrombophlebitis, varicose veins, and other conditions of impaired circulation of the lower extremities.

▶ ASSESSMENT

1. Assess the condition of the client's lower extremities, noting edema, color, temperature, intact skin, ulcers, or infections. **Establishes a baseline for comparison** (see Figure 10-4-1).

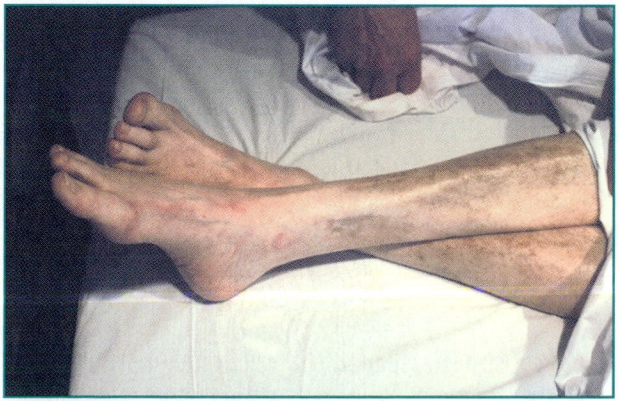

Figure 10-4-1 Assess the condition of the lower extremity prior to applying the antiembolic stocking.

2. Assess the quality and equality of peripheral pulses in the legs (either dorsalis pedis or posterior tibial pulses) **to determine circulatory status.**
3. Assess the client's understanding of the reasons for, and the use of, the antiembolic stockings **to determine the amount of client teaching required.**
4. Assess the client for signs and symptoms of deep vein thrombosis such as increased calf size or color change to determine **the appropriateness of the TED® hose placement.**

▶ DIAGNOSIS

Ineffective Tissue Perfusion

Risk for Impaired Skin Integrity

Risk for Peripheral Neurovascular Dysfunction

▶ PLANNING

Expected Outcomes:

1. The client will experience no signs or symptoms of deep venous thrombosis or thrombophlebitis.
2. The client's venous return will be improved.
3. The client's popliteal, posterior tibial, and dorsalis pedis pulses will remain intact while stockings are in place.
4. The client will have good circulation while stockings are in place, as evident by warm skin temperature, capillary return within normal limits, sensation present, and no edema present in both extremities.

Equipment Needed (see Figure 10-4-2):
- Antiembolic stockings and package directions (latex-free, if necessary)
- Tape measure

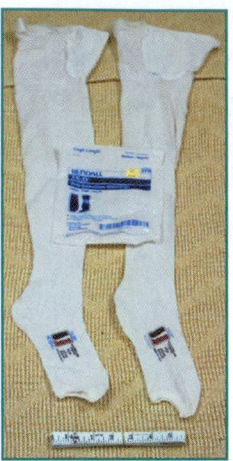

Figure 10-4-2 Antiembolic stockings and tape measure

▶ **CLIENT EDUCATION NEEDED:**

1. Client understands the purpose of antiembolic stockings.
2. Client understands that stockings must be in place and free of wrinkles to avoid skin breakdown and constraints of circulation.

Estimated time to complete the skill:
5–10 minutes

▶ **DELEGATION TIPS**

Ancillary personnel routinely remove and reapply antiembolic stockings. Instruction should be given to staff to apply stockings while client is supine in bed and to inspect and report any skin breakdown, impaired circulation, or excessive edema to the nurse.

IMPLEMENTATION—Action/Rationale

Action	Rationale
1. Wash hands.	1. Reduces the transmission of microorganisms.
2. Review the orders with the client, including the reason for the stockings and the type of stockings ordered; for example, knee or thigh high.	2. Facilitates compliance.
3. Explain the purpose of stockings and the procedure to the client.	3. Clients who understand the purpose may better comply with use.
4. With the client in a supine position in bed, measure the client's leg for the correct size: • Thigh-high stockings: from Achilles tendon to the gluteal fold and circumference of the midthigh • Below the knee stockings: from the Achilles tendon to the popliteal fold, and circumference of the midcalf	4. Supine position encourages venous return and decreases swelling, thereby allowing accurate measurement for size of stockings.
5. Compare the obtained measurements with the package insert to ascertain proper size.	5. Correct size is essential for stockings to apply the appropriate pressure for adequate venous return without compromise to circulation.

continues

Action	Rationale

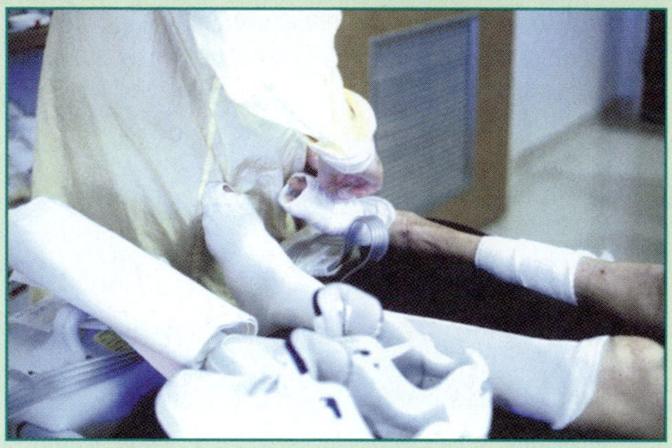

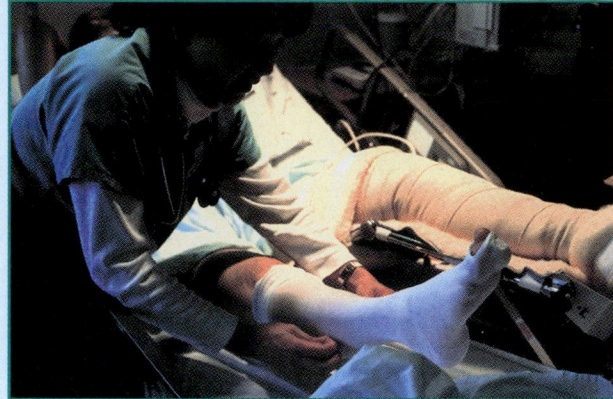

Figure 10-4-3 Place the stocking over the client's toes and foot.

Figure 10-4-4 Pull the stocking smoothly and evenly up the client's leg.

6. Apply stockings. The best time to apply stockings is early in the morning, before the client gets out of bed and before or immediately after surgery. Keep client in supine position until stockings are applied.

7. Insert hand and arm into stocking and grasp heel of stocking. Turn leg of stocking inside out to heel area. Do not turn heel or foot of stocking inside out.

8. Place foot of stocking over client's toes and foot.

9. Pull stocking over client's heel and ankle. Be sure client's heel is centered in heel pocket of stocking. Smooth any wrinkles in foot, heel or ankle.

10. Holding on to each side of stocking, firmly pull the stocking up the client's leg (see Figures 10-4-3 and 10-4-4).

11. Repeat with the other leg, if necessary.

6. Feet are less swollen in the morning because the feet have been in a nondependent position during the night and most venous return has occurred. This, of course, is not the case in a client who has been up frequently during the night.

7. Because stockings contain strong elastic, application can be difficult if not initiated from the bottom up and if stockings are not turned inside out. Wrinkles in stockings can also occur if a systematic approach is not used for application.

8. See Rationale 7.

9. See Rationale 7.

10. See Rationale 7.

11. See Rationale 7.

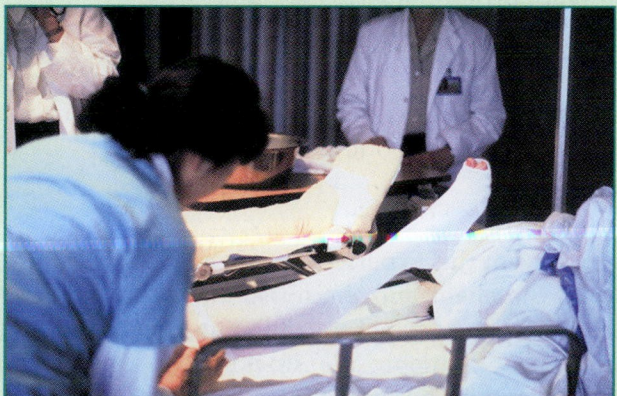

Figure 10-4-5 Smooth out any wrinkles and make sure the toes are comfortable.

continues

Action	Rationale
12. Smooth and remove any wrinkles in the stockings and smooth over (see Figure 10-4-5). Assess circulatory and neurostatus of feet. (CMS: circulatory, movement, sensation)	12. Wrinkles can create skin breakdown and can cause a tourniquet effect on the leg. Establishes baseline assessment.
13. Wash hands.	13. Reduces the transmission of microorganisms.

▶ REAL WORLD ANECDOTES

Mrs. Gooch is a home care client who wears antiembolic stockings to control lower leg edema. While making a home care visit the nurse noted that Mrs. Gooch's edema was worse. The nurse questioned Mrs. Gooch about any changes in diet or medication that might account for this, but Mrs. Gooch denied doing anything different. When the nurse asked Mrs. Gooch if she was wearing her antiembolic stockings, Mrs. Gooch stated that she was wearing them although she had removed them prior to the nurse's arrival to facilitate the visit. Noticing an indented circle around Mrs. Gooch's upper calf, the nurse asked Mrs. Gooch to apply her stockings while she observed. Mrs. Gooch successfully applied the stockings but, because they were too long, Mrs. Gooch then rolled the top band of the stockings down just below her knees. The rolled band corresponded to the indented area on Mrs. Gooch's leg. The nurse explained the need for stockings that fit correctly. She noted that rolling the tops of the stockings down interfered with venous return, leading to increased edema. The nurse measured Mrs. Gooch's legs and wrote the measurements out for Mrs. Gooch so she could obtain a pair of stockings in the correct size.

▶ EVALUATION

• The client has not experienced any signs or symptoms of deep venous thrombosis or thrombophlebitis.
• The client's venous return is improved.
• The client's popliteal, posterior tibial, and dorsalis pedis pulses remain intact while stockings are in place.
• The client has good circulation while stockings are in place, as evident by warm skin temperature, capillary return within normal limits, sensation within normal limits, and no edema in either extremities.

▶ DOCUMENTATION

Nurses' Notes

• Use of stockings
• Skin integrity, any presence of venous problems and circulatory status of extremities
• Equality of pedal pulses
• Size and length of stockings

Document on appropriate flow sheet or electronic medical record (EMR).

▶ CRITICAL THINKING SKILL

Introduction

Application of antiembolic stockings takes some planning.

Possible Scenario

A client has antiembolic stockings ordered; however, he has been up in the chair for several hours. His legs and ankles are swollen with edema.

Possible Outcome

Getting the stockings on will be an arduous task for both the nurse and the client. If the client's experience with the stockings is very negative, future compliance could be poor.

Prevention

To prevent this experience from being unpleasant for both the client and the nurse, have the client lie in bed for one hour before applying stockings. Remind the client to apply the stockings in the morning, before getting up from the bed.

▶ VARIATIONS

Geriatric Variations:
- *Elderly clients who have not used stockings in the past may find them uncomfortable and not keep stockings in place.*
- *Because elderly clients often have dry skin, they may find stockings irritating to use.*
- *Many elderly clients may have poor circulation in the extremities and, therefore, need to be assessed more frequently for compromised circulation and skin breakdown.*
- *Because of the strength of the elastic in the stockings, elderly clients generally need help with using stockings or need another person to put them on.*

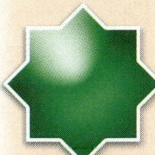

Pediatric Variation:
- *Elasticized stockings are generally not used on children.*

Home Care Variations:
- *Long-term use of stockings requires reinforcement of the problems of wrinkles, loosely fitted stockings, and/or stockings that roll and cause restricted circulation.*
- *Stockings need to be washed every few days and, therefore, more than one pair is needed.*
- *Clients should be encouraged to remove stockings at least twice a day and clean feet and legs.*
- *Clients and their family should be taught how to apply and remove the stockings and how to assess circulation.*

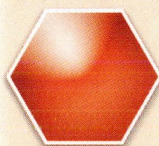

Home Care Variations:
- *Long-term use of stockings requires reinforcement of the problems of wrinkles, loosely fitted stockings, and/or stockings that roll and cause restricted circulation.*
- *Stockings need to be washed every few days and, therefore, more than one pair is needed.*
- *Clients should be encouraged to remove stockings at least twice a day and clean feet and legs.*
- *Clients and their family should be taught how to apply and remove the stockings and how to assess circulation.*
- *Stockings will stretch after long-term use and, therefore, size should be assessed periodically.*
- *Re-instruction may be necessary to reinforce problems associated with wrinkles and rolling of stockings.*
- *Clients may become careless with using stockings over long periods; therefore, reinforce purpose and proper use.*

▶ COMMON ERRORS

Possible Error:

The client's stockings are the wrong size.

Prevention:

Measure the client's legs according to the manufacturer's instructions. After applying the stockings, check the fit. Check later with client to verify stocking fit.

▶ **NURSING TIPS**

- Check stockings for proper placement at least every 2 hours or more often if needed.
- Stocking may roll and cause constrictions. Readjust periodically.
- Check lower extremities for circulatory status.
- If the client has peripheral vascular disease, check with the health care provider to ascertain that antiembolic stockings are not contraindicated.
- Remove stockings twice daily and have client exercise feet and toes.

▶ **SPECIAL CONSIDERATIONS**

- *Getting the correct size is key to applying antiembolic stockings. If there are problems with a pair currently in use, check size and change if needed.*
- *Some men feel embarrassed with stockings on. Be sensitive to this and stress the importance of compliance.*
- *Be sure to ascertain if the client has a latex allergy and use latex-free stockings accordingly.*
- *Some clients may choose to use powder for easier application of stockings. Avoid use of cornstarch and powder when decreased skin integrity or allergy is present.*
- *Replace or wash stockings when soiled. Wash frequently, especially if powder is used. It is best not to use powder; however, some clients find it easier to pull up stockings with use of powder.*
- *Antiembolic stockings generally are not used on clients with poor arterial perfusion.*
- *Extra precaution should be used with obese clients as stockings may roll and create a tight band around the legs and constrict perfusion. Check frequently and smooth out wrinkles.*
- *Latex-free stockings are available for use with clients with a history of latex allergy or contact dermatitis related to previous stocking use.*

Applying a Pneumatic Compression Device

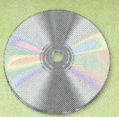

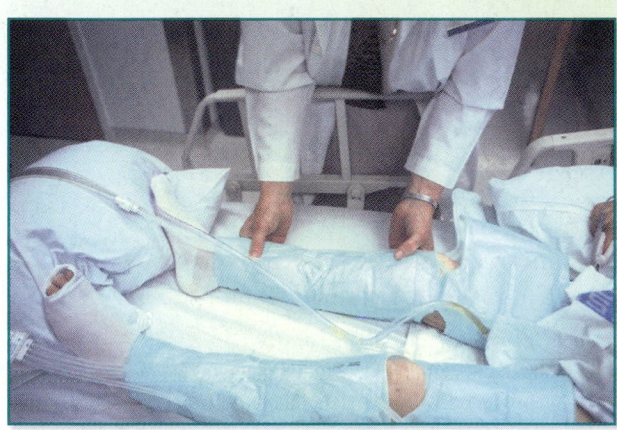

▶ OVERVIEW OF THE SKILL

Pneumatic compression devices (PCD), also known as sequential compression devices (SCD), are used to minimize lower extremity venous stasis. They are used in clients who are immobile for an extended period of time and who are at risk of developing deep venous thrombosis as well as in clients with lower extremity edema. Cuffs or stockings that inflate and deflate at alternating intervals are applied to the lower extremities. The stockings inflate in a sequence that promotes blood flow back to the heart and decreases pooling of the blood in the lower extremities. Because the cuffs cause compression of vessels they are contraindicated in disorders of arterial insufficiency and preexisting venous thrombosis.

▶ ASSESSMENT

1. Assess the condition of the client's lower extremities, noting edema, color, temperature, intact skin, ulcers, or infections. **Establishes a baseline for comparison.**
2. Assess the quality and equality of peripheral pulses in the legs (either dorsalis pedis or posterior tibial pulses) **to determine circulatory status.**
3. Assess the client's understanding of the reasons for, and the use of, sequential compression devices **to determine the amount of client teaching required.**
4. Assess the client for signs and symptoms of deep vein thrombosis such as calf pain and increased

calf size **to determine the appropriateness of the sequential compression device placement.**

▶ DIAGNOSIS

Impaired Physical Mobility

Ineffective Tissue Perfusion: Peripheral

▶ PLANNING

Expected Outcomes:

1. The client will not develop deep venous thrombosis as evident by lack of leg pain or tenderness, and lack of redness, warmth, or swelling to the extremity.
2. The client's skin will remain intact.
3. The client's circulation to the lower extremities will not be compromised.

Equipment Needed (see Figure 10-5-1A–C):

- Pneumatic sequential compression device and accompanying stockings
- Electrical outlet
- Tape measure

▶ CLIENT EDUCATION NEEDED:

1. Explain to the client that the compression device must be worn while lying down.
2. Demonstrate the correct method of putting the compression device on. Be sure to explain that the device must be snug but not so tight that it compromises circulation.

1339

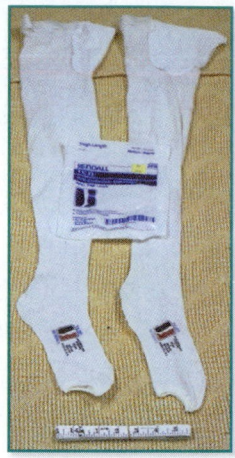

Figure 10-5-1A Antiembolic stockings and tape measure

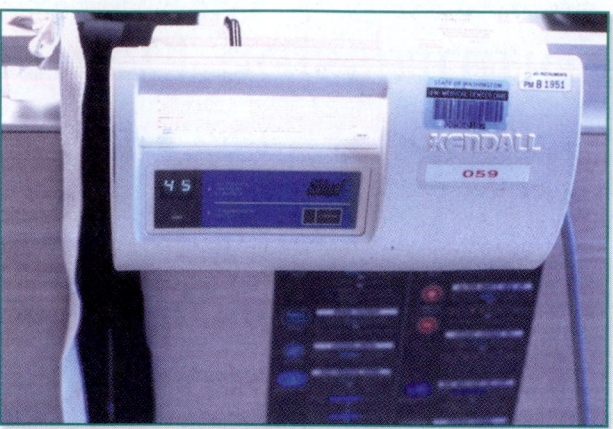

Figure 10-5-1B Pneumatic compression device

3. Reinforce the need for leg exercises to promote venous return despite the use of the compression device.

4. Educate the client to notify the nurse if he or she develops pain or tenderness in the calf or leg.

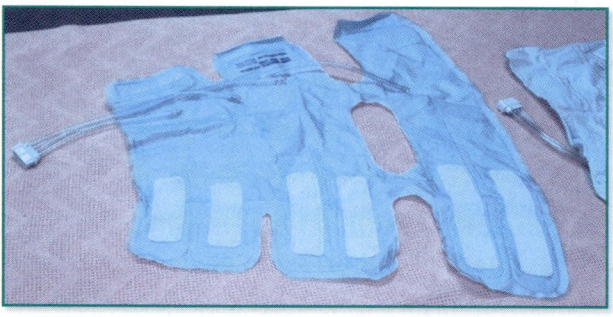

Figure 10-5-1C Pneumatic cuffs

Estimated time to complete the skill:
5–10 minutes

▶ **DELEGATION TIPS**

Ancillary personnel, once oriented to the equipment, can apply SCDs. Their performance of this skill should be monitored on an ongoing basis by the nurse once competency is established.

IMPLEMENTATION—Action/Rationale

Action	Rationale
1. Wash hands.	**1.** Reduces the transmission of microorganisms.
2. Explain procedure to client.	**2.** Client understanding promotes compliance.
3. Measure the leg according to manufacturer's recommendations.	**3.** Stockings must be the appropriate size to stay in place.
4. Check that pneumatic cuffs match the mechanical unit (see Figure 10-5-2).	**4.** If equipment is mismatched, a malfunction is likely.
5. Check if the client is wearing elastic stockings, and if so, check for wrinkles and folds.	**5.** Wrinkles and folds under pressure can cause skin breakdown.

continues

Action	Rationale

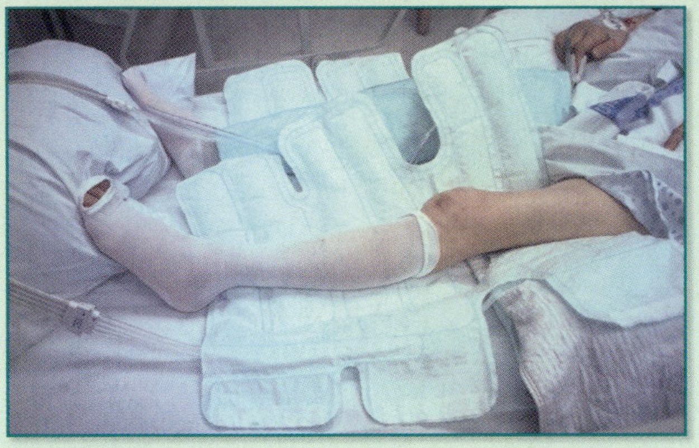

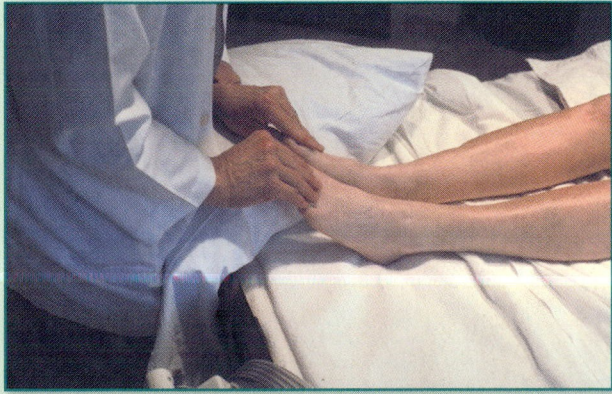

Figure 10-5-2 Make sure the correct size and type of pneumatic cuffs have been selected. If a client is wearing elastic stockings, make sure folds and wrinkles are smoothed out and toes are comfortable. The stocking in this photo needs to be adjusted.

6. Palpate both dorsalis pedis and posterior tibia pulses for presence and equality.
   • Perform baseline neurovascular assessment comparing both feet for color, movement, and sensation (see Figures 10-5-3 and 10-5-4).
   • Note if the client has evidence of skin irritation or breakdown, signs of infection, or arterial insufficiency (diminished pulses, loss of pedal and popliteal pulses, numbness, loss of hair on the legs, pain during exercise, or leg pallor).

7. Position the cuff flat on the bed next to the client's leg. Most manufacturers have markings for the position of the ankle and popliteal areas.

8. Place the client's leg directly in the center of the cuff with the back of the client's knee aligned with the opening in the back of the cuff (see Figure 10-5-5).

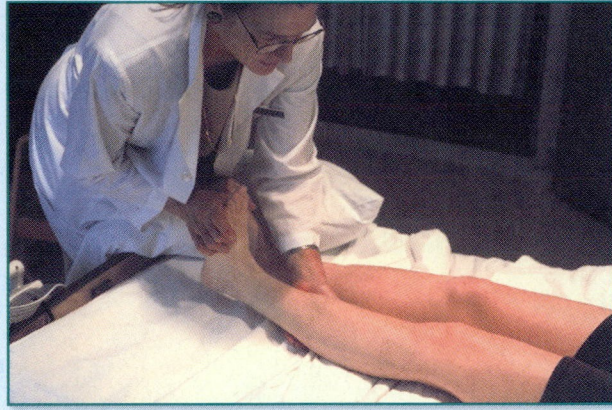

Figure 10-5-3 Perform a neurovascular assessment.

6. Need to assess the lower extremities for contraindications to compression device use. If contraindications are noted, the health care provider should be notified prior to placing the device.

7. Positioning is important for fit so that stockings will stay in place and function properly.

8. Proper positioning allows the cuff to stay in place and function properly.

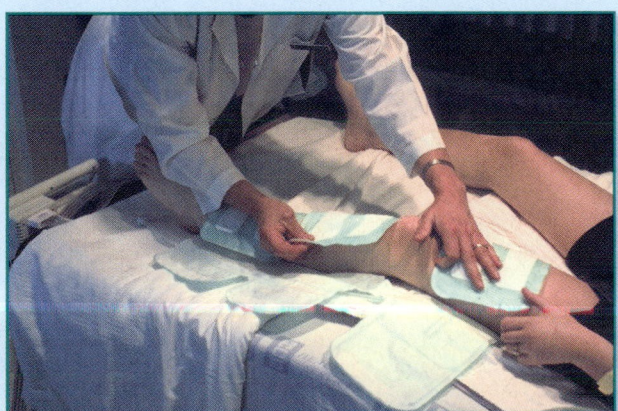

Figure 10-5-4 Check feet for pulse, warmth, color, movement, and sensation.

Figure 10-5-5 Position the cuff under the client's leg and wrap the cuff around the client's leg.

continues

Action	Rationale

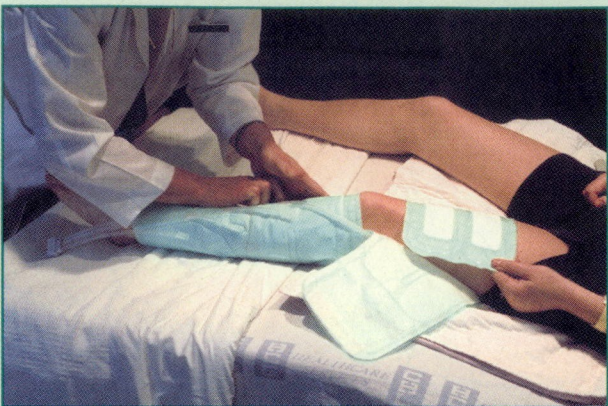

Figure 10-5-6   Secure the cuff in place.

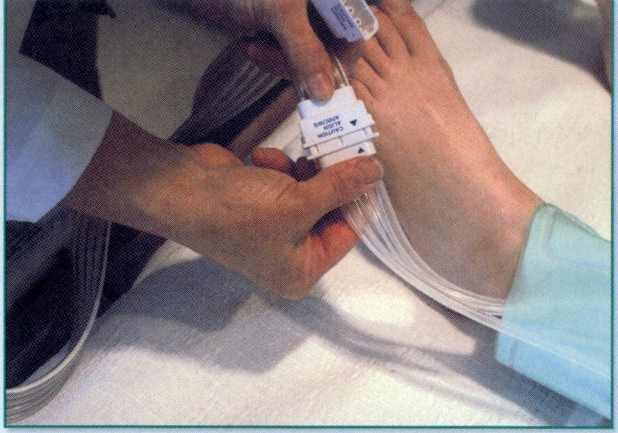

Figure 10-5-7   Attach the cuff to the pneumatic compression device.

9. Wrap the cuff around the client's leg with the opening in the front of the cuff over the client's knee (see Figure 10-5-6).

9. Proper positioning allows the cuff to stay in place and function properly.

10. Secure the cuff with the Velcro attachments, making sure two fingers fit between the client's leg and the cuff at both the ankle and knee.

10. Allows for expansion during inflation, while not slipping out of position during deflation.

11. Attach the cuff to the mechanical unit. Most manufacturers have arrows that line up on the mechanical unit tubing and the tubing on the cuff (see Figure 10-5-7).

11. If tubing is not tightly connected, the cuff will not properly inflate.

12. Turn the unit on and watch the movement of the cuff for one cycle to ensure proper inflation and deflation (see Figure 10-5-8).

12. It is important to watch for inflation and deflation because air leaks will cause the cuff to malfunction.

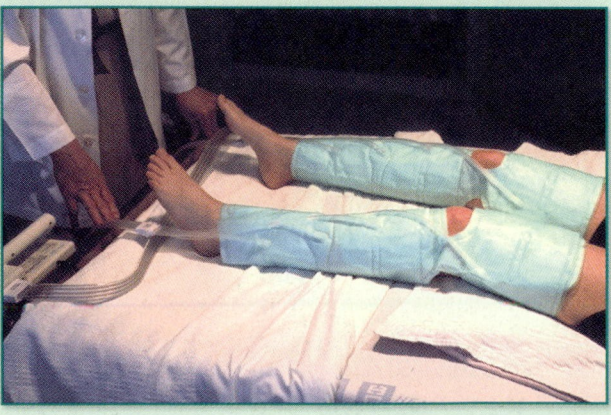

Figure 10-5-8   Observe the unit for one complete cycle of inflation and deflation.

continues

Action	Rationale
13. At regular intervals (at least every 4 hours) unplug the unit and remove the cuff after deflation. • Inspect the skin and provide skin care. • Perform a neurovascular assessment including CMS (color, movement, and sensation) and temperature of the skin, pulses, and capillary refill of the distal extremities. • Compare both extremities and compare with baseline assessment. • Avoid vigorous rubbing and massaging.	13. The plastic of the compression cuff can decrease air circulation to the skin leading to skin breakdown, especially in elderly clients. Inspecting the extremities at regular intervals is essential because deep venous thrombosis can occur even with the use of the compression cuff.
14. Wash hands.	14. Reduces the transmission of microorganisms.

▶ REAL WORLD ANECDOTES

During her change of shift assessment at 7:30 a.m., the nurse noted that Mrs. Rhinehart's pneumatic compression stockings were bunched down around her ankles, rendering them ineffective. The nurse removed the compression stockings, assessed Mrs. Rhinehart's lower extremities, and replaced the compression device in the proper position. As she was serving Mrs. Rhinehart's breakfast, the nurse noted that the compression stockings had slipped down around Mrs. Rhinehart's ankles again. Puzzled, she assessed Mrs. Rhinehart's legs and replaced the compression stockings. When the nurse returned to Mrs. Rhinehart's room to assist her with her bed bath she noted that Mrs. Rhinehart was not in bed. The nurse found Mrs. Rhinehart in the bathroom having a cigarette, despite orders for strict bed rest. The nurse noted that Mrs. Rhinehart's compression stockings were once more dangling around her ankles. The nurse assisted Mrs. Rhinehart back to bed and educated her regarding the need to stay in bed according to orders. The nurse also contacted Mrs. Rhinehart's physician regarding a prescription for a smoking cessation aid.

▶ EVALUATION

• The client does not exhibit any signs or symptoms of deep vein thrombosis.
• The skin on the client's lower extremities is intact.
• The circulation to the client's lower extremities is not compromised.

▶ DOCUMENTATION

Nurses' Notes

• The first time the compression device is placed, document the size and type of cuff used, assessment of the extremities, including neurovascular, capillary refill and skin condition, and the client's tolerance to the device

• Document subsequent assessments and any changes you have noted

Document on appropriate flow sheet or electronic medical record (EMR).

▶ CRITICAL THINKING SKILL

Introduction

Careful client assessment can prevent serious problems.

Possible Scenario

You are in Mrs. Flowers' room to put on her PCD. As you smooth the elastic stockings she will be wearing underneath the device to remove any wrinkles, she complains of pain in her left calf.

Possible Outcome

You assure Mrs. Flowers that she is just a little stiff from being in bed. You proceed to rub the area to relieve the pain. Mrs. Flowers begins to complain of shortness of breath and becomes cyanotic. You immediately request assistance and Mrs. Flowers is treated for an emergency. After she has been treated and transferred to the intensive care unit, you are told that Mrs. Flowers had deep vein thrombosis in her left calf and apparently a portion of the clot had broken off and migrated to her lungs.

Prevention

You should have stopped to assess her condition. You would have detected that she had developed deep venous thrombosis. You instruct Mrs. Flowers to remain in bed while you notify her physician regarding this new finding. In addition, it is contraindicated to rub or massage a client's lower extremities.

▶ VARIATIONS

Geriatric Variations:
- *Elderly clients may have wasting of the extremities so it is essential to carefully measure for size.*
- *Elderly clients who are not active may complain of pain with dorsiflexion because of stiff ankles. If the client has pain with dorsiflexion, check the back of the calf for redness, lumps, hardness, and increased size of calf of leg.*

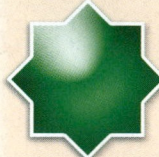

Pediatric Variations:
- *The sequential compression device is rarely used on children.*
- *On occasion it may be used to mobilize edema that has pooled in an extremity. If this is the case, children must be watched very closely for fluid overload because their tolerances are much lower than adults.*

Home Care Variations:
- *Pneumatic compression devices may be used in the home with clients who suffer from stasis pooling of fluids in their extremities.*
- *These clients generally suffer from congestive heart failure or some other fluid sensitive disorder. They must be watched closely for fluid overload when the device is first being used.*
- *These clients may have several gallons of water pooled in the lower extremities, and the sudden fluid shift could send them into cardiac failure.*

Long-Term Care Variations:
- *You should assess the equipment periodically for wear and tear.*
- *Pinhole leaks in the compression device can render it useless.*
- *If the plastic is stretched beyond elasticity from use, the stocking portion of the device must be replaced.*

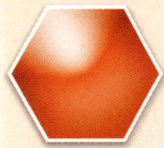

▶ COMMON ERRORS

Possible Error:
The compression stockings do not seem to be inflating properly.

Prevention:
Be sure the equipment is in good working order before starting the procedure. Is the machine turned on? Are the compression stockings connected properly to the machine? Are there any tears or holes in the compression stockings?

▶ **NURSING TIPS**

- Compression stockings may become loose when clients are restless and move in bed. Approximately every 2 hours check that stockings are tight enough and properly positioned.

- Check skin integrity and circulation every 4–8 hours.
- Be sure to monitor for deep vein thrombosis and fluid overload.

▶ **SPECIAL CONSIDERATIONS**

- *Some manufacturers have installed a cooling mechanism to decrease feelings of heat and dampness under the plastic sleeves. When available, this product may encourage compliance and increase tolerance of therapy.*
- *When using a sleeve that covers the calf and thigh in one piece, correct placement is very important to avoid constriction of the blood vessels around the knee.*

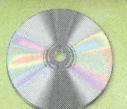
Applying Abdominal, T-, or Breast Binders

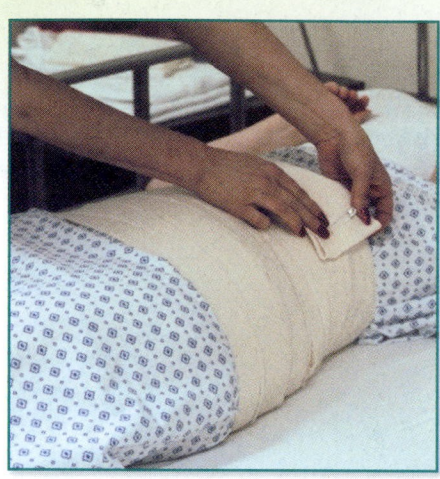

▶ OVERVIEW OF THE SKILL

In the past, abdominal binders were primarily used to provide support and comfort for an incision following abdominal surgical procedures. Today binders are most often used to hold dressings in place, to support soft tissue, or to suppress lactation. Single and double T-binders hold rectal or perineal dressings in place. Abdominal binders support the abdomen and hold abdominal dressings in place. Stretch net binders are not designed for support, but simply to hold dressings in place.

A breast binder or a tight bra is used as a nonpharmacologic device to aid in lactation suppression. In addition, a breast binder may be used after breast reduction surgery, a mastectomy, or breast reconstruction surgery. The binder is placed over the breast to prevent breast and nipple stimulation. Ice packs are used in conjunction with breast binders to relieve discomfort associated with breast engorgement.

Proper placement of any binder is essential for optimum comfort and effect. The binder must be smooth, the right size for the client, not interfere with circulation, or put too much pressure on the bound area.

▶ ASSESSMENT

1. Assess the reason the binder is needed **to determine the correct binder and correct placement.**

2. Assess the client's skin condition for rashes, inflammation, open areas, or dressings **to provide a baseline for future assessments.**
3. Assess and measure the client **to determine what size binder will be needed.**
4. Assess for any special circumstances that may affect the placement of the binder such as dressings, tubing, or catheters **to determine a plan for binder placement.**
5. Assess the client's understanding of the reasons for the binder and the method of placing the binder **to determine what types of client teaching will be needed.**

▶ DIAGNOSIS

Interrupted Breastfeeding

Impaired Physical Mobility

▶ PLANNING

Expected Outcomes:

1. For breast binder, lactation will be suppressed.
2. Binder will provide support for dressings or soft tissue.
3. Binder will not be too tight or compress the skin.
4. T-binder in a male client will not compress the testicles.
5. Client will assist in the placement of the binder as much as possible.

Equipment Needed (see Figure 10-6-1):

- Correct binder for intended purpose (latex-free, if indicated)
- Safety pins or fasteners

▶ **CLIENT EDUCATION NEEDED:**

1. Explain to the breast binder client that lactation may continue for up to 16 days.
2. Advise the breast binder client that, for adequate suppression and support, the binder should be worn 24 hours a day.
3. With a breast binder, allow the client to express her concerns regarding the cessation of lactation. It is important for her to voice questions or concerns, and to receive a satisfactory response.
4. With a breast binder, remind client of the signs and symptoms of both breast engorgement and mastitis.
5. Remind the client that if breathing is difficult with a binder on, the binder should be adjusted for a more comfortable fit.

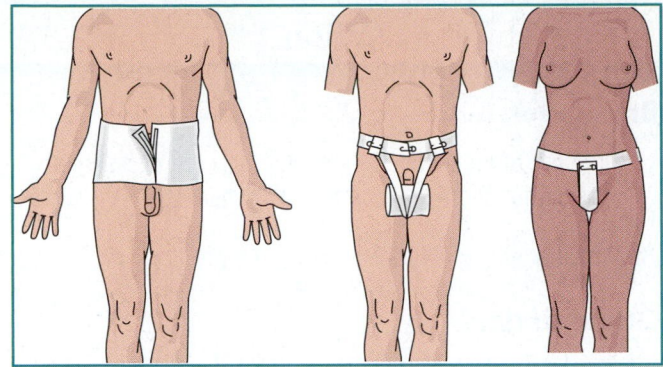

Figure 10-6-1 A. Abdominal Binder. B. T-Binders: Double and Single.

6. Discuss the signs and symptoms of skin breakdown, and encourage the client to report signs of skin irritation. Encourage the client to examine the skin beneath the binder each day that the binder is in use.

 Estimated time to complete the skill: **5–10 minutes**

▶ **DELEGATION TIPS**

Abdominal binder application may be performed by ancillary personnel after the nurse has assessed the client's tolerance of the binder. The client should be able to breathe effectively and move adequately. In addition, ancillary personnel should be instructed to ensure the client's skin is intact and to report any breakdown for nurse evaluation.

IMPLEMENTATION—Action/Rationale

Action	Rationale
Bra Binder	
1. Wash hands.	1. Reduces the transmission of microorganisms.
2. Assist the client to a sitting position.	2. Sitting will allow ease in placement of the bra. If not possible, turn client side-to-side while applying bra.
3. Apply bra, adjusting for a snug fit.	3. The tightness of the bra will be instrumental in adequate lactation suppression.
4. Adjust if necessary. Be sure that breast binder is not restricting breathing or causing skin irritation.	4. Bra binders that are too tight may make breathing difficult and/or may contribute to skin irritation or breakdown.

continues

Action	Rationale
Bra Binder *continued*	
5. Add use of adjunctive treatments (e.g., ice packs, analgesics) for additional comfort, if needed.	5. If breasts are engorged, adjunctive treatment may be required to increase client's level of comfort.
6. Wash hands.	6. Reduces the transmission of microorganisms.
Other Binders	
7. Wash hands.	7. Reduces the transmission of microorganisms.
8. Choose correct binder. If a stretch net binder is being used, select the correct circumference and cut length to fit.	8. Select the correct binder for the job. The correct size will make the binder most effective.
9. Help the client into the proper position to place the binder. • For abdominal binders, the client should lie supine and lift the hips, or, alternatively, position the client on one side, and roll the client onto the binder (see Figure 10-6-2). For stretch net binders, slide the net over the head and neck, or slide the net up from the feet, depending on which is easier for the client. • For T-binders, select a single-tail binder for a female, a double-tail binder for a male. Have the client lift the hips or, alternatively, position the client on one side and roll the client onto the binder. Place the waistband at the waist, with the single or double tails pointing downward along the spine.	9. Applying binders can be awkward if the client is not positioned correctly.
10. Apply the binder. • For abdominal binders, wrap binder snugly around the client's waist starting from the lower abdomen and working upward (see Figures 10-6-3 and 10-6-4).	10. Correct application allows the client to get the most benefit from the binder.

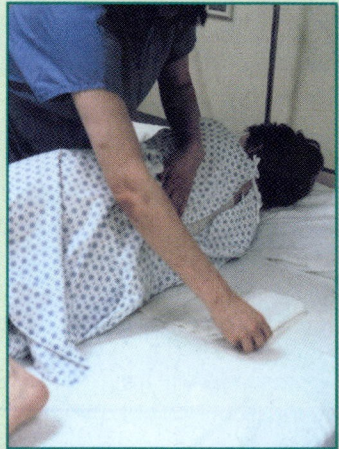

Figure 10-6-2 Place the binder under the client.

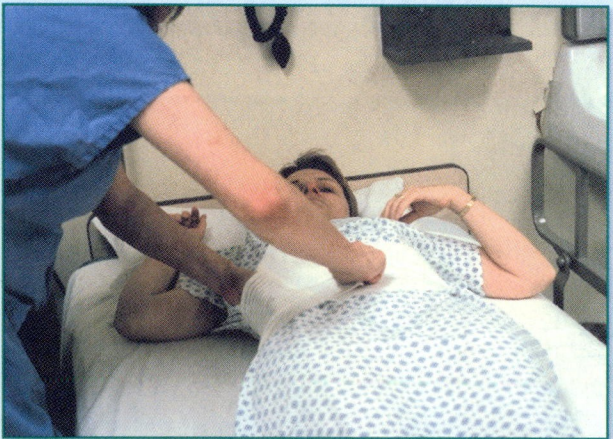

Figure 10-6-3 Wrap the binder snugly around the waist.

continues

Action	Rationale

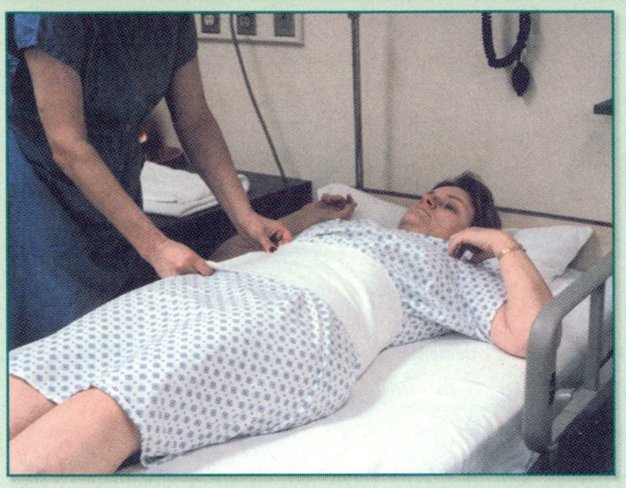

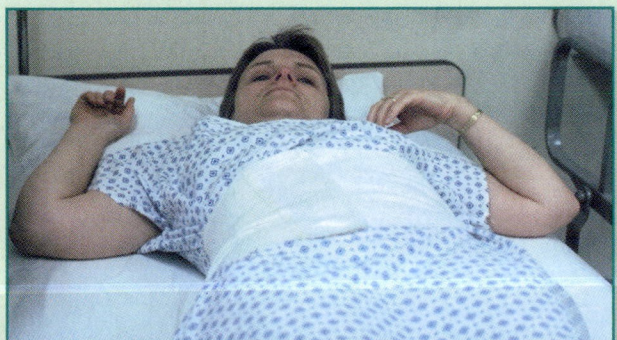

Figure 10-6-4   Secure the lower abdomen first and work upward.

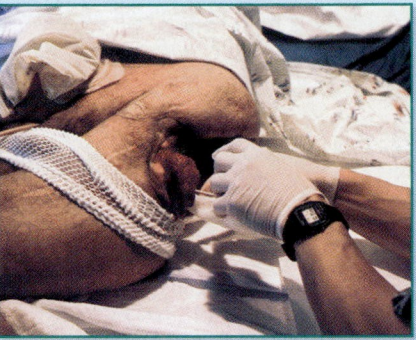

Figure 10-6-5   Stretch net binders are flexible and elastic. They cling and stretch over the body part that needs to be covered. In this case, the stretch net binder will be used to hold sterile dressings over the wound.

- For T-binders, bring the tail(s) up between the client's legs. For males, one tail should be placed on each side of the testicles. Join tails to the waistband and secure
- For stretch net binders, adjust to cover the dressings they will be holding in place.

11. Secure binders with fasteners. If the binder does not have Velcro fasteners, secure with safety pins. Stretch net binders cling and stretch over the body part and do not need additional fastening (see Figure 10-6-5). Check for snug fit.

12. Adjust if necessary. Be sure that binders are not restricting breathing or circulation (see Figure 10-6-6). Be sure that sterile dressings are in place between the binder and any wound (see Figure 10-6-7).

13. Wash hands.

11. Fasteners will keep binder in place. Be sure that all fasteners are closed securely to prevent possible client injury.

12. Binders that are too tight may make breathing difficult, and may contribute to skin irritation or breakdown. Binders are generally not sterile, so sterile dressings must be in place over the wound.

13. Reduces transmission of microorganisms.

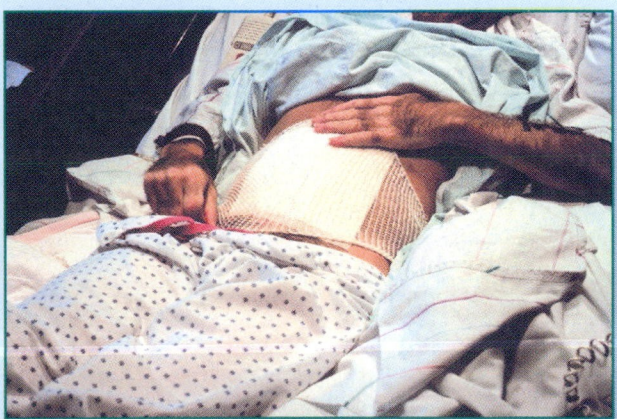

Figure 10-6-6   Assess the client to be sure the binder does not restrict breathing or circulation.

Figure 10-6-7   If a stretch net binder is used to cover a wound, make sure a sterile dressing is in place between the binder and the wound.

> **REAL WORLD ANECDOTES**

A nurse went to apply an abdominal binder to a very obese man recovering from an exploratory laparotomy. It took extensive struggling to move the equipment and visitors from the bedside, position the bed, roll the man to his side, and place the binder. When he rolled back to the supine position, the nurse began to adjust and fasten the binder. She then discovered that it was 6 inches too short to go around his middle. She had to start over. In her hurry, the nurse guessed at the correct size binder for this client, but was incorrect.

► EVALUATION

- For breast binder, lactation is suppressed.
- Binder provides support for dressings or soft tissue.
- Binder is not too tight and does not compress the skin.
- T-binder on a male client does not compress the testicles.
- Client assists in the placement of the binder as much as possible.

► DOCUMENTATION

Nurses' Notes

- Time, date, and type of binder
- Any difficulty that the client experienced with the procedure

Document on appropriate flow sheet or electronic medical record (EMR).

► CRITICAL THINKING SKILL

Introduction

Your client, a 13-year-old primipara, is complaining of sore, heavy breasts on postpartum day 2. You offer her a breast binder for comfort, but as you start to explain how it is applied, she bursts into tears. She states that she has tried to breast-feed, but her boyfriend (the baby's father) does not want her to continue. She is anxious and indecisive. What do you do?

Possible Scenario

Now is not a good time to discuss the need for a breast binder, because this client has not made up her mind regarding breast-feeding. This is a critical moment for additional nursing assessment. This client has psychosocial needs surrounding the birth of the child, changes to her relationship, and changes to her body. A visit by a psychosocial care provider may answer questions that she and her partner have regarding breast-feeding and other issues related to the pregnancy.

Possible Outcome

Your timely nursing intervention allows the client and her boyfriend to discuss their fears and uncertainties regarding the baby and the decision to breast-feed. Later that day, you continue with education regarding the breast binder and other methods to reduce discomfort.

Prevention

The stress of having a child, especially among very young mothers, may precipitate distress related to breast-feeding and/or the need for lactation suppression. Be alert for verbal and nonverbal cues and practice therapeutic communication as needed.

> **VARIATIONS**

Geriatric Variations:
- *If the elderly client is confused, try to avoid using safety pins to fasten binders.*
- *If safety pins are required, cover them with tape or dressing to discourage the client from unfastening the binder or sticking him- or herself with the pins.*

continues

▶ VARIATIONS (continued)

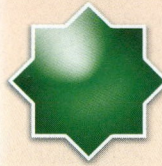

Pediatric Variations:
- Stretch net binders may need to be taped in place to help younger or more active children avoid dislodging the bandage underneath.
- When applying a stretch net binder, consider bringing another piece of stretch net in a smaller size so the child can "bandage" a doll or favorite toy.
- In young children, try to avoid using safety pins. If safety pins must be used, cover them with tape or a dressing to discourage the child from opening the pin.

Home Care Variations:
- When considering the use of breast binders, the decision to suppress lactation may be made after the client leaves the facility, or during a home birth, where the client is not admitted postpartum.
- The nurse may be advised of the desire for lactation suppression while the client is in the outpatient setting. In these cases, instructions may be given over the phone.
- The use of a bra binder may be more appropriate and easier for the client to manage in a home setting.
- Rather than use a commercially manufactured breast binder, it may be more cost-effective to encourage the client to use a sports bra or other snug-fitting bra from home.
- Abdominal and T-binders can be improvised in the home care setting, using readily available materials, such as safety pins, Velcro, elastic webbing, and strong, smooth material, such as cotton or muslin. Make sure the binder is large enough to bind the area without undue constriction.
- Make two or three binders if they will be used for more than a day, so one may be worn while the others are laundered.
- The use of a breast binder might be implemented in the home or for outpatient use. Similar teaching can be done over the telephone.

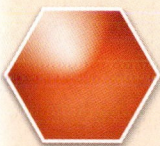

Long-Term Care Variations:
- Make sure any binders are checked regularly for comfort, skin irritation, shifting of the binder, or constriction of the area under the binder.
- If applicable, encourage the client to self-examine the skin beneath the binder each day that the binder is in use.
- If a client requires a binder for long-term use, teach the client to apply and monitor it independently, if possible, to encourage independence and self-care.

▶ COMMON ERRORS

Possible Error:
The binder does not fit.

Prevention:
Take the extra time to measure the binder and the client before you begin the procedure. Be sure the binder is large enough for the client but small enough to provide the necessary support.

▶ **NURSING TIPS**

- There are commercially made breast binders that can be ordered from medical or surgical supply companies. However, these may be a more costly alternative to using a bra binder or other type of breast binder.
- A good bra often provides both lactation suppression and support.
- If abdominal binders are used, periodically assess for tightness and adjust if the binder impedes respiration.
- If the stretch net binder rolls when the client moves about in bed, consider taping it to the skin with paper tape in one or two strategic places.
- A bra binder may be the most suitable choice for a woman without assistance in the home because of ease of care.

▶ **SPECIAL CONSIDERATIONS**

- *If safety pins are used as fasteners, pin the binder in a place where the client can reach them easily.*
- *In some obese clients an abdominal binder may have a tendency to roll or fold. In these cases, assess skin carefully for redness, irritation, or breakdown.*
- *Use latex-free binders if the client has a history of latex allergy or contact dermatitis related to binders.*

Applying Skin Traction—Adhesive and Nonadhesive

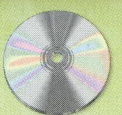

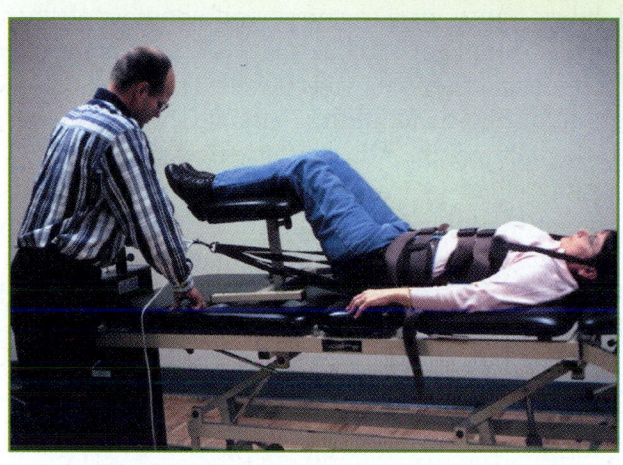

► OVERVIEW OF THE SKILL

Traction is designed to align or immobilize parts of the body. Traction may be used to reduce or immobilize fractures or to reduce muscle spasms. Traction is applied using weight or force to gently pull on the body parts. There are two basic types of traction—skin traction and skeletal traction. This skill deals with the application, use, and evaluation of various types of skin traction.

Skin traction uses the client's skin as the anchor point of the weight or force. The traction is anchored to the skin using either adhesive tapes, Velcro straps, or a fitted brace. Some types of skin traction employ a brace or other rigid garment to apply gentle force to the client's body. Others use weights, ropes, and pulleys to apply force to the client's body.

Traction often requires specialized equipment for support and proper alignment. Many hospitals employ technicians who are trained to set up and maintain traction equipment and to fit braces. The nurse may be called upon to measure and fit some types of traction, as well as assess and maintain traction devices.

Following are some of the more common types of skin traction:

Buck's traction: This is straight traction placed on the lower extremity to help reduce a hip or femur fracture. Buck's traction can also reduce or prevent muscle spasms caused by a hip or femur fracture. Buck's traction can be applied with adhesive tape secured with an elastic bandage and attached to a pulley and weight (see Figure 10-7-1). A manufactured "boot" is also available. The boot wraps around the leg and is secured with straps. It is then attached to the pulley and weight system in the same way as the adhesive traction. Care must be taken to maintain alignment and watch for any skin breakdown that may occur. Maintenance of the pulley system is very important. The line must not become tangled in the bed linen and the weights must hang freely.

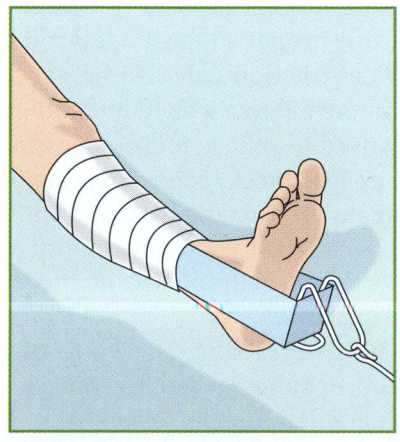

Figure 10-7-1 Buck's traction

Bryant's traction: This is very similar to Buck's traction and is used for reduction of femur fractures or to immobilize the hip joints in children who weigh less than 40 pounds. In Bryant's traction both of the child's legs are wrapped and a spreader bar is placed to separate the limbs. Two sets of pulleys and weights are then attached overhead to lift the child's buttocks off the mattress by about 1 to 2 inches. This traction maintains alignment, helps reduce any fracture, and immobilizes the child. Bryant's traction places the child's skin at risk in several areas. The client's back, elbow, coccyx, and head are vulnerable to skin irritation and breakdown and must be closely monitored. This position also raises concerns regarding elimination, feeding, and hydration. All these basic needs must be met, as well as the child's mental and emotional needs related to immobility, and the need for stimulation.

Russell's traction: This is a balanced traction arrangement of pulleys, lines, slings, and weights used to treat knee or hip injuries in adults and to reduce femur fractures in children. Russell's traction is applied to the client's lower leg. A sling is placed under the client's knee and two pulley and weight setups are applied to support the knee sling. Assessment of the skin is critical in this type of traction because of the possibility of skin breakdown on the coccyx, back, elbows, head, and parts of the noninjured extremity, especially the heel. Footdrop is also a risk and exercises as well as foot support should be used.

Cervical traction: Cervical traction can be applied in several different ways. Paramedics often apply a hard cervical collar on clients with suspected cervical injury. This type of collar is generally used only for short periods of time. Care must be taken to maintain good alignment when placing this type of collar. Care should be taken to properly fit this collar. It can cause skin breakdown if not fit correctly and will not provide proper support if it is too large or too small. Cervical traction can also be applied using a cloth collar attached to a weight and pulley system. It is primarily used to relieve muscle spasms and nerve compression in the neck. Neurologic assessment and skin assessment are extremely important in this type of traction because of the vulnerability of the area. The client is not usually placed in this traction for long periods of time.

Pelvic belt or girdle: This type of traction is used to relieve pain caused by muscle spasm or nerve impingement in the lower back. A girdle is placed around the client's hips and a pulley and weight system is then attached to the girdle, extending down over the foot of the bed. This maintains alignment of the back, hips, and legs and provides gentle pulling on the lower back. Pelvic traction can be used in the home setting. The nurse should reinforce client teaching regarding the proper use of this type of traction.

Humerus traction: Humeral traction is used to stabilize upper arm fractures and shoulder dislocations. The upper arm is held at a 90-degree angle from the body and the forearm is flexed. Traction is placed to pull on the hand and the elbow. This allows for a gentle pull to realign the fracture or dislocation.

Any client in traction is at risk for skin breakdown at the injury site and also in areas with a thin layer of skin over bony prominences such as the shoulder, back, coccyx, heels, and head. A thorough skin assessment must be performed regularly to prevent skin breakdown.

► ASSESSMENT

1. Assess skin integrity **to evaluate and treat any actual or potential skin breakdown in the traction area.**
2. Assess neurovascular status in the affected areas **to evaluate any potential or actual neurovascular compromise.**
3. Assess the client's understanding of and need for the treatment **to provide any client education and support needed.**
4. Assess for complications of traction and immobility **to determine a plan of treatment.**

► DIAGNOSIS

Acute Pain

Impaired Physical Mobility

Risk for Constipation

Risk for Disuse Syndrome

Risk for Impaired Skin Integrity

Risk for Peripheral Neurovascular Dysfunction

► PLANNING

Expected Outcomes:

1. The affected body part will have adequate neurovascular perfusion as evident by pulses, color, capillary refill, movement, and sensation.
2. The client will understand the reason for the traction and be able to cooperate in his or her care and treatment.

3. The client will experience a minimum of discomfort and trauma secondary to the traction.

Equipment Needed (see Figure 10-7-2):

- Pain medication, if necessary
- Overhead traction bars, if needed
- Weights in various pounds
- Traction line and pulleys
- Skin traction device as ordered by the health care provider
- Adhesive traction tape and elastic bandage, if appropriate
- Razor, if needed

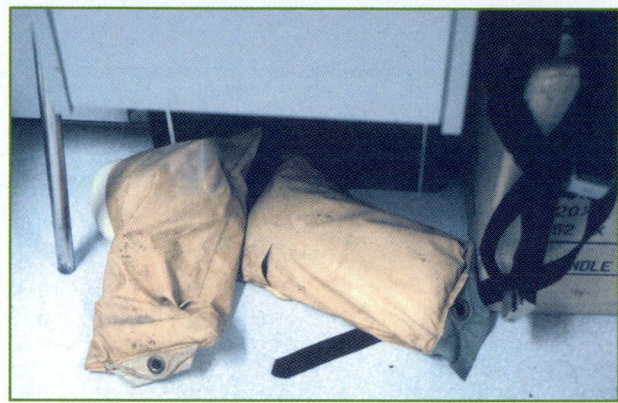

Figure 10-7-2 Sandbags provide weight for traction

▶ CLIENT EDUCATION NEEDED:

1. Explain the need for the traction. Discuss the continuing injury to the tissues, muscles, and blood supply that can occur without immobilization.
2. Assure the client that this is a necessary, but usually temporary, procedure that will aid in the healing process and that every measure will be taken to make the client as comfortable as possible during the procedure.
3. Explain the procedure step by step and ask questions. This will help the client anticipate what will occur. Asking questions will provide a sense of control and help alleviate anticipatory anxiety.
4. Explain that some discomfort may occur, and outline options for pain control.

5. Explain the possible complications of traction and prolonged immobilization. Teach the client to self-assess for these complications and to report them to the staff. This increases the client's sense of autonomy and control.
6. Teach the client appropriate range of motion exercises to prevent muscle atrophy and cramping as much as possible.

Estimated time to complete the skill:
30 minutes

▶ DELEGATION TIPS

Ancillary personnel may assist with applying skin traction with proper instruction and supervision. The nurse or physical therapist should perform the initial setup, ensuring proper body alignment, neurovascular integrity, and proper padding of skin surfaces.

IMPLEMENTATION—Action/Rationale

Action	Rationale
Applying Skin Traction	
1. Wash hands.	1. Reduces the transmission of microorganisms.
2. Assemble the overhead traction bars, if needed (see Figure 10-7-3).	2. Provides a stable foundation for the traction.

continues

Action	Rationale

Applying Skin Traction *continued*

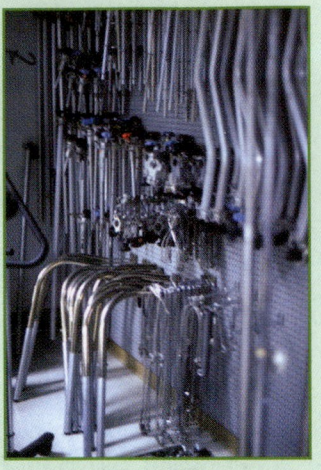

Figure 10-7-3 Overhead traction bars must be assembled before use.

3. Clean the skin area the traction will be applied to, assessing the area at the same time.

4. Know the type of traction being applied. Request assistance if you are working with unfamiliar equipment or if the task requires more than one person to accomplish (see Figure 10-7- 4).

Adhesive Traction

5. Shave the area as needed.

6. Place the adhesive traction tape on the body part to provide the appropriate direction of pull. Add any spreader bars or hooks needed to attach the tape to the traction rope and weights.

7. Wrap the body part and adhesive tape with the elastic bandage.

3. Clean skin will provide a better base for adhesive traction. Clean skin is less likely to break down.

4. Reduces the risk of injury to the client or nurse.

5. Provides better adhesion with the skin and prevents pain from hair pulling.

6. Placing the tape in the direction of pull allows for maximum traction from the weight used.

7. Provides support for the body part and holds the adhesive tape in place.

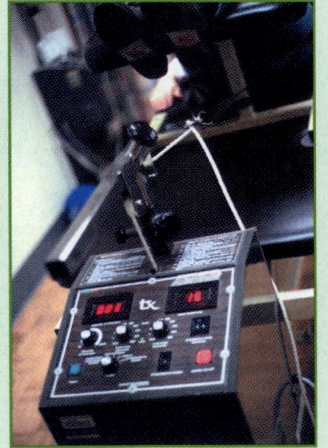

Figure 10-7-4 There are many types of traction devices. Understand how the device you are using works before applying traction to the client.

continues

Action	Rationale

Nonadhesive Traction

8. Apply the traction appliance to the appropriate body part (see Figure 10-7-5).

9. Secure it with the fasteners provided (Velcro, straps and buckles, ties) (see Figures 10-7-6 and 10-7-7). If no fastener is provided, an elastic bandage may be wrapped around the appliance or adhesive tape may be used. Be sure not to fasten the appliance too loose or too tight.

10. If the appliance is to be attached to weights, or a traction device, attach the appropriate spreader bars, hooks, or other hardware (see Figure 10-7-8).

11. Apply the amount of traction ordered for the correct amount of time.

Traction with Weights

12. Place pulleys on traction setup as needed. Be sure pulleys are aligned straight with body part in the desired direction of pull.

13. Using the proper weight setup, tie the traction rope around eyelets in weights or in a loop at the end of the rope to hang traction on, depending on the supplies available. Be sure the knot is nonslip so it will stay where it is tied.

14. Gently release rope with weights on it to apply traction to the body part.

15. Monitor the client for slipping, excessive pain, or weights that do not hang freely.

8. Nonadhesive traction requires a halter, corset, boot, or other device for the weight to pull against.

9. Keeps the appliance in the proper position. A loose appliance will decrease the effectiveness of the traction. A tight appliance will constrict circulation to the body part.

10. Provides a place to fasten the traction rope.

11. Provides the maximal therapeutic benefit.

12. Allows for proper body alignment.

13. Securely attaching weights to the rope will prevent sudden release from improper knots or fastening.

14. A gentle application of weight will prevent excessive pain and unnecessary jerking of the body part.

15. Ensures client safety and proper use of traction.

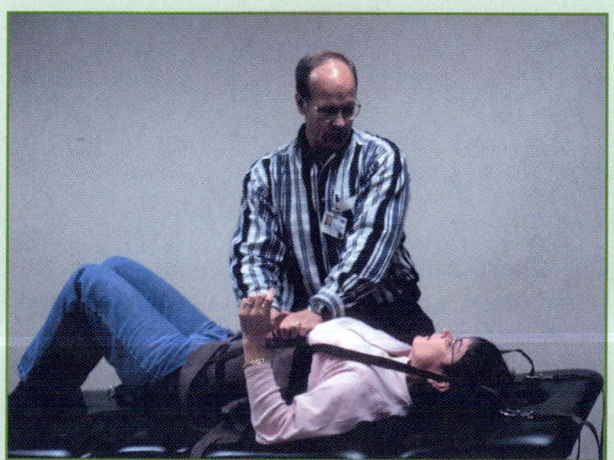

Figure 10-7-5 Apply the traction to the appropriate body part.

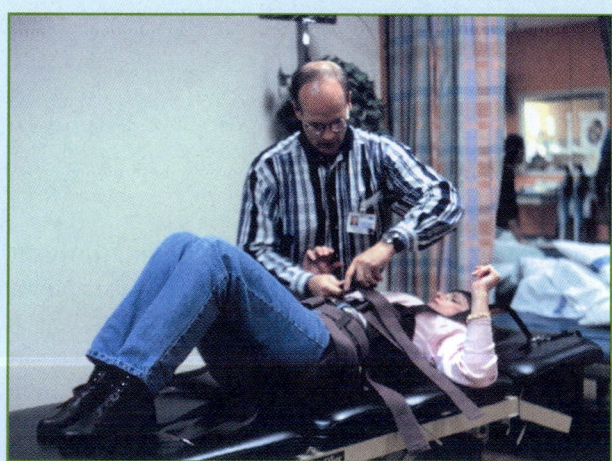

Figure 10-7-6 Secure the traction snugly to the body with the fasteners provided.

continues

Action	Rationale

Traction with Weights *continued*

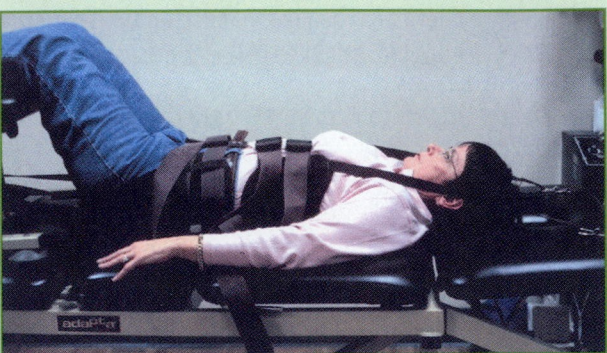

Figure 10-7-7 Traction device is properly applied and secured.

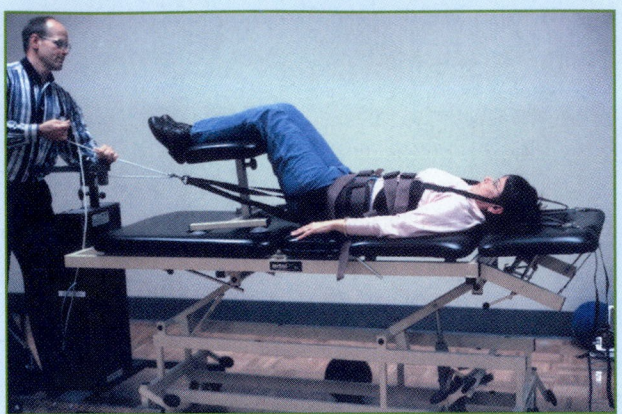

Figure 10-7-8 Connect the client to the source of traction.

16. Recheck circulatory and neurovascular status of the affected extremity for any changes.

17. Wash hands.

16. Monitors for any changes in circulation, possibly preventing further injury.

17. Reduces the transmission of microorganisms.

▶ REAL WORLD ANECDOTES

A client was placed in a plastic cervical collar because of an injury to his neck. The client was also a heavy smoker and after being outside for a considerable amount of time he returned to the unit with his C-collar on sideways and upside down. When questioned about this he completely denied any personal adjustment of his collar and stated that the nurse on the previous shift placed him in the collar exactly this way. The client was placed on strict bed rest, more X-rays were taken and, fortunately, the client suffered no ill effects. This incident shows the need for client education and for verification that the client understands the treatment.

▶ EVALUATION

- The affected body part has adequate neurovascular perfusion as evident by color, pulses, capillary refill, movement, and sensation.
- The client understands the reason for the traction and is able to cooperate in own care and treatment.
- The client experiences a minimum of discomfort and trauma secondary to the traction.

▶ DOCUMENTATION

Nurses' Notes

- The client's skin condition and neurovascular status as well as how the client is coping with the traction.
- Any client teaching done.

Document on appropriate flow sheet or electronic medical record (EMR).

▶ CRITICAL THINKING SKILL

Introduction

Client education is critical to client compliance.

Possible Scenario

A middle-aged female client is in pelvic traction for lower back pain. She has bathroom privileges and has been taught how to apply and remove the pelvic traction girdle by herself. Upon starting your shift, you note that this client is lying in bed, watching TV without her pelvic traction. When you ask her about it, she notes that her back does not hurt right now and she is tired of being pulled down in bed all the time.

Possible Outcome

You counsel the client regarding wearing her traction whenever she is in bed. She reapplies the pelvic girdle and you gently reapply the weight to the pelvic traction. The next time you check on the client she is once again lying in bed without her traction. She explains that she had just returned from the bathroom and was about to replace her traction. You note that she appears to have been lying in bed without her traction for some time. You assist the client to reapply the traction but you are concerned that she will remove it again after you have left the room. In report the next day you find out that this client has had an increase in lower back pain and is scheduled for a myelogram and possibly a lumbar laminectomy because of the exacerbation in her symptoms.

Prevention

Explain to the client the need for keeping the traction in place even if the symptoms have eased. The traction is probably the reason the symptoms initially decreased and discontinuing the traction could lead to a return of symptoms or possibly increased damage to the area.

▶ VARIATIONS

Geriatric Variations:
- *With older adults, skin breakdown is a concern and special emphasis is placed on checking for any redness over bony prominences. In this population special concerns regarding nutrition and elimination are important factors and have to be dealt with on an individual basis.*
- *Feelings of helplessness and hopelessness are prevalent in this age category and the need to bring in family, perhaps pastoral care, and even rehab psychology may be considered to help with this life transition to ensure a positive outcome.*

Pediatric Variations:
- *With children, traction is extremely difficult because of their inability to understand their limitations and the need to remain compliant with the plan of care.*
- *Special support from the parents is essential in treatment. Generally, involvement of the parents in the decision-making process increases understanding and compliance considerably.*

Home Care Variations:
- *Clients using traction at home should be reevaluated frequently for compliance, and proper placement and usage of the traction.*
- *Frequent evaluation of skin integrity and teaching the client to self-monitor is necessary.*

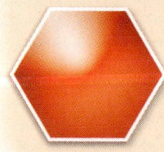

Long-Term Care Variation:
- *Equipment used for long-term care should be examined frequently for wear and tear, and replaced promptly if worn or frayed.*

▶ COMMON ERRORS

Possible Error:

The client's feet are resting on the foot of the bed.

Prevention:

If the client's feet are resting on the end of the bed, or if the traction weights are resting on the floor, the client is not receiving the traction ordered. Teach the client how to move up in bed safely. If not contraindicated and the client can tolerate it, raise the foot of the bed to prevent sliding down to the foot of the bed. Be sure the client understands the importance of maintaining the full weight of the traction for the prescribed time.

▶ NURSING TIPS

- Get adequate help when turning the client while in traction or in a supportive brace.
- Make certain that nutrition and elimination issues are addressed; many clients become constipated because of pain medication and inactivity, thereby adding to their discomfort.
- Adequate pain relief is essential in dealing with clients in traction. Muscle spasms and bone pain can be excruciating if the pain is not being properly addressed.
- The basic principle of traction is proper alignment.
- If the body part is not in alignment the pain will increase considerably. Make certain all lines are straight, weights are free to hang, all extremities are straight and, if indicated, client should be properly supported by pillows and other supportive devices.
- Make certain that body jackets or braces are properly fit and no skin is caught in the sides or pinched where the sides meet.
- Gain client compliance by teaching the important points of dealing with traction or a brace. Listen to their concerns and take time to answer the client's needs.
- Recreational therapy can offer diversional activities to clients who are in traction for long periods of time.

▶ SPECIAL CONSIDERATIONS

- *When moving or turning a client in traction, be certain to talk to the client throughout each step, and remind the client to take deep, slow breaths to relax. It is a protective mechanism to jerk against the movement of the health care team to avoid pain, but doing this only makes the transition worse.*
- *Some traction setups can be complicated. Ask for help if it is a new type of traction or if there are multiple pieces.*
- *Always have adequate help when adjusting any type of traction or brace.*

Maintaining and Monitoring Skeletal Traction

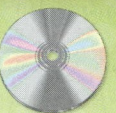

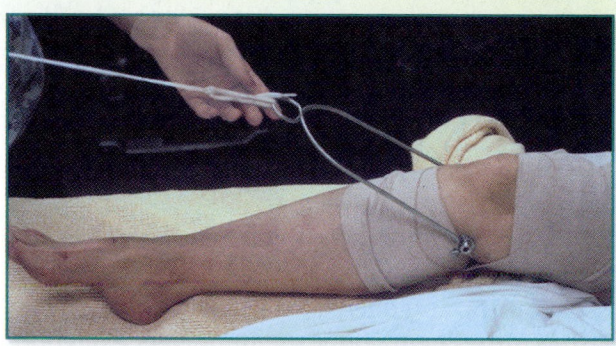

▶ OVERVIEW OF THE SKILL

Sometimes traction is applied directly to bone using special equipment such as Crutchfield tongs, or Steinman or Kirschner pins. This type of traction is called skeletal traction. Skeletal traction better immobilizes the affected bone and allows for more precise alignment of a fracture. It may also provide stronger and more consistent pull than skin traction. Skeletal traction can be used for a short-term treatment before surgery or can allow for an extended period of therapy when needed. There are several types of skeletal traction, including balanced suspension traction, halo traction, external fixation, and skull tongs.

When skeletal traction is in use, pain management and preventing complications are major nursing interventions. The client may experience pain during the placement of pins, when being moved, or with routine pin care. Nursing involvement in these times is essential to a good outcome for the client. Although an orthopedic surgeon or other qualified practitioner places pins and external fixators, nursing presence is important to support client needs. After the pins have been placed and the client is stable, the nurse must continually assess for complications and pain.

Complications that occur during traction are often caused by impaired mobility. These may include respiratory complications, constipation, decreased circulation in the lower extremities, diminishing muscle strength in the affected extremity, skin breakdown, and social isolation to name a few. Compartment syndrome, a medical emergency, can also occur after any fracture. This syndrome occurs when one or more compartments (a muscle group surrounded by a sheath of fascia that is innervated by nerves and blood vessels) in the area of the original fracture or pin insertion site is filled with blood or body fluid beyond the capacity of the surrounding fascia. This extensive swelling can cause nerve damage and muscle death by the increased pressure of veins, arteries, and nerves. This condition is serious and requires immediate intervention by a health care provider.

Monitoring pain, alignment, peripheral pulses, color, and CMS (circulation, movement, and sensation) becomes necessary and is an ongoing job of the nurse. Having a recorded baseline and watching for changes can save the client from further complications.

▶ ASSESSMENT

1. When assessing traction, assess the position, alignment, skin condition, overall health considerations, and CMS (circulation, movement, and sensation). **This can help determine changes from baseline, and help detect any emerging complications from traction.**
2. Assess pain location, intensity, and description. Discuss options for pain management. **Allows for client involvement in plan of care for pain and proper pain control.**
3. Determine from the chart what type of traction and how much weight is ordered for the client. **Allows the opportunity to make necessary adjustments to the traction.**
4. Assess general skin condition and pressure points. **It is important to record any changes and care for emerging pressure sores.**

▶ **DIAGNOSIS**

Acute Pain

Impaired Physical Mobility

Risk for Disuse Syndrome

Risk for Impaired Skin Integrity

Risk for Peripheral Neurovascular Dysfunction

▶ **PLANNING**

Expected Outcomes:

1. Client will maintain traction as ordered.
2. Neurovascular status will be maintained and monitored
3. Skin condition will be maintained intact and monitored.

Equipment Needed (see Figure 10-8-1):

• Pain medication
• Traction setup
• Weights as ordered

▶ **CLIENT EDUCATION NEEDED:**

1. Explain the need for traction, maintaining body alignment, and overall plan of care.
2. Explain what procedure will be performed (e.g., turning or transferring).

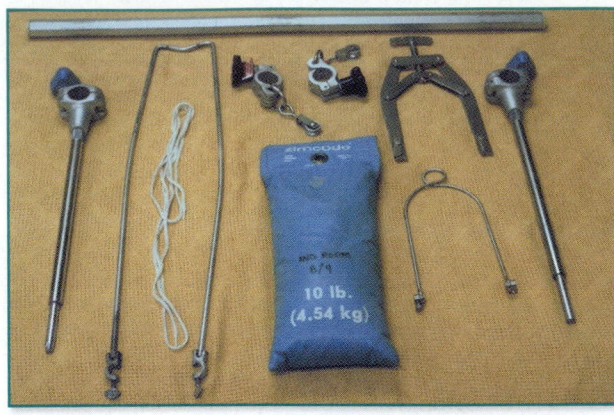

Figure 10-8-1 Traction equipment, pulleys, cords, and weights

3. Discuss common emotional manifestations of immobility, including sensory deprivation, loss of control, and decreased socialization.
4. Teach the client about the importance of good skin care and the importance of self-assessment when able.

 Estimated time to complete the skill: **10–15 minutes depending on the type of traction**

▶ **DELEGATION TIPS**

Skeletal traction is applied by the health care provider. Orthopedic technicians may be employed as ancillary personnel to assist in the application of the traction.

IMPLEMENTATION—Action/Rationale

Action	Rationale
Preparation for Moving a Client in Traction	
1. Assess CMS, body alignment, pain, and skin condition (see Figure 10-8-2).	1. Allows for a comparison, a baseline to determine any changes or emerging problems.
2. Acquire the necessary number of people to accomplish the task. This will be different depending on the kind of traction, how much the client can assist, and how recently post-op they are. Have plenty of pillows available for the turn.	2. Decreases the possibility of increased pain to the client and injuries to the staff.

continues

Action	Rationale

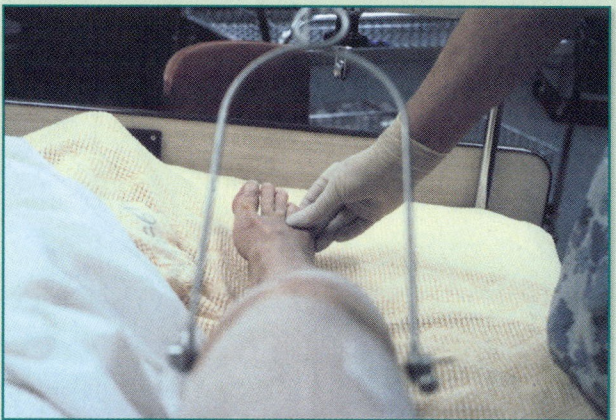

Figure 10-8-2 Assess skin circulation, movement, and sensation of extremities.

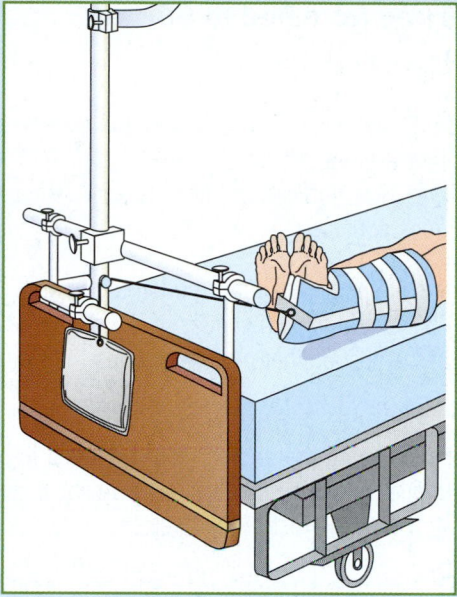

Figure 10-8-3 Make sure the traction weights hang freely.

3. Explain the procedure to the client throughout the entire procedure.

3. Decreases anxiety and increases client's ability to assist and cooperate.

4. Assess the traction setup. Be sure the lines and weights hang freely and the structural frame is secure (see Figure 10-8-3).

4. Assesses the effectiveness of the traction.

5. Wash hands.

5. Reduces the transmission of microorganisms.

Turning the Client

6. One person will monitor the traction and fractured extremity.

6. Allows for proper alignment and pull of the traction.

7. Turn the client.
   - For a client who is unable to assist with the move, two people are on the side that will lift the client's body, and one person is on the opposite side to stuff pillows.
   - For a client who is able to assist, leave the bed rail up so the client can use it to pull the upper body across. Another staff member will need to put pillows.

7. Accomplishes the task.
   - Decreases possibility of staff injury and client pain.
   - Allows for assessment of skin while the client accomplishes another task.
   - For a client with a fractured hip, be careful where pillows are placed beneath the fracture. There should be enough support without misaligning the bones. Keeping the broken hip abducted is usually more comfortable for the client.
   - Be sure to assess the skin of the back while client is up on side.

8. Once the client is settled, reassess CMS, body alignment, and pain.

8. A comparison assessment will recognize any problems that have arisen.

continues

Action	Rationale
Transferring from Bed to Gurney	
9. See Actions 1 to 5.	**9.** See Rationales 1 to 5.
10. Assess the gurney or bed to be sure the correct traction setup and equipment are available. *Note:* Most gurneys and beds require different sized posts for traction setup.	**10.** Allows for smooth transition and weight reapplication once in the new bed.
11. One person applies manual traction to the arch, the metal piece that joins the sides of the pin where the rope attaches, while another person removes the weights and rope.	**11.** This allows for removal of the weights and pulley until moved into the new bed.
12. Use a slide board to transfer client from bed to bed. Be certain one person is monitoring the broken extremity, moving it with the rest of the body.	**12.** Allows for smooth transition from bed to bed and minimizes pain.
13. Once the client is straight in the new bed, reapply traction slowly. The person holding manual traction should not let go until the weights are freely hanging.	**13.** This ensures that the transition from manual to weighted traction is smooth and allows the staff a chance to be sure the traction will hang freely before releasing the arch.
14. Once the client is settled, reassess CMS, body alignment, and pain.	**14.** A comparison assessment will recognize any new problems.
15. Wash hands.	**15.** Reduces the transmission of microorganisms.

► **REAL WORLD ANECDOTES**

Mrs. Gonzales was in 15 pounds of skeletal traction to the left femur. She had been called to go to surgery for an intermedullary rodding and would need to be moved to a gurney. After proper premedication, four staff put on gloves and the client's nurse explained what would happen. One nurse held manual traction while the others removed the weights and readied the setup on the gurney. Then using a slider board and the sheets on the bed, the rest of the staff moved the client smoothly onto the gurney. Although the client had muscle spasms almost immediately, the transition went well. After waiting for the muscle spasms to subside, the weights were reapplied and a CMS check was performed.

► **EVALUATION**

- Client maintained traction as ordered.
- Body alignment was maintained at all times.
- Neurovascular status was maintained and monitored.
- Skin condition was maintained intact and monitored.

► **DOCUMENTATION**

Nurses' Notes

- The type of weight, traction, and treatment done.
- Client's tolerance and involvement in the procedure.
- Number of people needed to accomplish the task.

Document on appropriate flow sheet or electronic medical record (EMR).

► **CRITICAL THINKING SKILL**

Introduction

Turning even when in traction is important to the overall health of the client.

Possible Scenario

After a car accident, Mr. John was in pain and was extremely reluctant to move even a muscle. After much discussion and encouragement, the client still refused. The nurse charted and left a note for the health care provider.

Possible Outcome

Client develops skin breakdown and blisters on the buttocks and heels. Client is in more pain than he was before because of increased muscle spasms from lack of movement and relaxation.

Prevention

Sometimes a client will refuse to move. Most often it is because of lack of knowledge and fear. Teaching and encouragement can sometimes convince a client to try to move. However, if even this cannot convince a person to turn, encourage ankle pumps (toes pull up towards the head and then push down like on a gas pedal). Sometimes a client will move himself rather than allowing someone else to do it. For instance, if the client is able to bend his good leg and use it to lift his hips and back, this should be encouraged and an overhead trapeze supplied where possible.

► **VARIATIONS**

Geriatric Variations:

- *Elderly clients may become confused at night and try to remove traction or get out of bed; frequent monitoring is important.*
- *Elderly clients may need reminders regarding why they are in traction and what to expect.*
- *Muscle atrophy occurs more rapidly in elderly clients. Teach and encourage exercises such as ankle pumps and range of motion in the unaffected extremities.*
- *Pain medication can sometimes have heightened effects in the elderly client.*

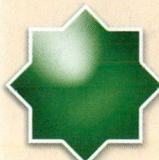

Pediatric Variations:

- *Pediatric clients may not be able to understand the need for traction or proper alignment. Education of the parents or caregiver is essential.*
- *Frequently, children are placed in skin or boot traction instead of skeletal traction.*
- *Be sure to find activities to occupy the child's attention and mind when possible as they will be unable to get out of bed while in traction.*

Home Care Variations:

- *Traction is not used frequently in the home care setting, but the basic principles of care are the same.*
- *Traction equipment attached to a bed frame will require a hospital bed.*

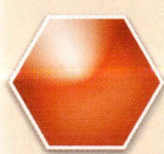

Long-Term Care Variation:

- *Traction is not used frequently in the long-term care setting, but the basic principles remain the same.*

> ▶ **COMMON ERRORS**

Possible Error:

The traction is ineffective.

Prevention:

Always check the pulleys, cords, weights, bed frame, and position of pillows.

Possible Error:

When moving an emergency room client into bed, posts from the gurney do not fit into the bed slots; therefore, traction has to be maintained manually for an extended period of time.

Prevention:

Be sure to assess the traction equipment and setup to be sure all the correct pieces are assembled for the transition.

> ▶ **NURSING TIPS**

- Always have enough people present to assist with moves or transfers.
- Have extra rope available when moving from gurney to bed in case the old rope is too short.
- Encourage ankle exercises to assist with muscle relaxation and decrease spasms.
- Pillows can be used to support the fractured limb, maintain the client's position, and promote comfort.

> ▶ **SPECIAL CONSIDERATIONS**

- *Discuss with the client what will happen and what to expect. Fear and anxiety are some of the main reasons for discomfort with traction and refusal to participate in care activities.*
- *Traction is used to counteract the pull muscles have. This pull is what causes fractured bones to rub together, thereby increasing pain. There should be a decrease in pain with traction. If there is not, be sure to consult the health care provider after reassessing the traction setup for errors.*
- *There are many types of traction; not all of them can be covered here in this section. If a setup is complicated or new to you, ask someone to assist with the initial assessment of the traction.*

External Fixation
or Skeletal Pin Care

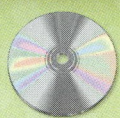

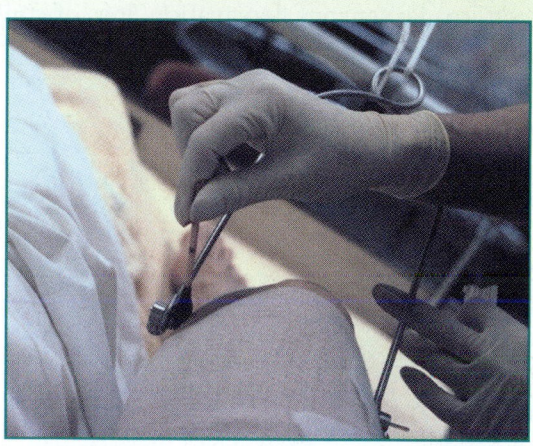

▶ OVERVIEW OF THE SKILL

Intervention is often needed after a fracture to achieve proper healing. Sometimes this includes traction or external or internal fixation (see Skill 10-8 for a description of skeletal traction). Whenever there is a break in the skin's surface, care must be taken to reduce infection risk and minimize future scarring.

External fixation uses pins implanted into the bone that are attached to an external metal frame to stabilize a fracture. Halo traction, one such fixation, provides support for cervical or basilar skull fractures. It consists of pins placed into the skull and attached to a metal ring that surrounds the head. This ring is then secured to a chest vest to hold it the head in place.

Pins for external fixation or to secure traction need to be kept clean and clear of scabs or skin overgrowth in order to reduce infection and scarring. This task should be done every 8 hours or as ordered by the health care provider. During this care, it is important to inspect the extremity or fracture site to ensure there are no changes in circulation, movement, or sensation, which could suggest a complication or change.

▶ ASSESSMENT

1. Assess client's knowledge of the procedure, its importance, and client's ability to assist. **Helps provide education about the procedure and reduces anxiety.**
2. Assess client for pain, proper alignment, positioning, skin condition, and overall health. Also assess for circulation, movement, and sensation (CMS). **This helps determine any changes from baseline and detect any emerging complications.**
3. Assess client's chart for anticipated length of treatment via traction or external fixation. A client or family member can be taught to assist or perform pin care if the client will be in therapy for an extended period. **Important for encouraging self-care and independence, as well as acceptance of current physical limitations and body image disturbances.**

▶ DIAGNOSIS

Acute Pain

Impaired Physical Mobility

Impaired Tissue Integrity

Risk for Infection

Risk for Peripheral Neurovascular Dysfunction

▶ PLANNING

Expected Outcomes:

1. Traction will be maintained throughout care.
2. Client will maintain proper body alignment.
3. Client will maintain good skin condition and circulation, movement, sensation in the affected extremity.
4. Client will show no signs or symptoms of infection.
5. Client will not experience excessive pain.

Equipment Needed:

- Pain medication
- Cotton tip applicators, at least 2–4 per pin site
- Gloves
- 4 × 4 gauze, two per pin site
- Cleaning solution as ordered. *Note:* There are few published research studies on the type of solution to be used to prevent infection at the pin site. The National Association of Orthopaedic Nurses recommends chlorhexidine 2 mg/mL solution. Check orders and institutional policy to know the correct solution to use.

▶ **CLIENT EDUCATION NEEDED:**

1. Explain to the client the importance of cleaning the pin sites regularly, maintaining alignment, and self-assessing skin condition.

2. If client or a caregiver can assist with pin care, teach proper technique, then watch a return demonstration.
3. Teach client to report any changes in circulation, sensation, or pain. Discuss options for proper pain control.
4. Discuss common emotional feelings associated with immobility. These may include disturbed body image, sensory deprivation, loss of control, and decreased socialization.

Estimated time to complete the skill:
5 minutes per pin

▶ **DELEGATION TIPS**

The assessment of an external fixation device or of external traction pins requires a nursing evaluation. Ancillary personnel should be instructed to immediately report any redness, drainage, change in color or temperature of the extremity, or looseness of the appliance to the nurse.

IMPLEMENTATION—Action/Rationale

Action	Rationale
1. Wash hands.	1. Reduces the transmission of microorganisms.
2. Premedicate with analgesics if necessary.	2. Proper medication can reduce discomfort and increase compliance.
3. Assess pulses, color, movement, sensation, and skin condition.	3. Determines if there are any changes from the baseline.
4. Assess for proper alignment, positioning, and traction lines that are free from the bed and linens.	4. Maintaining proper traction and alignment will facilitate proper healing and minimize pain.
5. Obtain prescribed solution.	5. Minimizes risk of infection.
6. Put gloves on and replace as needed if soiled.	6. Accomplishes body substance isolation.

continues

Action	Rationale

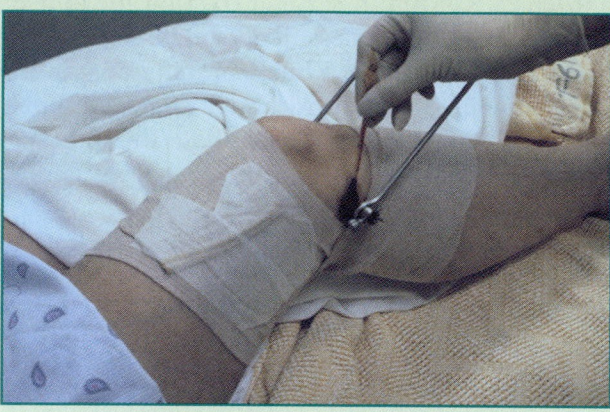

Figure 10-9-1   Perform pin care every 8 hours or as needed.

7. Remove current dressing around each pin site. Inspect skin condition. Notice if there is any skin growth on the pin, or scabbing. Note color, amount, and type of drainage. Also note any increasing size of the insertion site.

8. Soak cotton tip applicator with cleaning solution. Swipe around each pin site once per swab. Use as many swabs as needed until sites are clean. No skin should be attached to the metal pin, but should move freely around it. (see Figure 10-9-1).

9. Apply dressing if site is draining.

10. Remove gloves and wash hands.

7. Proper assessment and documentation of changes can expedite proper treatment and diagnosis.

8. Correct cleaning of each pin site will facilitate minimal scarring and decrease the risk of infection.

9. Protects the site and collects drainage.

10. Reduces the transmission of microorganisms.

▶ **REAL WORLD ANECDOTES**

Scenario 1

As the nurse attempts to remove the bandages from Mr. Frank's pin sites, he notes that there is moderate yellow purulent drainage and the old dressing seems to be attached to the pins and the skin around them. Using normal saline, the nurse soaks the dressing and is then able to pull it off. He notes that the skin around the site is reddened. After cleaning the sites as ordered, the nurse notifies the health care provider of the drainage and the condition of the pin site. The nurse documents the assessment and communicates the findings to the next nurse.

Scenario 2

After placement of an external fixator, a client and his partner were interested in going home as soon as possible. The nurse on each shift worked with the two to help them gain an understanding of how to care for the fixator and skin underneath. Once they were able to return-demonstrate the skill and the social worker was able to arrange for care in the home, the client was discharged to home.

▶ **EVALUATION**

- Traction was maintained throughout care.
- Client maintained proper body alignment.
- Client maintained good skin condition, circulation, movement, and sensation.
- Client showed no signs or symptoms of infection.

- Client maintained adequate pain control throughout procedure.

▶ DOCUMENTATION

Nurses' Notes

- Document assessment of the client to establish any occurring changes from baseline.
- Describe skin condition around pin site, drainage amount, color, and type.
- Document type of solution used and what time procedure was done.
- Document client tolerance of procedure and pain rating.

Document on appropriate flow sheet or electronic medical record (EMR).

▶ CRITICAL THINKING SKILL

Introduction

Chart findings after each cleaning in order to monitor for any changes.

Possible Scenario

The night shift nurse came into the room of a client who had been in skeletal traction for four days. As she does her assessment she notices that the dressings around the Kirschner pins are saturated with sanguineous fluid. Although she could not find any note from previous nurses about the status of the pin sites, she assumed that the drainage was normal and simply changed the dressings.

Possible Outcome

The hematocrit is found to be lower the next day, thus postponing the scheduled surgery.

Prevention

With proper charting the nurse would have been able to see that the bleeding was new. She would have been able to talk to the health care provider, possibly allowing surgery to take place on time.

▶ VARIATIONS

Geriatric Variations:
- *Some pain medications have heightened effects and increased side effects in elderly clients. Therefore, close monitoring is required.*
- *Confusion at night is not uncommon in elderly clients. During this time they may try to remove traction, get out of bed, or do things that could lengthen their healing time.*
- *Skin can be thin and fragile, making it more susceptible to breakdown.*
- *Elderly clients may need reminders regarding why they are in traction and what the expected outcomes are.*

Pediatric Variations:
- *Pediatric clients may not be able to understand the need for traction or cleaning of the pin sites. Reassurance and parental involvement may be useful.*
- *Frequent assessment of alignment and position may be needed because of the difficulty of explaining body alignment to children.*
- *In some serious fractures, children may be in traction for an extended period of time. Addressing social, school, and psychological implications is important to the child's health and well-being.*

Home Care Variations:
- *The basic principles are the same. Teaching the caregivers in the home is the most important nursing intervention.*
- *For traction attached to a bed frame, a hospital bed will be required.*

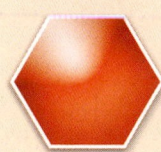

Long-Term Care Variations:
- *Traction is rarely used in long-term care facilities. However, should traction be ordered in the long-term care setting, continued care of pin sites, body alignment, and skin is important.*
- *Nutrition, immobility-related effects, and exercises of the unaffected limbs are important nursing considerations with long-term use of traction.*

► **COMMON ERRORS**

Possible Error:

Using a cotton tip applicator for more than one swipe.

Prevention:

Use as many cotton tip applicators as needed to clean the sites. Do not use an applicator for more than one swipe.

► **NURSING TIPS**

- Maintaining good pain control will assist in the healing process. The client will be able to move around better and assist more with self-care.
- Use of overhead trapeze aids the client in being more independent.
- If halo traction is in use, be sure to have the necessary equipment in the room or with the client at all times to remove the chest piece in an emergency, such as when CPR is needed.
- Client participation in this skill can allow for a feeling of usefulness and independence that is important while the client is limited in movement and activity.

► **SPECIAL CONSIDERATIONS**

- *Sometimes, just after surgery, there is a dressing or even a cast over an external fixator that renders the pin sites impossible to clean. Do not remove the dressing unless it is ordered.*
- *If there is a problem with the client touching the pin sites or removing the dressings, an Ace bandage can be wrapped around the entire setup to protect against this.*
- *Be sure the pin care is not skipped; the dressings can become stuck to the skin or pin and make the procedure more painful for the client.*

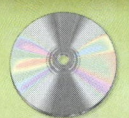
Assisting with Casting—
Plaster and Fiberglass

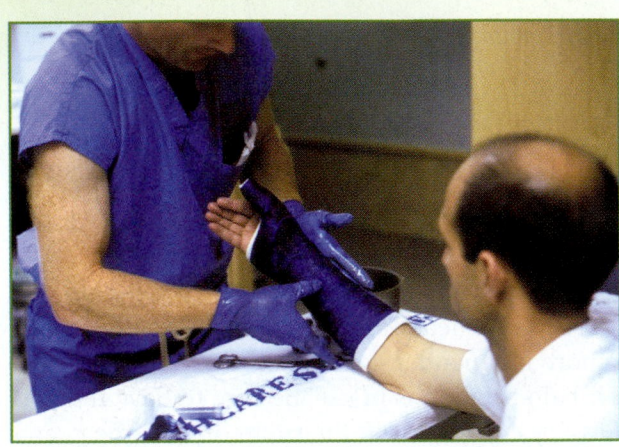

▶ OVERVIEW OF THE SKILL

Casts are placed to provide stability to a fracture, dislocation, or soft-tissue injury while it heals. Casts have traditionally been made of plaster of Paris but more and more are now made with fiberglass. The health care provider will decide which type of cast to use, depending on many factors, including the age of the client and the reason and location of the cast. The primary goals of the nurse assisting with the procedure and caring for a client with a new cast are to:

- Assist the health care provider or technician in rapid and correct placement of the cast, including assembling all necessary equipment at the bedside so the cast can be applied without interruption.
- Assess and intervene to reduce pain during reduction of the fracture and placement of the cast.
- Prevent vascular compromise from swelling after the cast is placed.
- Provide intravenous access, if necessary, so the client can be medicated for pain.
- Give clear information as to what the client should expect during the procedure.

▶ ASSESSMENT

1. Assess the client for acute pain or anxiety **to determine the need for medications or possible conscious sedation during the procedure.**
2. Assess the neurovascular status of the injured area before and after the cast is applied **to determine**

changes in status. Neurovascular checks include skin color, skin temperature, capillary refill, pulses, touch, movement, and sensation.
3. Understand the kind of injury and the type of cast being applied. **Helps recognize potential complications to watch for.**
4. Assess the skin that will soon be inaccessible under the cast. Note any bruising, abrasions, incisions, or skin conditions **that might contribute to discomfort, infection, drainage, or skin break-down after the cast is applied.**
5. Assess the client's understanding of the injury and the casting procedure **to determine what teaching is needed.**

▶ DIAGNOSIS

Acute Pain

Anxiety

Impaired Physical Mobility

Risk for Impaired Skin Integrity

Risk for Ineffective Tissue Perfusion

Risk for Peripheral Neurovascular Dysfunction

▶ PLANNING

Expected Outcomes:

1. The cast will maintain good bone alignment.
2. A cast will be applied to the fracture rapidly with minimal pain and anxiety to the client.

3. There will be no vascular compromise to the client during or after the procedure.

Equipment Needed (see Figure 10-10-1):

- Appropriate size cotton (for plaster) or synthetic (for fiberglass) cast padding such as Webril
- Stockinette, cut approximately 6 inches longer than the part to be casted
- Appropriate size plaster or sealed fiberglass rolls
- For plaster casts: Ace wraps, 2- or 3-inch sizes, 2 to 3 rolls
- For plaster casts: bucket of warm water
- For plaster casts: roll of 3- to 4-inch tape
- Protective clothing for yourself
- Nonsterile gloves

▶ CLIENT EDUCATION NEEDED:

1. Instruct the client on the need to help maintain correct alignment and positioning of the affected body part during the procedure.
2. Inform the client that when the casting material is placed, it will feel warm as it sets.
3. Instruct the client not to bear weight on the cast while it is drying. Plaster casts take up to 48 hours to dry. Fiberglass casts dry in about 1 hour.
4. Remind the client to communicate any pain during the procedure so pain intervention can be provided.
5. Provide instruction on cast care after the procedure is completed.

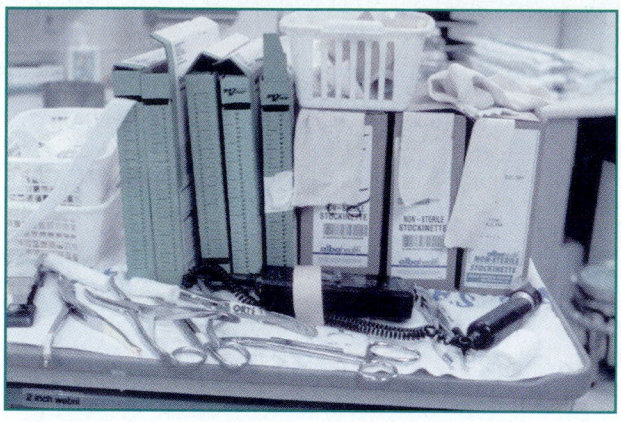

Figure 10-10-1 Casting supplies, including stockinette, tape, and casting tools

6. Instruct the client receiving a plaster cast that the plaster will feel warm for several minutes as it sets, then cool for several hours as it dries.
7. After the cast is applied, provide instructions on the following: care of the cast, elevation of the affected extremity, keeping the cast dry, checking for warmth, sensation, and movement of the exposed extremity, observing the color of the exposed extremity, and comfort and pain measures that can be used by the client.

Estimated time to complete the skill: **30–60 minutes**

▶ DELEGATION TIPS

Orthopedic technicians may be employed as ancillary personnel to assist the health care provider in the application of a cast. A complete assessment of the client should be performed by the nurse following cast application.

IMPLEMENTATION—Action/Rationale

Action	Rationale
1. Introduce yourself to the client. Assess current neurovascular status.	1. Makes the client aware of who is caring for him or her during the casting.
2. Communicate with client during the procedure.	2. Decreases client's anxiety level and promotes cooperation.

continues

Action	Rationale
3. Prepare all equipment.	**3.** Facilitates an efficient practice.
4. Protect the bed and client, if necessary, from water and casting residue.	**4.** Promotes client comfort.
5. Have the client in the proper position for reduction and casting.	**5.** Facilitates the casting procedure.
6. Wash hands. Wear gloves and protective clothing as needed.	**6.** Keeps nurse's hands and uniform clean and dry while working with wet and sticky substances.
7. For a plaster cast, place the plaster roll into the warm water on its end until the bubbles stop rising from the roll. Remove it from the water and squeeze gently to remove the excess water (see Figure 10-10-2). Hand the roll to the person applying the cast.	**7.** Preparing the plaster facilitates rapid and smooth application of the cast.
8. For a fiberglass cast, open the sealed fiberglass rolls as needed, and hold the package so the person applying the cast can remove the roll.	**8.** Facilitates rapid and smooth application of the cast.
9. Assist the person applying the cast. This person will: • Position the part to be casted (see Figure 10-10-3). Place stockinette over the skin (see Figure 10-10-4). Wrap the site with cast padding (see Figure 10-10-5). • Place the fiberglass or plaster over the fracture (see Figure 10-10-6), extending the coverage above and below the fracture site (see Figure 10-10-7). • Edges will be trimmed and finished and any supports or reinforcements to the cast will be applied (see Figure 10-10-8).	**9.** Allows rapid placement of cast.

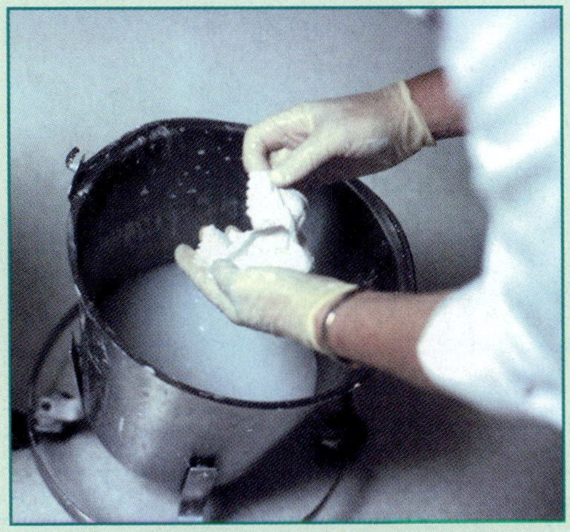

Figure 10-10-2 Place the plaster roll in warm water until it stops bubbling. Remove the plaster roll from the water and squeeze gently to remove excess moisture.

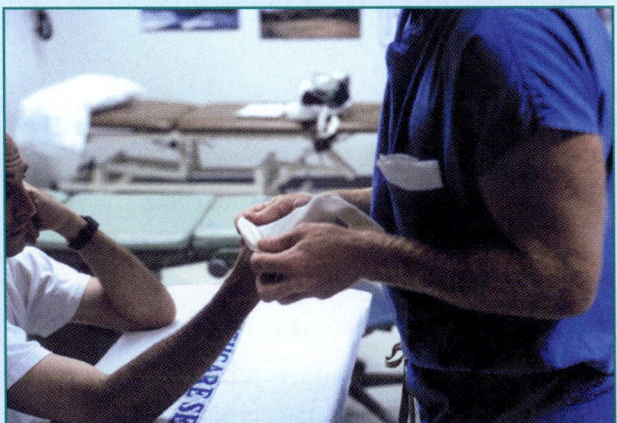

Figure 10-10-3 Position the extremity to be casted.

continues

Action	Rationale

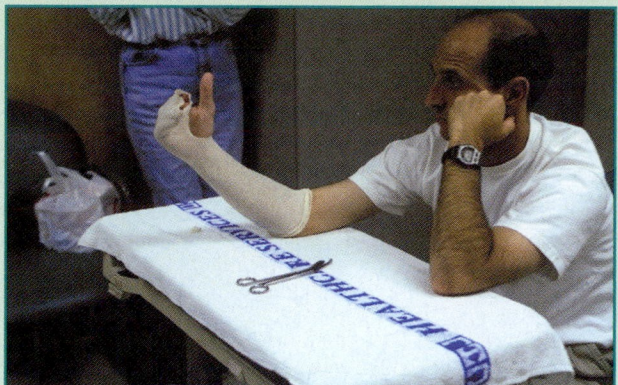

Figure 10-10-4   Place stockinette over the skin where the casting material will be applied.

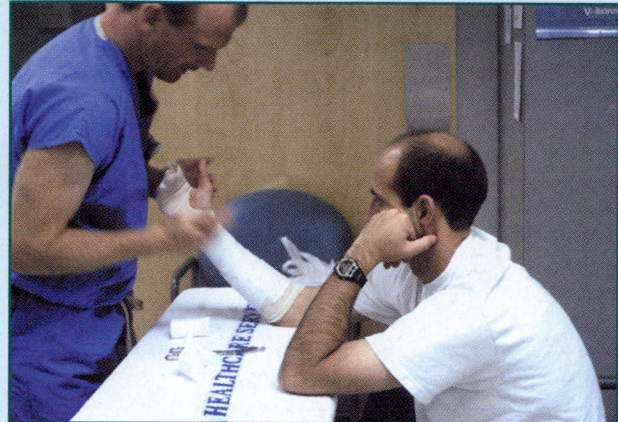

Figure 10-10-5   Apply the cast padding.

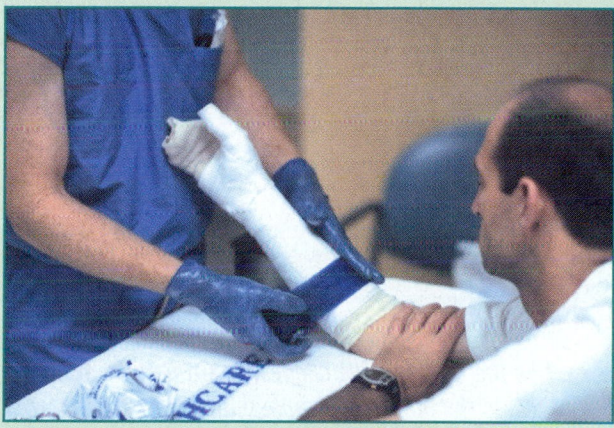

Figure 10-10-6   Apply the casting material.

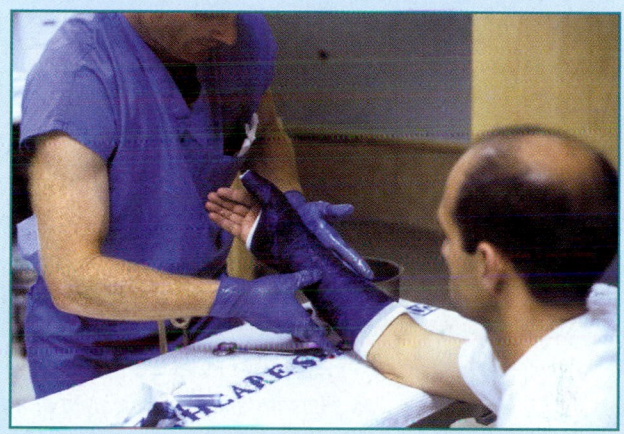

Figure 10-10-7   The casting material must extend above and below the fracture site.

10. Elevate cast site when complete.

11. Leave the cast uncovered while it is drying. Be sure there are no pressure or resting areas where the damp cast could change shape while drying.

12. Reassess neurovascular status.

13. Swelling may occur after the cast is applied. The cast may be bivalved, or cut in half, to allow for swelling. If this is done, wrap the cast in Ace wraps to hold it in place.

14. A window may be cut in the cast to relieve pressure or to monitor the skin at that location under the cast.

10. Prevents cast swelling.

11. Facilitates drying time. Flattening or indentations in the cast could apply pressure to underlying tissue.

12. Prevents neurovascular complications.

13. Prevents neurovascular compromise or discomfort.

14. Prevents neurovascular compromise or discomfort.

continues

Action	Rationale

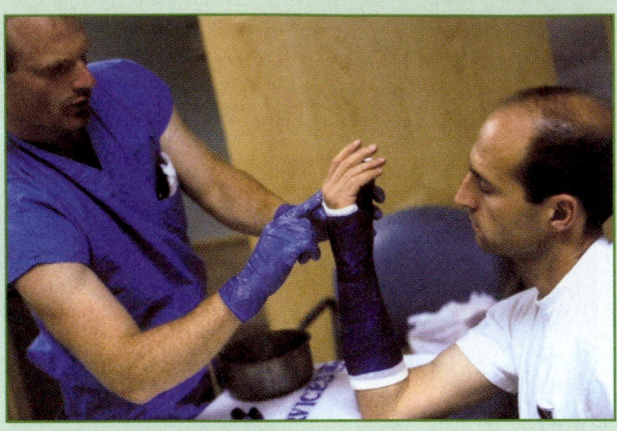

Figure 10-10-8 Edges are finished by pulling the first layer of stockinette back around the padding and adhering it to the fiberglass.

15. Clean the bed and remove casting materials, if needed. Check for bits of dried plaster or fiberglass cuttings and packaging material that could cause skin irritation.

16. Prepare client for postreduction X-ray as necessary.

17. Remove gloves and wash hands.

15. Promotes client comfort.

16. Assesses bone alignment.

17. Reduces the transmission of microorganisms.

► **REAL WORLD ANECDOTES**

Scenario 1

A nurse was assisting in the application of a fiberglass cast on the forearm. The client was sitting on a stretcher with his forearm bent at the elbow, resting on an overbed table. As the physician wrapped the cast from the wrist downward, the nurse held the wrist tightly to support the client's hand in the proper position. The tight pressure on the soft cast pressed the fiberglass into the ulnar styloid process. When the client returned for a follow-up visit and cast change, the skin over this bony prominence had broken down.

Scenario 2

A nursing student working in the emergency room learned about the properties of plaster of Paris the hard way. Setting up for a casting session, she soaked all the rolls of plaster ahead of time and laid them out on the casting table. When the physician and client arrived for the procedure, the rolls were rock hard.

► **EVALUATION**

- The cast maintains good bone alignment.
- A cast was applied to the fracture rapidly with minimal pain and anxiety to the client.
- There is no vascular compromise to the client during or after the procedure.

► **DOCUMENTATION**

Nurses' Notes

- The type of cast and where it was applied
- Any medications used during the procedure
- Any specific aids used after the cast was applied, for example, use of crutches or slings

- Client teaching
- Pre- and postprocedure neurovascular status

Document on appropriate flow sheet or electronic medical record (EMR).

▶ CRITICAL THINKING SKILL

Introduction

Nurses must be able to evaluate effective and adequate circulatory status, thus preventing vascular compromise.

Possible Scenario

A cast has been placed on the arm of an accident client newly transferred to the floor. The nurse's initial assessment showed a warm extremity, good movement of the fingers, and good capillary refill. The nurse concluded that the client had adequate circulatory status.

It was a busy night, and she did not get back for a second assessment for almost three hours. By then the client was complaining of severe pain and cold fingers.

Possible Outcome

The client developed compartmental syndrome and needed surgical intervention.

Prevention

The client sustained vascular compromise to the extremity. This could have been prevented by proper elevation of the affected part after casting and placing ice on the area of the fracture. More frequent evaluation of the client's circulatory status, especially knowing that the client had a recent injury and a new cast, would have alerted the nurse to the worsening vascular status in the limb.

▶ VARIATIONS

Geriatric Variations:

- *Older clients often do not have the muscle tone and/or balance to walk with crutches or support the weight of the cast for long periods. This needs to be taken into account prior to placing the cast.*
- *An older client may not be able to maintain the desired position during casting. Plan ahead to make position modifications or provide extra support if necessary.*
- *Older clients may be more susceptible to drug toxicity and drug sensitivity because of impaired liver and renal functions. Keep this in mind when medicating for pain.*

Pediatric Variations:

- *Remember to review comparison X-ray views of fractures in children. Be sure you are aware of the growth plate and problems arising in fractures in the growth plate in children.*
- *Fiberglass casts are often used in children when possible. The bright colors and greater durability of the fiberglass cast make it a preferred choice.*
- *Allow the child to choose the color of the cast if the cast is fiberglass and if different colors are available.*
- *A child may be more prone to "exploring," that is, inserting objects under the cast while it is drying. This increases the risk of skin trauma and breakdown and can rearrange the cast padding, creating pressure points and discomfort.*

Home Care Variations:

- *If the client is going directly home with the cast, educate about such tasks as toileting, feeding, and other self-care activities.*
- *Discuss clothing modifications needed to wear clothes over casted limbs. Pants and shirts can be cut up the seam, and Velcro closures can be sewn on the fabric. Loose-fitting clothes made of stretchy fabrics will often go over the cast, but may be stretched out of shape over time. Remind clients that the fiberglass cast will snag nylon and finely woven knit fabrics.*

continues

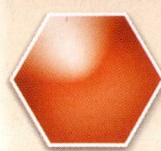

▶ VARIATIONS *(continued)*

Long-Term Care Variations:
- *Casts should be assessed regularly for fit.*
- *Clients who will be wearing a long-term cast should be taught how to keep the cast dry while bathing.*

▶ NURSING TIPS

- To promote good body mechanics, and for comfort, be sure the bed or stretcher is at a comfortable height during the procedure.
- Have all supplies prepared in advance of the cast application.
- Overestimate the amount of materials to have on hand; often the person applying the cast will use extra supplies to shape or reinforce the cast.
- Be sure that sharp scissors are available to cut the plaster if needed.
- If client complains of tingling, numbness, pain, or odor at the site of the cast, report these immediately to the health care provider.

- Continue to talk to the client during the procedure to assess response to the procedure and to decrease anxiety.
- If family or friends stay with the client, educate them in advance on what to expect during the procedure. Keep an eye on client for signs of dizziness or emotional upset, and assist as needed. Remind client to stay sitting down during the procedure, and to request help if they start to feel "funny."
- Do not dispose of plaster or plaster water in a regular sink, as it can clog the plumbing. Dispose of it following institutional policy.

▶ SPECIAL CONSIDERATIONS

- *Do not try to speed the drying process with a blow-dryer and teach clients not to as well.*
- *Explain the risk of skin breakdown and infection associated with using powders or creams inside a cast. Objects should never be placed inside a cast as this will cause pressure and, eventually, skin breakdown.*
- *For some casts, such as a spica cast, toileting and hygiene must be carefully explained. The cast should be assessed to be sure it will accommodate such tasks. Frequent monitoring to ensure cleanliness of the cast and the client is essential.*

Cast Care and Comfort

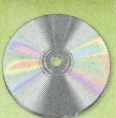

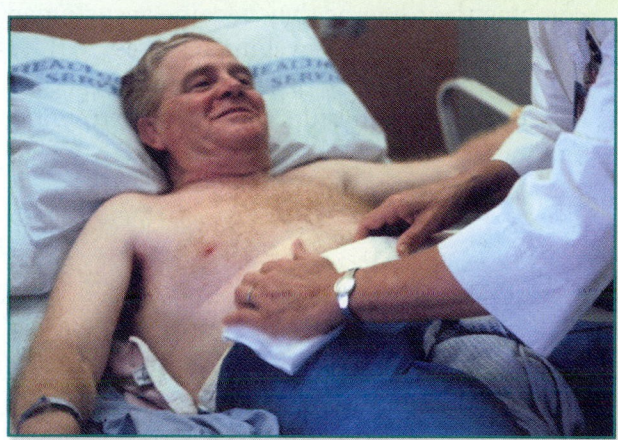

▶ OVERVIEW OF THE SKILL

A cast is placed for 6–8 weeks to provide stabilization for healing. Casts are made of plaster of Paris or of fiberglass. Casts covering forearms or lower legs are called short-arm or short-leg casts. A long-leg cast covers the entire leg and a hanging cast covers the entire arm. A body cast covers the chest and abdomen and the Minerva cast covers the chest, neck, and head with openings for the ears, face, and arms. The spica or hip spica cast covers the hips and one or both legs.

A cast should fit snugly and support the fracture. It may be changed several times during the healing process if reduction in swelling or loss of muscle tone causes it to become too loose. During the first 24 hours after the application of a cast, edema can create a tourniquet effect and inhibit circulation to the tissue, which can cause irreversible damage. The abdominal area can also expand as a result of eating or drinking. The nurse should assess the cast site for healing and/or irritation to the skin.

A window can be cut in the cast to facilitate skin care, to relieve discomfort over a bony prominence, to relieve nerve compression, or to reduce the weight of the cast.

▶ ASSESSMENT

1. Assess the circulation, movement, and sensation every 8 hours **because changes in circulation,** **sensation, and movement may signal the** **development of compartmental syndrome,** **a medical emergency.**
2. Assess for color, temperature, edema, pain, skin irritation, capillary refill, and drainage. **These** **changes may indicate that edema is causing** **restriction of circulation.**
3. Assess for severe pain over bony prominences **to prevent the risk of skin ulceration.**
4. Assess the condition of the cast **to determine** **need for client education.**
5. Assess the client's understanding of the cast and its care **so that client education can be** **tailored to his or her needs.**

▶ DIAGNOSIS

Acute Pain

Impaired Physical Mobility

Impaired Tissue Perfusion: Peripheral

Risk for Impaired Skin Integrity

Risk for Ineffective Tissue Perfusion

Risk for Peripheral Neurovascular Dysfunction

▶ PLANNING

Expected Outcomes:

1. There will be no vascular compromise to the client while the cast is in place.
2. The skin around the cast remains intact.

3. The cast will remain intact.
4. The client will be comfortable while the cast is in place.

Equipment Needed:

- Tape
- Pen to mark drainage
- Padding

▶ CLIENT EDUCATION NEEDED:

1. Teach isometric exercises to prevent muscle atrophy.
2. Instruct client regarding skin care while the cast is in place.
3. Instruct the client to keep the cast dry.
4. Teach the client to report a cast that "doesn't feel right." Ignoring it may lead to skin breakdown.
5. Teach the client to report any foul odor because it may indicate skin breakdown or infection under the cast.

6. Suggest that the client use an oversized cotton glove on a forearm fiberglass cast when doing gardening or housework to keep the edges clean.
7. Teach client never to try to clean the edges of a cast or remove dirty edges because of the risk of removing the necessary padding.
8. Reassure clients that they may be able to do more activities such as tying their shoes or combing their hair as they become accustomed to the cast and as the swelling resolves.
9. Remind the client that premature removal of a cast can lead to dysfunction of the extremity and increased pain by delaying healing.

Estimated time to complete the skill:
10 minutes

▶ DELEGATION TIPS

Assessment of the client, including the status of the casted extremity, is the responsibility of the nurse. Ongoing cast care may be delegated to properly trained ancillary personnel, who should be instructed to report any abnormal findings such as changes in extremity circulation, sensation, color, movement, or an increase in pain to the nurse for evaluation.

IMPLEMENTATION—Action/Rationale

Action	Rationale
1. Wash hands.	1. Reduces the transmission of microorganisms. Establishes baseline assessment.
2. Check circulation, movement, and sensation (CMS) (see Figure 10-11-1). • Note color and temperature of skin. • Pinch finger or toe and watch for capillary refill within 2 to 4 seconds. • Ask client to wiggle fingers or toes if possible. • Ask client to tell you if he or she feels you touching the extremity (see Figure 10-11-2). Be aware of possible hypersensitive or neuropathic sensation of the extremities, which changes normal baseline.	2. Prevents complications such as nerve or muscle damage, skin ulceration, and pain.

continues

Action	Rationale

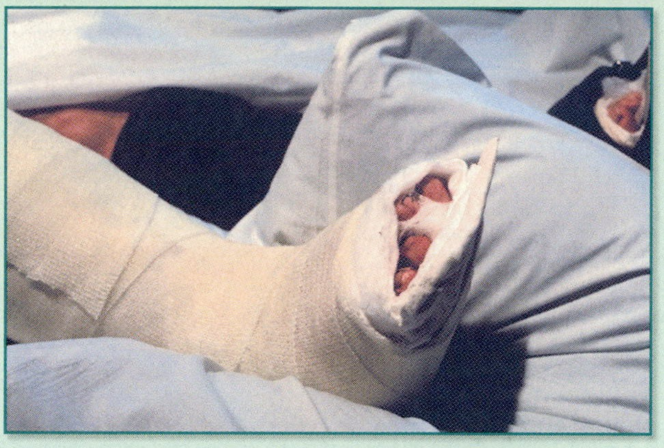

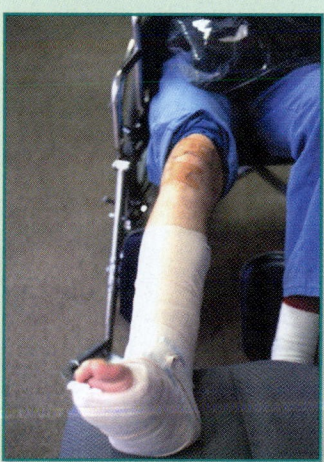

Figure 10-11-1 Assess circulation, movement, and sensation in the toes.

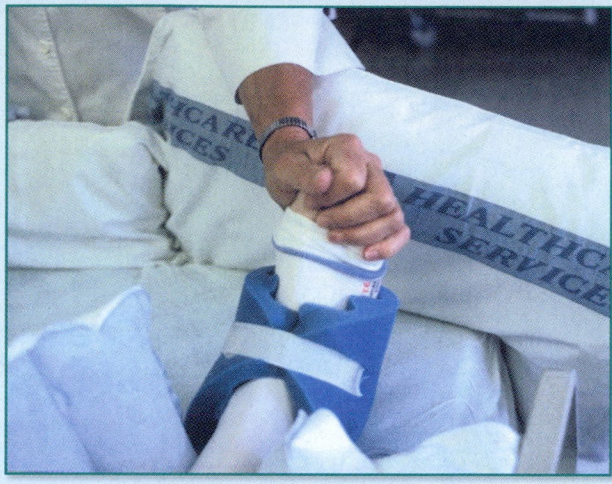

Figure 10-11-2 Ask the client if he or she can feel you touching the extremities distal to the immobilized area.

3. Assess skin.
   - Tell client not to put objects into the cast.

   - Use powders or creams only outside the cast.

4. Assess pain or soreness.
   - Reposition the extremity every 2 hours.

   - Elevate the extremity (see Figure 10-11-3) and apply ice.

5. Assess cast for intact cotton padding. Pad or add additional padding to areas of redness or irritation (see Figure 10-11-4).

3. Prevents skin from becoming irritated or ulcerated.
   - Objects under the cast may cause damage to skin and the cast material.
   - Powder inside the cast can cake and cause irritation.

4. Pain may be related to surgery or edema.
   - Relieves pain over bony prominence such as wrist or ankle.
   - Elevation and ice can decrease swelling and pain.

5. Wadded cotton padding may cause pressure in the cast and irritate the skin. Flattened or missing padding can cause the hard cast to abrade or irritate the skin.

Figure 10-11-3 Elevate the extremity to help relieve swelling and discomfort.

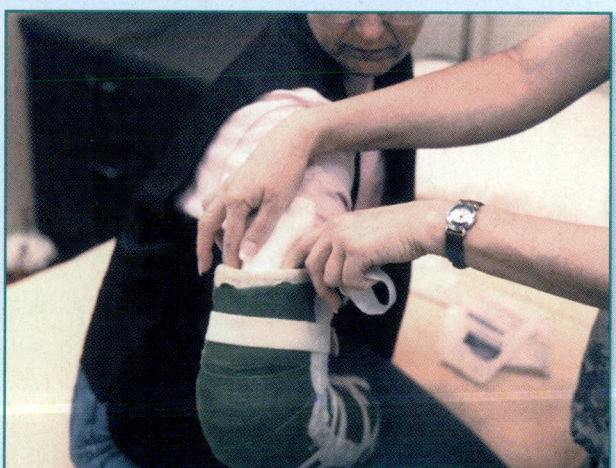

Figure 10-11-4 Add additional padding to areas where the cast is rubbing against the skin.

continues

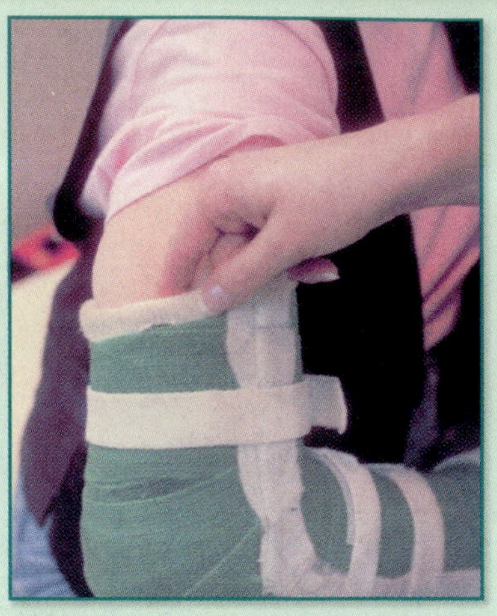

Action	Rationale

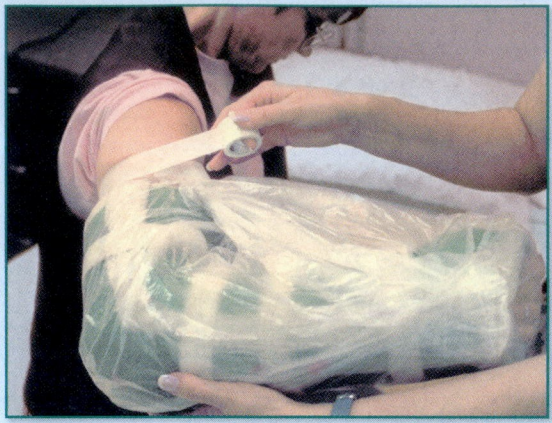

Figure 10-11-6 Keep the cast as dry as possible. Cover the cast with plastic wrap prior to bathing.

Figure 10-11-5 Gently run your fingers along the inside of the cast to detect plaster crumbs or sharp edges.

6. Assess cast for intact edges.
   - If edges are crumbling or peeling, or if the cast has been bivalved or windowed, use tape to petal the edges (see Figure 10-11-5).
   - Do not allow the cast to get wet. Teach the client how to cover the cast when bathing or showering (see Figure 10-11-6).

7. Assess safety. If cast is on a lower extremity and the client is to ambulate, provide a cast boot for protection and safety (see Figure 10-11-7).

8. Instruct client and caregiver about symptoms to report to the health care provider:
   - An increase in swelling.
   - A tingling or burning sensation.

6. Reduces skin irritation.
   - Prevents skin irritation from pieces of plaster falling into cast.

   - Wetness may cause weakness in the cast and maceration of the skin underneath the cast.

7. Reduces risk of injury.

8. Prompt reporting of symptoms will decrease risk of complications such as infection or compartmental syndrome.

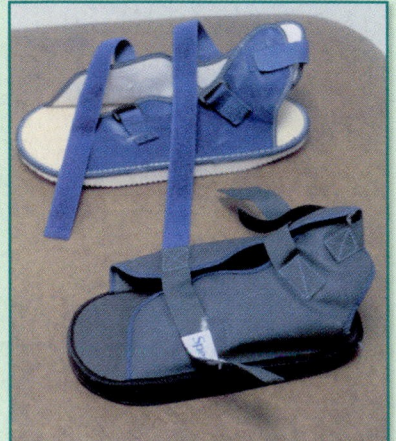

Figure 10-11-7 If the cast is on a lower extremity and the client will be ambulating, provide a cast boot for protection and safety.

continues

Action	Rationale

• An inability to move muscles around the cast.
• A foul odor around the edges of the cast.
• Any drainage, which may show through the cast.
• Any cracks or breaks in the cast.
 	
9. Support the cast.
   • Use pillows for arms and legs.
   • Use a bed board under the mattress for a spica cast.
 	
10. Assess for infection.
   • Check for foul odor under cast.
   • Check for drainage on cast.
   • Mark drainage and date on cast.
 	
11. Synthetic casts should be kept dry. If the health care provider does permit bathing or swimming, the wet cast should be dried quickly and thoroughly. Dry the cast with a towel. Allow to dry until the padding underneath does not feel cold or damp to the skin.
 	
12. Wash hands.
	
	9. Reduces risk of complications and increases client comfort.
	   • Elevating the extremity decreases edema.
	   • Provides firm support for a large cast.
	
	10. Early detection of infection will lead to appropriate treatment.
	
	11. Even though the synthetic or fiberglass can be wet, wet padding underneath the cast may macerate the skin and promote skin breakdown.
	
	12. Reduces transmission of organisms.

► REAL WORLD ANECDOTES

George was 92 years old when he fell and broke his wrist. George resisted going to the emergency department. He said, "There is nothing wrong with my arm; it just hurts a little. It will be fine tomorrow." His wife finally talked him into having a cast put on "for just a few days." About a week later, he was found in the garage at his workbench trying to saw it off. "I don't need this thing on my arm" was his response when questioned. His wife coaxed him into the house, but 2 days later he managed to cut it off. His wife called the doctor and they agreed that it would be fruitless to try to put on another cast. Fortunately, it was not a bad break and it seemed to heal without complication.

► EVALUATION

- There is no neurovascular compromise to the client while the cast is in place.
- The skin around the cast remains intact.
- The cast remains intact.
- The client is comfortable while the cast is in place.

► DOCUMENTATION

Nurses' Notes

- Document condition of skin, circulation, and neurovascular assessment.

Document on appropriate flow sheet or electronic medical record (EMR).

► CRITICAL THINKING SKILL

Introduction

Clients may complain of itching of the skin under a cast. Care should be taken to prevent skin breakdown while attempting to relieve the itching.

Possible Scenario

A man with a cast complained of itching of the skin under his short-arm cast, so he tied cotton twill tape to a wire and ran it through the cast. He removed the wire and then looped the twill tape and tied the ends together. When the itching bothered him, he tugged on the tape to pull it in a circle so it would gently scratch the itchy spot.

Possible Outcome

The wire scratched his skin slightly as he pulled it through the cast, and the twill tape irritated the skin more as he pulled it to relieve the itching. The skin began to break down and the padding curled up with the tape movement.

Prevention

Clients should be instructed about not inserting objects between the skin and the cast. Medication may be needed to control itching.

▶ VARIATIONS

Geriatric Variations:

- *Elderly clients may have fragile skin and need careful assessment to prevent breakdown.*
- *Vascular deficiency in older clients may lead to decreased circulation.*
- *Elderly clients benefit from lightweight casts so they can maintain balance and keep active.*
- *Older clients may have reduced sensation and be unable to identify pressure points.*

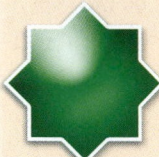

Pediatric Variations:

- *Allow children to choose the color of their fiberglass cast.*
- *Children may have curiosity about what can be put into the cast such as coins, straws, or Popsicle sticks.*
- *Infants may indicate pain in affected limb through restlessness or crying.*
- *Infants or young children in casts for club feet will have decreased mobility and require frequent cast changes.*
- *Children with spica casts will need plastic shielding over the perineum to keep the cast dry while urinating.*
- *Help children think about what clothes would be comfortable to wear over their cast.*

Home Care Variations:

- *Clients in spica casts should be turned every 2 hours to avoid pressure on skin.*
- *A bed board should be placed between the frame and mattress to provide firm support.*
- *Assess the client with a long leg cast or spica for ability to get in and out of small bathroom stalls, cars, or low chairs.*
- *Keep plastic bags and rubber bands in bathroom and kitchen for "emergency" use.*
- *Do not dispose of crumbled plaster in a sink because it can clog the plumbing.*
- *Pillows or chairs should be available to elevate the affected extremity in order to prevent edema.*
- *Pants and shirts can be cut along a seam and Velcro closures sewn in to accommodate a cast.*
- *Fiberglass casts may snag nylon or finely woven fabrics.*

▶ COMMON ERRORS

Possible Error:

The cast cracks from improper drying or stress.

Prevention:

Support the cast with pillows and allow it to dry uncovered. Use the palm of your hands, not the fingertips, when handling the cast in order to prevent indentations. If indentations occur, notify the health care provider immediately. Reassure the client and instruct not to move the casted area until the health care provider assesses it.

▶ **NURSING TIPS**

- Place a bed board under the mattress of a client with a spica cast to provide firm support.
- Use a pen to mark drainage on the cast and write the date and time.
- Check cast protection devices such as rubber bands used around plastic bags to be sure they do not act like a tourniquet.

▶ **SPECIAL CONSIDERATIONS**

- *Sometimes after surgery, a client may have a nerve block or local anesthetic in place for pain management. This will hinder movement as well as sensation for a period of time. Be aware of the types of analgesics in use with each client when performing a postoperative assessment.*

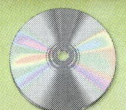

Cast Bivalving and Windowing

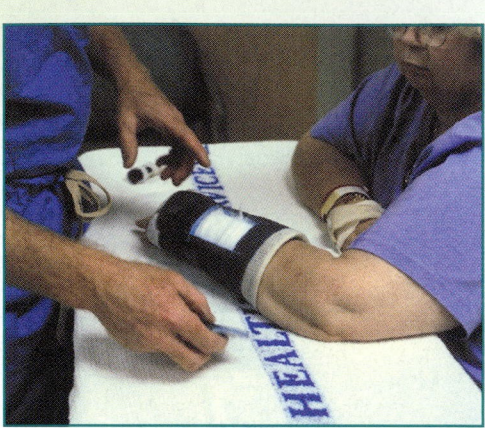

▶ OVERVIEW OF THE SKILL

Bivalving or windowing a cast is done to improve circulation, allow for skin care, and relieve pressure while continuing to maintain alignment of the bones for proper healing. Bivalving or windowing can occur immediately, or with an older cast on a fracture that is partially healed. Edema is very common after surgery or after a traumatic injury to a limb. During the first 24 hours after the application of a cast, edema can create a tourniquet effect and inhibit circulation to the tissue. This can cause irreversible damage. The abdominal area can also expand as a result of eating. Sometimes the skin under a cast needs care—an open wound, an infection, or a surgical incision, for example. Finally, discomfort and skin breakdown over a bony prominence, nerve compression, and discomfort caused by the weight of the cast are all reasons for bivalving or cutting a window in the cast.

▶ ASSESSMENT

1. After a cast has been applied, assess circulation, movement, and sensation q 1 hour × 4, q 2 hour × 4, q 4 hours × 4, then q 8 hours. **Changes in circulation, movement, and sensation may indicate the development of compartment syndrome, which would require immediate medical attention.**
2. Pain that is severe and unrelieved by medication or by repositioning, and is not proportional to the severity of the injury, requires immediate investigation by the health care provider. **This could signal the development of a compartment syndrome.** Calling the health care provider immediately if any changes occur is crucial to prevent further tissue damage.
3. Assess for severe pain over bony prominences (which can be a warning signal of a pressure sore), odor, or drainage on the cast. **These symptoms can indicate skin breakdown or infection under the cast.**

▶ DIAGNOSIS

Acute Pain

Anxiety

Ineffective Tissue Perfusion: Peripheral

Risk for Impaired Skin Integrity

Risk for Peripheral Neurovascular Dysfunction

▶ PLANNING

Expected Outcome:

1. If the purpose of the procedure is to relieve pressure, complaints and signs of pressure will diminish.
2. If the purpose of the procedure is to expose underlying skin, then the correct area will be exposed.
3. The cast will not be cracked or damaged during the procedure.

Equipment Needed (see Figure 10-12-1):
- Cast cutter
- Cast spreaders
- Bandage scissors
- Surgical or plaster knife

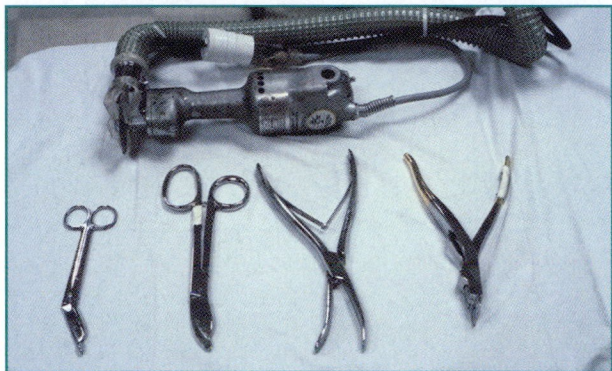

Figure 10-12-1   Cast cutter, cast spreaders, and bandage scissors

▶ **CLIENT EDUCATION NEEDED:**

1. Inform the client why the cast is being modified.
2. Explain that the cast cutter sounds and looks like a small saw, but is only a vibrating machine and will not cut the skin or do painful damage. Explain that the scissors being used are designed not to cut the skin.
3. Demonstrate the action of the blade against the palm of your hand to show that it will not hurt. Demonstrate the scissors being used.
4. Explain that after the cast is modified, it will not harm the alignment of the fracture and will continue to give proper support so that healing will occur.

Estimated time to complete the skill:
15–20 minutes

▶ **DELEGATION TIPS**

The health care provider may choose to delegate modifying the client's cast by bivalving or creating a window to a properly trained technician or the nurse practitioner. The nurse is responsible to monitor the client for improvement after the procedure. Ongoing cast care may be delegated to properly trained ancillary personnel who should be instructed to report any abnormal findings such as changes in extremity circulation, sensation, color, movement, or an increase in pain to the nurse for evaluation.

IMPLEMENTATION—Action/Rationale

Action	Rationale
1. Wash hands.	1. Reduces transmission of microorganisms.
2. Assess the client for intact cotton padding underneath the cast.	2. Even though the cast cutter will not cut the skin, heat from the cutting of the plaster and pieces of crumbling plaster can irritate the skin.
3. Remind the client that the blade will not cut and the procedure will reduce the pain.	3. Reassurance is important when the client is in pain and anxious about any procedure that involves electrical equipment or sharp instruments next to the skin.
4. Medicate the client with adequate pain medication.	4. Reducing the pain may also reduce the anxiety associated with the procedure.
5. Assist the client in placing the extremity in a comfortable position.	5. Encourages the client to relax during the procedure.

continues

Action	Rationale

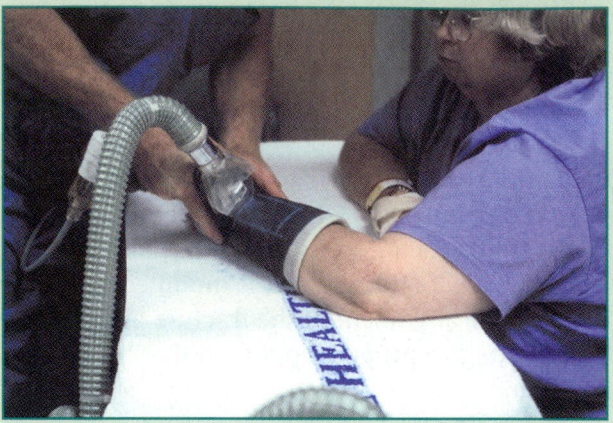

Figure 10-12-2   Use the cast cutter to cut a window out of the cast. Use a light touch, but make sure the fiberglass is cut through.

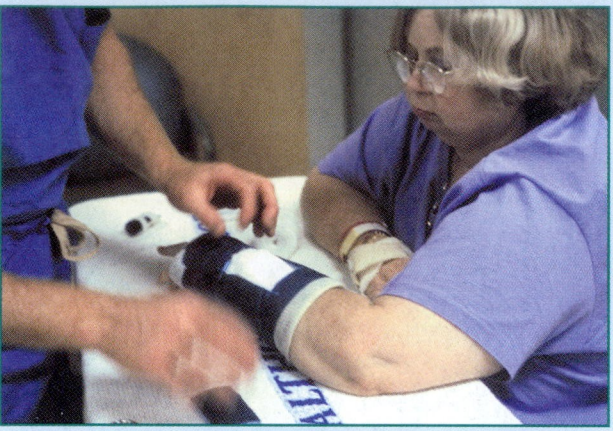

Figure 10-12-3   Remove the fiberglass window.

6. Assist in cutting the cast as requested.

6. Facilitates the procedure.

7. To window a cast, use a very light touch with the cast cutter over the appropriate area. Make sure the cast is cut through (see Figure 10-12-2).

7. Bearing down too hard will cause the blade to inflict pain to the client. The cast must be cut through for the window to be removed.

8. Remove the window (see Figure 10-12-3).

8. Exposes the padding.

9. Cut the padding away to expose the skin (see Figure 10-12-4).

9. Allows for assessment of the skin.

10. When bivalving a cast, the technician will cut along the length of the cast on each side of the limb. Assist in using cast spreaders to spread the edges of the cast, and cut the padding underneath with bandage scissors.

10. Aides in a clean cut.

11. Petal the edges of the new window or bivalve edges to prevent irritation (see Figure 10-12-5). If the edges of the new window will be exposed to drainage, urine, or feces, protect the edges of the window with plastic wrap.

11. Prevents skin irritation and maintains a clean cast.

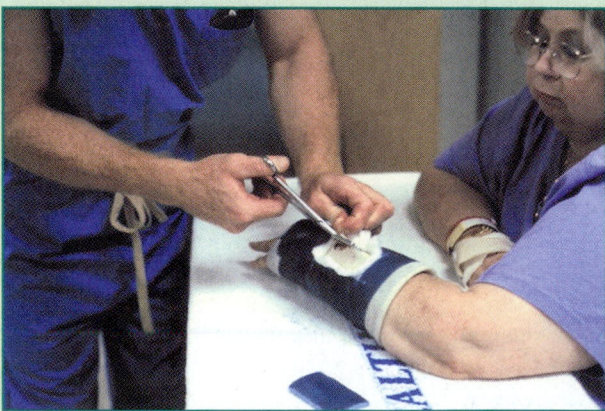

Figure 10-12-4   Cut the padding and stockinette away to inspect the skin.

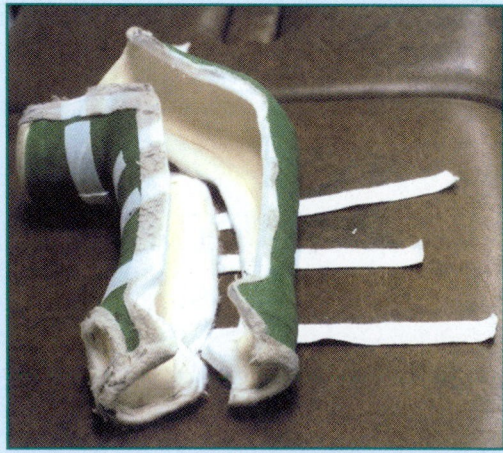

Figure 10-12-5   The edges of this bivalved cast have been protected with additional padding to reduce skin irritation.

continues

Action	Rationale

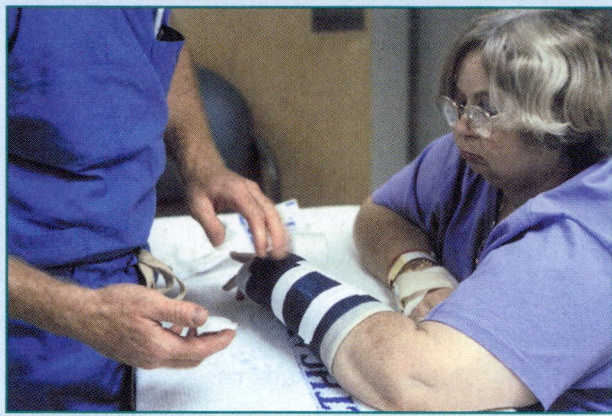

Figure 10-12-6 The window has been replaced and is held in place by tape.

Figure 10-12-7 The bivalved cast maintains immobilization of the area, but pressure has been released.

12. Secure the cast together with Velcro, Ace wrap, or tape (see Figures 10-12-6 and 10-12-7).

13. Assess neurovascular status.

14. Wash hands.

12. Maintains cast stability and immobilization of the area. Establishes baseline assessment.

13. Establishes baseline assessment

14. Reduces the transmission of microorganisms.

▶ **REAL WORLD ANECDOTES**

Bob fell off a ladder at work and was admitted to the hospital with a diagnosis of a right calcaneal fracture. After a lengthy operation, Bob arrived on the unit with his right foot and leg in a large plaster cast, with only his toes showing. Over the next 4 hours, things went fine. Bob had some pain but it was easily relieved by the use of prescribed medications. During the night, he started complaining of increased pain that was severe and unrelenting even after taking his pain medications. Efforts to reposition his leg did not relieve this excruciating pain. Referring to the flow sheets that were started by the previous shift, it appeared that Bob's toes were cool instead of warm, which was recorded. On assessment, it was noted that a disparity existed between toes on his left foot and those on his right. When Bob was asked to move his toes, he was barely able to extend them. When the nurse extended his toes, Bob cried out in agony. This was quite different from only a few hours before when he had no trouble at all moving his toes. The physician was notified and came to assess the situation. The physician decided to bivalve Bob's cast to relieve the pressure. Bob was premedicated, the procedure was explained, and the cast was bivalved. The client reported that he was much more comfortable. His toes were pink, and he continued to improve.

▶ **EVALUATION**

- If the purpose of the procedure was to relieve pressure, complaints and signs of pressure have diminished.
- If the purpose of the procedure was to expose the underlying skin, then the correct area was exposed.

- The cast was not cracked or damaged during the procedure.

▶ **DOCUMENTATION**

Nurses' Notes

- Indicate the signs and symptoms that preceded the cast cutting, and the neurovascular and skin evaluation following the event.

- Record the circulation, movement, and sensation checks before and after the procedure.
- Document the type of cut made and how the client tolerated the procedure.

Document on appropriate flow sheet or electronic medical record (EMR).

▶ CRITICAL THINKING SKILL

Introduction

Decisions regarding cast alterations must be made on the basis of all available information.

Possible Scenario

The client complained of postsurgical pain in the right lower extremity, which increased significantly after getting up to ambulate 48 hours after surgery. Assessments were made including capillary refill, ability to move toes, color of toes, temperature, drainage, sensation, and edema, which all appeared to be normal and unchanged. The pain was relieved by elevation and ice. The nurse practitioner, erring on the side of caution, bivalved the cast anyway.

Possible Outcome

The cast was bivalved unnecessarily. The physician opted to replace the cast prior to the client's discharge the next day.

Prevention

Assessment must include all the information available. The surgical report, neurovascular status, fever, pain, drainage, and the overall condition of the client must be taken into consideration to form an overall picture prior to implementing any procedure. If the pain did not subside and there were other abnormal findings upon assessment, then further investigation by the physician or nurse practitioner would have been necessary.

▶ VARIATIONS

Geriatric Variations:
- *Older adults may need more reassurance that the procedure is not painful.*
- *More care must be taken when using the cast saw. A very light touch should be used because the skin in an older adult may be more fragile.*

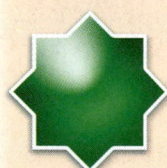

Pediatric Variations:
- *Pediatric clients may not be able to verbally express themselves regarding increased pain when assessing a cast that may be too tight. Use of other assessment skills is imperative.*
- *Pediatric clients' fear of the unknown and a noisy cast saw can be extremely frightening. Having a parent to aid in comforting the child is important.*
- *Demonstration of the instrument as well as allowing the child to touch them when appropriate may help in alleviating some anxiety.*
- *Pediatric clients can also develop compartmental syndrome, which is why it is important to assess these clients even more frequently than adults.*

Home Care Variations:
- *Instruct the client not to remove the bivalved cast without specific orders from the health care provider.*
- *See cast care instructions in Skill 10-11 for the home care client.*

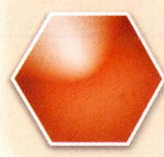

Long-Term Care Variations:
- *In a windowed cast the exposed skin may swell through the window, causing pressure sores and circulatory compromise. Teach the client to watch for this.*
- *See cast care in Skill 10-11 for the long-term care client.*

▶ COMMON ERRORS

Possible Error:

Failing to reassure the client that the saw will cut the cast but not the skin.

Prevention:

Be sure the client understands that the saw will not cut the skin before starting the procedure. Demonstrate on yourself to ease the client's fears. Small children may need extra assurance.

▶ NURSING TIPS

- Make sure cast is lined with soft material before cutting it.
- Fully describe the procedure to the client.
- Premedicate as needed.

- Familiarize yourself with all the tools and equipment prior to implementing the procedure.
- Assessment of the client is imperative.

▶ SPECIAL CONSIDERATIONS

- *Many times a window is cut during the initial placement of the cast. Postprocedural management of windows includes assessment of the neurovascular status and assessment of the skin under the window.*
- *Maintain padding around window as well as petal the edges of the cast as needed for client comfort.*
- *Monitor a bivalved cast to be sure it does not loosen and become ineffective.*

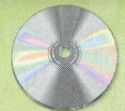

Cast Removal

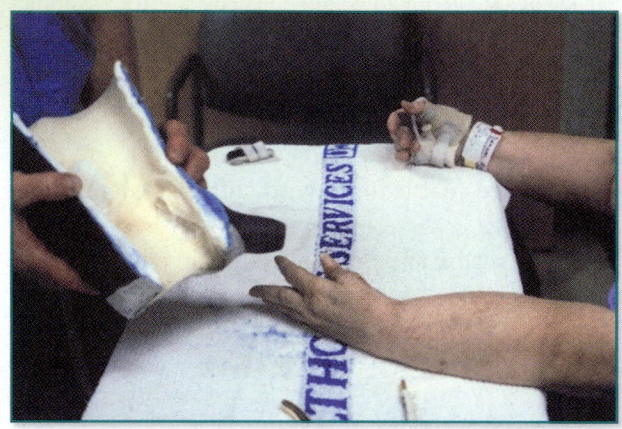

▶ OVERVIEW OF THE SKILL

After a period of 6 to 8 weeks, or as needed, a cast may be removed. This involves taking off the cast and instructing clients what to expect when the cast is removed (and possible replacement of the cast). Assess the cast site for healing and/or irritation to the skin. If the cast is fairly new and is being replaced, assess for condition, length of time the cast has been on, and the need for further client education in the care of the cast. If the cast has been replaced several times already and is now being removed permanently, the client will already be familiar with the procedures, while clients with new casts being replaced will need information on what procedures will be done. Once the case is off, assess the skin under the cast and assess the injury site for signs of healing or complications.

▶ ASSESSMENT

1. Determine whether the client is having the cast removed permanently or whether a new cast is being applied. **Knowing this information will assist you in having the proper supplies available during the cast removal and the amount of information the client will need about the procedures.**
2. Determine if there is any suspected disruption in skin integrity under the cast. **This will determine how carefully the cast needs to be**
removed, and what skin care will be needed. **It may affect how a cast is reapplied.**
3. Determine how many weeks the fracture has been healing. **This will determine how carefully the cast needs to be removed.**
4. Determine the condition of the cast. **This will tell you how much additional client education is necessary if the cast is being replaced and was not being properly cared for.**
5. If this is a final cast removal, do a range of motion and muscle strength test. **This will give you an idea of what further care and rehabilitation the client will need. The client may need assistance moving without the cast.**

▶ DIAGNOSIS

Acute Pain

Anxiety

Impaired Physical Mobility

Impaired Skin Integrity

▶ PLANNING

Expected Outcomes:

1. The cast will be removed successfully from the client.
2. Client will remain safe after the removal of the cast.
3. Proper equipment will be given to the client on discharge.

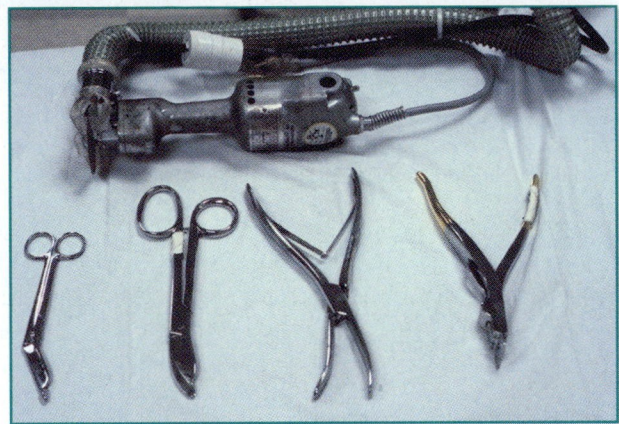

Figure 10-13-1   Cast cutter, cast spreaders, and bandage scissors

Equipment Needed (see Figure 10-13-1):

- Cast removal saw
- Protective towel or waterproof pad
- Bandage scissors
- Cast splitter
- Water, washcloth, towels, basin, or sink

▶ CLIENT EDUCATION NEEDED:

1. Educate the client that the saw is noisy.
2. Educate the client that he or she will feel warmth and vibration, but the saw will not cut the skin.
3. Demonstrate by holding the saw against the skin.
4. Educate the client on the need to hold the cast still.
5. Educate the client on how the affected limb will look and feel after the cast is removed. Remind the client that the skin will be pale and thin looking, hair growth may have occurred, and there might be a buildup of dead skin cells.
6. Caution the client that the area might feel tender and the muscles previously under the cast might feel weak.
7. Review cast care instructions with the client if there is any evidence of improper care or signs that the client has tampered with the cast.
8. Educate the client after cast removal on the care of the skin and the use of the affected area.
9. During early stages of healing, cast manipulation may cause the injury to ache, even though it has not been painful before manipulation. Discuss pain control techniques, elevation, and restricting range of movement with the client.

Estimated time to complete the skill: **5–20 minutes, depending on the size of the cast**

▶ DELEGATION TIPS

Assisting the health care provider with cast removal may be delegated to properly trained ancillary personnel. After cast removal, client education is the responsibility of the nurse.

IMPLEMENTATION—Action/Rationale

Action	Rationale
1. Wash hands.	1. Reduces the transmission of microorganisms.
2. Introduce yourself to client and explain the planned procedure.	2. Educates the client.
3. Assess neurovascular status.	3. Establishes a baseline for post removal comparison.
4. Communicate with the client during the entire process.	4. Decreases client's anxiety level.

continues

Action	Rationale
5. Prepare equipment and have it at bedside.	5. Facilitates an efficient practice.
6. Prepare environment and client.	6. Have client in proper position for cast removal.
7. Wear protective clothing as needed.	7. Practices clean technique.
8. Prepare client for how extremity will look after reduction. Extremity will look thinner than nonfractured site. Mobility will be less than nonfractured site.	8. Prepares client for what to expect and decreases anxiety.
9. Client may need to continue to use crutches or immobilizer until full mobility of extremity is regained.	9. Client education helps prevent reinjury of fracture.
10. The cast removal technician will cut the cast with the saw (see Figure 10-13-2). Support the limb in the proper position as requested.	10. Ensures a safe and smooth cut.
11. The cast technician will split the cast with a cast splitter, and cut the padding underneath (see Figure 10-13-3).	11. Splitting the cast and cutting the padding allows the cast to be removed.

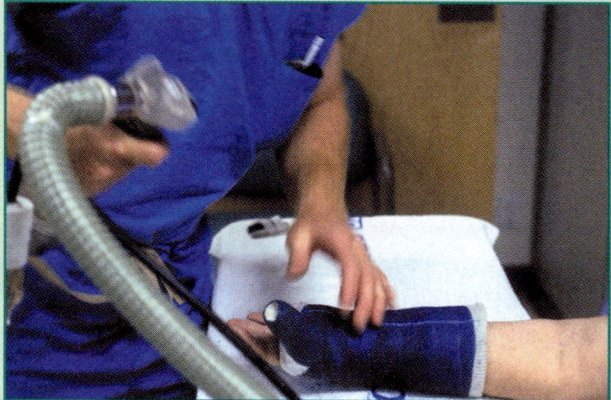

Figure 10-13-2   The cast is cut with the cast cutter down opposite sides.

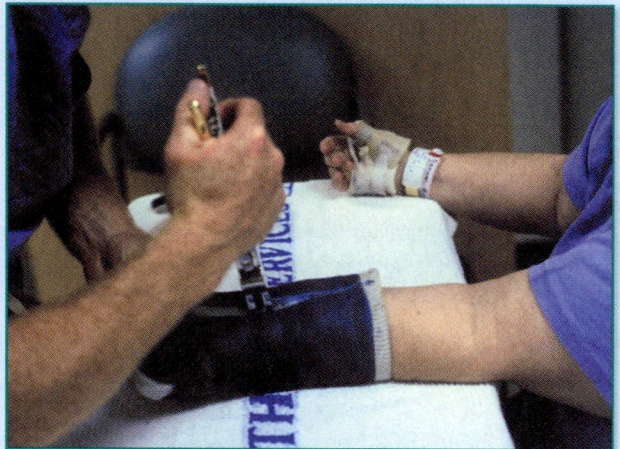

Figure 10-13-3   After the cast has been split apart with the cast splitter, the padding and stockinette underneath are cut apart.

Action	Rationale
12. The cast technician will then pull the cast apart and remove it. Support the limb and reassure the client, as this step can be anxiety producing and sometimes uncomfortable (see Figure 10-13-4).	12. Reduces client anxiety.
13. Assess the skin underneath the cast. Gently clean the skin with warm water. Do not rub or use friction on the skin.	13. Provides comfort, hygiene, and allows for detection of pressure sores or marks under the skin.
14. Apply Ace wrap after cast removal as needed.	14. Supports injured joint.

continues

Action	Rationale

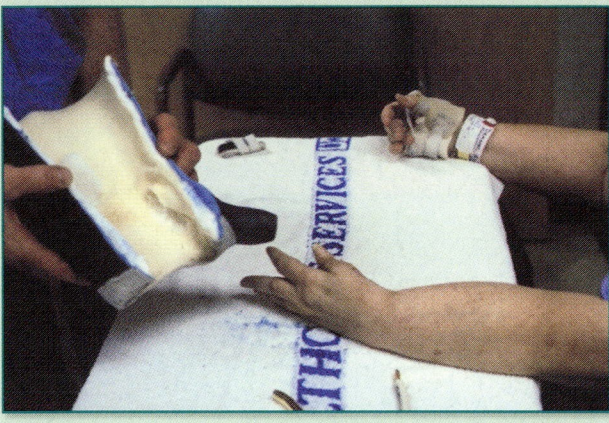

Figure 10-13-4   The cast has been pulled apart and removed from the limb.

15. Document the cast removal, include the extremity where the cast was removed, assessment of the extremity, and assessment of the skin underneath the cast.

16. Wash hands.

15. Records implementation of intervention and provides baseline data.

16. Reduces the transmission of microorganisms.

▶ REAL WORLD ANECDOTES

Jerry had a series of casts on his left wrist for 10 weeks. He was so excited about getting his cast off, he planned a full day of golf with his golfing buddies. The next day, he was back in the physician's office complaining of severe muscle pain. His left forearm hurt so badly he was sure he had refractured the bone. Like many clients, Jerry expected to have full range of motion and use of the extremity after the cast was removed. Protect your client from further injury by preventing him from full use of the extremity before he is ready. Good education at cast removal time could have saved Jerry a great deal of pain and inconvenience.

▶ EVALUATION

- Cast was removed successfully from the client.
- Client remains safe after the removal of the cast.
- Proper equipment was given to the client on discharge.

▶ DOCUMENTATION

Nurses' Notes

- Document what type of cast was removed and where it was removed.
- Make a notation on how the extremity looks, its range of motion, strength, and skin assessment.

- Document any specific aids that the client will use after cast removal, for example, slings, immobilizers, and crutches.

Document on appropriate flow sheet or electronic medical record (EMR).

▶ CRITICAL THINKING SKILL

Introduction

Nurses must be able to evaluate range of motion and muscle strength of an extremity.

Possible Scenario

Your client has a cast removed from his leg. You are called out of the room before you can assess the range of motion or strength of the extremity.

The client decides he needs a drink of water and gets off the table.

Possible Outcome
The client falls and refractures the leg.

Prevention
Client education about decreased use of the fractured extremity is important. You should evaluate strength and range of motion of extremity and communicate results with the client.

▶ VARIATIONS

Geriatric Variation:
- *Elderly clients may take longer to recover muscle function.*

Pediatric Variations:
- *Children will be afraid of the cast saw and need extra support and extra time for education.*
- *Allow children to help, if possible.*
- *Allow children to keep the cast.*
- *The saw used to take off the cast is loud. Show it to the child before it is used. Show them how it works and the sound it makes. If possible, show the child that it will not hurt or cut them.*
- *Children may use sharp objects to scratch under the cast. Assess for this carefully.*

Home Care Variation:
- *Caution clients who are tempted to remove a cast at home to not do so. A cast taken off too early can lead to long-term dysfunction in the limb, excess pain, and more trips to the doctor.*

▶ COMMON ERRORS

Possible Error:
Not preparing the client for the sound and feel of the cast saw.

Prevention:
Demonstrate the use of the saw. Explain the sight, sounds, and sensations.

▶ NURSING TIPS
- The saw is loud; prepare your client for its sound.
- Assure the client that the saw will not cut him or her.
- Save the cast, especially for children; they may want it for a souvenir.

▶ SPECIAL CONSIDERATIONS
- *After removal of a cast, muscles will be weak. Education about therapy exercises and plan for continuing care is important to decrease risk of further injury.*
- *Educate the client to the appearance of a previously casted body part, including changes in color, shape, and skin, to reduce client anxiety.*

Assisting with a Continuous Passive Motion Device

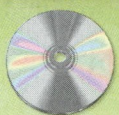

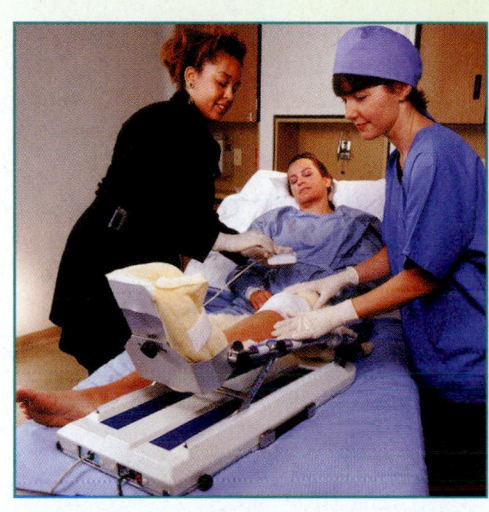

▶ OVERVIEW OF THE SKILL

Clients recovering from surgical procedures to synovial joints, fractures, contractures, and general immobility may benefit from continuous passive motion (CPM). CPM facilitates joint range of motion (ROM), promotes wound healing, prevents formation of adhesions, decreases edema, and decreases the effects of immobility.

The parameters of the CPM device include the amount of time it is to be used each day, the amount of ROM prescribed, and the speed of passive movement generated by the unit. The CPM device includes a single-use client softgoods kit to comfortably position the involved extremity in the unit. The unit also has a stop-and-go switch so the client can turn off the unit if extreme discomfort is produced. There are many different types and models of CPM units available, so be sure to familiarize yourself with the softgoods kit and the control parameters of your unit before attempting to apply it to the client.

Neurovascular assessment of the client using the CPM unit is essential. This assessment confirms that the client's vascular and neural structures are not compromised by postsurgical complications, client positioning in the unit, or by excessive ROM positions during the procedure.

The presence of edema in the involved extremity may greatly limit the ability of the client to achieve prescribed ROM goals. Therefore edema must be monitored and adjustments made accordingly to unit control settings. Any indications of vessel disease, thrombophlebitis, or infections must be noted and cleared with the health care provider before administration.

▶ ASSESSMENT

1. Assess orders for CPM usage including frequency, duration, degree of range of motion (ROM), and restrictions to ROM for the involved extremity **to verify that the correct procedure is being followed.**
2. Neurovascular assessment of the involved extremity before the start of CPM usage includes sensation, skin color, temperature, and presence of pulses. **Establishes a baseline for future comparisons.**
3. Assess movement of the involved extremity **to determine whether the procedure is appropriate.**
4. Pay attention to client's report of pain and discomfort. **Pain assessment is helpful in reports to the health care provider to determine whether treatment is appropriate.**

► **DIAGNOSIS**

Activity Intolerance

Acute Pain

Impaired Physical Mobility

Risk for Impaired Skin Integrity

Risk for Peripheral Neurovascular Dysfunction

► **PLANNING**

Expected Outcomes:

1. Will facilitate joint range of motion.
2. Will promote wound healing.
3. Will prevent formation of adhesions.
4. Edema, both peripheral and central, will decrease.
5. Effects of immobility will decrease.

Equipment Needed:

- CPM device
- CPM softgoods
- Tape measure

► **CLIENT EDUCATION NEEDED:**

1. Client should understand reason for and use of CPM.
2. Client should understand plan to increase duration, speed, and ROM of CPM.
3. Client should understand use of CPM stop-and-go button.
4. Client should understand signs and symptoms to report related to effects or changes in physical condition.

Estimated time to complete the skill: **15 minutes**

► **DELEGATION TIPS**

The application of the CPM machine is the responsibility of the nurse. A neurovascular assessment and proper setting of the machine according to the health care provider's orders is required. Ancillary personnel may be instructed in techniques for client care while the machine is in place and to report any increase in pain or any changes in the affected extremity to the nurse.

IMPLEMENTATION—Action/Rationale

Action	Rationale
1. Wash hands.	1. Reduces transmission of microorganisms.
2. Explain procedure to client and instruct regarding reportable signs and symptoms or untoward effects.	2. Decreases anxiety; improves client compliance and cooperation.
3. Raise bed to comfortable working height and lower side rails.	3. Protects caregiver from back injury or muscle strain.
4. Position CPM device on the bed and install client softgoods kit to unit. For client comfort and safety make sure kit extends over metal support tubes of device.	4. Protects client from skin chafing on exposed metal.
5. Set CPM controls according to health care provider's order: check for ROM limitations, speed, and duration of movement. Ensure CPM stops are properly adjusted to settings.	5. Provides for client safety and maximizes therapeutic outcomes.

continues

Action	Rationale
6. Measure client from the hip joint to the knee and from knee to slightly beyond the bottom of the foot. Adjust length of CPM device to correspond to upper and lower leg measurements.	6. Provides for proper fit and positioning of CPM device.
7. Confirm that CPM device is adjusted to accept appropriate extremity.	7. Some CPM devices may be set up for various extremities.
8. Position client in the middle of the bed with involved extremity slightly abducted to accommodate CPM device. Lock knee control on bed in the straight position so the knee section will not bend when the head of the bed goes up or down.	8. Provides for proper positioning of CPM device and prevents the effects of poor or improper positioning.
9. Place client's extremity in unit, maintaining proper anatomic placement of extremity in relation to CPM device. Align knee joint with corresponding hinge point on unit. Make sure leg is not internally or externally rotated. Best adjustment can be made with the CPM in its fully extended position (see Figure 10-14-1).	9. Provides for client safety through proper positioning of involved extremity in CPM device.
10. Make appropriate adjustments to the foot pad so the client's foot rests comfortably against the pad and the remainder of his leg is well supported (see Figure 10-14-2).	10. Provides for client safety and comfort.
11. Apply CPM restraining straps so that client's extremity maintains position in device. Be sure not to apply straps too snugly so that circulation will not be compromised (see Figure 10-14-3).	11. Provides for client safety and comfort.

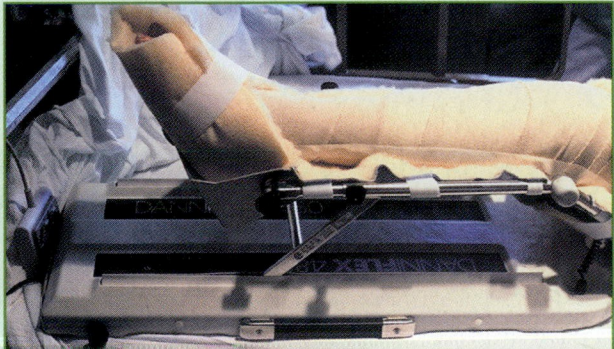

Figure 10-14-1 Make sure the knee lines up with the hinge and the leg is not internally or externally rotated.

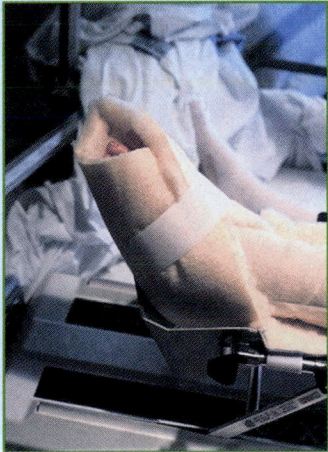

Figure 10-14-2 Adjust the foot pad so the foot rests comfortably. Add protective padding if needed.

continues

Action	Rationale
12. If you are satisfied with the CPM control settings and the client's position, start the CPM by turning the unit on. The operation of the unit should be closely monitored for the first several cycles to make sure the client is comfortable. The speed of the CPM is determined by the client's comfort. To maximize client comfort, start slowly and increase speed as client tolerates (see Figure 10-14-4).	12. Provides for client safety, comfort, and appropriate therapeutic outcome.
13. Give the client the CPM stop-and-go switch so he or she can turn off the unit in case of extreme discomfort.	13. Provides for client safety. Provides for sense of self-care and control if untoward effects occur.
14. Replace side rails to their upright position as well as lowering bed to starting height.	14. Provides for client safety.
15. Place the call light within reach of the client. Move the bedside table close to the bed and place items of frequent use within reach of the client.	15. Provides for client safety and comfort.
16. Wash hands.	16. Reduces the transmission of microorganisms.
17. Chart the specifics of the treatment and the response of the client.	17. Provides documentation of care and evidence of client response.

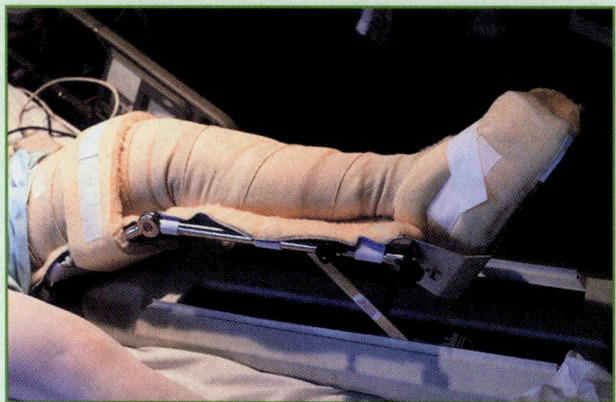

Figure 10-14-3 Apply the restraining strap snugly, but do not restrict circulation.

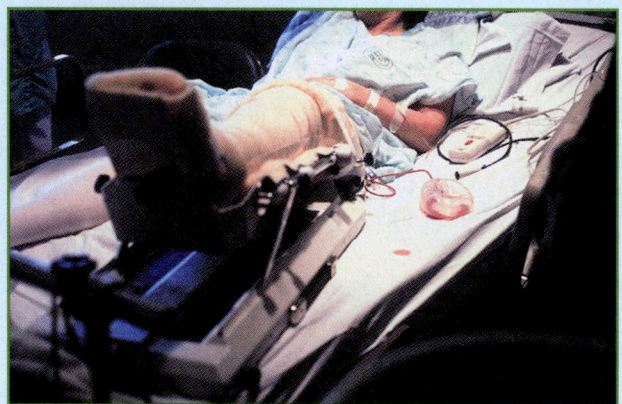

Figure 10-14-4 Observe the unit closely for the first several cycles to make sure the unit is working properly and the client is comfortable.

▶ REAL WORLD ANECDOTES

After knee surgery, Mr. Mason was discharged home with a CPM machine to prevent adhesions and provide gentle movement. When the home health nurse stopped by the next day Mr. Mason was not using the CPM machine. When asked about it, Mr. Mason became angry, shouting about the machine not working right. He told the nurse that it was a waste of time to use it. When the nurse examined the CPM machine it appeared to be in working order. The nurse then asked Mr. Mason to place his leg and knee in the machine so she could evaluate its function. Mr. Mason placed the machine correctly and turned it on. Within seconds Mr. Mason was exclaiming that the machine obviously didn't work, that it wasn't moving. While the nurse had Mr. Mason watch carefully she pointed out that the CPM machine was not supposed to provide vigorous exercise, just slow, constant motion. Once Mr. Mason realized that the CPM machine was indeed working the way it was supposed to, he used it successfully.

► EVALUATION

- Facilitated joint range of motion.
- Promoted wound healing.
- Prevented formation of adhesions.
- Edema, both peripheral and central, was decreased.
- Effects of immobility were decreased.

► DOCUMENTATION

Nurses' Notes

- Duration of CPM usage, including start and stop time
- CPM control parameters used, including ROM achieved
- Client's tolerance of procedure
- Neurovascular status of client's involved extremity
- Skin integrity

Document on appropriate flow sheet or electronic medical record (EMR).

► CRITICAL THINKING SKILL

Introduction

Client understanding and cooperation is essential to the use of the CPM machine.

Possible Scenario

Mrs. Frank has just returned to the unit following knee surgery with orders for a CPM machine. As you place the machine and explain its purpose you note that Mrs. Frank is still sleepy. Mrs. Frank's knee and leg remain in good alignment during the routine postoperative checks and she is resting quietly. After the routine postoperative checks are completed, another client returns from surgery, and it is several hours before you check on Mrs. Frank again. When you do return to check on Mrs. Frank, you find that she has tried to roll over in her sleep. Because she is still groggy, she did not realize the CPM machine was in place and she has twisted her leg sideways in the machine. Her leg is now out of alignment and rubbing against the hinge of the machine.

Possible Outcome

Mrs. Frank has an open area where her leg has been rubbing against the hinge, which results in a prolonged recovery time and unnecessary pain.

Prevention

Be sure the client is capable of understanding the reasons for the CPM machine and cooperating with its use. Wait until the client is more attentive or have a family member stay at the bedside to watch the client.

► VARIATIONS

Geriatric Variations:

- *With aging, neurologic and concomitant neurosensory responses, including reduced sensations of pain, must be noted.*
- *The skin of the elderly is sensitive and more easily "gouged," so attention to skin integrity is paramount. Breaks in skin integrity naturally lead to a compromised state of possible infection.*

Pediatric Variations:

- *Explanations of the device in understandable, analogous terms is essential to decrease anxiety in the child, such as utilizing a doll or stuffed animal to share the experience with the child.*
- *During the treatment, arrangements for social or creative activities that are developmentally appropriate will also facilitate the effect of the treatment; for example, relaxed muscles improve circulation, which enhances movement.*

continues

▶ VARIATIONS *(continued)*

Home Care Variations:
- *Adaptations include posturing and positioning in the home based on bed heights or other reclined positions to properly administer the treatment.*
- *Special attention to the stability of the machinery is important.*
- *It is important to monitor and educate the client about skin care.*

Long-Term Care Variations:
- *Clients (children, adults, or the elderly) who are participants in long-term care services must be attended to with equivalent concerns, that is, safe, correct, effective care to provide appropriate treatment followed by proper posturing, positioning, and careful skin care.*
- *Pay attention to individual responses, for example, sensory, motor, pain, or discomfort.*

▶ COMMON ERRORS

Possible Error:

Not anatomically aligning client's knee joint properly with hinge joint of CPM.

Prevention:

Align knee joint with corresponding hinge point on unit. Make sure leg is not internally or externally rotated. Best adjustment can be made with the CPM in its fully extended position.

▶ NURSING TIPS

- Familiarize yourself with the CPM unit prior to applying it to a client.
- Make sure client's involved extremity is correctly and comfortably positioned in CPM unit.
- Make sure client's joints correctly align with the CPM's hinge joints.
- Check control settings prior to applying CPM to client.
- Regularly monitor neurovascular status of client's involved extremity.
- Flexion should be increased until maximum flexion ordered has been reached. Do not decrease flexion unless ordered.
- After time, the CPM machine may move towards the foot of the bed, or the extremity may slip out of alignment with the motion; readjust as needed to maintain proper body alignment.

▶ SPECIAL CONSIDERATIONS

- *Sometimes a health care provider will order a degree of flexion that is too much for the client to begin with. Start at a lower flexion and increase periodically throughout therapy. Consult with health care provider regarding goal.*
- *In large or obese clients the adjustment knobs at the hip end of the machine may rub the scrotum or perineum. Be sure to monitor skin and pad knobs as needed.*
- *After a long period without use, the affected joint may become stiff and more painful with movement.*
- *During therapy session start slowly. Do not allow too much time between therapy sessions. This practice may alleviate some pain at the start of each session.*
- *Remember that the degrees marked by the machine are a rough estimate. The knee never goes completely flat while in the machine; therefore it is necessary for the extremity to be out of the machine for a period of time each day to maintain full extension and flexion.*

Assisting with Crutches, Cane, or Walker

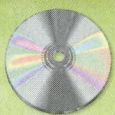

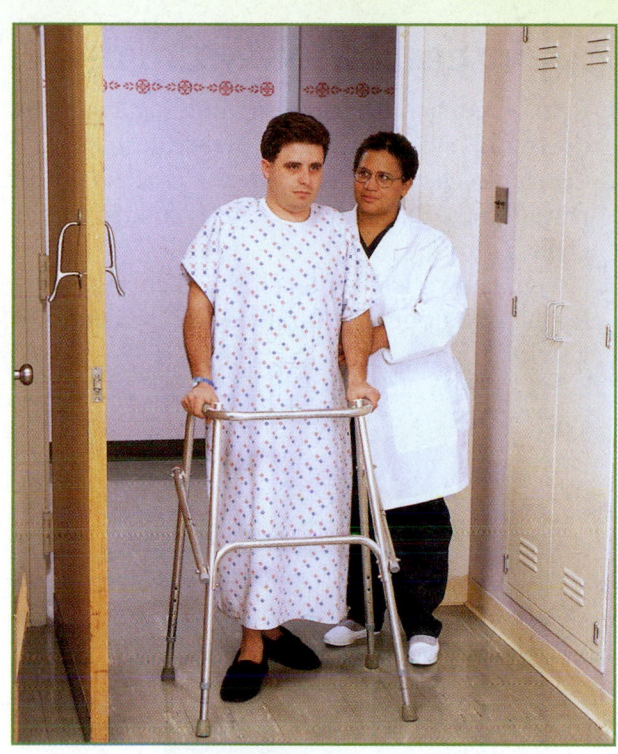

▶ **OVERVIEW OF THE SKILL**

Independence is an important part of a client's recovery process. Being able to move about in the environment can be the difference between living at home and living in a health care facility. Being able to move independently improves a client's emotional, mental, and physical well-being.

Clients who cannot safely walk unassisted can use devices designed to aid them in walking independently. The three most common devices used are crutches, canes, and walkers.

The appropriate device for each client is determined by the client's health care provider, physical therapist, or nurse. Often these caregivers work together to determine which device will be best for the client. This decision is based on the client's ability to bear weight on the legs, upper arm strength, stamina, and the presence or absence of unilateral weakness.

Crutches can be used by clients who cannot bear any weight on one leg, clients who can only bear partial weight on one leg, and clients who have full weight bearing ability on both legs. There are several types of crutches available, depending on the length of time the client will require the assistance and the client's upper body strength.

A cane is used by clients who can bear weight on both legs but one leg or hip is weaker or impaired. There are several types of canes as well. The standard, straight cane is used most often. There are also canes with three or four legs on the end, called quad canes, to increase a client's stability when walking.

Walkers are used by clients who require more support than a cane provides. Walkers are available with or without wheels. Walkers without wheels provide the most stability but they must be lifted with each step. Walkers with wheels are somewhat less stable but a client who does not have the upper body strength to lift the walker repeatedly can push it along while walking. Mobility is an important part of everyone's life. The ability to get around can contribute greatly to a client's well-being.

▶ ASSESSMENT

1. Assess the reason the client requires an assistive device. Is the need long-term or a short-term one? **This helps determine which device to use.**
2. Assess the client's physical limitations. How much weight is the client able to bear? Can the client bear weight on both legs or just one? Is the upper body strength good? Does the client tire easily? **Assesses safety and comfort.**
3. Assess the client's physical environment. Is the client at home or in a medical facility? Is the environment suited to assistive needs and the assistive device the client will be using? Are the hallways wide enough? Well lit? Are the doorways wide enough? Are there stairs used frequently and, if so, how many? Do the doors swing open far enough? **Assesses safety and comfort.**
4. Assess the client's ability to understand and follow directions regarding use of an assistive device. Can the client understand the instructions? Can he or she remember them? Has the client used this device in the past? Is there a language barrier that might limit understanding? **Assesses safety, educational, comfort, and effectiveness.**

▶ DIAGNOSIS

Activity Intolerance

Deficient Knowledge

Impaired Physical Mobility

Risk for Falls

▶ PLANNING

Expected Outcomes:

1. The client will be able to demonstrate safe and independent ambulation with the assistance of crutches, a cane, or a walker.

2. The client will feel confident and safe while using the assistive device.

Equipment Needed (see Figure 10-15-1):

- Gait belt
- Assistive device: crutches, cane, or walker
- Tape measure
- Nonslip footwear

▶ CLIENT EDUCATION NEEDED:

1. Reinforce teaching regarding holding a cane on the "good" side rather than the weak side.
2. Teach the client not to allow the crutch pad to rest in the axilla. This can cause damage to the client's arm.
3. When using a walker, teach the client not to let the walker get too far ahead of the center of gravity.

Estimated time to complete the skill: **30 minutes**

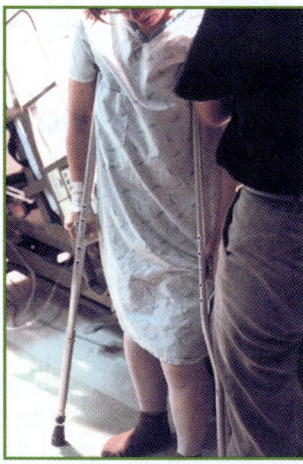

Figure 10-15-1 Crutches, braces, and walkers are used to assist ambulation.

▶ DELEGATION TIPS

Ambulation of clients with assistive devices is frequently delegated to ancillary personnel. The initial teaching of and ongoing assessment of the proper use of the device is not delegated. The nurse or physical or occupational therapist is responsible to observe the client's technique, to demonstrate it again if necessary, and document the client's proficiency.

IMPLEMENTATION—Action/Rationale

Action	Rationale
Crutch Walking	
1. Inform client that you will be assisting with ambulation using the device chosen.	1. Reduces anxiety and helps increase comprehension and cooperation.
2. Assess client for strength, mobility, range of motion, visual acuity, perceptual difficulties and balance. *Note:* The nurse and physical therapist often work together on assessment and choosing the correct assistive equipment of ambulation.	2. Helps determine the client's capabilities and amount of assistance required.
3. Measure client for size of crutches and adjust crutches to fit. While supine, measure client from heel to axilla.	3. Correct fit increases client safety and comfort.
4. Provide a robe or other covering as well as nonslip foot coverings or shoes.	4. Provides for privacy and safety.
5. Lower the height of the bed.	5. Allows client to sit with feet on the floor and increases safety.
6. Dangle the client at the side of the bed for several minutes. Assess for vertigo or nausea.	6. Allows for stabilization of blood pressure, thus preventing orthostatic hypotension; also increases client comfort.
7. Apply gait belt around the client's waist if balance and stability are unknown or unreliable. It is good practice to use a gait belt the first time the client is out of bed.	7. Provides support and promotes safety.
8. Instruct client on method of holding crutches while he or she remains seated. This should be with elbows bent 30 degrees while hands are on the hand grips and pads 1.5 to 2 inches below the axilla (see Figure 10-15-2). Instruct client to position crutches 4 to 5 inches laterally and 4 to 6 inches in front of feet. This skill can be demonstrated on yourself to increase client understanding.	8. Increases comprehension and cooperation, decreases anxiety.

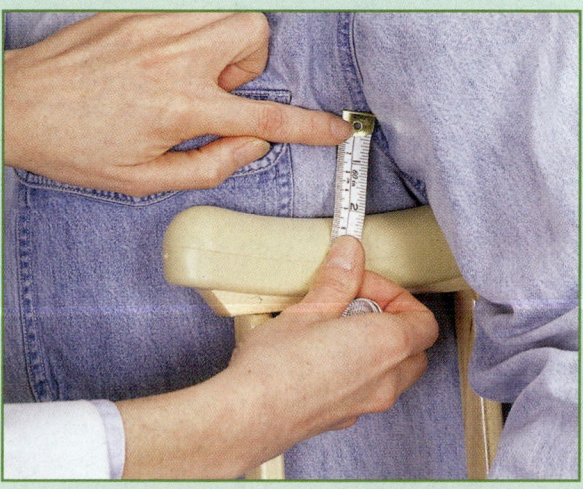

Figure 10-15-2 Adjusting the crutches to fit the client will increase comfort and stability.

continues

Action	Rationale
Crutch Walking *continued*	
9. Assist the client to a standing position by placing both crutches in the nondominant hand. Then, using the dominant hand, push off from the bed while using the crutches for balance. Once erect, the extra crutch can be moved into the dominant hand.	9. Allows for stability while promoting independence.
10. Instruct the client to remain still for a few seconds while assessing for vertigo or nausea. Stand close to the client to support as needed. While client remains standing, check for correct fit of the crutches. The client's body weight should be supported on the hands and arms, not in the axillary area.	10. Promotes client comfort, support, and safety. If the client becomes dizzy, sit client back down and wait before trying again. Pressure in the axillary area can cause damage to nerves and blood vessels.
Four-Point Gait (see Figure 10-15-3)	
11. Position the crutches 4.5 to 6 inches to the side and in front of each foot. Move the right crutch forward 4 to 6 inches and move the left foot forward, even with the left crutch. Move the left crutch forward 4 to 6 inches and move the right foot forward, even with the right crutch. Repeat the four-point gait.	11. The four-point gait (used for partial or full weight bearing) provides greater stability. Weight bearing is on three points (two crutches and one foot or two feet and one crutch) at all times. The client must be able to bear weight with both legs.
Three-Point Gait (see Figure 10-15-4)	
12. Advance both crutches and the weaker leg forward together 4 to 6 inches. Move the stronger leg forward, even with the crutches. Repeat the three-point gait.	12. The three-point gait (used for partial or nonweight-bearing) provides a strong base of support. This gait can be used if the client has a weak or nonweight-bearing leg.
Two-Point Gait	
13. Move the left crutch and right leg forward 4 to 6 inches. Move the right crutch and left leg forward 4 to 6 inches. Repeat the two-point gait.	13. The two-point gait (used for partial weight bearing) provides a strong base of support. The client must be able to bear weight on both legs. This gait is faster than the four-point gait.

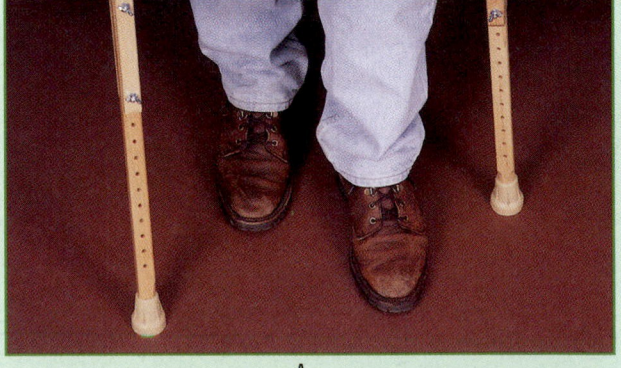

A.

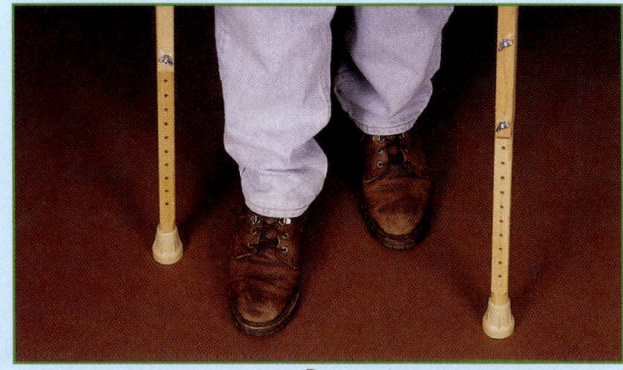

B.

Figure 10-15-3   Crutch walking, four-point gait: **A.** Moving right crutch forward and left foot forward; **B.** Moving left crutch forward and right foot forward, even with right crutch.

continues

Action	Rationale

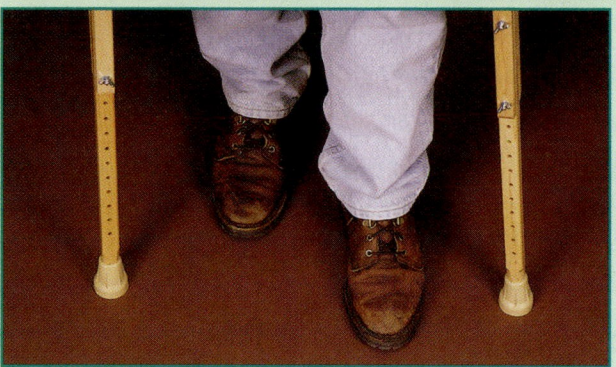

Figure 10-15-4 Crutch walking, three-point gait: advancing both crutches and weaker leg forward together.

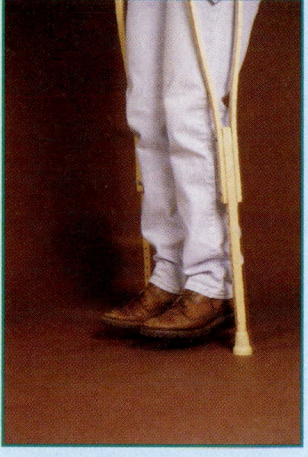

Figure 10-15-5 Crutch walking; swing-through gait

Swing-Through Gait (see Figure 10-15-5)

14. This step is basically the same as the three-point gait. The difference is that on the swing, whichever leg is moving will go past the stationary point and set down in front.

14. The swing-through gait permits a faster pace. This gait requires greater balance, strength, and more practice. Usually used only after a client has become comfortable with the swing-through gait.

Walking Upstairs

15. Stand beside and slightly behind client. Instruct client to position the crutches as if walking. Place body weight on hands. Place the strong leg on the first step. Move the crutches and the weak leg up to the first step. Repeat the pattern for all steps.

15. Prevents weight bearing on the weaker leg. When ascending stairs, crutches should follow the legs, thereby allowing stability if the client's weight shifts down the stairs while moving. This allows the client to catch him- or herself instead of falling backward.

Walking Downstairs

16. Position the crutches as if walking. Place weight on the strong leg. Move the crutches down to the next lower step. Place partial weight on hands and crutches. Move the weak leg down to the step with the crutches. Put total weight on arms and crutches. Move strong leg to same step as weak leg and crutches. Repeat for all steps. A second caregiver standing behind the client holding on to the gait belt will further decrease the risk of falling.

16. Prevents weight bearing on the weaker leg. Crutches in front of the legs while descending stairs allow the client more forward stability if his or her weight shifts down the stairs while client is moving. This allows client to catch him- or herself before falling forward.

17. Set realistic goals and opportunities for progressive ambulation using crutches.

17. Crutch walking takes up to 10 times the energy required for unassisted ambulation.

18. Consult with a physical therapist for clients learning to walk with crutches.

18. The physical therapist is the expert on the health care team for crutch-walking techniques.

19. Wash hands.

19. Reduces the transmission of microorganisms.

Sitting with Crutches

20. Instruct client to back up to chair until it is felt with the back of the legs.

20. Allows for less turning, better stability, and increased safety.

continues

Action	Rationale
Sitting with Crutches *contnuied*	
21. Place both crutches in the nondominant hand and use the dominant hand to reach back to the chair.	21. Increases safety by giving the client an idea of how far away he or she is from the seat.
22. Instruct client to lower slowly into the chair.	22. Lowering slowly decreases pain and possible injuries.
Walking with a Cane	
23. Repeat Actions 1 to 7.	23. See Rationales 1 to 7.
24. Have the client hold the cane in the hand opposite the affected leg. Explain the safety and body mechanics underlying use of a cane on the strong side.	24. Promotes safety and cooperation. Promotes client autonomy. By holding the cane on the stronger side the client has more control and strength for using it.
25. Have the client push up from the sitting position while pushing down on the bed with arms.	25. Promotes autonomy as well as increases upper body strength.
26. Have the client stand at the bedside for a few moments.	26. Allows the client to gain balance. The nurse can check for strength and balance.
27. Assess the height of the cane. With the cane placed 6 inches ahead of the client's body, the top of the cane should be at wrist level with the arm bent 25% to 30% at the elbow.	27. A 25–30% bend at the elbow provides for better muscle strength and support than if the arm is straight.
28. Walk to the side and slightly behind the client, holding the gait belt if needed for stability.	28. Allows the nurse to provide stability or assistance if the client needs it.
The Cane Gait	
29. Move the cane and the weaker leg forward at the same time for the same distance (see Figure 10-15-6). Place weight on the weaker leg and the cane. Move the strong leg forward. Place weight on the strong leg.	29. The cane helps to provide a wide base of support for the body when the weight is on the weaker leg.

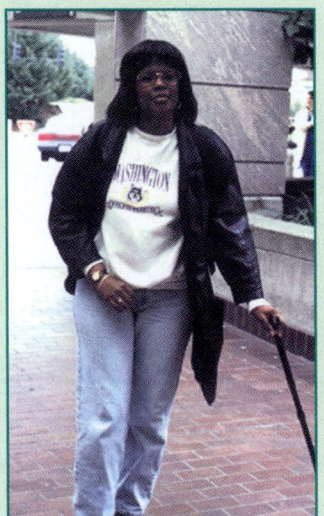

Figure 10-15-6 Move the cane and the weaker leg forward. *Note:* Client is misusing cane; it should be in alignment with client.

continues

Action	Rationale
Sitting with a Cane	
30. Have client turn around and back up to the chair. Have client grasp the arm of the chair with the free hand and lower self into the chair. Be sure to place the cane out of the way but within reach.	30. The cane provides additional support as client lowers self into the chair.
31. Set realistic goals and opportunities for progressive ambulation using a cane.	31. Walking with a cane takes practice.
32. Consult with a physical therapist for clients learning to walk with a cane.	32. The physical therapist is the expert on the health care team for cane-walking techniques.
33. Wash hands.	33. Reduces the transmission of microorganisms.
Walking with a Walker	
34. Repeat Actions 1 to 7.	34. See Rationales 1 to 7.
35. Place the walker in front of the client.	35. Positions the walker for use and allows for stability when the client is standing.
36. Have the client put the nondominant hand on the front bar of the walker or on the handgrip for that hand, whichever is more comfortable. Then, using the dominant hand to push off from the bed and the nondominant hand for stabilization, help the client to an erect position.	36. Uses upper body strength and encourages independence.
37. Have the client transfer hand to the walker handgrips.	37. Allows the client to maintain balance while transferring weight.
38. Be sure the walker is adjusted so the handgrips are just below waist level and the client's arms are slightly bent at the elbow.	38. Provides maximum support from the arms while ambulating.
39. Walk to the side and slightly behind the client, holding the gait belt if needed for stability.	39. Allows the nurse to provide stability or assistance if the client needs it.
Walker Gait	
40. Move the walker and the weaker leg forward at the same time (see Figure 10-15-7). Place as much weight as possible or as allowed on the weaker leg, using the arms for supporting the rest of the weight. Move the strong leg forward and shift the weight to the strong leg (see Figure 10-15-8).	40. Provides support for a weak or nonweight-bearing leg by using arm and upper body strength.
Sitting with a Walker	
41. Have the client turn around in front of the chair and back up until the back of the legs touch the chair. Have client place hands on the chair armrests, one hand at a time, then lower self into the chair using the armrests for support.	41. Using the armrests of the chair is a more stable support than using the walker.

continues

Action	Rationale

Sitting with a Walker *continued*

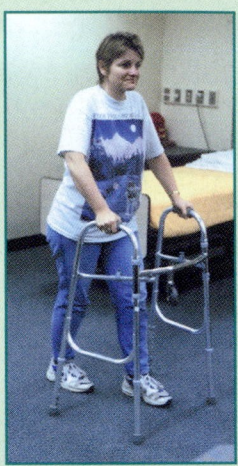

Figure 10-15-7   Move the walker and the weaker leg forward.

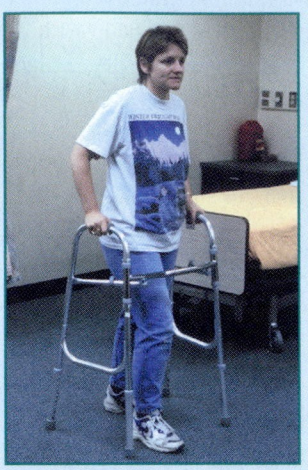

Figure 10-15-8   Use the arms to support the rest of the weight and move the strong leg forward.

42. Set realistic goals and opportunities for progressive ambulation using a walker.

42. Walking with a walker takes practice.

43. Consult with a physical therapist for clients learning to walk with a walker.

43. The physical therapist is the expert on the health care team for walker techniques.

44. Wash hands.

44. Reduces the transmission of microorganisms.

► REAL WORLD ANECDOTES

Nurse Mwangi was doing a home follow-up with Mrs. Munson. Mrs. Munson had recently been discharged from rehabilitation following a stroke. She had one-sided weakness and had been taught to use a walker in rehab. While talking, Nurse Mwangi noted that Mrs. Munson was not using her walker. To get around in the house Mrs. Munson was holding onto furniture and the walls. The nurse noted that Mrs. Munson was quite unsteady using this method of ambulation. Upon questioning, Mrs. Munson claimed that she did not need the walker, that she was doing just fine without it. The nurse found the walker folded up, leaning against the wall. She brought it out to reinforce Mrs. Munson's teaching regarding use of the walker. When the nurse handed the walker to Mrs. Munson she became angry and blurted out, "I can't use that thing. I can't even get it open." Upon further questioning, Nurse Mwangi discovered that the rehab nurses had always folded and unfolded Mrs. Munson's walker for her. After returning home, Mrs. Munson had discovered that she could not get it folded and unfolded on her own. As a result she had simply stopped using it.

Nurse Mwangi discussed several options with Mrs. Munson, including simply leaving the walker unfolded and available or possibly getting a different walker that was easier for her to manipulate.

Be sure the client really knows how to do the task. Do not mindlessly perform it for the client. Do not take things at face value. Be sure to dig deep enough to get the real answer regarding a situation.

▶ EVALUATION

- The client was able to demonstrate safe and independent ambulation with the assistance of crutches, a cane, or a walker.
- The client was confident and safe while using the assistive device.

▶ DOCUMENTATION

Nurses' Notes

- Document the type of device the client is using, the level of understanding regarding the use of the device, how far the client is able to walk using the device, and the client's response to the activity.

Document on appropriate flow sheet or electronic medical record (EMR).

▶ CRITICAL THINKING SKILL

Introduction

Cane to good side not bad side.

Possible Scenario

While assisting Mr. Lujan to ambulate using his cane, you note that he is holding the cane on his weaker side.

Possible Outcome

If Mr. Lujan also has weakness in his arm on that side, he is at greater risk for falling. His weaker arm will tire more easily and is more likely to give way. By keeping the cane close to the weaker foot, Mr. Lujan is using the cane as a substitute limb. This does not help strengthen the weak leg through use. It also negates any wide-stance stabilizing effect from the cane. This is a safety concern as it puts Mr. Lujan at risk of falling.

Prevention

The cane is present to increase stability, not to act as a replacement limb. By holding the cane on the stronger side, the client has more control and strength for using it. Also, the client has a three-point, wider stance with the cane and the affected leg farther apart. The wider stance promotes stability and good body mechanics.

By using the cane as a replacement limb, Mr. Lujan does not get any strengthening benefit in his weaker leg. By using the cane for stability, Mr. Lujan's weaker leg can gain strength through use.

▶ VARIATIONS

Geriatric Variations:
- *Elderly clients may not have sufficient upper body strength to lift a walker prior to each step. They may need a rolling walker.*
- *If an elderly client tends to tire easily, walkers with fold-down seats built in are available so clients can sit and rest.*
- *To foster independence, a basket or an apron with pockets on the front of a walker can help the client carry small items.*
- *Using walkers outdoors can pose special hazards to elderly clients. Wheels and tips can become stuck in the mud, grass, or cracks in the pavement.*

Pediatric Variations:
- *Be sure to get the correct size device for a child. Children grow quickly and will need to be assessed more often regarding the size of the device.*
- *If a child is very young, he or she may revert to crawling or creeping rather than try to use a device to assist with walking. Try to make using the device fun.*
- *Children may feel more comfortable with a walker they can "customize" with decals and decorations. Make sure these do not pose a safety hazard.*

continues

► **VARIATIONS** (continued)

Home Care Variations:
- *Assess the home for narrow hallways, doorways, and steps. Advise the client regarding ways to negotiate around the home.*
- *Mark the front edge of steps with tape or paint so it is highly visible to clients walking with assistive devices.*
- *Advise clients to remove or fasten down throw rugs that might slide and cause the client to fall.*
- *Make sure handrails on stairs are securely fastened to the wall.*

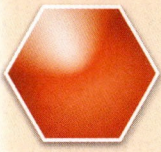

Long-Term Care Variations:
- *Be sure to check the rubber tips on assistive devices for wear. With the rubber worn away the client is at risk of slipping and falling.*
- *Clients who use an assistive device frequently may need hand protection such as gloves or padding on the handgrip.*

► **COMMON ERRORS**

Possible Error:

Leaning on the top of the crutch with the axilla when walking.

Prevention:

Clients who walk leaning on the crutch with their axilla are at risk of damage to the nerves, blood vessels, and muscles. This is called crutch palsy.

► **NURSING TIPS**

- Be sure there is about 2 inches or 3 fingers' width of distance between the client's axilla and the top of the crutch.
- Be sure the client is holding the cane on the good side for optimal effect.
- Be sure that the client's walker is just below waist level. This allows the client's arms to be slightly bent when standing in the walker. This is a stronger arm position than with the arms totally straight.
- Check the rubber tips on all assistive devices frequently. They can become worn quickly and lead to instability and falls.
- When measuring the height of a cane be sure the client stands erect, not hunched or bent over.
- Provide a robe or other covering and shoes with firm, nonslip soles to provide for modesty and safety.
- Label the client's equipment.

► **SPECIAL CONSIDERATIONS**

- *When ascending or descending stairs with handrails, the rail should be used on the good side, and the crutch or cane on the weak side to further increase stability.*
- *Sometimes at night or after long periods of inactivity, clients may become more unstable than usual. Be aware of this and be present as needed.*
- *Clients with more than one injury (especially those with arm injuries as well) may need special equipment to assist with ambulation. Physical or occupational therapists will usually provide them with this equipment. Contact the therapists with any questions.*
- *Sitting up and then standing can often present problems with vertigo and nausea. Instruct the client to do these steps slowly and allow time in between.*
- *For clients who are having difficulty ambulating with or without a device, consider asking for a physical therapist consultation if one is not ordered.*
- *Padding on crutches may contain latex. Cover padding if client has a history of latex allergy or contact dermatitis.*

Special Procedures

Administering an Electrocardiogram

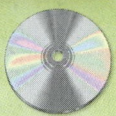

SKILL 11-1

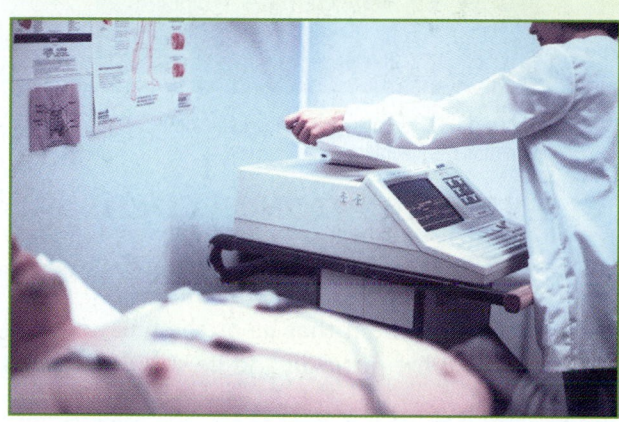

▶ OVERVIEW OF THE SKILL

The 12-lead electrocardiogram (ECG or EKG) is a standardized noninvasive diagnostic tool used to record the electrical activity of the heart. Electrodes are placed in designated positions on the surface of the body and attached to a monitor that allows for visualization of electrical activity of the heart, primarily of the left ventricle. As the ECG measures electrical changes of the cardiac muscle with a graph tracing, it can be used to identify rhythm disturbances and many types of cardiac abnormalities, such as myocardial ischemia or infarction, structural changes such as hypertrophy, axis deviation, certain drug effects, and electrolyte imbalances, all of which affect the electrical activity of the cardiac muscle. The ECG offers only initial screening information for cardiac abnormalities that result in aberrations of the flow of electrical activity in the heart and little information regarding the contractile or hemodynamic function. Nonetheless, the ECG is the most frequently used screening tool, other than pulse and blood pressure determination. The placement of 10 electrodes (4 on the limbs and 6 on the chest) in standardize locations provides "views" of cardiac activity from 12 different vantage points on the body surface. It is noninvasive, painless, and can be obtained within a few minutes. Training is required to identify placement of the electrodes and proper operation of ECG machines. Even

though most current machines provide a computer-derived interpretation simultaneous with the graph tracing, this preliminary data should be sent to a cardiologist or trained provider who "overreads" and professionally interprets the tracing.

▶ ASSESSMENT

1. Assess age, sex, and current medication history for any medications with possible cardiac or hemodynamic effects. Gather other data that may be required by unit/institution protocol (e.g., height, weight, recent blood pressure, operator identification). **Reference standards are tailored to age and gender. Some medications cause abnormalities in portions of the ECG complex that must be recognized as medication effect.**
2. Determine that the client is able to tolerate a supine position and that adequate exposure of chest and limbs is possible for electrode placement. **Correct location of electrodes is enhanced by a comfortable, stable position.**
3. Determine presence of neck, arm, jaw, or other pain with possible cardiac origin. **Chest or other pain may provide additional information useful in serial comparison of ECGs.**

4. Assess client's need for information about the procedure, purpose, and requirements, and ability to cooperate. The client should lie still and refrain from talking. Electrode attachment and procedure lasts only a few minutes and is painless. **Anxiety may be relieved by simple explanation of intent, duration, and purpose.**

5. Assess whether the client has a pacemaker **as the pacemaker function will be evident on the ECG and interfere with the diagnostic ability of the ECG.**

▶ DIAGNOSIS

Deficient Knowledge

Anxiety

Decreased Cardiac Output

Risk for Impaired Skin Integrity

▶ PLANNING

Expected Outcomes:

1. The client will be able to lie quietly and cooperate with procedure.
2. The client will not be anxious.
3. The client will be able to describe the reason for the ECG.

Equipment Needed (see Figure 11-1-1):

• Twelve-lead ECG machine with charged batteries, cables and leads, and the correct recording paper for the machine
• Disposable electrodes and gel or paste, if not already on the electrodes
• Alcohol wipes
• Pillows
• Sheet or drape
• Towel and washcloth
• Disposable razor

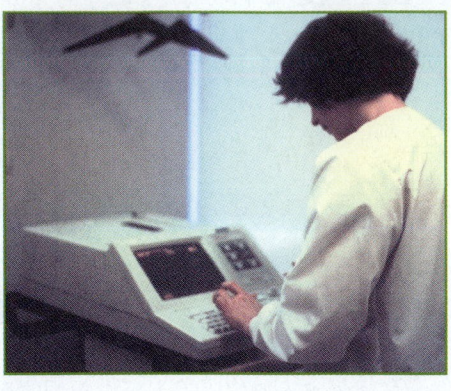

Figure 11-1-1 Enter the demographic data into the ECG machine.

▶ CLIENT EDUCATION NEEDED:

1. Assure the client that no electrical current goes through the body from the machine.
2. Explain to the client that he or she will need to be in the supine position and lie still during this test.
3. Explain to client that he or she will need to breathe normally and refrain from talking.
4. Instruct the client to report chest pain or other symptoms to the nurse or physician.
5. Explain to client that it may be necessary to shave body hair at some sites where electrodes are to be placed to provide good contact.
6. Tell the client that he or she will have to remove clothes from the waist up and expose arms and legs during the procedure.
7. Assure the client that his or her privacy will be guarded.

Estimated time to complete the skill: **10 minutes**

▶ DELEGATION TIPS

Specially trained technicians may perform electrocardiograms. The nurse should explain the procedure to the client before the technician performs the examination and assure the client the health care provider will inform him or her of the test results.

IMPLEMENTATION—Action/Rationale

Action	Rationale
1. Wash hands.	1. Reduces the transmission of microorganisms.
2. Close door and curtains.	2. Provides privacy.
3. Explain the procedure and rationale for ECG.	3. Decreases anxiety and promotes cooperation.
4. Review machine operation requirements. Bring ECG machine to the bedside and open electrode packages.	4. Ensures smooth procedure.
5. Enter all demographic data into the machine (see Figure 11-1-1).	5. Ensures accurate diagnosis for correct client.
6. Position the client in a supine and relaxed position (see Figure 11-1-2).	6. Provides comfort and privacy and ensures accurate ECG.
7. Remove moisture, oil, and excess hair from site at electrode sites.	7. Promotes adherence of leads to chest and extremities.
8. Attach four electrodes to the extremities—1 on each arm and 1 on each leg; attach 6 electrodes to the chest (Figure 11-1-3 and Figure 11-1-4). • V_1—4th intercostal space (ICS) at right sternal border. Females: Choose a site as close to standard position as possible. • V_2—4th ICS at left sternal border. • V_3—Midway between V_2 and V_4. • V_4—5th ICS at midclavicular line. • V_5—Left anterior axillary line at level of V_4 horizontally. • V_6—Left midaxillary line at level of V_4 horizontally (see Figure 11-1-2).	8. Proper placement of electrodes allows for proper recording of electrical activity of the heart on ECG paper. • In women and sometimes obsese men, breast tissue obscures sternal border.
9. Attach electrodes to the chest (Figure 11-1-5).	9. Promotes proper display of chest leads on graph.

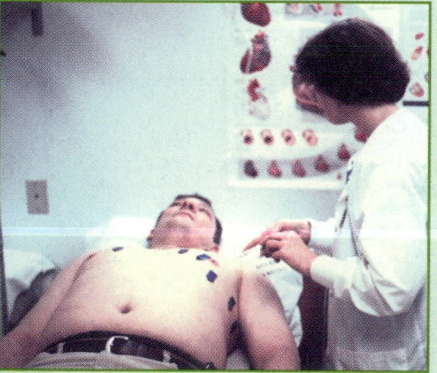

Figure 11-1-2   Position client in relaxed position before placing electrodes.

continues

Action	Rationale

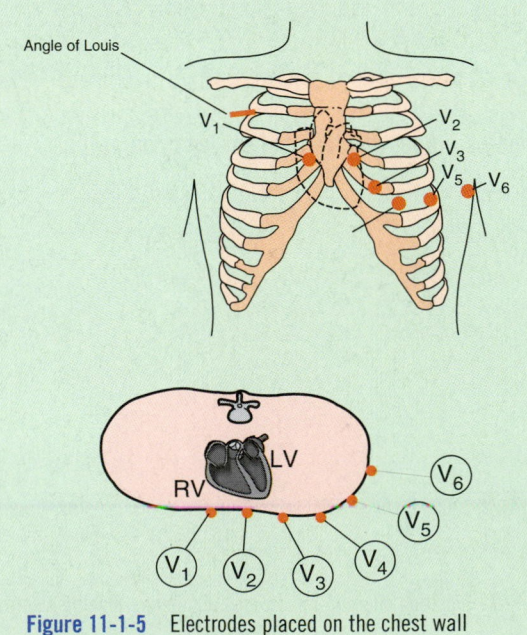

Figure 11-1-3 ECG placement for standard 12-lead ECG.

Angle of Louis

Figure 11-1-5 Electrodes placed on the chest wall comprise the 6 recordial leads.

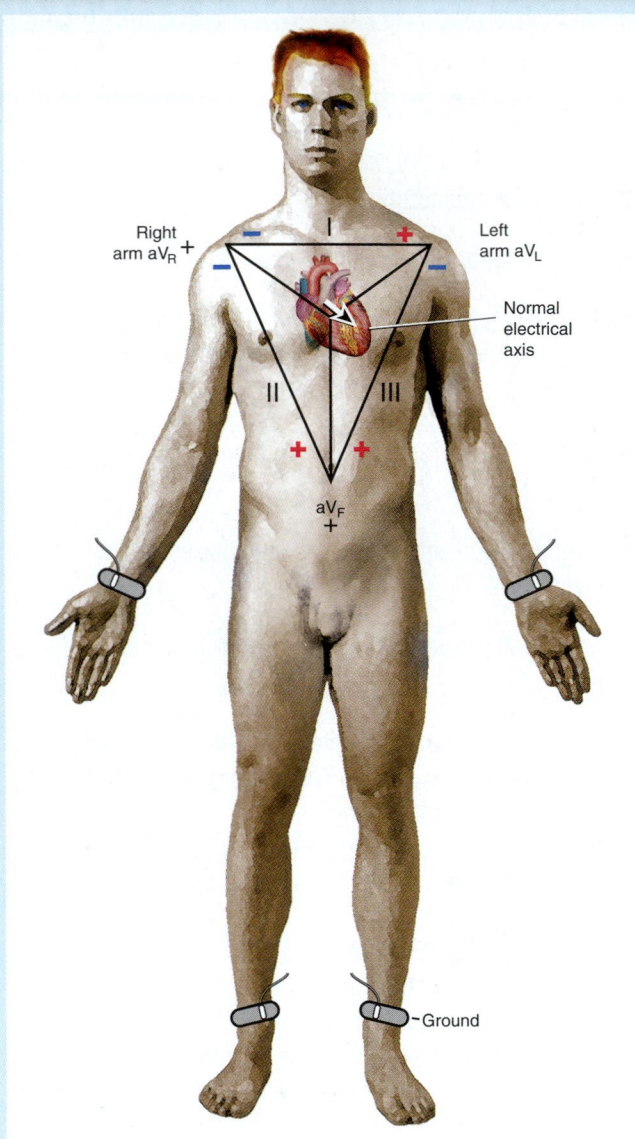

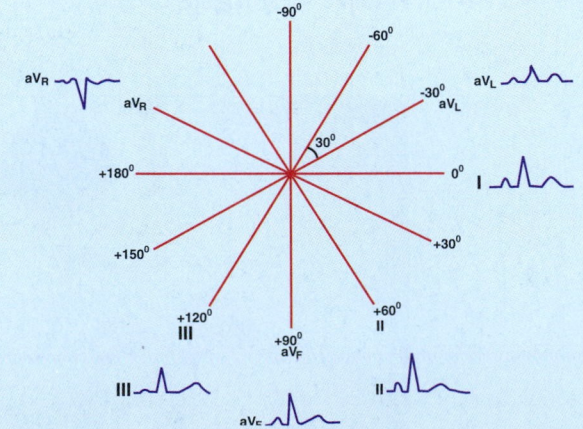

Figure 11-1-4 Bipolar frontal plate leads (I, II, III) and unipolar frontal plane leads (aV$_R$, aV$_L$, and aV$_F$) comprise the 6 limb leads by using 4 electrodes

continues

Action	Rationale
10. Obtain tracing by following the instructions from the physician or qualified practitioner. In general, a 2.5-second strip from each lead, plus a 10-second rhythm strip, is required.	**10.** Data are gathered and transferred onto paper for analysis.
11. Inspect tracing for adequate quality.	**11.** Muscle movements may cause "fuzzy" waveforms.
12. Remove leads and electrodes. Wipe paste from skin.	**12.** Promotes comfort and hygiene and minimizes skin irritation.
13. Notify physician or qualified practitioner of abnormalities.	**13.** Certain changes may require prompt treatment.
14. Wash hands.	**14.** Reduces the transmission of microorganisms.
15. Return machine and replace supplies.	**15.** Ensures equipment is ready for next use.

▶ REAL WORLD ANECDOTES

Scenario 1

Alonzo, a 73-year-old client with known coronary artery disease, hypertension, and chronic obstructive pulmonary disease, was admitted to the cardiac care unit 12 hours earlier with chest pain and pneumonia. He now notified the nurse that he was having chest pain and felt lightheaded. In assessing him, the nurse found his apical pulse to be 160 and irregular, blood pressure 134/92. He admitted that his chest pain had returned approximately 10 minutes earlier when he began to feel slightly dizzy. The nurse took an ECG, the protocol for recurrent chest pain, which confirmed a rate of 145 to 175 beats/minute, and a rhythm interpretation confirmed atrial fibrillation with premature ventricular contractions. Alonzo's physician was notified and Alonzo was given medication to control his tachycardia and dysrhythmias.

Scenario 2

Esther, a 58-year-old woman with history of non–insulin-dependent diabetes mellitus, obesity, chronic low back pain, and mild congestive heart failure, was admitted 24 hours earlier for continuous IV heparin therapy for deep vein thrombosis in her left leg. The nurse's aide now reports that Esther is sitting up in bed, is "sweaty," and has pain in her chest and is breathing rapidly. The nurse finds that Esther is tachycardic, short of breath, and extremely diaphoretic with a blood pressure of 94/62 and pulse oximetry of 84%. Breath sounds are clear throughout all lung fields. Oxygen by mask is started, and a 12-lead ECG is obtained while the physician is paged. The ECG reveals sinus tachycardia, rate 132 beats/minute. Her QRS axis has changed from 300 to +1100 and computer interpretation reveals nonspecific ST changes. The nurse reported all these findings to the physician when he arrived at the client's bedside.

▶ EVALUATION

- The client tolerated the ECG procedure.
- The client is able to state purpose of ECG.
- An accurate tracing was obtained for analysis.

▶ DOCUMENTATION

Nurses' Notes

- Note the date and time of the ECG.
- Describe the reason for the ECG and any significant findings.

• Record the time the tracing results were reported to the physician or qualified practitioner.

Document on appropriate flow sheet or electronic medical record (EMR).

Medication Administration Record

• Note the date and time of any cardiac medication.

▶ CRITICAL THINKING SKILL

Introduction

Quick response to any cardiac symptoms or complaints is essential in giving appropriate and timely treatment. Taking an ECG should be second nature to staff in emergency rooms, medical units, and cardiac care units.

Possible Scenario

A woman being treated for recently diagnosed diabetes on the medical unit had just eaten her lunch when she mentioned to the nurse that she had heartburn. She said she often got it after eating and it always went away when she reclined in her chair. The nurse noted that she looked comfortable and went to the next client.

Possible Outcome

An hour later, the client put on her call light and told the nurse that her heartburn had not disappeared as it usually did. The nurse then took her vital signs and called the doctor. He ordered an ECG and the nurse called the ECG technician. The preliminary result showed possible cardiac ischemia. When the doctor was notified, he ordered the client to be transferred to the cardiac care unit for further evaluation.

Prevention

The nurse should have listened to the client's complaint and acted immediately by calling the doctor or doing the ECG him- or herself if the institution policy allowed it.

▶ VARIATIONS

Geriatric Variations:
• *Elderly clients may have difficulty lying on their backs.*
• *Older clients with respiratory problems may have the ECG taken while sitting.*
• *Some clients may have had amputation of a limb, so the extremity electrodes will require adjustment of the electrode placement.*
• *An elderly client with surgical dressings or appliances may require repositioning of the electrodes.*
• *The skin of older clients may be fragile, so care should be taken when applying and removing the electrodes and cleaning the skin of the gel.*

Pediatric Variations:
• *Infant or pediatric electrodes should be the appropriate size.*
• *Reassure the child that the ECG will not hurt and that it will take only a few minutes.*
• *Young children may need to be offered a pacifier or bottle so they can relax and breathe normally.*
• *Children may be distracted by a video or a story read to them.*
• *Careful electrode placement is essential as ECG computers recognize age and include age-appropriate algorithms in the computer interpretation.*

Home Care Variation:
• *ECGs are not commonly done in the home setting; however, clients with arrhythmia or other symptoms that occur intermittently may use portable units at home. Cardiac event recorders, such as King of Hearts, or a portable ECG machine, such as a Holter monitor, record ECG data at home. Clients transmit the data over the telephone or take the units to the facility.*

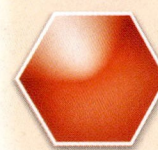

Long-Term Care Variation:
• *Clients in long-term care facilities may have skin or musculoskeletal disturbances that will need special attention when doing an ECG.*

▶ **COMMON ERRORS**

Possible Error:

You attach the electrodes for the arms onto the legs and the electrodes for the legs onto the arms, causing a faulty interpretation.

Prevention:

Read the labels or look at the color coding on each electrode and verify that they are attached to the correct extremity. If you believe the electrodes are incorrectly placed, remove the electrodes and start over again.

Possible Error:

You attach the lead wires to the wrong chest electrodes, causing a misinterpretation.

Prevention:

Pay close attention to the electrodes and wires as you prepare to attach them to the client. Laying them out on the bed or client so you can see them will make it easier to identify the correct leads.

▶ **NURSING TIPS**

- Gain the client's cooperation so he or she will lie still and be relaxed so as to minimize artifact caused by muscle movement.
- Use diagrams and instructions for correct electrode placement.
- Palpation of ribs and intercostal spaces and visual references to clavicle and axilla are necessary to place electrodes correctly.
- Dry diaphoretic skin before the ECG as it may hinder attachment of electrodes; one loose lead can cause the tracing to be faulty.

- Shave body hair in any area where it prevents good skin contact of the electrode.
- Attach the lead wire to button-type electrodes first so you do not have to press it into the client.
- Use the ECG machine's display messages to guide you during the ECG.
- Remember that skeletal muscle tremors interfere with detection of cardiac electrical activity and may produce artifact in the tracing.
- If a client has a pacemaker, the ECG may not be diagnostic of a myocardial infarction.

▶ **SPECIAL CONSIDERATIONS**

- *Placement of the electrodes with good contact may be difficult in women with large breasts. Be sure they are as close to standard position as possible.*
- *If a rhythm looks unexpectedly abnormal, check lead placement/attachment and contact the health care provider if life-threatening abnormalities are present.*

Magnetic Resonance Imaging (MRI)

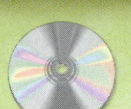

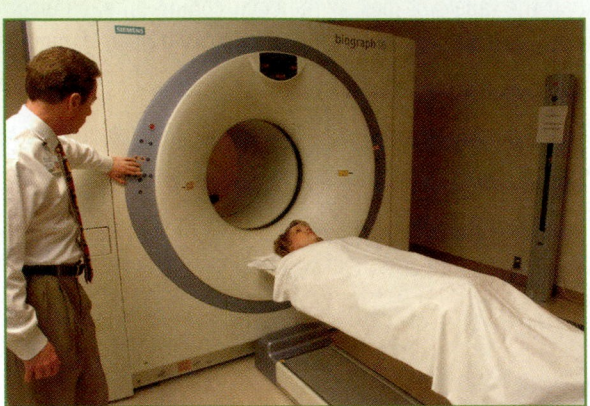

▶ OVERVIEW OF THE SKILL

Magnetic resonance imaging (MRI) is a scanning technique performed by a specially trained technologist. It allows internal organs and structures to be seen by means of magnetic forces rather than by radiation. The large electromagnet in which the client is placed senses the change in alignment of the hydrogen atoms in the body and sends this information to a computer where billions of mathematical calculations are made that produce clear images on a television monitor.

MRI is useful in diagnosing pathologic lesions in any organ or tissue, contrasting normal and abnormal tissue, and distinguishing white and gray matter of the brain.

▶ ASSESSMENT

1. Assess the client's knowledge of the purpose and plan of the procedure **so he or she will cooperate and not be anxious.**
2. Review the client's signature on the informed consent form. **It is a legal requirement.**
3. Assess the client's weight **as the procedure is contraindicated in clients weighing more than 300 pounds.**
4. Assess the client for cardiac pacemaker, aneurysm clips, and history of valve replacement or other metal objects in the body **as the magnet may cause movement of metal or electronic objects**.

5. Assess the client for claustrophobia as the electromagnet is a large tube that does not allow for any movement. **Sedation may be necessary.**
6. Asses the client for pregnancy. **An MRI is contraindicated, especially in the first trimester.**
7. Assess the client's ability to remain still for 30–90 minutes during the procedure. **Movement may produce unreliable images.**
8. Assess the client for allergies to dye or contrast medium **to avoid an anaphylactic reaction.**
9. Assess the client for adequate venous access **for injection of the contrast medium.**

▶ DIAGNOSIS

Anxiety

Fear

Deficient Knowledge

Risk for Allergy Response

▶ PLANNING

Expected Outcomes:

1. The client will tolerate the procedure without anxiety.
2. The client will remain still during the procedure.
3. Successful images will be obtained for diagnosis.
4. If contrast medium is used, the client will not experience a reaction to it.

Equipment Needed:

- Contrast medium ordered by physician or qualified practitioner
- MRI scanner
- Intravenous access

▶ **CLIENT EDUCATION NEEDED:**

1. The client should be taught the rationale for the procedure and how it will be performed.
2. Recommend that clients limit their fluid intake so they will not have to urinate for 30–90 minutes during the test.
3. The client should void just before the procedure as he or she will not be able to move during the lengthy procedure.
4. Explain to the client that no metallic objects, including makeup (contains metallic particles), should be worn. Metal may be affected by the strong magnet and can disrupt the images.
5. Although the study is painless, there may be a slight discomfort if a contrast dye is injected intravenously.
6. Tell the client that the machine will make various humming and loud thumping noises.
7. Ask the client to verbalize his or her knowledge and feelings about the procedure.

Estimated time to complete the skill:
30–90 minutes

▶ **DELEGATION TIPS**

Assessment of the client before and after diagnostic testing is the responsibility of the nurse. Vital signs after an MRI procedure may be delegated; ancillary personnel should be instructed to report any symptoms of respiratory distress or allergic reactions to the nurse.

IMPLEMENTATION—Action/Rationale

Action	Rationale
1. Provide teaching regarding the MRI machine.	1. Reduces anxiety and fear of the unknown.
2. Assess the client for contraindications in having an MRI, such as pacemakers, artificial valves, orthopedic hardware, aneurysm clips, shrapnel, or metal plates in the head.	2. The presence of any of these objects would prohibit the client from having an MRI.
3. Have client remove all metallic objects, such as watch, rings, coins, keys, hair pins, credit cards, dentures containing metal, and external prostheses.	3. Reduces artifacts on the scan. Avoids damage to some metal objects by the magnetic field.
4. Instruct client to void.	4. Ensures client comfort and avoids movement during procedure.
5. Assist client onto padded table beside electromagnet. • Secure client on table with Velcro straps. • Provide client with earplugs, intercom, or earphones.	5. Provides correct positioning for study. • Keeps client from moving during study. • Decreases noises of machine and provides communication between client and technologist. • If the head is to be scanned, place special helmet around head.

continues

Action	Rationale
6. Give sedation to client, if ordered.	**6** Sedation may be necessary to complete the procedure, particularly for clients who are claustrophobic or have difficulty lying still.
7. Observe client for signs of claustrophobia or inability to remain still (see Figure 11-2-1).	**7.** May necessitate the administration of a sedative during the procedure.
8. If contrast medium is injected during procedure, assess for an allergic reaction (see Figure 11-2-2).	**8.** Provides immediate detection of a life-threatening emergency.
9. Technologist performs MRI (see Figure 11-2-3): • Provides accurate imaging.	**9.** The technologist is trained to perform this procedure.
10. After study is completed, assist client to sitting position. When client is ready, assist to a standing position.	**10.** Decreases risk of orthostatic hypotension.
11. Wash hands.	**11.** Reduces the transmission of microorganisms.

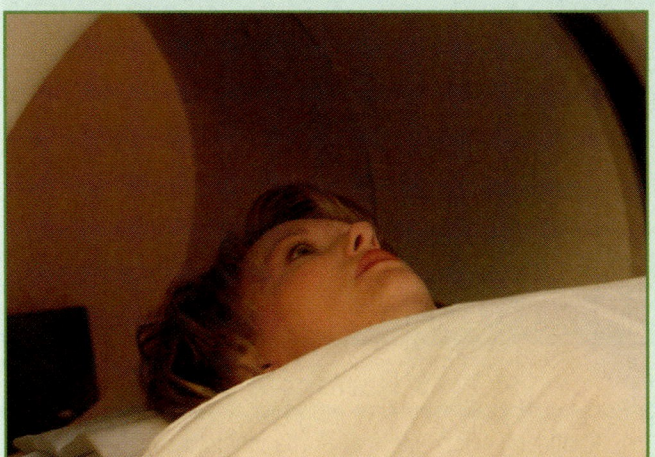

Figure 11-2-1 Observe client for signs of claustrophobia or inability to remain still.

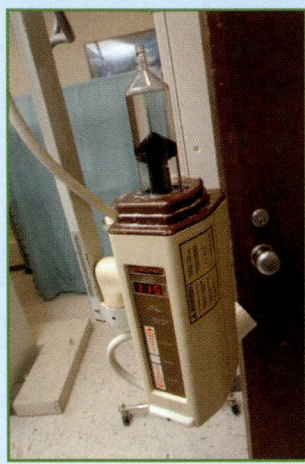

Figure 11-2-2 Contrast dye may be given during the procedure.

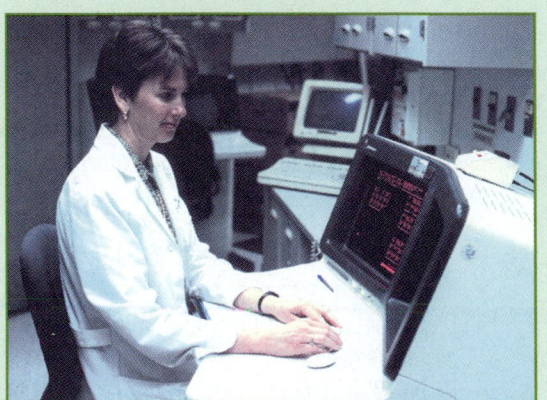

Figure 11-2-3 The MRI technologist performs the procedure.

► **REAL WORLD ANECDOTES**

Martha was admitted to the hospital to evaluate her abdominal pain. The nurse explained the MRI to her, but Martha confided that she was afraid of closed spaces. The nurse asked the physician for a sedative order. After giving the medication to Martha, the nurse sat with her, held her hand, and taught her a simple imagery exercise to practice while she was in the MRI tube.

► **EVALUATION**

- The client tolerated the procedure without anxiety.
- The client remained still during the procedure.
- Successful images were obtained for diagnosis.
- If contrast medium was used, the client did not experience a reaction to it.

► **DOCUMENTATION**

Nurses' Notes

- Note the date, time, length, and place the procedure was done.
- Describe the client's tolerance of the procedure.
- If contrast medium was used, describe the client's response.
- Document the client's status after the procedure.

Document on appropriate flow sheet or electronic medical record (EMR).

Medication Administration Record

- Record medications administered before or during the procedure, such as diazepam (Valium) or midazolam (Versed).

► **CRITICAL THINKING SKILL**

Introduction

Metallic objects can create false images on the scan and some can even damage the magnetic fields. All jewelry, coins, watches, keys, hair pins, credit cards, prostheses, and dentures containing metal must be removed.

Possible Scenario

A devoutly religious woman was scheduled for an MRI. She removed her watch and rings but refused to remove a metallic religious object.

Possible Outcome

She could be allowed to hold the object in her hand until she is positioned on the table and ready to be placed into the tube. She would be assured that a relative could hold the object during the procedure and would return it to her as soon as the test was finished.

Prevention

The nurse could have discussed the reason for the removal of metallic objects in more detail after assessing the woman's beliefs.

► **VARIATIONS**

Geriatric Variations:

- *Elderly clients who are confused may have difficulty remaining still during the procedure.*
- *Clients need to be questioned in detail about metallic objects (e.g., they may not realize a prosthesis or dentures contain metal).*

Pediatric Variations:

- *Children may need their parents nearby during the procedure. This is allowed as there is no radiation exposure.*
- *Children may need to be sedated if they are not able to remain still during the procedure.*
- *Children can be shown the machine and allowed to play in it before the actual procedure in order to become familiar with it.*

continues

▶ VARIATIONS *(continued)*

Home Care Variation:
- *Coordination with client's primary physician or qualified practitioner may increase home care nurses' knowledge of client's condition. Having this information will allow clients and family a greater benefit of coordinated services.*

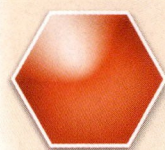

Long-Term Care Variation:
- *Ensure that debilitated clients have adequate nutrition, pain medications, or other symptom management.*

▶ COMMON ERRORS

Possible Error:

The client was extremely agitated when placed in the tube.

Prevention:

If the client is oriented, ask whether he or she suffers from claustrophobia or has any fears regarding the procedure. Check with the client frequently regarding anxiety or a feeling of being closed in. If the client is frightened or confused, sedation may be necessary.

▶ NURSING TIPS

- Give earplugs to clients who may be uncomfortable with the noise of the electromagnet.
- Assist the client into a comfortable position using a pillow under the knees if possible.
- Assure the client that there is no danger of radiation.
- Assist the client into a comfortable position after the test.

▶ SPECIAL CONSIDERATIONS

- *Some facilities offer an "open" MRI, which does not totally enclose the client. This may eliminate or decrease the claustrophobia associated with MRI procedures; however, the image may not be as optimal as with the traditional machines. Newer versions of MRI equipment may include microphones, which may help to decrease anxiety. Learn what a particular facility offers and what options are available for clients within the community.*
- *Clients with a past history of claustrophobia or a history of being trapped in a fire or automobile accident may require complete sedation to administer an MRI.*
- *Monitor for complications postprocedure if contrast medium was given. Complications may include a reaction to the contrast medium, constipation, or an adverse reaction to current medication.*
- *Metal objects inside clients, for example, orthopedic hardware, intrauterine devices, pacemakers, aneurysm clips, or artificial valves, can malfunction, be dislodged, or absorb heat during the procedure. Inform client and practitioners appropriately before the MRI.*

Assisting with Computed Tomography (CT) Scanning

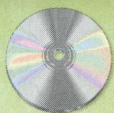

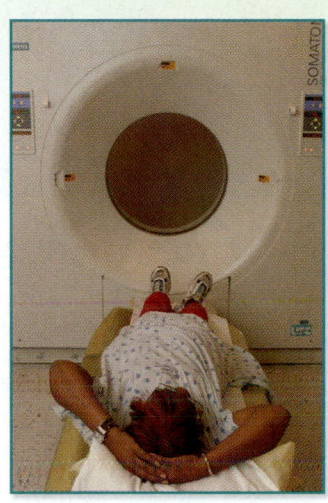

▶ OVERVIEW OF THE SKILL

Computed tomography (CT) employs a narrow beam of X-ray to sweep transverse planes or sections of the body and a computerized analysis to reconstruct images of the irradiated tissues. The X-ray beam is in motion in relation to the subject and the film or sensor; the result is a selective blurring of areas not within a specific slice of tissue and a focused image of tissue within that plane. The resulting images are sharp and detailed, and considered to be far superior to images obtained by conventional X-rays. The primary purpose for the use of CT scans is to image structures or masses within body organs. The technique is useful in obtaining images of the brain, liver, lung, abdomen, chest, and certain vascular spaces. The difference in tissue density can be used to identify tumors, brain infarctions, displacement of cerebral ventricles, and cortical atrophy. Whole-body scans allow visualization of the spinal cord and tumors or lesions in organs. A pregnant woman may have a CT scan in her first trimester to confirm the pregnancy.

The scan is itself noninvasive but uses ionizing radiation, and some techniques include use of injected contrast agents. Because the CT scan makes multiple images, the procedure is not instantaneous like most X-rays, but takes 30–60 minutes to complete, depending on the tissues or organs studied and the number of "slices" to be made. A CT scan is contraindicated in clients weighing more than 300 pounds.

In order to obtain clear images, the client must remain motionless during the procedure. The client is immobilized and partially confined in a narrow chamber while lying on a hard surface. This position, along with the clicking and clanging noises of the machine, may cause the client to become anxious and claustrophobic. Sedation is sometimes required to obtain immobility in addition to counteracting feelings of claustrophobia.

▶ ASSESSMENT

1. Confirm client's identity and knowledge level concerning the procedure and purpose for the CT scan **so teaching can be tailored to needs.**
2. Determine the need for informed consent and witness the signing of the consent **so institutional and legal regulations are followed.**
3. Determine the client's ability to lie still, supine for up to 1 hour, **as this position is necessary for the procedure.**
4. Assess the client for feelings of claustrophobia **as some clients feel confined in the scanner during the procedure.**
5. Assess the client for an allergy to iodine or other contrast agents if CT is to be an "enhanced"

study or contrast agents will be used **so an allergic reaction will be avoided.**

6. Determine whether the client has a history of compromised renal function **to avoid renal complication if contrast agents are used.**

7. Assess the client's need for sedation during procedure **as anxiety or claustrophobia may prevent the client from being able to lie still.**

▶ DIAGNOSIS

Disturbed Sensory Perception

Deficient Knowledge

Anxiety

Risk for Allergy Response

▶ PLANNING

Expected Outcomes:

1. The client will cooperate, be comfortable, and free of anxiety during the procedure.
2. Satisfactory images will be obtained for diagnosis.
3. The client will understand the purpose of the scan and when he or she will be informed of the results.

Equipment Needed:

- Sterile needle and syringe for administering contrast dye, if ordered
- CT scanner
- Intravenous access

▶ CLIENT EDUCATION NEEDED:

1. Inform the client that the procedure will take 30 minutes to 1 hour.
2. Reassure the client that a CT scan is a noninvasive procedure unless intravenous (IV) contrast dye is used.
3. If a contrast agent is used, inform the client he or she may feel warm or flushed and experience a metallic or salty taste momentarily.

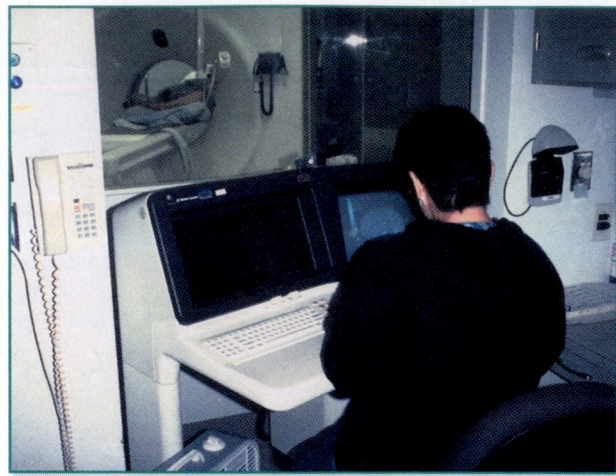

Figure 11-3-1 Instruct the client that although alone in the room where the test is being performed, he or she can speak with the technician at any time through an intercom.

4. Inform the client about the image.
5. Instruct the client he or she will need to lie still in a supine position on a hard surface.
6. Instruct the client that a restraint or belt will be used to hold hips, abdomen, or head in place on the table.
7. Reassure the client that the amount of radiation used is similar to having several chest X-rays.
8. Tell the client that while alone in the scanner, he or she can talk to a technician through an intercom (see Figure 11-3-1).
9. Reassure the client that family can wait nearby.
10. Tell the client that the machine will make clicking and whirring noises.
11. Reassure the client that he or she will be made comfortable after the test.

 Estimated time to complete the skill: **30–90 minutes**

▶ DELEGATION TIPS

Assessment of the client and administration of contrast medium are the responsibility of the nurse. Vital signs after a CT scanning procedure may be delegated; ancillary personnel should be instructed to report any signs of respiratory distress or allergic reactions to the nurse.

IMPLEMENTATION—Action/Rationale

Action	Rationale
1. Wash hands.	1. Reduces the transmission of microorganisms.
2. Confirm identity of client. If contrast medium is to be used, assess for client allergies.	2. Essential for diagnosis and treatment decisions and client safety.
3. Explain procedure and rationale to client.	3. Decreases anxiety and promotes cooperation.
4. Confirm that client has signed informed consent.	4. Ensures physician or qualified practitioner has informed client of expected benefits and risks of procedure and that client has given consent.
5. Assist the client onto the CT table and position as appropriate (arms above the head if it is a chest or abdominal CT; see Figure 11-3-2).	5. Assures client is as comfortable as possible during procedure.
6. Give sedation to client if ordered.	6. Sedation may be necessary to complete procedure, particularly for clients who are claustrophobic or have difficulty lying still.
7. Start IV contrast dye if it is to be given (see Figure 11-3-3).	7. Gives dye time circulate in the body prior to the start of the CT.

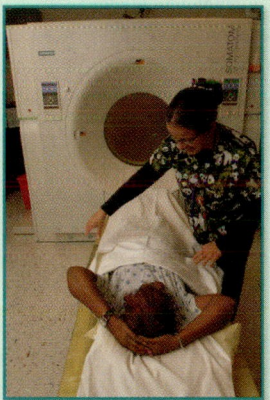

Figure 11-3-2 Assist client onto CT table in the appropriate position for the type of scan.

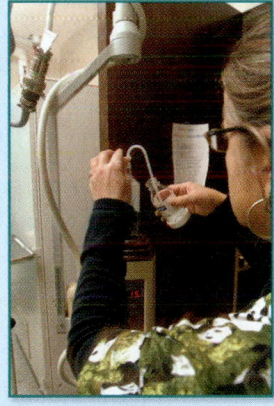

Figure 11-3-3 The radiology technician prepares the IV contrast dye.

Action	Rationale
8. Instruct client about the procedure. Tell the client to: *Lie still* *Do not be afraid of whirring and clicking noises* (see Figure 11-3-4) *Breathe deeply and relax*	8. Promotes client comfort and safety and ensures adequate images.
9. Assist client to a comfortable position after the scan.	9. Ensures client safety and comfort.

continues

Action	Rationale
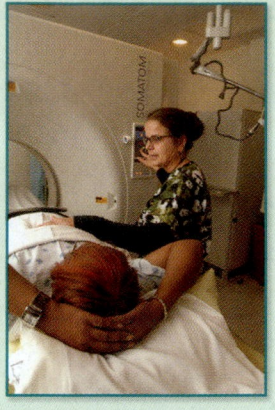	
	Figure 11-3-4 Instruct client that whirring and clicking sounds may be heard during the procedure.
10. Assess client for possible allergic reaction if dye was given.	**10.** Ensures client receives appropriate and immediate intervention if a reaction is suspected.
11. Return client to wheelchair or bed.	**11.** Ensure client comfort and safety.

▶ **REAL WORLD ANECDOTES**

Randy was a high school senior when he injured his knee playing football. He was scheduled for a CT scan of his knee so his physician could plan his treatment. Randy was hearing impaired and wore hearing aids. When his nurse told him about the loud noises he might hear inside the scanner, he said that he would simply remove the aids and then it would not bother him. Otherwise, the noises might be abnormally amplified. He was able to relax while in the scanner and had no need to communicate with the technician during the procedure. The nurse allowed this, but the nurse was careful to discuss hand signals and how to communicate in the event of an emergency.

▶ **EVALUATION**

- The client cooperated during the procedure and was free from anxiety.
- The client was as comfortable as possible during and after the procedure.
- Satisfactory images were obtained for diagnosis.
- The client understands the general nature of the information to be obtained and when and how he or she will be informed of the results of the CT scan.

▶ **DOCUMENTATION**

Nurses' Notes

- Document the date, time, and length of the procedure.
- Document the date and time the contrast dye was given.
- Describe the response of the client to the procedure.

Document on appropriate flow chart or electronic medical record (EMR).

Medication Administration Record

- Document date and time of sedation.
- Document date and time contrast dye was given.

▶ **CRITICAL THINKING SKILL**

Introduction

The reason for lying still during a CT scan is to produce clear images of the organs or structures being examined.

Possible Scenario

An elderly gentleman was scheduled for a CT scan of his abdomen. He had been confused at times but was generally cooperative. He was sent to radiology for his CT scan without the benefit of any sedation. He seemed to understand when the nurse told him about not moving during the test.

Possible Outcome

When the client was placed into the scanner, he immediately became agitated and tried to get out. After attempting to calm him with soothing words and touch, the nurse realized she was not succeeding. The nurse called his physician for an order for sedation. The test had to be postponed until he was sedated.

Prevention

A careful assessment of the client's ability to understand the procedure and need to remain still is necessary before a CT scan. Sedation can be given prior to the procedure to ensure an accurate examination.

▶ VARIATIONS

Geriatric Variations:
- *Confused elderly clients may have difficulty remaining still during the procedure.*
- *Older clients may be reluctant to voice their anxiety.*
- *Clients may have arthritis or back pain that could make them uncomfortable while lying on a hard surface.*

Pediatric Variations:
- *Children may need reassurance that their parents are nearby and can talk to them during the procedure.*
- *Allowing a child to take a favorite stuffed animal or toy may reduce anxiety.*
- *Children may need to be sedated if they are not able to remain still during the procedure.*

Home Care Variations:
- *Not applicable*

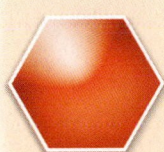

Long-Term Care Variations:
- *Not applicable*

▶ COMMON ERRORS

Possible Error:

The client having a CT scan was in extreme pain from a back injury.

Prevention:

Check the medical record for the previous time pain medication was given and medicate the client to achieve pain relief; complete the CT scan when the client is more comfortable.

Possible Error:

A contrast dye was ordered for a client with an allergy to iodine.

Prevention:

Assess the medical record for client's allergy history. Ask the client if he or she has any allergies, especially to shellfish, iodine, or dye. If so, do not administer the contrast dye. Notify the physician or qualified practitioner and proceed with the test if it is to be done without contrast.

► **NURSING TIPS**

- Give earplugs to clients who may be uncomfortable with the noise of the CT scanner.
- Assure the client that the risk of radiation is the same as several routine X-rays.

- Assist the client into a comfortable position after the test.
- Monitor the client for level of consciousness, oxygenation, and hydration, particularly if contrast agents were used for the procedure.

► **SPECIAL CONSIDERATIONS**

- *Many clients have back pain when lying supine, and lying on a flat hard surface may exacerbate this. Adequate pain control should facilitate obtaining clear images.*
- *Monitor the client for the possible occurrence of postprocedure complications resulting from the use of contrast medium.*

Assisting with a Liver Biopsy

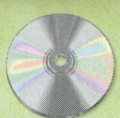

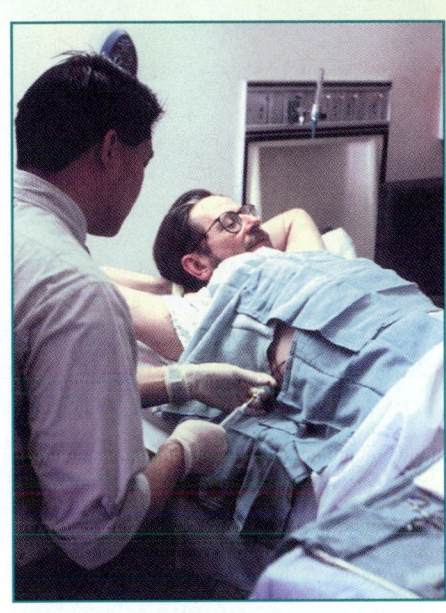

▶ OVERVIEW OF THE SKILL

A liver biopsy is a test to diagnose disorders of the liver, confirm the infiltration of cancer, or assess the effects of hepatotoxic drugs. In clients with hepatitis, a biopsy can document treatment response. Most liver biopsies are done at the bedside using a percutaneous needle to obtain the sample. The physician or qualified practitioner performs the biopsy while staff assist and support the client.

▶ ASSESSMENT

1. Assess the client's knowledge of the purpose and plan of the procedure **so he or she will cooperate, have decreased anxiety, and lie still during the procedure.**
2. Review the client's signature on the informed consent form. **It is a legal requirement.**
3. Assess the client's ability to remain still in both the supine position used during the procedure, and the right lateral position required 2 hours after the procedure. **These positions are required to access the liver and control bleeding after the procedure.**
4. Assess the client for ability to cooperate and hold breath for 15 seconds during the procedure as the liver **can be accessed best when the client has exhaled.**
5. Assess vital signs as baseline data **to compare with postprocedural vital signs.**
6. Review the medical record for client's risk of bleeding, including use of anticoagulants, prothrombin time, and platelet count. **These factors may affect the risk of bleeding.**
7. Review the medical record for a history of allergic reactions to antiseptic or anesthetic solutions **to avoid an allergic reaction.**
8. Assess the client for massive ascites **as fluid in the abdominal cavity increases the risk of laceration of the liver's surface.**
9. Assess the client for pneumonia **as an infection in the right pleural space could contaminate the biopsy needle at it passes through to the liver.**
10. Assess client's understanding of risk and ability to sign consent form.

▶ DIAGNOSIS

Anxiety

Fear

Deficient Knowledge

Acute Pain

Risk for Infection

Risk for Injury

Risk for Fluid Volume Deficit

▶ PLANNING

Expected Outcomes:

1. The client will understand the rationale for the procedure and tolerate it without anxiety.
2. The client will assume the required position and remain still during and after the procedure.
3. The client will experience minimal pain.
4. There will be no bleeding or infectious complications.
5. The client will not experience complications such as pneumothorax, puncture of blood vessel in the liver, perforation of the gallbladder, bacteremia, or septic shock.

Equipment Needed (see Figure 11-4-1):

- Liver biopsy tray, including:
  - Antiseptic solution (povidone-iodine)
  - Gauze sponges (4 × 4)
  - Sterile towels
  - Local anesthetic solution (lidocaine)
  - Sterile syringes: two 3-mL with 23- to 25-gauge needles for anesthetic and two 10-mL for biopsy
  - Three 5-mL vials of normal saline
  - One biopsy needle
  - One number 11 scalpel
  - Specimen containers with formalin
  - Povidone-iodine ointment
  - Sterile gauze and tape
  - Gloves
- Sterile gloves

▶ CLIENT EDUCATION NEEDED:

1. The client should be taught the rationale for the procedure.
2. Assure the client that the actual biopsy takes only 5–10 seconds.

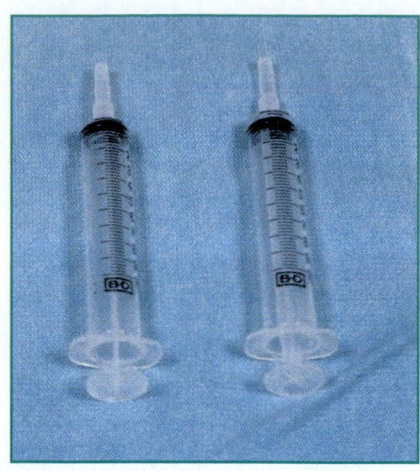

Figure 11-4-1 Two 10-mL syringes

3. The client should be told about the need for sterile technique.
4. The client should be instructed on the position to be assumed and the importance of remaining still.
5. The client should be instructed to practice breathing and holding the breath for the procedure.
6. The client should be instructed to not eat or drink anything for 6 hours *before* or 2 hours *after* the biopsy.
7. Encourage the client to take slow, deep breaths and use imagery to promote relaxation.
8. The client should be assured that a local anesthetic will be given to dull the pain.
9. The client should be encouraged to ask questions and verbalize fears or anxiety.
10. The client should be told that he or she will need to remain in bed for 6 hours after the procedure, the first 2 hours in the lateral position on the right side.
11. Instruct the client to report any severe pain, shortness of breath, or fever immediately.
12. The client should be instructed to refrain from coughing or straining for 4 hours after the procedure and to avoid lifting heavy objects or strenuous activities for 1 week.

Estimated time to complete the skill:
30 minutes

▶ DELEGATION TIPS

Assessment for bleeding, pain, shortness of breath, and proper postprocedure position is the responsibility of the nurse. Measurement of vital signs may be delegated to ancillary personnel.

IMPLEMENTATION—Action/Rationale

Action	Rationale
1. Have client void.	1. Promotes client comfort.
2. Wash hands.	2. Reduces the transmission of microorganisms.
3. Administer medication for sedation or pain.	3. Promotes cooperation, comfort, and remaining still during procedure.
4. Take vital signs and record in nurses' notes.	4. Postprocedure vital signs will be compared with the baseline values.
5. Set up sterile tray.	5. Maintains sterile technique.
6. Biopsy site is midway between upper and lower borders of hepatic dullness, in 8th or 9th intercostal space. The physician or qualified practitioner may use a pen to mark this site with an "X." Assist client in maintaining correct position: • Have client place the right arm under head. • Have client place left arm at side, under head, or as instructed by the physician or qualified practitioner. • Advise the client to lie quietly (see Figure 11-4-2).	6. Biopsy site is midway between upper and lower borders of hepatic dullness, in 8th or 9th intercostal space. Assisting client in maintaining correct position decreases risk of complications during procedure by misplacement of needle.
7. Inform the client that the physician or qualified practitioner will ask him or her to hold breath during the procedure. A typical scenario would have the client: • Take several deep breaths • Take a deep breath in • Blow all the air out and hold breath • Hold breath for 15 seconds or until the physician or qualified practitioner indicates the procedure is completed • Breathe normally	7. Breathing out places the liver in the proper position snug against the chest wall and ensures the liver and diaphragm do not move while the biopsy needle is inserted.
8. Nurse supports the client and assists the physician or qualified practitioner during the procedure: • Reassure client while explaining each step of procedure. • Assess client's condition during the procedure. • Coach client on breathing and holding the breath when physician or qualified practitioner is ready to insert needle.	8. • Increases client comfort and relaxation. • Provides for treatment of a potential complication. • Ensures a successful, nontraumatic biopsy.
9. Physician or qualified practitioner performs the aspiration; the nurse assists as needed as the following are done: • Wash hands. • Put on mask and goggles if required by institution policy, apply sterile gloves, and drape the client with sterile towels (see Figure 11-4-3).	9. • Maintains surgical asepsis. • Reduces the number of microorganisms on the skin.

continues

Action	Rationale

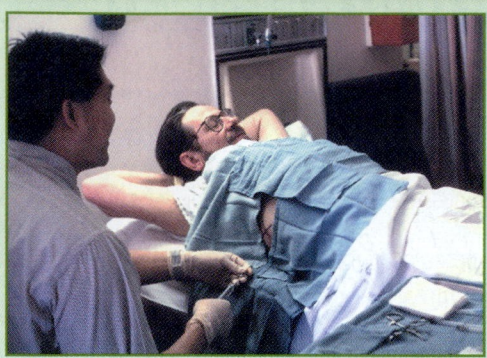

Figure 11-4-2 The client must lie quietly through the procedure. Make sure the client is comfortable and in the proper position prior to beginning the procedure.

- Disinfect client's skin with antiseptic solution
- Inject local anesthetic to the subcutaneous tissue and the capsule of the liver and ask client when it has taken effect.
- Ask the client to take a deep breath, exhale completely, and hold the breath. Assist the client to do this.
- Insert the biopsy needle attached to a syringe into the liver (see Figure 11-4-4).
- Aspirate the liver tissue quickly and withdraw the needle. Help the client to remain still and provide support and information.
- Instruct the client to take a breath and breathe normally.
- After removing the biopsy needle, apply pressure to the incision (see Figures 11-4-5 and 11-4-6).
- Apply antiseptic ointment and a pressure dressing.
- Place specimen in the sterile container with formalin (see Figures 11-4-7 and 11-4-8).
- Discard used supplies appropriately

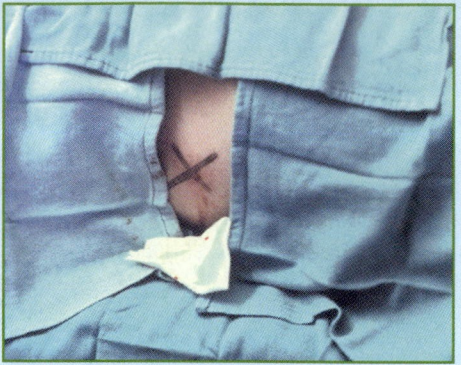

Figure 11-4-3 Note how the sterile drape protects the biopsy site from contamination from the gown or bedding.

- Provides anesthesia during the aspiration.
- Facilitates insertion of biopsy needle.

- Ensures the liver is immobilized during biopsy.

- Ensures a sample of liver tissue is obtained.

- Reassures the client while the procedure is performed.

- Restores normal respirations.

- Prevents bleeding at biopsy site.

- Reduces risk of infection.
- Allows specimen to be examined in the laboratory.

- Prevents transmission of microorganisms and accidental needle punctures.

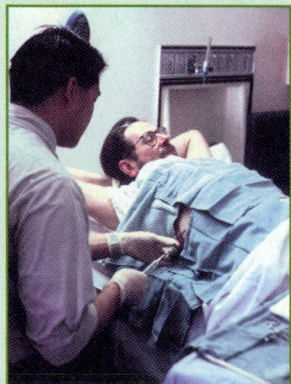

Figure 11-4-4 The biopsy needle is inserted through the incision and into the liver.

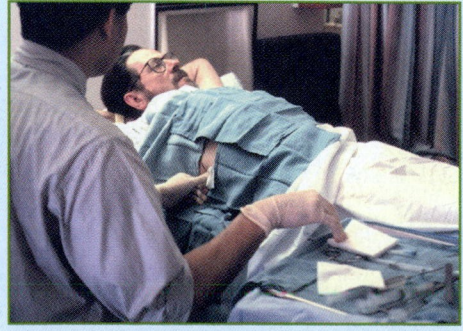

Figure 11-4-5 After removing the needle, pressure is applied to the site.

continues

Action	Rationale

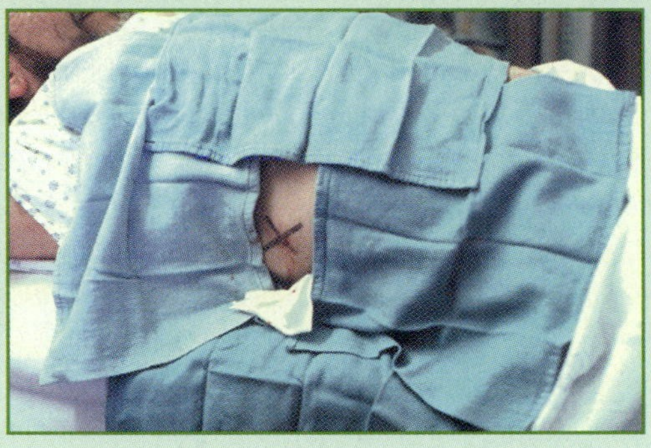

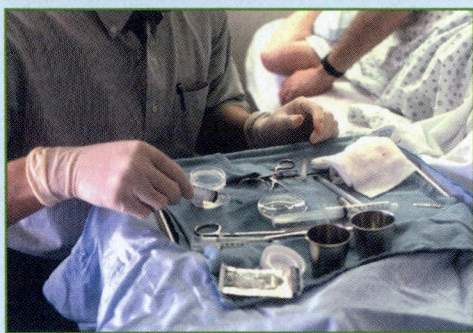

Figure 11-4-6 Applying pressure prevents bleeding at the biopsy site.

Figure 11-4-7 The specimen is removed from the needle.

10. Continue to apply pressure to biopsy site:
    • Instruct client to roll onto the right side and remain in that position for 2 hours (see Figure 11-4-9).

11. Label the specimen with client's name and send specimen to laboratory.

12. Assess vital signs every 15 minutes for the first hour, every 30 minutes for the next 2 hours, then every hour for 4 hours, and then every 4 hours until stable.

13. Remove gloves and wash hands.

10. Controls bleeding.
    • Ensures the liver capsule is compressed against the chest wall at the biopsy site.

11. Ensures results will be reported for correct client.

12. Promotes early detection of a bleeding complication.

13. Reduces the transmission of microorganisms.

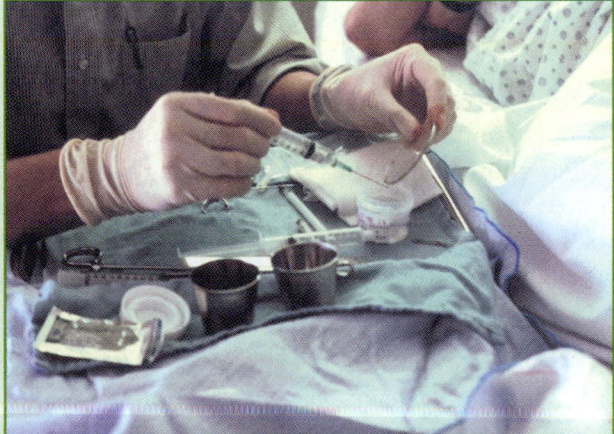

Figure 11-4-8 The specimen has been placed in a sterile container with formalin.

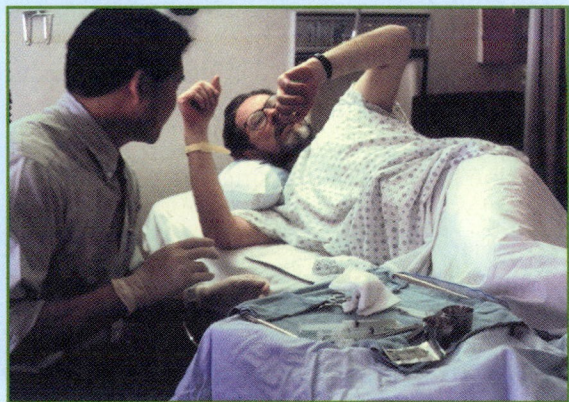

Figure 11-4-9 The client will roll on the right side and remain in that position for 2 hours to compress the liver against the chest wall at the biopsy site.

> ► **REAL WORLD ANECDOTES**
>
> *Harry noticed that his eyes were yellow so he made an appointment to see his doctor. After some baseline blood tests were done, the doctor told Harry that he needed a liver biopsy to be able to make a diagnosis and treatment plan.*
> *Harry had never heard of sticking a needle in a liver; in fact, he had never had very many needles stuck in him at all in his 56 years. He lived simply and worked as a janitor and did not understand very much about medicine. So the nurse sat with him to explain the procedure the day before it was scheduled to be done. She had a diagram of where the liver was located and how the ribs surrounded it. Then she assured him that he would receive medication to numb the skin; however, he would probably feel some pain when the doctor did the biopsy. She told him how to breathe during the biopsy and practiced the routine several times with him to see how long he could hold his breath.*
> *He was cooperative and rather interested in learning about what was going to happen to him. She gave him an illustrated booklet about the liver biopsy so he could read it at home*
> *The next day, Harry had the biopsy without any complications and thanked the nurse for helping him.*

► EVALUATION

- The client understood the rationale for the procedure and tolerated it without anxiety.
- The client assumed the required position and remained still during and after the procedure.
- The client experienced minimal pain.
- There were no bleeding complications.
- The client did not experience complications such as pneumothorax, puncture of blood vessel in the liver, perforation of the gallbladder, bacteremia or septic shock.

► DOCUMENTATION

Nurses' Notes

- Note date, time, and site of the liver biopsy.
- Describe how the client tolerated the procedure.
- Document laboratory tests ordered and when specimen was sent.
- Describe the type of dressing and ointment applied.
- Record vital signs before and after the procedure.
- Document the presence of any bleeding at the site.

Document on appropriate flow sheet or electronic medical record (EMR).

Medication Administration Record

- Document the date and time of pain medication or sedative.

► CRITICAL THINKING SKILL

Introduction

The most common but serious complication after a liver biopsy is bleeding, either externally or internally. Maintaining pressure over the biopsy site will usually prevent this from occurring.

Possible Scenario

The client was resting comfortably on his side after the biopsy was done. There was no sign of bleeding in the first 30 minutes, but the client became tired of lying on his right side so he turned over onto his left side. The nurse came in to take his 45-minute vital signs and noticed the gauze dressing had a large amount of bloody drainage on it that was not there at the previous check.

Possible Outcome

The nurse applied direct pressure for a few minutes, applied another dressing over the old dressing, and assisted the client onto his right side again. The nurse took his vital signs and noted that his blood pressure was slightly lower than previously, then reported the bleeding to the physician.

Prevention

The client should have been assessed for his understanding of the required position after the procedure and his ability to cooperate.

► VARIATIONS

Geriatric Variations:
- Older clients may have difficulty assuming the position necessary for the procedure. Help them by positioning with a pillow prior to the procedure and holding them in position, using proper body mechanics during the procedure.
- Older clients may have difficulty holding their breath during the biopsy and need to practice their breathing.
- Some elderly clients may have coagulation alterations that may increase their risk of bleeding after a liver biopsy.

Pediatric Variations:
- Small children or infants will probably need general anesthesia for a liver biopsy in order to remain still during the procedure.
- Children may need sedation so they will remain quiet for 6 hours after the procedure.

Home Care Variations:
- This procedure is not applicable in the home care setting.
- The care giver should be aware of complications that may occur postprocedure. These include bleeding, pain, and shortness of breath.

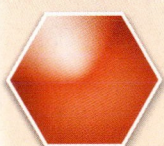

Long-Term Care Variations:
- This procedure is not applicable in the long-term care setting.
- Staff providing long-term care should be aware of complications that may occur postprocedure. These include bleeding into the biliary tract, pain, pneumothorax, or bile peritonitis.

► COMMON ERRORS

Possible Error:
The client is not able to hold his or her breath for long enough during the biopsy and takes a deep breath.

Prevention:
The client should have practiced the breathing necessary for the procedure and been evaluated for how long he could hold his or her breath. If it is not long enough, the physician or qualified practitioner will have to determine if one can still obtain the tissue sample, and may have to pull out the needle so it does not damage the lung, gallbladder, or nearby blood vessels.

► NURSING TIPS

- Use pillows, rolled towels, or blankets to assist the client into a comfortable position.
- Remember that severe pain in the upper right quadrant or in the right shoulder could be a symptom of peritoneal hemorrhage.
- Have the client practice the breathing pattern that will be required during the biopsy.
- Monitor the client for internal bleeding (pain, distention, abdominal tenderness, changes in vital signs, color, or mentation).

▶ **SPECIAL CONSIDERATIONS**

- Explain to the client what to expect after a liver biopsy and have emergency numbers readily available.
- A minimal amount of pain is expected after a liver biopsy; however, any increase in temperature, dizziness, pain, or a "tender-to-touch" abdomen should be reported to the health care provider. The most common complications after a liver biopsy are bleeding and peritonitis. As the functions of the liver affect clotting, most clients who have a liver biopsy are at increased risk for bleeding tendencies and need to be informed regarding identification of excessive bleeding. The presence of ascites, often observed in liver failure, complicates the health care provider's assessment of a tense abdomen; therefore, pain and temperature should be monitored carefully to evaluate for the presence of peritonitis.

Assisting with a Thoracentesis

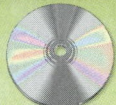

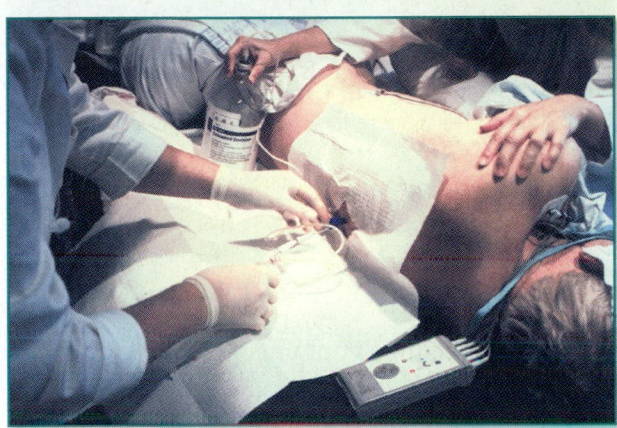

▶ **OVERVIEW OF THE SKILL**

Thoracentesis is the process of inserting a large-bore needle through the chest wall into the pleural cavity (utilizing sterile technique) for the purpose of removing fluid or administering medications intrapleurally. Fluid accumulating in the pleural cavity is usually the result of infection, trauma, or a disease process such as a malignancy. Excess fluid in the pleural cavity can cause pain, dyspnea, or significant cardiopulmonary compromise, and result in a life-threatening emergency. The primary purpose of thoracentesis is either to eliminate these potential symptoms or to diagnose an effusion of unknown etiology. The need for and location of the site for thoracentesis is most commonly determined by chest X-ray, although physical examination, ultrasound, and fluoroscopy are also employed to determine the presence and location of a pleural effusion.

Fluid removed from the pleural cavity is assessed for quality and quantity as well as analyzed in the laboratory for cell count and differential, protein, glucose, lactic dehydrogenase (LDH), and specific gravity. In the event of a suspected malignancy or infection, samples are sent to cytology for definitive diagnosis.

Thoracentesis may be performed as an inpatient, emergency room, or outpatient procedure in an ambulatory clinic or physician's or qualified practitioner's office. Key to the success of the procedure is the proper positioning of the client. The client is either sitting at the edge of the bed or exam table with the arm of the affected side elevated over a bedside stand or sitting straddled in a chair with arms resting on the back of the chair. Infants and small children and clients who are unable to tolerate a sitting position or are on a ventilator are usually positioned supine with the affected side elevated.

▶ **ASSESSMENT**

1. Determine the necessary pretests needed and their purpose prior to the thoracentesis, **to determine the proper positioning of the client and the exact location of the pleural effusion.**
2. Obtain consent per institution policy. **This protects against legal action and provides an opportunity to inform the client and family about the procedure.**
3. Obtain baseline vital signs and medical history. **Baseline vital signs are necessary to determine tolerance during and changes in health status following the procedure.**
4. Determine client's knowledge of and prior experience with thoracentesis. **This helps determine knowledge base to tailor teaching. Client may have a routine that is used to prepare, such as relaxation, guided imagery, or the use of transdermal numbing medication.**

5. Assess the need for sedation, premedications, or restraints. Some pediatric and adult clients may be unable to cooperate with a thoracentesis. **Proper positioning and lack of movement are important to prevent complications or damage to the lungs or other internal organs or tissue.**

6. Assess client's ability to sign a consent form.

▶ DIAGNOSIS

Anxiety

Ineffective Breathing Pattern

Impaired Gas Exchange

Deficient Knowledge

Risk for Injury

Risk for Infection

Acute Pain

▶ PLANNING

Expected Outcomes:

1. The client's pain will decrease or cease.
2. Respiratory status will remain stable during the procedure.
3. Arterial blood gases, pulse oximetry, and other diagnostic tests will improve.
4. The client will experience minimal discomfort with the procedure.
5. The client will not experience any complicating injury or infection related to procedure.

Equipment Needed (see Figure 11-5-1):

- Thoracentesis tray (may be disposable kit, or reusable tray from central supply). In addition, there are specific trays available for infants and small children. If a thoracentesis tray is not available in a prepackaged form, then the following equipment is necessary:
  - Antiseptic solution
  - Sterile gauze sponges (4 × 4 in. and 2 × 2 in.)
  - Sterile towels and drapes
  - Local anesthetic (e.g., lidocaine 1%)
  - Sterile syringes and needles: two 3- to 5-mL with 23- to 25-gauge needles for administration of local anesthetic medication; two 20- to 50-mL syringes with 14- to 17-gauge needles 5 to 7 cm in length for fluid drainage
  - Three-way stopcock/two-way stopcock with extension tubing

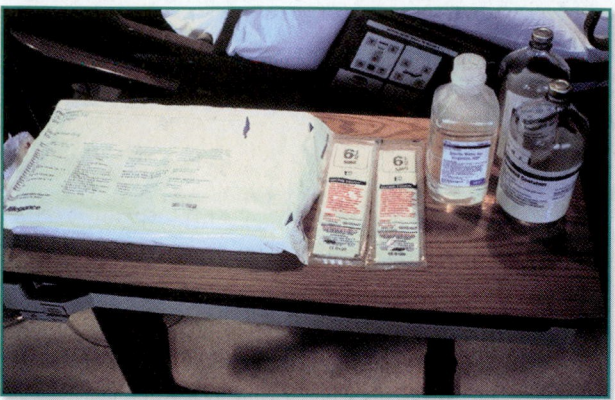

Figure 11-5-1   Thoracentesis tray, sterile gloves, and sterile fluid receptacle

- Hemostat
- Fluid receptacle
- Sterile specimen containers
- Items needed for Standard Precautions (mask/face shield, gown, gloves), as needed
- Sterile gloves in appropriate size for physician or qualified practitioner and anyone assisting in the sterile field
- Laboratory specimen container with labels and requisitions (a specimen container with a preservative may be needed for biopsy purposes)
- Premedications (e.g., sedation, pain medication, cough suppressant)

▶ CLIENT EDUCATION NEEDED:

1. Explain the purpose and approximate length of the test.
2. Review the body position the client will need to assume and emphasize the need to remain immobile throughout the procedure.
3. Provide an opportunity for the client to practice the position required for the procedure.
4. Describe the sensations the client will experience with the local anesthesia and the pressure from the needle insertion.
5. Review all pre- and posttests required to assist the client in knowing what to expect.
6. Provide timeline to client for when to expect laboratory test results and state who will communicate results.
7. Teach relaxation or guided imagery, which can often minimize the anxiety related to the procedure.
8. Instruct the client to void before the procedure.

9. Help the client determine the necessary supports needed (e.g., pillows) to assume the ideal body positioning for a thoracentesis.
10. Review the need to remain immobile and not to move suddenly or cough during the thoracentesis as this could cause injury.
11. Describe routine tests (e.g., chest X-ray) and monitoring required after the thoracentesis.
12. Review delayed complications of the procedure (e.g., spleen or liver perforation) and instruct client to report dyspnea, chest pain, or cough.
13. Review both early-onset and delayed complications of thoracentesis, and ask client to repeat information back before discharge from the

hospital, clinic, or office. Provide written information.
14. Instruct client that there is usually no need to remain nothing per mouth (NPO) before or after the procedure. If anxiety usually makes the client queasy, he or she may wish to not eat or to eat lightly to reduce the risk of nausea, vomiting, and aspiration during the procedure.

Estimated time to complete the skill: **30 minutes**

▶ DELEGATION TIPS

Assessment for bleeding, pain, shortness of breath, and proper postprocedure position is the responsibility of the nurse. Measurement of vital signs may be delegated to ancillary personnel.

IMPLEMENTATION—Action/Rationale

Action	Rationale
1. Wash hands before baseline assessment and as necessary throughout the preparation, procedure, and follow-up.	1. Reduces the transmission of microorganisms.
2. Identify client and obtain baseline assessment and medical history of client paying close attention to respiratory status and vital signs.	2. Prevents performing an invasive procedure on the wrong client. Provides a baseline for comparison after procedure to assess tolerance and improvement in clinical status.
3. Be sure a signed consent has been completed.	3. Reduces the legal risk to the nurse, physician, or qualified practitioner and hospital and ensures the client has been informed of procedure and risks.
4. Review necessary pretests (e.g., X-ray) and have information available at the bedside.	4. Enables the physician or qualified practitioner to identify the appropriate site to perform the thoracentesis. Assists the nurse in proper positioning of the client.
5. Prepare necessary client-specific laboratory/cytology labels and requisitions. Check that the client's correct name and identification number are listed on each label and requisition.	5. Reduces risk of incorrect labeling or handling of specimens obtained during the procedure. Sample is correctly identified with client's name and identification number.
6. Review client teaching and assess anxiety.	6. Provides reinforcement of prior teaching and opportunity for anxiety-reducing techniques (e.g., relaxation, guided imagery).

continues

Action	Rationale
7. Re-identify client, assess allergy history, and premedicate him or her as ordered.	7. Ensures medication is administered to the proper client and that there is no history of allergic reaction to the medication. Premedications for a thoracentesis are usually for either sedation, pain control, or cough-suppressant purposes.
8. Prepare the necessary equipment and sterile field. Make sure any prepackaged trays have all necessary supplies.	8. Provides a safe, organized approach to the procedure and prevents introduction of microorganisms into the pleural cavity.
9. Assist in client positioning: • Sitting at the edge of the bed with arms on the bedside table. • Straddling the back of a chair, with arms supported on the back of the chair. • Lying on the unaffected side.	9. Ensures the diaphragm is dependent and facilitates access to the pleural cavity through intercostal spaces.
10. Assist throughout procedure with client positioning (see Figure 11-5-2), assessment of vital signs, client reassurance, management of supplies, and maintenance of sterile field and technique. • The physician or qualified practitioner will perform the procedure (see Figures 11-5-3 to 11-5-6).	10. Decreases risk of complications (e.g., client moving, sterile field becoming contaminated) and monitors client's tolerance.
11. Physician or qualified practitioner performs the procedure; the nurse assists as needed as the following are done: • Wash hands. • Put on mask and goggles if required by institution policy, apply sterile gloves, and drape the client with sterile towels. • Disinfect client's skin with povidone-iodine solution (see Figure 11-5-3). • Inject local anesthetic to the subcutaneous tissue.	11. • Reduces the transmission of microorganisms. • Maintains surgical asepsis. • Reduces the number of microorganisms on client's skin. • Provides anesthesia during the procedure.

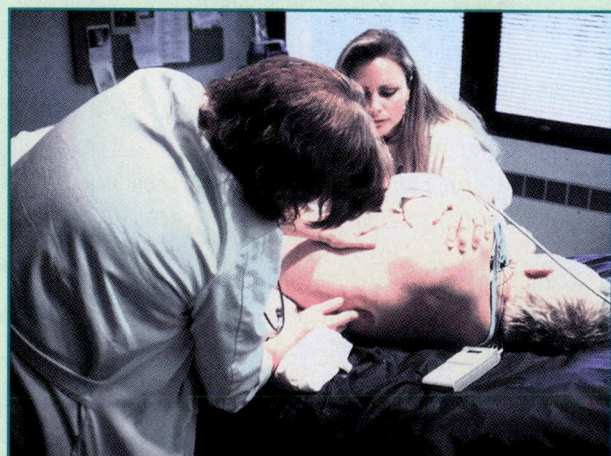

Figure 11-5-2 The client is positioned on the unaffected side. The nurse assists the client to maintain the proper position.

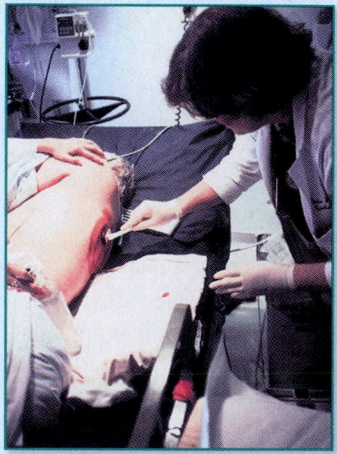

Figure 11-5-3 The site is cleaned with povidone-iodine solution.

continues

Action	Rationale

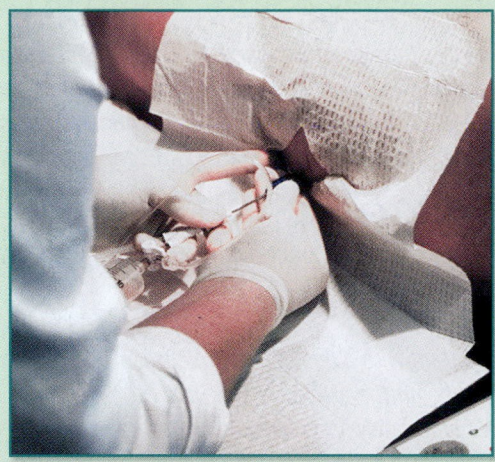

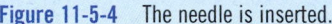
Figure 11-5-4   The needle is inserted.

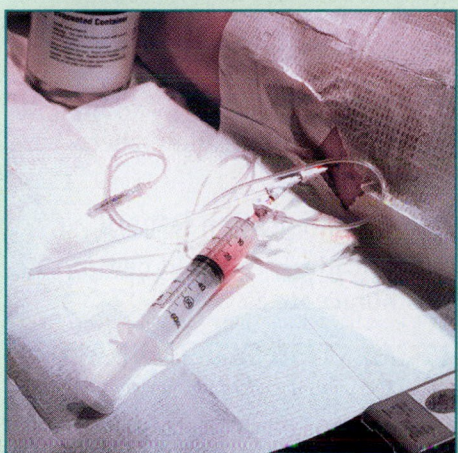

Figure 11-5-5   Fluid is removed from the pleural cavity.

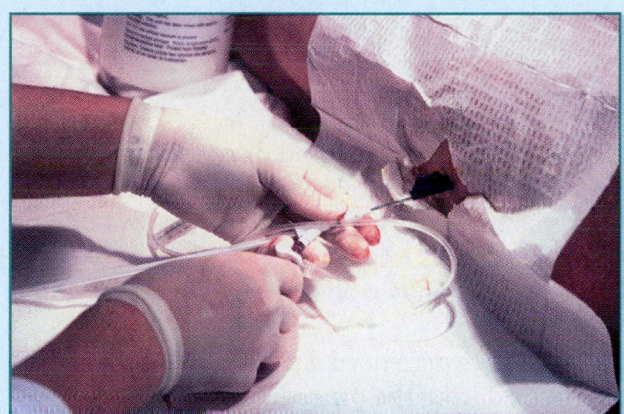

Figure 11-5-6   The needle is stabilized as fluid is drained from the pleural cavity.

Action

- Needle is inserted into pleural space (see Figure 11-5-4).
- Fluid is removed from the pleural space (see Figure 11-5-5).
- Needle is stabilized as fluid is drained from pleural space (see Figure 11-5-6).

12. Upon completion of procedure:
- Apply occlusive sterile dressing to thoracentesis site.

- Position client in comfortable position on unaffected side.
- Appropriately dispose of contaminated disposable and reusable supplies and equipment.
- Label and send out specimens for testing as ordered.

13. Remove gloves and wash hands.

14. Assess vital signs every 15 minutes for 1 hour, or as ordered.

15. Assess client for complications.

Rationale

- Provides access to pleural space.
- Prevents movement of needle during procedure.

12.
- Prevents the entry of microorganisms into the pleural cavity.
- Bed rest is recommended for at least 1 hour following a thoracentesis.
- Practices infection control and proper disposal of contaminated items.
- Ensures availability of laboratory data necessary to evaluate client's health status.

13. Reduces the transmission of microorganisms.

14. Monitors the client for complications of hemorrhage or shock.

15. Prevents complications and adverse sequelae.

Scenario 1

The nurse went into Mr. Rudder's room and began to prepare him for a thoracentesis. The physician arrived and was about to begin the procedure when none of the study results (e.g., chest X-ray) indicating a presence of a pleural effusion could be found. It took an additional 15 minutes to locate test results to determine the most appropriate site for needle insertion. During this time Mr. Rudder became increasingly anxious, began to hyperventilate, and fainted. The procedure had to be delayed until the client was stabilized. He required sedation and several health care team members to assist in positioning him to prevent movement during the thoracentesis when it was finally performed. The nurse should have made sure all the information and equipment needed were available prior to beginning the procedure.

Scenario 2

Special arrangements were made to provide conscious sedation to an infant with a documented pleural effusion of unknown origin in an ambulatory operating room suite. As the physician was about to begin the procedure, he noted that an adult thoracentesis tray had been ordered, and the procedure had to be delayed until the appropriately sized needles were obtained. This interrupted the flow of the outpatient procedures scheduled, prolonged the period of time the child was sedated, and increased parental anxiety.

► **EVALUATION**

- The client's pain decreased or ceased.
- Respiratory status showed no evidence of distress.
- Arterial blood gases, pulse oximetry, and other diagnostic tests improved.
- Pleural effusion was absent on follow-up diagnostic tests.
- The client experienced a minimal amount of discomfort during the procedure.
- The client has not experienced any complicating injury or infection related to the procedure.

► **DOCUMENTATION**

Nurses' Notes

- Record pre- and post-assessments, including vital signs and other physiologic parameters.
- Document the length of and client's tolerance to the procedure.
- Describe the location and type of dressing placed after the thoracentesis.
- Describe the color, quantity, and quality of fluid obtained from the pleural cavity.
- Describe the color, quality, and quantity of fluid on the postthoracentesis dressing.
- Document laboratory tests sent and pending.
- Record any adverse events that would indicate complications from the procedure and reports given to the physician or qualified practitioner.
- Document laboratory tests sent and pending.
- Document follow-up chest X-ray.

Document on appropriate flow sheet or electronic medical record (EMR).

Medication Administration Record

- Record medications required before, during, and after the thoracentesis.

► **CRITICAL THINKING SKILL**

Introduction

A thoracentesis is an invasive procedure that requires a thorough medical history as well as baseline vital signs.

Possible Scenario

An adult client presented with a pleural effusion of unknown etiology in significant respiratory distress. The nurse was informed that a thoracentesis would be required and quickly prepared the client for the procedure. Unfortunately, neither the nurse nor the physician assessed the client for current medications, and the client was on anticoagulant therapy for a history of a mesenteric thrombus. The procedure was done.

Possible Outcome

Failure to fully assess this medical history led to significant bleeding and a potential hemothorax. The client's recovery was complicated by the incomplete assessment prior to the procedure.

Prevention

Clients undergoing a thoracentesis should have a complete medical history, including medication profile and any history of clotting abnormalities. They should have a baseline physical assessment, including vital signs.

► VARIATIONS

Geriatric Variations:

- *Age-related changes in the musculoskeletal system (e.g., osteoporosis) might limit positioning of the geriatric client.*
- *Geriatric clients may have age-related changes in their respiratory status, which result in ineffective breathing patterns that can compound the problems being caused by a pleural effusion.*
- *Evaluation of blood pressure along with pulse and respirations are important because changes in chest pressures may significantly affect cardiac function in the geriatric population.*
- *The geriatric client may require oxygen therapy during the procedure and may need a longer period of bed rest following a thoracentesis to adjust to the fluid shift.*

Pediatric Variations:

- *Infants and small children may need adjustment in their positioning as well as sedation to maintain immobility.*
- *Special procedure trays are usually available for infants and very small children.*
- *Transdermal numbing medications currently available are often useful as initial preparation of the thoracentesis site.*
- *If a child is in the hospital and is mobile, procedures should be performed in a procedure area away from the child's room to maintain the hospital room as a "safe haven."*
- *Many children may need a special toy, blanket, or parent to assist in their comfort with the procedure.*
- *The teaching involved should be directed at either the parent or guardian as well as at an age-appropriate level for the child.*

Home Care Variations:

- *This procedure is not done in the home. Instruct the client and caregiver to report any signs of dyspnea, chest pain, dizziness, fever, or cough after returning home.*
- *Clearly outline the follow-up plans and when test results can be expected.*
- *Be sure the client has 24-hour access to a telephone and a number to reach help in case of a problem.*

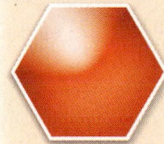

Long-Term Care Variations:

- *Long-term care clients may either be ventilator-dependent, cognitively impaired, or elderly. In each of these scenarios, it is important to assess procedure changes required for client positioning, teaching, and geriatric considerations.*
- *It is essential to be sure all health care staff (e.g., aides) in long-term settings are trained to identify potential signs of complications.*
- *Many of the high-technology physiologic assessment tools, such as pulse oximetry and arterial blood gas monitoring, may not be available in the long-term setting; therefore, careful assessment of the respiratory status is imperative.*

► COMMON ERRORS

Possible Error:

Not monitoring for maintenance of a sterile field.

Prevention:

Make all participants (physician, health care workers, and client) aware of the importance of this requirement and aggressively enforce this practice.

continues

► **COMMON ERRORS** *(continued)*

Possible Error:

Not assessing client for tolerance to position required for procedure.

Prevention:

Make client positioning part of your initial assessment in preparing a client for a thoracentesis. If the client has difficulty, assist the client with positioning to determine which of the possible positions will be tolerated and support the client as necessary with pillows or have other health care team members help to maintain immobility during the thoracentesis.

► **NURSING TIPS**

- Identify that you have all the necessary pretest results, premedication orders, and a signed consent form before proceeding with the procedure.
- Check all supplies to be sure you have the appropriate thoracentesis tray, laboratory specimen tubes, and labels.
- Assess client's tolerance to positioning requirements before the actual procedure.
- Inform another nurse of the procedure in progress to obtain assistance in the event of an unexpected outcome.
- Provide comfort measures (e.g., blanket, toy) to a child and whenever possible allow parent(s) to remain with the child to reduce anxiety.
- Employ techniques that clients have used with past invasive procedures to decrease anxiety and promote relaxation. Talking to the client while the procedure is being performed may help decrease anxiety and increase cooperation.

- Approach the client with confidence and reassure the client that you will remain with him or her throughout the procedure.
- After the procedure, monitor the client for signs and symptoms of complications, which may include:
  - Pneumothorax (shortness of breath, decreased breath sounds, decreased chest movement with inspiration, asymmetric chest wall movement, tachypnea)
  - Shock (hypotension, syncope, tachycardia, peripheral vasoconstriction)
  - Infection/sepsis (fever, chills, tachycardia, tachypnea)
  - Hemothorax (tachypnea, diminished breath sounds, dullness to percussion)
  - Subcutaneous emphysema (soft tissue swelling, crepitation palpable in affected area)

► **SPECIAL CONSIDERATIONS**

- *In the presence of a large pleural effusion, a supine position will be difficult for a client who may become dyspneic. The client may need to be in a semi-Fowler's position to breathe adequately. Prior to the thoracentesis assess the most comfortable position and alert the health care practitioner accordingly.*
- *Rarely, a tension pneumothorax, pulmonary embolus, or pulmonary edema can occur following a thoracentesis. Be alert for signs and symptoms of tension pneumothorax (deviation of the trachea, asymmetry of respiratory movement, tachycardia, dyspnea, hypoxemia, and extreme anxiety); pulmonary embolus (shortness of breath, anxiety, hemoptysis, syncope, or tightness/pain in the chest); or pulmonary edema (blood-tinged mucus, dyspnea, decreased breath sounds with rales).*

Assisting with an Abdominal Paracentesis

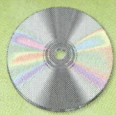

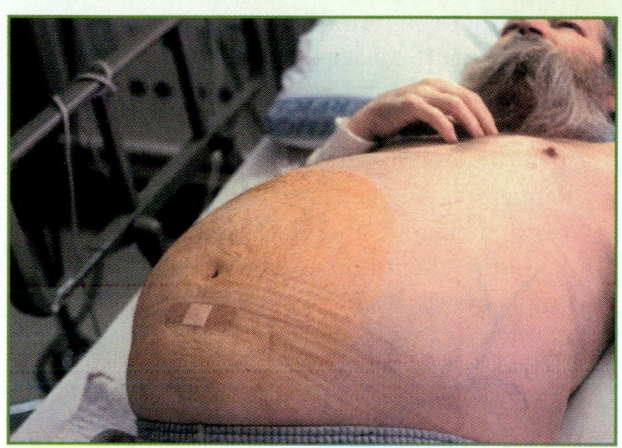

▶ OVERVIEW OF THE SKILL

The abdomen usually contains a minimal amount of fluid. In certain conditions, fluid can accumulate in the abdominal cavity. The abdominal paracentesis (abdominal tap) is a sterile procedure in which a needle is inserted through the abdominal wall to obtain a sample of any fluid that is present or to drain a larger volume of fluid to relieve pressure. Paracentesis is used before surgery, radiography, or ascites reinfusion or to remove fluid to relieve pressure on the diaphragm.

Abdominal paracentesis can be done in an office, treatment room, or the hospital. The presence of bloody fluid after internal injury suggests internal organ bleeding. Other findings may indicate infection, a tumor, appendicitis, cirrhosis of the liver, disease of the pancreas, kidney, or heart, or a damaged bowel. During abdominal paracentesis, there is a slight chance of the needle puncturing the bowel, bladder, or a blood vessel in the abdomen. If a large quantity of fluid is removed, there is a slight risk of hypotension. There is also a slight risk of infection.

▶ ASSESSMENT

1. Identify the purpose for the abdominal paracentesis. **This allows the nurse to anticipate effects of the abdominal paracentesis and to observe the client's response.**

2. Check allergies to medications or anesthetic, bleeding problems, medications currently using, (including aspirin), or if the client might be pregnant. **This will decrease the chance of complication during the procedure.**

3. Assess client's knowledge regarding the abdominal paracentesis. **Determines need for education and assists in identifying questions and concerns.**

4. Assess the client for bleeding tendencies to determine the risk of bleeding during and after the procedure.

5. Assess client's ability to sign a consent form.

▶ DIAGNOSIS

Pain

Excess Fluid Volume

Deficient Fluid Volume

Risk for Infection

▶ PLANNING

Expected Outcomes:

1. Client will experience minimal discomfort during abdominal paracentesis procedure.

2. Client will not suffer any adverse effects such as cardiovascular distress, shock, infection, or internal bleeding following the procedure.

3. Client will experience relief of symptoms of excessive abdominal fluid, such as increased respiratory rate and decreased respiratory volume.

Equipment Needed (see Figures 11-6-1A and B):

- Disposable paracentesis tray *or* 16-gauge 3.5-inch aspiration needle
- Ampule of 1% lidocaine, 5 mL
- Needles for local anesthetic, 25-gauge, 5/8 inch
- Needle, 21-gauge 1.5 inches
- Syringe, 5-mL
- Syringe, 50-mL
- Prep tray
- Prep applicators
- Sterile drapes
- Sponges
- Two-way valve
- Specimen tubes
- Drainage bag or bottles
- Adhesive bandage
- Sterile gloves
- Masks (optional)
- Biohazard bag

▶ CLIENT EDUCATION NEEDED:

1. Explain purpose of abdominal paracentesis and risks. Reinforce verbal teaching with written instructions.
2. Instruct the client that there will be a stinging sensation from the anesthetic and a feeling of pressure as the needle is inserted.
3. Explain positioning during procedure and ensure that client understands.
4. Explain that if a large amount of fluid is withdrawn, the client may experience dizziness or lightheadedness.
5. Client understands the need to report any changes in symptoms, such as shortness of breath, dizziness, and increased perspiration.
6. Make sure client knows who to call if any complications arise after the procedure is completed.

Estimated time to complete the skill: **5–15 minutes**

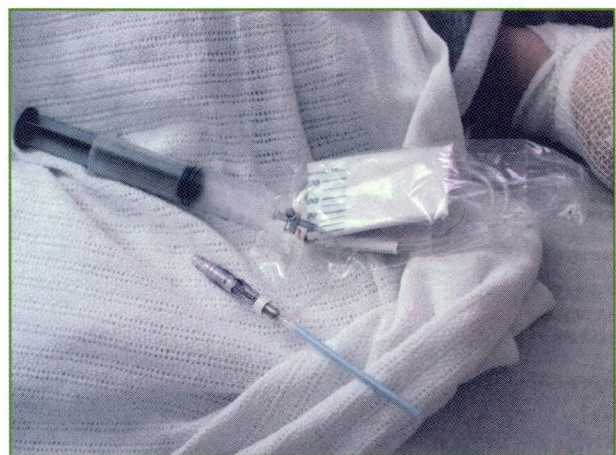

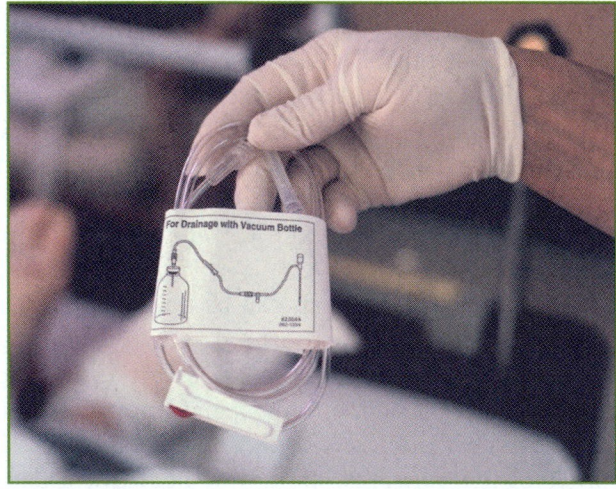

Figure 11-6-1 **A.** Aspiration needle, tubing, and syringe.

B. Drainage tubing

▶ DELEGATION TIPS

Assessment for bleeding, pain, shortness of breath, and proper postprocedure position is the responsibility of the nurse. Measurement of vital signs may be delegated to ancillary personnel.

IMPLEMENTATION—Action/Rationale

Action	Rationale
1. Wash hands.	1. Reduces the transmission of microorganisms.
2. Ask the client if he or she has ever undergone the procedure previously. Describe the procedure and tell the client that the procedure is usually not painful.	2. Paracentesis is an invasive procedure. Explanation of the procedure should clarify any questions the client may have.
3. Check the physician's or qualified practitioner's order for the reason for the test and clarify diagnosis.	3. By understanding the reasons, the nurse can better clarify procedure for clients. This also allows the nurse to have available the correct collection container. If the procedure is for a cell count, a test tube for a small amount of fluid will be needed to send a specimen to the laboratory.
4. Verify that a consent form has been signed by the client.	4. This is a surgical procedure and requires that the client understand the potential associated risks. The consent also legally protects the hospital, client, physician or qualified practitioner, and nurse.
5. Assess the client's allergic status to local anesthetics or antiseptic solutions.	5. Protects the client from an avoidable allergic reaction.
6. Ask the client to void as completely as possible.	6. Decreases the potential of inadvertently piercing the client's bladder. If urination is not possible, catheterization will be necessary.
7. Measure the client's abdominal girth and weight.	7. Allows for assessment of the amount of fluid removed and serves as a comparison if fluid reaccumulates.
8. Help the client to assume a fully supported upright position in the bed or chair, if possible. If the client can sit in a chair, support his or her feet.	8. In a sitting position, the client's intestines will float away from the paracentesis site and the danger of punctured intestines will be lessened.
9. Wash your hands again.	9. Decreases the transmission of microorganisms.
10. Assemble equipment. Open the sterile abdominal paracentesis tray using sterile technique, if requested by the person performing the procedure.	10. Maintains sterile procedure.
11. Place a blood pressure cuff on one of the client's arms (see Figure 11-6-2).	11. Allows you to assess the client's blood pressure continuously as the removal of excessive fluid or removal that is too fast can cause a decrease in blood pressure and, potentially, shock.
12. As the physician or qualified practitioner performs the procedure (see Figure 11-6-3), help the client maintain position. The nurse may assist the physician or qualified practitioner as needed when the following are done: • Wash hands	12. Proper positioning lessens the danger of punctured intestines. • Reduces the transmission of microorganisms.

continues

Action	Rationale
• Put on masks and goggles if required by institution policy, apply sterile gloves and drape the client with sterile towels.	• Maintains sterile technique.
• Disinfect the client's skin with antiseptic solution.	• Reduces the number of microorganisms on client's skin.
• Inject local anesthetic agent to subcutaneous tissue.	• Provides anesthesia to site during procedure.
• Needle is inserted into peritoneal space.	• Provides access to peritoneal space.
• Fluid is removed from peritoneal space.	• Prevents entry of microorganisms into peritoneal space.
• Needle is removed and sterile dressing applied.	
13. Reassure the client during the procedure.	13. Helps the client cope with the situation and reduces anxiety.
14. Record the client's blood pressure readings and pulse rate at 15-minute intervals and observe the client for signs of pallor or sweating.	14. Indicates if the client is experiencing vascular collapse.
15. When the procedure is completed, assist the client to assume a comfortable position.	15. Enables the client to relax after the procedure.
16. Obtain measurements of the client's abdominal girth and weight (see Figure 11-6-4).	16. Serves as a comparison with the preparacentesis.
17. Monitor the client's vital signs, urine output, and dressing drainage or bleeding every 15 minutes for 1 hour or as ordered.	17. Monitors the client for complications of shock or hemorrhage.
18. Label the fluid specimen, place in biohazard bag, and send to the laboratory as soon as possible.	18. If the fluid is for culture and sensitivity, overgrowth of microorganisms will occur if the fluid is allowed to sit. Label identifies specimen. Bag protects you from contact with body fluids.

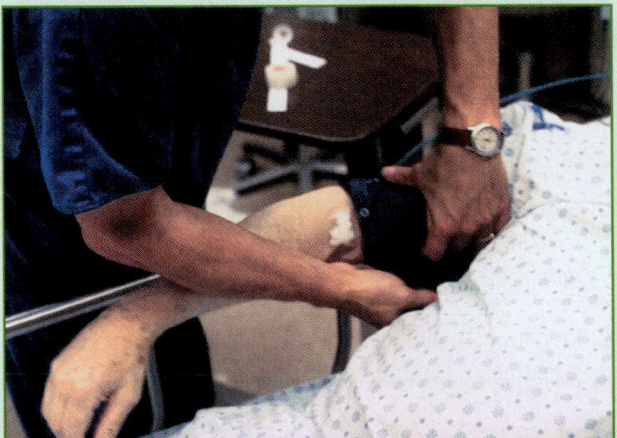

Figure 11-6-2 Place the blood pressure cuff on the arm.

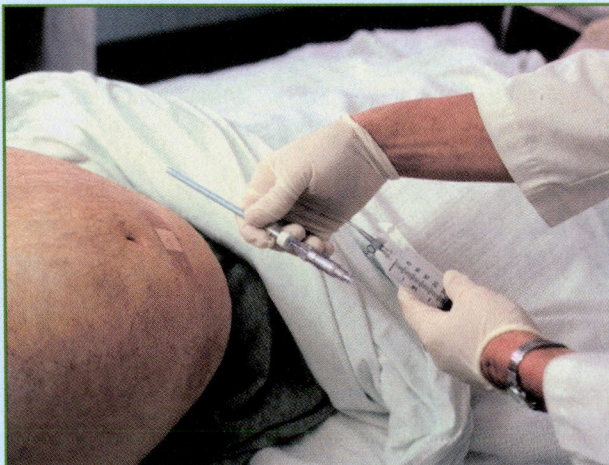

Figure 11-6-3 The physician or qualified practitioner prepares to perform the procedure.

continues

Action	Rationale
19. Record and describe the amount of fluid drained. Describe consistency, color, and opacity of the fluid (see Figure 11-6-5).	**19.** Communicates the findings to the other members of the health care team and contributes to the legal record by documenting the care given to the client.
20. Apply gloves and dispose of equipment according to your agency guidelines.	**20.** Decreases the transmission of microorganisms.
21. Remove gloves and wash hands.	**21.** Reduces the transmission of microorganisms.
22. Assess the laboratory results.	**22.** Based on the results, further medical intervention may be necessary.

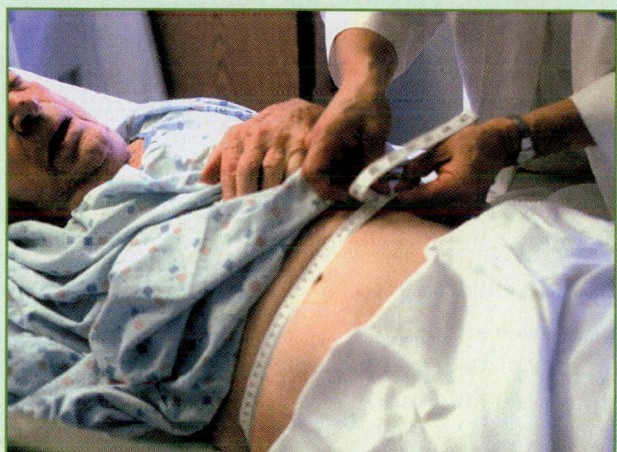

Figure 11-6-4   Measure the abdominal girth.

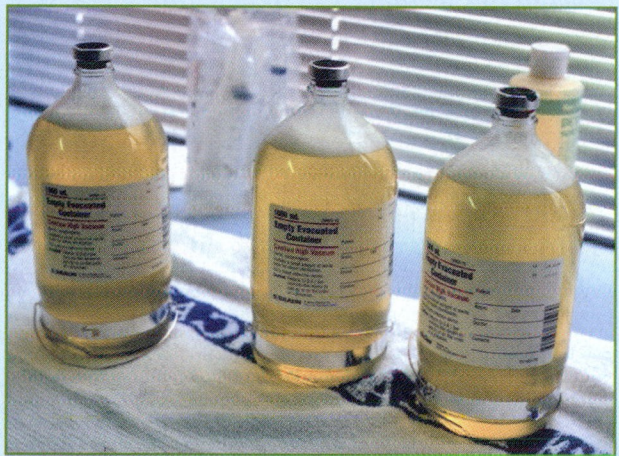

Figure 11-6-5   Record and describe the amount of fluid drained.

▶ REAL WORLD ANECDOTES

Jim is scheduled for an abdominal paracentesis this afternoon. His nurse orders the supplies, explains the procedure to him, and assists the physician with the procedure. Once the needle is removed, a dressing is placed over the puncture site. The nurse checks on Jim 10 minutes after the procedure and notes that the dressing is saturated with blood and blood is oozing from the site. Jim mentions that he has been taking aspirin regularly for an injured knee and wonders if this has anything to do with the bleeding. Although the nurse asked the client about medication usage, it was not clear to Jim that this included over-the-counter medications. It is important to obtain an in-depth, accurate health history.

▶ EVALUATION

- Client experienced minimal discomfort during abdominal paracentesis procedure.
- Client did not suffer any adverse effects such as cardiovascular distress, shock, infection, or internal bleeding following the procedure.
- Client experienced relief of symptoms of excessive abdominal fluid, such as increased respiratory rate and decreased respiratory volume.

▶ DOCUMENTATION

Nurses' Notes:

- Note the time the abdominal paracentesis procedure was performed.
- Record the anatomic site of puncture.
- Document laboratory analysis ordered for sample of fluid.
- Document the client's response to procedure.
- Document the specimens collected and where they were sent.
- Record the vital signs during procedure and every 15 minutes up to 4 times after the procedure or until the client is stable.
- Describe the pressure dressing and assessment of drainage.
- Record urinary output (may be covered in the intake and output record).
- Record abdominal girth and weight before and after the procedure.
- Record urinary output.
- Record the amount of fluid removed from the abdominal cavity.

- Record the anatomical site of puncture.
- Document laboratory analysis ordered for sample of fluid.

Document on appropriate flow sheet or electronic medical record (EMR).

▶ CRITICAL THINKING SKILL

Introduction

Abdominal paracentesis is sometimes performed to remove fluid from the peritoneal cavity. If a large volume of fluid is drained during abdominal paracentesis, the client may become dizzy or lightheaded.

Possible Scenario

Janet is a 48-year-old woman with metastatic breast cancer involving her liver and bones. She has noticed increasing weight and abdominal bloating and is very uncomfortable. She is scheduled to have an abdominal paracentesis to remove some fluid and relieve her abdominal pressure. During the procedure, Janet becomes very dizzy and lightheaded. Her blood pressure drops from 140/80 to 100/62 after removal of one and a half liters of fluid.

Possible Outcome

The physician decides to stop the procedure and consider placement of a catheter into the abdomen to remove the fluid more slowly over time.

Prevention

Careful monitoring of blood pressure during removal of large volumes of fluid and diligent assessment of symptoms can help detect this side effect more quickly.

▶ VARIATIONS

Geriatric Variations:

- *Elderly clients tend to have slower return to normal of cardiovascular status.*
- *Elderly clients may not be able to sit for long periods; therefore, organization is critical so the procedure can be performed quickly and smoothly.*

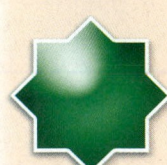

Pediatric Variation:

- *Even small amounts of fluid can cause rapid vascular shifts in pediatric clients.*

continues

► **VARIATIONS** *(continued)*

Home Care Variation:
- *This procedure is not done in the home care setting. Instruct the client and caregiver to report abdominal pain, bleeding, drainage from paracentesis site, and elevated temperature. Make sure the client knows who to contact if complications occur after returning home.*

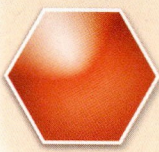

Long-Term Care Variation:
- *Clients who experience buildup of ascites may require repeated paracentesis and are at increased risk for complications.*

► **COMMON ERRORS**

Possible Error:

Adequate number of collection containers are not available for abdominal fluid collection.

Prevention:

Check supplies before procedure begins. Ask the physician, qualified practitioner, or nurse practitioner what is expected volume of fluid to be removed.

► **NURSING TIPS**

- Always check the equipment and supplies before the procedure begins.
- Explain the procedure thoroughly to the client to ensure that he or she understands and knows what symptoms to report during the procedure.
- Client should be designated as NPO (nothing per mouth) at midnight the night before the procedure or receiving only clear liquids the morning of the procedure.
- Keep long needle out of sight, if possible.

- Return within appropriate time (5–10 minutes) to evaluate client's response to abdominal paracentesis procedure.
- Assess for pain, dizziness, and lightheadedness.
- Report signs and symptoms of complications immediately.
- Assess paracentesis site for bleeding and drainage.
- Assess for internal bleeding (increased abdominal pain, changes in vital signs and color).
- Monitor for peritonitis (increased temperature, abdominal pain, and tense abdomen) following the procedure.

► **SPECIAL CONSIDERATIONS**

- *For clients with large amounts of fluid in the abdomen, positioning may be difficult. Before the health care practitioner arrives to perform the paracentesis, find a position tolerable for the client.*
- *After fluid has been removed from the client's abdomen, monitor respirations and oxygen saturations.*
- *Wean the client off oxygen as there is more room for the lungs to exchange gas.*
- *Shock is of concern for clients who have had more than 1,000 to 1,500 cc of fluid removed. Monitor vital signs closely and watch for syncope, change in mental status, skin color or temperature change, and hypoxemia.*
- *Clients requiring a paracentesis may have liver failure, along with vitamin K deficiency, and, therefore, may have an increased bleeding tendency.*
- *Clients may have an enlarged liver; therefore, risk of puncturing the organ is present.*

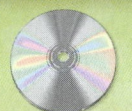

Assisting with a Bone Marrow Biopsy/Aspiration

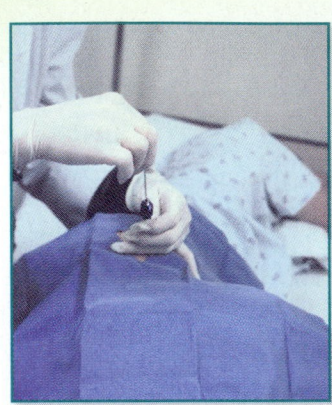

▶ OVERVIEW OF THE SKILL

A bone marrow biopsy and a bone marrow aspiration are two distinct procedures. Bone marrow aspiration is the removal of a small amount of organic material from the medulla of certain bones by a large-bore needle. This spongy bone is where hematopoiesis (formation of blood cells) takes place. The sternum and posterior iliac crests are the most commonly used sites. A bone marrow biopsy is the removal of a core of bone marrow cells by a biopsy needle. The cells are then examined in the laboratory to describe the number, size, shape, and development of the erythrocytes and megakaryocytes. The procedure is usually performed by a physician or qualified practitioner assisted by a nurse; however, in hematology/oncology clinics, advanced practice nurses may perform bone marrow aspirations.

The biopsy or aspiration is used to diagnose leukemia, anemia, thrombocytopenia, and other malignancies such as non-Hodgkin's lymphoma or multiple myeloma. It may also be used to monitor the response to therapy for certain cancers.

▶ ASSESSMENT

1. Assess the client's knowledge of the purpose and plan of the procedure **so he or she will cooperate and not be anxious.**
2. Review the client's signature on the informed consent form. **It is a legal requirement of the institution.**

3. Assess the client's ability to remain still in the supine, prone, or lateral position during the procedure. **This is required in order to assess the bone marrow properly.**
4. Assess vital signs as baseline data **to compare with postprocedural vital signs.**
5. Review the medical record for the client's risk of bleeding, including use of anticoagulants, prothrombin time, and platelet count. **These factors may affect the risk of bleeding.**
6. Review the medical record for a history of allergic reactions to antiseptic or anesthetic solutions **to avoid an allergic reaction.**
7. Assess client's ability to sign a consent form.

▶ DIAGNOSIS

Anxiety

Deficient Knowledge

Acute Pain

Risk for Injury

Risk for Infection

▶ PLANNING

Expected Outcomes:

1. The client will understand the rationale for the procedure and tolerate it without anxiety.
2. The client will assume the required position and remain still during the procedure.
3. The client will experience minimal pain.

4. There will be no extensive bleeding or infectious complications.
5. The aspiration or biopsy will be sufficient for diagnostic testing.

Equipment Needed (see Figure 11-7-1):

- Bone marrow aspiration/biopsy tray, including:
  - Antiseptic solution (povidone-iodine)
  - Gauze sponges (4 × 4)
  - Sterile towels
  - Local anesthetic solution (lidocaine)
  - Sterile syringes: two 3-mL with 23- to 25-gauge needles for anesthetic
  - Two 10-mL syringes for marrow aspiration
  - Two bone marrow needles with inner stylus
  - One biopsy needle
  - Test tubes and glass slides
  - Povidone-iodine ointment
  - Sterile gauze and tape or Band-Aid®
- Sterile gloves
- Masks and goggles for physician or qualified practitioner and nurse, if required
- Pain medication or sedative as ordered (to be given before procedure)

► CLIENT EDUCATION NEEDED:

1. The client should be taught the rationale for the procedure.

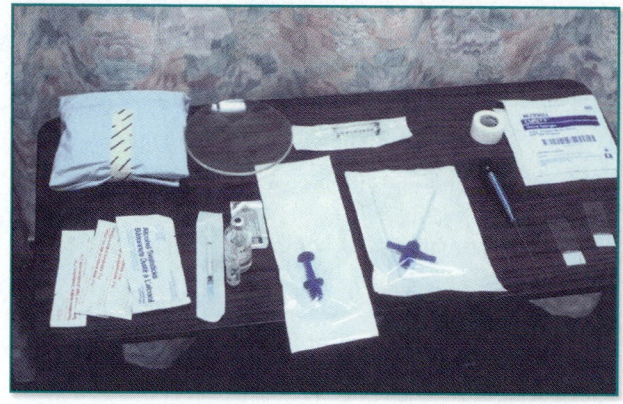

Figure 11-7-1 Glass dish, syringe, gauze, tape, povidone-iodine, lidocaine, bone marrow needle, and slides

2. The client should be told about the need for sterile technique.
3. The client should be instructed on the position to be assumed and the importance of remaining still.
4. Encourage the client to verbalize fears or anxiety.
5. The client should be encouraged to ask questions.
6. Assure the client that the actual aspiration takes only a minute or two.
7. Encourage the client to take slow, deep breaths and use imagery to promote relaxation.

Estimated time to complete the skill:
15 minutes

► DELEGATION TIPS

Assessment for bleeding, pain, shortness of breath, and proper postprocedure position is the responsibility of the nurse. Measurement of vital signs may be delegated to ancillary personnel.

IMPLEMENTATION—Action/Rationale

Action	Rationale
1. Have the client void.	1. Promotes client comfort.
2. Administer medication for sedation or pain. Be alert to medications that may alter clot formation.	2. Promotes comfort and assurance of remaining still during procedure. Bleeding is a risk factor of this procedure.
3. Wash hands.	3. Reduces the transmission of microorganisms.

continues

Action	Rationale
4. Set up sterile tray.	**4.** Maintains sterile field.
5. Assist client in maintaining correct position for site to be aspirated: • Sternum—supine • Posterior iliac crests—prone or lying on side	**5.** Decreases risk of complications during procedure by misplacement of needle.
6. Reassure client while explaining each step of procedure. A sharp sting usually occurs with the local anesthetic and a brief dull pain when the needle enters the bone.	**6.** Increases client comfort and relaxation. Informs client of what to anticipate.
7. Assess client's condition during the procedure.	**7.** Provides for treatment of a potential complication.
8. Physician or qualified practitioner performs the aspiration or biopsy: • Select the site to be used • Wash hands. • Put on mask, goggles if required, and sterile gloves (see Figure 11-7-2). • Drape client with sterile towels or drape (see Figure 11-7-3). • Disinfect client's skin with antiseptic solution (see Figure 11-7-4) and dry with cotton swab (see Figure 11-7-5).	**8.** • These can be the anterior or posterior iliac spine or iliac crest of the pelvic bones or the body of the sternum. • Reduces the transmission of microorganisms. • Maintains surgical asepsis. • Maintains sterile field. • Maintains sterile field.

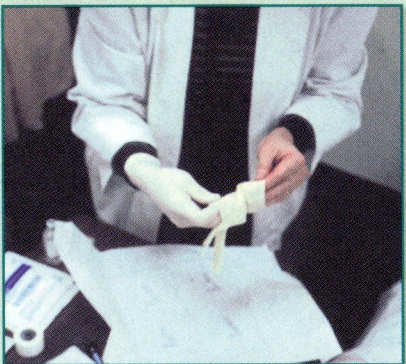

Figure 11-7-2 Apply sterile gloves.

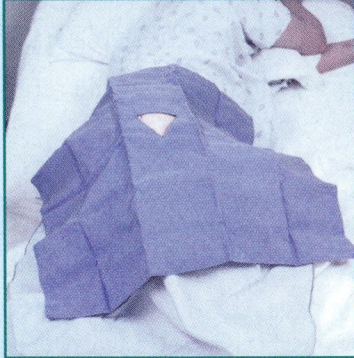

Figure 11-7-3 The posterior iliac crest draped with a sterile drape.

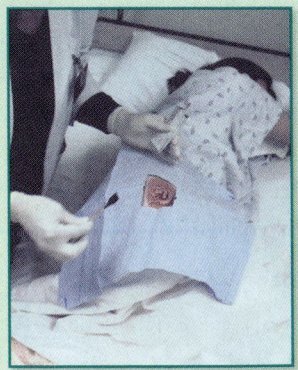

Figure 11-7-4 Disinfect the skin.

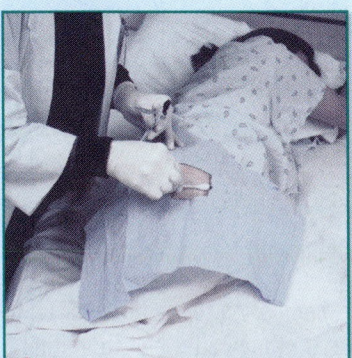

Figure 11-7-5 Dry the area with a sterile cotton swab.

continues

Action	Rationale
• Inject local anesthetic to the site and ask client when it has taken effect (see Figure 11-7-6).	• Provides anesthesia during the aspiration.
• Bone marrow aspiration: Insert the needle with inner stylus into the bone (see Figure 11-7-7), then advance the needle until it reaches the area of softer, spongy bone and remove the stylus (see Figure 11-7-8). Attach the 10-mL syringe to the needle and aspirate bone marrow (see Figure 11-7-9).	• The inner stylus is stiffer than the needle and has a longer bevel to enter the bone. Approximately 1 to 2 ml of bone marrow is needed for laboratory examination.
• Bone marrow biopsy: Screw the core biopsy instrument into the bone and remove a plug of tissue.	• A long core of marrow is needed for more detailed examination.
• Place specimens into appropriate containers for transfer to the laboratory.	• Certain fixatives and preparations are needed for aspirate and bone samples.
• Label specimens with client name and date.	• Assures proper identification in laboratory.
• After removing the needle or biopsy corer, apply pressure to the puncture site (see Figure 11-7-10).	• Prevents bleeding at puncture site.
• Apply antiseptic ointment and a gauze dressing.	• Reduces risk of infection
• Place specimen on glass slides or in a test tube.	• Allows specimen to be examined in the laboratory.
• Remove gloves and wash hands.	• Reduces the transmission of microorganisms.

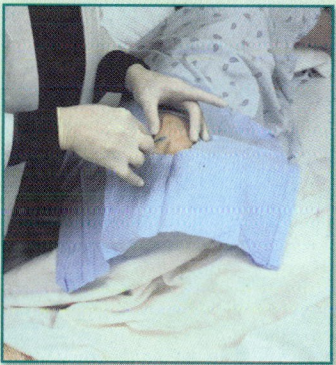

Figure 11-7-6   Inject a local anesthetic.

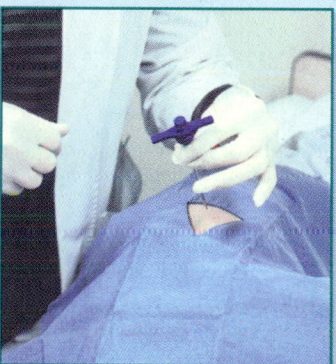

Figure 11-7-7   Insert the needle with the inner stylus into the bone.

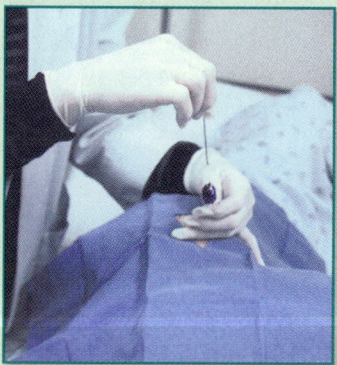

Figure 11-7-8   Advance the needle until it reaches softer bone and remove the stylus.

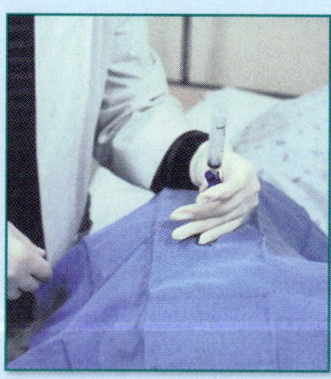

Figure 11-7-9   Attach a 10-mL syringe to the needle and aspirate the sample.

continues

Action	Rationale
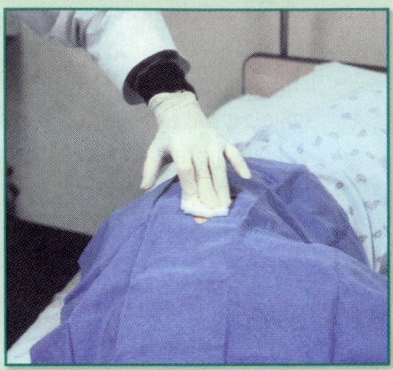	Figure 11-7-10 After the needle is removed, apply pressure to the site.

9. Apply gloves and apply pressure to the site and apply dressing as per institution protocol. The nurse or a technologist may prepare the slides or test tubes with the specimen and label them with client's name. Send specimens to laboratory.

9. Reduces the transmission of microorganisms and reduces risk of bleeding.

10. Assist client into a comfortable position.

10. Promotes comfort after the procedure.

11. Put on gloves and discard supplies appropriately.

11. Reduces the transmission of microorganisms and risk of accidental needle punctures.

12. Remove gloves and wash hands.

12. Reduces the transmission of microorganisms.

▶ REAL WORLD ANECDOTES

Scenario 1
Jessica was 14 years old when her doctor suspected aplastic anemia. He needed to do a bone marrow biopsy to make a definitive diagnosis. Jessica had never heard of a bone marrow biopsy so her nurse calmly explained the procedure to her and her mother. Jessica asked whether the puncture would hurt more or less than a blood test. The nurse honestly told her that the needle stick to give the local anesthetic would be similar but that aspirating the bone marrow could be more painful. When Jessica started to cry, the nurse gave her a tissue, held her hand, and assured her that she would receive a tranquilizer to help her relax. She said that the actual aspiration usually takes only a minute or two and that her mother could be with her if she wanted.

Scenario 2
Marge was a large woman from a rural area who came to a large medical center for a bone marrow transplant for acute myelogenous leukemia. Even though she appeared to be brave, she had never been sick before and was afraid. She had some tranquilizers at home and took several pills before coming to the clinic for her test but did not tell her doctor or nurse. She was given short-acting conscious sedation before the bone marrow aspiration and suddenly became apneic. The doctors and nurse used an Ambu®-bag to revive her and coached her to take deep breaths while the doctor finished doing the aspiration. The nurse needed to assess if she had taken medications prior to coming to the clinic for her test.

► EVALUATION

- The client understood the rationale for the procedure and tolerated it without anxiety.
- The client assumed the required position and remained still during the procedure.
- The client experienced minimal pain.
- There was no extensive bleeding or infectious complications.
- Reduces risk of infection.
- Allows specimen to be examined in the laboratory.
- Reduces the transmission of microorganisms.
- The aspiration or biopsy was sufficient for diagnostic testing.

► DOCUMENTATION

Nurses' Notes

- Record the date, time, and site of the bone marrow aspiration or biopsy.
- Describe the amount and color of bone marrow aspirated.
- Document laboratory tests ordered and when specimens were sent.
- Document the type of dressing and ointment applied.
- Record vital signs before and after the procedure.
- Note complications or pain.
- Note the presence of any bleeding at the site.
- Describe the condition of the skin at the site.

Document on appropriate flow sheet or electronic medical record (EMR).

Medication Administration Record

- Record the date and time of pain medication or sedative.

► CRITICAL THINKING SKILL

Introduction

The prone position can be difficult for clients with respiratory compromise or joint pain.

Possible Scenario

The client was obese and had asthma that required bronchodilators at times. She became somewhat anxious before her bone marrow aspiration and was experiencing some difficulty breathing when she was asked to lay prone on the bed.

Possible Outcome

The nurse assisted the client into a latero decubitus position with the superior leg resting in front of the inferior leg. This enabled her to breathe with more ease and allowed the subcutaneous tissue to fall away from the iliac crest so the bone was easier to access.

Prevention

The client could have been assessed for her respiratory history, pain, and anxiety.

► VARIATIONS

Geriatric Variations:
- *Older clients with arthritis may have difficulty assuming the position necessary for the procedure.*
- *Bones may be either very hard or brittle.*

Pediatric Variations:
- *A child could practice the procedure on a doll before his or her test.*
- *A parent should be allowed to stay with the child.*
- *Sedation may be necessary for young children.*

Home Care Variation:
- *This procedure is not done in the home care setting. The home health nurse who may be caring for a client after a bone marrow aspiration or biopsy procedure needs to assess for possible bleeding or infection.*

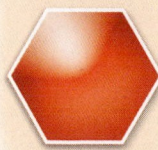

Long-Term Care Variation:
- *Long-term cancer clients may be immunosuppressed and require regular assessments for personal hygiene, bleeding, and infection after the procedure.*

▶ **COMMON ERRORS**

Possible Error:

A young client suddenly jerks and starts crying after the physician or qualified practitioner has inserted the needle into the bone.

Prevention:

Assess the client's need for sedation, effective teaching, and preparation. If an error occurs, stop the procedure and calm the client by softly assuring him or her. Ask parents to comfort the child. Ask the physician or qualified practitioner for sedation orders and give the medication. When the client is sedated, resume the procedure.

▶ **NURSING TIPS**

- Use pillows, rolled towels, or blankets to assist the client into a comfortable position.

- If a sternal puncture is being done, the semi-Fowler's position may be more comfortable.

▶ **SPECIAL CONSIDERATIONS**

- *Because a bone marrow biopsy is used to diagnose various types of cancer or monitor response to therapy for leukemia, clients are already in a compromised state and may need additional psychological support, comfort measures, and assistance in maintaining self-esteem.*

Assisting with a Lumbar Puncture

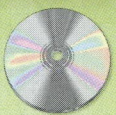

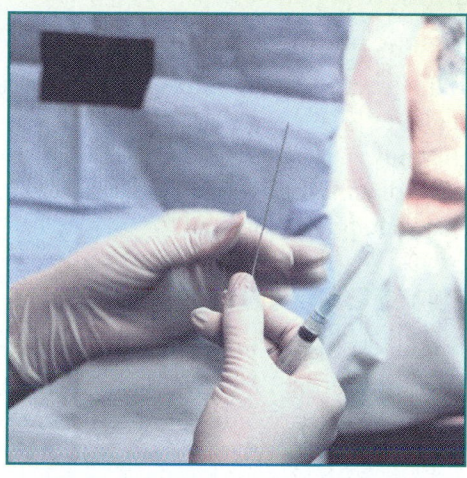

▶ OVERVIEW OF THE SKILL

A lumbar puncture, also called a spinal tap or a spinal puncture, is the introduction of a needle into the subarachnoid space of the spinal column. The purposes of a lumbar puncture are to measure the pressure in the subarachnoid space, to obtain cerebral spinal fluid (CSF) for laboratory examination, or to inject anesthetic, diagnostic, or therapeutic agents. A lumbar puncture is useful in the diagnosis of meningitis, encephalitis, brain or spinal cord tumors, and cerebral hemorrhage. The procedure is done by a physician or other qualified health care provider; the nurse is needed to assist him or her and to provide care and support of the client.

A lumbar puncture can also be used to treat various conditions such as increased intercranial pressure through removal of excess CSF, or infections through intrathecal placement of antibiotics. The same basic nursing methods are used for these procedures as when placing an epidural at the bedside during labor.

One common side effect from lumbar punctures is headache associated with the decrease in CSF pressure and circulating volume. This occurs in less then half the people undergoing a lumbar puncture, usually within 2 days, but resolves spontaneously after 2 weeks. There is much research and controversy about treatment and nursing intervention for these clients. The most commonly advised conservative treatment is to encourage bed rest, increased fluid intake, and pain medications as needed.

▶ ASSESSMENT

1. Assess the client's ability to understand and follow instructions necessary to assume and maintain the proper position **to avoid trauma of the spinal canal by the needle.**
2. Assess the client's musculoskeletal condition and ability to assume the lateral decubitus position necessary **to place the spinal needle into the subarachnoid space.**
3. Assess the ability of the client to maintain the fetal position **as movement can cause injury from the spinal needle.**
4. Review the medical record for signs of increased intracranial pressure or degenerative joint disease that **are contraindicated in this procedure.**
5. Review the medical record to see if the client has an allergy to any local anesthetic agents **to prevent an allergic reaction.**
6. Check for informed consent form—**a legal requirement for most invasive diagnostic procedures.**
7. Assess the client's knowledge about the procedure **to provide tailored client education.**

8. Assess vital signs and neurologic reactions of legs, specifically movement, sensation, and muscle strength, **to compare baseline assessment with postprocedure assessment.**
9. Assess client's ability to sign a consent from.

▶ DIAGNOSIS

Anxiety

Deficient Knowledge

Pain

Risk for Injury

Risk for Peripheral Neurovascular Dysfunction

▶ PLANNING

Expected Outcomes:

1. Client will understand the procedure and its rationale.
2. Client will be comfortable and not anxious.
3. There will be minimal bleeding or leakage of cerebral spinal fluid.
4. The client will not experience a postprocedure headache.
5. The test results of the CSF will be normal.

Equipment Needed:

- Lumbar puncture tray (see Figure 11-8-1), including:
  - Antiseptic solution (povidone-iodine)
  - Ten gauze sponges (4 × 4)
  - Sterile towels
  - Spinal needles of various sizes (5 to 12.5 cm long) with inner obturators

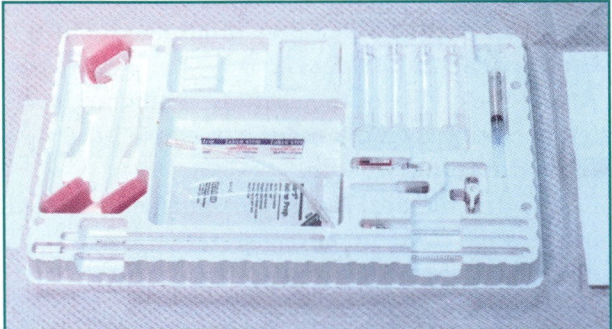

Figure 11-8-1 Lumbar puncture tray

- Alcohol swabs
- Anesthetic agent (lidocaine)
- Syringes (3- to 5-mL)
- Needles (⅝ to 1½ inches, 21- to 25-gauge)
- Glass or plastic manometer with three-way stopcock
- Four test tubes
- Antiseptic ointment
- Band-Aid® or 2 × 2 gauze dressing and tape
- Sterile gloves
- Straight chair
- Pillow for placing between client's knees
- Masks and goggles (optional)

▶ CLIENT EDUCATION NEEDED:

1. The client should be taught the reason for the lumbar puncture.
2. Explain how the procedure will be done and the need to remain in the fetal position without moving so that no injury will be caused by the needle.
3. The client should be informed that local anesthetic will be used but that he or she might experience some pain.
4. Assure the client that the procedure should not cause paralysis or spinal cord injury because the needle is inserted below the spinal cord.
5. The importance of lying flat after the procedure to prevent a headache should be stressed.
6. Provide written or illustrated instructions about the procedure.
7. A diagram can be used to show adult clients where the needle will be placed.
8. Tell the client to ask for assistance the first time he or she gets up after the procedure.

Estimated time to complete the skill: **30–45 minutes**

▶ DELEGATION TIPS

Assessment for bleeding, pain, shortness of breath, and proper postprocedure position is the responsibility of the nurse. Measurement of vital signs may be delegated to ancillary personnel.

IMPLEMENTATION—Action/Rationale

Action	Rationale
1. Explain the procedure to client (see Figure 11-8-2): • To assume the fetal position and remain still. • To breathe slowly and deeply; do not cough. • To be aware of possible discomfort.	1. Decreases anxiety from lack of knowledge. • Avoids movement of needle. • Prevents false reading of CSF pressure. • Eliminates sudden movement caused by surprise pain.
2. Obtain informed consent.	2. Client gives consent for the procedure.
3. Have the client void before the procedure.	3. Prevents interruption of the procedure.
4. Prepare labels and requisitions for specimens. Label specimen bottles, if possible. If the tubes are in the sterile tray, take labels to bedside for immediate placement when the procedure is complete.	4. Decreases chance of mislabeling tubes or delaying the testing of CSF.
5. Position client in the fetal position. Turn on the side with back facing you (see Figure 11-8-3): • Flex head and neck (see Figure 11-8-4). • Bring arms and knees toward each other (see Figure 11-8-5). Have client clasp knees with hands if this helps maintain the position. • Place pillow between knees.	5. Allows ease of access to spinal canal. • Allows maximum space between vertebrae. • Allows maximum space between vertebrae. • Prevents upper leg from rolling forward.
6. Expose the spine.	6. Allows for cleaning and draping before the procedure.

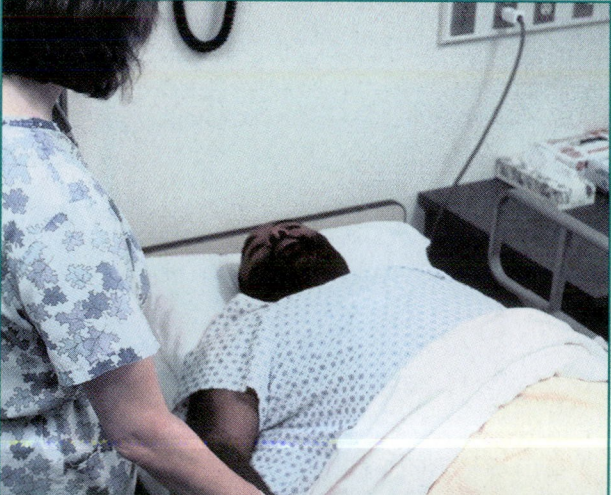

Figure 11-8-2 Explain the procedure to the client and answer questions prior to beginning the procedure.

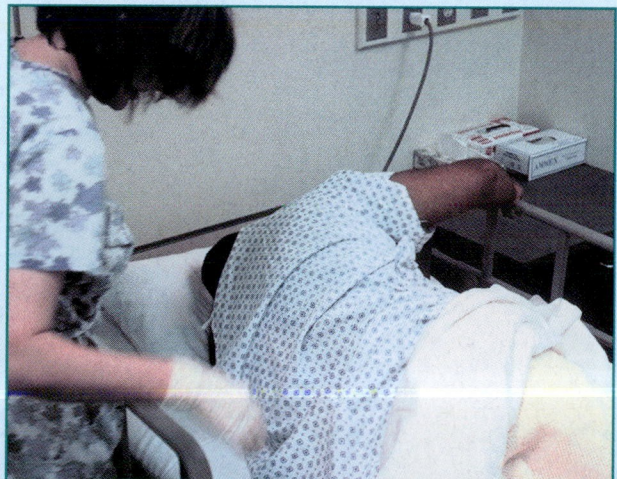

Figure 11-8-3 Turn the client on side with back facing you.

continues

Action	Rationale

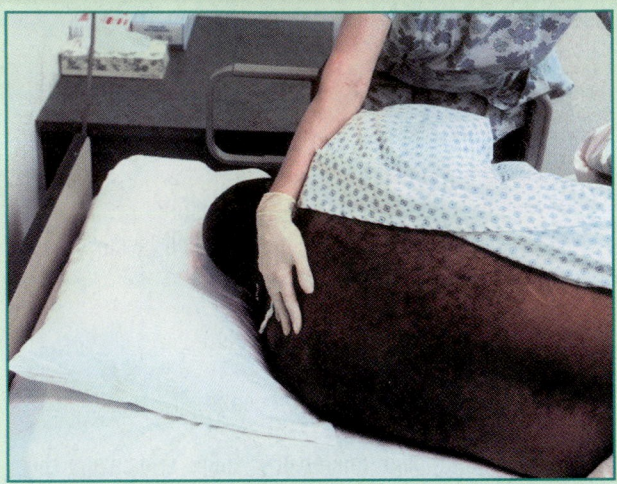

Figure 11-8-4   Flex the neck and head.

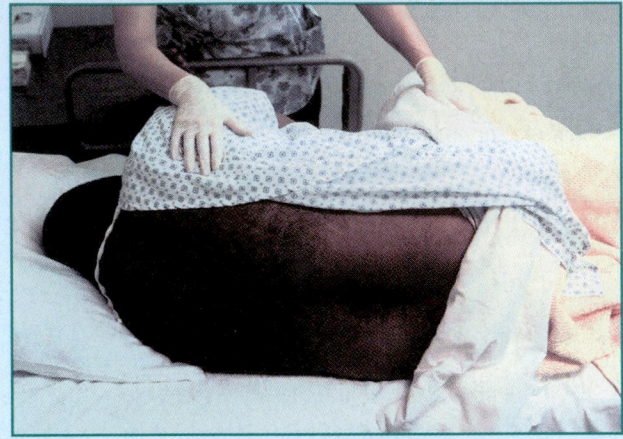

Figure 11-8-5   Bring the knees up tightly toward the arms.

7. The qualified practitioner performs the following steps:
- Wash hands, set up sterile lumbar puncture tray, and put on sterile gloves (see Figure 11-8-6).
- Clean skin of lower spine with povidone-iodine swabs (see Figure 11-8-7).
- Drape with sterile drape (see Figure 11-8-8).
- Inject local anesthetic agent.
- Insert spinal needle with inner obturator into spinal canal between L3 and L4 (see Figure 11-8-9).
- Remove obturator and attach manometer with stopcock and read pressure on manometer as it is opened (see Figure 11-8-10).
- Turn stopcock to collect CSF.
- Inject diagnostic or therapeutic agent, if indicated.
- Remove spinal needle and apply pressure on insertion site.
- Apply antiseptic ointment and Band-Aid® or gauze dressing to insertion site (see Figure 11-8-11).

7.
- Reduces the transmission of microorganisms.

- Reduces the transmission of microorganisms.

- Reduces the transmission of microorganisms.
- Reduces pain in the skin at the site.
- Decreases the chance of trauma to the spinal cord since it ends at L2.
- Allows CSF to flow from subarachnoid space. Manometer is calibrated in centimeters of water.

- Allows for laboratory examination of CSF.
- Allows direct access, bypassing the blood-brain barrier.
- Stops CSF from leaking out of spinal canal and decreases bleeding at site.
- Prevents organisms from entering skin at site.

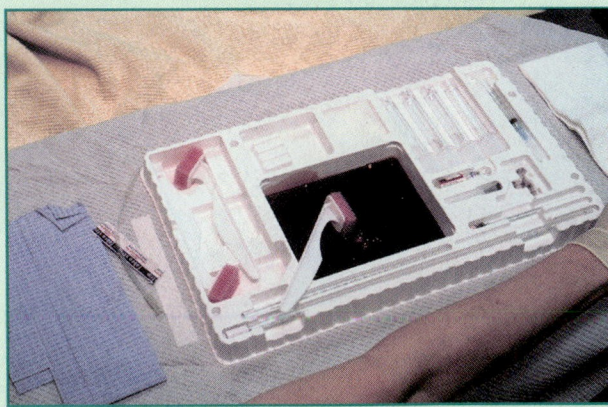

Figure 11-8-6   Set up the lumbar puncture tray.

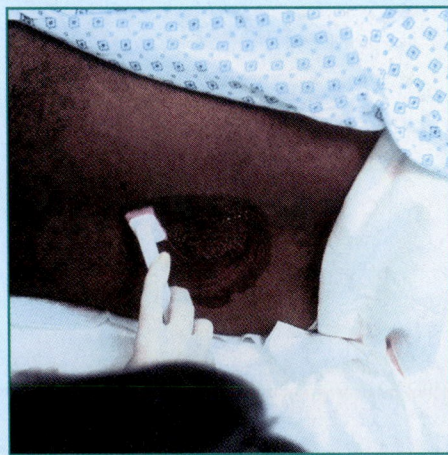

Figure 11-8-7   Clean the skin over the lower spine with povidone-iodine.

continues

Action	Rationale

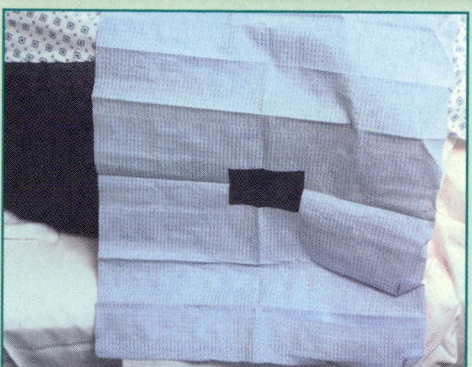

Figure 11-8-8 Cover the site with a sterile drape.

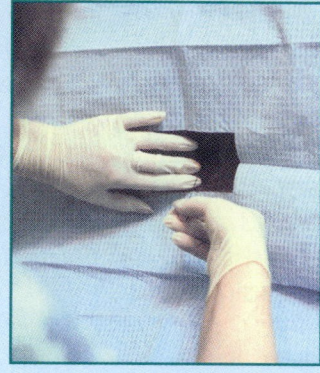

Figure 11-8-9 The physician or qualified practitioner will insert the spinal needle with inner obturator.

8. Observe client during and after procedure for neurologic changes such as:
   - Change in level of consciousness, pupil size, or pupil reaction.
   - Vital signs, or respiratory status.
   - Numbness, tingling, or pain in the legs or lower back.

9. Assist client in maintaining position while talking to client throughout the procedure.

10. Put on gloves.

11. Assist with direct pressure and application of antibiotic ointment and dressing as needed.

12. Label specimens with name, date, and time, as well as order specimens were taken.

13. Assist client to a comfortable position flat in the bed. Client may turn from side to side as desired. Educate the client to remain flat for 12–24 hours.

14. Encourage fluid intake and assess and manage pain as needed.

15. Wash hands.

8. Detects increased intracranial pressure or possible spinal nerve irritation.

9. Allows for safe placement of the needle and decreases anxiety.

10. Decreases risk of contamination.

11. Helps to accomplish the procedure.

12. Avoids error in testing or results.

13. Decreases CSF pressure in the caudal area where the needle insertion occurred and decreases the risk of leakage.

14. Replaces fluid loss and increases client comfort.

15. Reduces the transmission of microorganisms.

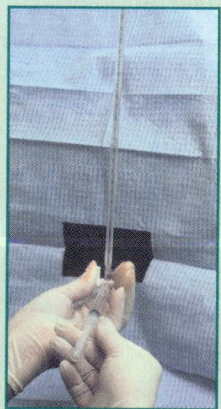

Figure 11-8-10 The physician or qualified practitioner will attach the manometer and read the cerebral spinal pressure.

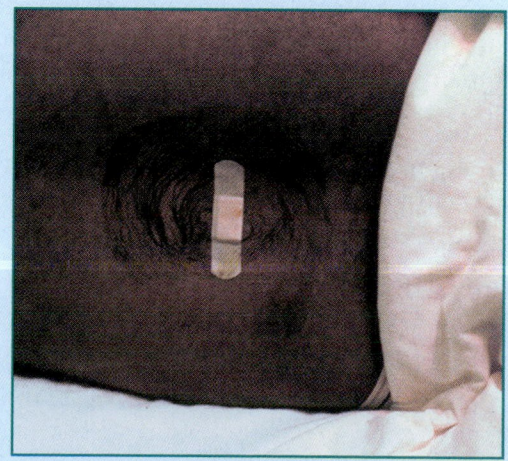

Figure 11-8-11 After applying pressure, apply a bandage to the site.

► **EVALUATION**

• The client understood the procedure and its rationale.
• The client was comfortable and not anxious.
• There was minimal bleeding or leakage of cerebral spinal fluid.
• The client did not experience a postprocedure headache.

► **DOCUMENTATION**

Nurses' Notes

• Document the date and time lumbar puncture was performed.
• Document name of physician or qualified practitioner performing the procedure.
• Describe how client tolerated the procedure.
• Record initial pressure.
• Note color of CSF.
• Document specimens sent for laboratory examination.
• Note presence of any bleeding or CSF leakage at the site.
• Document occurrence of a headache or other pain.

Document on appropriate flow sheet or electronic medical record (EMR).

Flow Sheet

• Record vital signs.
• Record neurologic signs.

• Document respiratory status before, during, and after the procedure.

► **CRITICAL THINKING SKILL**

Introduction

The most important part of the lumbar puncture is maintaining the client in a fetal position so that the needle can be placed correctly and not cause trauma.

Possible Scenario

A child needs to have a diagnostic lumbar puncture because of symptoms of meningitis. She is feeling very sick and afraid because of all the tests she has had done. She begins to cry and hiccough right after the local anesthetic is given. She is inconsolable even by her mother.

Possible Outcome

The procedure is delayed until the child can be calmed because of the danger of trauma if the spinal needle is inserted. The nurse administers a short-acting sedative that the doctor orders; the doctor waits for it to calm the child before proceeding.

Prevention

The nurse will document the anxiety of the child and assess for anxiety before another procedure is needed. Other coping skills may be taught to the child and parents to prepare her for future procedures.

► VARIATIONS

Geriatric Variations:
- *Client with osteoarthritic or other joint pain may find it difficult or impossible to assume the position required for the procedure.*
- *Older clients may have respiratory deficits that make breathing more difficult in the fetal position.*

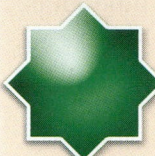

Pediatric Variations:
- *A child may need sedation to tolerate the procedure.*
- *A child may benefit from having a parent hold him or her behind the knees and neck.*
- *It may be comforting for a child to hug a favorite stuffed animal while lying on the side during the procedure.*

Home Care Variations:
- *Home health nurses need to be advised when a client has had a lumbar puncture so they can assess for possible spinal headache and neurologic changes.*
- *Teach the client commonly used treatments to prevent postprocedural headaches (e.g., lie flat, increase fluid intake, avoid aspirin and caffeine, keep lights in the room dimmed, avoid excessive stimulation, avoid Valsalva maneuvers, and use pain medications as ordered).*
- *Teach the client to monitor for neurologic changes (e.g., dizziness, blurred vision, changes in mentation, and lethargy). Be sure the client has telephone number for emergency contact.*

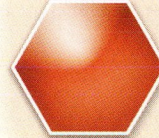

Long-Term Care Variation:
- *Postprocedural symptoms, such as a severe headache, can manifest hours after the procedure is completed. Nurses need to monitor debilitated clients for 24–48 hours.*

► COMMON ERRORS

Possible Error:
The client was not assessed for ability to assume the knee-chest position.

Prevention:
When a physician or qualified practitioner orders a lumbar puncture, ask the client to demonstrate ability to assume this position. Then assess the client and report to the physician or qualified practitioner if client is able to maintain the position. If the client is unable to assume the proper position, inform the practitioner and discuss alternate positions.

Possible Error:
The spinal needle on the sterile tray becomes contaminated.

Prevention:
Have extra spinal needles of various sizes available, so if the spinal needle becomes contaminated, you can quickly obtain another spinal needle and give it to the physician or qualified practitioner using sterile technique.

▶ **NURSING TIPS**

- Use pillows or rolled towels to position the client comfortably.
- Headaches can be treated with bed rest, an ice-pack applied to the head, analgesia, and forcing fluids.
- Have the tubes labeled and requisition forms prepared before the procedure.
- Keep needles and other instruments out of sight in order to decrease anxiety.
- Assess the needle insertion site for bloody drainage or CSF leakage (look for clear fluid drainage). If there is excessive CSF leakage, the physician or qualified practitioner must be notified immediately.
- Ask the client to notify the nurse if he or she experiences a headache.

- Evaluate for signs and symptoms of local irritation, such as swelling or pain from a hematoma and meningeal irritation (nuchal rigidity).
- Monitor for neurologic changes such as headache, visual changes (blurring), dizziness, changes in mentation, or lethargy.
- Educate the client before discharge regarding commonly used treatments to prevent postprocedural headaches (e.g., lie flat, increase fluid intake, avoid aspirin and caffeine, keep lights in the room dimmed, avoid excessive stimulation, avoid Valsalva maneuvers, and use pain medication as ordered). Before discharge be sure the client has an emergency telephone number to call in case of problems or questions.

▶ **SPECIAL CONSIDERATIONS**

- *Depending on the physician or practitioner's preference, a client may be asked to assume a hunched sitting position over a table with a pillow. The nurse can assist by putting a hand on the head or neck of the client to remind him or her to remain still and bend forward.*
- *There is a general fear surrounding a lumbar puncture related to spinal cord injury. Educate and assess for anxiety before the procedure begins. Reassure the client and answer questions.*
- *If a post-lumbar puncture headache occurs, notify the health care provider, decrease stimulus in the room, and administer pain and/or nausea medications as ordered. Some practitioners recommend a flat, prone position while others recommend lying flat on the back to prevent CSF leakage.*
- *In cases of severe headache associated with CSF leakage, a "patch" procedure may be used to stop leakage.*
- *Clients with a history of back or spinal cord injury have an increased risk of CSF leakage.*

Assisting with Amniocentesis

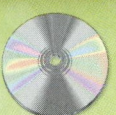

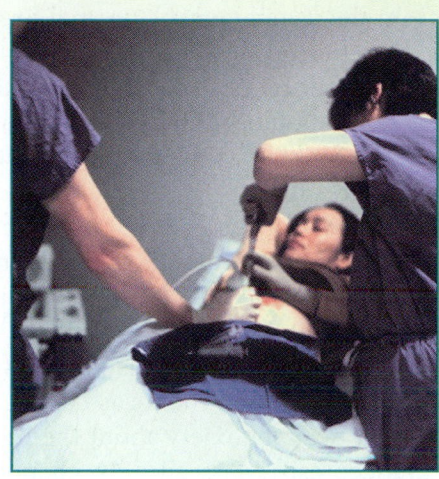

▶ OVERVIEW OF THE SKILL

An amniocentesis is a procedure performed on a pregnant woman to obtain amniotic fluid for diagnostic analysis or therapeutic effects. Following a complete ultrasound examination, amniocentesis is performed using visualization by ultrasound. A needle is inserted through the abdomen, through the uterine wall, and into a "pocket" of amniotic fluid. Amniotic fluid is then withdrawn and sent to the laboratory for analysis. Local anesthetic may or may not be used, depending on the practitioner.

▶ ASSESSMENT

1. Assess gestational age of the infant. **Care during and after amniocentesis will depend on the baby's gestational age.**
2. Ascertain the family's understanding of the reasons for the procedure. **Amniocentesis is not a routine procedure.**
3. Assess client's emotional status. **Often, amniocentesis is performed when a problem is suspected in either the infant or the mother.**
4. Assess fetal heart rate and long-term variability before procedure **to establish a baseline for monitoring changes.**
5. Assess maternal vital signs **to establish a baseline for monitoring changes.**
6. Assess client's ability to sign a consent form.

▶ DIAGNOSIS

Risk for Injury

Risk for Deficient Fluid Volume

Risk for Infection

Anxiety

▶ PLANNING

Expected Outcomes:

1. The client will not experience lightheadedness or diaphoresis.
2. The client will tolerate the procedure with minimal discomfort.
3. The client will not experience bleeding.
4. If contractions are present following amniocentesis, these will subside by 1 hour postprocedure.
5. The fetal heart rate, variability, and periodic changes will remain stable compared to baseline.
6. The family will be told when to expect a report of findings.

Equipment Needed (see Figure 11-9-1):

- Ultrasound equipment
- Amniocentesis tray with extra needles
- Sterile towels
- Sterile gloves

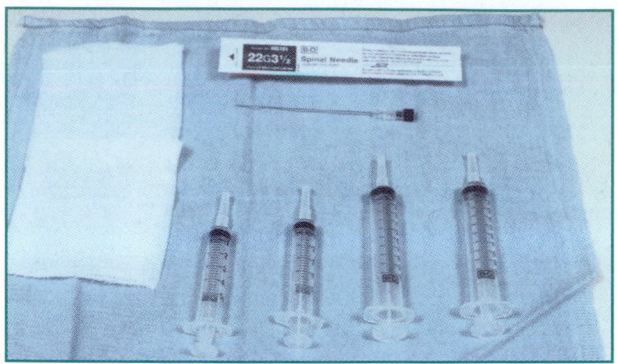

Figure 11-9-1 Amniocentesis tray includes syringes, needle, and gauze.

- Specimen containers (Check with laboratory in your institution for each test anticipated. Consider having extra containers available.)
- Pillows
- Warmed ultrasonic gel
- Towels
- Fetal monitor, if indicated, or per agency policy

► CLIENT EDUCATION NEEDED:

1. The reasons for doing an amniocentesis and the implications of having the results should be discussed by the physician or genetic counselor with clients and their families at length.
2. The physician or qualified practitioner will discuss the procedure, risks, and alternatives with the client and her family.
3. Remind the client that amniocentesis is performed with constant visualization of the needle and the baby so the needle will not hurt the baby.
4. Reassure the client that once the pocket of fluid is found, the procedure itself is quick, usually about 30 seconds.
5. Agree upon a plan for distraction or relaxation at the time of needle insertion for women who are afraid they will jump as the needle is being inserted.
6. Include partners in the teaching and preparation for the amniocentesis and respect their level of participation or support during the procedure.

7. Mild cramping may be normal for the first 24 hours after amniocentesis. Clients should be instructed to report bleeding, cramping, loss of fluid from the vagina, or other problems.
8. Instruct the client to report cramping that does not diminish as some clients may experience mild cramping even if labor is progressing.
9. Tell the client that a small amount of leakage of fluid from the vagina may be normal but that it should be reported.
10. Results of amniocentesis tests may be available in 1 day to several days, and clients should be aware of the length of time they will have to wait for the results.
11. Inform client it may be necessary to rest quietly for 30 to 60 minutes with electronic monitoring of the fetal heart rate (FHR) before leaving the health care facility.
12. Give written postprocedure instructions and write down any appointments as the client may have a great deal of anxiety about the results of the amniocentesis. Make sure the client understands what signs and symptoms to report as not all complications occur while the client is in the clinic.
13. Instruct the client to take acetaminophen or apply a warm pack if the needle insertion site is painful. Reassure her that the pain will resolve in a short time.

Estimated time to complete the skill:

30–60 minutes (can vary because of length of time for complete ultrasound examination and performance of the amniocentesis)

► DELEGATION TIPS

Assessment for bleeding, pain, shortness of breath, and proper postprocedure position is the responsibility of the nurse. Measurement of vital signs may be delegated to ancillary personnel.

IMPLEMENTATION—Action/Rationale

Action	Rationale
1. Wash hands.	1. Reduces the transmission of microorganisms.
2. Arrange amniocentesis equipment and specimen containers.	2. Equipment should be in a convenient arrangement for the physician or qualified practitioner who will manage the sterile field.
3. Position client in left lateral tilt (if greater than 20 weeks' gestation) with several pillows, if needed for support.	3. Client will be recumbent throughout procedure. If client is greater than 20 weeks' gestation, lateral tilt will prevent vena cava syndrome. Pillows will allow client to comfortably tolerate position.
4. Provide ultrasound technologist with warm ultrasound gel.	4. Often, a large amount of gel is used, and warmed gel is more comfortable for the client.
5. When the physician or qualified practitioner is ready to start the amniocentesis, encourage the client to relax. Provide comfort as required. Individualize this for each client (see Figure 11-9-2).	5. Minimizes stress response.
• Explain to the client the steps of the procedure as they are being performed.	• Understanding the procedure reduces client anxiety and promotes cooperation.
• The ultrasound technologist will determine the fetus's position within the uterus (see Figure 11-9-3).	• Determines where the needle will be inserted to avoid damage to the fetus.
• While monitoring the fetus via ultrasound, the physician or qualified practitioner will insert the amniocentesis needle.	• Allows the practitioner to guide the needle and avoid the fetus.
• The physician or qualified practitioner will then withdraw 3–4 syringes' worth of amniotic fluid (see Figure 11-9-4).	• The amniotic fluid will be sent for analysis.

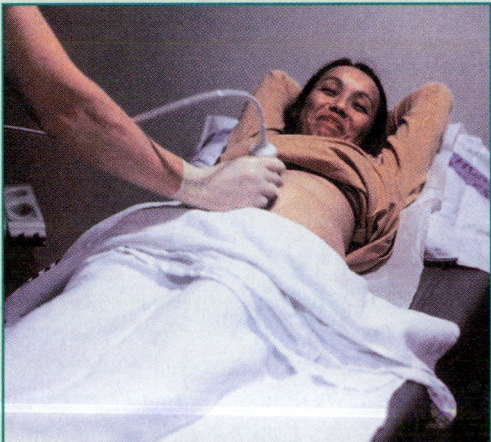

Figure 11-9-2 Position the client comfortably, encourage her to relax, and answer questions before beginning the amniocentesis.

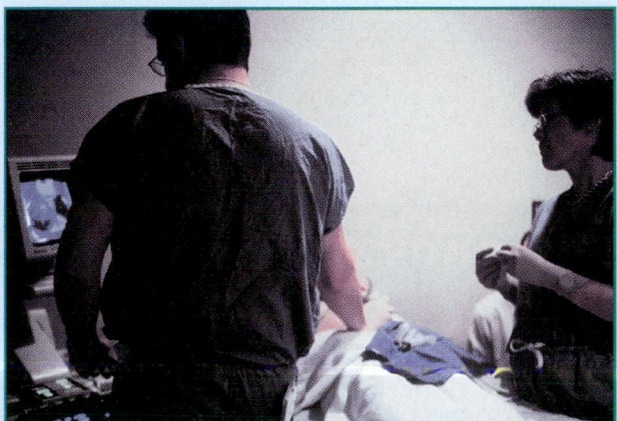

Figure 11-9-3 The ultrasound technologist determines the fetus's position.

continues

Action	Rationale

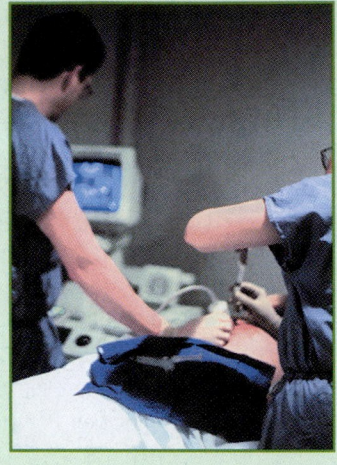

Figure 11-9-4   Withdraw three to four syringes of amniotic fluid.

6. After the procedure, clean excess gel from the client's abdomen. Physician or qualified practitioner may apply a Band-Aid® to site.

6. Ultrasound gel is sticky and dries to a flaky white film that may be itchy. Protects insertion site from microorganisms.

7. Label specimens, fill in laboratory requisition form completely, and transport to laboratory according to hospital protocol.

7. Laboratory specimens must be handled according to hospital/clinic protocol.

8. If indicated, monitor fetal heart rate (FHR) per physician's or qualified practitioner's order or hospital protocol.

8. If the client requires FHR monitoring after amniocentesis, the nurse must be trained in FHR interpretation.

9. Ascertain that client understands signs and symptoms to report after discharge.

9. Cramping, uterine contractions, bleeding, or loss of vaginal fluid indicate complications and should be reported. Clients can expect some mild cramping and tenderness at the insertion site.

10. Arrange for follow-up for client to learn the results of the procedure.

10. Test results may take 24 hours to several days to complete. Clients should have a date for test results to help minimize the anxiety of waiting.

11. Apply gloves and discard supplies.

11. Reduces the transmission of microorganisms.

12. Remove gloves and wash hands.

12. Reduces the transmission of microorganisms.

▶ REAL WORLD ANECDOTES

Donna's due date was 4 weeks away. Her fundal height did not increase as expected from 2 weeks before. Her doctor sent her to the ultrasound clinic for an ultrasound examination. There was not a lot of amniotic fluid or many fetal breathing movements. Her doctor was concerned about the baby's growth and the condition of the placenta. As the due date was still 4 weeks away, an amniocentesis was performed to ascertain fetal lung maturity. A mature lung would be indicated by amniotic fluid with a lecithin/sphingomyelin (LS) ratio of 2:1 or better with phosphatidyl glycerol (Pg) present. The ultrasound showed a pocket of fluid large enough to aspirate that was

continues

> **REAL WORLD ANECDOTES** *(continued)*

away from the baby's face, placenta, and cord. Under ultrasound guidance, the doctor inserted the needle into the pocket of fluid. The baby moved and the doctor withdrew the needle at once before a sample was obtained. After a few minutes, the doctor tried again. When a pocket appeared, the doctor used a new needle to obtain enough fluid for an LS ratio. She performed a "shake test," which was positive for stable bubbles (probable maturity). Donna stayed in the hospital overnight on fetal monitoring in anticipation of an induction. Laboratory results showed the LS ratio was positive with Pg present. Donna's labor was complicated by frequent fetal heart rate variable decelerations relieved with intra-amniotic fluid transfusion after artificial rupture of the membranes. The baby was born with an Apgar score of 8 to 9. Examination revealed a newborn small for his gestational age.

> **EVALUATION**

- The client did not experience lightheadedness or diaphoresis.
- The client tolerated the procedure with minimal discomfort.
- The client did not experience bleeding.
- If contractions were present, following amniocentesis, these subsided by 1 hour post-procedure.
- The fetal heart rate, variability, and periodic changes remained stable when compared to baseline.
- The family was told when to expect a report of findings.

> **DOCUMENTATION**

Nurses' Notes

- Record date and time of procedure.
- Record amount and appearance of fluid.
- Document tests ordered for specimens obtained.
- Describe client tolerance of procedure (presence or absence of complications).
- Note fetal heart rate characteristics before and following procedure, if applicable.
- Document client teaching done.
- Record arrangements for follow-up visit.

Document on appropriate flow sheet or electronic medical record (EMR).

> **CRITICAL THINKING SKILL**

Introduction

Sometimes tests during an amniocentesis are for a chromosome analysis to rule out Down's syndrome as a follow-up of abnormally low alpha-fetoprotein levels. Some clients may not be aware of why they are having the procedure and may not understand the implications of the test.

Possible Scenario

Anna Scott and her husband, Dale, arrive at your ultrasound clinic for a scheduled amniocentesis. You do not know her history except that Anna is 32 years old and this is her first pregnancy. Anna states she is excited to find out if the baby is a boy or a girl. During the time before the obstetrician and the ultrasound technician arrive, you talk to Anna and Dale about their pregnancy experience so far. They tell you that they had a low result on a routine test but otherwise everything in the pregnancy was just fine.

Possible Outcome

If you have reason to believe that parents do not understand the test or the implications of a procedure, bring this to the primary care provider's attention. Parents may be experiencing levels of anxiety that may make it difficult to interpret information they receive. Moreover, clients may find it difficult to ask questions of their physician. In Anna and Dale's case, you contact their physician. She thanks you for bringing this to her attention. She arranges to come early and discuss the test again with Anna and Dale. After their discussion, Anna and Dale express surprise that this test was so serious. They decide to proceed with the amniocentesis. They decide that knowing about any genetic anomaly would help them prepare emotionally for a baby with special needs and they do want to know.

Prevention

This scenario raises ethical concerns about the use of technology in pregnancy. Parents may not understand the implications of all the tests that are offered and the ways in which information obtained through certain tests may affect their choices and lives. Care providers must not assume that all parents understand the implications of technology. In addition, even though the practitioner may believe he or she has adequately explained a test, variables such as anxiety, cultural beliefs, or educational level may interfere with or enhance a client's understanding.

Using a team approach and active communication, health care professionals can enhance the client's ability to make the best choices.

► VARIATIONS

Geriatric Variations:
- *Not applicable.*

Pediatric Variation:
- *Adolescents dealing with a pregnancy will often be very frightened and uneducated about aspects of the pregnancy. This fear and lack of information can translate into reticence to keep appointments and to follow through with necessary care. It is important to offer nonjudgmental support and careful teaching before, during, and after the procedure.*

Home Care Variation:
- *Cramping or discomfort may be experienced for a few hours after the procedure. Instruct the client to report any unusual symptoms such as fever, chills, or excess tenderness at the puncture site.*

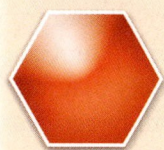

Long-Term Care Variation:
- *Clients with disabilities still need routine prenatal care, but this care must be modified to accommodate their disabilities. Clients in a long-term care setting because of disabilities that make independent living unfeasible may not have access to prenatal resources available to others in the community. Use the amniocentesis appointment as an opportunity to assess the overall needs and resources available to the long-term care client.*

► COMMON ERRORS

Possible Error:
You have only one specimen container for the amniotic fluid and the doctor orders three separate tests.

Prevention:
Before the procedure ask the physician or qualified practitioner which tests he or she wants done. Call the laboratory to be sure you have the correct containers. If you are low on containers, immediately obtain the correct ones and prepare them for the physician or qualified practitioner. Label the containers correctly and fill out the requisition forms before sending them to the laboratory.

▶ NURSING TIPS

- Use guided imagery or progressive relaxation to help minimize the client's anxiety.
- Make sure the client is in a comfortable position with pillows to support her.
- If the client is accompanied by her partner, include the partner in conversation and position where partner may also see the ultrasound images, if possible.

- Consider having the partner remain seated during the procedure in case of lightheadedness.
- Use encouragement and touch to help the client relax.
- Demonstrate your confidence in the client's ability to relax during the procedure.

▶ SPECIAL CONSIDERATIONS

- *After the procedure, the fetal heart rate should be assessed sonographically and documented.*
- *Inform the client that she may experience uterine cramping, transient spotting, and vaginal loss of a few drops of amniotic fluid immediately after the procedure. She should be instructed to report any persistent loss of amniotic fluid or bleeding, severe uterine cramping lasting for several hours, or fever.*
- *Instruct the client to rest on the day of the procedure; however, she may resume normal activities and sexual intercourse the next day.*

Assisting with Bronchoscopy

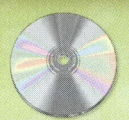

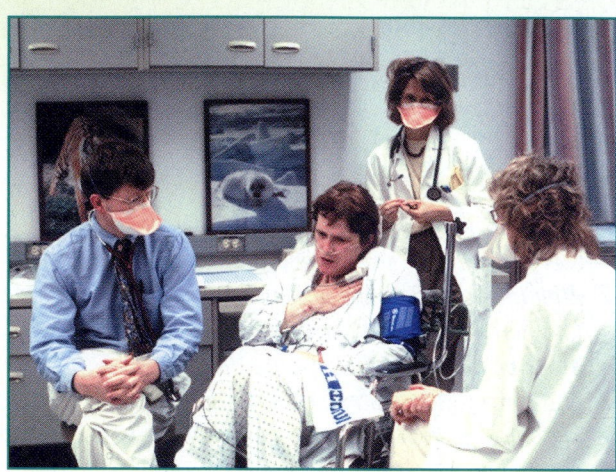

▶ OVERVIEW OF THE SKILL

Flexible fiberoptic bronchoscopy is used for direct visualization of the upper and lower respiratory tract to diagnose and manage infections and malignant and inflammatory diseases of the lungs (see Figure 11-10-1). Flexible fiberoptic bronchoscopy may involve obtaining cell washings (bronchoalveolar lavage); the taking of tissue samples (biopsies by brushing, needles, or bites of the lung tissue); removing abnormal tissue with the use of laser; removal of a foreign body; or removal of secretions.

Indications for Bronchoscopy

- Abnormal chest X-ray: presence of a lesion, persistent atelectasis, infiltrates in the lung fields
- Hemoptysis
- Unexplained cough, localized wheeze, or stridor
- Need to obtain lower respiratory tract secretions or tissue for diagnostic purposes
- To assess and/or evaluate airways
- To perform difficult intubations
- To remove a foreign body

Complications

- Hypoxemia
- Hypercarbia
- Hypotension
- Laryngospasm
- Bradycardia
- Pneumothorax
- Hemoptysis
- Adverse effect of medication used before and during the bronchoscopy

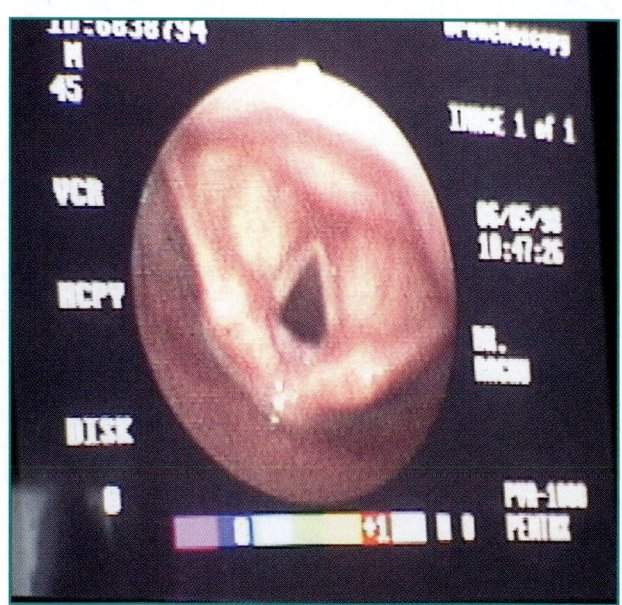

Figure 11-10-1 Bronchoscopy is used to visualize the respiratory tract.

Contraindications

- Inability to adequately oxygenate the client during the bronchoscopy
- Clients with severe obstructive lung disease
- Unstable hemodynamic status
- Lack of client consent
- Low platelet count

Note: The safety of asthmatic clients during a bronchoscopy procedure is a concern, but the presence of asthma does not preclude the use of bronchoscopy.

▶ ASSESSMENT

1. Determine whether the client has been NPO for 4–8 hours. **The bronchoscopy will have to be postponed if the client has been receiving nothing per mouth (NPO) because of the danger of aspiration.**
2. Determine the presence of a current chest X-ray and blood work (especially bleeding times). **The act of inserting the scope and obtaining the samples needed can cause bleeding, so bleeding times must be known. Viewing the chest X-ray just prior to, and during, the procedure will help obtain good samples.**
3. Assess where the procedure is to be performed (in a hospital room or in the bronchoscopy suite) **to determine that the area is available and where to set up the equipment.**
4. Identify the drugs ordered: action, purpose, normal dosage, common side effects, time of onset and peak action, duration of action and implications. **This allows you to anticipate effects of the drug and to observe client's response.**
5. Assess the client's vital signs, including lung sounds and blood oxygen levels, **to establish baseline values.**
6. Assess the client's chart for a signed consent form **to conform with institutional and legal requirements.**
7. Assess the client's level of understanding regarding the procedure as well as the client's level of anxiety **to determine the amount and type of client teaching needed.**
8. Assess client's ability to understand risks and sign a consent form.

▶ DIAGNOSIS

Ineffective Breathing Pattern

Risk for Suffocation

Risk for Aspiration

Deficient Knowledge

Impaired Gas Exchange

Anxiety

Ineffective Airway Clearance

Risk for Injury

▶ PLANNING

Expected Outcomes:

1. The client will express understanding of the procedure prior to the bronchoscopy.
2. The client will tolerate the procedure with a minimum of anxiety or discomfort.
3. The purpose of the bronchoscopy will be achieved.
4. Usable samples will be obtained, correctly processed, and correctly labeled.
5. The client will not suffer any adverse effects from the procedure.

Equipment Needed (see Figure 11-10-2):

- Bronchoscope (The scope size will be determined by the physician or qualified practitioner based on the client and the procedures to be performed.)
- Light source for the bronchoscope and any related video or photographic equipment
- Brushes (cytology brushes, protected for microbiology tissue samples)
- Specimen traps
- Syringes of various sizes for bronchoalveolar lavage, drug delivery, and needle aspiration
- Bite block (to protect the scope)
- Intubation tray
- Intravenous supplies
- Resuscitation bag
- Monitoring devices: pulse oximeter, ECG monitor, sphygmomanometer
- Oxygen delivery equipment: cannula, masks
- Suction supplies for scope and/or mouth

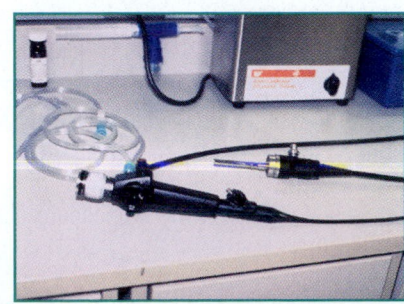

Figure 11-10-2 Bronchoscope with oxygen supply line

- Fluoroscopy equipment, including personal protection and radiation badge
- Adequate ventilation, to prevent the spread of infection
- Ultraviolet light, to prevent transmission of tuberculosis
- Cleaning, disinfection, and sterilizing equipment

▶ CLIENT EDUCATION NEEDED:

1. Review the indications for the bronchoscopy.
2. Remind the client that he or she must be NPO at least 4 hours before the bronchoscopy.
3. It is a good idea to call the client the day before the bronchoscopy to instruct not to drive self to the hospital and to stay NPO after midnight.
4. Explain to the client the reasons for wearing a gown and removing neck jewelry.

5. Make sure you review what to expect postprocedure with the client and the escort or caregiver.
6. Review hand signals to signal pain or discomfort when the client is unable to talk.
7. Give instructions not only verbally, so the client can ask questions, but also in writing. Written instructions should include what to expect, when to be concerned, what to do, and whom to contact and how.

Estimated time to complete the skill:
The time from setup to cleanup can vary with the indications for the bronchoscopy, from 1 to 2.5 hours.

▶ DELEGATION TIPS

Assessment for bleeding, pain, shortness of breath, and proper postprocedure position is the responsibility of the nurse. Measurement of vital signs may be delegated to ancillary personnel.

IMPLEMENTATION—Action/Rationale

Action	Rationale
1. Wash hands.	1. Reduces the transmission of microorganisms.
2. Set up for the bronchoscopy. Plug the appropriate bronchoscope in a light source and connect the suction tubing.	2. Setting up ahead of time helps reduce mistakes or forgotten items. Watching a nurse set up the procedure can increase the client's anxiety.
• Set up an emergency oral suction.	• Decreases the risk of aspiration. It is a good idea to have an oral suction set up at all times, especially when the danger of hemoptysis is present.
3. Draw up medication per physician's or qualified practitioner's orders and label each syringe with drug and dosage per milliliter.	3. Ensures accuracy in the administration of the medication.
4. Ready syringes of saline for the bronchoalveolar lavage and saline washes.	4. Decreases the possibility of contaminating the saline and helps the bronchoscopy flow more smoothly.

continues

Action	Rationale
5. Lay out traps, biopsy forceps, cytology brushes, and protected brushes as needed. Have everything ready for an intravenous (IV) placement (if an outpatient client; an inpatient client should already have an IV).	5. Provides easy access to give conscious sedation, drugs, and emergency medications.
6. Make sure all the required paperwork is filled out and ready for the client and the physician or qualified practitioner. This should include, but not be limited to, bronchoscopy consent form, drug forms, and laboratory request.	6. Documents procedure to prevent mistakes.
7. Check that emergency medications and supplies are available.	7. Ensures that needed equipment is available.
8. Verify client's identity.	8. Ensures correct client.
9. Have client put on a gown if an outpatient client (see Figure 11-10-3).	9. Protects clothing; increases radiology view of chest.
10. Place monitoring devices for vital signs. Record baseline vital signs and continue to monitor every 5–15 minutes depending on institution policies.	10. Assesses how the client is tolerating the procedure and medications (too much/too little or adverse reactions). Monitors oxygenation status.
11. For outpatient clients, confirm the presence of a family member or caregiver to provide transportation after the procedure.	11. It is not safe for the client to drive for at least 6 hours after receiving sedation for the bronchoscopy.
12. Obtain informed consent from the client prior to the bronchoscopy procedure.	12. Ensures that the client understands what the procedure involves and all the possible risks.
13. Start supplemental oxygen (see Figure 11-10-4).	13. The suctioning during the bronchoscopy will decrease oxygenation.
14. Have client remove false teeth (if appropriate).	14. Prevents choking, aspiration, or damage to teeth and/or scope.

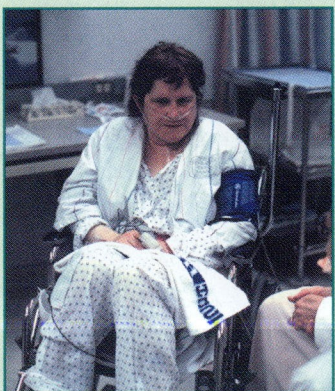

Figure 11-10-3 Have the client put on a gown and robe.

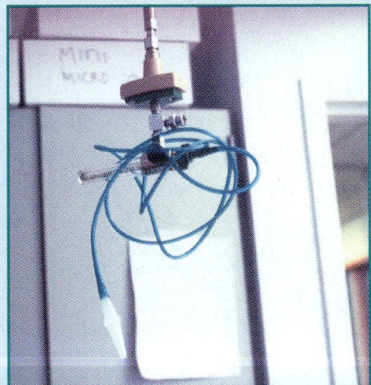

Figure 11-10-4 Obtain supplemental oxygen. Administer oxygen to the client during the bronchoscopy.

continues

Action	Rationale
15. Give the anticholinergic agent if the physician or qualified practitioner has ordered it. Watch the heart rate closely.	**15.** Reduces secretions and minimizes vasovagal reflexes. Can increase the heart rate significantly.
16. The physician or qualified practitioner may also want a nebulizer given with a bronchodilator diluted with lidocaine.	**16.** Starts the numbing process and relaxes the airway, minimizing bronchospasm.
17. Anesthetize the nares and the throat with topical lidocaine and cocaine (see Figure 11-10-5).	**17.** Helps to decrease the gag reflex and make the client more comfortable.
18. Give first dose of IV sedation; may be required prn prior to and during procedure depending on client's tolerance to the drugs and comfort level.	**18.** Helps the client to relax. Increases comfort level.
19. Lubricate the distal end of the scope using a water-soluble lubricant.	**19.** Helps the passage of the scope through the airways. Any substance going into the lungs should be water soluble.
20. If you are introducing the scope orally, place a mouth guard or airway in client's mouth. Secure if possible.	**20.** Maintains airway and prevents damage to scope.
21. As the physician or qualified practitioner passes the scope into the airways (see Figure 11-10-6), the assistant will inject lidocaine into the scope, numbing the airways as they go. This is usually 2 mL of 2% lidocaine (no preservatives) with 3 mL of air in the syringe.	**21.** Minimizes cough and gag reflexes. Using air to push the lidocaine through the scope helps decrease the amount of lidocaine, thus decreasing medication side effects.
22. Instruct the client not to talk. If client needs something, have him or her use the prearranged hand signals.	**22.** Talking with the scope in place bruises the vocal cords and can damage them.

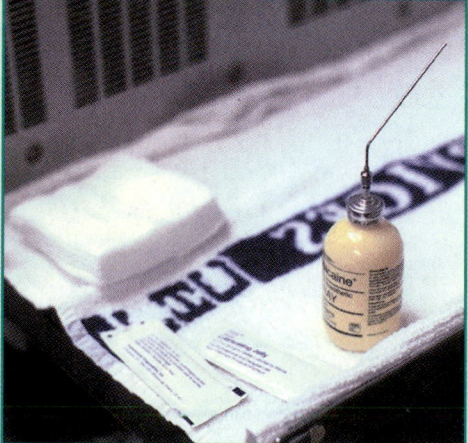

Figure 11-10-5 Anesthetize the client's nose and throat.

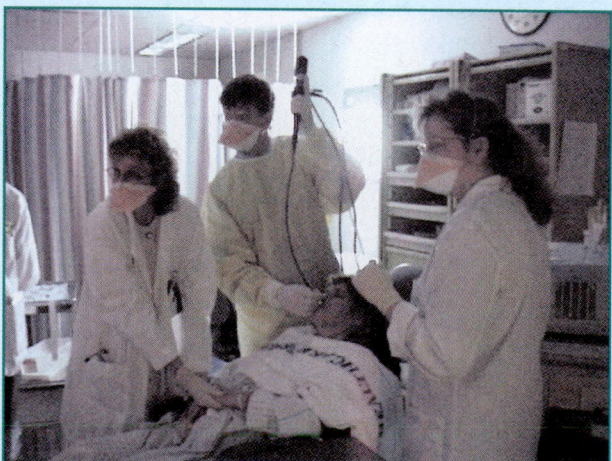

Figure 11-10-6 The physician or qualified practitioner passes the scope into the airway and observes the monitor.

continues

Action	Rationale
23. Assist the physician or qualified practitioner in obtaining the type of samples needed:	**23.**
Bronchoalveolar lavage	
• With the scope wedged in an airway, place a large suction trap on the suction port of the scope, being careful not to touch the sterile connector ends. Reconnect the suction connecting tubing.	• Maintains sterility of trap.
• In 30-mL aliquots, introduce sterile nonbacteriostatic saline through the biopsy port into the lung.	• Bacteriostatic saline would destroy the bacteria and defeat the purpose of the bronchoscopy.
• Monitor the return suctioned back into the trap.	• You do not get all the lavage back.
• Repeat the preceding two bulleted actions until an adequate sample is obtained.	
• Remove the suction trap from the scope carefully. Avoid touching the connector ends and cap them off (usually done by hooking them together). Be careful with the suction when removing the trap or the sample may be lost.	• Maintains sterility of sample.
Cytology brush	
• Remove the brush from the package, uncoil, and make sure the brush is inside the protective sheath.	• If the brush is not in the protective sheath, it could damage the scope or pick up contaminants.
• Carefully push the brush down through the biopsy port on the scope 1 to 2 cm at a time.	• Carefully advancing the brush prevents damage to the brush and the scope.
• Once the brush is through the port, slowly advance it until the physician or qualified practitioner tells you to stop.	• Trying to push the brush too fast may damage the brush or scope.
• Push the brush out and move it back and forth inside the airway 3 or 4 times.	• Ensures there are enough cells from the suspect area that a diagnosis may be obtained.
• Pull the brush back into the protective sheath and carefully pull the brush and sheath out of the scope.	• Maintains sample and protects from contaminants.
• Prepare the sample according to hospital policy. This may include cutting the brush end off and placing it in saline, rubbing the brush onto slides, or placing it in a fixative.	• Do this quickly as cells exposed to air lose their integrity and the cell walls are destroyed, thus making them unrecognizable.
Protective brush	
• Used for microbiology samples; the brush is double sheathed and has a wax plug in the end.	• Maintains sterility. The wax plug keeps contaminants from coming in contact with the brush.
• Remove from packaging and carefully uncoil.	• Maintains sterility.
• Carefully push the brush down through the biopsy port on the scope 1 to 2 cm at a time.	• Trying to push brush too fast may damage brush and scope.
• Once through the port, slowly advance until the physician tells you to stop.	• Pushing the brush too fast may damage the brush or the scope.
• Pull the two sheaths together and push out the wax plug. Push the brush out and move it back and forth inside the airway 3 or 4 times.	• Ensures there are enough cells from the suspect area that a diagnosis may be obtained.

continues

Action	Rationale
Protective brush (continued) • Pull the brush back into the protective sheath and carefully pull the brush and sheath out of the scope. • Carefully advance the brush out of the sheath and, using sterile wire cutters, cut the brush end off into a sterile vial containing 1 mL of sterile nonbacteriostatic saline (or follow hospital procedure).	• Maintains sample and protects form contaminants. • Maintains sterility. Bacteriostatic saline would destroy the bacteria and defeat the purpose of the bronchoscopy.
Biopsies • Often done under fluoroscopy. • Remove the biopsy forceps from the package, and test them while they are still looped in a circle. Testing them involves opening and closing them. If they work while in a loop, they should work well in the lungs. If they do not open and close easily, get another pair. • The physician or qualified practitioner may want to instill 3 to 5 cc of a 1:10,000 solution of epinephrine at this time. • Carefully push the closed biopsy forceps down through the biopsy port on the scope 1 to 2 cm at a time. • Once through the end, slowly advance until the physician or qualified practitioner tells you to stop. • Open the forceps and push forward; close firmly and hold when told to by the physician or qualified practitioner and give a sharp, hard tug, pulling the forceps out of the scope. • Place biopsy in a container of formalin. • Rinse the forceps off in alcohol if you placed them in the formalin while removing the biopsy sample. Repeat actions for another biopsy.	• Biopsy areas may be too far out into the lungs to be visualized any other way. • Testing while the forceps are still looped will let you know if they will work when they are twisted in the airway. • Often used as a preventive against hemoptysis. • Pushing the forceps down faster may bend the forceps, which then may not work correctly and could damage the scope. • Pushing the forceps too fast may damage the forceps or the scope. • Ensures collection of a good specimen. The client should not feel any pain. • Preserves the tissue. • Formalin is a carcinogen.
24. While obtaining the samples, make sure to label all of them immediately with client's name, ID number, date, time, and location in lung.	24. More than one sample type is taken from any given area/segment and often more than one site is used. If samples are not labeled immediately, they can be confused or mislabeled.
25. After the bronchoscopy, rinse the scope by suctioning approximately 240 mL of soapy water through the working channel of the scope (see Figure 11-10-7).	25. Cleaning the scope immediately ensures it will not be damaged by dried secretions.
26. During the recovery period (at least 30 minutes), wean the client off oxygen (if none was required before the procedure).	26. The saline introduced into the lungs during the bronchoscopy can decrease the client's oxygenation. This can take several hours to be absorbed by the body. The client may also experience a low-grade fever during this time.
27. Remember to keep a close watch on the oxygen saturation and the vital signs.	27. The recovering client may fall into deep sleep with a decreased respiratory rate and blood pressure.

continues

Action	Rationale

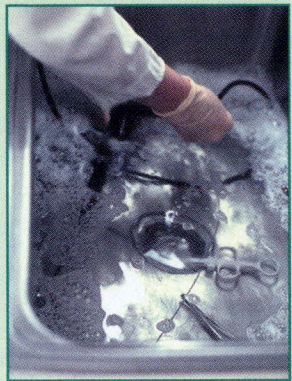

Figure 11-10-7   Clean the scope immediately after the bronchoscopy to prevent secretions from drying.

28. When client is awake and vital signs have returned to baseline, take out the IV and instruct the client or the caregiver to withhold food and liquids for at least 2 hours after the procedure.

28. There is a danger of aspiration because the airways may still be a little numb.

29. Instruct the client and/or caregiver about common side effects to expect following the bronchoscopy.
- Outpatient clients should not drive for at least 6 hours after the bronchoscopy.
- For inpatient clients, call a report to the floor if the physician or qualified practitioner has not already done so.

29. Since the sedation is in effect, it is a good idea to reinforce the verbal instructions with written ones.
- The sedation may remain in the client's system even though the client feels awake.
- Increases communication; provides better client care.

30. Deliver samples to the various laboratories if you have not already done so.

30. The longer a specimen sits, the more likely it will become unusable.

31. Check the scope for any leaks or damage sustained during the procedure.

31. Moisture will damage fiberoptic fibers of the scope. Anywhere there is moisture there is the possibility of bacterial growth.

32. If there are no leaks or damage, clean the scope inside and out with soft brushes. Rinse well and sterilize.

32. If there is any particulate matter left on the scope, it is not going to be sterile after processing.

33. Periodic postprocedure follow-up monitoring of client condition is advisable for 24 to 48 hours for inpatients. Outpatients should be instructed to contact the physician or qualified practitioner regarding fever, chest pain or discomfort, dyspnea, wheezing, hemoptysis, or any new findings presenting after the procedure has been completed.

33. Ensures continuity of care.

34. Wash hands.

34. Reduces the transmission of microorganisms.

▶ REAL WORLD ANECDOTES

Martha McPeek, a normally healthy middle-aged woman, presented one evening to the emergency department (ED) with decreased level of consciousness, nearly comatose. Despite the ED staff's best efforts, Martha died. The ED doctors had not been able to determine the reason for Martha's sudden decline and demise. The coroner's investigation revealed a potentially fatal level of lidocaine in Martha's blood. The morning before her death, she had undergone a bronchoscopy as part of a research study. The bronchoscopy records indicated that Martha had not tolerated the procedure well. To suppress her coughing and gagging during the procedure, the physician had administered a larger-than-usual amount of lidocaine. Martha had apparently recovered from the bronchoscopy without complications and had been discharged to home a few hours before her visit to the ED.

Lidocaine is commonly used in many procedures and is not considered to be a dangerous drug. This case illustrates that every client is unique and underscores the need for careful assessment and teaching. Client and family members must feel comfortable calling to report any symptoms or questions they may have following discharge.

▶ EVALUATION

- The client expressed understanding of the procedure prior to the bronchoscopy.
- The client tolerated the procedure with a minimum of anxiety or discomfort.
- The purpose of the bronchoscopy was achieved.
- Usable samples were obtained, correctly processed, and correctly labeled.
- The client did not suffer any adverse effects from the procedure.

▶ DOCUMENTATION

Nurses' Notes

- A detailed record should be kept of the procedure from the time the client is admitted to your care for the bronchoscopy procedure, including but not limited to:
  - Level of consciousness
  - Medications administered, dosage route, and time of delivery
  - Subjective response to procedure (e.g., pain, discomfort, dyspnea)
  - Vital signs: blood pressure, respiratory rate, heart rate, rhythm, and changes in cardiac status
  - SpO_2 and FIO_2
  - Lavage volumes (delivered and retrieved)
  - Site of biopsies and washings and tests requested on each sample
  - Tidal volume, peak inspiratory pressure, adequacy of inspiratory flow, and other ventilation parameters if the subject is being mechanically ventilated.

Document on appropriate flow sheet or electronic medical record (EMR).

▶ CRITICAL THINKING SKILL

Introduction

A careful client history can help avoid complications during a procedure.

Possible Scenario

You are admitting and preparing Mr. Larson for an outpatient bronchoscopy. During the intake process, you ask Mr. Larson if he has had breakfast. He denies eating before admission, and you proceed with the preparation for the bronchoscopy. As you are setting Mr. Larson up in the bronchoscopy chair, you notice a white chalky color on his tongue and mouth.

Possible Outcome

If you do not follow up on this finding and question Mr. Larson as to the cause of the white residue, Mr. Larson is at risk for vomiting and aspiration of the Maalox he took before arriving at the facility. Because he did not eat breakfast, he was experiencing heartburn and he took several doses of Maalox to combat it. In this case, you did ask Mr. Larson about the white residue, and Mr. Larson's bronchoscopy was delayed until later in the day.

Prevention

When questioning clients regarding eating or drinking prior to a procedure, be sure to ask about all oral intake. Clients often do not consider coffee or medications when asked about eating breakfast.

▶ VARIATIONS

Geriatric Variations:
- *As people age, their metabolism slows; older clients need to be watched closely for any reaction to sedation and/or reaction to the vagal stimulation of the bronchoscopy.*
- *The medication dosages should also take into account the client's age.*

Pediatric Variations:
- *Most bronchoscopies done on children are done in surgery under general anesthesia.*
- *Place in lateral position postprocedure.*

Home Care Variations:
- *Clients who will be returning home should be instructed to contact their physician or qualified practitioner regarding fever, chest pain or discomfort, dyspnea, wheezing, hemoptysis, or any new findings presenting after the procedure has been completed.*
- *Clients should not drive for at least 6 hours after the bronchoscopy.*

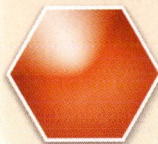

Long-Term Care Variation:
- *Periodic postprocedure follow-up monitoring of client's condition is advisable for 24–48 hours for clients in an institutional setting.*

▶ COMMON ERRORS

Possible Error:

Specimens become mixed up and the nurse is unsure where each sample was taken.

Prevention:

Specimens need to be labeled as soon as they are obtained. More than one sample type is taken from any given area/segment and often more than one site is used. If samples are not labeled immediately, they can be confused or mislabeled. If samples are not correctly identified, the procedure will need to be repeated.

▶ NURSING TIPS

- Try to set up as much as possible before the client arrives. This helps instill confidence in the client and will make the procedure go more smoothly.
- Always set up for two suctions: one for the suction to the scope and one to help clear secretions from the client's oropharynx.
- Fill out as much paperwork and labels as you can before the procedure so you can quickly label all specimens as they are obtained to prevent any mix up.

- Check vital signs frequently. For some people there is a fine line between conscious and unconscious sedation. The goal is to make the client comfortable and not put the client out completely, as the physician or qualified practitioner may need the client's help in obtaining samples.
- If you are assisting with or administering a topical anesthetic, remember the better the vocal cords are anesthetized, the better the client will tolerate the procedure and the less sedation will be needed. Remember that lidocaine is a drug too

and it is possible to administer an overdose, so keep track of how much you are using.

- Review the side effects of the procedure with the client and caregiver, along with what needs to be done if there are any reactions. Give them a written copy of these instructions.
- Observe client for a minimum of 30 minutes after the bronchoscopy procedure. Watch for any side effects of the procedure, including:

  – Any shortness of breath, which could indicate bronchospasm or a pneumothorax

  – An adverse reaction to any of the drugs given

  – Changes in vital signs

  – Amount of coughing postprocedure and any hemoptysis

▶ **SPECIAL CONSIDERATIONS**

- *Bronchoscopy is generally safe; however, the client may experience a mild fever or sore throat after the procedure. Mild fever, which lasts approximately 24 hours, is caused by an inflammatory response from the residual saline instilled into the lungs during the procedure. Call the physician or nurse practitioner if the temperature is over 102° F as the client may have developed an infection. A sore throat is caused by irritation from the scope insertion or trying to talk while the scope is in place. Hypoxemia and bronchospasm may also occur during the procedure. On rare occasions clients experience hemoptysis from irritation caused by scope insertion especially if biopsies or brushings were done during the procedures. Pneumothorax rarely occurs and is usually associated with clients who had biopsies taken or experienced severe coughing during the procedure. Perforation is a possibility, although extremely rare.*
- *Proper care of the bronchoscope is essential. Contamination of bronchoscopes has been associated withthe transmission of infection. Follow institution protocol for proper care and cleaning of equipment. Scopes must have a leak and pressure test prior to cleaning. If air escapes and a leak is present, the equipment should be cleaned and sent back to the manufacturer for repairs. Under no circumstances should faulty equipment be used because bacteria can harbor in areas of leakage.*

Assisting with a Gastrointestinal Endoscopy

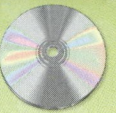

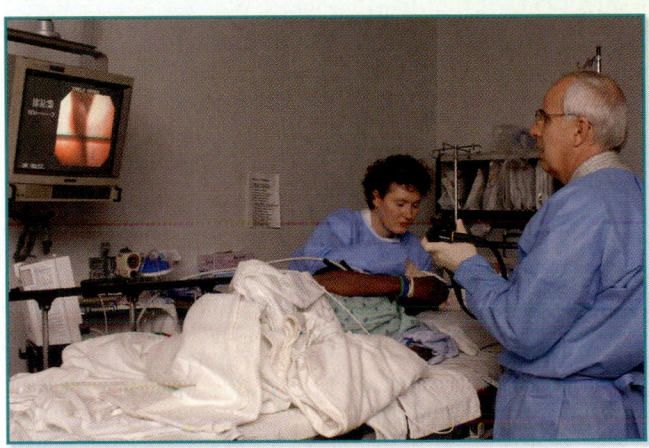

▶ OVERVIEW OF THE SKILL

Endoscopy is the visualization of a body organ or cavity via a lighted, flexible scope. Gastrointestinal (GI) endoscopy allows assessment of the GI tract. The scope is inserted via the rectum for a colonoscopy or sigmoidoscopy or via the mouth for an esophagogastroduodenoscopy (EGD) or endoscopic retrograde cholangiopancreatography (ERCP). After the endoscope is inserted, biopsies and photographs can be taken to aid in diagnosis, foreign objects and polyps can be removed, and internal bleeding can be identified and controlled. Other procedures that can be done with the endoscope are listed in Table 11-11-1.

Clients undergoing endoscopic exams, except for a sigmoidoscopy, receive intravenous (IV) medications to sedate and control pain during the procedure. Use of conscious sedation for procedures requires frequent monitoring of vital signs, level of consciousness, oxygenation, and heart rhythms. Other than the ERCP, which is typically performed in radiology for X-ray access, most endoscopic procedures are performed in a special laboratory or clinic, often serving both inpatient and outpatient clients. Nurses who work in the GI-endoscopy laboratory may be required to start IVs when indicated, give IV medications, monitor a client undergoing conscious sedation,

assist the physician or qualified practitioner, prepare specimens for the laboratory, monitor clients after the procedures, and provide discharge instructions for the procedure and after sedation.

There are several physiologic and psychologic factors the nurse needs to consider in the care of the client undergoing this procedure. Prior to endoscopic exams, most clients experience some anxiety. Some willingly state that they are anxious and ask for additional information. Often clients who are anxious will have elevated blood pressures and heart rates. Preparing for the colonoscopy procedure may cause the client to be dehydrated secondary to the frequency of diarrhea stools. Low blood pressure, pale and clammy skin, tachycardia, and tachypnea may indicate the client is dry in the intravascular space.

During upper endoscopies, the risk of aspiration is a possibility secondary to conscious sedation, anesthetizing the back of the throat prior to passing the scope and the passage of the scope into the esophagus. Clients may exhibit gagging, restlessness, and a decrease in oxygenation if aspirating. Also, the client is unable to speak because the scope is inserted via the mouth. Assessing body language (grimacing, trying to pull at the scope) and elevation in heart rate and blood pressure can assist the nurse in identifying

Table 11-11-1   Endoscopic Procedures

PROCEDURE/AREA STUDIED	PREPARATION/POSITION	CLINICAL SIGNIFICANCE
Colonoscopy—examines the large intestine	Instruct client to maintain a clear liquid diet for 48 hours before the test; take the prescribed laxative the evening before the examination. Place client on left side with knees flexed and drape.	Identify origin of bleeding or lesions; evaluate inflammatory and ulcerative bowel disease and recurrence of polyps or malignant lesions.
Esophagogastroduodenoscopy (EGD)—examines the esophagus, stomach, and upper duodenum	Instruct client to remain NPO for 8–12 hours before the test. An IV sedation may be given, then a local anesthetic is sprayed into the back of the throat to decrease the gag reflex (swallowing will seem difficult). Place client in left side-lying position.	Identify diverticula, varices, Mallory-Weiss syndrome, esophageal rings and hiatal hernia, and esophageal and gastric stenoses. When combined with histologic and cytologic tests, may indicate acute or chronic ulcers, benign or malignant tumors, and inflammatory disease.
Endoscopic retrograde cholangiopancreatography (ERC)—examines the liver, gallbladder, and pancreas visually and radioscopically. An endoscope is inserted orally into the duodenum. A small catheter is inserted into the common bile duct and pancreatic duct. A radiographic dye is injected to visualize the liver, gallbladder, and pancreas. The physician may also remove gallstones, dilate strictures, or obtain tissue samples for biopsy.	Instruct client to remain NPO for 8–12 hours before the test. An IV sedation may be given, then a local anesthetic is sprayed into the back of the throat to decrease the gag reflex (swallowing will seem difficult). Place client in left side-lying position.	Identify blockage of bile duct by gallstone, cancer, or strictures. Obtain biopsy of tumors. Diagnose pancreatic pseudocysts.
Sigmoidoscopy—examines the rectum and sigmoid colon.	Instruct client to have clear liquid diet 12–24 hours before the test. Take the prescribed enema before the test. Place client in left side-lying position or knee-chest position.	Identify polyps, tumors, fissures, or hemorrhoids.
Proctosigmoidoscopy—three steps: 1. Digital examination to dilate the anal sphincters to detect obstruction that might hinder passage of the endoscope. 2. A sigmoidoscope to examine the distal sigmoid colon and rectum. 3. A proctoscope to examine the lower rectum and anal canal.	Instruct client according to physician or qualified practitioner's orders relative to dietary restrictions and bowel preparation (these are usually based on physician or qualified practitioner preference). If the client has rectal inflammation, a local anesthetic agent is applied to decrease discomfort. Secure the client to a tilting table that rotates into horizontal and vertical positions.	Identify internal hemorrhoids, hypertrophic anal papillae, polyps, fissures, fistulae, and rectal and anal abscesses.

pain. Depending on the client's underlying medical condition, age, the procedure, and the dosage and type of medications given, the client will have an altered sensory response. Usually, the client is sleepy and unable to clearly process information. Return of the gag reflex in clients who have undergone an EGD is an indication that the medication effect is diminishing.

Although rare, there is always a risk for bleeding after the exam, particularly if biopsies were taken or polyps removed. In addition, esophageal varices may bleed. Unusual chest or abdominal pain, difficulty swallowing or moving the neck, or rectal or oral bleeding experienced by the client even after discharge should be immediately reported to the physician or qualified practitioner.

Potentially perforating the GI tract during the procedure is a rare occurrence. Signs and symptoms of diagnosing a perforation include an elevated temperature, chills, unusual chest, abdominal, or shoulder pain, abdominal tenderness, guarding, rectal or oral bleeding, and hypovolemic shock.

▶ ASSESSMENT

1. Assess the client's knowledge of, preparation for, anxiety level concerning, and readiness to undergo the endoscopic procedure. **Accurate assessment will allow the nurse to provide more information if needed about the endoscopic procedure. Proper preparation for the exam (i.e., nothing per mouth [NPO] status, laxatives, enemas) will influence whether the procedure can be performed and the quality of the exam.**

2. Perform a brief health assessment, focusing on identifying whether a client has underlying heart, liver, or kidney disease. Specifically, it is helpful to know about implanted prosthetic devices, hepatitis, insulin-dependent and non–insulin-dependent diabetes mellitus (IDDM/NIDDM), hypertension, bleeding, seizure disorders, or pregnancy. **Knowledge about the general health of the client, in addition to assessing for certain conditions, can better prepare the health practitioners to care for the client during the endoscopic exam. Clients who have diabetes, for example, should have their blood sugars monitored and be observed for hypo- or hyperglycemic reactions. Clients with a history of pulmonary and coronary disease should be monitored closely for excessive sedation or dysrhythmias during medication administration. Extra caution must be taken with the electrosurgical equipment if the client has a pacemaker. Clients with liver or kidney disease should be carefully assessed regarding the extent of their illness because their tolerance of medications may be impaired.**

3. Determine the need for informed consent and the need for signatures of the client and a witness. Assess the client's ability to sign a consent form. **Endoscopic procedures require informed consent. The physician or qualified practitioner must explain the purpose of the procedure, risk, and benefits prior to the client signing the consent form.**

4. Check for allergies to drugs. **During most endoscopic exams, IV medications are given, which may include fentanyl, morphine, meperidine, hydromorphone, midazolam, lorazepam, diazepam, hydroxyzine, and promethazine. Also, check for an allergy to the "caine" family if the client is undergoing an EGD because the back of the throat may be sprayed with Cetacaine or other anesthetic before insertion of the scope.**

5. Ask about current medications, specifically whether the client has taken Coumadin, aspirin, nonsteroidal anti-inflammatory drugs (NSAIDS), heparin, or other anticoagulants recently (within the last 5 days). **These medications cause anticoagulation of the blood and can contribute to bleeding during the procedure, especially if biopsies are indicated.**

6. Check for dentures, removable dental plates, and/or loose teeth if client is undergoing EGD and ERCP. **Because the endoscope is inserted through the mouth, removal of dentures and dental plates is essential prior to the procedure.**

7. Verify plans for transportation home if client is an outpatient. **For 24 hours after the completion of the procedure, it is recommended that the client not operate moving machinery if conscious sedation was utilized.**

▶ DIAGNOSIS

Anxiety

Acute Pain

Risk for Aspiration

Risk for Deficient Fluid Volume

Risk for Injury

Deficient Knowledge

Disturbed Sensory Perception

▶ PLANNING

Expected Outcomes:

1. Client will have no signs of bleeding or perforation.
2. Client will have a stable airway and respiratory status (respiratory rate and O_2 saturation within normal limits).

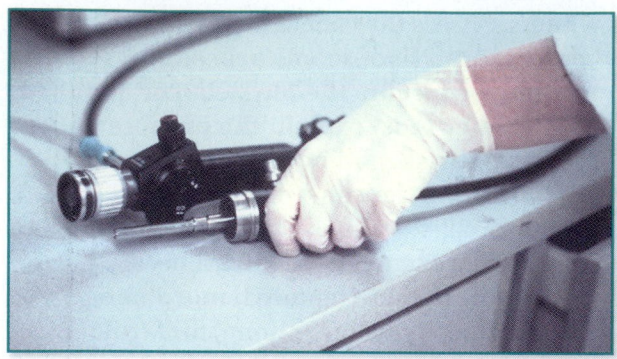

Figure 11-11-1 Endoscope

3. Client will have stable cardiovascular status (blood pressure and heart rate within normal limits).
4. Client will be easily aroused and able to talk.
5. Gag reflex will be intact.
6. Client will be able to move with minimal assistance.

Equipment Needed:

- Blood pressure monitoring equipment
- Continuous pulse oximeter and cardiac monitoring
- IV start equipment
- Suction
- Emergency equipment
- IV medications, properly labeled
- Oxygen
- Endoscope (see Figure 11-11-1) and related equipment
- Gloves

▶ CLIENT EDUCATION NEEDED:

1. Before the procedure, explain preparation needed (i.e., NPO from midnight or 8 hours prior to the procedure for most endoscopy procedures; laxatives and/or enemas for lower endoscopy).
2. Explain the procedure, including when the client will be asked to move or to swallow, what sounds he or she may hear, how the procedure will progress, how long the procedure will take, and what sensations he or she may feel.
3. Explain to the client that he or she will be connected to monitoring equipment during the procedure to observe vital signs. Reassure the client that this is a normal part of the procedure.
4. If used, explain the use of conscious sedation and what the client will experience.
5. After the procedure, discuss discharge instructions with the client and also provide written discharge instructions. It is important that the client clearly understands instructions.
6. Explain to the client undergoing a colonoscopy or sigmoidoscopy that feelings of mild abdominal fullness or cramping after the procedure are normal.
7. Instruct the client to report symptoms of acute abdominal pain, fever, chills, or bleeding immediately.

Estimated time to complete the skill:
1–2 hours

▶ DELEGATION TIPS

Assessment for bleeding, pain, shortness of breath, gag reflex, and proper postprocedure position is the responsibility of the nurse. Measurement of vital signs may be delegated to ancillary personnel.

IMPLEMENTATION—Action/Rationale

Action	Rationale
1. Wash hands.	1. Reduces the transmission of microorganisms.
2. Check equipment, including endoscope, to be sure it is functioning.	2. Properly working equipment is essential.
3. Prepare for possible biopsies, polyp removal, photos.	3. It is preferable to set up all equipment before the case starts because the room will be darkened during the procedure and the nurse may be unable to leave the client.
4. Check that emergency equipment is available, including emergency medications such as naloxone (opioid antagonist) and flumazenil (benzodiazepine antagonist).	4. Having ready access to emergency equipment will assist the nurse in providing appropriate care when necessary.
5. Verify client identification.	5. Ensures the correct client.
6. Perform brief nursing assessment.	6. Provides information about the general health of the client, focusing on areas that may place a client at risk from the procedure or the medications.
7. Check for drug allergies or unusual reactions to medications.	7. Helps to determine which medications to give, including the dosage.
8. Verify client's readiness for the procedure; include the last time the client had anything to eat or drink. Also, ask about the type of bowel prep and the results if the client is undergoing lower endoscopic exams.	8. It is important to maintain NPO status before EGD and ERCP to minimize risks of aspiration as the endoscope will be inserted through the mouth after the client's throat is numb and the gag reflex is suppressed. Thorough cleansing of the bowel via the prep will enable the physician or qualified practitioner to see the lining of the GI tract.
9. Verify that the consent form for the procedure is signed.	9. Clients must give consent prior to endoscopic exams. Ensures that client has been educated about procedure; also protects nurse, qualified practitioner, and institution.
10. Verify client has a ride home if undergoing conscious sedation.	10. Clients who receive conscious sedation should not drive for approximately 24 hours as their judgment may be impaired.
11. Answer any questions.	11. Often clients have questions about the exam that should be addressed prior to starting the procedure.
12. Start IV and IV fluids, if indicated.	12. IV site is needed for IV conscious sedation. IV fluids are usually given to clients undergoing colonoscopy because they have lost fluids during the bowel prep and are NPO. No IV site is usually needed for a flexible sigmoidoscopy because clients do not usually receive conscious sedation.

continues

Action	Rationale
13. Connect to electrocardiographic, blood pressure, and oximetry monitoring systems.	**13.** Because of the immediate sedative effect of the medications, it is essential to monitor the client during conscious sedation.
14. Check baseline vital signs, heart rhythm, respiratory rate, O_2 saturation, and level of consciousness.	**14.** Establishing a baseline allows the nurse a point of comparison to better evaluate the effect of medications during the procedure.
15. Start oxygen via nasal cannula or tracheostomy collar, if applicable.	**15.** Providing supplemental oxygen during the procedure is easier if the oxygen is already in place on the client.
16. Wear appropriate protective garb as indicated. This may include goggles, masks, face shields, gown, and gloves.	**16.** Appropriate protective garb prevents the health professional from exposure to secretions.
17. Position client on left side with head of bed as flat as tolerated.	**17.** For the EGD, colonoscopy, and flexible sigmoidoscopy, the client is positioned on the left side for better tube insertion. For the ERCP, the client begins the procedure lying on the left side but is moved onto the stomach, facing right, after the endoscope is inserted.
18. Ensure client privacy and dignity during the exam.	**18.** Privacy will help maintain respect.
19. For an EGD and ERCP, instruct client that the throat will be numbed either by a spray or gargle and a plastic mouthpiece inserted (see Figure 11-11-2 and Figure 11-11-3).	**19.** Numbing the throat will help minimize discomfort to the client when the endoscope is passed into the stomach. The mouthpiece allows the endoscope a clear passage to the back to the mouth, protecting the teeth.
20. Per the physician's or qualified practitioner's orders, administer IV medications for sedation.	**20.** Usually two types of medications are given, an opioid and a benzodiazepine, in order to sedate a client adequately to pass the endoscope.
21. While giving IV medications for sedation, continually monitor vital signs, O_2 saturation, heart rhythm, airway, and level of consciousness.	**21.** Medications given for conscious sedations can adversely affect vital signs and oxygen saturation. A client's level of consciousness should decrease from an alert state to a state in which the client is sleepy but able to be aroused and able to follow some commands.

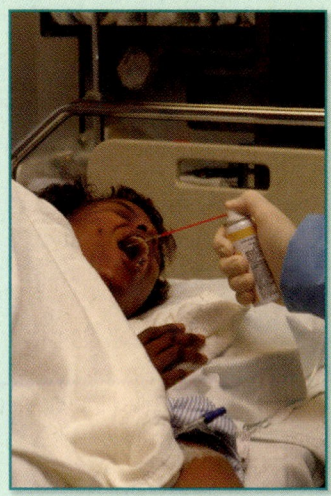

Figure 11-11-2   The client's throat is numbed with a spray.

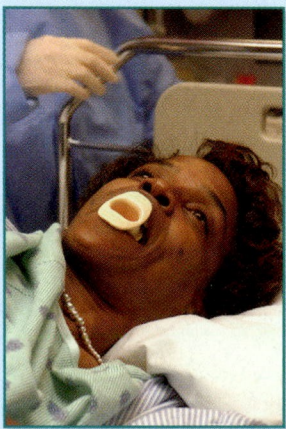

Figure 11-11-3   Note the plastic mouthpiece inserted to allow the endoscope clear passage and to protect the teeth.

continues

Action	Rationale
22. Document vital signs, O₂ saturation, and level of consciousness within 2 minutes of giving medications and at least every 15 minutes (may be more frequent as indicated) and at the end of the procedure.	**22.** Frequency and type of documentation during conscious sedation are determined by hospital policy but must be done to maintain client safety.
23. Notify the physician or qualified practitioner of any changes in vital signs, O₂ saturation, or heart rate/rhythm.	**23.** Although the physician or qualified practitioner is in the room during the procedure, he or she may be focused on the endoscope and the monitor and not the monitoring equipment. Prompt notification of changes in vital signs, heart rhythm, and oxygenation is essential.
24. If cautery is used, apply a grounding pad to the thigh or hip.	**24.** Ensures client safety.
25. Assist with biopsies or other specimen as needed (see Figure 11-11-4).	**25.** Often biopsies, polyps, or other tissue specimen may be obtained during the procedure.

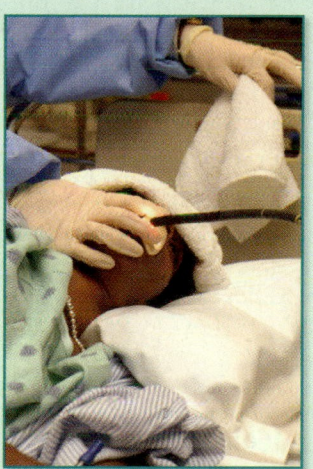

Figure 11-11-4   The nurse is assisting with the procedure by holding the mouth guard in place.

Action	Rationale
26. Following the procedure, ensure client safety by keeping side rails up until sedation has worn off, monitor airway, and assess the gag reflex (especially if upper endoscopy is performed).	**26.** Ensures client safety.
27. Document all medications given, including name, dosage, route, time, and administrator.	**27.** Properly documents administration.
28. Assess for signs of bleeding and perforation, that is, unusual abdominal pain, guarding, tenderness, rectal or oral bleeding, or hypovolemic shock.	**28.** Although a rare complication, the lumen of the GI tract could have been perforated during the exam and bleeding could occur. If noted, the physician or qualified practitioner should be informed immediately.
29. After the procedure, monitor vital signs, level of consciousness, and O₂ saturation every 15 minutes for at least 1 hour and until within 20% of the baseline readings.	**29.** Monitoring until the effects of conscious sedation have worn off indicates when the client can safely leave the area.
30. Provide written discharge instructions, including phone numbers of the GI clinic and appropriate staff who are able to answer questions after hours.	**30.** Written discharge instructions specific to each procedure provide the client with reference information.
31. If an outpatient client, discontinue IV access prior to discharge, observe site, and apply dressing.	**31.** In outpatient clients, IV access is no longer needed once the procedure is completed.

► REAL WORLD ANECDOTES

Scenario 1

Bob has completed an EGD 1 hour previously and is resting in the recovery area. All vital signs are stable and have returned to baseline. Bob is much more alert and is expressing a desire to leave for home. Prior to discontinuing the IV, the nurse assists Bob to a sitting position and rechecks the blood pressure, which is stable. After sitting up for 3–4 minutes, Bob became nauseated and flushed and collapsed back on the bed. The nurse assesses Bob and rechecks the blood pressure and vital signs. The blood pressure is lower than normal, and Bob's heart rate is only in the 40s. The heart rhythm reveals a third-degree atrioventricular (AV) block with nonconducted P waves. On admission, Bob had reported that he had an AV block but it had been relatively asymptomatic. On further assessment, the nurse learns that Bob had a syncopal episode several months ago, reported to the emergency room, but received no medical treatment. After returning to bed rest, Bob reports that he feels better, but his heart rate is still in the 40s. The physician is notified and orders are received to start IV fluids, obtain a stat ECG, and notify the referring physician. After further assessment, Bob is admitted to the hospital for a cardiac work-up.

Scenario 2

In this small rural hospital, sigmoidoscopies were done in the emergency department (ED) in the quiet morning hours between 6:00 a.m. and 7:00 a.m. When Mack arrived at the ED, his eyes were downcast, he was hunched up in his coat, and he would not make eye contact with the receptionist. The nurse, sensing his discomfort, brought him to a private room and spoke with him. He admitted that he was extremely embarrassed about the procedure and "where they would be poking around." The prep for the procedure had been extremely embarrassing as well, as his family "knew" what he had to do, and he felt like they were watching him. The nurse reassured him that these feelings were very normal. She discussed with him the ways his privacy and dignity would be protected during the procedure and provided education about the procedure. She listened to his concerns, and together they discussed ways he could cope with his feelings and things he could do to reduce his sense of embarrassment.

► EVALUATION

- The client had no signs of bleeding or perforation.
- Client had a stable airway and respiratory status (respiratory rate and O_2 saturation within normal limits).
- Client had a stable cardiovascular status (blood pressure and heart rate within normal limits).
- Client was easily aroused and able to talk.
- Client was able to move with minimal assistance.

► DOCUMENTATION

Flow Sheet

- Record the client's vital signs, before, during, and after the procedure.
- Record oxygen saturation, before, during, and after the procedure.
- Document assessments of level of consciousness.
- Note IV fluids given; include rate, type of fluid, time started, and time discontinued.

Document on appropriate flow sheet or electronic medical record (EMR).

Medication Administration Record

- Record the time, name, dosage, route, and initials of administrator for any medications given to the client.

Nurses' Notes

- Describe overall tolerance to procedure, including biopsies, polypectomy, and dilation.
- Note the IV site.
- Document admission assessment for outpatient clients.
- Document health assessment for outpatient clients.
- Document escort available at discharge for outpatient clients.
- Note client allergies.
- Note current medications.
- Document preparation for procedure.
- Document the presence and handling of dentures, glasses, and other personal items.
- Document the presence of an interpreter, if needed.
- Document client teaching and time of discharge.

- Note follow-up information provided, including prescription and return appointment.

► CRITICAL THINKING SKILL

Introduction

A client with end-stage renal failure and GI bleeding undergoes an EGD to isolate the source of bleeding. During the procedure, he is given too much sedation and becomes difficult to arouse.

Possible Scenario

Jim is an inpatient referred to the GI clinic to locate the source of GI bleeding manifested as tarry stools. Although the client was given shorter-acting medications for the procedure, the client was difficult to arouse at the conclusion of the exam. In addition, Jim's oxygenation dropped to the high 80s. His blood pressure was also lower than normal. A bolus of normal saline was started, oxygen was increased to 4–5 liters per nasal cannula, the head of the bed was elevated, and naloxone was given to reverse the effects of the opioids. The nurse continues to monitor Jim's vital signs, respiratory status, and level of consciousness, administering more naloxone and possibly flumazenil IV, if indicated.

Possible Outcome

Jim may not respond to naloxone, flumazenil, and increased oxygen flow rate. His vital signs may continue to worsen, prompting a need for intubation if he is unable to sustain an adequate airway. Or Jim may respond well to the naloxone and support measures, waking up enough to breathe adequately under his own power, without further medical intervention.

Prevention

Careful assessment of the client's underlying health status is very important prior to giving the client IV narcotics and sedatives. Examining the current laboratory values, researching medications given during prior procedures, and assessing the current medical record may provide helpful information. Also, be sure that emergency equipment and medications are readily available during the procedure.

► VARIATIONS

Geriatric Variations:
- *Some medications are absorbed differently in older adults. You may need to use smaller amounts.*
- *Be sure to assess whether the older client has taken aspirin, NSAIDS, or Coumadin prior to the exam.*

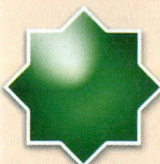

Pediatric Variation:
- *A young pediatric endoscopy client may not be able to verbally describe symptoms that might indicate complications. Be especially vigilant when assessing for nonverbal communication of pain or distress, as well as other symptoms of perforation or sepsis.*

Home Care Variation:
- *This procedure is not done in the home care setting. Clients should be taught what symptoms to watch for, including nausea, vomiting, bleeding and abdominal pain, and who to call to report symptoms and ask questions.*

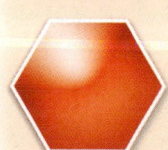

Long-Term Care Variation:
- *This procedure is not done in the long-term care setting. Staff providing care should be aware of complications that may occur postprocedure. These include bleeding, abdominal pain, and difficulty breathing.*

> ▶ **COMMON ERRORS**

Possible Error:

Inadequate preparation for the exam by the client.

Prevention:

Be sure that the client has received accurate and easily understandable preparation instructions. Provide phone numbers of the clinic and after-hour contact if the client has any questions prior to the exam. Emphasize the importance of following the instructions.

▶ **NURSING TIPS**

- Check all equipment before beginning the procedure. It is very difficult to set up equipment once the procedure has started because of the darkness of the room.
- Be sure emergency equipment and medications are available.

- Be familiar with medications commonly given and their respective antidotes.
- Wear appropriate protective gear (i.e., goggles, face shields, gown, shoe covers, and gloves, as indicated).

▶ **SPECIAL CONSIDERATIONS**

- *Before the exam, the client should be instructed not to eat or drink anything for 6–8 hours. Inform the client that it is important for the stomach to be empty at the time of the endoscopy to allow the endoscopist to complete a thorough examination without the risk of aspiration.*
- *Clients generally are very concerned about how they will feel after the test. The best method of relieving anxiety is to provide information. Let the client know that the most common discomforts associated with endoscopy are a feeling of bloating from the air introduced during the examination and a sore throat, both of which usually resolve shortly after the procedure. The client may eat a few hours after the exam, unless advised otherwise. Subsequent to endoscopy the client may feel lethargic and must not drive a car. Arrangement should be made prior to the endoscopy for transportation. Depending on the amount of sedation used, most clients will sleep for several hours after the procedure and should not anticipate returning to work on the day of the test.*
- *Inform clients of risk of perforation and to report signs and symptoms of complications to the physician or health care provider. General symptoms of perforation are bleeding, fever, or dysphagia. Even though perforation is rare, the client must report abdominal pain, tense abdomen, or fever. Cervical perforation would be exhibited by neck or throat pain, dysphagia, and/or crepitus (cracking under the skin) around the neck area. Epigastric or shoulder pain could be the result of esophageal perforation. Evaluate for cyanosis, dyspnea, and pleural effusion, the result of perforation affecting the respiratory system.*

Assisting with a Proctosigmoidoscopy

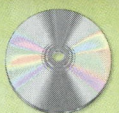

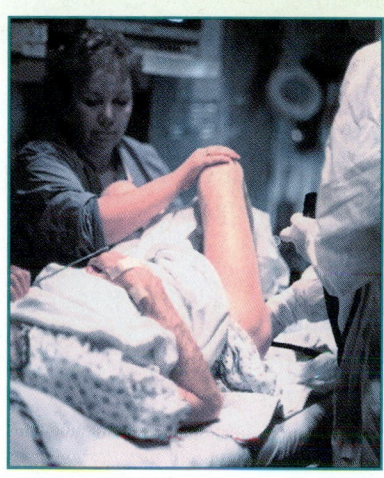

▶ OVERVIEW OF THE SKILL

A proctosigmoidoscopy is the insertion of a rigid or flexible scope into the lower gastrointestinal tract through the anus to examine the distal sigmoid colon, rectum, and anal canal. This endoscopic examination is performed to diagnose malignant and benign tumors and for the detection of hemorrhoids, polyps, fissures, fistulas, and abscesses within the rectum and anal canal. The American Cancer Society recommends that persons older than 50 years of age should have a proctosigmoidoscopy every 3–5 years to detect and prevent colon cancer.

The client requires enemas the night before and the day of the procedure so that the colon can be unobstructed and visualized. The most common enema is a Fleet Enema (see Skill 6-19).

Note: The nurse will be assisting the physician or qualified practitioner unless the nurse has received education and training in techniques of flexible sigmoidoscopy. Gastrointestinal nurses can only perform this procedure for the purpose of colorectal cancer screening.

▶ ASSESSMENT

1. Auscultate the abdomen for bowel sounds. **This will allow the nurse to determine if the client is experiencing any alteration in gastrointestinal function.**

2. Assess client's understanding of the procedure. **This will enable the nurse to determine possible educational needs immediately before the procedure.**

3. Assess client's compliance with bowel preparation prior to the start of the procedure. **This will enable the nurse to determine if the bowel is free of stool to allow visualization of colon.**

4. Inspect the perianal skin. **This will allow the nurse to determine whether there is a pre-existing alteration in skin integrity.**

5. Assess client's ability to sign a consent form.

▶ DIAGNOSIS

Risk for Injury

Pain

Anxiety

Fear

Risk for Compromised Human Dignity

Bowel Incontinence

▶ PLANNING

Expected Outcomes:

1. The client will tolerate the procedure without undue fear or anxiety.

2. The client will not experience pain related to the procedure.
3. The client will not experience any injury related to the procedure.
4. The procedure will successfully visualize the client's distal colon, rectum, and anal canal.

Equipment Needed (see Figure 11-12-1):

- Rigid or flexible proctosigmoidoscope
- Water-soluble lubricant
- Clean gloves
- Intravenous access

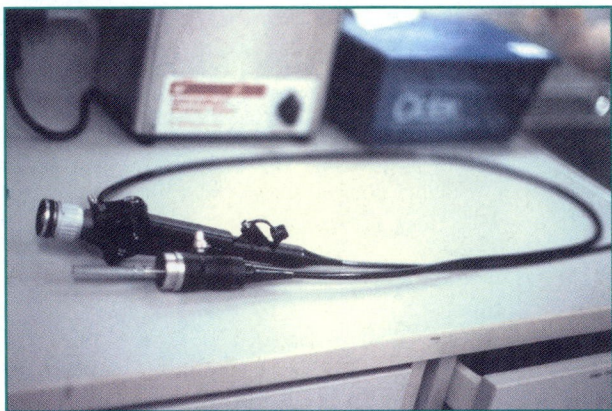

Figure 11-12-1 Endoscope

▶ CLIENT EDUCATION NEEDED:

1. Provide the client with an explanation of procedure, including any sensations the client may experience.
2. Explain the reasons for not eating or drinking after midnight the night before.
3. Instruct the client regarding the bowel preparation procedure.
4. Review the positions the client may be asked to assume during the procedure.
5. Tell the client when he or she can expect the test results and who will be providing them.
6. Explain rationale for the initial and follow-up examinations, if required.

Estimated time to complete the skill: **10–15 minutes**

▶ DELEGATION TIPS

Assessment for bleeding, pain, shortness of breath, and proper postprocedure position is the responsibility of the nurse. Measurement of vital signs may be delegated to ancillary personnel.

IMPLEMENTATION—Action/Rationale

Action	Rationale
1. Obtain informed consent and ensure IV access.	1. Invasive procedures require that the client should understand the purpose, risks, benefits, and client permission.
2. Wash hands.	2. Practices aseptic technique.
3. Assemble equipment (see Figures 11-12-2 and 11-12-3).	3. Ensures that all equipment is ready to use.
4. Explain procedure to client.	4. Decreases client's anxiety in relation to an invasive process

continues

Action	Rationale

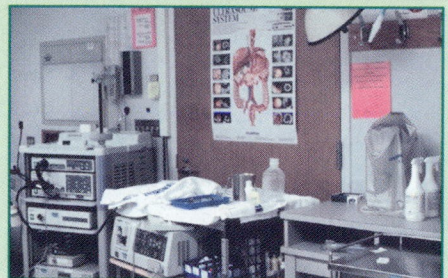

Figure 11-12-2 Endoscopy procedure room with endoscopy equipment

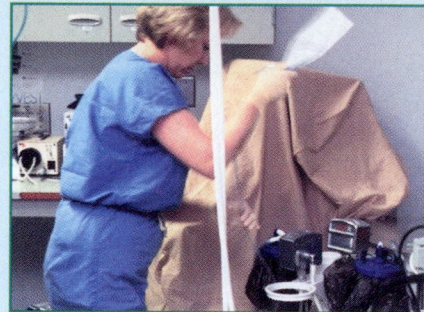

Figure 11-12-3 Assemble equipment.

5. Instruct client to undress and don hospital gown. Cover to protect privacy. Place clothes under gurney (see Figure 11-12-4) or as per hospital policy.

5. Keeps clothes safe and prevents clothes from interfering with procedure.

6. Apply monitoring equipment.

6. Allows close monitoring of the client during the procedure.

7. Position client in the knee-chest position. If client is aged, weak, or ill, the left lateral Sim's position is acceptable.

7. Allows the sigmoid colon to straighten.

8. Administer sedation to client as ordered.

8. Sedation is used to make the client comfortable during the procedure but allows the client to remain conscious during the procedure.

9. Assist or secure assistance helping the client maintain position (see Figure 11-12-5).

9. Allows the procedure to proceed without interruption.

10. Apply gloves.

10. Practices aseptic technique.

11. Continue to explain the procedure to the client as it progresses (see Figure 11-12-6).

11. Provides information to the sedated but aware client.

12. Apply lubricant to a gloved finger.

12. Protects fragile mucosa from injury.

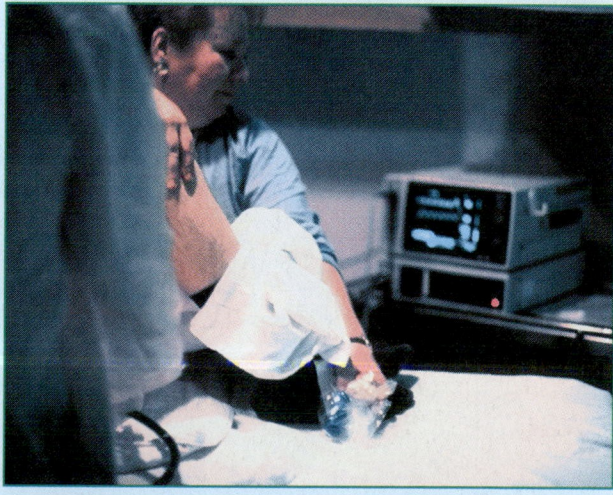

Figure 11-12-5 Note how the nurse is assisting the client to maintain the proper position.

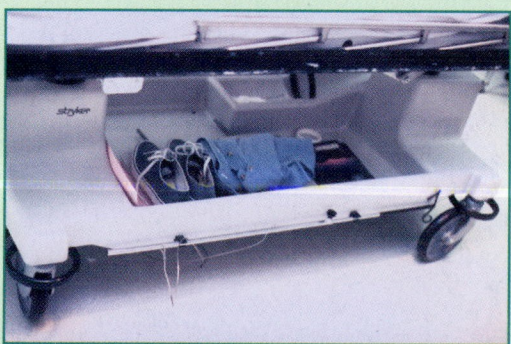

Figure 11-12-4 Place the client's clothes under the gurney.

continues

Action	Rationale

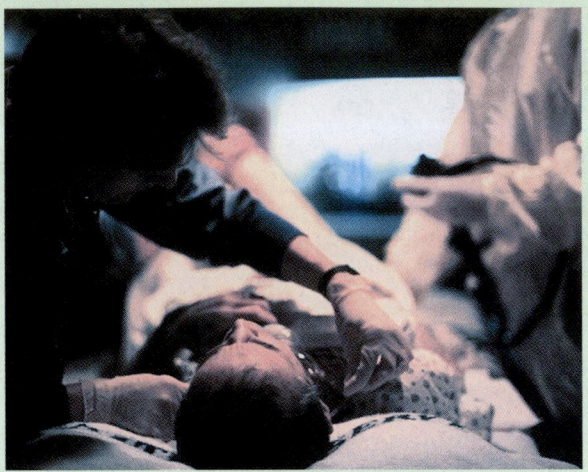

Figure 11-12-6 The client is sedated but aware. The nurse explains the procedure to the client as it progresses.

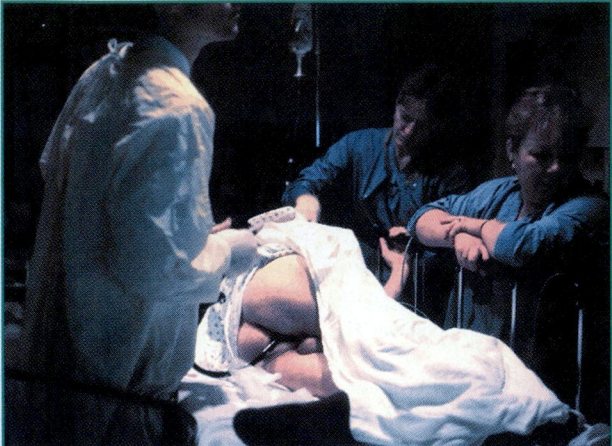

Figure 11-12-7 The endoscope is inserted in the anal canal.

13. Insert lubricated finger into rectum to check for possible obstructions prior to insertion of rectal tube.

13. Prevents possible injury to bowel mucosa from a blind entry.

14. Lubricate end of endoscope.

14. Facilitates entry of endoscope into anal canal.

15. A physician or qualified practitioner gently inserts endoscope into anal canal and gradually increase depth of insertion into colon (see Figure 11-12-7).

15. Facilitates slow access into colon and allows for visualization of mucosa.

16. Examine the distal sigmoid colon, rectum, and anal canal as required (see Figure 11-12-8). If cramping occurs, the client may require more medication or a temporary pause in the forward movement of the scope.

16. Completes the purpose of the exam. Relieves client's pain and allows evaluation of cramping.

17. Slowly remove endoscope at completion of exam.

17. Prevents injury to mucosa and client discomfort.

18. Place endoscope in appropriate container and cleaning solution.

18. Practices infection control standards.

19. Remove soiled gloves and place in appropriate receptacle.

19. Practices infection control standards.

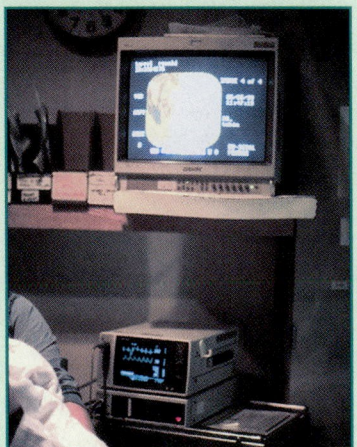

Figure 11-12-8 The intestinal tract is examined.

continues

Action	Rationale
20. Wash hands.	**20.** Practices aseptic technique.
21. Apply gloves	**21.** Prevents transmission of microorganisms.
22. Cleanse perianal area with soap and water.	**22.** Decreases risk of transmission of microorganisms and provides for client comfort after the procedure.
23. Continue to monitor vital signs until client is fully awake and responsive.	**23.** Ensures that client has stable vital signs since sedation was administered.
24. Assist client to a comfortable position.	**24.** Provides for client comfort.
25. Transfer client back to hospital room or recovery area.	**25.** Ensures the client will continue to be monitored.

► REAL WORLD ANECDOTES

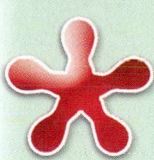

A 50-year-old white male client calls into the office to schedule his annual physical and is informed that a proctosigmoidoscopy will be performed as part of his examination. He quickly becomes very agitated and anxious and starts to cancel the appointment. The receptionist keeps him on the line until the consulting nurse can speak to him about the procedure. He is still very anxious. The consulting nurse offers to fax him information and makes an appointment with him the next day to answer his questions over the phone. As a result of the nurse's supportive intervention, the client completes his exam.

► EVALUATION

- The client tolerated the procedure without undue fear or anxiety.
- The client did not experience pain related to the procedure.
- The client did not experience any injury related to the procedure.
- The procedure successfully visualized the client's distal colon, rectum, and anal canal.

► DOCUMENTATION

Nurses' Notes

- Describe client's tolerance of procedure.
- Document insertion and removal of endoscopic tube.
- Note appearance of perianal skin, if alteration was observed.
- Describe bowel mucosa, if the procedure was performed by nurse.

Document on appropriate flow sheet or electronic medical record (EMR).

► CRITICAL THINKING SKILL

Introduction

Look at a scenario in which the client is experiencing changes in bowel habits and rectal bleeding. She needs this procedure but is dissuaded by her preprocedure care.

Possible Scenario

A 50-year-old white client has been experiencing rectal bleeding on and off for 6 months that she attributes to hemorrhoids. Her physician schedules a proctosigmoidoscopy to rule out rectal cancer. The client is seen by the nurse to be instructed on bowel preparation and diet before the procedure.

Possible Outcome

The consultation with the nurse is less than optimal. The nurse is rushed and starts to discuss the enema regimen in the hall as she is walking with the client back to her office. She is carrying the Fleet Enema box and gesturing the motions of insertion. Her voice carries to other people in the hall. Once in her office, she uses jargon and hurries the meeting. The client is embarrassed and confused. The client cancels the test the next day, saying that she needs emergency dental work and will reschedule in a few months.

Prevention

An astute nurse would realize that this is the client's first experience with a proctosigmoidoscopy and that the client is fearful of a possible diagnosis of rectal cancer. The client is also experiencing deficient knowledge in relation to the procedure. Providing instruction about the procedure and the bowel preparation in a private and supportive setting helps to decrease the client's anxiety related to the procedure. By decreasing the client's anxiety, the procedure will be less uncomfortable. The client should also be told when to expect the results of the test, and her concerns should be heard and discussed.

▶ VARIATIONS

Geriatric Variation:
- *Older or debilitated clients may be unable to assume the knee-chest position but can be placed in the Sim's position for the examination.*

Pediatric Variation:
- *Small children require scopes of a different size.*

Home Care Variation:
- *Home care nurses must be made aware of the client's procedure so that they may reinforce teaching and be prepared for the client's having some residual diarrhea or slight bleeding after the procedure.*

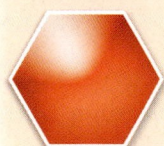

Long-Term Care Variation:
- *Long-term facility staff must be made aware of the client's procedure so that they may reinforce teaching and be prepared for the client's having some residual diarrhea or slight bleeding after the procedure.*

▶ COMMON ERRORS

Possible Error:

Missing the cues of the client's anxiety and/or fear level.

Prevention:

Ask client questions appropriate to ascertaining both knowledge and comfort level for having this procedure performed (i.e., "Have you ever had this procedure done before?" "Do you understand how the doctor will be examining your colon?" "Can you repeat to me how you will be doing the bowel prep?"). Always take the time to speak with the client in an unhurried manner and use active listening skills.

► **NURSING TIPS**

- Use visual aids when instructing the client on the procedure.
- Provide client with a quiet place to rest following the procedure.
- Provide client with written instructions on bowel preparation and signs/symptoms that necessitate calling the physician or qualified practitioner.

► **SPECIAL CONSIDERATIONS**

- *Clients often complain about the bowel preparation when they are required to drink a prep prior to proctosigmoidoscopy. It is often helpful to ice the drink to make it more palatable.*
- *Encourage the client to drink plenty of fluids after the procedure to avoid dehydration.*

Assisting with Arteriography

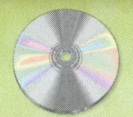

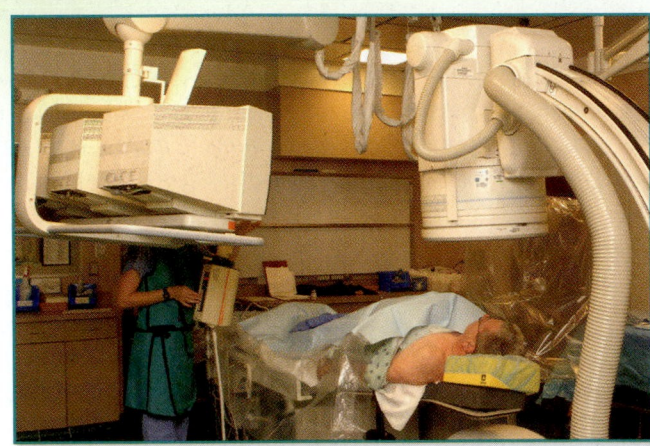

▶ OVERVIEW OF THE SKILL

An arteriogram is a radiologic procedure intended to provide morphologic visualization of the arterial lumen. Arteriograms are one type of angiogram (a radiologic study of blood vessels), but the terms arteriogram and angiogram are often used interchangeably. Arteriograms are usually performed by a radiologist and involve inserting an intra-arterial catheter percutaneously (see Figure 11-13-1) and advancing it with fluoroscopic visualization to a position near the arterial bed of interest. Radiopaque contrast material is injected (see Figure 11-13-2) to permit optimal visualization of the arteries (see Figure 11-13-3). Arteriograms are the most commonly

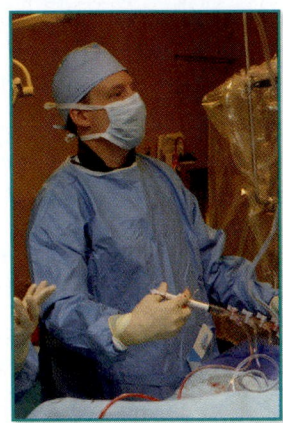

Figure 11-13-2 Radiopaque contrast material is injected.

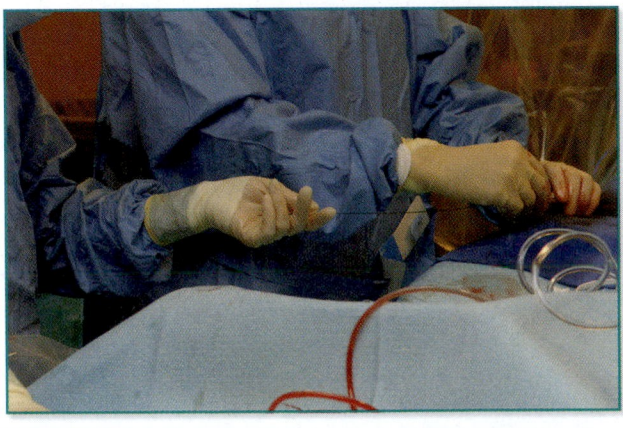

Figure 11-13-1 An intra-arterial catheter is inserted percutaneously.

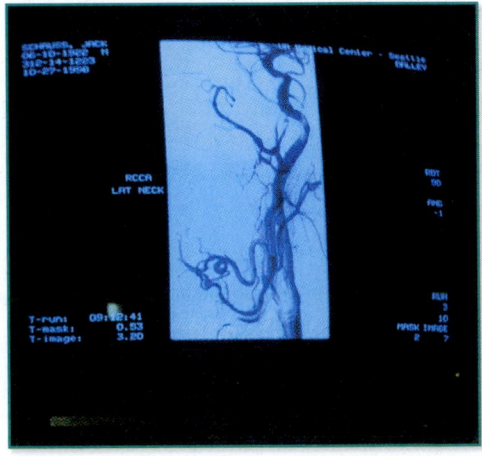

Figure 11-13-3 The arteries are visualized.

used diagnostic procedures to determine the presence and extent of arterial obstruction, occlusion, aneurysm formation, or site of bleeding. However, arteriograms may be combined with therapeutic measures such as balloon dilation of a stenosed artery and/or stent insertions (intended to "splint" or hold open the problematic section of artery). Arterial circulations frequently studied with arteriographic procedures include carotid or cerebral circulations, the aorta (aortogram), renal arterial beds, the coronary circulation (coronary arteriogram or angiogram), and femoral and distal lower extremity circulations.

Because vascular disease or trauma can occur in many body areas, variations will be encountered in artery access sites and arterial beds studied. Access sites must be near the body surface and of sufficient caliber and alignment to permit passage of the catheter to the arterial bed of interest. Sites encountered are femoral arteries, brachials and, rarely, the carotid arteries. The access site variations need to be considered to determine if shaving or other site preparation is to be done by the nurse.

Postprocedure care will follow the same general guidelines, with some variations in size and amount of pressure applied and methods used to secure pressure dressings. Variations in technique to effect relative immobilization of the access site will also be seen and may include use of sandbags over accessed site (groin or brachial). Occasionally, the nurse may encounter a commercial pressure device such as Fem-stop that is used to apply pressure directly over the artery puncture site. These devices are used for only brief periods in order to bring about hemostasis and usually require specific training in application, usage, and removal. These devices are usually applied immediately following withdrawal of the catheter and are removed prior to return of the client to the nursing unit.

► **ASSESSMENT**

1. Confirm the client's identity, knowledge level concerning the procedure, and purpose for the arteriogram. **Proper identification is a priority safety measure; client knowledge must be assessed so that a specific plan may be made to provide necessary teaching that enhances client comfort and allays anxiety.**

2. Determine the need for informed consent and the need for signatures of client and witness. Assess the client's ability to sign a consent form. **Arteriography is an invasive procedure and is associated with risks that must be explained to the client by the physician or qualified practitioner.**

3. Determine allergy or reaction to iodine or contrast agents. **Products containing iodine or similar agents are frequently used to prepare the skin over intravenous (IV) and artery access sites. Radiopaque contrast agents are used in the study, and the client may have to be premedicated with medications such as diphenhydramine or methylprednisolone to decrease allergic response to the contrast agents.**

4. Determine baseline vital signs, if these have not been obtained previously. **Baseline vital signs, including temperature, are necessary to determine change.**

5. Determine the presence, characteristics, and symmetry of peripheral pulses, particularly the brachials, radials, femorals, and dorsalis pedis and posterior tibial pulses. **Baseline pulse determinations are imperative for postprocedure comparisons.**

6. Determine need for baseline renal function tests (blood-urea-nitrogen [BUN] and creatinine) prior to the study. **The use of radiopaque contrast agents may be nephrotoxic, particularly to a client with existing, impaired kidney function, and special attention to hydration is a priority for clients with impaired renal function.**

7. Determine last oral intake of client. **Oral intake of fluids and a "light" meal is often permitted before angiography, but heavy recent intake may require a delay in the procedure if a lengthy procedure is planned or client is to be sedated, thus increasing risk of aspiration.**

8. Ask about current medications, specifically whether the client is taking anticoagulants (Coumadin), aspirin, or nonsteroidal anti-inflammatory drugs. **These medications cause anticoagulation of the blood and can contribute to bleeding during the procedure.**

► **DIAGNOSIS**

Risk for Fluid Volume Deficit

Risk for Peripheral Vascular Dysfunction

Deficient Knowledge

Anxiety

Acute Pain

► PLANNING

Expected Outcomes

1. Client will be able to identify general purpose and nature of procedure.
2. Client will be able to verbalize presence of anxiety and will inform staff if feeling unable to cope with anxiety or if anxiety symptoms are increasing.
3. Client will be able to verbalize any pain and obtain a level of relief that is tolerable for rest/sleep following pain interventions.
4. The client will not experience bleeding or vascular dysfunction, such as decrease in peripheral pulses.

Equipment Needed:
Preprocedure

- Towel, washcloth, warm water, disposable razor (if shaving over access site is desired and site is known)
- Indelible marking pen for marking pulse sites on distal extremities (if desired)

Postprocedure

- Sandbag(s) or other mobility-restricting devices such as soft restraints
- Standard monitoring equipment for vital signs, including pulse oximeter and pulse-Doppler, if needed

► CLIENT EDUCATION NEEDED:

1. Inform client that the procedure is invasive and the discomfort is similar to that of having a large IV started.
2. Inform client that there is a relatively low level of pain, usually on placement of the vascular catheter.
3. Inform client that the procedure is usually performed while the client is awake and able to follow simple directions, but the client may be sedated or treated with pain medications.

4. Inform client that he or she may feel warm or flushed at the time of dye administration and may briefly experience a metallic, salty taste.
5. Inform client to alert persons in the room if experiencing pain or difficulty at any time.
6. Inform client that he or she will be transported to and from the radiology department via a stretcher.
7. Inform client that a tight, compressive bandage may be placed over the artery access site and he or she may have to lie with accessed site in a straight position for several hours (if located in groin area or inside the elbow).
8. Inform client that vital signs, pulses, and the insertion site will be monitored frequently for several hours.
9. Emphasize the importance of resting with minimal flexion of involved artery access site for the prescribed number of hours following the procedure. Inform client that you will assist with back rubs, turning side to side within prescribed limits, and positioning for meals, drinking, and elimination concerns.
10. Emphasize intake of liquids in the immediate postprocedure period (4 to 8 hours). Explain the diuretic action of the contrast materials used and the need to drink (or for IV fluids) to ensure hydration and to prevent hypotension.
11. Advise the client that assistance will be required the first few times he or she gets out of bed.
12. Ask the client to report any unusual sensations such as pain, numbness, or temperature variations.
13. If Doppler is used to monitor pulses, either before or after the procedure, reassure the client that the equipment makes use of sound waves that are painless.

Estimated time to complete the skill:
Preprocedure: 10–15 minutes
Postprocedure: 4–8 hours

► DELEGATION TIPS

Assessment for bleeding, pain, shortness of breath, and proper postprocedure position is the responsibility of the nurse. Measurement of vital signs may be delegated to ancillary personnel.

IMPLEMENTATION—Action/Rationale

Action	Rationale
1. Confirm identity of client.	1. Ensures client safety.
2. Explain procedure and rationale for procedure.	2. Allays anxiety and promotes cooperation.
3. Confirm the presence of a signed consent.	3. Ensures physician or qualified practitioner has informed client of expected benefits and risks of procedure and that client has consented.
4. Confirm presence of any allergies, particularly to iodine or contrast agents, and label chart prominently.	4. Allergic reactions to contrast "dyes" are not uncommon. Premedication with diphenhydramine or methylprednisolone or use of other contrast agents may be required.
5. Wash hands.	5. Reduces the transmission of microorganisms.
6. Clip and shave arterial access site, if site is known and part of protocol.	6. May be required for access and saves expensive radiology suite time.
7. Obtain baseline vital signs.	7. Baseline determinations are necessary for postprocedure comparisons.
8. Obtain baseline pulses, characteristics, and mark sites with X.	8. Baseline determinations of peripheral pulses are necessary for postprocedure comparisons; marks assist in locating pulses if client is hypotensive or complication occurs. Frequent "downstream" determination of pulses is necessary to immediately detect and treat sudden occlusions by spasm or clot or other pathologic problem.
9. Arrange for transport to the radiology department.	9. Transport should be arranged according to institution policy.
10. The procedure will be performed by a physician as follows: • A small incision is made in the groin or the arm. • Using a fluoroscope to visualize the path, a radiopaque guidewire is inserted into the blood vessel through the skin and threaded through the access site to the area to be examined. • A catheter is threaded over the guidewire and the guidewire is removed. • Contrast dye is injected.	10. • Provides access to the artery. • Allows proper placement of the guidewire. • Guides the catheter to the area to be evaluated. • Makes the arteries and any stenosis visible on the fluoroscope. • After evaluating the results, the radiologist and the client's physician will decide on a course of treatment. That treatment may be done at this time and may include angioplasty or placement of a stent. Other interventions may include open heart surgery at a later time, management using medications, or continued observation. • Following the evaluation and treatment, the catheter is removed and pressure is applied to the insertion site. • Making the decision before the catheter is removed allows some interventions to be performed promptly. • Application of pressure prevents arterial bleeding.

continues

Action	Rationale
11. Gather postprocedure equipment and position near client's room or bed.	11. Postprocedure care may require use of pulse oximeter, sandbags, 4 × 4 gauze, and limb-restraint devices to maintain the limb in an unflexed position so that the client's artery can be assessed. Accessed limb should remain unflexed to prevent flow-obstructing clot formation, permit hemostasis, and lessen risk of complications such as pseudoaneurysm formation.
12. Wash hands and apply gloves, as needed.	12. Reduces the transmission of microorganisms.
13. Obtain vital signs, level of consciousness, and a pain assessment. Assess the vascular access site and downstream circulation adequacy by performing downstream pulse checks and assessing for warmth, sensation, blanching with pressure, and capillary refill.	13. Ensures client safety and comfort. Monitoring arterial site is vital, assuring continued hemostasis. Downstream pulse checks give clues to continued adequacy of circulation beyond the manipulated segment of artery.

▶ REAL WORLD ANECDOTES

Frances Baird, a 73-year-old female client, returned to the nursing unit after an aortogram and bilateral femoral arteriogram. Her blood pressure is noted to be 94/58 on admission to the unit, all pulses are palpable, 2+, and her limbs are slightly cool but blanch with pressure and refill in less than 2 seconds. She admits "some" discomfort at the right femoral arterial access site; the dressing is dry and intact; and the femoral pulse is 2+. She has an IV saline lock in place and patent in her left forearm. She reports nausea and refuses any oral fluids. At 1 hour after return to the unit, all findings are unchanged, except her blood pressure is now 88/54. The nurse suspects that this hypotension may be caused by relative hypovolemia, as she gives history of little intake in 24 hours and has received a contrast agent during the arteriographic procedure. She takes only sips of water and reports nausea remains. The nurse phones the physician with a report of client's condition. After obtaining an order, the nurse administers 1 liter of normal saline and begins the infusion of normal saline at approximately 100 mL/hour, medicates the client for nausea, and monitors intake and output.

▶ EVALUATION

1. Client was able to identify general purpose and nature of procedure.
2. Client was able to verbalize anxiety and informed the staff if feeling unable to cope with anxiety or if anxiety symptoms increased.
3. Client was able to verbalize any pain and obtained a level of relief that was tolerable for rest/sleep following pain interventions.
4. The client did not experience bleeding or vascular dysfunction, such as decrease in peripheral pulses.

▶ DOCUMENTATION

Nurses' Notes

- Document vital signs pre- and postprocedure.
- Note the presence of peripheral pulses, equality, and strength in the client before and after the procedure.
- Record the color and temperature of the client's extremities, before and after the procedure.
- Note any site preparation.
- Record the condition of the dressing at the insertion site and any weights or pressure applied.

Document on appropriate flow sheet and electronic medical record (EMR).

Medication Administration Record

- Record medications given before and after the procedure for pain or anxiety.

▶ CRITICAL THINKING SKILL

Introduction

The hardest part of the procedure is often holding still afterward.

Possible Scenario

Your 71-year-old male client has just returned to the floor after an arteriogram. You check the arterial access site in his groin. The dressing is secure and a sandbag is in place over the dressing. He is awake but sleepy and not in the best of moods. He complains that the last time he had to lie still on his back for 8 hours his back hurt for a week from the "lousy hospital bed." His wife and two coworkers are with him in the room, joking with him and tossing a stuffed animal back and forth. When you come back for a check in 15 minutes, the coworkers are gone. The wife is reading a magazine by the window. The client is lying on his left side, in a fetal position, snoring. The sandbag is on the floor.

Possible Outcome

You wake him and check his dressing, which is soaked with blood. You apply direct pressure and, when the bleeding has stopped, reapply the pressure dressing and the sandbag. You notify the nurse practitioner and instruct the client and his partner on the importance of remaining supine with the leg straight. The next week, the client comes by after his outpatient visit to show you the bruise, which extends from his groin to below his knee.

Prevention

In this case, education and understanding for both the client and the partner might have improved his compliance. Recognizing and intervening to increase comfort, including distraction, positioning, wrinkle-free linen, or other padding or skin protection, may have helped him tolerate the period of inactivity. Regular reminders and supportive statements when he was complying may have helped him stay motivated to maintain this uncomfortable position.

▶ VARIATIONS

Geriatric Variation:
- *Geriatric skin is thin and more fragile. Geriatric clients may have significant bruising at the insertion site.*

Pediatric Variation:
- *It is difficult for parents to have an invasive procedure performed on their child. Provide information and support for the parent. Base your teaching on the parents' most pressing concerns. These may include how long the procedure will last, how the child will be sedated, any pain the child may experience, and when the parent will be able to be with the child. Make sure the parents have the opportunity to ask questions directly with appropriate staff members prior to the procedure.*

Home Care Variations:
- *This procedure is not done in the home care setting.*
- *Arteriography and related procedures can cause anxiety and fear. The home care setting can provide a good opportunity for teaching and support for both the client and family members prior to the procedure.*
- *The caregiver should be aware of complications that may occur postprocedure. These include bleeding, reduced circulation distal to the insertion site, embolism, and bruising at the catheter insertion site.*

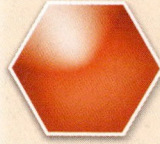

Long-Term Care Variations:
- *This procedure is not done in the long-term care setting.*
- *Staff providing long-term care should be aware of complications that may occur postprocedure. These include bleeding, reduced circulation distal to the insertion site, embolism, and bruising at the catheter insertion site.*

▶ COMMON ERRORS

Possible Error:

Pressure dressings may be so tight as to impede arterial flow and cause diminished pulses downstream, or pressure dressings may be too loose, permitting "oozing" of blood from the artery into tissues and subsequent hematoma formation. Frank surface oozing of blood into dressing may be seen or frank pulsatile bleeding may be apparent.

Prevention:

Be careful when applying pressure dressings. If the dressing is found to be too tight, release some pressure caused by dressing or device while maintaining access site hemostasis and palpate or use Doppler for pulses again. Two persons may be necessary. Notify physician or qualified practitioner for confirmed absent or diminished pulse and document steps taken and person notified. If the dressing is too loose, treat oozing or bleeding by reapplication of direct pressure (manual) and reapplication of pressure dressing once ooze or bleeding has been controlled. Notify physician or qualified practitioner and document steps taken and person notified.

▶ NURSING TIPS

- Marking the site of downstream pulses prior to the procedure or on first postprocedure assessment facilitates subsequent assessments with minimal disturbance of the client. Rate the pulse (downstream) for quality according to the institution's protocol in order to ensure use of same scale in comparisons of pulse quality (0 to 4 is a common scale).

- Offer/encourage oral fluid intake with each site check/vital sign check. Offer fluid of client's preference.
- Encourage family members to stay with client while relatively immobilized. Use hip flexion limits and knee-Gatch flexion limits on electric beds if designed controls are available on control panel.

▶ SPECIAL CONSIDERATIONS

- *Angiography has been considered the "gold standard"; however, it is not without risk and is an expensive procedure. Health care providers may order a combination of carotid ultrasound and MRI to assess clients with carotid artery disease instead of angiography.*
- *It is important to encourage the client to drink large amounts of water following the procedure to decrease the risk of complications, especially renal.*
- *Dysrhythmias may occur and need treatment. As many clients undergoing arteriography have underlying cardiac conditions, be alert to medications that may not have been taken while the client was NPO prior to the procedure. Some ectopic beats may occur. Be alert for life-threatening arrhythmias and know proper protocol to follow.*
- *Be sure the client voided prior to the arteriography. A vasovagal reaction, consisting of nausea, hypotension, and bradycardia, may be precipitated by distended bladder. If this should occur, intervention may be necessary with positioning the client supine and administration of cardiac medications.*

Positron-Emission Tomography Scanning

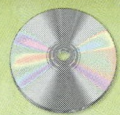

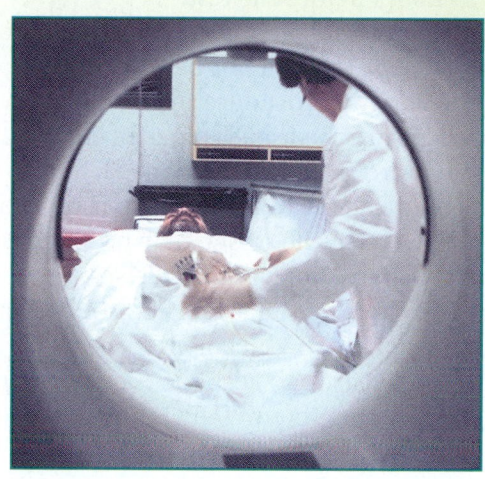

▶ OVERVIEW OF THE SKILL

Positron-emission tomography (PET) offers a way to study the metabolism occurring in an organ, instead of just the anatomy of the organ. The PET scans are most commonly used to study the brain and the heart when an invasive procedure is not possible. PET scans are used to measure many physiologic components that affect metabolism (e.g., blood flow, glucose uptake, and oxygen extraction and perfusion); and, therefore, can be used to monitor clients with epilepsy, Alzheimer's or Parkinson's disease, head injuries, brain tumors, schizophrenia, and manic-depressive disorders, and they are especially useful in monitoring clients during and following strokes. In a PET scan, isotopes are injected into a client. These isotopes are absorbed into the tissue and then emit radioactivity in the form of positrons (electrons with a positive charge) that are converted into a calculation of energy emitted and a color image by a computer. A short-lived radionuclide such as oxyglucose is either inhaled by the client or injected intravenously. When the brain is being imaged, the client may be asked to perform basic mental exercises. These help stimulate the brain.

Clients need to be able to lay still for 60–90 minutes for the test and might need to avoid taking certain medications and other substances such as alcohol, caffeine, sedatives, tranquilizers, or tobacco in the 24 hours prior to the test. Diabetic clients should ask their physicians or qualified practitioners about special dietary instructions for the PET scan preparation.

▶ ASSESSMENT

1. Assess the client's knowledge of the purpose and plan of the procedure **so he or she will cooperate and not be anxious.**
2. Review the client's signature on the informed consent form. **It is a legal requirement of the institution.**
3. Assess the client's use of alcohol, caffeine, sedatives, tranquilizers, or tobacco within 24 hours of the test. **These substances can alter test results.**
4. Assess the client's veins **for adequate venous access for injection of the radioisotope.**
5. Assess for the possibility of pregnancy if the client is female, **as women who are pregnant should not have a PET scan.**
6. Assess recent glucose intake, **as PET scans use glucose uptake as a marker and the client's blood sugar must be as low as safely possible.**

▶ **DIAGNOSIS**

Anxiety

Fear

Deficient Knowledge

▶ **PLANNING**

Expected Outcomes:

1. The client will tolerate the procedure without anxiety.
2. The client will maintain the required positions during the procedure.
3. Successful images will be obtained for diagnosis.
4. The client will not experience any adverse effects secondary to being NPO.

Equipment Needed (see Figure 11-14-1):

- Band-Aid® or gauze dressing for intravenous (IV) site
- IV setup and materials, or inhaler

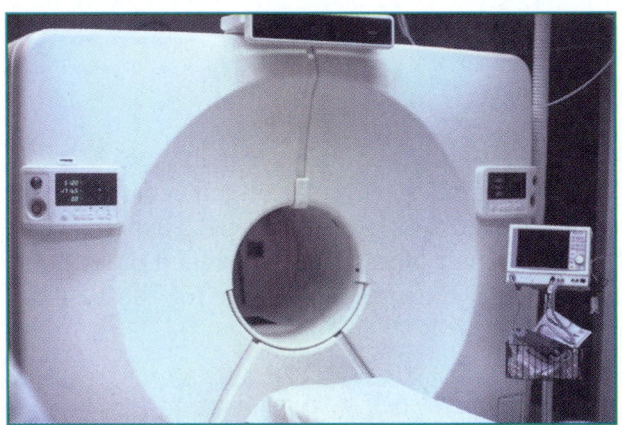

Figure 11-14-1 Positron-emission tomography scanner

▶ **CLIENT EDUCATION NEEDED:**

1. The client should be taught the rationale for the procedure and how it will be performed. Provide written or illustrated instructions about the procedure.
2. The client should be instructed not to use alcohol, caffeine, sedatives, tranquilizers, or tobacco for 24 hours before the test.
3. The client should void just prior to the procedure as he or she will not be able to move during the lengthy procedure.
4. The client may be asked to perform several mental exercises during a brain PET scan.
5. Prepare the client with sample questions or mental exercises he or she may be asked to perform if undergoing a brain PET scan.
6. Reassure the client that the test is not painful except where the IV needle is inserted.
7. Explain the reason to keep the client from ingesting anything per mouth (NPO) before the test, including IV fluids that contain glucose.
8. The client will be able to return home after the procedure if not hospitalized.

Estimated time to complete the skill: **60–90 minutes**

▶ **DELEGATION TIPS**

Assessment for bleeding, pain, shortness of breath, and proper postprocedure position is the responsibility of the nurse. Measurement of vital signs may be delegated to ancillary personnel.

IMPLEMENTATION—Action/Rationale

Action	Rationale
1. Wash hands.	1. Reduces the transmission of microorganisms.
2. Cover the scanner bed with a clean sheet (see Figure 11-14-2), and prepare a pillow.	2. Provides comfort and hygiene.

continues

Action	Rationale

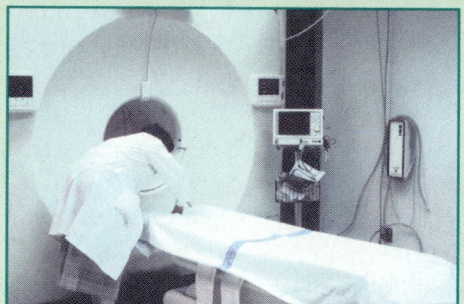

Figure 11-14-2 Cover the scanner bed with a clean sheet.

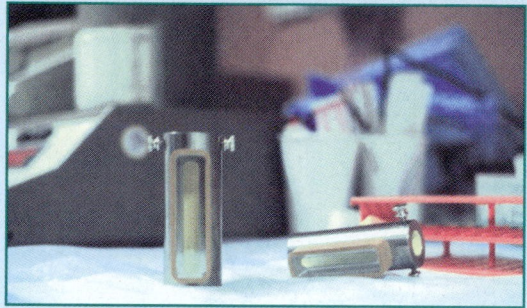

Figure 11-14-3 Radioisotope containers

3. Provide teaching regarding the PET scan and the scanner.

4. Ask client if he or she has used alcohol, caffeine, sedatives, tranquilizers, or tobacco in the last 24 hours. Ask the client when he or she last ate or drank.

5. Instruct client to void.

6. Start an IV or perform venipuncture. Do not use IV fluids that contain glucose. A small amount of radioactive material is administered through the IV or venipuncture 30 to 45 minutes prior to the procedure (see Figure 11-14-3). A blood sample or blood samples are collected from the other arm.

7. Assist client into the scanning bed (see Figure 11-14-4).

8. Secure the client and apply a thermal plastic mask to reduce head movement, or use other stabilizing devices as needed or ordered (see Figure 11-14-5).

3. Reduces anxiety and fear of the unknown.

4. These substances can alter test results.

5. Ensures client comfort and avoids movement or interruption during procedure.

6. Using glucose in the IV will alter the test results. Radioactive material enables PET images to be created. Blood samples are used to obtain information on the amount of radioactive material in the blood.

7. Provides comfort for the client and correct positioning for study.

8. Helps the client hold the proper position for long periods of the scan.

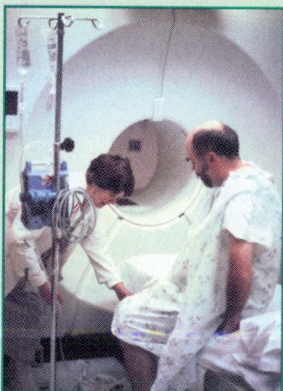

Figure 11-14-4 Assist the client onto the scanning bed.

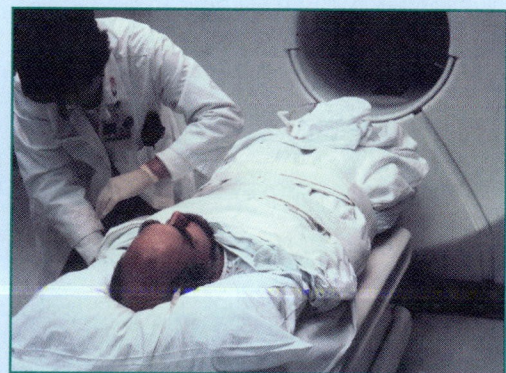

Figure 11-14-5 Secure the client.

continues

Action	Rationale

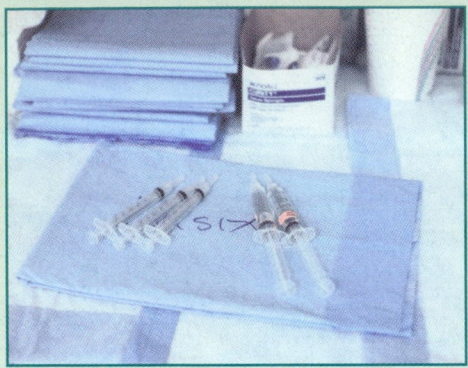

Figure 11-14-6 Have additional medications or injections prepared and ready.

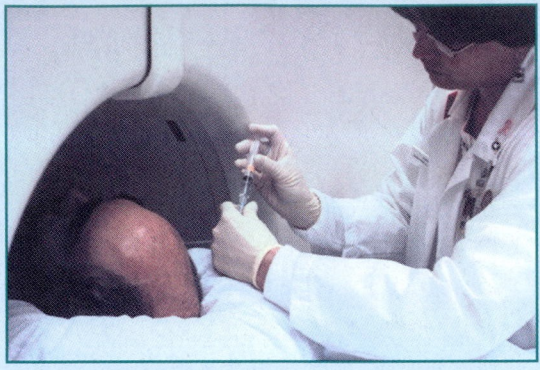

Figure 11-14-7 Administer additional radioactive material as required.

9. Administer radioactive material by inhaler or IV injection as ordered (see Figures 11-14-6 and 11-14-7).

9. Orders differ for different procedures. Injections or inhalations of additional radioactive material allow the test to proceed as ordered.

10. The PET scan generally takes 1 to 2 hours (see Figure 11-14-8), during which time the client must lie quietly in the PET scanner.

10. Ensures that the test is being accurately performed.

11. If the brain is being scanned, ask the client to perform various mental exercises such as reasoning and remembering. The client's eyes may be covered and the client's ears plugged after the injection to minimize sensory stimulation.

11. Measures brain activity changes as various areas of the brain are used.

12. After the test is completed, remove the IVs, unless otherwise ordered by the physician or qualified practitioner, and apply gauze dressing or Band-Aid®.

12. Applies pressure to prevent bleeding.

13. Assist the client to a sitting and then standing position.

13. Decreases risk of orthostatic hypotension.

14. Encourage client to drink fluids.

14. Promotes excretion of radioactive material from body.

15. Dispose of all IV equipment or syringes in appropriate radioactive waste containers (see Figure 11-14-9).

15. Equipment is contaminated with radioactive isotopes.

16. Wash hands.

16. Reduces the transmission of microorganisms.

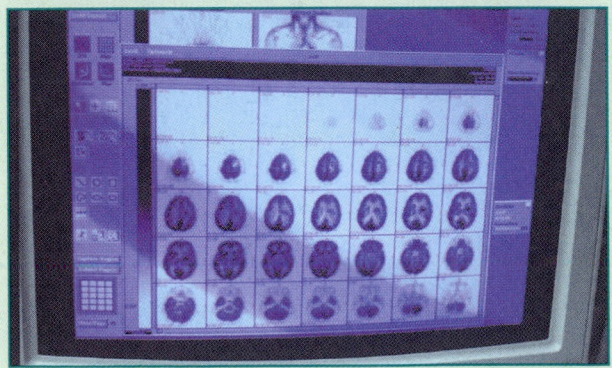

Figure 11-14-8 PET scan output images

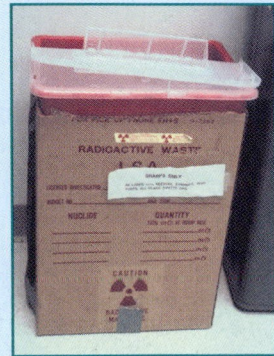

Figure 11-14-9 Dispose of IV equipment and syringes in radioactive waste containers.

► **EVALUATION**

- The client's status and comfort is confirmed after the procedure.
- Assess the IV sites for bleeding or hematoma.

► **DOCUMENTATION**

Nurses' Notes

- Record the date, time, length, and place the procedure was done.
- Note the client's tolerance of the procedure.
- Note the client's status after the procedure.

Document on appropriate flow sheet or electronic medical record (EMR).

Medication Record

- Record the date, time, and route the radioactive material was administered.

► **CRITICAL THINKING SKILL**

Introduction

Alcohol, caffeine, sedatives, tranquilizers, or tobacco ingested within 24 hours prior to the test can alter the test results because of changes in metabolism.

Possible Scenario

An older client did not understand the written instructions he was given a week before the PET scan and he took his sleeping pill as usual the night before his appointment. He did not realize that a sleeping pill was the same as a sedative or tranquilizer.

Possible Outcome

When the client was assessed by the nurse before the test, he listed all the pills he had taken in the last 24 hours, including the sleeping pill. The test was postponed until the following day and the nurse instructed him to omit that evening's dose of the sedative.

Prevention

The written instructions could have specific names of medications rather than classifications. The nurse giving the instructions could review all medications at the time of scheduling the test.

► **VARIATIONS**

Geriatric Variations:

- *Elderly clients may have impaired hearing or vision, which might make it difficult to understand the purpose of the test and to cooperate with the test.*
- *Elderly clients may have poor venous access and fragile veins. Care must be taken when giving IV medications.*
- *Elderly clients who are restless, confused, or in pain might find it difficult to lie still, or may find the enclosed space too confining. If you suspect the client might have trouble cooperating for the length of the procedure, discuss this concern with the physician or qualified practitioner before beginning the test.*

continues

▶ **VARIATIONS** *(continued)*

Pediatric Variations:
- *Children may need distraction so they will be able to lie down for 60 to 90 minutes. Age-appropriate recorded stories or music may help.*
- *Children may need sedation so they can relax during the procedure. Double check that this is a medication that will not alter the test results.*
- *Children will need careful placement of an IV so it can be used for the PET scan.*
- *Children may be frightened of the equipment or confined space. Take time to show the child the equipment and to explain the procedure. Answer any questions.*

Home Care Variations:
- *Not applicable.*

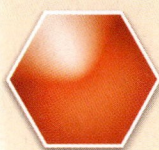

Long-Term Care Variations:
- *Not applicable.*

▶ **COMMON ERRORS**

Possible Error:

While attempting to inject the isotope, the nurse was unable to aspirate blood. The test had to be delayed while a new IV was started.

Prevention:

Assess the venous access before starting the test. Choose the optimal location to start the IV. If this error does occur, start a new IV and be sure it remains patent. A slow infusion of normal saline may be required to keep the vein open.

▶ **NURSING TIPS**

- Be sure venous access will allow for infusion of the isotope and drawing of blood samples.
- Use pillows, rolled blankets, or towels to increase client comfort during the test.
- Do not use IV fluids that contain glucose as this will interfere with the test results.

> ▶ **SPECIAL CONSIDERATIONS**

- *Sedation is sometimes required to obtain immobility in addition to counteracting feelings of claustrophobia. The chamber of the scanner is a narrow, confining tube with a hard surface on which to lie. Clients with Parkinson's disease may have difficulty controlling involuntary movements and lying still and, hence, require premedication. Clients with Alzheimer's disease may not understand the procedure and have increased agitation and require sedation.*

- *Clients may be asked questions or given small calculation problems to stimulate the brain and brain metabolism, and, hence, increase cerebral perfusion. Inform clients of this exercise and examples of questions that may be asked (e.g., "subtract 7 from 92"). Alert the client that these are not to test intelligence but rather to study brain perfusion and metabolism.*

- *If the client is diabetic, blood-glucose levels should be below 150 g/dl as the scanner is used to measure glucose metabolism, and hyperglycemia will impede accurate measurements.*

- *PET scan is an expensive test and may not be covered by conventional insurance.*

- *Pregnancy and breast feeding are contraindications with PET scanning. Premenopausal women should practice birth control prior to the procedure. Breast-feeding women should stop nursing for several days after the scan and consult the nuclear medicine department for exact guidelines.*

References

CHAPTER 1 – PHYSICAL ASSESSMENT

Anderson, G., Myunghee, J., & Kyungsook, C. (2007). Breast cancer screening for Korean women must consider traditional risks as well as two genetic risk factors: Genetic polymorphisms and inheritable gene mutations. *Cancer Nursing, 30*(3), 213–222.

Anderson, P. (2007). Health check: Breast cancer strikes in men. *Men in Nursing, 2*(6), 8–10.

Anthony, A. (2006). Red flags: When the blood glucose level takes a dive. *Nursing Made Incredibly Easy! 4*(6), 15–17.

Barron, M. A., & Fishel, R. S. (2007). Talk to your patients about breast disease. *The Nurse Practitioner: The American Journal of Primary Health Care, 32*(10), 22–32.

Beaumont, C. (2006). Acoustic or electronic: Which stethoscope works best for you? *Men in Nursing, 1*(1), 6–7.

Beaumont, C. E. (2007) Choosing the best stethoscope. *Nursing, 37*(Suppl. 10: Med/Surg Insider), 12–13.

Bushing, J. (2007). Clinical do's and don'ts: Obtaining a throat culture. *Nursing2007, 37*, 20.

Carter-Templeton, H. (2006). Red flags: Temperatures rising. *Nursing Made Incredibly Easy! 4*(4), 10–11.

Cleveland Clinic, Stein DW (reviewer, n.d.). *Hypertension: In-home blood pressure monitoring.* Retrieved December 28, 2007, from *WebMD* Web site: www.webmd.com/hypertension-high-blood-pressure/guide/hypertension-home-monitoring

Clinical rounds: Sputum test detects cancer earlier. (2006) *Nursing2006 36*, 34–34.

Dale, L. (2007). Make a point about alternate site blood glucose sampling. *Nursing2007, 36*, 52–53.

DeLaune, S. C., Ladner, P. K. (2006) *Fundamentals of nursing: Standards & practice.* (3rd ed.). Clifton Park, NY: Thomson Delmar Learning.

Editors of *Nursing* (2007). Taking care with tympanic temperature readings. *Nursing2007, 37*, 52–53.

Foran, C. K. (2007). Heartbeats: Recognize supraventricular tachycardia. *Nursing Critical Care, 2*(6), 14–17.

Fry M. (2006). Assessment of reproductive function. In Daniels, R., Nosek, L., Nicoll, L., *Contemporary medical-surgical nursing* (pp. 2077–2080). Clifton Park, NY: Thomson Delmar Learning.

Goertz, S. (2006). Eye on diagnostics: Gauging fluid balance with osmolality. *Nursing2006, 36*(10), 70–71.

Greenwald, B. (2005). From guaiac to immune fecal occult blood tests: The emergence of technology in colorectal cancer screening. *Gastroenterology Nursing, 28*(2), 90–96.

Hemoccult slide test home instructions: Health facts for you. Department of Nursing. Retrieved January 12, 2008, from the University of Wisconsin Hospitals and Clinics Authority Web site: www.uwhealth.org/servlet/Satellite?cid=112665035

Infant heel puncture. Retrieved January 15, 2008, from the Quest Diagnostics Web site: www.labreference.com/pdfs/Infant_Heel_Puncture.pdf

Kamienski, M. (2007). Emergency: When sore throat gets serious: Three different cases, three very different causes. *American Journal of Nursing, 107*(10), 35–38.

Livingston, M. W., & Overton, D. T. (2007) *Bradycardia.* Retrieved January 2, 2008, from the *Medicine* Web site: www.emedicine.com/emerg/topic534.htm

Maddox, T., & Parker, D. M. (2006). Peak technique: Don't let hypertension sneak by you. *Nursing Made Incredibly Easy! 4*, 9–11.

McCormick, M.. (2007). Every breath you take: Making sense of breath sounds. *Nursing Made Incredibly Easy! 5*, 7–11.

Midthun, S., Paur, R., Bruce, A. W., & Moore, K. N. (2006). A protocol for the urine dipstick/pad method. *Journal of Wound, Ostomy, and Continence Nursing, 33*, 396–400.

Obtaining a clean catch urine specimen (female). Retrieved January 14, 2008, from the Landstuhl

Regional Medical Center Web site: www.landstuhl.
healthcare.hqusareur.army.mil/departments/lab/
instr/clean_catch_f.aspx

Obtaining a clean catch urine specimen (male).
Retrieved January 14, 2008, from the Landstuhl
Regional Medical Center Web site: www.landstuhl.
healthcare.hqusareur.army.mil/departments/lab/
instr/clean_catch_f.aspx

Raymen, S. (2007). Health assessment. In Daniels,
R., Nosek, L., Nicoll, L., *Contemporary Medical-
Surgical Nursing* (pp. 174–196). Clifton Park, NY:
Thomson Delmar Learning.

Roe, B., & Moore, K. N. (2006). Commentary: Awareness of urine flow in people with long-term urinary catheters. *Journal of Wound, Ostomy, and
Continence Nursing, 33,* 174–174.

Shindler, D. M. (2007). Practical cardiac auscultation.
Critical Care Nursing Quarterly, 30, 166–180.

Skin puncture with fingerstick or heelstick lancet.
Retrieved January 15, 2008, from the University
of California at San Francisco Clinical Laboratories Web site: http://labmed.ucsf.edu/labmanual/
mftlng-mtzn/dnld/Fingerstick.pdf

Spector, N., Connolly, M. A., Carlson, K. K., &
Carison, K. K. (symposium editor, 2007). Dyspnea:
Applying nursing research to bedside practice.
AACN Advanced Critical Care, 18(1), 45–58.

Urine culture: Clean catch. Retrieved January 12,
2008, from the University of California, San
Francisco (UCSF) Web site: www.ucsfhealth.org/
adult/adam/data/003751.html

Wahis, T. (2007). Diagnostic errors and abnormal
diagnostic tests lost to follow-up: A source of
needless waste and delay to treatment. *Journal of
Ambulatory Care Management, 30*(4), 338–343.

CHAPTER 2 – SAFETY AND INFECTION CONTROL

Allen, M., Clement, M. A., Fowler, K. A., & Harne-
Britner S. (2007). Improving hand hygiene:
Adherence among healthcare providers. *Clinical
Nurse Specialist: The Journal for Advance Nursing
Practice, 21*(2), 101–102.

Aragon, D., Sole, M. L., Brown, S., & Kleinpell, R.
M. (2005). Outcomes of an infection prevention
project focusing on hand hygiene and isolation
practices. *AACN Advanced Critical Care, 16*(2),
121–132.

Fralick, S. L. (2007). Restraint utilization project.
Nursing Administration Quarterly, 31(3), 219–225.

Gustafson, S. E. (2007). Assess for fall risk, intervene—and bump up patient safety. *Nursing2007,
27*(12), 24–25.

Hendrich, A. (2007). Predicting patient falls: Using
the Hendrich II fall risk model in clinical practice.
Am Journal of Nursing, 102(11), 50–59.

Hughes, N. L. (2006). Handwashing: Going back to
basics in infection control. *American Journal of
Nursing, 106*(7), 96.

Jasniewski, J. (2006). Take steps to protect your
patient from falls. *Nursing2006, 30,* 24–25.

Markwell, S. K. (2005). Long-term restraint
reduction: One hospital's experience with restraint
alternatives. *Journal of Nursing Care Quality, 20*(3),
253–260.

Mincer, A. B. (2007). Assistive devices for the adult
patient with orthopaedic dysfunction: Why physical therapists choose what they do. *Orthopaedic
Nursing, 26*(4), 226–231.

Poe, S. S., Cvach, M., Dawson, P. B., Straus, H., &
Hill, E. E. (2007). The John Hopkins fall assessment
tool: Postimplementation evaluation. *Journal of
Nursing Care Quality, 22*(4), 293–298.

*Restraint use for psychiatric patients in the pediatric
emergency department.* (2006). *Pediatric Emergency Care, 22*(1), 7–12.

Rushing, J. (2006). Wearing personal protective gear.
Nursing2006, 36(10), 56–57.

Santulli, E. (2007). Liquid gel vs. hand sanitizers. *American Journal of Nursing, 107*(10), 72CC–72DD.

Siegel, J. D., Rhinehart, E. Jackson, M., & Chiarello,
L., for the Healthcare Infection Control Practice
Advisory Committee. (2007). *2007 Guideline for
isolation precautions: Preventing transmission of
infectious agents in healthcare settings.* Retrieved
December 2, 2007, from the Centers for Disease
Control Web site: www.cdc.gov/ncidod/dhqp/pdf/
isolation2007.pdf

Wilson, P., & Rodger, B. (2006). Research briefs: Research on falls prevention and physical activity
in older adults and a notice of a new web-based
quality system by the agency for Healthcare Research and Quality. *Home Healthcare Nurse, 24*(10),
632–633.

CHAPTER 3 – CLIENT CARE AND COMFORT

Anderson, P. G., & Cutshall, S. M. (2007). Massage therapy: A comfort intervention for cardiac
surgery patients. *Clinical Nurse Specialist, 21*(3),
161–165.

Barrere, C. C. (2007). Discourse analysis of nurse-patient communication in a hospital setting: Implications for staff development. *Journal for Nurses in Staff Development, 23*(3), 114–122.

Beider S, Mahrer N. E., & Gold J. I. (2007). Pediatric massage therapy: An overview for clinicians. *Pediatric Clinics of North America, 54*(6), 1025–1041.

Campos de Carvalho, E., Martins, F. T., & dos Santos, C. B. (2007). A pilot study of a relaxation technique for management of nausea and vomiting in patients receiving cancer chemotherapy. *Cancer Nursing, 30*(2), 163–167.

Daniels, R., Nosek, L., & Nicoll, L. (2007). Complementary and alternative therapies. In *Contemporary medical-surgical nursing* (pp. 375–399). Clifton Park, NY: Delmar, Cengage Learning.

Delaune, S. C., & Ladner, P. K. (2006). Complementary and alternative modalities. In *Fundamentals of nursing: standards and practice* (3rd ed., pp. 864–890). Clifton Park, NY: Delmar, Cengage Learning.

Delaune, S. C., & Ladner, P. K. (2006). Skin integrity and wound healing. In *Fundamentals of nursing: standards and practice* (3rd ed., pp. 1224–1230). Clifton Park, NY: Delmar, Cengage Learning.

Ernst, E., Pittler, M. H., Wider, B., & Boddy, K., (2007). Mind-body therapies: Are the trial data getting stronger? *Alternative Therapies in Health and Medicine, 13*(5), 62–64.

Holmgren, C., Carlsson, T., Mannheimer, C., & Edvardsson, N. (2008). Risk of interference from transcutaneous electrical nerve stimulation on the sensing function of implantable defibrillators. *Pacing and Clinical Electrophysiology: PACE, 31*(2), 151–158.

Maramkhah, F. (2006). Device safety: Don't let radiant warmers overheat infants. *Nursing2006, 36*(3), 28.

McCaffrey, R., & Taylor, N. (2005). Effective anxiety treatment prior to diagnostic cardiac catheterization. *Holistic Nursing Practice, 19*(2), 70–73.

Morone, N. E., & Greco, C. M. (2007). Mind-body interventions for chronic pain in older adults: A structured review. *Pain Medicine, 8*(4), 359–375.

Pullen, R. L. (2005). Clinical do's & don'ts: Tips for using dry heat therapy. *Nursing2005, 35*(12), 18.

Sheldon, L. K., Barrett, R., & Ellington, L. (2006). Difficult communication in nursing. *Journal of Nursing Scholarship, 38*(2), 141–147.

Sully, P., Dallas, J., & Nicol, M. (2005). *Essential communication skills for nursing practice.* Edinburgh, UK: Mosby.

Tejirian, T., & Abbas, M. A. (2005). Sitz bath: Where is the evidence? Scientific basis of a common practice. *Diseases of the Colon and Rectum, 48*(12), 2336–2340.

Wagner, D., Byrne, M., & Kolcaba, K. (2006). Effects of comfort warming on preoperative patients. *AORN Journal, 84*(3), 427–448.

Wehmer, M. A. (2007). Warm up to your patients: Hypothermia management. *OR Nurse 2007, 1* (1), 21–30.

CHAPTER 4 – BASIC CARE

Ayello, E. A., & Lyder, C. H. (2007). Protecting patients from harm: Preventing pressure ulcers in hospital patients. *Nursing2007*, 37(10), 36–40.

Baptiste, A. (2007). Technology solutions for high-risk tasks in critical care. *Critical Care Nursing Clinics of North America, 19*(2), 177–186.

Boyd-Monk, H. (2005). The eyes have it: Understanding problems of the aging eye. *Nursing Made Incredibly Easy, 3*(5), 34–45.

Chichester, M. (2007). Requesting perinatal autopsy: Multicultural considerations. *MCN, The American Journal of Maternal/Child Nursing, 32*(2), 81–86.

Critical care extra: Preoperative hair removal and surgical site infection: Long-accepted practices aren't always best. (2006). *AJN, American Journal of Nursing, 106*(5), 64II–64NN.

Critical care extra: Eye care for patients in the ICU. (2006). *AJN, American Journal of Nursing, 106*(1), 72AA–72DD.

Daniels, R., Nosek, L. & Nicoll, L. (2007). Preoperative nursing management. In *Contemporary medical-surgical nursing* (pp. 608–651). Clifton Park, NY: Thomson Delmar Learning.

Daniels, R., Nosek, L. & Nicoll, L. (2007). Postoperative nursing management. In *Contemporary Medical-Surgical Nursing* (pp. 691–732). Clifton Park, NY: Thomson Delmar Learning.

Delaune, S. K., & Ladner, P. K. (2006). Safety, infection control and hygiene. In *Fundamentals of nursing: standards and practice* (3rd ed., pp. 668–771). Clifton Park, NY: Delmar, Cengage Learning.

Delaune, S. K., & Ladner, P. K. (2006). Infection control and hygiene. In *Fundamentals of nursing: standards and practice* (3rd ed., pp. 746–755). Clifton Park, NY: Delmar, Cengage Learning.

Delaune, S. K., & Ladner, P. K. (2006). Nutrition. In *Fundamentals of nursing: standards and practice* (3rd ed., pp. 1034–1084). Clifton Park, NY: Delmar, Cengage Learning.

Delaune, S. K., & Ladner, P. K. (2006). Mobility. In *Fundamentals of nursing: standards and practice* (3rd ed., pp. 1158–1163). Clifton Park, NY: Delmar, Cengage Learning.

Delaune, S. K., & Ladner, P. K. (2006). Mobility. In *Fundamentals of nursing: standards and practice* (3rd ed., pp. 1164–1207). Clifton Park, NY: Thompson

Delaune, S. K., & Ladner, P. K. (2006). Elimination. In *Fundamentals of nursing: standards and practice* (3rd ed., pp. 1279–1347). Clifton Park, NY: Delmar, Cengage Learning.

Delaune, S. K., & Ladner, P. K. (2006). Nursing care of the preoperative client. In *Fundamentals of nursing: standards and practice* (3rd ed., pp. 1348–1391). Clifton Park, NY: Delmar, Cengage Learning.

Dreger, V. A., & Tremback, T. F. (2006). Management of preoperative anxiety in children. *AORN Journal, 84*(5), 778–804.

Fehder, W. P., (2008). Nursing care and management of pathological oral conditions among women and children. *MCN, The American Journal of Maternal/Child Nursing, 33*(1), 38–44.

Flori, L. (2007). Healthier aging: Don't throw in the towel. Tips for bathing a patient who has dementia. *Nursing2007, 37*(7), 22–23.

Gardner, J. (2006). Health matters: What you need to know about genital herpes. *Nursing2006, 36*(10), 26–27.

Garg, A., Miholland, S., Deckow-Schaefer, G., & Kapellusch, J. M. (2007). Justification for a minimal lift program in critical care. *Critical Care Nursing Clinics of North America, 16*(2), 187–196.

Gray, M., Bliss, D. Z., Doughty, D. B., Ermer-Seltun, J., Kennedy-Evans, K. L., Palmer, M. H., et al. (2007). Incontinence-associated dermatitis: A consensus. *Journal of Wound, Ostomy and Continence Nursing, 34*(1), 45–54.

Griffiths, H., & Gallimore, D. (2005). Positioning critically ill patients in hospital. *Nursing Standard, 19*(42), 56–64.

Grimalt, R. (2007). A practical guide to scalp disorders. *Journal of Investigative Dermatology Symposium Proceedings, 12*(2), 4–10.

Hess, J. A., Kincl, L. D., & Mandeville, D. S. (2007). Comparison of three single-person manual patient techniques for bed-to-wheelchair transfers. *Home Healthcare Nurse, 25*(9), 577–579.

Kiely, C. I., Crestodina, L., & Ramundo, J. M., (2006). Diabetic foot care education: It's not just about the foot. *Journal of Wound, Ostomy and Continence Nursing, 33*(4), 416–421.

Mallory, J. L., & Allen, C. L. (2006). Care of the dying: A positive nursing experience. *Medsurg Nursing, 15*(4), 217–222.

Myers, N. E., Compliment, J. M., Post, J. C., & Buchinsky, F. D. (2006). Clinical case report: Tonsilloliths a common finding in pediatric patients. *The Nurse Practitioner: The American Journal of Primary Health Care, 31*(7), 53–54.

Odom-Forren, J. (2006). Preventing surgical site infections. *Nursing2006, 36*(6), 59–63.

Palmer, J. L., & Metheny, N. A. (2008). How to try this: Preventing aspiration in older adults with dysphagia. *AJN, American Journal of Nursing, 108*(2), 40–48.

Pellino, T. A., Owen, B., Knapp, L., & Noack, J. (2006). The evaluation of mechanical devices for lateral transfers on perceived exertion and patient comfort. *Orthopaedic Nursing, 25*(1), 4–10.

Photo Guide: Performing passive range-of-motion exercises. (2006). *Nursing2006, 36*(3), 50–51.

Plauntz, L. M. (2007). Preoperative assessment of the surgical patient. *Nursing Clinics of North America, 42*(3), 361–377.

Powers, J., Brower, A., & Tolliver, S. (2007). Impact of oral hygiene on prevention of ventilator-associated pneumonia in neuroscience patients. *Journal of Nursing Care Quality, 22*(4), 316–321.

Rader, J., Barrick, A. L., Hoeffer, B., Sloane, P. D., McKenzie, D., Talerico, K. A., et al. The bathing of older adults with dementia. *AJN, American Journal of Nursing, 106*(4), 40–48.

Ratliff, C. & Dixon, M. (2007). Treatment of incontinence-associated dermatitis (diaper rash) in a neonatal unit. *Journal of Wound, Ostomy and Continence Nursing, 34*(2), 158–161; discussion 161–162.

Richards, J., & Hubbert, A. O. (2007). Experiences of expert nurses in caring for patients with postoperative pain. *Pain Management Nursing, 8*(1), 17–24.

Robinson, S. B., Weitzel, T., & Henderson, L. (2005). The sh-h-h-h project: Nonpharmacological interventions. *Holistic Nursing Practice, 19*(6), 263–266.

Rushton, C. H., Reina, M. L., & Reina, D. S. (2007). Building trustworthy relationships with critically ill patients and families. *AACN Advanced Critical Care, 18*(1), 19–30.

Sevim, C., & Doughty, D. (2007). Surgical wound infections in the intensive care unit: The nurse's role. *Journal of Wound, Ostomy and Continence Nursing, 34*(5), 499–504.

Strauss, M. B., (2007). Objective evaluation, management, and prevention tools to meet the challenge – Addressing foot and toenail concerns in diabetes. *Journal of Musculoskeletal Medicine, 24*(7), 312–319.

Wardell, H. (2007). Reduction of injuries associated with patient handling. *AAOHN Journal, 55*(10), 407–412.

Xia, C., & McCutcheon, H. (2006). Mealtimes in hospital—who does what? *Journal of Clinical Nursing, 15*(10), 1221–1227.

CHAPTER 5 – MEDICATION ADMINSTRATION

Al-Showair, R. A., Pearson, S. B., & Chrystyn H. (2007). The potential of a 2Tone Trainer to help patients use their metered-dose inhalers. *Chest, 131*(6), 1776–1782.

Anderson, M. R., McKee, D., Yukes, J., Alvarez, A., & Karasz A. (2008). An investigation of douching practices in the botánicas of the Bronx. *Culture, Health, & Spirituality, 10*(1), 1–11.

Berry, P. H., & Dahl, J. L. (2007). Advanced practice nurse controlled substances prescriptive authority: A review of the regulations and implications for effective pain management at end-of-life. *Journal of Hospice and Palliative Nursing, 9*(5), 238–245.

Bower, L. M. (2005). Photo guide: Is your patient's inhaler technique up to snuff? *Nursing2005, 35*(8), 50–51.

Bradshaw, A., & Price, L. (2007). Rectal suppository insertion: the reliability of the evidence as a basis for nursing practice. *Journal of Clinical Nursing, 16*(1), 98–103.

Brown, M. (2005). Optimize IV safety with a comprehensive approach. *Nursing Management, 36*(10-Supplement IV Solutions), 19–22.

Caesar, B. R. (2006). Reducing medication errors by using technology. *Nursing2006, 36*(8), 24–25.

Clinical rounds: Do you use the Z-tract method? (2005). *Nursing2005, 35*(23), 34–34.

Clinical rounds: IM Injections: Pick your site. (2006). *Nursing2006, 36*(6), 34–34.

Cohen, M. R. (2006). Medication errors: Splitting pills. *Nursing2006, 36*(8), 13.

Cohen, M. R. (2007). Medication errors: Eardrop medications. *Nursing2007 37*(1), 14.

Cohen, M. R. (2007). Medication errors: Nasal medications. *Nursing2007, 37*(4), 18.

D'Arcy, Y. (2006). Which analgesic is right for my patient? *Nursing2006 36*(7), 50–55.

D'Arcy, Y. (2007). Pain pointers: Safe pain relief at the push of a button. *Nursing Made Incredibly Easy! 5*(6), 9–12.

D'Arcy, Y. (2008). Keep your patient safe during PCA. *Nursing2008, 38*(1), 50–55.

DeLaune, S. C., & Ladner, P. K. (2006). *Fundamentals of Nursing: Standards & Practice* (3rd ed., pp. 811). Clifton Park, NY: Thomson Delmar Learning.

DeLaune, S. C., & Ladner, P. K. (2006). *Fundamentals of Nursing: Standards & Practice* (3rd ed., pp. 848–851). Clifton Park, NY: Thomson Delmar Learning.

Earhart, A. (2007). Evidence-based practice in infusion nursing. *Clinical Nurse Specialist: The Journal for Advanced Nursing Practice, 21*(2), 107–107.

Evans, E., & Gray, M. (2005). Do topical analgesics reduce pain associated with wound dressing changes or debridement of chronic wounds? *Journal of Wound, Ostomy and Continence Nursing, 32*(5), 287–290.

Fields, M., & Peterman J. (2005). Intravenous medication safety system averts high-risk medication errors and provides actionable data. *Nursing Administration Quarterly, 29*(1), 78–87.

Friedman, M. (2005). Medication safety: Look-alike/sound-alike drugs in home care. *Home Healthcare Nurse, 23*(4), 243–253.

Gaunt, M. J., & Johnston, J. (2007). Safety monitor: Automated dispensing cabinets. *American Journal of Nursing, 107*(8), 27–28.

Gold, K., & Schumann, J. (2007). Dangers of used sharps in household trash: Implications for home care. *Home Healthcare Nurse, 25*(9), 602–607.

Grimley, D. M., Annang, L., Foushee, H. R., Bruce, F. C., & Kendrick, J. S. (2006). Vaginal douches and other feminine hygiene products: Women's practices and perceptions of product safety. *Maternal and Child Health Journal, 10*(3), 303–310.

Guide to care for patients: Asthma. (2005). *The Nurse Practitioner: The American Journal of Primary Health Care, 30*(4), 49–50.

Gupta, P. J. (2007). Suppositories in anal disorders: A review. *European Review for Medical and Biological Sciences, 11*(3), 165–170.

Hadaway, L. (2007). Infiltration and extravasation. *American Journal of Nursing, 107*(8), 64–72.

Hadaway, L. C. (2005). IV rounds: Administering parenteral nutrition with other IV drugs. *Nursing, 35*(2), 26–26.

Hader, C. F. (2007). Epidural analgesia in the critically ill. *Nursing Critical Care, 2*(5), 20–30.

Hicks, R. W., & Becker, S. C. (2006). An overview of intravenous-related medication administration errors as reported to MEDMARX®, a national medication error-reporting program. *Journal of Infusion Nursing, 29*(1), 20–27.

Higgens, D. (2007). Administering a suppository. *Nursing Times, 103*(10), 26–27.

Intramuscular injection (IM). Retrieved January 11, 2008, from the Cincinnati Children's Hospital Medical Center Web site: www.cincinnatichildrens.org/health/info/medication/f-i/intramuscular-injection.htm

IV pump: Gaps in home infusion therapy coverage could spark policy debate. (2007). *Journal of Infusion Nursing, 30*(4), 201–202.

Jacobs, B. (2006). High tech/high care: Pump away high-risk infusion errors. *Men in Nursing, 1*(2), 6–9.

Kirmse, J. (2006). Subcutaneous administration of immunoglobulin. *Journal of Infusion Nursing, 29*(3), Suppl. pp. S15–S20.

Levitt, F. C. (2006). Lidocaine versus guided imagery: Patient preferences for pain management during IV insertion. *Clinical Nurse Specialist: The Journal for Advanced Nursing Practice, 20*(3), 156–156.

Love, G. H. (2006). Administering an intradermal injection. *Nursing2006, 30*(6), 5–9.

Mager, D. (2007). Medication errors and the home care patient. *Home Healthcare Nurse, 25*(3), 151–155.

Marshall, K. M. (2006). Are patients in labor satisfied with PCEA? *Nursing2006, 36*(6), 18–19.

Milano, C. (2006). In the news: Narcotics abuse in correctional facilities: Is pain medication being used inappropriately? *American Journal of Nursing, 106*(2), 22–22.

Nicholas, P. K., & Agius, C. R. (2005). Toward safer IV medication administration: The narrow safety margins of many IV medications make this route particularly dangerous. *American Journal of Nursing, 105*(3-Supplement: State of the science on safe medication administration), 25–30.

Nisbet, A. C. (2006). Intramuscular gluteal injections in the increasingly obese population: Retrospective study. *British Medical Journal, 332*, 637–638.

Pasero, M. S., Manworren, R. C. B., & McCaffery, M. (2007). Pain control: IV opioid range orders for acute pain management. *American Journal of Nursing, 107*(2), 52–59.

Pasero, M. S., & McCaffery, M. (2005). Pain control: Authorized and unauthorized use of PCA pumps: Clarifying the use of patient-controlled analgesia,

in light of recent alerts. *American Journal of Nursing, 105*(7), 30–32.

Patient/Family Education. *IV medications at home (IV push method).* Retrieved January 10, 2008, from the Children's Hospitals and Clinics of Minnesota Web site: http://xpedio02.childrenshc.org/stellent/groups/public/@Manuals/@PFS/@HomeCare/documents/PolicyReferenceProcedure/018700.pdf

Peak technique: Are you on track with Z-tract injections? (2005). *Nursing Made Incredibly Easy! 3*(1), 58–59.

Polzien, G. (2007). Prevent medication errors: Teaching patients about their medications. *Home Healthcare Nurse, 25*(1), 59–62.

Pullen, R. L. (2005). Clinical Do's & Don'ts: Administering medication by the Z-tract method. *Nursing2005, 35*(7), 24–24.

Research report: Intranasal and IV morphine equally effective. (2006). *Nursing Critical Care, 1*(3), 55–56.

Rokosky, J. M. (2005). Teaching correct use of inhaled medications. *Home Healthcare Nurse. 23*(12), 766–744.

Rosenthal, K. (2006). Intravenous fluids: The whys and wherefores. *Nursing2006, 36*(7), 26–27.

Rosenthal, K. (2006). Dangerous drug interactions: One size doesn't fit all... and other perils of IV administration. *Nursing Made Incredibly Easy! 4*(6), 18–21.

Rosenthal, K. (2007). Are you up to date with the infusion nursing standards? *Nursing2007, 37*(7), 15.

Rosenthal, K. (2007). IV essentials: What's new in the infusion nursing standards? *Nursing Made Incredibly Easy! 5*(1), 12–13.

Rushing, J. (2007). Administering eyedrops. *Nursing2007, 37*(3), 18.

Schulmeister, L. (2005). Transdermal drug patches: Medicine with muscle. *Nursing2005, 35*(1), 48–62.

Schultz, W. B. (2007). Bolstering the FDA's drug safety authority. *The New England Journal of Medicine, 357*(22), 2217–2219.

Schwartz, A. J. (2006). Learning the essentials of epidural anesthesia. *Nursing2006, 36*(1), 44–49.

Shores, J. T., Gabriel, A., & Gupta, S. (2007). Skin substitutes and alternatives: A review. *Advances in Skin and Wound Care: The Journal for Prevention and Healing, 20*(9), 493–508.

Springer, R. (2006). Managing controlled substances in the office surgical setting. *Plastic Surgical Nursing, 25*(2), 100–104.

Thomson MICROMEDEX (2007). *How to give an intramuscular injection.* Retrieved from the Healthtouch Online for Better Health Web site: www.healthtouch.com/bin/EContent_HT/cnote-ShowLft

Vandervoort, J., & Ludwig, A. (2008). Microneedles for transdermal drug delivery: A minireview. *Frontiers in Bioscience, 1*(13), 1711–1755.

Warren Grant Magnuson Clinical Center. *Giving a subcutaneous injection. Patient Information Publications.* Retrieved January 8, 2008, from the National Institutes of Health Web site: www.cc.nih.gov/ccc/patient_education/pepubs/subq.pdf

Wynaden, D., Landsborough, I., Chapman, R., McGowan, S., Lapsley, J., & Finn M. (2005). Establishing best practice guidelines for administration of intramuscular injections in the adult: A systematic review of the literature. *Contemporary Nurse, 20*(2), 267–277.

CHAPTER 6 – NUTRITION AND ELIMINATION

Best, C. (2007). Nasogastric tube insertion in adults who require enteral feeding.*Nurs Stand, 21*(40), 39–43.

Clinical evaluation of a flexible fecal incontinence management system. (2007). *Am J Crit Care, 16*(4), 384–393.

'Condom' catheter can improve outcomes. (2006). *Healthcare Benchmarks Qual Improv, 13*(10), 113–115.

Cochran, S. (2007). Care of the indwelling urinary catheter: Is it evidence based? *J Wound Ostomy Continence Nurs, 34*(3), 282–288.

de Aguilar-Nascimento, J. E., & Kudsk, K. A. (2007). Use of small-bore feeding tubes: Successes and failures. *Curr Opin Clin Nutr Metab Care, 10*(3), 291–296.

Falagas, M. E., & Vergidis, P. I. (2005). Urinary tract infections in patients with urinary diversion. *Am J Kidney Dis, 46*(6), 1030–1037.

Fogg, L. (2007). Home enteral feeding part 1: An overview. *Br J Community Nurs, 12*(6), 246, 248, 250–252.

Garcia, M. M., Gulati, S., Liepmann, D., Stackhouse, G. B., Greene, K., & Stoller, M. L. (2007). Traditional Foley drainage systems—do they drain the bladder? *J Urol. 177*(1), 203–207; discussion 207.

Gouëffic, Y., Rozec, B., Sonnard, A., Patra, P., & Blanloeil, Y. (2005) Evidence for early nasogastric tube removal after infrarenal aortic surgery: A randomized trial. *J Vasc Surg, 42*(4), 654–659.

Hautmann, R. E. (2003). Urinary diversion: Ileal conduit to neobladder. *J Urol, 169*(3), 834–842.

Hyde, S. J., Coulthard, M. G., Jaffray, B., Vallely, M. E., & Harding, S. M. (2008). Using saline solutions for ACE washouts. *Arch Dis Child, 93*(2), 149–150.

Kralik, D., Seymour, L., Eastwood, S., & Koch, T. (2007). Managing the self: Living with an indwelling urinary catheter. *J Clin Nurs 16*(7B), 177–185.

Kyle, G., Prynn, P., & Oliver, H. (2005). A procedure for the digital removal of faeces. *Nurs Stand, 19*(20), 33–39.

Melvin, W., & Fernandez, J. D. (2005). Percutaneous endoscopic transgastric jejunostomy: A new approach. *Am Surg, 71*(3), 216–218.

Moss, G. (2005) Enteral feeding monitor/manager. *Biomed Instrum Technol, 39*(2), 151–154.

Nakagawa, T., & Toguri, A. G. (2006). Early catheter removal following transurethral prostatectomy: A study of 431 patients. *Med Princ Pract, 15*(2), 126–130.

Padmanabhan, A., Stern, M., Wishin, J., Mangino, M., Richey, K., & DeSane, M. (2007).

Pomfret, I., Bavait, F., Mackenzie, R., Wells, M., Winder, A. (2004). Using bladder instillations to manage indwelling catheters, *Br J Nurs,* 13(5):261–267.

Pullen, R, L, Jr. (2006). Teaching your patient to irrigate a colostomy. *Nursing, 36*(4), 22.

Rabindranath, K. S., Adams, J., Ali, T. Z., Daly, C., Vale, L., & Macleod, A. M. (2007). Automated vs continuous ambulatory peritoneal dialysis: A systematic review of randomized controlled trials. *Nephrol Dial Transplant, 22*(10), 2991–2998.

Roodhouse, A., & Wellsted, A. (2006). Safety in urine sampling: Maintaining an infection-free environment. *Br J Nurs, 15*(16), 870–872.

Saint, S., Kaufman, S. R., Rogers, M. A., Baker, P. D., Ossenkop, K., & Lipsky, B. A. (2006). Condom versus indwelling urinary catheters: A randomized trial. *J Am Geriatr Soc, 54*(7), 1055–1061.

Toth, P. E. (2006). Ostomy care and rehabilitation in colorectal cancer. *Semin Oncol Nurs, 22*(3), 174–177.

Turi, M. H., Hanif, S., Fasih, Q., & Shaikh, M. A. (2006). Proportion of complications in patients practicing clean intermittent self-catheterization (CISC) vs indwelling catheter. *J Pak Med Assoc 56*(9), 401–404.

Walsh, S. R., Tang, T., & Gaunt, M. E. (2006). Regarding "Evidence for early nasogastric tube removal after infrarenal aortic surgery: A randomized trial." *J Vasc Surg, 43*(3), 644–645; author reply 645.

CHAPTER 7 – OXYGENATION

Abramov, D., Yeshaaiahu, M., Tsodikov, V., Gatot, I., Orman, S., & Gavriel, A. (2005). Timing of chest tube removal after coronary artery bypass surgery. *J Card Surg, 20*(2), 142–146.

Akça, O. (2007). Endotracheal tube cuff leak: Can optimum management of cuff pressure prevent pneumonia? *Crit Care Med, 35*(6), 1624–1626.

Baser, S., Ozkurt, S., Topuz, B., Kiter, G., Karabulut, H., & Akdag, B. (2007). Peak expiratory flow monitoring to screen for asthma in patients with allergic rhinitis. *J Invest Allergol Clin Immunol, 17*(4), 211–215.

Bjessmo, S., Hylander, S., Vedin, J., Mohlkert, D., & Ivert, T. (2007). Comparison of three different chest drainages after coronary artery bypass surgery—a randomised trial in 150 patients. *Eur J Cardiothorac Surg 31*(3), 372–375.

Bourgault, A. M., Brown, C. A., Hains, S. M., & Parlow, J. L. (2006). Effects of endotracheal tube suctioning on arterial oxygen tension and heart rate variability. *Biol Res Nurs, 7*(4), 268–278.

Chowdhuri, S. (2007). Continuous positive airway pressure for the treatment of sleep apnea. *Otolaryngol Clin North Am, 40*(4), 807–827.

Christopher, K. L. (2005). Tracheostomy decannulation. *Respir Care, 50*(4), 538–541.

Cornforth, B. M. (2007). Difficulty in deflating a tracheostomy tube cuff. *Anaesthesia, 62*(3), 298–299.

Fessler, H. E., Derdak, S., Ferguson, N. D., Hager, D. N., Kacmarek, R. M., & Thompson, B. T. (2007). A protocol for high-frequency oscillatory ventilation in adults: Results from a roundtable discussion. *Crit Care Med, 35*(7), 1649–1654.

Hess, D. R. (2005). Tracheostomy tubes and related appliances. *Respir Care, 50*(4), 497–510.

Krachman, S. L., Nugent, T., Crocetti, J., D'Alonzo, G. E., & Chatila, W. (2005). Effects of oxygen therapy on left ventricular function in patients with Cheyne-Stokes respiration and congestive heart failure. *J Clin Sleep Med, 1*(3), 271–276.

Lehwaldt, D., & Timmins, F. (2007). The need for nurses to have in service education to provide the best care for clients with chest drains. *J Nurs Manage, 15*(2), 142–148.

Mair, H., Sodian, R., & Daebritz, S. (2007). Modern drainage techniques for pain reduction during chest tube removal. *Heart Lung, 36*(3), 232–233.

Naylor, J. M., McLean, A., Chow, C. M., Heard, R., Ting, I., & Avolio, A. (2006). A modified postural drainage position produces less cardiovascular stress than a head-down position in patients with severe heart disease: A quasi-experimental study. *Aust J Physiother, 52*(3), 201–209

O'Neill, J. F., & Deakin, C. D. (2007). Do we hyperventilate cardiac arrest patients? *Resuscitation, 73*(1), 82–85.

Ramirez, P., Ferrer, M., & Torres, A. (2007). Prevention measures for ventilator-associated pneumonia: A new focus on the endotracheal tube. *Curr Opin Infect Dis, 20*(2), 190–197.

Rechner, J. A., Loach, V. J., Ali, M. T., Barber, V. S., Young, J. D., & Mason, D. G. (2007). A comparison of the laryngeal mask airway with facemask and oropharyngeal airway for manual ventilation by critical care nurses in children. *Anaesthesia, 62*(8), 790–795.

Rieger, K. M., Wroblewski, H. A., Brooks, J. A., Hammoud, Z. T., & Kesler, K. A. (2007). Postoperative outpatient chest tube management: Initial experience with a new portable system. *Ann Thorac Surg 84*(2), 630–632.

Robert, D., & Argaud, L. (2007). Non-invasive positive ventilation in the treatment of sleep-related breathing disorders. *Sleep Med, 8*(4), 441–452.

Schallom, L., Sona, C., McSweeney, M., & Mazuski, J. (2007). Comparison of forehead and digit oximetry in surgical/trauma patients at risk for decreased peripheral perfusion. *Heart Lung, 36*(3), 188–194.

Thompson, R., Delfino, R. J., Tjoa, T., Nussbaum, E., & Cooper, D. (2006). Evaluation of daily home spirometry for school children with asthma: New insights. *Pediatr Pulmonol, 41*(9), 819–828.

Torres, H. A., Hanna, H. A., Graviss, L., Chaiban, G., Hachem, R., & Chemaly, R. F. (2006). Chest tube-related empyema due to methicillin-resistant *Staphylococcus aureus*: Could the chest tube be coated with antiseptics? *Infect Control Hosp Epidemiol, 27*(2), 195–197.

Westerdahl, E., Lindmark, B., Eriksson, T., Friberg, O., Hedenstierna, G., & Tenling, A. (2005). Deep-breathing exercises reduce atelectasis and improve pulmonary function after coronary artery bypass surgery. *Chest, 128*(5), 3482–3488.

Wynne, R., Botti, M., Copley, D., & Bailey, M. (2007). The normative distribution of chest tube drainage volume after coronary artery bypass grafting. *Heart Lung, 36*(1), 35–42.

CHAPTER 8 – CIRCULATORY

Alisky, J. M. (2007). Implantable central venous access ports for minimally invasive repetitive drainage of pleural effusions. *Med Hypotheses, 68*(4), 910–911.

Bakdash, S., & Yazer, M. H. (2007). What every physician should know about transfusion reactions. *CMAJ, 177*(2), 141–147.

Bankhurst, A. D. (2007). Needle phobia and stress-reducing medical devices in pediatric and adult chemotherapy patients. *J Pediatr Oncol Nurs, 24*(1), 20–28.

Banks, A. (2007). Innovations in postoperative pain management: Continuous infusion of local anesthetics. *AORN J, 85*(5), 904–914.

de Andrade, D., & Ferreira, V. (2007). Central venous access for haemodialysis: Prospective evaluation of possible complications. *J Clin Nurs, 16*(2), 414–418.

De Carolis, M. P., Costa, S., Polimeni, V., Di Stasi, C., Papacci, P., & Romagnoli, C. (2007). Successful removal of catheter fragment from right atrium in a premature infant. *Eur J Pediatr, 166*, 617–618.

Dillon, P. A., & Foglia, R. P. (2006). Complications associated with an implantable vascular access device. *J Pediatr Surg, 41*(9), 1582–1587.

Gülcü, N., Karaaslan, K., Koçoğlu, H., & Gümüş, E. (2007). A new method for epidural catheter fixation. *Agri, 19*(2), 33–37.

Hadaway, L. (2006). Technology of flushing vascular access devices. *J Infus Nurs, 29*(3), 129–145.

Hicks, R. W., & Becker, S. C. (2006). An overview of intravenous-related medication administration errors as reported to MEDMARX, a national medication error-reporting program. *J Infus Nurs, 29*(1), 20–27.

Hofmann, R., Steinwender, C., Kammler, J., Kypta, A., & Leisch, F. (2005). Effects of a high dose intravenous bolus amiodarone in patients with atrial fibrillation and a rapid ventricular rate. *Int J Cardiol 110*(1), 27–32.

Jacobson, A. F. (2006). Cognitive-behavioral interventions for IV insertion pain. *AORN J, 84*(6), 1031–1048.

Jacobson, A. F., & Winslow, E. H. (2005). Variables influencing intravenous catheter insertion difficulty and failure: An analysis of 339 intravenous catheter insertions. *Heart Lung, 34*(5), 345–359.

Kettwich, S. C., Sibbitt, W. L. Jr., Brandt, J. R., Johnson, C. R., Wong, C. S., & Kogon, B., Voss, J., Villari, C., Shah, N., Spitzer, K., & Moore, M. (2007). Utility of intravenous catheters for femoral arterial cannulation in infants having complicated sternal re-entry. *J Thorac Cardiovasc Surg, 134*(3), 746–749.

Kolbeck, K. J., Stavropoulos, S. W., & Trerotola, S. O. (2006). Aerostasis during central venous access: Updates in protective sheaths. *J Vasc Interv Radiol, 17*(7), 1155–1163.

Kuo, Y. S., Schwartz, B., Santiago, J., Anderson, P. S., Fields, A. L., & Goldberg, G. L. (2005). How often should a port-A-cath be flushed? *Cancer Invest, 23*(7), 582–585.

Magder, S. (2006). Central venous pressure: A useful but not so simple measurement. *Crit Care Med, 34*(8), 2224–2227.

Marra, A. R., Opilla, M., Edmond, M. B., & Kirby, D. F. (2007). Epidemiology of bloodstream infections in patients receiving long-term total parenteral nutrition. *J Clin Gastroenterol, 41*(1), 19–28.

McBeth, C. L., McDonald, R. J., & Hodge, M. B. (2004). Antibiotic sampling from central venous catheters versus peripheral veins. *Pediatr Nurs, 30*(3), 200–202.

Mermel, L. A. (2007). Prevention of central venous catheter-related infections: What works other than impregnated or coated catheters? *J Hosp Infect, 65*(Suppl 2), 30–33.

Mok, E., Kwong, T. K., Chan, M. F. (2007). A randomized controlled trial for maintaining peripheral intravenous lock in children. *Int J Nurs Pract, 13*(1), 33–45.

Lindsey, T., Watts-Tate, N., Southwood, E., Routhieaux, J., Beatty, J., & Diane, C. (2005). Chronic blood transfusion therapy practices to treat strokes in children with sickle cell disease. *J Am Acad Nurse Pract, 17*(7), 277–282.

Little, M. A., Hussein, T., Lambert, M., & Dickson, S. J. (2007). Percutaneous venepuncture practice in a large urban teaching hospital. *Clin Med, 7*(3), 243–249.

Ozasa, H., Ishibashi, N., Ikeda, S., Imaizumi, T., Miyagi, M., & Yano, S. (2006). Clinical examination of the water-soluble vitamin levels in blood during peripheral parenteral nutrition. *Kurume Med J 53*(3–4), 79–87.

Ozyuvaci, E., & Kutlu, F. (2006). Totally implantable venous access devices via subclavian vein: A retrospective study of 368 oncology patients. *Adv Ther,* *23*(4), 574–581.

Pieger-Mooney, S. (2005). Innovations in central vascular access device insertion. *J Infus Nurs, 28*(3 Suppl), S7–12.

Plumb, T. J., Adelson, A. B., Groggel, G. C., Johanning, J. M., Lynch, T. G., & Lund, B. (2007). Obesity and hemodialysis vascular access failure. *Am J Kidney Dis, 50*(3), 450–454.

Sümpelmann, R., Osthaus, W. A., Irmler, H., & Hernandez, C. (2006). Prevention of burns caused by transillumination for peripheral venous access in neonates. *Paediatr Anaesth, 16*(10), 1097–1098.

Stewart, S., (2006). Review: routine changes of IV administrations sets (not containing lipids or blood products) at intervals 96 hours do not affect infusate or catheter related bloodstream infection. *Evid Based Nurs.* 9(3), 81.

Tilton, D. (2006). Central venous access device infections in the critical care unit.*Crit Care Nurs Q, 29*(2), 117–122.

Wilson, G. J., van Noesel, M. M., Hop, W. C., & van de Ven, C. (2006).The catheter is stuck: complications experienced during removal of a totally implantable venous access device. A single-center study in 200 children. *J Pediatr Surg, 41*(10), 1694–1698.

Zavorsky, G. S., Cao, J., Mayo, N. E., Gabbay, R., & Murias, J. M. (2007). Arterial versus capillary blood gases: A meta-analysis. *Respir Physiol Neurobiol, 155*(3), 268–279.

CHAPTER 9 – SKIN INTEGRITY AND WOUND CARE

Bishop, L., Dougherty, L., Bodenham, A., Mansi, J., Crowe, P., & Kibbler, C. (2007). Guidelines on the insertion and management of central venous access devices in adults. *Int J Lab Hematol, 29*(4), 261–278.

Campton-Johnson, S. & Wilson, J. (2001). Infected wound management: Advanced technologies, moisture-retentive dressings, and die-hard methods. *Critical Care Nursing Quarterly, 24*(2) 64–77.

Dedmond, B. T., Kortesis, B., Punger, K., Simpson, J., Argenta, J., & Kulp, B. (2006). Subatmospheric pressure dressings in the temporary treatment of soft tissue injuries associated with type III open tibial shaft fractures in children. *J Pediatr Orthop, 26*(6), 728–732.

Dykes, P. J. (2007). The effect of adhesive dressing edges on cutaneous irritancy and skin barrier function. *J Wound Care, 16*(3), 97–100.

Erol, F. S., Topsakal, C., Faik Ozveren, M., Kaplan, M., & Tiftikci, M. T. (2005). Irrigation vs. closed drainage in the treatment of chronic subdural hematoma. *J Clin Neurosci, 12*(3), 261–263.

Heal, C., Buettner, P., Raasch, B., Browning, S., Graham, D., & Bidgood, R. (2006). Can sutures get wet? Prospective randomised controlled trial of wound management in general practice. *BMJ, 332*(7549), 1053–1056.

Horrocks, A. (2007). Prontosan wound irrigation and gel: management of chronic wounds. *Br J Nurs, 15*(22), 1222, 1224–1228.

Hughes, S. A., Ozgur, B. M., German, M., & Taylor, W. R. (2006). Prolonged Jackson-Pratt drainage in the management of lumbar cerebrospinal fluid leaks. *Surg Neurol, 65*(4), 410–414, discussion 414–415.

Macmillan, M. S., Wells, M., MacBride, S., Raab, G. M., Munro, A., & MacDougall, H. (2007). Randomized comparison of dry dressings versus hydrogel in management of radiation-induced moist desquamation. *Int J Radiat Oncol Biol Phys, 68*(3), 864–872.

Montalvo, I. (2007). Pressure ulcer prevention. *Am J Nurs, 107*(7), 15.

Motta, G. J., & Trigilia, D. (2005). The effect of an antimicrobial drain sponge dressing on specific bacterial isolates at tracheostomy sites. *Ostomy Wound Manage, 51*(1), 60–62, 64–66.

Niezgoda, J. A., & Mendez-Eastman, S. (20060. The effective management of pressure ulcers. *Adv Skin Wound Care, 19*(Suppl 1), 3–15.

Paddle-Ledinek, J. E., Nasa, Z., & Cleland, H. J. (2006). Effect of different wound dressings on cell viability and proliferation. *Plast Reconstr Surg, 117*(7 Suppl), 110S-118S; discussion 119S–120S.

Pierce, M., Rice, M., & Fellows, J. (2006). Wet colostomy and peristomal skin breakdown. *J Wound Ostomy Continence Nurs, 33*(5), 541–546; discussion 546–548.

Pullen, R. L. Jr. (2007). Replacing a urostomy drainage pouch. *Nursing, 37*(6), 14.

Raja, S. G., & Berg, G. A. (2007). Should vacuum-assisted closure therapy be routinely used for management of deep sternal wound infection after cardiac surgery? *Interact Cardiovasc Thorac Surg, 6*(4), 523–527.

Sakurai, A., Hashikawa, K., Yokoo, S., Terashi, H., & Tahara, S. (2007). Simple dressing technique using polyurethane foam for fixation of skin grafts. *Dermatol Surg, 33*(8), 976–979.

Shetty, A. A., Kumar, V. S., Morgan-Hough, C., Georgeu, G. A., James, K. D., & Nicholl, J. E. (2004). Comparing wound complication rates following closure of hip wounds with metallic skin staples or subcuticular Vicryl suture: A prospective randomised trial. *J Orthop Surg (Hong Kong), 12*(2), 191–193.

Talbot, T. R., Peters, J., Yan, L., Wright, P. F., & Edwards, K. M. (2006). Optimal bandaging of smallpox vaccination sites to decrease the potential for secondary vaccinia transmission without impairing lesion healing. *Infect Control Hosp Epidemiol, 27*(11), 1184–1192.

Weinrauch, P. (2005). Diagnostic value of routine drain tip culture in primary joint arthroplasty. *ANZ J Surg, 75*(10), 887–888.

CHAPTER 10 – IMMOBILIZATION AND SUPPORT

Baldwin, T. M., Bruker, C. T., Gibbs, A. E., & Sekiya, J. K. (2006). Isolated anterior interosseous nerve palsy following sling immobilization. *Orthopedics, 29*(6), 543–545.

Brown, R., DiMarco, A. F., Hoit, J. D., & Garshick, E. (2006). Respiratory dysfunction and management in spinal cord injury. *Respir Care, 51*(8), 853–868; discussion 869–870.

Carmichael, K. D., & Westmoreland, J. (2005). Effectiveness of ear protection in reducing anxiety during cast removal in children. *Am J Orthop, 34*(1), 43–46.

Cebesoy, O., Kose, K. C., Kuru, I., Altinel, L., Gul, R., & Demirtas, M. (2007). Use of a splint following open carpal tunnel release: a comparative study. *Adv Ther, 24*(3), 478–484.

Egol, K. A., Paksima, N., Puopolo, S., Klugman, J., Hiebert, R., & Koval, K. J. (2006). Treatment of external fixation pins about the wrist: A prospective, randomized trial. *J Bone Joint Surg Am, 88*(2), 349–354.

Haley, C. A., DeJong, E. S., Ward, J. A., & Kragh, J. F. Jr. (2006). Waterproof versus cotton cast liners: a randomized, prospective comparison. *Am J Orthop, 35*(3), 137–140.

Kahn, S. R., Shbaklo, H., Shapiro, S., Wells, P. S., Kovacs, M. J., & Rodger, M. A. (2007). Effectiveness of compression stockings to prevent the post-thrombotic syndrome (the SOX Trial and Bio-SOX biomarker substudy), a randomized controlled trial. *BMC Cardiovasc Disord, 7*, 21.

Kavros, S. J. (20050) The efficacy of a pneumatic compression device in the treatment of plantar fasciitis. *J Appl Biomech, 21*(4), 404–413.

Kazakos, K., Lyras, D. N., Verettas, D., Galanis, V., Psillakis, I., and Xarchas, K. (2007). External fixation of intertrochanteric fractures in elderly high-risk patients. *Acta Orthop Belg 73*(1), 44–48.

Lee, Y. H., Lim, K. B., Gao, G. X., Mahadev, A., Lam, K. S., & Tan, S. B. (2007). Traction and spica casting for closed femoral shaft fractures in children. *J Orthop Surg (Hong Kong), 15*(1), 37–40.

Lynch, D., Ferraro, M., Krol, J., Trudell, C. M., Christos, P., & Volpe, B. T. (2005). Continuous passive motion improves shoulder joint integrity following stroke. *Clin Rehabil, 19*(6), 594–599.

Panchbhavi, V. K., Rowell, M., & Trevino, S. G. (2006). Technique tip: Bivalving a below knee cast with a stable notch. *Foot Ankle Int, 27*(1), 64–65.

Parker, M. J., & Handoll, H. H. (2006). Preoperative traction for fractures of the proximal femur in adults. *Cochrane Database Syst Rev, 19;3*: CD000168.

Smith, G. D., Hart, R. G., & Tsai, T. M. (2005). Fiberglass cast application. *Am J Emerg Med, 23*(3), 347–350.

Walker, L., & Lamont, S. (2007). Use and application of graduated elastic compression stockings. *Nurs Stand, 21*(42), 41–45.

Zhou, T., Liu, Z. J., Zhou, S. H., Shen, X. Q., Liu, Q. M., & Fang, Z. F. (2007). Treatment of post-catheterization femoral arteriovenous fistulas with simple prolonged bandaging. *Chin Med J (Engl), 120*(11), 952–955.

Zorowitz, R. D. (2005). Ambulation in a wheelchair-bound stroke survivor using a walker with body weight support: A case report. *Top Stroke Rehabil, 12*(4), 50–55.

CHAPTER 11 – SPECIAL PROCEDURES

Augustyniak, P. (2007). Reliability-based rearrangement of ECG automated interpretation chain. *Anadolu Kardiyol Derg, 7*(Suppl 1), 148–152.

Cingoz, F., Gunay, C., Ozal, E., & Tatar, H. (2007). Repeated paracentesis for treatment renal failure after heart transplantation in patient with ascites. *J Card Surg, 22*(2), 147–148.

Di Domenico, S., Simonassi, C., & Chessa L. (2007). Inexpensive anatomical trainer for bronchoscopy. *Interact Cardiovasc Thorac Surg, 6*(4), 567–569.

Dobrow, M. J., Cooper, M. A., Gayman, K., Pennington, J., Matthews, J., & Rabeneck, L. (2007). Referring patients to nurses: Outcomes and evaluation of a nurse flexible sigmoidoscopy training program for colorectal cancer screening (review). *Can J Gastroenterol, 21*(5), 301–308.

Fisher, J. C., & Guarrera, J. V. (2007). Modified thoracentesis technique using a triple-lumen catheter. *Am J Surg, 194*(3), 406–408.

Goernig, M., De Melis, M., Paolo, D. D., Tedeschi, W., Liehr, M., & Figulla, H. R. (2007). Stress testing in coronary artery disease by magnetic field imaging: A 3D current distribution model. *Anadolu Kardiyol Derg, 7*(Suppl 1), 191–192.

Gould, K. L., Pan, T., Loghin, C., Johnson, N. P., Guha, A., & Sdringola, S. (2007). Frequent diagnostic errors in cardiac PET/CT due to misregistration of CT attenuation and emission PET images: A definitive analysis of causes, consequences, and corrections. *J Nucl Med, 48*(7), 1112–1121.

Ishikawa, S., Aoki, J., Ohwada, S., Takahashi, T., Morishita, Y., & Ueda, K. (2007). Mass screening of multiple abdominal solid organs using mobile helical computed tomography scanner—a preliminary report. *Asian J Surg, 30*(2), 118–121.

Kikushige, Y., Takase, K., Sata, K., Aoki, K., Numata, A., & Miyamoto, T. (2007). Repeated relapses of acute myelogenous leukemia in the isolated extramedullary sites following allogeneic bone marrow transplantations. *Intern Med, 46*(13), 1011–1014.

Kim, K. W., Romero, R., Park, H. S., Park, C. W., Shim, S. S., Jun, J. K., & Yoon, B. H. (2007). A rapid matrix metalloproteinase-8 bedside test for the detection of intraamniotic inflammation in women with preterm premature rupture of membranes. *Am J Obstet Gynecol, 197*(3), 292.e1–e5.

Shah, K. H., McGillicuddy, D., Spear, J., & Edlow, J. A. (2007). Predicting difficult and traumatic lumbar punctures. *Am J Emerg Med, 25*(6), 608–611.

Stacul, F., Pozzi-Mucelli, F., Lubin, E., Gava, S., Cuttin-Zernich, R., Grisi, G., & Cova, M. A. (2006). MR angiography versus intra-arterial digital subtraction angiography of the lower extremities: Activity-based cost analysis (in Italian). *Radiol Med (Torino), 111*(1), 73–84.

Stecco, A., Saponaro, A., & Carriero, A. (2007). Patient safety issues in magnetic resonance imaging: state of the art. *Radiol Med (Torino), 112*(4), 491–508.

Veronesi, G., Bellomi, M., Veronesi, U., Paganelli, G., Maisonneuve, P., & Scanagatta, P. (2007). Role of positron emission tomography scanning in the management of lung nodules detected at baseline computed tomography screening. *Ann Thorac Surg, 84*(3), 959–965; discussion 965–966.

Vettoretto, N., Romessis, M., Di Gaspare, A., Pettinato, G., Arru, L., & Giovanetti, M. (2007). Hemoperitoneum after percutaneous liver biopsy. Video-laparoscopic management. *Ann Ital Chir, 78*(1), 65–67.

Williams, C., Tonkin, S., (2003) Blocked urinary catheters: solutions are not the only solution. *Br J Community Nurs.* 8(7): 321–326.

Williams, J., Russell, I., Durai, D., Cheung, W. Y., Farrin, A., Bloor, K., Coulton, S., & Richardson, G. (2006). What are the clinical outcome and cost-effectiveness of endoscopy undertaken by nurses when compared with doctors? A Multi-Institution Nurse Endoscopy Trial (MINuET). *Health Technol Assess, 10*(40), iii–iv, ix–x, 1–195.

Note: Figures and tables are indicated by "f" or "t," respectively, following page numbers.